Gastrointestinal and Liver Pathology

Gastrointestinal and Liver Pathology

THIRD EDITION

A Volume in the Series Foundations in Diagnostic Pathology

Edited By

Amitabh Srivastava, MD
Member, Memorial Hospital
Attending, Memorial Hospital for Cancer and Allied Diseases
Memorial Sloan Kettering Cancer Center
New York, New York

Daniela S. Allende, MD, MBA
Co-Section Head, Gastrointestinal and Hepatobiliary Pathology
Vice Chair of Research
The Cleveland Clinic

Associate Professor of Pathology
Cleveland Clinic Lerner College of Medicine at Case Western Reserve University
Cleveland, Ohio

Series Editor

John R. Goldblum, MD, FCAP, FASCP, FACG
Chairman
Department of Pathology
The Cleveland Clinic;
Professor of Pathology
Cleveland Clinic Lerner College of Medicine at Case Western Reserve University
Cleveland, Ohio

ELSEVIER

Elsevier
1600 John F. Kennedy Blvd.
Ste 1800
Philadelphia, PA 19103-2899

GASTROINTESTINAL AND LIVER PATHOLOGY,
THIRD EDITION

ISBN: 978-0-323-52794-1

Executive Content Strategist: Michael Houston
Content Development Manager: Somodatta Roy Choudhury
Content Development Specialist: Rishi Arora
Publishing Services Manager: Shereen Jameel
Project Manager: Haritha Dharmarajan
Design Direction: Patrick Ferguson

Printed in India

Last digit is the print number: 9 8 7 6 5 4 3 2 1

To my mentors and my family

—AS

To my wonderful sons and husband for their love and support

—DA

Contributors

Daniela S. Allende, MD, MBA
Co-Section Head, Gastrointestinal and Hepatobiliary Pathology
Vice Chair of Research
The Cleveland Clinic;
Associate Professor of Pathology
Cleveland Clinic Lerner College of Medicine at Case Western Reserve University
Cleveland, Ohio
Non-Neoplastic Disorders of the Liver; Liver Neoplasms, and Pathology of the Liver; and Small Bowel and Pancreas Transplantation

Lodewjk A.A. Brosens, MD, PhD
Associate Professor of Pathology
Gastrointestinal and Endocrine Pathology
UMC Utrecht, Netherlands
Non-Neoplastic and Neoplastic Pathology of the Pancreas

James Conner, MD, PhD
Assistant Professor
Department of Laboratory Medicine & Pathobiology
University of Toronto
Toronto, Canada
Pathology of the Gallbladder and Extrahepatic Bile Ducts

Michael Cruise, MD, PhD
Associate Professor of Pathology
Gastrointestinal and Hepatobiliary Pathology Staff
Informatic Systems Medical Director
Department of Pathology
Cleveland Clinic
Cleveland, Ohio
Gastrointestinal Lymphoma

Leona Doyle, MD
Associate Professor of Pathology
Harvard Medical School
Department of Pathology
Brigham and Women's Hospital
Boston, Massachusetts
Gastrointestinal Mesenchymal Tumors

Ilyssa O. Gordon, MD, PhD
Associate Professor of Pathology
Co-Section Head, Gastrointestinal and Hepatobiliary Pathology
Cleveland Clinic
Cleveland, Ohio
Non-Neoplastic Disorders of the Esophagus

Catherine Hagen, MD
Consultant, Division of Anatomic Pathology
Assistant Professor of Laboratory Medicine and Pathology
Mayo Clinic
Rochester, Minnesota
Tumors of the Esophagus

Bence Kövari, MD, PhD
Assistant Professor
Department of Pathology
University of Szeged
Albert Szent-Györgyi Medical School,
Hungary Department of Pathology
H. Lee Moffitt Cancer Center & Research Institute
Tampa, FL
Epithelial Polyps and Neoplasms of the Stomach

Gregory Y. Lauwers, MD, PhD
Professor of Pathology
Moffit Cancer Center
Tampa, Florida
Non-Neoplastic Disorders of the Stomach and Epithelial Polyps and Neoplasms of the Stomach

Mikhail Lisovsky, MD
Associate Professor of Pathology and Laboratory Medicine
Geisel School of Medicine, Dartmouth
Department of Pathology
Dartmouth Hitchcock Medical Center
Lebanon, New Hampshire
Pathology of the Anal Canal

Mari Mino-Kenudson, MD
Professor of Pathology
Pulmonary Pathology Director
Gastrointestinal Pathology Staff
Massachusetts General Hospital
Boston, Massachusetts
Non-Neoplastic and Neoplastic Pathology of the Pancreas

Reetesh K. Pai, MD
Professor of Pathology
Anatomic Pathology Director
UPMC Presbyterian
Gastrointestinal Pathology Center of Excellence Director
Pittsburgh, PA, USA
Neoplasms of the Small Bowel

Rish K. Pai, MD, PhD
Professor of Laboratory Medicine and Pathology
Department of Laboratory Medicine and Pathology
Consultant
Mayo Clinic Arizona
Phoenix, Arizona
Non-Neoplastic Disorders of the Colon

Nicole C. Panarelli, MD
Associate Professor of Pathology
Albert Einstein College of Medicine
Section Head, Gastrointestinal Pathology
Director of Anatomic Pathology Research
Montefiore Medical Center
New York, New York
Infectious Diseases of the Gastrointestinal Tract

David Papke, MD, PhD
Instructor in Pathology
Department of Pathology
Brigham and Women's Hospital
Boston, Massachusetts
Gastrointestinal Mesenchymal Tumors

Deepa T. Patil, MBBS, MD
Associate Professor of Pathology
Harvard Medical School
Pathologist
Brigham and Women's Hospital
Boston, Massachusetts
Non-Neoplastic and Inflammatory Disorders of the Small Bowel; Non-Neoplastic and Neoplastic Disorders of the Appendix; Epithelial Neoplasms of the Colorectum, Molecular Testing of Colorectal Carcinoma; and Pathology of the Liver, Small Bowel, and Pancreas Transplantation

Scott Robertson, MD, PhD
Assistant Professor of Pathology
Research Analytics Medical Director
Gastrointestinal Pathology Staff
Cleveland Clinic
Cleveland, Ohio
Non-Neoplastic and Inflammatory Disorders of the Small Bowel

Safia Nawazish Salaria, MD, MMHC
Section Chief and Fellowship Director
Division of GI, Liver and Pancreas Pathology
Diversity, Equity, and Inclusion Officer
Associate Professor, Pathology, Microbiology and Immunology
Vanderbilt University Medical Center
Nashville, Tennessee
Liver Neoplasms

Amitabh Srivastava, MD
Member, Memorial Hospital
Attending, Memorial Hospital for Cancer and Allied Diseases
Memorial Sloan Kettering Cancer Center
New York, New York
Tumors of the Esophagus, Gastrointestinal Polyposis Syndromes, Pathology of the Gallbladder and Extrahepatic Bile Ducts, and Liver Neoplasms

Sarah E. Umetsu, MD
Assistant Professor
Department of Pathology
University of California San Francisco
San Francisco, California
Non-Neoplastic Disorders of the Stomach

Kwun Wah Wen, MD, PhD
Associate Professor
Department of Pathology
University of California San Francisco
San Francisco, California
Epithelial Polyps and Neoplasms of the Stomach

Laura D. Wood, MD, PhD
Associate Professor of Pathology & Oncology
Department of Pathology
Johns Hopkins University School of Medicine
Baltimore, Maryland
Non-Neoplastic and Neoplastic Pathology of the Pancreas

Lisa M. Yerian, MD
Chief Improvement Officer
Associate Professor of Pathology
Gastrointestinal and Hepatobiliary Pathology Staff
Cleveland Clinic
Cleveland, Ohio
Non-Neoplastic Disorders of the Liver and Pathology of the Liver, Small Bowel, and Pancreas Transplantation

Foreword

The study and practice of anatomic pathology are both exciting and overwhelming. Surgical pathology, with all of the subspecialties it encompasses, and cytopathology have become increasingly complex and sophisticated, particularly with the incorporation of molecular pathology. It is simply not possible for any single individual to master all of the skills and knowledge required to perform these tasks at the highest level. Simply being able to make a correct diagnosis is challenging enough, but the standard of care has far surpassed merely providing a diagnosis. Pathologists are now asked to provide large amounts of ancillary information, both diagnostic and prognostic, often on small amounts of tissue, a task that can be daunting even to the most experienced surgical pathologist.

Although large general surgical pathology textbooks are useful resources, by necessity, they could not possibly cover many of the aspects that pathologists need to know and include in their diagnostic reports. As such, the concept behind the *Foundations in Diagnostic Pathology* series was born. *Foundations in Diagnostic Pathology* is designed to cover the major areas of surgical and cytopathology, and each edition is focused on one major topic. The goal of every book in this series is to provide the essential information that any pathologist, whether general or subspecialized, in training or in practice, would find useful in the evaluation of virtually any type of specimen encountered.

I am pleased that Drs. Daniela S. Allende and Amitabh Srivastava agreed to edit this edition of their book. Both of these individuals are superb gastrointestinal pathologists from major academic centers (Cleveland Clinic and Memorial Sloan Kettering Cancer Center, respectively), and they have edited an outstanding, state-of-the-art book on gastrointestinal pathology, which cuts to the essentials of what all pathologists want and need to know about diseases of the tubular gut, biliary tree, pancreas, and liver. The list of contributors is impressive and includes nationally and internationally renowned pathologists who excel in their areas of expertise. The content in each chapter is practical, well organized, and well written, focusing on the thorough evaluation of biopsy and resection specimens and culminating in an accurate diagnosis using traditional morphology supported by immunohistochemical and molecular genetic techniques.

This edition of *Gastrointestinal and Liver Pathology* is organized into 20 chapters, covering all of the major problems encountered in gastrointestinal pathology. There are separate chapters that describe the non-neoplastic and neoplastic conditions of the esophagus, stomach, small intestine, appendix, colon, and anus. Superb separate chapters on mesenchymal tumors of the gastrointestinal tract, infectious diseases of the colon, and polyps and polyposis syndromes allow for the necessary depth to cover these broad topics. In addition, pathology of the gallbladder, extrahepatic bile ducts, and pancreas are covered in separate chapters, each of which provides the essential information and nuances of the organ that is covered. The last four chapters of the book cover non-neoplastic liver pathology, transplantation, liver neoplasms, and gastrointestinal lymphomas. I know of no other book in the literature that covers all of these aspects of gastrointestinal pathology in such a concise manner. Moreover, many of the photomicrographs are new to this edition.

I wish to extend my sincere appreciation to Drs. Allende and Srivastava, as well as all of the authors who contributed to this outstanding edition in the *Foundations in Diagnostic Pathology* series. I sincerely hope you enjoy this volume in the *Foundations in Diagnostic Pathology* series.

John R. Goldblum, MD

Preface

The practice of gastrointestinal, hepatobiliary, and pancreatic pathology has undergone significant changes since the publication of the second edition of this book. To keep up with the ever-expanding pool of knowledge, addition of multiple new entities and the increasing integration of molecular pathology into anatomic pathology can be incredibly challenging. This is more so in an environment of increasing daily workloads, physician stress, and burnout that applies not just to pathologists in practice but also those in residency or fellowship training. We are delighted to have this opportunity to put together the third edition of *Gastrointestinal and Liver Pathology* for the *Foundations in Diagnostic Pathology* series for all of you. Each chapter in this edition retains the novel structured format of the prior editions that is complemented by numerous tables and illustrations. This should allow rapid skimming through any chapter or section to gather the most relevant information that may be of interest to a particular reader. We are deeply grateful to the editors of the previous editions for giving us a wonderful template to work with and even more to all the authors who contributed time, effort, and expertise while submitting chapters for this third edition. We would not have been able to bring this book to fruition without their invaluable support. Our hope is that this book will provide a concise yet valuable sign out resource for all those interested in gastrointestinal pathology.

Amitabh Srivastava, MD
Daniela S. Allende, MD, MBA

Acknowledgments

The editors acknowledge the tireless support and patience at Elsevier of Michael Houston, who has kept us on track, and Rishi Arora and Haritha Dharamrajan, who went through each and every page of the text with great care.

Amitabh Srivastava, MBBS
Daniela S. Allende, MD, MBA

Contents

1 Non-Neoplastic Disorders of the Esophagus 1
Ilyssa O. Gordon, MD, PhD

2 Tumors of the Esophagus 29
Catherine Hagen, MD and Amitabh Srivastava, MD

3 Non-Neoplastic Disorders of the Stomach 53
Sarah E. Umetsu, MD and Gregory Y. Lauwers, MD

4 Epithelial Polyps and Neoplasms of the Stomach 91
Bence Kövari, MD, PhD, Kwun Wah Wen, MD, PhD, and Gregory Y. Lauwers, MD, PhD

5 Non-Neoplastic and Inflammatory Disorders of the Small Bowel 119
Scott Robertson, MD, PhD and Deepa T. Patil, MD

6 Neoplasms of the Small Intestine 151
Reetesh K. Pai, MD

7 Gastrointestinal Mesenchymal Tumors 169
David Papke, MD, PhD and Leona Doyle, MD

8 Non-Neoplastic and Neoplastic Disorders of the Appendix 211
Deepa T. Patil, MD

9 Infectious Diseases of the Gastrointestinal Tract 243
Nicole C. Panarelli, MD

10 Non-Neoplastic Disorders of the Colon 299
Rish K. Pai, MD, PhD

11 Gastrointestinal Polyposis Syndromes 337
Amitabh Srivastava, MD

12 Epithelial Neoplasms of the Colorectum 363
Deepa T. Patil, MD

13 Molecular Testing of Gastrointestinal Neoplasms 395
Daniela S. Allende, MD, MBA and Amitabh Srivastava, MD

14 Pathology of the Anal Canal 407
Mikhail Lisovsky, MD

15 Pathology of the Gallbladder and Extrahepatic Bile Ducts 435
James Conner, MD, PhD and Amitabh Srivastava, MD

16 Non-Neoplastic and Neoplastic Pathology of the Pancreas 455
Lodewijk A.A. Brosens, MD, PhD, Mari Mino-Kenudson, MD, and Laura D. Wood, MD, PhD

17 Non-Neoplastic Disorders of the Liver 489
Daniela S. Allende, MD, MBA and Lisa M. Yerian, MD

18 Liver Neoplasms 557
Safia N. Salaria, MD, Amitabh Srivastava, MD, and Daniela S. Allende, MD, MBA

19 Gastrointestinal Lymphoma 613
Michael Cruise, MD, PhD

20 Pathology of Liver, Small Bowel, and Pancreas Transplantation 657
Daniela S. Allende, MD, MBA, Lisa M. Yerian, MD, and Deepa T. Patil, MD

Index 691

1

Non-Neoplastic Disorders of the Esophagus

Ilyssa O. Gordon, MD, PhD

The esophagus is designed to simply serve as a conduit to carry food into the stomach. It does not have any digestive, endocrine, or metabolic role. As a result, most non-neoplastic disorders affecting the esophagus are a result of mechanical, chemical, or immune-mediated injury to the relatively resilient nonkeratinizing squamous mucosa. These disorders can be broadly categorized into inflammatory, infectious, congenital and acquired structural abnormalities; motility, traumatic, and vascular disorders; and those associated with systemic diseases. Inflammatory disorders and infections are by far the most common disorders encountered in daily practice. The remainder of the disorders usually require a combination of clinical, radiographic, and endoscopic examinations for accurate diagnosis, and histologic examination often does not yield specific diagnostic findings.

This chapter is organized based on broad categories of non-neoplastic esophageal disorders. It is, however, essential to note that inflammatory disorders are a manifestation of several common types of stimuli, such as reflux, infections, drugs, and systemic disorders, among others. Therefore, based on the predominant inflammatory cell, these disorders can also be categorized into neutrophil-rich esophagitis, eosinophil-rich, lymphocyte-rich, and paucicellular esophagitis. Neutrophil-rich disorders are most commonly caused by reflux disease and infections (see Chapter 9 for details). Eosinophil-rich disorders include eosinophilic esophagitis (EoE), reflux, parasitic infections, Crohn's disease, drug hypersensitivity, hypereosinophilic syndrome, celiac disease, vasculitis, and collagen vascular disorders. Lymphocytes are a predominant component of inflammation in patients with chronic reflux, drugs or medications, Crohn's disease (pediatric), achalasia or motility disorders, autoimmune diseases, immunodeficiency (human immunodeficiency virus [HIV], common variable immunodeficiency [CVID]), celiac disease, and dermatologic conditions. Last, some conditions, such as corrosive injury, sloughing esophagitis, graft-versus-host disease (GVHD), CVID, and certain medications may not show a significant inflammatory component and thus manifest as paucicellular esophagitis.

ESOPHAGITIS

Inflammatory Disorders

Reflux Esophagitis

Reflux esophagitis, also known as *gastroesophageal reflux disease* (GERD), is one of the most common non-neoplastic disorders of the esophagus. Its prevalence ranges between 5% and 22% and depends on the geographic location. The reported prevalence of GERD is 22% in the United States. Pregnant women have a higher incidence. The pathophysiologic hallmark of reflux is the presence of lower esophageal sphincter (LES) dysfunction. Nonerosive reflux disease (NERD) is defined as patients with classic GERD symptoms but no evidence of mucosal injury on endoscopy.

Clinical Features

Reflux occurs at all ages and in both genders. Typical symptoms include heartburn and regurgitation. Other uncommon or atypical symptoms include dysphagia, angina-like chest pain, chronic hoarseness or cough, asthmatic episodes, and protracted hiccups. If left untreated, reflux may lead to complications such as erosive esophagitis, strictures, Barrett's esophagus (BE), and malignancy. Importantly, a number of individuals with reflux do not manifest symptoms, although the risk for adenocarcinoma arising from BE remains. GERD may be a secondary complication of other disorders affecting the esophagus, such as systemic sclerosis.

Gastroesophageal reflux disease is a clinical diagnosis and is often classified as *erosive* or *nonerosive* based on endoscopic or pathologic findings. The current recommendations from the American Society of Gastrointestinal Endoscopy do not support using endoscopy and biopsy to diagnose typical GERD but rather to exclude other pathologies in complicated or refractory cases. Furthermore, the degree of histologic damage may not correlate with clinical symptoms, and histologic findings alone have a low sensitivity and specificity for diagnosing GERD.

Pathologic Features

Gross Findings

Endoscopic examination in cases of reflux is variable, depending on the severity and the chronicity of the symptoms. Some patients may have erythema, erosions, or ulceration. Deep ulcerations, bleeding, and peptic strictures are seen in severe cases (Fig. 1.1). Patients with NERD by definition have normal white-light endoscopy, although high-definition endoscopy or narrow-band imaging may reveal subtle changes, including prominent vascularity and irregularity of the gastroesophageal junction (GEJ), creating a group of patients with so-called minimal change esophagitis.

Microscopic Findings

Histologic findings are usually localized to the lower esophagus and taper off or are virtually absent in the proximal segment of esophagus. The typical histologic features include basal cell hyperplasia (thickening of the basal layer to >15% of the total epithelial thickness or more than four to six basal cell layers in well-oriented sections), elongation of the papillae (>60% of the total epithelial thickness), and spongiosis (Fig. 1.2). Inflammatory changes include increased numbers of lymphocytes (Fig. 1.3), neutrophils, and eosinophils (Fig. 1.4). Erosions or ulcers are typically associated with severe GERD. Intraepithelial lymphocytes are predominantly T cells, which tend to acquire an elongated shape ("squiggly lymphocytes") while traversing between the intercellular spaces. Additional findings including balloon cell change (Fig. 1.5) and hyperkeratosis.

The presence of dilated intercellular spaces (spongiosis; see Fig. 1.3) was once considered to be a promising histologic marker of early GERD. It may be the predominant histologic finding in a patient with GERD; however, given the low interobserver agreement in assessing this feature, it remains less helpful compared with other

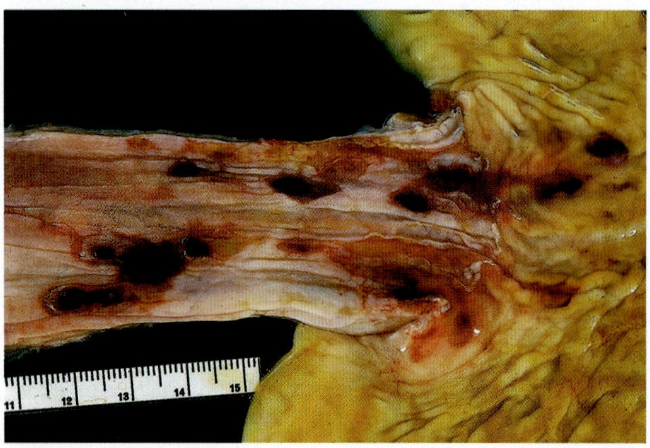

FIGURE 1.1
Esophagitis. Severe, with hemorrhagic erosions. (Courtesy of Dr. P. Vasallo.)

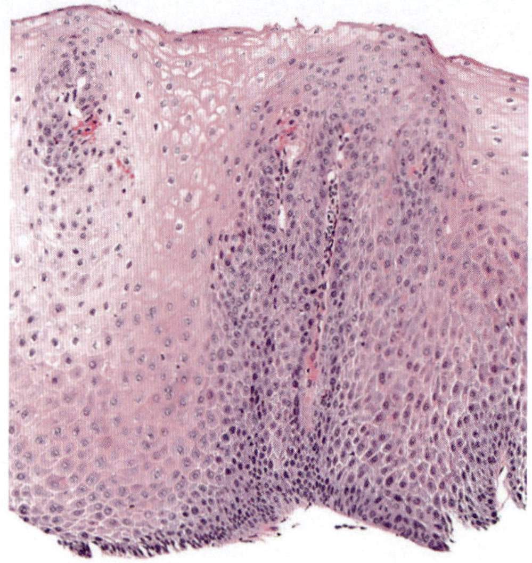

FIGURE 1.2
Reflux esophagitis. Basal cell hyperplasia, elongation of papillae, and spongiosis.

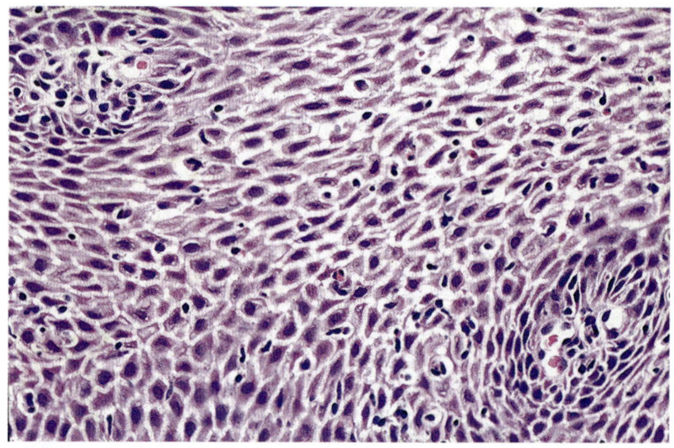

FIGURE 1.3
Reflux esophagitis. Increased numbers of intraepithelial lymphocytes are present among dilated intercellular spaces (spongiosis).

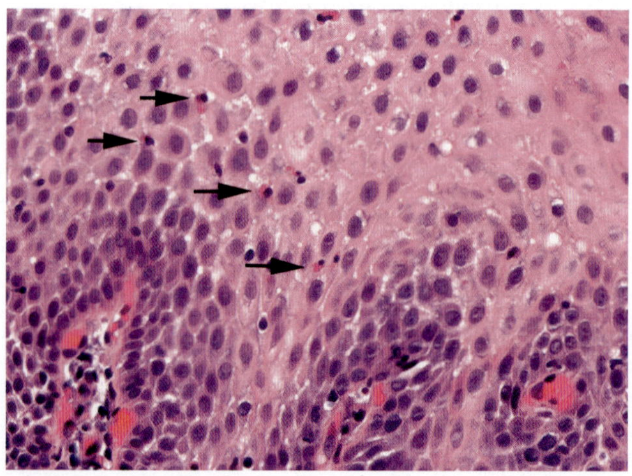

FIGURE 1.4
Reflux esophagitis. Intraepithelial eosinophils *(arrows)*.

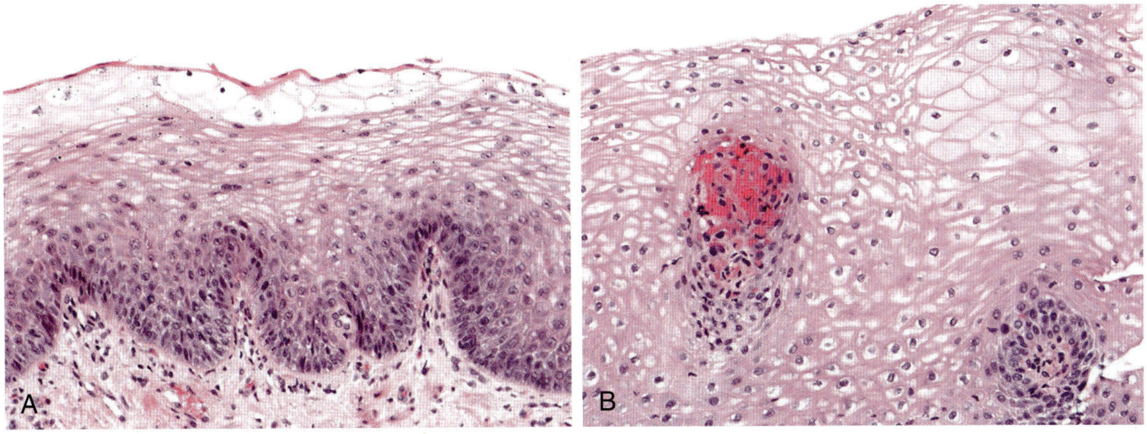

FIGURE 1.5
Reflux esophagitis. Balloon cells can be present along the luminal aspect (**A**) or within (**B**) the squamous epithelium.

typical features of GERD described already. It should be noted that many patients undergoing endoscopic biopsy have been on a trial of proton pump inhibitors (PPIs) and may have been asked to discontinue the medications 1 or 2 weeks or before endoscopy. In this setting, the most common histologic features are increased intraepithelial lymphocytes, basal layer hyperplasia, and elongation of the papillae. The finding of basal layer hyperplasia, elongation of the papillae, and a few eosinophils within 1 to 2 cm of the GEJ may also represent physiologic reflux. This finding is of no clinical significance. In a recent prospective evaluation of 336 patients with clinical symptoms of GERD, Vieth et al. (2016) found that total epithelial thickness of 400 µm or greater at 0.5 cm and 430 µm or greater at 2.0 cm above the Z line was the best histologic feature to reliably identify patients with GERD.

Although endoscopically normal, patients with NERD may have dilated intercellular spaces (spongiosis), as well as basal layer hyperplasia and elongation of the papillae of the squamous epithelium, often grouped together as reactive epithelial change, without significant inflammation. Reporting these findings may be helpful to distinguish patients with NERD from those with functional heartburn.

Differential Diagnosis

Eosinophilic esophagitis, infectious esophagitis, and pill esophagitis are in the differential diagnosis. In EoE, there is an increased density of eosinophils per high-power field (hpf) along with eosinophil microabscess formation and superficial layering of eosinophils. More importantly, EoE affects both the distal as well as proximal segments of the esophagus, is associated with characteristic rings and furrows on endoscopy, and is resistant to PPI therapy.

Infectious esophagitis, such as that caused by *Candida*, herpes simplex virus (HSV), and cytomegalovirus (CMV) shows specific features. *Candida* esophagitis reveals yeast and pseudohyphal forms that invade the mucosa and are accompanied by severe acute inflammation. Squamous epithelial cells infected with HSV show multinucleation, nuclear molding, and margination of chromatin. Viral cytopathic effect of CMV is best appreciated in stromal and endothelial cells within granulation tissue where large, infected cells show intranuclear and intracytoplasmic eosinophilic inclusions.

Pill esophagitis can be associated with prominent eosinophilia, spongiosis, and ulceration. These changes are nonspecific and need to be analyzed in light of the clinical presentation. Polarizable crystalline material may be seen in alendronate-related injury, and crystalline stainable iron can be found in ferrous sulfate-induced esophagitis. Lymphocytic esophagitis (LE), skin disorders such as lichen planus, and esophageal dysmotility states, such as achalasia and strictures, are in the differential diagnosis when increased intraepithelial lymphocytes are present. Esophagitis can also be seen in Crohn's disease, sarcoidosis, GVHD, collagen vascular disease, or Stevens-Johnson syndrome.

Prognosis and Therapy

Prognosis depends on the degree of LES pressures. Extremely low pressures (6 mm Hg) predict a more severe degree of reflux and worse prognosis. Early diagnosis, before the onset of extensive ulcers and strictures, is essential for best patient outcome. Conservative therapy includes significant lifestyle modifications, such as elevation of the head of the bed, avoiding recumbence after meals, weight loss in obese patients, avoiding dietary triggers, and avoiding tobacco and alcohol consumption. PPIs, histamine 2 receptor antagonists, and antacids are the mainstay medical therapy for GERD. Nissen fundoplication and laparoscopic sphincter augmentation are surgical options for those who have failed medical or endoscopic therapy,

REFLUX ESOPHAGITIS—FACT SHEET

Definition

- Inflammation of the lower esophagus resulting from damage caused by acid reflux from the stomach

Incidence and Location

- The most common form of esophagitis, with prevalence of about 22% in the United States
- Localized to the distal esophagus

Gender and Age Distribution

- Affects both sexes and all age groups

Clinical Features

- Heartburn and regurgitation are the typical symptoms; dysphagia also occurs
- Atypical presentation includes angina-like pain, hoarseness, cough, asthma, and hiccups
- Some individuals are asymptomatic

Prognosis and Therapy

- Prognosis depends on the degree of lower esophageal sphincter pressure
- Early detection prevents complications
- If left untreated, severe ulcerations, strictures, Barrett's esophagus, and adenocarcinoma may develop
- Treatment includes lifestyle modifications, proton pump inhibitors, and surgical procedures (Nissen fundoplication) in severe cases

REFLUX ESOPHAGITIS—PATHOLOGIC FEATURES

Gross Findings

- Half of symptomatic patients have normal endoscopic examinations
- Erythema, erosions, or ulceration can be seen
- Deep ulcers are followed by strictures in severe disease
- Barrett's esophagus (salmon-colored mucosal tongues) may be present in long-standing cases

Microscopic Findings

- Architectural changes of basal cell layer hyperplasia, elongation of papillae, and spongiosis
- Increased numbers of intraepithelial eosinophils, lymphocytes, and/or neutrophils
- Erosion or ulceration
- Balloon cell change, hyperkeratosis, and increased total epithelial thickness may be seen

Differential Diagnosis

- Eosinophilic esophagitis has proximal esophageal involvement and often has more severe eosinophilic infiltrates, superficial eosinophil layering, and eosinophilic microabscesses
- Infectious esophagitis (*Candida*, herpes simplex virus, and cytomegalovirus) can be assessed on hematoxylin and eosin and confirmed by special stains and immunohistochemical stains
- Lymphocytic esophagitis and lymphocyte-rich skin disorders typically have only lymphocytes without neutrophils or eosinophils but require clinical correlation
- Pill esophagitis and Crohn's disease require clinical correlation

EOSINOPHILIC ESOPHAGITIS

CLINICAL FEATURES

Eosinophilic esophagitis is a primary clinicopathologic disorder of the esophagus that has been associated with an increasing prevalence and has gained significant recognition over the past few years. It is defined as a chronic immune and antigen-mediated esophageal disease characterized clinically by symptoms related to esophageal dysfunction and histologically by eosinophil-predominant inflammation. Three specific criteria are required to diagnose EoE: symptoms related to esophageal dysfunction, a peak eosinophil count of at least 15 eosinophils/hpf on esophageal biopsy, and eosinophilia limited to the esophagus with other causes of esophageal eosinophilia excluded. Although one of the clinical features of EoE is the lack of response to PPIs, recent studies have shown that one-third or more patients with esophageal eosinophilia can show response to PPIs. This phenomenon has been termed *PPI-responsive esophageal eosinophilia*. A recent transcriptome analysis study by Wen et al. (2015) found significant molecular overlap between PPI-responsive esophageal eosinophilia and EoE, suggesting these two entities represent a diagnostic continuum or that PPI-responsiveness is a subphenotype of EoE. However, this relationship is yet to be fully characterized.

Eosinophilic esophagitis occurs in all age groups but is seen more frequently in young children with atopic symptoms such as eczema, asthma, and food allergies. Symptoms manifest differently in different age groups: whereas infants and children often present with feeding difficulties, regurgitation, dyspepsia, abdominal pain, and vomiting, adults usually describe dysphagia and food impaction with or without chest or abdominal pain. If not recognized early, EoE can progress to odynophagia and stenosis.

EOSINOPHILIC ESOPHAGITIS—FACT SHEET

Definition

- A form of allergic esophagitis associated with atopic symptoms
- Can present alone or as part of eosinophilic gastroenteritis

Incidence and Location

- 1% to 2% of patients undergoing esophageal biopsy
- The entire esophagus is involved; proximal eosinophil count may be higher than distal; eosinophils may be patchy in distribution

Gender and Age Distribution

- Occurs in all age groups but is more common in the children and young adults
- Men are more frequently affected than women

Clinical Features

- Symptoms in children include vomiting, abdominal pain, dyspepsia, and solid food impaction
- Symptoms in adults include dysphagia, food impaction, and chest and abdominal pain
- Associated with food allergies and atopic symptoms

Prognosis and Therapy

- Best outcome if diagnosed and treated early
- May lead to severe esophageal strictures if untreated
- Elimination of food allergens and topical corticosteroids are the treatments of choice
- When strictures occur, dilation is indicated

Pathologic Features

Gross Findings

Classic endoscopic findings include mucosal rings, furrows (also known as "trachealization" of the esophagus), granularity, exudates, and mucosal fragility (Figs. 1.6 and 1.7). However, in some patients, the endoscopic findings can be completely normal. In long-standing cases, stricture formation may be seen.

Microscopic Findings

Biopsies show increased intraepithelial eosinophils (≥15 eosinophils/hpf) with concentration of eosinophils toward the luminal aspect of the epithelium (superficial layering). Eosinophilic microabscesses and degranulation of eosinophils (Fig. 1.8) are frequently present. The density of eosinophils can vary with anatomic location of biopsy and within biopsy fragments. In general, biopsies from the proximal segment reveal more eosinophilia than the distal segment. It is therefore recommended that the total number of eosinophils per high-power field be generated by examining the fragments at low magnification and selecting the high-power field with maximum number of eosinophils (Fig. 1.9). Care should be taken to avoid counting eosinophils within the papillae. Other findings include basal cell hyperplasia, elongation of the papillae to greater than 50% the thickness of the squamous epithelium, spongiosis, lamina propria, and submucosal fibrosis. In patients who have received diet elimination or steroid therapy, follow-up biopsies may be performed to evaluate response to therapy, in which case, giving the exact eosinophil count may be helpful.

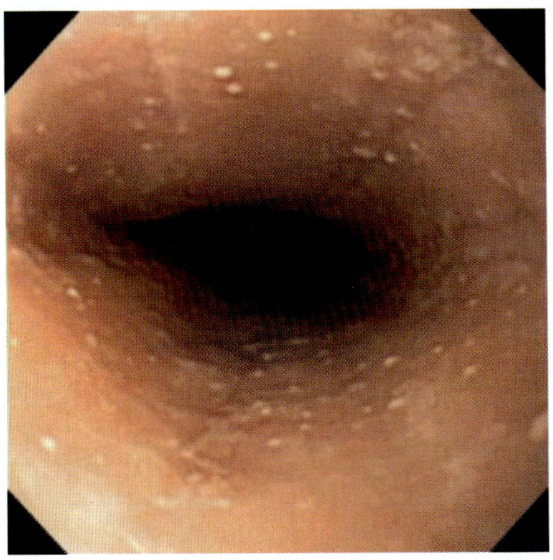

FIGURE 1.6

Eosinophilic esophagitis—endoscopy. Mucosal granularity. (Courtesy of Dr. J. Gramling.)

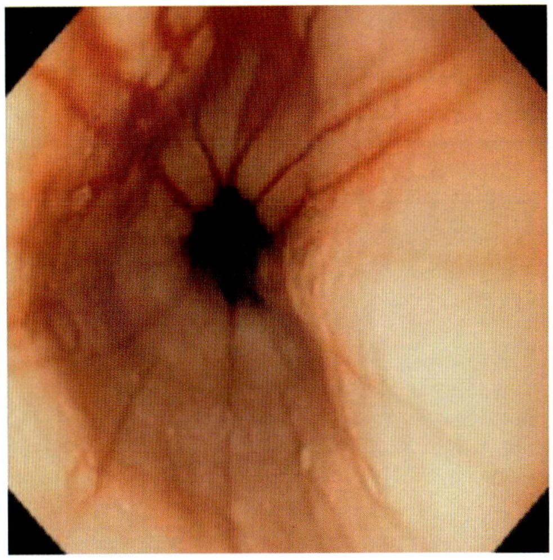

FIGURE 1.7

Eosinophilic esophagitis—endoscopy. Typical furrows and rings. (Courtesy of Dr. J. Gramling.)

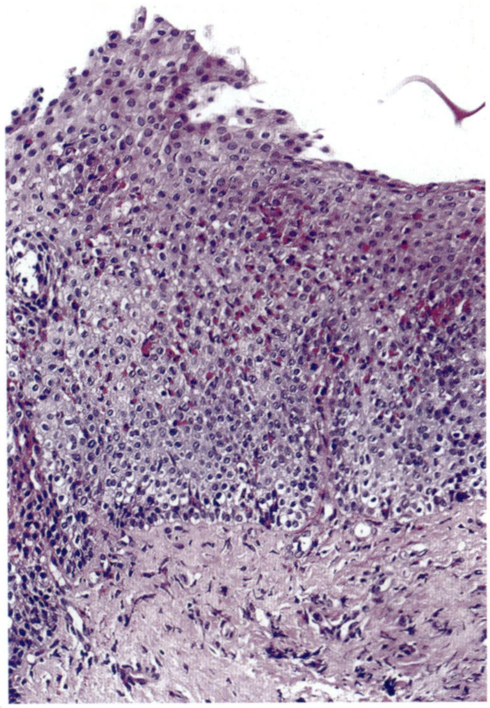

FIGURE 1.8

Eosinophilic esophagitis. Intense eosinophilic infiltrate.

EOSINOPHILIC ESOPHAGITIS—PATHOLOGIC FEATURES

Gross Findings

- Endoscopic examination reveals mucosal rings, furrows ("trachealization" of esophagus), erythema, and granularity
- In long-standing cases, strictures are seen

Microscopic Findings

- Marked increase in intraepithelial eosinophils (≥15/hpf)
- Eosinophil infiltrates may be more prominent in the proximal than in the distal esophagus
- Superficial layering of eosinophils, eosinophilic microabscesses, and degranulation
- Additional findings include basal cell hyperplasia, elongation of the papillae, spongiosis, and fibrosis of the lamina propria and submucosa

Differential Diagnosis

- Reflux esophagitis changes are mostly seen in biopsy samples from the distal esophagus or gastroesophageal junction
- In eosinophilic gastroenteritis, eosinophils are also present in other segments of the gastrointestinal tract
- Drug-induced injury to the esophagus requires clinicopathologic correlation
- Parasitic infections do not typically affect the entire esophagus. Biopsy specimens may show parasitic organisms

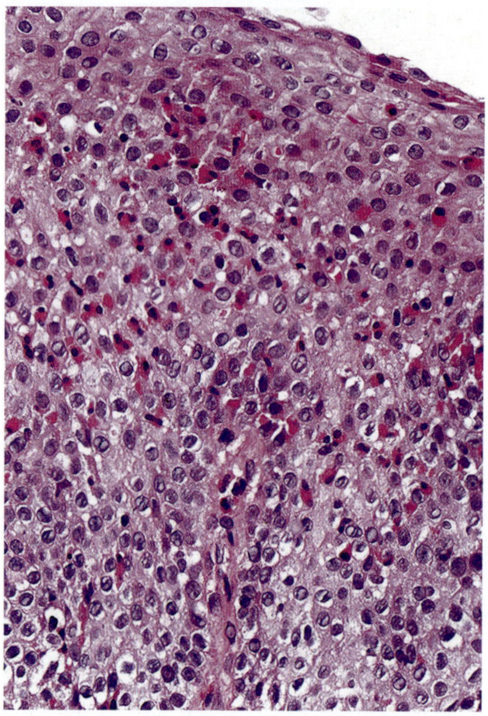

FIGURE 1.9
Eosinophilic esophagitis. Intraepithelial eosinophils (>20/hpf).

DIFFERENTIAL DIAGNOSIS

Eosinophilic esophagitis must be distinguished from reflux esophagitis, pill-induced esophagitis, eosinophilic gastroenteritis, and parasitic infections. It is important to note that any of the histologic features of EoE can also be seen in patients with reflux esophagitis. Distal esophagus-predominant mucosal changes with unremarkable proximal esophageal biopsy favors a diagnosis of reflux esophagitis. Pill-induced esophagitis is often accompanied by ulcer and granulation tissue. Some medications (alendronate, iron supplements) can be visualized on light microscopy. However, confirmation of drug-induced injury requires clinicopathologic correlation. Eosinophilic gastroenteritis is usually associated with peripheral blood eosinophilia and affects the rest of the gastrointestinal (GI) tract. Parasitic infections tend to be a localized phenomenon, and deeper levels may reveal the organism.

PROGNOSIS AND THERAPY

The prognosis is excellent when treatment is given promptly. Dietary elimination of the six common offending foods (milk, egg, wheat, soy, peanuts and tree nuts, and seafood) and topical steroids leads to dramatic improvement in symptoms and histology. Rarely, patients refractory to steroid therapy may show disease progression in the form of esophageal strictures that require repeated dilation procedures.

LYMPHOCYTIC ESOPHAGITIS

Lymphocytic esophagitis is a poorly defined clinicopathologic entity. A variety of clinical diagnoses may be associated with increased intraepithelial lymphocytes on biopsy; therefore, *lymphocytic esophagitis pattern of injury* is the preferred diagnostic terminology used by many pathologists. Some studies have demonstrated that the increased intraepithelial lymphocytes of LE in patients with dysmotility are predominantly CD4+ T cells, in contrast to the normally present scattered intraepithelial lymphocytes, which are CD8+ T cells. In patients with LE and normal motility, both CD4+ and CD8+ T cells are increased.

CLINICAL FEATURES

Symptoms include dysphagia, chest pain, heartburn, nausea, and odynophagia. Symptoms can lead to a clinical impression of EoE. Adults and children both can be affected, and most patients are diagnosed in the fifth or sixth decade of life. Men and women are equally affected. Many patients diagnosed with LE also have potentially confounding diagnoses, including GERD, inflammatory bowel disease (IBD), hypothyroidism, allergies or asthma, history of radiation or chemotherapy, and connective tissue disease.

Pathologic Features

Gross Findings

In about a quarter of patients, the endoscopic impression of the mucosa is normal. Endoscopic findings can mimic those seen in EoE and include esophageal rings, esophagitis, and strictures. Findings suggestive of motility disorder may be identified. Erythema, nodularity, plaques, furrows, and webs have also been reported.

Microscopic Findings

The esophageal biopsy shows increased intraepithelial lymphocytes, predominantly in a peripapillary distribution, with spongiosis of the associated peripapillary squamous epithelium (Fig. 1.10). Similar to EoE, the distribution of intraepithelial lymphocytes is usually patchy and can vary between different biopsy fragments, with some papillae being unaffected. Neutrophils or eosinophils are rare or even absent. There may be accompanying basal cell hyperplasia and spongiosis. Unfortunately, there is no standard number of intraepithelial lymphocytes to diagnosis LE, and studies have included various minimum cut-offs of 20 lymphocytes, 30 lymphocytes, or 50 lymphocytes per high-power field. It is therefore appropriate to render a descriptive diagnosis of “LE pattern of injury” with a comment consisting of the various conditions that may result in this pattern of injury.

Differential Diagnosis

Increased intraepithelial lymphocytes can be seen in reflux esophagitis, which typically shows more neutrophils and eosinophils. Esophageal Crohn’s disease is characterized by increased intraepithelial lymphocytes, especially in the pediatric population. Granulomas may be seen in some cases. However, involvement of the rest of the GI tract is helpful in confirming a diagnosis of Crohn’s disease. Achalasia and other motility disorders can have increased intraepithelial lymphocytes on biopsy but usually show radiographic and endoscopic evidence of dysmotility. Inflammatory disorders of the skin, including lichen planus, can affect the esophagus resulting in increased intraepithelial lymphocytes. The presence of interface activity, hyperkeratosis, parakeratosis, dyskeratotic keratinocytes, or a history of inflammatory skin disease can be helpful.

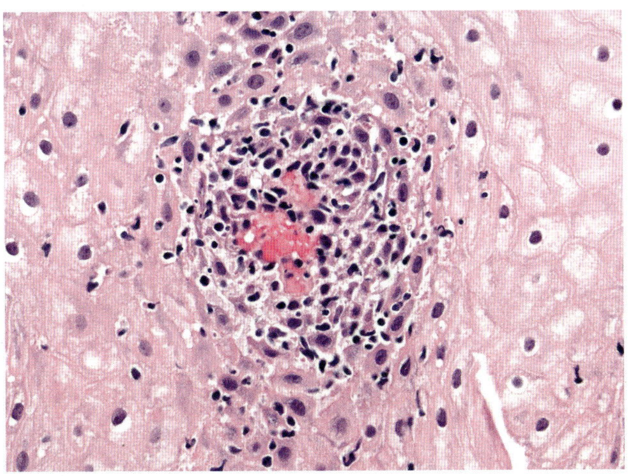

FIGURE 1.10

Lymphocytic esophagitis. Peripapillary lymphocytosis with spongiosis.

Prognosis and Therapy

More than half of patients have symptomatic improvement with treatment, which most often includes a PPI. Patients with IBD may benefit from immunomodulatory therapy. Dilation is often helpful in patients with strictures. Follow-up endoscopic biopsies with the LE pattern of injury have shown persistence of LE, progression to reflux or Crohn’s disease, or complete resolution of histologic findings.

LYMPHOCYTIC ESOPHAGITIS—FACT SHEET

Definition

- Increased number of intraepithelial lymphocytes, predominantly peripapillary, within the squamous esophageal mucosa, with associated spongiosis, and rare to no neutrophils or eosinophils

Incidence and Location

- Incidence has been increasing over time
- Can be seen anywhere along the esophagus

Gender and Age Distribution

- Men and women are equally affected
- Any age can be affected; most patients are diagnosed in the fifth to sixth decade of life

Clinical Features

- Symptoms include dysphagia, odynophagia, chest pain, and heartburn
- Patients may also carry a diagnosis of gastroesophageal reflux disease, inflammatory bowel disease, or allergy

Prognosis and Therapy

- Most patients have symptomatic improvement with proton pump inhibitors
- Dysphagia is likely to resolve
- Gastrointestinal symptoms and histologic findings persist in some patients

Lymphocytic Esophagitis—Pathologic Features

Gross (Endoscopic) Findings

- Normal mucosa, esophageal rings, esophagitis, strictures, features of motility disorder, erythema, nodularity, plaques, furrows, and webs

Microscopic Findings

- Increased peripapillary lymphocytes associated with spongiosis and rare to no neutrophils or eosinophils on biopsy of esophageal squamous mucosa
- The lymphocytosis is patchy, with some unaffected papillae

Differential Diagnosis

- Gastroesophageal reflux disease has more than rare granulocytes
- Crohn's disease may have granulomas and almost always has involvement of other gastrointestinal sites
- Motility disorders have radiographic and endoscopic evidence of dysmotility
- Inflammatory disorders of skin may have interface activity, hyperkeratosis, and dyskeratotic keratinocytes

LICHEN PLANUS AND LICHENOID ESOPHAGITIS

Clinical Features

Lichen planus of the esophagus, or lichen planus esophagitis, can occur with or without concurrent cutaneous lichen planus. For both lichen planus and lichenoid esophagitis pattern of injury, girls and women are affected about three times more often than boys and men. Adults and children can be affected, with a median age of about 64 years. Clinical symptoms include dysphagia and stricture and less commonly, esophagitis, heartburn, chest pain, and hiatal hernia. Whereas comorbidities including viral infections (HIV, hepatitis B, and hepatitis C) have been reported in patients with lichenoid esophagitis, hypothyroidism and rheumatologic diseases have been reported in patients with lichen planus esophagitis. Polypharmacy is associated with both conditions.

Pathologic Features

The squamous epithelium and lamina propria are involved by a dense band of predominantly T-cell lymphocytic infiltrates. Lymphocytic inflammation can be patchy or diffuse and affect the upper and lower esophagus. Apoptotic or otherwise degenerating squamous cells (Civatte bodies) in a lichenoid background are diagnostic of lichen planus esophagitis. The background squamous epithelium can be atrophic. Other inflammatory cell types are not prominent. Direct immunofluorescence demonstrates globular immunoglobulin M (IgM) deposits at the squamous–subsquamous interface in lichen planus and cases with negative direct immunofluorescence but with the other histologic features of lichen planus have been termed *lichenoid esophagitis pattern of injury*.

Differential Diagnosis

Graft-versus-host disease, achalasia and other motility disorders, Crohn's disease, and reflux esophagitis with increased intraepithelial lymphocytes are prominent. LE has a peripapillary lymphocytosis, rather than bandlike, and lacks Civatte bodies.

Prognosis and Therapy

Lichen planus is a chronic progressive disease that can result in esophageal stricture or even squamous cell carcinoma (SCC). Immunomodulatory medications are the mainstay of treatment.

CROHN'S DISEASE

Clinical Features

Esophageal involvement in Crohn's disease is uncommon, affecting about 6% of patients with Crohn's disease.

Pathologic Features

Esophageal biopsies may show increased intraepithelial lymphocytes, especially in pediatric patients (Fig. 1.11). Well-formed, non-necrotizing epithelioid granulomas may also be present. Active inflammation consisting of intraepithelial neutrophils, erosion, or ulceration can be seen.

Differential Diagnosis

Knowledge of a patient's diagnosis of Crohn's disease, by demonstrated involvement in other organs, is useful when considering the differential diagnosis. Granulomatous esophagitis and LE are the main considerations if there is no other evidence of Crohn's disease

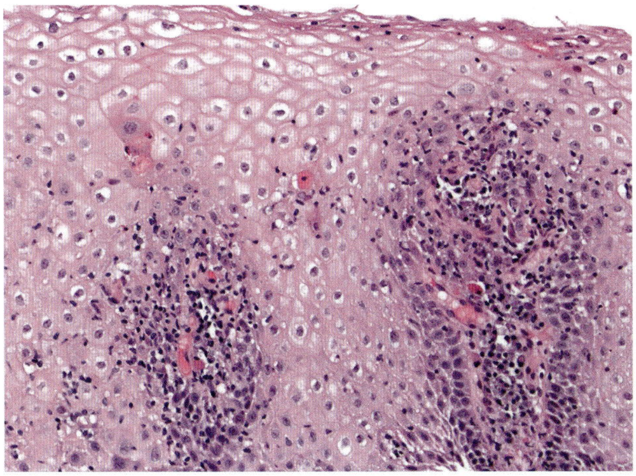

FIGURE 1.11

Crohn's disease. Inflammation is predominantly lymphocytic with a few eosinophils and dyskeratotic keratinocytes.

in other organs. Granulomatous esophagitis can be caused by infections, such as mycobacteria and fungus, sarcoidosis, Wegener's granulomatous, chronic granulomatous disease, or some medications.

Prognosis and Therapy

Patients with Crohn's disease who have esophageal involvement are treated similar to those with disease elsewhere in the GI tract, including antiinflammatory agents and immunomodulators. There is no reported difference in prognosis for patients with Crohn's disease who have esophageal involvement.

GRAFT-VERSUS-HOST DISEASE

Clinical Features

Esophageal involvement is uncommon in patients with GVHD and usually accompanies involvement of other parts of the GI tract. Symptoms of esophageal involvement include dysphagia and chest pain. On endoscopy, the mucosa appears friable and may be ulcerated. Rarely, severe cases may show prominent sloughing of the esophageal mucosa.

Pathologic Features

A lichenoid pattern of intraepithelial lymphocytosis along with scattered apoptosis manifested as dyskeratotic keratinocytes is characteristic. In acute GVHD, neutrophilic inflammation, including erosions or ulcers and rarely sloughing, can be seen. Chronic GVHD may affect the esophagus with lamina propria fibrosis, although this may be difficult to detect on biopsy.

Differential Diagnosis

Infectious esophagitis, pill esophagitis, sloughing esophagitis, LE, cutaneous lichenoid disorders affecting the esophagus, and mycophenolate injury are all in the differential diagnosis and can be excluded by clinical history and special stains.

IGG4-RELATED ESOPHAGEAL DISEASE

Similar to other organ systems, a rare subset of patients with IgG4-related disease can show esophageal involvement. The clinical presentation can be quite variable and includes strictures, posttreatment achalasia, erosive esophagitis, and submucosal esophageal nodule. The diagnostic criteria for IgG4-esophagitis include the presence of IgG4-positive plasma cells (≥50 IgG4-positive plasma cells per high-power field or a ratio of IgG4 to IgG-positive plasma cells ≥50%) and two of the three major histologic features: prominent lymphoplasmacytic inflammation, storiform pattern of fibrosis, and obliterative phlebitis. Needless to say, these changes are best appreciated on esophageal resection specimens. The biopsy findings tend to be quite variable and nonspecific. Whereas some cases may show ulceration with a marked increase in intraepithelial lymphocytes and plasma cells, others show an esophagitis dissecans superficialis–like pattern. Immunohistochemical stain is helpful in highlighting a dominant population of IgG4-positive plasma cells. A study by Clayton et al. (2014) found IgG4-positive plasma cells to be prominent in adults with EoE, raising the possibility for a role of the IgG4 pathway in the pathophysiology of EoE. At this time, there is no standard recommendation as to when to perform an IgG4 immunohistochemical stain, especially on biopsy specimens.

THERAPY OR TOXIN-RELATED INJURY RADIATION OR CHEMOTHERAPY ESOPHAGITIS

Clinical Features

Esophageal symptoms in radiation injury depend on factors such as total dose, time period, and previous surgery. At doses of 60 Gy (6000 rads), the esophagus suffers irreversible damage. Acute radiation injury develops after 2 weeks of therapy and consists of dysphagia, odynophagia, and sometimes hematemesis and chest pain. These symptoms subside after radiation stops. Sequelae of radiation include strictures with dysmotility and dysphagia.

Symptoms are similar with different chemotherapeutic agents. When chemotherapy and radiation therapy are given, their synergistic effect results in more severe damage and more serious symptoms. The incidence of severe acute esophagitis in patients with lung cancer receiving chemoradiotherapy is 14%.

Pathologic Features

Gross Findings

In acute cases, endoscopic examination reveals friable mucosa with edema and coalescent ulcers (mucositis). In chronic cases, strictures develop 13 to 21 months after therapy (Fig. 1.12).

Microscopic Findings

Biopsies are not often procured in the acute stage, but when examined, they show mucosal necrosis and edema. Histologic examination in chronic radiation or chemotherapy esophagitis shows significant atypia in epithelial and stromal cells. The cells are enlarged with hyperchromatic nuclei and a smudged chromatin pattern. Multinucleation as well as abundant vacuolated cytoplasm is common (Fig. 1.13). The nuclear-to-cytoplasmic ratio is usually preserved. More superficial biopsies show active esophagitis, granulation tissue, or both.

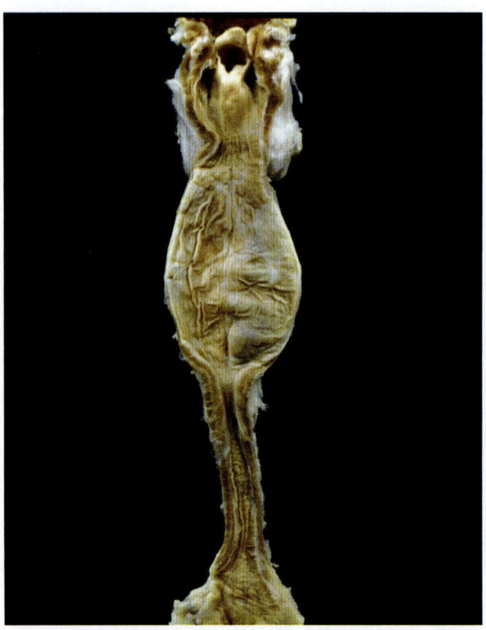

FIGURE 1.12

Esophageal stricture. (From Turk JL, ed. Royal College of Surgeons of England. *Slide Atlas of Pathology. Alimentary Tract System*. London, Gower Medical, 1986, with permission.)

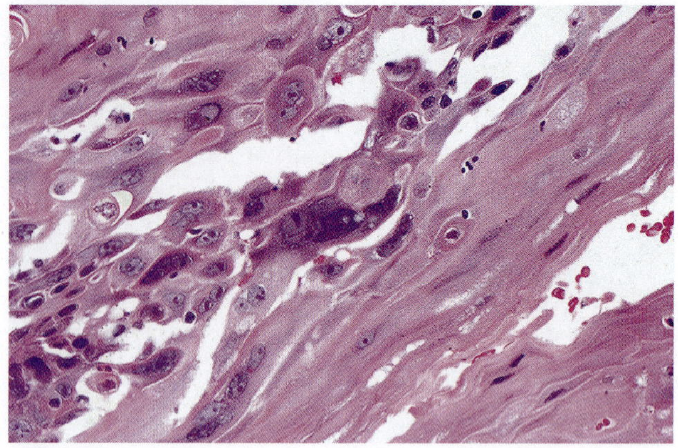

FIGURE 1.13

Radiation esophagitis. Cytomegaly with pale nuclei, abundant cytoplasm, and multinucleation.

Resection specimens of posttreatment esophageal carcinomas often show atrophic mucous glands, squamous metaplasia of esophageal ducts, submucosal and mural fibrosis, and hyalinized vessels. These atrophic glands should not be misinterpreted as residual tumor and can be identified by their location and lobular configuration. The mural fibrosis may alter the wall architecture sufficiently to make staging of residual tumor difficult. A localized ulcer may also be present.

Differential Diagnosis

The most important entities in the differential diagnosis are malignancy and viral esophagitis. Malignant epithelial cells and radiation- or chemotherapy-induced damage can mimic each other and sometimes coexist in the same patient. Malignant cells show an increased nuclear-to-cytoplasmic ratio, hyperchromatic nuclei, irregular nuclear membranes, and mitotic activity. Malignant glands may be simplified but are often angulated and do not form a lobule as an atrophic gland would. Atypical stromal cells are usually single cells with ill-defined cell borders, smudged nuclear chromatin, and elongated cell processes. It can mimic therapy-related changes in an isolated malignant cell, which usually has a well-defined cell border and denser eosinophilic cytoplasm. A cytokeratin immunostain can be helpful to confirm the presence of a malignant cell versus an atypical stromal cell. Multinucleation can be confused with herpes infection, but there is no molding or margination of chromatin. Special immunostains for HSV are indicated to help in this differential diagnosis.

Prognosis and Therapy

Reversible damage occurs in doses lower than 6000 rads. There prognosis is more severe when the damage is a result of both radiation and chemotherapy. Esophageal dilation is indicated when stricture develops.

RADIATION OR CHEMOTHERAPY ESOPHAGITIS—FACT SHEET

Definition

- Damage to the esophagus as a result of radiation, chemotherapy, or both

Incidence and Location

- The incidence of severe acute esophagitis in patients with lung cancer receiving chemoradiotherapy is 14%
- Any part of the esophagus exposed to the therapy may be affected

Clinical Features

- Acute radiation injury occurs after 2 weeks of therapy, and symptoms include dysphagia, odynophagia, hematemesis, and chest pain
- Chronic radiation injury resulting in stricture leads to dysmotility and dysphagia
- Symptoms from chemotherapy are similar

Prognosis and Therapy

- Damage is reversible if exposure is less than 6000 rads
- The prognosis is worse when damage is from a combination of radiation and chemotherapy
- Dilation is indicated for therapy of esophageal stricture

RADIATION OR CHEMOTHERAPY ESOPHAGITIS—PATHOLOGIC FEATURES

Gross (Endoscopic) Findings

- Acute injury includes friable mucosa with edema and ulceration
- Chronic injury is characterized by stricture

Microscopic Findings

- Mucosal necrosis and edema are seen in the acute stage on biopsy
- Atypia of stromal cells and epithelial cells are seen in the chronic stage
- Enlarged, hyperchromatic nuclei with smudged chromatin and multinucleation
- Vacuolated cytoplasm and preserved nuclear-to-cytoplasmic ratio
- In posttreatment resection specimens, there are atrophic mucous glands, squamous metaplasia of esophageal ducts, fibrosis within the wall (sometimes distorting the normal wall organization and architecture), and hyalinized vessels. Localized ulceration can also be seen

Differential Diagnosis

- Malignancy can coexist with radiation- or chemotherapy-induced damage or can be missed if the clinical history is not known
- Multinucleation or atypia of viral esophagitis can be confused with radiation- or chemotherapy-induced damage and atypia. Immunohistochemical stains for viral entities should be used

PILL ESOPHAGITIS

Clinical Features

Pill esophagitis is a result of esophageal injury that occurs because of prolonged direct mucosal contact with tablets or capsules taken in therapeutic doses. Commonly implicated agents include antibiotics (particularly doxycycline), potassium chloride, ferrous sulfate, quinidine, and alendronate, among others.

Although the older adult population is more often affected, pill esophagitis can occur at any age. The main symptoms are sudden retrosternal pain and painful swallowing. The patient often gives a history of having taken the medication with little or no fluid just before going to bed and was aware that the pill had "stuck" in the chest. Some patients present with atypical symptoms, suggesting a myocardial infarction or reflux disease. Some medications such as sodium valproate, ferrous sulfate, and aspirin–caffeine compounds have been associated with esophageal perforation and mediastinitis.

Pathologic Features

Gross Findings

Endoscopic examination reveals the presence of one or more discrete ulcers, often containing residual pill fragments. The lesions are more commonly seen at the level of the aortic arch.

Microscopic Findings

Histologic findings are nonspecific and include superficial erosions or ulcerations with marked acute inflammation and florid granulation tissue (Figs. 1.14 and 1.15). However, many patients have prominent eosinophilia, spongiosis, and necrosis of the squamous epithelium. Polarizable crystalline material (alendronate) or stainable crystalline iron can be demonstrated in the ulcer bed.

Differential Diagnosis

Severe GERD, infections, and EoE can mimic pill esophagitis. Fungal or viral infection can be excluded

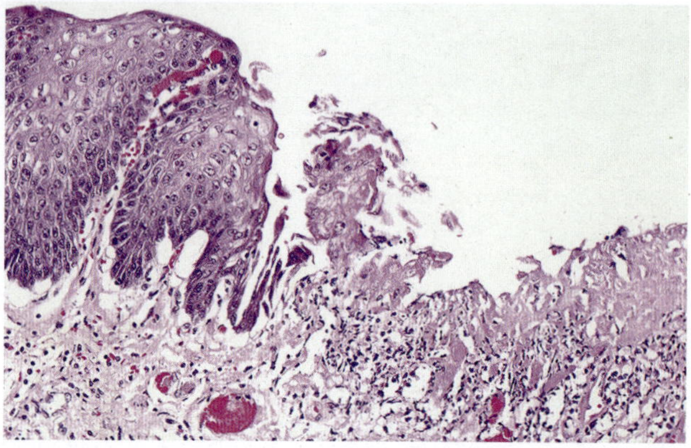

FIGURE 1.14

Pill esophagitis. Esophageal mucosa with ulceration.

by special stains. GERD and EoE are typically associated with other salient histologic findings of basal cell hyperplasia, spongiosis, and history of prior clinical symptoms.

Prognosis and Therapy

Most patients have an uneventful recovery after discontinuing use of the medication. Antireflux medication and topical anesthetics may also be helpful to relieve symptoms.

PILL ESOPHAGITIS—FACT SHEET

Definition

- Esophageal injury that occurs because of prolonged direct mucosal contact with tablets or capsules taken in therapeutic doses

Gender and Age Distribution

- Any age can be affected but more common in older adults

Clinical Features

- Antibiotics are among the common medications that cause pill esophagitis
- Feeling of a pill being stuck in the esophagus after taking the pill with little or no fluid, especially just before lying down
- Atypical symptoms can mimic myocardial infarction or reflux

Prognosis and Therapy

- Recovery occurs after stopping the medication
- Antireflux medication or topical anesthetic may help alleviate symptoms

Pill Esophagitis—Pathologic Features

Gross Findings

- One or more discreet ulcers, which may contain pill fragments, most commonly at the level of the aortic arch

Microscopic Findings

- Nonspecific erosions or ulcerations
- Prominent eosinophilia, spongiosis, and necrosis of the squamous epithelium
- Pill fragments or polarizable or stainable crystalline material can sometimes be seen

Differential Diagnosis

- Severe gastroesophageal reflux disease and eosinophilic esophagitis have basal cell hyperplasia, spongiosis, and prior typical clinical symptoms
- Fungal or viral infections can be excluded by special stains and immunohistochemistry

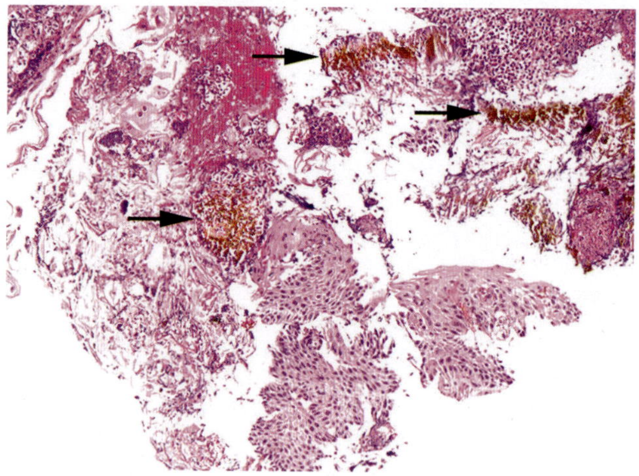

FIGURE 1.15

Pill esophagitis. Refractile brown iron pill material *(arrows)* is present among inflamed squamous epithelium.

ESOPHAGITIS DISSECANS SUPERFICIALIS OR SLOUGHING ESOPHAGITIS

Clinical Features

Sloughing esophagitis is a recently described entity that has also been reported in the literature as esophagitis superficialis dissecans. It is unclear whether these are two distinct entities or represent a spectrum of the same disease process. Patients are typically middle aged, debilitated, and taking multiple (five or more) medications (especially bisphosphonates, potassium chloride, nonsteroidal antiinflammatory drugs [NSAIDs]), often including a central nervous system depressant. Consumption of hot beverages, chemical irritants, smoking, and collagen vascular diseases have also been associated with this condition. Clinical symptoms include upper GI bleed, dysphagia, and nausea and vomiting.

Pathologic Features

Gross Findings

Endoscopically, necrosis of the superficial squamous epithelium is seen as white plaques or membranes, the edges of which may be detached from the underlying tissue, creating the appearance of linear ulcers (Fig. 1.16). The distal esophagus is most often affected. Involvement of the mid and proximal esophagus can be seen when the process is more diffuse.

Microscopic Findings

The most striking feature is a two-toned appearance of the squamous mucosa at low power, with the superficial necrotic aspect being markedly eosinophilic compared with the viable basal aspect (Fig. 1.17). A distinct demarcation between the two layers is present, and neutrophils and apoptotic debris may be present along this line of demarcation. In some cases, the superficial layer shows parakeratosis and sloughing of the necrotic squamous epithelium.

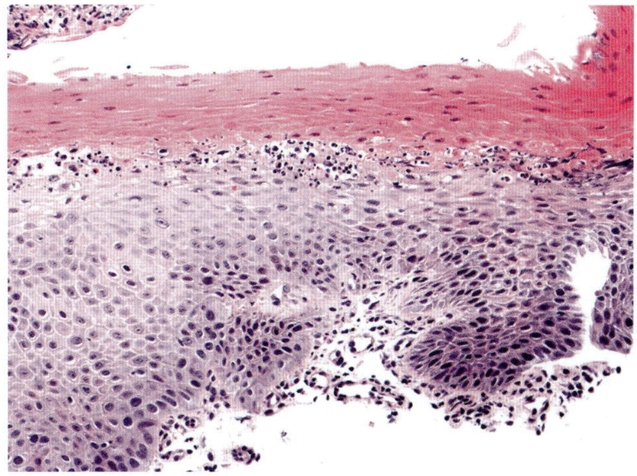

FIGURE 1.17

Sloughing esophagitis. Superficial necrosis is seen as an eosinophilic luminal aspect and a basophilic basal aspect. This case has degenerative nuclei in between the layers.

Differential Diagnosis

Fungal esophagitis, pill esophagitis, and caustic esophageal injury can all result in necrosis of the esophageal epithelium. Clinical history of ingestion and special stains for fungal elements can help distinguish these entities.

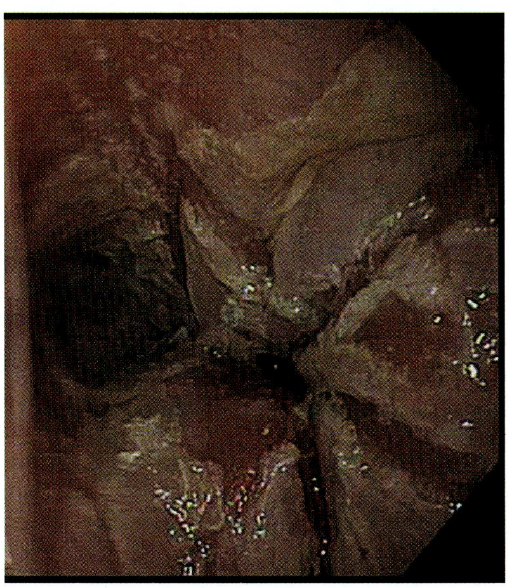

FIGURE 1.16

Sloughing esophagitis. Endoscopically, white plaques with detached edges characterize the superficial epithelial necrosis.

Bullous skin lesions affecting the esophagus should also be considered and can be distinguished by their characteristic histologic features and immunofluorescence. Acute esophageal necrosis may have a similar endoscopic appearance, but histologically, the characteristic features include diffuse and deep ulceration with fibrinopurulent exudate and full-thickness mucosal necrosis.

Prognosis and Therapy

The lesion tends to heal with acid suppressants, topical anesthetics, and discontinuation of the offending agents. A high death rate of patients with sloughing esophagitis is attributed to the comorbid conditions.

ESOPHAGITIS DISSECANS SUPERFICIALIS OR SLOUGHING ESOPHAGITIS—FACT SHEET

Definition

- A recently described entity that may be a spectrum of the same disease process, characterized by detachment of the superficial squamous epithelium

Clinical Features

- Affects middle-aged debilitated patients taking five or more medications, which often include a central nervous system depressant, bisphosphonates, potassium chloride, and nonsteroidal antiinflammatory drugs
- Also can occur in the setting of hot beverage consumption, chemical irritant exposure, smoking, and collagen vascular disease
- Symptoms include upper gastrointestinal tract bleeding, dysphagia, nausea, and vomiting

Prognosis and Therapy

- Lesions heal with acid suppressants, topical anesthetics, and discontinuation of the offending agents
- High death rate attributed to comorbid conditions

Esophagitis Dissecans Superficialis or Sloughing Esophagitis—Pathologic Features

Gross (Endoscopic) Findings

- White plaques or membranes, the edges of which are detached from the underlying tissue, creating the appearance of a linear ulcer
- Distal esophagus most often affected, but diffuse cases can involve the mid and proximal esophagus

Microscopic Findings

- Two-toned appearance of the squamous mucosa at low power: superficial aspect is markedly eosinophilic and sharply demarcated from the viable basal aspect
- Neutrophils and apoptotic debris may be present along the line of demarcation

Differential Diagnosis

- Fungal esophagitis can have acute inflammation and some sloughing; fungal elements can be highlighted by special stains
- Pill esophagitis often has more an ulcer and a typical clinical history
- Caustic esophageal injury can be considered based on the clinical history
- Bullous skin lesions affecting the esophagus have characteristic histologic features and immunofluorescence
- Acute esophageal necrosis has diffuse and deep ulceration with fibrinopurulent exudates

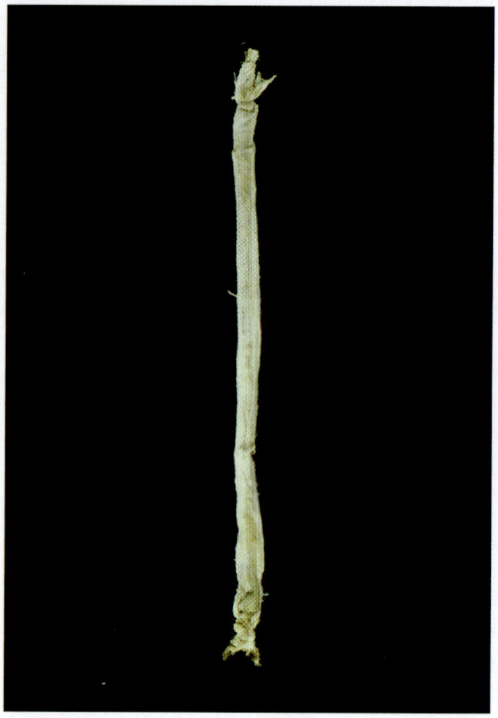

FIGURE 1.18

Esophageal mucosal cast. (From Turk JL, ed. Royal College of Surgeons of England. *Slide Atlas of Pathology. Alimentary Tract System*. London, Gower Medical, 1986, with permission.)

CAUSTIC ESOPHAGEAL INJURY

Clinical Features

Caustic injuries in children are a public health problem, with more than 5000 cases reported yearly in the United States. It is less common in adults, with an incidence of 1 in 100,000; the majority are the result of suicidal attempts. Children younger than 3 years are the most frequent victims of accidents involving common household products such as bleaches, detergents, and alkalis.

The symptoms are quite variable, and there is little correlation between the severity of symptoms and the degree of esophageal damage. Dysphagia and odynophagia are the main symptoms, with chest and back pain presenting to a lesser extent. In severe cases, the entire esophageal mucosal cast is extruded (Fig. 1.18). In the most extreme cases, esophageal and gastric perforation with mediastinitis and peritonitis occur. Alkali ingestions are less common but more severe than those caused by acids.

Pathologic Features

Gross Findings

Endoscopic findings vary depending on the severity of mucosal injury. A grading system exists similar to the one in skin burns. First-degree cases have superficial edema and erythema. Second-degree cases have muscular involvement with ulceration and necrosis. Third-degree cases have transmural lesions with possible extraesophageal extension (Fig. 1.19).

Microscopic Findings

Variable degrees of injury occur depending on the offensive agent. Lesions caused by alkali are more severe than those caused by acids. Areas of coagulative necrosis, diffuse ulceration, and hemorrhage are characteristic. Transmural ulceration and necrosis are seen in third-degree lesions.

Differential Diagnosis

When the clinical history is not available, other entities enter into the differential diagnosis, including reflux and infectious esophagitis. Extensive and diffuse coagulative necrosis is uncommon in reflux esophagitis. Infectious processes are usually associated with discrete esophageal ulcers or esophageal plaques with characteristic viral cytopathic effect (CMV or HSV) or fungal forms (*Candida*), respectively.

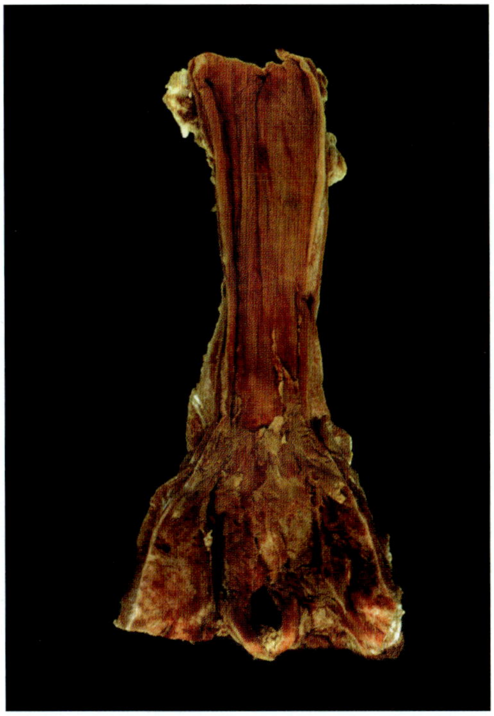

FIGURE 1.19

Caustic esophagitis. Necrosis and perforation. (From Turk JL, ed. Royal College of Surgeons of England. *Slide Atlas of Pathology. Alimentary Tract System*. London, Gower Medical, 1986, with permission.)

Prognosis and Therapy

Cases are always fatal when more than 6 mL of concentrated alkaline material is ingested. Intravenous (IV) fluids, total parenteral nutrition (if patients are unable to swallow), steroid therapy, and antibiotics are used for conservative management. Esophageal dilation is required if strictures develop. Because patients with corrosive strictures have an increased risk of developing SCC, patients should be evaluated, especially if they develop dysphagia or poor response to dilation after a latent period of negligible symptoms.

MISCELLANEOUS LESIONS

Miscellaneous lesions include lesions discovered incidentally during upper GI endoscopy. The differential diagnosis includes fungal esophagitis, esophageal neoplasm, or metastatic malignancy.

INLET PATCH

Heterotopic gastric mucosa of the proximal esophagus, also called a gastric or cervical inlet patch, is an asymptomatic salmon-colored mucosal patch just distal to the upper esophageal sphincter, found in 1% to 18% of endoscopic studies. Cervical inlet patch consists of benign gastric cardiac, antral, or fundic mucosa surrounded by esophageal squamous mucosa (Fig. 1.20). Complications of cervical inlet patch include involvement by *Helicobacter pylori* infection, ulceration, stricture, IM, and dysplasia.

HETEROTOPIC SEBACEOUS GLANDS

Heterotopic sebaceous glands are found in the mid to distal esophagus. They are seen endoscopically as single or multiple small 1- to 2-mm yellow to white mucosal plaques or nodules. Heterotopic sebaceous glands are mature clusters of sebaceous glands interspersed among the esophageal squamous mucosa (Fig. 1.21). Heterotopic sebaceous glands have no clinical significance.

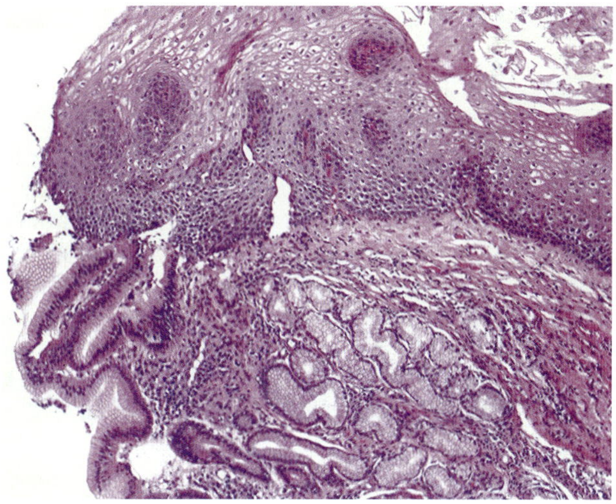

FIGURE 1.20

Gastric heterotopia inlet patch. Cardiac-type mucosa with inflammation.

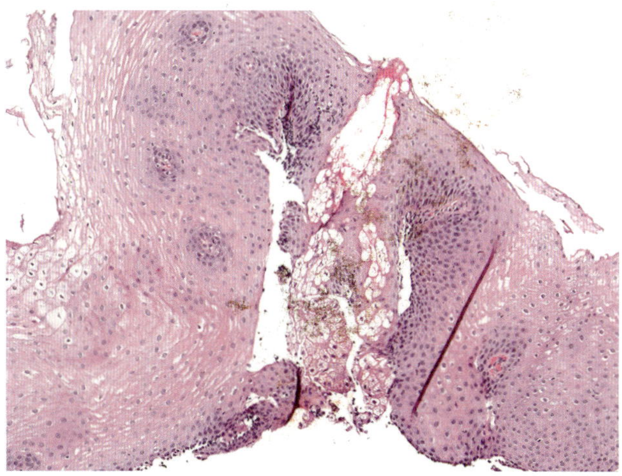

FIGURE 1.21

Heterotopic sebaceous glands. A mature sebaceous gland is present surrounded by esophageal squamous mucosa.

GLYCOGENIC ACANTHOSIS

Glycogenic acanthosis is seen as multiple, slightly elevated, rounded nodules less than 1 cm in diameter. Eighty percent of patients with Cowden syndrome (a PTEN hamartoma tumor syndrome) have a characteristic diffuse glycogenic acanthosis. Biopsy of incidentally identified esophageal lesions is performed to confirm the benign nature of the lesion and to exclude a neoplastic process. Glycogenic acanthosis may be seen as a subtle hyperplasia of the esophageal squamous mucosa at low power. At higher magnification, squamous cells in the involved area have abundant glycogen-filled cytoplasm, which can be confirmed by periodic acid–Schiff stain (Fig. 1.22). Sporadic glycogenic acanthosis may be related to GERD. The presence of diffuse glycogenic acanthosis should prompt further work-up for Cowden syndrome.

ESOPHAGEAL HYPERKERATOSIS AND EPIDERMOID METAPLASIA

In esophageal hyperkeratosis, a white plaque, which may be circumferential, is seen on endoscopy. Biopsy of the plaque reveals hyperkeratosis with a prominent granular layer, with or without a few neutrophils or eosinophils. This lesion has been reported in association with gastroesophageal reflux and vitamin A deficiency and has been reported in adults and children. Although the findings may persist with antireflux therapy, there are no reported long-term sequelae. In patients being seen at a specialty cancer center, Taggart et al. (2013) reported an incidence on esophageal biopsy of 2%. In 62% of these patients, hyperkeratosis was found within squamous mucosa associated with BE or adenocarcinoma. In the remaining 38% of patients, hyperkeratosis was more often multifocal, involved the midesophagus, was associated with endoscopic leukoplakia 24% of the time, and was seen more often in patients with current or former alcohol use. The presence of hyperkeratosis outside of BE or adenocarcinoma was associated with squamous neoplasia of the esophagus and with squamous carcinoma of the oropharynx.

Epidermoid metaplasia is a rare entity, seen endoscopically as a white to tan well-demarcated and slightly elevated mucosal patch or scaly plaque of variable size (from 1 cm to 24 cm, with a median of 8.5 cm), within the proximal to middle third of the esophagus. On biopsy, there are thickening of the basal layer, acanthosis, and a prominent granular cell layer, not usually found in the esophageal squamous mucosa. The luminal aspect shows hyperorthokeratosis. Epidermoid metaplasia is associated with synchronous or metachronous esophageal SCC. Targeted next-generation sequencing has revealed epidermoid hyperplasia to be a precursor to esophageal dysplasia and carcinoma, harboring gene mutations in *TP53, PIK3CA, EGFR*, and others. Similar to esophageal squamous carcinoma, epidermoid metaplasia is seen in patients with history of significant tobacco smoking and alcohol intake. Interestingly, although inflammation is not a characteristic of epidermoid metaplasia of the esophagus, patients can have concurrent histologic features of lichenoid esophagitis or esophageal lichen planus.

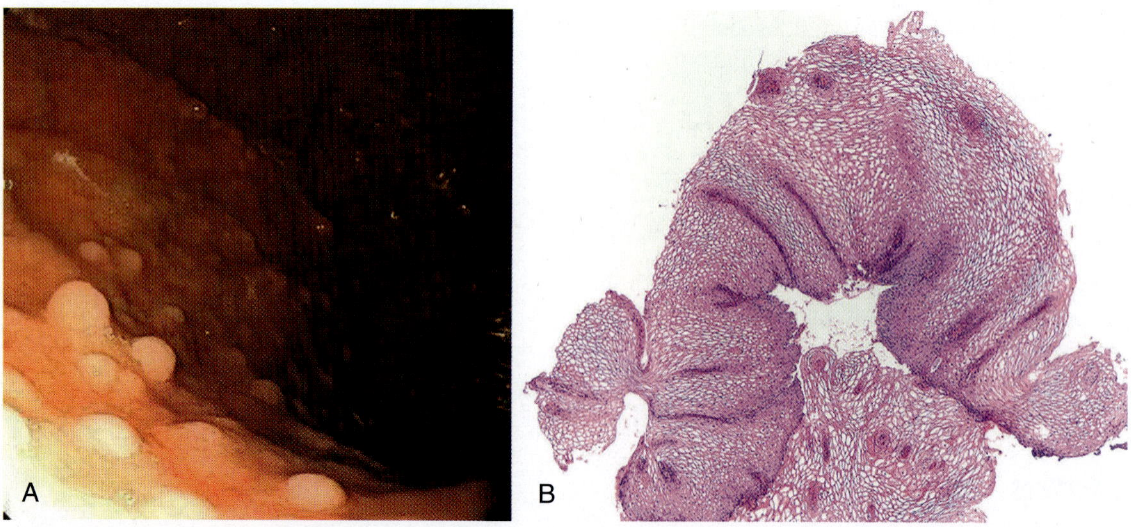

FIGURE 1.22

Glycogenic acanthosis. Multiple small round nodules are seen on endoscopy (**A**). Squamous cells in involved areas have abundant glycogen-filled cytoplasm (**B**).

INFLAMMATION AND INTESTINAL METAPLASIA OF THE GASTROESOPHAGEAL JUNCTION

The GEJ mucosa usually shows some degree of chronic inflammation within the lamina propria. This can either be attributed to physiologic or pathologic GERD. In the setting of inflamed GEJ, the main differential diagnoses are *H. pylori*–induced gastritis versus reflux disease. On its own and without other more specific findings, such as accompanying antral *Helicobacter* gastritis or reflux squamous esophagitis, the cause of inflammation of gastric-type mucosa in this region cannot be ascertained.

Intestinal metaplasia (IM) at the GEJ similarly has been a subject of an ongoing debate as to whether metaplastic columnar epithelium in biopsy samples taken from the GEJ is caused by reflux disease–induced BE or *H. pylori*–induced intestinalized pangastritis. To date, the clinical significance of these distinctions is unknown because long-term prospective follow-up data are lacking. As a practical matter, at present, if the biopsy shows the presence of submucosal or mucosal esophageal glands, squamous-lined ducts, multilayered epithelium, or hybrid glands, the biopsy is derived from the tubular esophagus rather than gastric cardia (see Chapter 2 for details). Fortunately, given that the current American College of Gastroenterology guideline defines BE when there is extension of salmon-colored mucosa into the tubular esophagus extending 1 cm or more proximal to the GEJ with biopsy confirmation of IM, the problem of IM at GEJ perhaps is less relevant to daily practice.

STRUCTURAL ABNORMALITIES

CONGENITAL (ESOPHAGEAL ATRESIA, TRACHEOESOPHAGEAL FISTULA, DUPLICATION, AND DEVELOPMENTAL CYSTS)

Clinical Features

Esophageal atresia and tracheoesophageal fistula typically occur together and result from failure of the foregut to completely divide into the esophagus and trachea. This separation occurs in the fourth week of gestation. One of every 3500 live births is affected. The affected babies have food regurgitation, salivation, cyanosis, and aspiration. Sometimes they are associated with a trisomy (21, 18, and partial 13) or with the VACTERL (vertebral abnormalities, anal atresia, cardiac abnormalities, tracheoesophageal fistula and/or esophageal atresia, renal agenesis and dysplasia, and limb defects) association.

Esophageal duplications and developmental cysts are not always easy to differentiate from one another. Esophageal duplication accounts for 10 % to 20 % of all GI duplications and is the result of a morphogenetic abnormality occurring around the fifth to eighth week of gestation. Cysts can be classified as bronchogenic, enteric, or neuroenteric. Patients experience feeding difficulties or respiratory distress during childhood. In some cases, the anomaly remains asymptomatic and is discovered during a routine chest x-ray examination.

Pathologic Features

Gross Findings

Esophageal atresias, with or without tracheoesophageal fistulas, are of five different types (Fig. 1.23). Type C is the most common, accounting for 85 % of the cases (Figs. 1.24 and 1.25). The E type (also known as H because of its shape) may be overlooked and diagnosed in older children with repeated bouts of pneumonia.

Duplications occur in the lower esophagus in 60 % of cases; they are usually intramural and do not communicate with the esophageal lumen. Bronchogenic cysts present anteriorly and contain a rim of cartilage. Enteric or neuroenteric cysts sometimes have an hourglass shape, with one portion in the posterior mediastinum and the other inside the vertebral canal.

Microscopic Findings

Duplications are located within the esophageal wall and have distinct layers of muscularis propria containing nerve plexuses (Fig. 1.26). In contrast, other

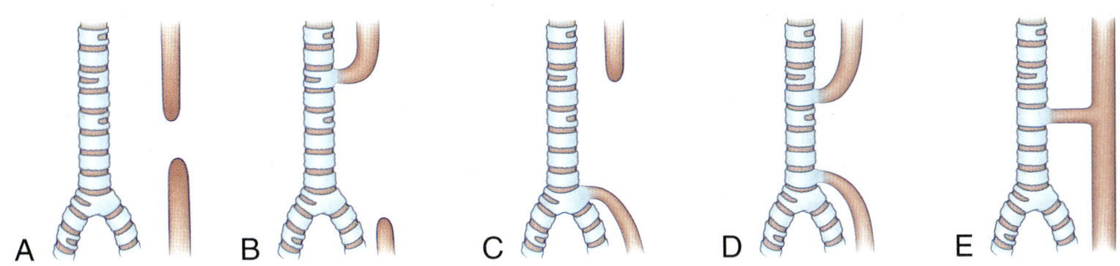

FIGURE 1.23
The five types (**A–E**) of esophageal atresias.

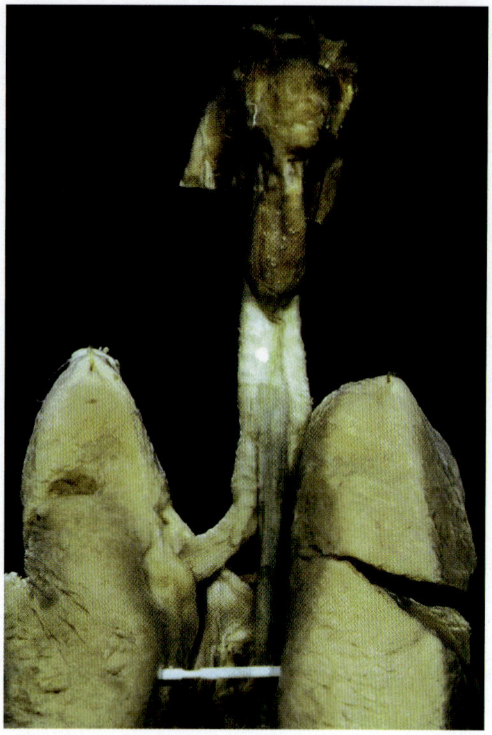

FIGURE 1.24

Esophageal atresia with tracheoesophageal (TE) fistula (posterior view). Blind pouch in the upper esophagus and distal TE fistula at the tracheal bifurcation. (From Turk JL, ed. Royal College of Surgeons of England. *Slide Atlas of Pathology. Alimentary Tract System*. London, Gower Medical, 1986, with permission.)

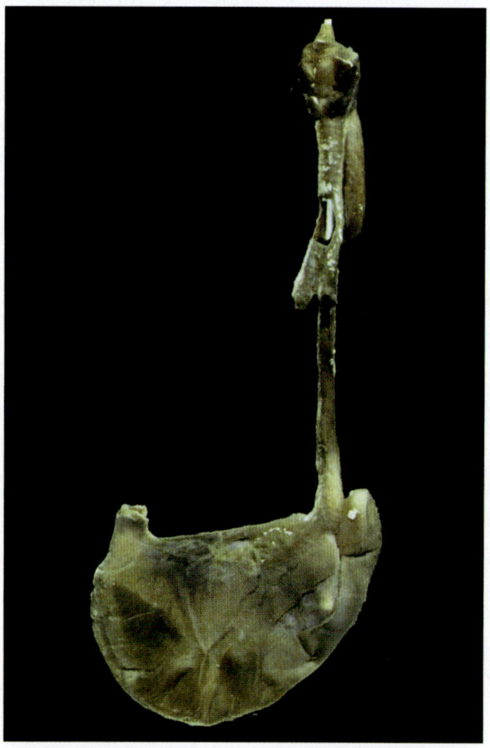

FIGURE 1.25

Esophageal atresia with tracheoesophageal fistula. The stomach and distal esophagus connect with the fistula at the tracheal bifurcation. (From Turk JL, ed. Royal College of Surgeons of England. *Slide Atlas of Pathology. Alimentary Tract System*. London, Gower Medical, 1986, with permission.)

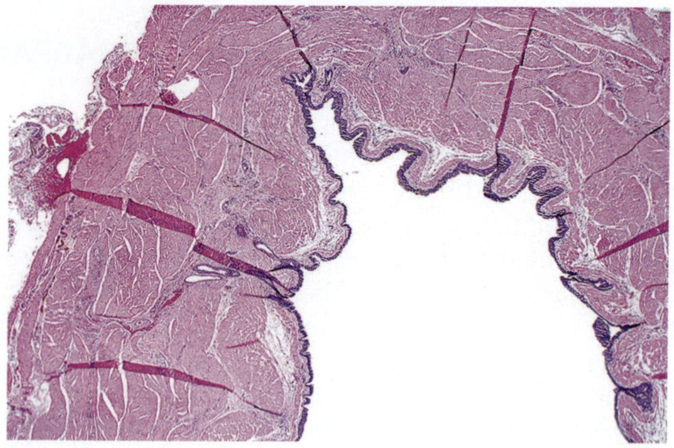

FIGURE 1.26

Esophageal duplication. Intact muscularis propria and cuboidal epithelium.

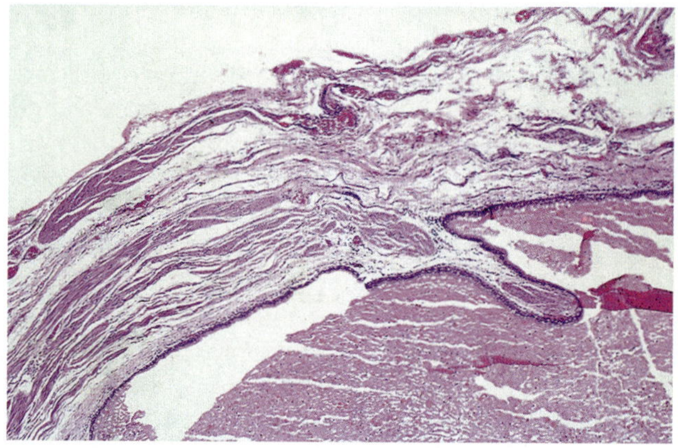

FIGURE 1.27

Esophageal cyst with columnar epithelium, luminal secretions, and attenuated muscle layer.

developmental cysts show an attenuated single layer of smooth muscle. The epithelial lining of either duplications or cysts may have squamous, cuboidal, or ciliated epithelium (Fig. 1.27). Most bronchogenic cysts contain cartilage in their walls.

Differential Diagnosis

Esophageal atresia and tracheoesophageal fistula should be differentiated from the less common congenital esophageal stenosis (Fig. 1.28), which demonstrates a significant narrowing of the midesophagus resulting from a web or muscular hypertrophy. Congenital pyloric stenosis presents with projectile vomiting, and radiographs show esophageal integrity with air trapped in the stomach. Acquired diverticula occur in adults and always communicate with the esophageal lumen. The squamous epithelial lining may show erosions and ulcerations.

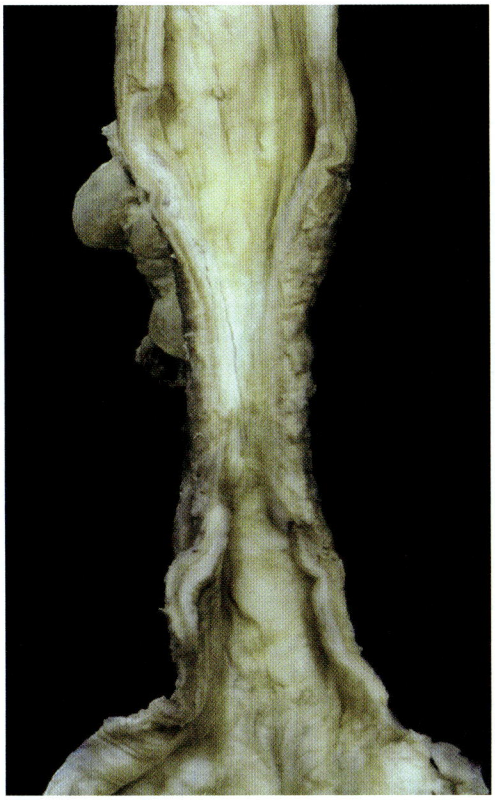

FIGURE 1.28

Esophagus with congenital esophageal stenosis. Note the narrowing of the middle segment. (From Turk JL, ed. Royal College of Surgeons of England. *Slide Atlas of Pathology. Alimentary Tract System*. London, Gower Medical, 1986, with permission.)

Prognosis and Therapy

Early diagnosis with prompt surgical repair confers an excellent prognosis. Additional anatomic anomalies and chromosomal alterations are associated with poor outcomes in patients with esophageal atresia and tracheoesophageal fistula.

CONGENITAL STRUCTURAL ABNORMALITIES—FACT SHEET

Definition

- Esophageal atresia and tracheoesophageal fistula are congenital anomalies resulting from failure of the foregut to divide into trachea and esophagus during the fourth week of embryonic development
- Duplications and developmental cysts are congenital anomalies caused by failure of normal development around the fifth to eighth week of gestation

Incidence and Location

- Esophageal atresia and tracheoesophageal fistula occur in 1 of every 3500 live births
- Duplications are seen in 1 in 8000 autopsies
- Located in lower third of esophagus, duplications protrude into the posterior mediastinum
- Bronchogenic cysts protrude into the anterior mediastinum
- Enteric or neuroenteric cysts occupy the posterior mediastinum
- Neuroenteric cysts can have an hourglass configuration

Gender and Age Distribution

- Newborn through early childhood
- Some cases remain asymptomatic and are discovered on routine chest radiography

Clinical Features

- Food regurgitation, drooling, and aspiration in newborns
- Older children with repeated bouts of pneumonia

Prognosis and Therapy

- Excellent prognosis with early diagnosis and surgical correction
- Patients with associated anomalies have poorer outcomes

Congenital Structural Abnormalities—Pathologic Features

Gross Findings

- There are five types of atresia, most occur with tracheoesophageal fistula (see Fig. 1.23)
- The most common is type C, which occurs in 85% of cases
- Duplication appears as an intramural mass in the lower esophagus
- Bronchogenic cysts may show a rim of cartilage on gross examination
- Neuroenteric cysts may have an hourglass appearance with one component in the posterior mediastinum and the other inside the vertebral canal

Microscopic Findings

- Duplications have a complete muscle layer with neural plexuses
- Developmental cysts usually contain an attenuated single muscle layer
- Bronchogenic cysts contain cartilage in their walls
- Duplications as well as developmental cysts can be lined by squamous, cuboidal, or ciliated epithelium
- Neuroenteric cysts are lined with intestinal epithelium or gastric mucosa

Differential Diagnosis

- Congenital esophageal stenosis and congenital pyloric stenosis may mimic atresia and can be distinguished by radiologic examination
- Acquired diverticula communicate with the esophageal lumen and are lined by squamous epithelium

ACQUIRED (DIVERTICULA, WEBS, AND RINGS)

Clinical Features

Diverticula are outpouchings of the esophagus containing one or more layers of the esophageal wall.

Three major types are recognized based on location: upper esophagus (Zenker's and Killian-Jamieson), level of tracheal bifurcation (midesophageal), and lower esophagus (epiphrenic). Zenker's diverticulum is associated with symptoms of dysphagia, regurgitation, halitosis, and aspiration in middle-aged and older adults. A gurgling sound upon swallowing and a neck mass may be present. Midesophageal diverticula may be asymptomatic and are often associated with mediastinal inflammation. The epiphrenic diverticulum is symptomatic because of its coexistence with hiatal hernia.

Esophageal webs and rings are common and are mostly acquired, except for the rare cases of congenital esophageal stenosis. They are concentric or eccentric narrowings of the esophageal lumen. Webs are found in 4% to 10% of autopsies. Clinically, they are observed in 5% to 15% of patients presenting with dysphagia and choking sensation. The now rare Plummer-Vinson syndrome consists of iron-deficiency anemia, glossitis, cheilosis, and an upper esophageal web (Fig. 1.29). Rings are found in 0.7% to 16% of autopsies. Their pathogenesis is unclear. Rings are usually localized to the lower esophagus, and the most common type of ring associated with reflux disease and hiatal hernia is *Schatzki's ring*.

Pathologic Features

Gross Findings

Zenker's diverticulum is a pouch located at the level of the pharyngoesophageal junction, a weak point in the wall between the inferior constrictor muscle of the pharynx and the fibers of the cricopharyngeal muscle. This triangular area is known as the *triangle of Killian* (Fig. 1.30). The diverticula vary in size and may be filled with necrotic debris. The midesophageal diverticulum (also called *traction diverticulum*) is located at the level of the tracheal bifurcation (Figs. 1.31 and 1.32). The epiphrenic diverticulum lies close to the diaphragm and is seen in association with a hiatal hernia. Endoscopic examination reveals rings and webs as mucosal folds or indentations. Ulceration may be present. Webs are usually noncircumferential.

Microscopic Features

Esophageal diverticula are true diverticula because they are lined by squamous epithelium and contain a muscular wall that can be attenuated (Fig. 1.33). SCC has been reported in 0.3% of Zenker's diverticula cases. Webs are lined by squamous mucosa with edematous

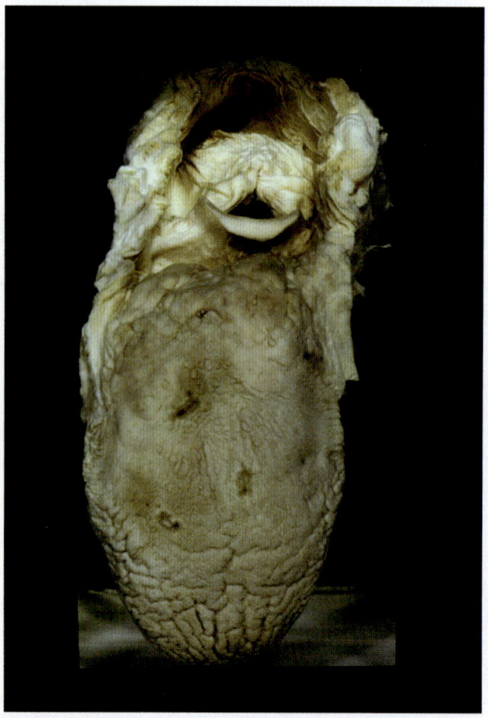

FIGURE 1.29

Upper esophageal web with glossitis. (From Turk JL, ed. Royal College of Surgeons of England. *Slide Atlas of Pathology. Alimentary Tract System*. London, Gower Medical, 1986, with permission.)

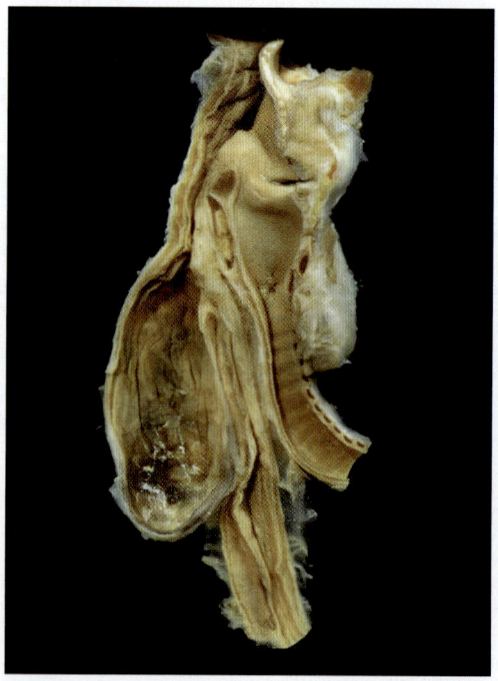

FIGURE 1.30

Zenker's diverticulum. Thin wall and luminal debris. (From Turk JL, ed. Royal College of Surgeons of England. *Slide Atlas of Pathology. Alimentary Tract System*. London, Gower Medical, 1986, with permission.)

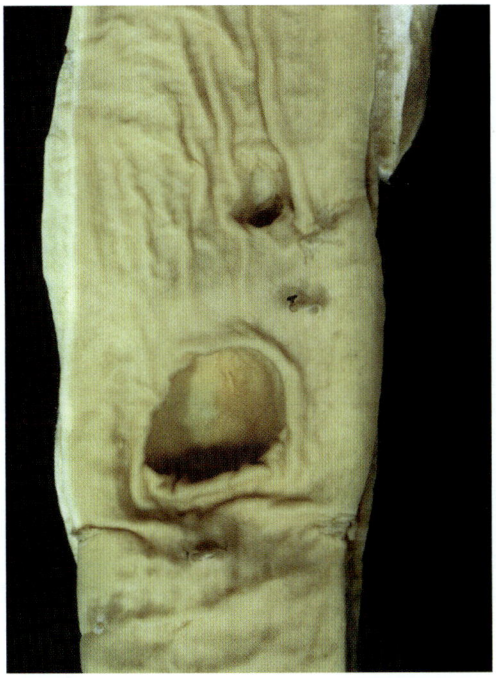

FIGURE 1.31

Midesophageal diverticulum (traction diverticulum; inside view). (From Turk JL, ed. Royal College of Surgeons of England. *Slide Atlas of Pathology. Alimentary Tract System*. London, Gower Medical, 1986, with permission.)

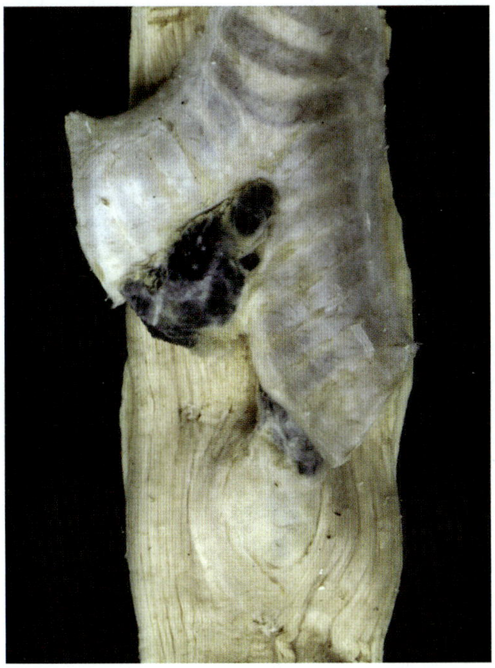

FIGURE 1.32

Midesophageal diverticulum (traction diverticulum; outside view). Adhesions between the lymph nodes and diverticulum. (From Turk JL, ed. Royal College of Surgeons of England. *Slide Atlas of Pathology. Alimentary Tract System*. London, Gower Medical, 1986, with permission.)

and inflamed submucosa. Lower esophageal rings and webs have squamous epithelium on the proximal side and columnar epithelium on the distal side. Some rings are a result of localized annular muscular thickening.

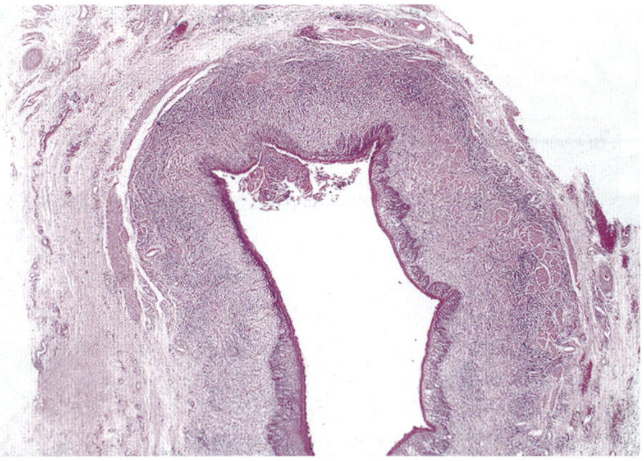

FIGURE 1.33

Zenker's diverticulum. Muscularis propria and squamous epithelial lining.

Differential Diagnosis

Diverticula should be differentiated from pseudodiverticula, which are cystic dilations of submucosal glands, lack involvement of the entire esophageal wall. A unique entity called *diffuse esophageal intramural pseudodiverticulosis* is also in the differential diagnosis. The radiologic examination with contrast media shows multiple minute outpouchings within the esophageal wall. This entity is associated with diabetes, alcoholism, candidiasis, and chronic granulomatous disease. Esophageal rings and webs must be distinguished from postinflammatory stenosis, which can be consequence of long-standing reflux disease or exposure to corrosive agents. Stenosis resulting from these conditions is characterized by marked submucosal fibrosis.

Prognosis and Therapy

Prognosis depends on the size of the diverticulum and on whether it is complicated by ulceration, hemorrhage, or superimposed infection. Large diverticula are treated with diverticulectomy and esophagomyotomy. Esophageal rings and webs can be treated with dietary modifications, dilation, or surgery in refractory cases.

ACQUIRED STRUCTURAL ABNORMALITIES—FACT SHEET

Definition

- Diverticula are acquired outpouchings in the upper, middle, and lower esophagus
- Rings and webs are folds causing concentric or eccentric narrowing of the esophageal lumen

Incidence and Location

- Zenker's diverticulum is the most common (70%)
- Zenker's diverticulum is located on the posterior wall at the junction between the pharynx and esophagus in an area called the *Killian triangle*
- Killian-Jamieson diverticulum is located in the upper esophagus on the anterolateral wall
- Midesophageal diverticulum is less common and occurs at the level of tracheal bifurcation
- Epiphrenic diverticulum is located in the lower esophagus and commonly associated with hiatal hernia
- Rings and webs are common; Schatzki ring is most common
- Webs are more common in the upper esophagus; rings are common in the lower esophagus

Gender and Age Distribution

- Middle-aged and older adults
- No gender preference

Clinical Features

- Small diverticula may be asymptomatic
- In large Zenker's diverticulum, dysphagia, a gurgling sound, and a neck mass may develop
- Regurgitation of food eaten several hours before is quite characteristic
- Inflammatory diseases of the mediastinum accompany the midesophageal diverticulum
- Hiatal hernia is seen in association with epiphrenic diverticulum
- Motility abnormalities are the most likely causes of upper and epiphrenic diverticula
- Rings and webs are mostly asymptomatic but may have dysphagia and odynophagia
- Upper esophageal webs are associated with the now rare Plummer-Vinson syndrome

Prognosis and Therapy

- Prognosis depends on the size of the lesion and associated conditions
- Large diverticula are treated with surgical resection and myomectomy
- Rings and webs are treated with dietary modifications, dilation, or surgery in refractory cases

Differential Diagnosis

- Pseudodiverticula, either single or multiple (diffuse esophageal intramural pseudodiverticulosis), are dilations of submucosal glands and lack involvement of the entire esophageal wall
- Postinflammatory stenosis, occurring after long-standing reflux, or stenosis secondary to corrosive agents, such as lye

Acquired Structural Abnormalities—Pathologic Features

Gross Findings

- Zenker's diverticulum is a sac located at the pharyngoesophageal junction
- Mid-diverticulum occurs at the level of bifurcation of the trachea
- Epiphrenic diverticulum occurs in the lower 10 cm of the esophagus
- Rings are seen as stenosis of the distal esophagus on endoscopy
- Webs are seen as thin mucosal folds on endoscopy

Microscopic Findings

- Diverticula contain all layers of the esophagus, but the muscle layer is attenuated
- Diverticula and webs are lined by stratified squamous epithelium which may be inflamed or ulcerated
- Squamous cell carcinoma rarely develops in Zenker's diverticulum
- Rings have squamous mucosa on the proximal side and columnar epithelium on the distal side

MOTILITY DISORDERS

Normal esophageal motility is a complex mechanism requiring intact, coordinated autonomic innervation. Inadequate function leads to motility disorders, which can be divided into the spastic variety and achalasia. Motility disorders are relatively uncommon. The prevalence of achalasia is 10 cases per 10^5 population. Spastic motility disorders include diffuse esophageal spasm (DES) and hypercontraction and are reported to occur in 4% to 12% of patients tested for typical symptoms.

Clinical Features

Dysphagia for liquids and solids occurs in DES, which is associated with impaired inhibitory innervation affecting the distal esophagus. Unexplained chest pain and psychiatric conditions are associated with hypercontraction, which includes hypertensive peristalsis (also referred to as *nutcracker esophagus*) and hypertensive LES. Diagnosis is based on esophageal manometry and esophageal pressure topography after excluding other esophageal disorders by endoscopic biopsy.

In achalasia, the abnormality consists of aperistalsis, lack of LES relaxation, and increased intraesophageal pressure. Patients are 25 to 60 years of age and have symptoms of progressive dysphagia, regurgitation, and aspiration. Systemic disorders such as systemic sclerosis, muscular dystrophies, amyloidosis, chronic idiopathic intestinal pseudo-obstruction, chronic gastroesophageal reflux, eosinophilic gastroenteritis, and Chagas disease also affect the normal peristaltic mechanism. The incidence of SCC is increased in patients with achalasia.

Pathologic Features

Gross Findings

Endoscopic examination in patients with achalasia shows dilation of the lumen, prominent vascularity, and pooled debris adherent to the wall (Figs. 1.34 and 1.35). In some cases, reflux changes and strictures are present.

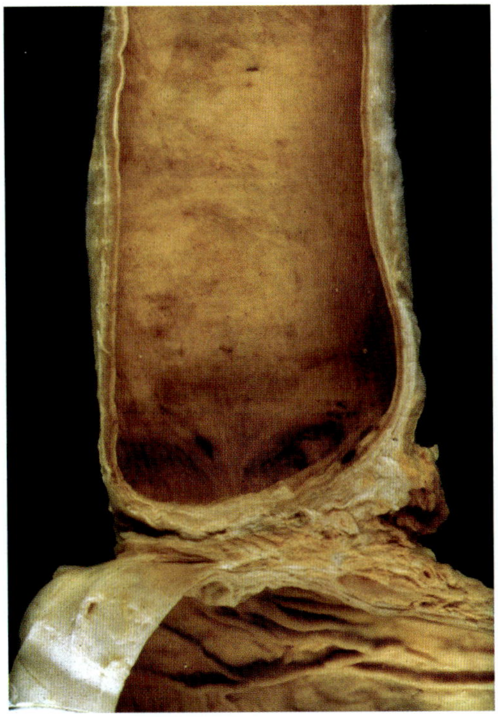

FIGURE 1.34

Achalasia. Marked lumen dilation. (From Turk JL, ed. Royal College of Surgeons of England. *Slide Atlas of Pathology. Alimentary Tract System*. London, Gower Medical, 1986, with permission.)

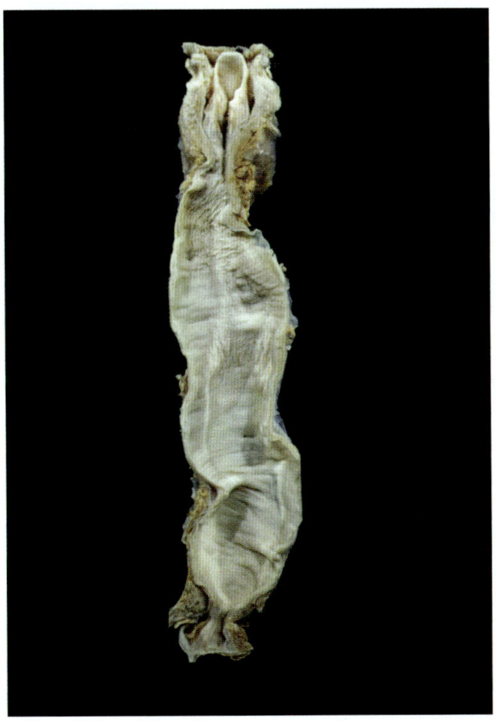

FIGURE 1.35

Achalasia. Tortuous esophagus and narrow distal segment. (From Turk JL, ed. Royal College of Surgeons of England. *Slide Atlas of Pathology. Alimentary Tract System*. London, Gower Medical, 1986, with permission.)

Microscopic Changes

Mucosal biopsies may appear normal or involved by inflammation and ulceration secondary to stasis. Although resection is not a standard therapy for achalasia, autopsy examination reveals characteristic findings of loss of myenteric plexus associated with chronic inflammation of the ganglion cells (Fig. 1.36). Similar morphologic changes can be seen in esophagomyotomy specimens from patients with achalasia. The LES also shows a decrease in the number of these cells but to a lesser degree and hypertrophic muscle. Mucosal changes are nonspecific and appear to be related to stasis. They consist of hyperplasia, papillomatosis, and increased intraepithelial lymphocytes. P53 immunoreactivity and increased CD3+ T cells have been demonstrated and may be related to SCC risk.

Differential Diagnosis

Spastic disorders can mimic angina pectoris. Idiopathic achalasia should be differentiated from secondary achalasia resulting from systemic sclerosis (Fig. 1.37), amyloidosis, muscular dystrophy, chronic idiopathic intestinal pseudo-obstruction, chronic gastroesophageal reflux, eosinophilic gastroenteritis, and Chagas disease (Fig. 1.38). In systemic sclerosis, marked intimal fibrosis of blood vessels is associated with atrophy and fibrosis of the muscularis propria. Amyloidosis reveals deposits of congophilic amyloid deposits in arterioles of the lamina propria. In the chronic phase of Chagas disease, there is complete destruction of myenteric plexuses, resulting in megaesophagus. The trypomastigotes and amastigote forms, however, are seldom present during this stage.

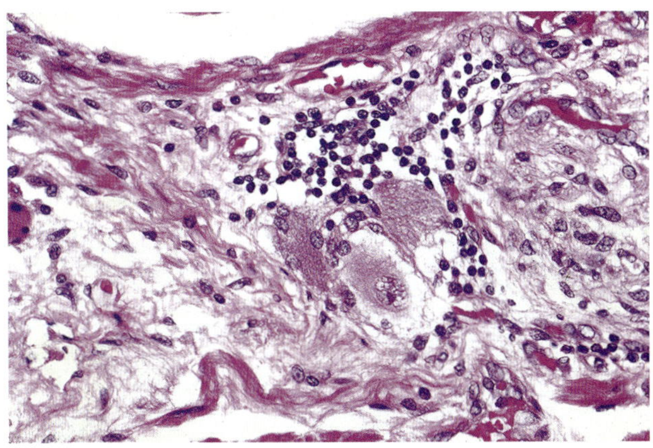

FIGURE 1.36

Achalasia. Myenteric plexus with chronic inflammation (ganglionitis).

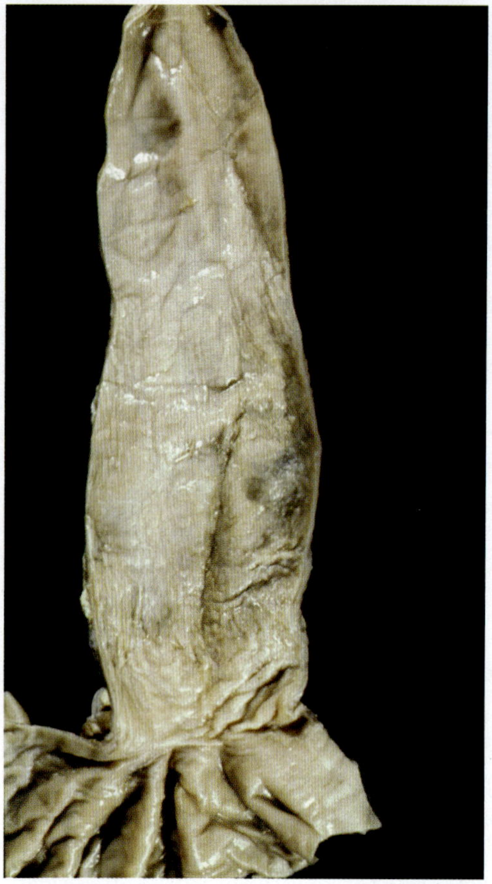

FIGURE 1.37

Scleroderma. Luminal dilation and thinning of muscle wall. (From Turk JL, ed. Royal College of Surgeons of England. *Slide Atlas of Pathology. Alimentary Tract System*. London, Gower Medical, 1986, with permission.)

Prognosis and Therapy

The treatment options for patients with achalasia include botulinum toxin injections and pneumatic dilation. Heller myotomy is an effective surgical therapy for those who do not respond to nonsurgical options. Achalasia is associated with increased risk for developing esophageal SCC. Treatment modalities for spastic disorders include calcium channel blockers, sedatives, nitrates, and pneumatic dilation.

MOTILITY DISORDERS—FACT SHEET

Definition

- Disease entities affecting the normal coordination of swallowing and peristalsis

Incidence and Location

- Motility disorders affect the entire esophageal length
- Spastic disorders are recognized with the use of manometric studies in patients with noncardiac chest pain
- Achalasia is an uncommon disorder with a prevalence of 10 cases per 10^5 population

Gender and Age Distribution

- Patients with achalasia are 25 to 60 years of age
- Men and women are equally affected

Clinical Features

- Severe episodic dysphagia and angina-type chest pain are typical of spastic disorders
- Achalasia presents with progressive dysphagia, regurgitation, aspiration, and weight loss

Prognosis and Therapy

- Prognosis depends on early diagnosis and treatment
- Treatment modalities for achalasia include botulinum toxin injections, pneumatic dilation, and Heller's myotomy
- Treatment for spastic disorders includes nitrates, sedatives, botulinum toxin, and pneumatic dilation
- Patients with achalasia have increased risk of developing squamous cell carcinoma

Motility Disorders—Pathologic Features

Gross Findings

- In achalasia, endoscopic examination reveals a dilated lumen, pooled debris, prominent vascularity, and a lack of normal relaxation of the lower esophageal sphincter (LES)
- Spastic disorders reveal abnormal motility on endoscopic examination

Microscopic Findings

- Chronic ganglionitis with myenteric plexus destruction in the dilated portion of the esophagus is seen in achalasia
- Thickened LES is common
- Mucosal biopsies may show hyperplasia, papillomatosis, and lymphocytic esophagitis

Differential Diagnosis

- Primary achalasia should be differentiated from secondary achalasia caused by systemic sclerosis, Chagas disease, and amyloidosis, among others

SYSTEMIC SCLEROSIS

Clinical Features

Systemic sclerosis, or scleroderma, commonly involves the GI tract, though not all patients are symptomatic. Symptoms include dysphagia, heartburn, choking sensation, and hoarseness. Most symptoms are caused by chronic gastroesophageal reflux associated with esophageal hypomotility and LES incompetence.

Pathologic Features

Gross Findings

Endoscopic findings can include reflux esophagitis, infection such as fungal or viral esophagitis, BE, and stricture. Biopsy can show corresponding findings.

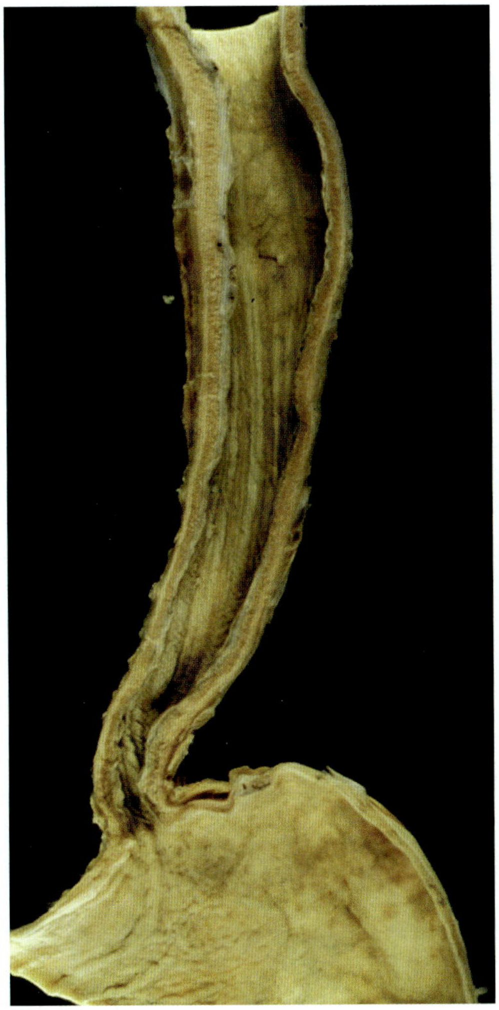

FIGURE 1.38

Chagas disease. Moderate luminal dilation. (From Turk JL, ed. Royal College of Surgeons of England. *Slide Atlas of Pathology. Alimentary Tract System*. London, Gower Medical, 1986, with permission.)

Microscopic Findings

Specific histologic features of systemic sclerosis are usually seen on esophageal resection specimen or at autopsy and include atrophy of the distal esophageal muscularis propria fibers and intimal proliferation of arterioles, without evidence of ischemic injury or significant myenteric plexus inflammation. Smooth muscle atrophy affects the circular layer more so than the longitudinal layer (Fig. 1.39) and the central fiber bundles more so than the peripheral fiber bundles. Fibrosis is not a significant finding, although this was once thought to be the mechanism of esophageal involvement. In patients with known systemic sclerosis, biopsies of the esophagus show proliferative and inflammatory gene expression profiles consistent with involvement by systemic sclerosis despite the lack of significant or specific histologic features and resulting in molecular subsets independent of skin subtype or serum autoantibodies.

Prognosis

The major complication from esophageal involvement is microaspiration, which can result in and exacerbate interstitial lung disease in these patients.

ESOPHAGEAL VARICES, PERFORATIONS, AND TEARS

Clinical Features

Esophageal varices can be subdivided radiographically into uphill or downhill types. Uphill esophageal varices are a manifestation of portal hypertension. Downhill

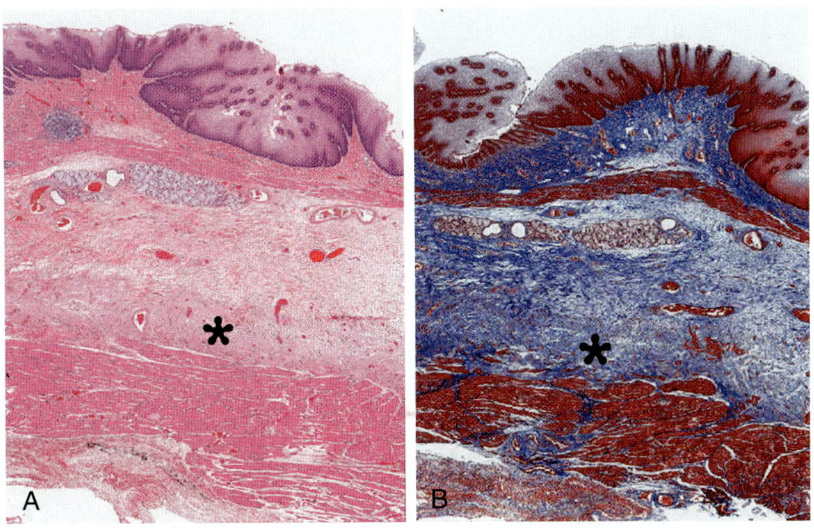

FIGURE 1.39

Scleroderma. **A**, Smooth muscle atrophy affects the inner circular layer *(asterisk)* of esophageal muscularis propria more so than the outer longitudinal layer. **B**, Fibrosis is not a significant finding, as seen on the accompanying trichrome stain.

esophageal varices are a result of superior vena cava obstruction caused by bronchogenic carcinoma with mediastinal metastasis. Patients with esophageal varices may be completely asymptomatic. However, rupture of varices results in massive hematemesis, melena, shock, and subsequent hepatic coma.

Esophageal perforations can be subdivided into spontaneous (Boerhaave's syndrome), iatrogenic, and posttraumatic. A sudden increase in intraesophageal pressure can cause "spontaneous" perforation. Boerhaave's syndrome typically occurs in middle-aged men after alcohol and food overindulgence. Esophageal tears are commonly iatrogenic in origin, resulting from surgical trauma. Endoscopic dilations and blunt trauma are other causes of perforation. Penetrating injuries result from knife or gunshot wounds (11%–17%) or from trauma related to foreign bodies (7%–14%). Symptoms and signs include severe chest and upper abdominal pain, nausea, subcutaneous emphysema, and shock. Esophageal (Mallory-Weiss) tears occur spontaneously or as a result of repeated episodes of vomiting in patients with alcoholism. Hematemesis and melena are the most common symptoms.

Pathologic Features

Gross Findings

Endoscopic examination reveals tortuous bluish mucosal elevations secondary to dilated submucosal veins (Figs. 1.40 and 1.41). Mallory-Weiss tears appear as longitudinal mucosal tears surrounded by hemorrhage extending across the Z line.

Microscopic Findings

Specimens from postmortem examination show ectatic submucosal veins and venules (Fig. 1.42) with occasional thrombosis. In fatal perforations, there is extensive intramural hemorrhage with or without serosal or adventitial fibroinflammatory reaction.

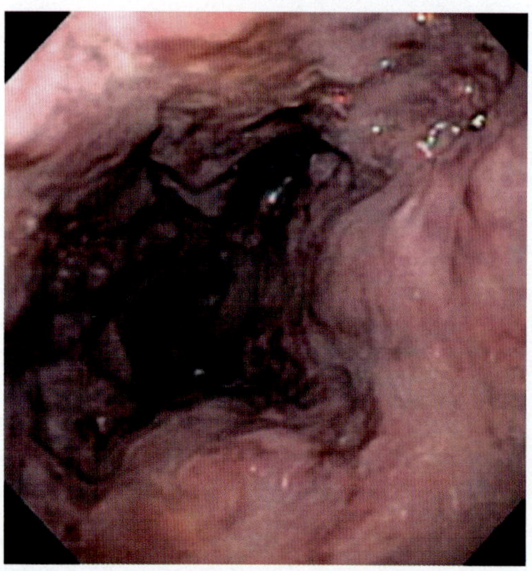

FIGURE 1.40

Esophageal varices—endoscopy. Varices with impending bleed. (Courtesy of Dr. E. Frizzell.)

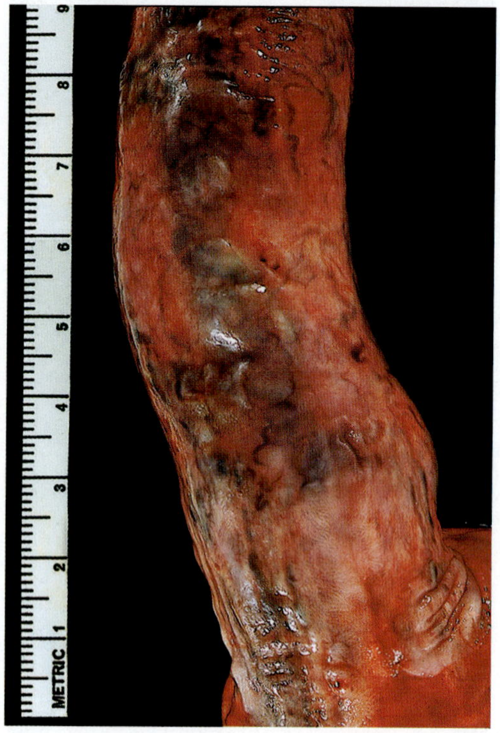

FIGURE 1.41

Esophageal varices. Prominent tortuous veins. (Courtesy of Dr. P. Vasallo.)

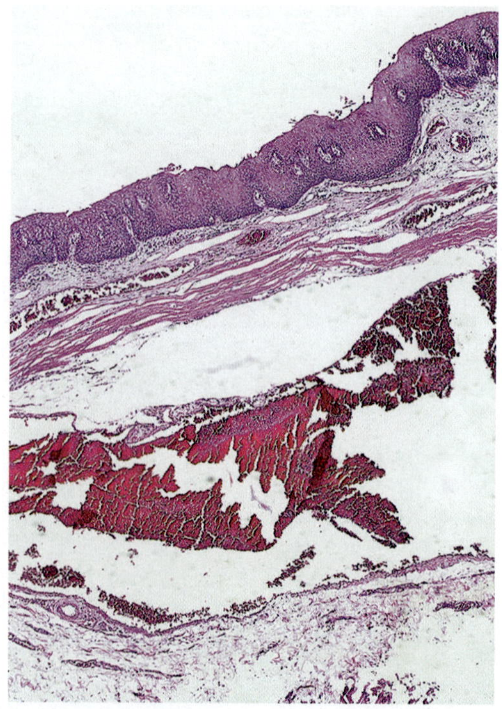

FIGURE 1.42

Esophageal varices. Dilated vessel beneath hyperplastic mucosa.

Differential Diagnosis

Mallory-Weiss tears need to be distinguished from severe GERD. Clinically, a large number of diseases can be confused with rupture, including perforated peptic ulcer, myocardial infarct, pancreatitis, and mesenteric thrombosis.

Prognosis and Therapy

In 60% of cases, the first episode of ruptured varices is fatal. Sclerotherapy is the treatment of choice for patients awaiting liver transplant for cirrhosis. In cases with delayed diagnosis, spontaneous and iatrogenic perforations are associated with a high mortality rate (15%–24%). Most patients are treated with surgery within 24 hours of diagnosis. Some, however, are treated conservatively with IV fluids and antibiotics if the perforation is contained. Patients with Mallory-Weiss tears are treated conservatively with thermal therapy and have a good prognosis.

ESOPHAGEAL VARICES, PERFORATIONS, AND TEARS—FACT SHEET

Definition

- Varicose veins in the lower esophagus are the result of portal hypertension caused by cirrhosis (uphill varices)
- Varicose veins in the upper esophagus are the result of superior vena cava obstruction (downhill varices)
- Spontaneous, iatrogenic, or traumatic lesions that result in perforation or tears in the esophagus

Incidence and Location

- Varices are a frequent complication of alcoholic cirrhosis in the United States
- Iatrogenic cases account for almost half of all perforations
- Tears (Mallory-Weiss syndrome) probably have a higher incidence than perforations
- Varices, perforations, and tears occur most commonly in the lower esophagus

Gender and Age Distribution

- Varices occur in men and women
- Boerhaave's syndrome occurs in men after consuming excessive alcohol, food, or both
- Iatrogenic perforations occur at any age and in both sexes
- Mallory-Weiss syndrome presents in adults with a history of alcoholism

Clinical Features

- A patient with esophageal varices may be asymptomatic
- Ruptured varices are associated with massive hematemesis and a high mortality rate
- Symptoms and signs of perforation include severe chest pain, vomiting, and subcutaneous emphysema
- Hematemesis and melena are characteristic of Mallory-Weiss syndrome

Prognosis and Therapy

- The prognosis of esophageal varices is poor if it is associated with cirrhosis and better if it is associated with portal vein thrombosis
- Sclerotherapy is the treatment of choice for varices
- There is a high mortality rate (15%–29%) in spontaneous or iatrogenic perforations if the diagnosis is delayed
- Treatment in most cases of perforation is surgical repair
- Endoscopic hemostasis and thermal therapy are treatments of choice in Mallory-Weiss syndrome

Esophageal Varices, Perforations, and Tears—Pathologic Features

Gross (Endoscopic) Findings

- Varices appear as bluish veins protruding into the esophageal lumen; red spots on the mucosal surface are associated with a high risk for rupture
- Perforations average 2 cm with surrounding hematoma or abscess
- Endoscopic findings in Mallory-Weiss syndrome show longitudinal mucosal tears extending across the Z line

Microscopic Findings

- Postmortem histology shows markedly ectatic veins and venules in the submucosa in cases of varices
- In fatal cases of Mallory-Weiss syndrome, the tears demonstrate mucosal dehiscence, edema, and mural hemorrhage

Differential Diagnosis

- No other entity looks like esophageal varices, but radiologically, they may be confused with submucosally infiltrating esophageal carcinomas
- Endoscopically, Mallory-Weiss syndrome may be confused with severe reflux. Reflux shows basal cell hyperplasia, elongation of papillae, and intramucosal neutrophil, eosinophils, and lymphocytes
- Clinically, the differential diagnosis of a perforation includes perforated peptic ulcer, myocardial infarct, pancreatitis, and mesenteric thrombosis

REFERENCES

1. Chong VH. Clinical significance of heterotopic gastric mucosal patch of the proximal esophagus. *World J Gastroenterol.* 2013;19:331–338.
2. Tsai SJ, Lin CC, Chang CW, et al. Benign esophageal lesions: endoscopic and pathologic features. *World J Gastroenterol.* 2015;21:1091–1098.

3. Pilarski R, Burt R, Kohlman W, et al. Cowden syndrome and the PTEN hamartoma tumor syndrome: systematic review and revised diagnostic criteria. *J Natl Cancer Inst*. 2013;105:1607–1616.
4. Dunbar KB, Agoston AT, Odze RD, et al. Association of Acute Gastroesophageal Reflux Disease With Esophageal Histologic Changes. *JAMA*. 2016;315:2104–2112.
5. Mikami DJ, Murayama KM. Physiology and pathogenesis of gastroesophageal reflux disease. *Surg Clin North Am*. 2015;95:515–525.
6. Grin A, Streutker CJ. Esophagitis: old histologic concepts and new thoughts. *Arch Pathol Lab Med*. 2015;139:723–729.
7. Schneider NI, Plieschnegger W, Geppert M, et al. Validation study of the Esohisto consensus guidelines for the recognition of microscopic esophagitis (histoGERD Trial). *Hum Pathol*. 2014;45:994–1002.
8. Raheem M, Leach ST, Day AS, et al. The pathophysiology of eosinophilic esophagitis. *Front Pediatr*. 2014;2:41.
9. Falk GW. Clinical presentation of eosinophilic esophagitis in adults. *Gastroenterol Clin North Am*. 2014;43:231–242.
10. Almashat SJ, Duan L, Goldsmith JD. Non-reflux esophagitis: a review of inflammatory diseases of the esophagus exclusive of reflux esophagitis. *Seminars in diagnostic pathology*. 2014;31:89–99.
11. Karabulut YY, Savas B, Kansu A, et al. Diagnosing oesophagitis in children: how discriminative is histology? *Acta Gastroenterol Belg*. 2013;76:300–305.
12. Dellon ES, Gonsalves N, Hirano I, et al. ACG clinical guideline: Evidenced based approach to the diagnosis and management of esophageal eosinophilia and eosinophilic esophagitis (EoE). The. *American journal of gastroenterology*. 2013;108:679–692. quiz 693.
13. Basseri B, Vasiliauskas EA, Chan O, et al. Evaluation of peripapillary lymphocytosis and lymphocytic esophagitis in adult inflammatory bowel disease. *Gastroenterol Hepatol (N Y)*. 2013;9:505–511.
14. Purdy JK, Appelman HD, McKenna BJ. Sloughing esophagitis is associated with chronic debilitation and medications that injure the esophageal mucosa. *Mod Pathol*. 2012;25:767–775.
15. Maguire A, Sheahan K. Pathology of oesophagitis. *Histopathology*. 2012;60:864–879.
16. Kidambi T, Toto E, Ho N, et al. Temporal trends in the relative prevalence of dysphagia etiologies from 1999-2009. *World J Gastroenterol*. 2012;18:4335–4341.
17. Kandulski A, Malfertheiner P. Gastroesophageal reflux disease--from reflux episodes to mucosal inflammation. Nature reviews. *Gastroenterology & hepatology*. 2012;9:15–22.
18. Haque S, Genta RM. Lymphocytic oesophagitis: clinicopathological aspects of an emerging condition. *Gut*. 2012;61:1108–1114.
19. Cohen S, Saxena A, Waljee AK, et al. Lymphocytic esophagitis: a diagnosis of increasing frequency. *J Clin Gastroenterol*. 2012; 46:828–832.
20. Liacouras CA, Furuta GT, Hirano I, et al. Eosinophilic esophagitis: updated consensus recommendations for children and adults. *J Allergy Clin Immunol*. 2011;128:3–20. e6; quiz 21-2.
21. Ebach DR, Vanderheyden AD, Ellison JM, et al. Lymphocytic esophagitis: a possible manifestation of pediatric upper gastrointestinal Crohn's disease. *Inflamm Bowel Dis*. 2011;17:45–49.
22. Noffsinger AE. Update on esophagitis: controversial and underdiagnosed causes. *Arch Pathol Lab Med*. 2009;133:1087–1095.
23. Allende DS, Yerian LM. Diagnosing gastroesophageal reflux disease: the pathologist's perspective. *Adv Anat Pathol*. 2009; 16:161–165.
24. Kahrilas PJ, Shaheen NJ, Vaezi MF. American Gastroenterological Association Institute technical review on the management of gastroesophageal reflux disease. *Gastroenterology*. 2008;135: 1392–1413. 1413 e1-5.
25. Gong B, Jiang N, Yan G, et al. Predictors for severe acute esophagitis in lung cancer patients treated with chemoradiotherapy: a systematic review. *Curr Med Res Opin*. 2016:1–8.
26. Chandan VS, Murray JA, Abraham SC. Esophageal lichen planus. *Arch Pathol Lab Med*. 2008;132:1026–1029.
27. Purdy JK, Appelman HD, Golembeski CP, et al. Lymphocytic esophagitis: a chronic or recurring pattern of esophagitis resembling allergic contact dermatitis. *Am J Clin Pathol*. 2008;130: 508–513.
28. Rubio CA, Sjodahl K, Lagergren J. Lymphocytic esophagitis: a histologic subset of chronic esophagitis. *Am J Clin Pathol*. 2006;125:432–437.
29. Vieth M., Mastracci L., Vakil N., et al. Epithelial thickness is a marker of gastroesophageal reflux disease. *Clin Gastroenterol Hepatol*. 2016;14(11):1544–1551.
30. Muthusamy VR, Lightdale JR, Acosta RD, et al. The role of endoscopy in the management of GERD. *Gastrointest Endosc*. 2015;81:1305–1310.
31. Camilleri M, Dubois D, Coulie B, et al. Prevalence and socioeconomic impact of upper gastrointestinal disorders in the United States: results of the US Upper Gastrointestinal Study. *Clin Gastroenterol Hepatol*. 2005;3:543–552.
32. Yerian L, Fiocca R, Mastracci L, et al. Refinement and reproducibility of histologic criteria for the assessment of microscopic lesions in patients with gastroesophageal reflux disease: the Esohisto Project. *Dig Dis Sci*. 2011;56:2656–2665.
33. Salaria SN, Abu Alfa AK, Cruise MW, et al. Lichenoid esophagitis: clinicopathologic overlap with established esophageal lichen planus. *Am J Surg Pathol*. 2013;37:1889–1894.
34. Abraham SC, Ravich WJ, Anhalt GJ, et al. Esophageal lichen planus: case report and review of the literature. *Am J Surg Pathol*. 2000;24:1678–1682.
35. Taggart MW, Rashid A, Ross WA, et al. Oesophageal hyperkeratosis: clinicopathological associations. *Histopathology*. 2013;63:463–473.
36. Kisloff B, McGrath KM, Davison JM. Esophageal hyperkeratosis in a healthy adult. *Clin Gastroenterol Hepatol*. 2011;9:A20.
37. Lehman MB, Clark SB, Ormsby AH, et al. Squamous mucosal alterations in esophagectomy specimens from patients with end-stage achalasia. *Am J Surg Pathol*. 2001;25:1413–1418.
38. Triantos C, Koukias N, Karamanolis G, et al. Changes in the esophageal mucosa of patients with non erosive reflux disease: How far have we gone? *World J Gastroenterol*. 2015;21:5762–5767.
39. Wen T, Dellon ES, Moawad FJ, et al. Transcriptome analysis of proton pump inhibitor-responsive esophageal eosinophilia reveals proton pump inhibitor-reversible allergic inflammation. *J Allergy Clin Immunol*. 2015;135:187–197.
40. Rouphael C, Gordon IO, Thota PN. Lymphocytic esophagitis: Still an enigma a decade later. *World J Gastroenterol*. 2017;23:949–956.
41. Hershcovici T, Fass R. Nonerosive Reflux Disease (NERD) - An Update. *J Neurogastroenterol Motil*. 2010;16:8–21.
42. Ezoe Y, Fujii S, Muto M, et al. Epidermoid metaplasia of the esophagus: endoscopic feature and differential diagnosis. *Hepatogastroenterology*. 2011;58:809–813.
43. Kirby DF, Chatterjee S. Evaluation and management of gastrointestinal manifestations in scleroderma. *Curr Opin Rheumatol*. 2014;26:621–629.
44. Obiorah I, Hussain A, Palese C, et al. IgG4-related disease involving the esophagus: a clinicopathological study. *Dis Esophagus*. 2017;30:1–7.
45. Clayton F, Fang JC, Gleich GJ, et al. Eosinophilic esophagitis in adults is associated with IgG4 and not mediated by IgE. *Gastroenterology*. 2014;147:602–609.
46. Dumas-Campagna M, Bouchard S, Soucy G, et al. IgG4-Related Esophageal Disease Presenting as Esophagitis Dissecans Superficialis With Chronic Strictures. *J Clin Med Res*. 2014;6:295–298.
47. Odze RD. Pathology of the gastroesophageal junction. *Seminars in diagnostic pathology*. 2005;22:256–265.
48. Soucy G, Onstad L, Vaughan TL, et al. Histologic Features Associated With Columnar-lined Esophagus in Distal Esophageal and Gastroesophageal Junction (GEJ) Biopsies From GERD Patients: A Community-based Population Study. *Am J Surg Pathol*. 2016;40:827–835.
49. Roberts CG, Hummers LK, Ravich WJ, et al. A case-control study of the pathology of oesophageal disease in systemic sclerosis (scleroderma). *Gut*. 2006;55:1697–1703.
50. Taroni JN, Martyanov V, Huang CC, et al. Molecular characterization of systemic sclerosis esophageal pathology identifies inflammatory and proliferative signatures. *Arthritis Res Ther*. 2015;17:194.

2

Tumors of the Esophagus

■ **Catherine Hagen, MD and Amitabh Srivastava, MD**

■ SQUAMOUS PAPILLOMAS

Clinical Features

These are uncommon, incidental findings at endoscopy that usually occur in women in the fifth decade of life. The vast majority are solitary; some may present as a papillomatosis. They are thought to be a reactive proliferation secondary to gastroesophageal reflux disease (GERD). In the Western population, most lesions arise in the distal esophagus, whereas mid-esophagus is the most common site of involvement reported in Japan.

Pathologic Features

Gross Findings

The lesions are typically seen as tiny well-demarcated polyps at endoscopy. Mucosal biopsy samples appear as small whitish nodules.

Microscopic Findings

These lesions are composed of bland polypoid squamous mucosa with fibrovascular cores (Fig. 2.1). Exceptional cases may display viral cytopathic effect, and these appear to be more prevalent in the upper esophagus.

Ancillary Studies

Immunohistochemistry

The majority of squamous papilloma are negative for human papillomavirus (HPV) by both immunohistochemistry and in situ hybridization. A subset of patients with HPV-associated laryngeal papillomatosis are reported to also have concurrent HPV-related squamous papillomatosis of the esophagus (Fig. 2.2).

Differential Diagnosis

The differential diagnosis includes squamous dysplasia, but squamous papillomas show no epithelial atypia, and the diagnosis is usually straightforward.

Prognosis and Therapy

Squamous papillomas have no risk of recurrence or malignant transformation.

SQUAMOUS PAPILLOMA OF THE ESOPHAGUS—FACT SHEET

Definition

- Small, incidental nodules of the esophagus composed of proliferative benign squamous epithelium

Incidence and Location

- Uncommon (<0.5%); usually involve the distal esophagus

Morbidity and Mortality

- None; other than rare examples associated with laryngeal papillomatosis, which may cause obstruction

Gender, Race, and Age Distribution

- Squamous papillomas are more common in white women, usually in their early 40s

Clinical Features

- Incidental smooth nodular lesions on endoscopy

Squamous Papilloma of the Esophagus—Pathologic Features

Gross Findings

- Small nodule with a smooth surface seen at endoscopy

Microscopic Findings

- Small nodular squamous proliferation aligned in a papillary configuration with fibrovascular cores

Immunohistochemistry

- Results from immunohistochemical, polymerase chain reaction, and in situ hybridization studies for human papillomavirus are negative in most series

Differential Diagnosis

- Papillary squamous neoplasia (low or high grade)

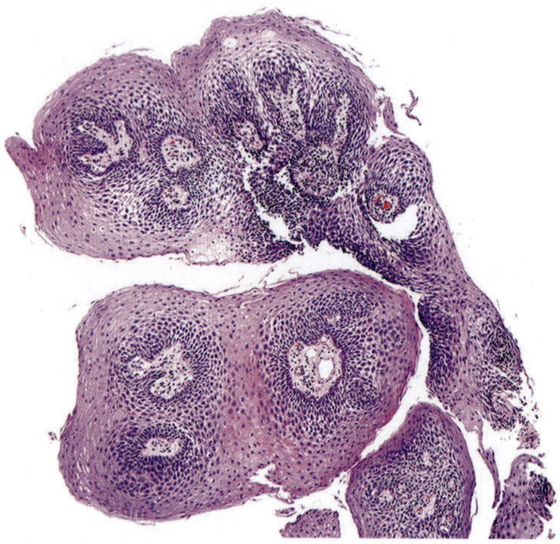

FIGURE 2.1

Squamous papilloma of the esophagus. Most such tumors are incidental and not associated with human papillomavirus infection.

ATYPICAL LIPOMATOUS TUMOR ("GIANT FIBROVASCULAR POLYP" OF THE ESOPHAGUS)

Clinical Features

Fibrovascular polyps are extremely rare submucosal tumors of the esophagus that have been variably classified as *lipomas, fibromas*, and *fibrolipomatous polyps*. Most patients described in literature are middle-aged or older men, although children, infants, and women may also be affected. Presenting complaints include dysphagia, substernal discomfort, and sensation of a mass. Recent data suggest these lesions are almost universally positive for MDM2 and CDK4 and show *MDM2* amplification on fluorescence in situ hybridization, suggesting that the so-called "giant fibrovascular polyp" is actually a unique macroscopic appearance of atypical lipomatous tumor involving the esophagus.

Pathologic Features

Gross Findings

On gross examination, these are sausage-like pedunculated polyps arising in the upper third of the esophagus and attached to the wall with a narrow stalk. Their surface is covered by squamous mucosa, and their cores consist of an admixture of grossly identifiable adipose tissue and firm white connective tissue.

Microscopic Findings

The lesions are composed of variable amount of mature adipose tissue, often separated by thick fibrous bands

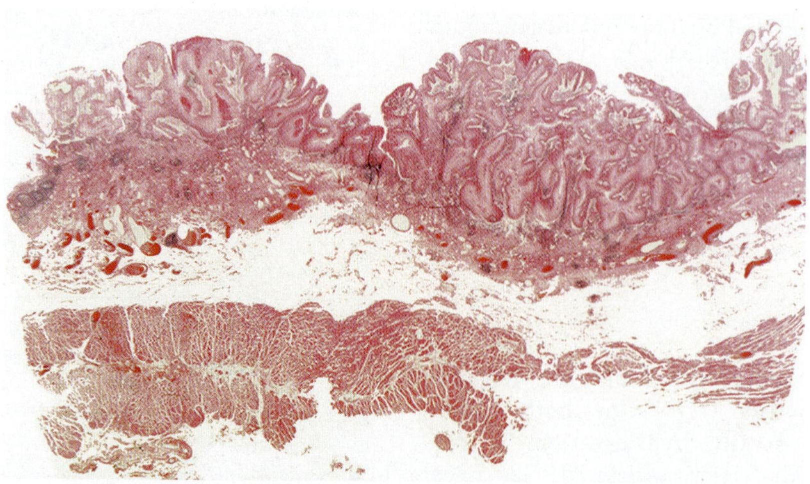

FIGURE 2.2

Esophageal papillomatosis in a young patient with tracheal papillomatosis associated with human papillomavirus.

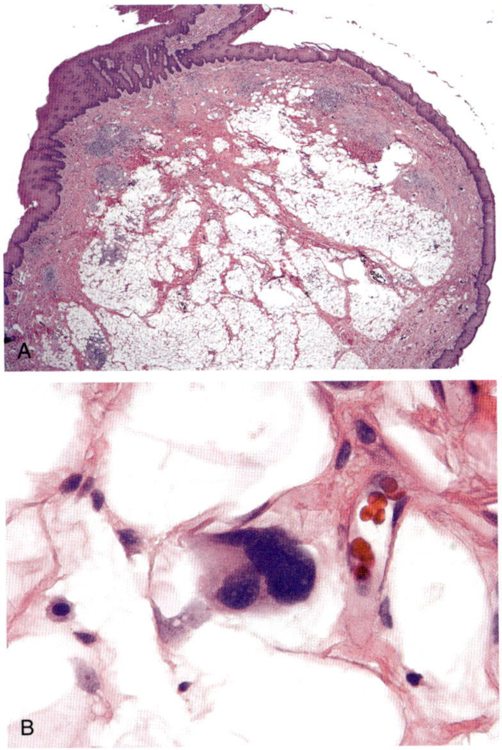

FIGURE 2.3

Giant fibrovascular polyp, low magnification. It consists of fat, fibrous tissue, and vessels (**A**). Almost all such lesions reported in literature represent atypical lipomatous tumors involving the esophagus. Careful evaluation for nuclear atypia in adipocytic and stromal components (**B**), and immunohistochemistry for MDM2 and CDK4 is helpful in making the diagnosis.

or sometimes a myxoid stroma and prominent vasculature, all surrounded by mature squamous epithelium (Fig. 2.3A). Scattered, large, atypical cells with hyperchromatic nuclei and classic atypical multivacuolated lipoblasts may also be seen (Fig. 2.3B). Rarely, dedifferentiated foci may also occur, similar to atypical lipomatous tumors of soft tissue.

ANCILLARY STUDIES

IMMUNOHISTOCHEMISTRY

MDM2 and CDK4 show positive staining in the adipocytic component and the atypical stromal cells in almost all cases.

MOLECULAR FINDINGS

Fluorescence in situ hybridization shows MDM2 amplification and ring chromosome involving chromosome 12q have been described in these lesions, similar to atypical lipomatous tumors of somatic soft tissue.

DIFFERENTIAL DIAGNOSIS

The main differential diagnosis is secondary esophageal involvement of the esophagus by contiguous extension of a primary mediastinal liposarcoma. The latter typically presents as a large mural mass while primary esophageal atypical lipomatous tumors presents as a slender elongated polyp with a narrow base. Inflammatory polyps of the esophagus usually occur in the distal third and show a fibromuscular stroma without an adipocytic component. The diagnosis of a "giant fibrovascular polyp" should not be made unless careful microscopic evaluation and ancillary work-up have completely excluded the possibility of an atypical lipomatous tumor.

PROGNOSIS AND THERAPY

Complete excision is curative in most cases, although local recurrences have also been described. Excision can be accomplished by endoscopic ligation or surgical excision when the base of the lesion is poorly visualized by endoscopy. Metastasis has not yet been reported from these lesions.

ATYPICAL LIPOMATOUS TUMOR ("GIANT FIBROVASCULAR POLYP") OF THE ESOPHAGUS—FACT SHEET

Definition

- Submucosal-based esophageal tumor composed of adipocytes and atypical stromal cells, thick-walled blood vessels and a fibrocollagenous or myxoid stroma similar to atypical lipomatous tumor of soft tissue

Incidence and Location

- Very rare; usually in the upper third of the esophagus

Morbidity and Mortality

- May cause morbidity and rare mortality based on obstruction of the esophagus or aspiration

Gender, Race, and Age Distribution

- Male predominance
- Typically middle aged to older

Clinical Features

- Present with dysphagia, mass sensation, retrosternal discomfort, or regurgitation of the mass

Prognosis and Therapy

- Local excision is curative

Atypical Lipomatous Tumor ("Giant Fibrovascular Polyp") of the Esophagus —Pathologic Features

Gross Findings

- Long, slender, finger-like lesion with a narrow stalk arising from the esophageal wall and protruding into the lumen

Microscopic Findings

- Mature squamous mucosa with underlying adipose tissue with adipocytes of variable size, atypical stromal cells, multivacuolated atypical lipoblasts in a fibrocollagenous or myxoid stroma rich in blood vessels

Ancillary studies

- Positive for CDK4 and MDM2
- MDM2 amplification on FISH
- Ring chromosomes involving chromosone 12q

Differential Diagnosis

- Inflammatory polyps
- Secondary involvement by mediastinal liposarcoma

BARRETT'S ESOPHAGUS

Clinical Features

Barrett's esophagus (BE) arises as a complication of chronic GERD. Its incidence is rising in the Western Hemisphere and parallels the increase in esophageal adenocarcinoma. Other risk factors for BE include male sex, white race, advanced age, and truncal obesity; cigarette smoking is a minor contributor. The presence of Barrett's mucosa in the esophagus does not cause symptoms, which makes it hard to screen the population for this precursor lesion of significant clinical consequence. The major importance of BE is the marked predisposition it confers on patients for subsequent development of esophageal adenocarcinoma through inflammation to metaplasia to dysplasia to adenocarcinoma sequence. However, most patients with esophageal adenocarcinoma present with cancer and do not carry a prior diagnosis of BE. Periodic surveillance and biopsy for early detection of neoplasia is the current standard of care for BE patients, but only a small minority of those under surveillance develop adenocarcinoma.

The 2011 American Gastroenterology Association (AGA) guidelines defined BE as intestinal-type metaplastic epithelium that replaces stratified squamous mucosa in the esophagus and predisposes to cancer development, requiring both endoscopic evidence of columnar metaplasia and histologic demonstration of goblet cells. However, in Japan and much of Europe and the United Kingdom, goblet cells are not required to diagnose BE. The term *columnar lined esophagus* is used instead of BE, emphasizing the endoscopic rather than histologic definition of the entity. The requirement for goblet cells is still used in the United States because population-based studies have shown a much higher risk of esophageal adenocarcinoma in patients with intestinal metaplasia than in those without intestinal metaplasia. Including patients without goblet cells into the periodic surveillance pool has major implications for cost of care and cannot be justified unless the risk in non-goblet metaplastic columnar epithelium is shown to be significant and comparable to those with goblet cells in longitudinal outcome studies. Detection of goblet cells is susceptible to sampling error. At least eight random biopsies or four biopsies per centimeter of columnar epithelium are recommended to obtain the maximum yield of intestinal metaplasia on histologic examination. According to the recently published 2016 American College of Gastroenterology guidelines, BE should only be diagnosed if there is extension of metaplastic columnar epithelium 1 cm or greater proximal to the GEJ. This change was recommended because patients with less than 1 cm of metaplastic columnar epithelium have a very low risk of esophageal adenocarcinoma in long-term follow-up studies, which does not justify routine surveillance. However, the AGA criteria do not have a length requirement and only require definite columnar mucosa lining the distal esophagus with intestinal metaplasia detected on biopsies from this segment.

Pathologic Features

Gross Findings

Barrett's esophagus appears as tongues and patches of red salmon-colored mucosa that extend up from the gastroesophageal junction (GEJ) for variable distance into the tubular esophagus and contrasts with the pearly gray-pink color of the normal squamous epithelium (Figs. 2.4 and 2.5). Traditionally, short-segment BE is defined as less than 3 cm of metaplastic columnar epithelium, and long-segment BE is defined as greater than 3 cm of metaplastic columnar epithelium. This distinction is important because although short-segment BE is more common, it is less likely than long-segment BE to give rise to esophageal adenocarcinoma.

Microscopic Findings

A majority of patients with BE have a concurrent hiatal hernia, and biopsies from the columnar segment in the distal esophagus may show a cardia- or oxyntocardiac-type glandular epithelium or an intestinalized epithelium with goblet cells. Goblet cells are readily identifiable on hematoxylin and eosin–stained slides, and ancillary stains are unnecessary (Fig. 2.6). Typically, these goblet cells are admixed with gastric-type lining cells, and this type of metaplasia is termed *incomplete*.

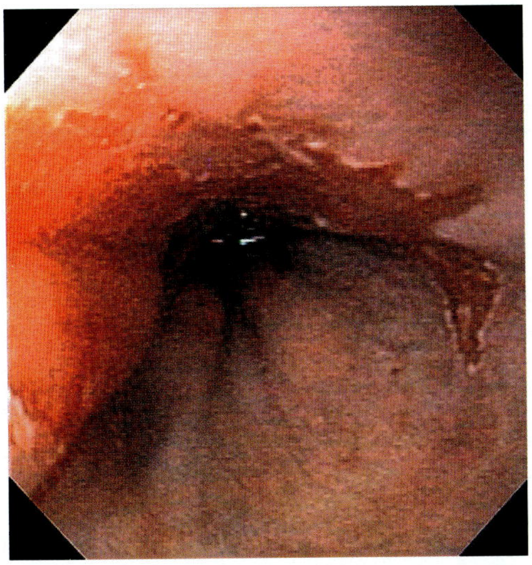

FIGURE 2.4

Barrett's esophagus, endoscopic appearance. Note the tongues of salmon-colored epithelium extending into the gray squamous mucosa to a variable extent.

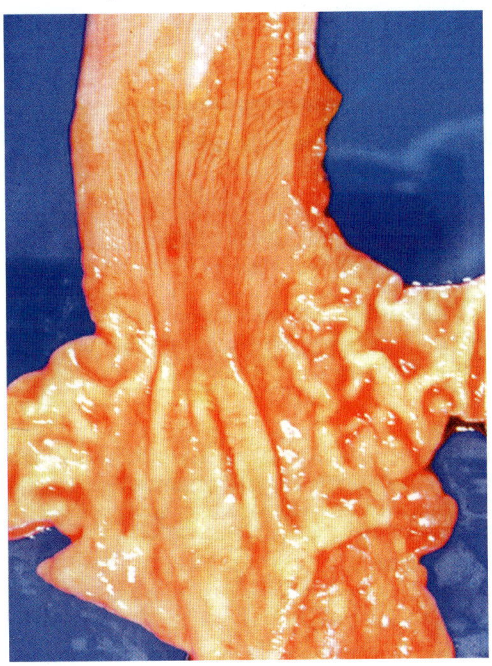

FIGURE 2.5

Long-segment Barrett's esophagus, resection specimen, showing velvetlike mucosa above the anatomic gastroesophageal junction which is defined by the proximal limit of the gastric rugal folds. This esophagus was excised in 1996 because of extensive high-grade columnar epithelial dysplasia. Today, such patients are managed endoscopically by radiofrequency ablation.

Multilayered epithelium is a hybrid epithelium consisting of mucin-containing glandular cells and basally located squamous cells, frequently seen in patients with GERD and may be a precursor of BE (Fig. 2.7). Its presence is not routinely reported in GEJ or esophageal biopsies, and it should not be considered to represent BE. The metaplastic intestinalized mucosa often lays down a new muscularis mucosae, resulting in two distinct

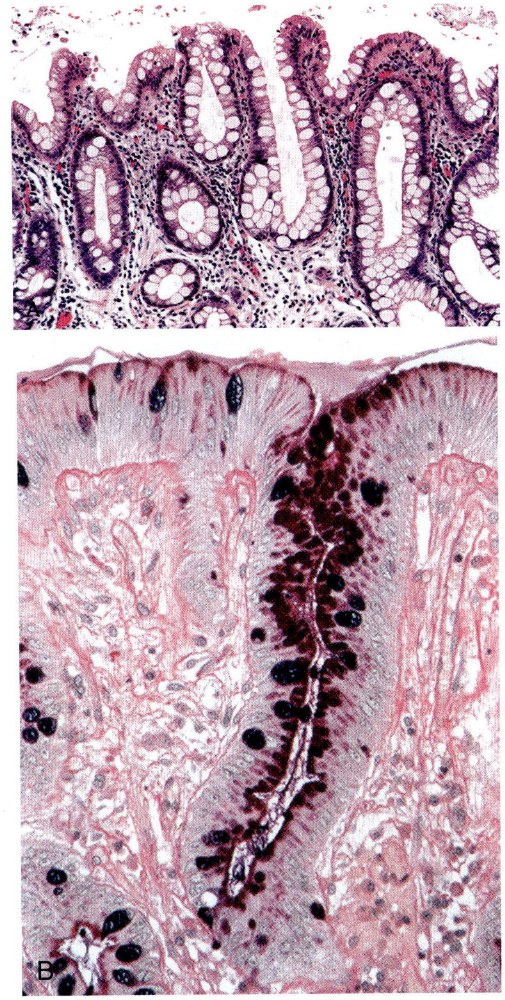

FIGURE 2.6

Barrett's esophagus. This biopsy specimen came from the tubular esophagus and shows intestinal metaplasia (**A**). Periodic acid–Schiff (PAS) and Alcian Blue (AB) stains can be used to highlight goblet cells but are not necessary in routine practice. Note the blue goblet cells with interposed cells displaying neutral mucin, imparting a magenta color on the PAS AB stain. This pattern is similar to gastric foveolar cells rather than intestinal absorptive cells. This combination of cell types is termed incomplete intestinal metaplasia (**B**).

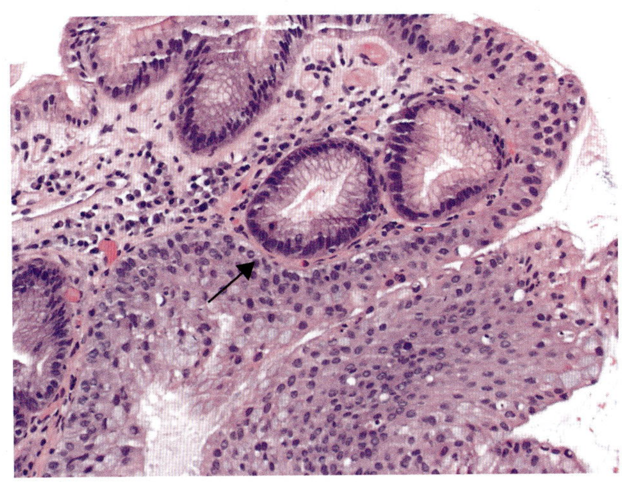

FIGURE 2.7

Multilayered epithelium (hematoxylin and eosin) is a hybrid epithelium demonstrating features of both squamous and columnar differentiation and suggested by may be a precursor of Barrett's esophagus.

layers: a delicate, frayed, superficial layer and a deep, thick, compact, native muscularis mucosae. The latter can be mistaken for muscularis propria because of its thickness.

Differential Diagnosis

The differential diagnosis of BE includes gastric carditis with intestinal metaplasia (CIM), seen in approximately 30% of patients with an abnormal squamocolumnar junction. CIM is most often associated with *Helicobacter pylori* infection and has a lower incidence of dysplasia compared with BE. Autoimmune gastritis may also cause CIM and should be considered in the differential diagnosis when only GEJ biopsies are available. Certain histologic features have been described to help distinguish BE from CIM. These include metaplastic crypts buried underneath squamous mucosa, hybrid glands consisting of cardia-type and intestinalized glands, and esophageal glands and ducts. The presence of esophageal glands or ducts adjacent to foci of intestinal metaplasia is diagnostic of BE (Fig. 2.8); other features are suggestive but not definitive.

Prognosis and Therapy

Barrett's esophagus is a preneoplastic precursor lesion with the risk of adenocarcinoma being approximately 0.5% per year. Patients with nondysplastic BE are therefore recommended periodic endoscopic surveillance at 3- to 5-year intervals. Therapy is largely based on treating GERD, typically with proton pump inhibitor therapy.

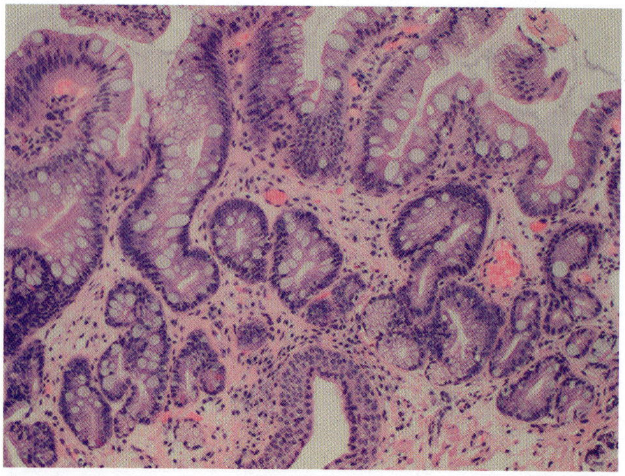

FIGURE 2.8

In biopsies obtained from the gastroesophageal junction, the presence of esophageal gland ducts (bottom of field) within the focus of intestinal metaplasia is diagnostic of Barrett's esophagus.

BARRETT'S ESOPHAGUS—FACT SHEET

Definition

- Columnar epithelium in the tubal esophagus with intestinal metaplasia on biopsy (US definition). In addition, some gastroenterology societies in the United States have also included a length (>1 cm) requirement. Goblet cells are not part of the definition in many parts of Europe and Japan (*columnar-lined esophagus* used as a synonym for Barrett's esophagus [BE])

Incidence and Location

- 5% of individuals with gastroesophageal reflux disease

Morbidity and Mortality

- Strong risk factor for esophageal adenocarcinoma, with an estimated annual rate of progression of approximately 0.5%

Gender, Race, and Age Distribution

- White male predominance with a median age in the early 50s

Clinical Features

- Usually asymptomatic; reflux symptoms may lead to screening for BE
- Well-defined criteria for screening patients for BE are lacking

BARRETT'S ESOPHAGUS—PATHOLOGIC FEATURES

Gross Findings

- Salmon-colored mucosa in the esophagus
- May appear as a markedly irregular Z-line, a visible tongue of columnar epithelium, or a discrete island of columnar epithelium surrounded on all sides by squamous mucosa

Microscopic Findings

- Admixture of cardia-type, oxyntocardiac-type, and intestinalized glands
- Intestinal metaplasia is typically of incomplete type, which shows goblet cells interspersed gastric foveolar-type cells
- Double muscularis mucosae may be present

Ancillary Studies

- PAS-AB stain highlights goblet cells but is not recommended for routine diagnosis

Differential Diagnosis

- Intestinal metaplasia of the gastric cardia secondary of *Helicobacter pylori* or autoimmune gastritis
- Esophageal glands or ducts, when present, are helpful in establishing a diagnosis of Barrett's esophagus. Endoscopic correlation needed in the remaining cases

RISK FACTORS FOR ESOPHAGEAL CARCINOMA

Barrett's esophagus arises as a complication of chronic reflux disease and is the major predisposing risk factor for esophageal adenocarcinoma. Other risk factors include obesity, older age, and to a lesser extent, smoking and alcohol intake. Any condition that causes chronic local irritation and inflammation of the esophageal mucosa appears to predispose to squamous cell carcinoma (SCC). Significant alcohol intake, especially in combination with smoking, greatly increases the risk of SCC. Other predisposing factors include achalasia and esophageal diverticula in which food retention leads to local release of chemical irritants, frequent consumption of extremely hot beverages, and ingestion of lye or other caustic liquids. SCC is also linked to low socioeconomic status and to nutritional deficiency syndromes, such as the Plummer-Vinson syndrome (dysphagia, iron-deficiency anemia, and esophageal webs).

Nonepidermolytic palmoplantar keratoderma (tylosis), a rare autosomal dominant disorder defined by a genetic abnormality at chromosome 17q25, is a familial syndrome that predisposes patients to SCC. It is characterized by hyperkeratosis of the palms and soles and thickening of the oral mucosa. It confers up to a 95% risk for SCC of the esophagus by the age of 70 years. A polymorphism that increases the risk for esophageal squamous carcinoma has also been identified in individuals with inactive aldehyde dehydrogenase.

DYSPLASIA IN BARRETT'S ESOPHAGUS

GRADING DYSPLASIA IN BARRETT'S ESOPHAGUS

Surveillance biopsies from patients with BE are classified as negative for dysplasia, indefinite for dysplasia (IND), low-grade dysplasia (LGD), and high-grade dysplasia (HGD) (Table 2.1). Histologic features that are helpful in evaluation of BE biopsies include the presence of architectural complexity, cytologic atypia involving the surface epithelium, and the presence of lamina propria inflammation, erosions, or ulcers. Surface maturation is key to diagnosis of nondysplastic BE. The proliferating nuclei in the basal part of the intestinalized crypts are larger, more hyperchromatic, and more stratified than those at the surface, which are generally arranged in a monolayer with polarized basal nuclei. Architectural abnormalities include gland crowding, crypt branching and budding, and villiform change. Cytologic features of dysplasia include nuclear enlargement and hyperchromasia, irregular nuclear contours, coarse chromatin with prominent nucleoli, and loss of polarity. In "normal polarity," the long axis of the nucleus remains perpendicular to the basement membrane and the nuclei are aligned parallel one to another, whereas "loss of nuclear polarity" refers to loss of this perpendicular and parallel orientation. Inflammation with consequent reparative changes can impart worrisome cytologic alterations that can be mistaken for dysplasia. An abrupt morphologic change from adjacent mucosa favors a diagnosis of dysplasia.

BARRETT'S ESOPHAGUS, NEGATIVE FOR DYSPLASIA

In BE without dysplasia, the glands tend to be straight with smooth contours, crypt budding or branching is minimal, and abundant lamina propria is present between glands. The cytologic atypia, if any, is confined to the basal aspect of the crypts, while the surface epithelium shows maturation with small basally located nuclei and abundant cytoplasm (Fig. 2.9). Mitoses may be present but are localized to the basal crypt epithelium. Nuclei have smooth nuclear membranes with fine chromatin and inconspicuous nucleoli. In the setting of reactive changes, epithelial cells in the zone of inflammation may display nuclear enlargement, and nucleoli

TABLE 2.1
Features for Classifying Dysplasia in Barrett's Esophagus

Dysplasia	Surface Maturation	Architecture	Cytology	Inflammation	Nuclear Polarity
Negative	+	Normal; abundant lamina propria between glands	Nuclear stratification and mitoses limited to gland base; smooth nuclear contours and inconspicuous nucleoli	−/+	Maintained
Indefinite	+/−	Normal to slight crowding of glands	Nuclear irregularity and hyperchromasia or mitoses typically limited to gland base	+/−	Maintained
Low grade	−	Mild to marked crowding of glands	Pencillate, stratified, hyperchromatic nuclei extending to surface epithelium (resemble colonic tubular adenoma)	−/+	Maintained
High grade	−	Marked crowding of glands; villiform architecture	Enlarged hyperchromatic nuclei, coarse clumped chromatin, nucleoli may be prominent; loss of polarity, frequent mitoses	−/+	Lost

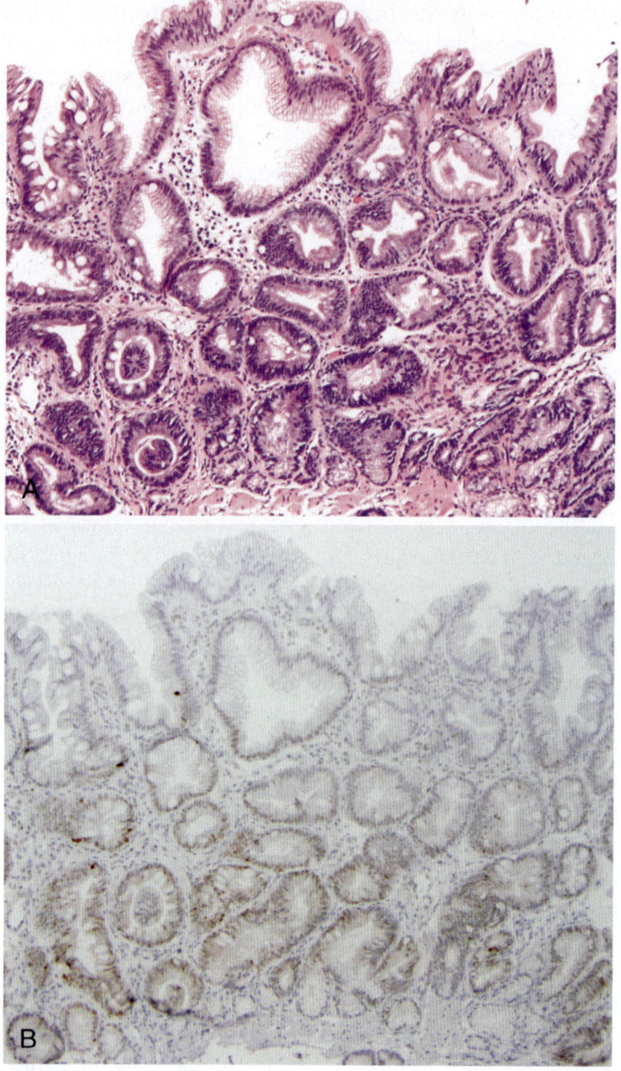

FIGURE 2.9

Barrett's esophagus, negative for dysplasia (**A**). The basal aspect of the crypts often appears regenerative and may be mistaken for dysplasia. The presence of surface maturation, as illustrated in this case, argues against a diagnosis of dysplasia. A "wild-type" pattern of p53 immunoreactivity shows scattered nuclei with weak positive staining (**B**) and can sometimes be useful in confirming the morphologic impression. Routine use of p53 immunostain in all surveillance biopsies is not recommended.

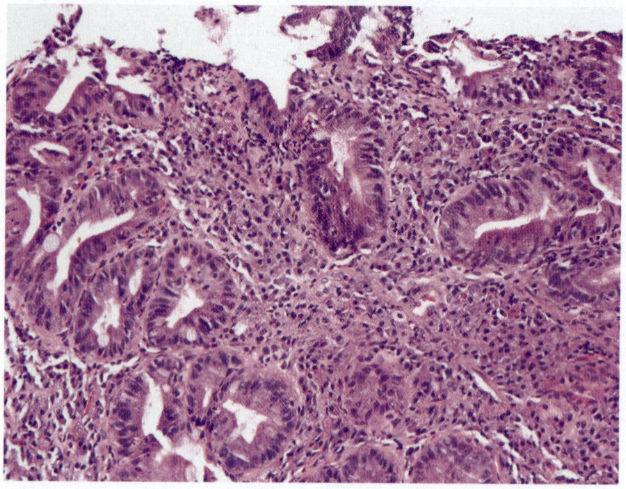

FIGURE 2.10

Barrett's esophagus, indefinite for dysplasia. The crypts show both pencillate and round nuclei with some hyperchromasia and gland crowding, but the lamina propria is densely inflamed, and multiple foci of cryptitis are present. Although the cytologic alterations are worrisome, these changes are best classified as indefinite for dysplasia in the setting of marked inflammation.

may become more prominent, but nuclear contours are generally smooth with a vesicular chromatin, small nucleoli and the overall nuclear-to-cytoplasmic ratio is preserved. There may be loss of cytoplasmic mucin, but surface maturation is preserved.

Barrett's Esophagus, Indefinite for Dysplasia

The indefinite for dysplasia (IND) category is a provisional category that should only be used in specific situations. Most often, these are either cases that show cytologic changes suggestive of dysplasia in deeper aspects of the crypt but also show surface maturation or those that show epithelial changes worrisome for dysplasia but significant inflammation is present and precludes an unequivocal diagnosis of dysplasia (Fig. 2.10). Cases in the IND category may have normal architecture or show some degree of glandular crowding. On cytologic evaluation, nuclei may be irregular and hyperchromatic, small nucleoli may be present, but surface maturation is usually preserved. Architectural abnormalities can be striking if the atypical focus is next to an ulcer. The presence of an abrupt "clonal" demarcation of the atypical from adjacent epithelium can be helpful in favoring a diagnosis of dysplasia. "Mutant" pattern of p53 expression (diffuse strong staining or complete loss of staining) on immunohistochemistry may be useful in this setting to suggest close surveillance but should not be used to upgrade the morphological diagnosis to low- or high-grade dysplasia.

Barrett's Esophagus, Low-Grade Dysplasia

Barrett's esophagus with low-grade dysplasia resembles a colonic adenoma (Fig. 2.11). The architecture shows mild distortion with glandular crowding, but lamina propria is still identifiable between glands. The nuclei are pencillate and hyperchromatic, stratified, and perpendicular to the basement membrane, and the changes extend to the surface epithelium. Nucleoli are not prominent, and the cells still retain their nuclear polarity. Both "wild-type" and mutant patterns of p53 staining can be seen in LGD. Therefore, p53 immunohistochemistry should not be performed upfront or routinely to determine the presence or grade of dysplasia without taking into account the histologic findings, which are still considered to be the gold standard for dysplasia diagnosis.

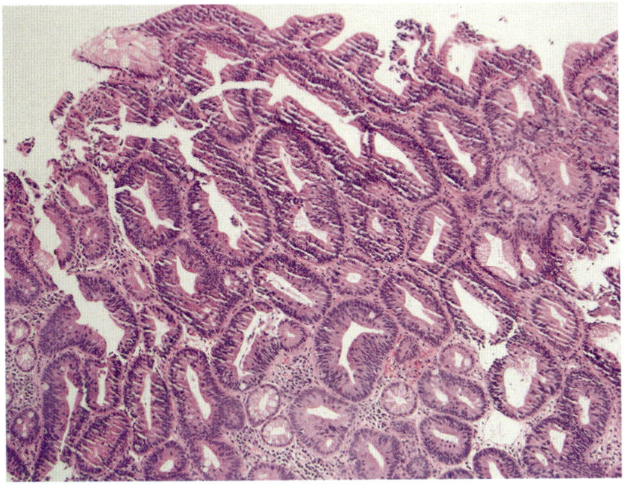

FIGURE 2.11

Low-grade dysplasia in Barrett's esophagus. Pencillate, stratified hyperchromatic nuclei uniformly involve the entire crypt from the base to the surface epithelium.

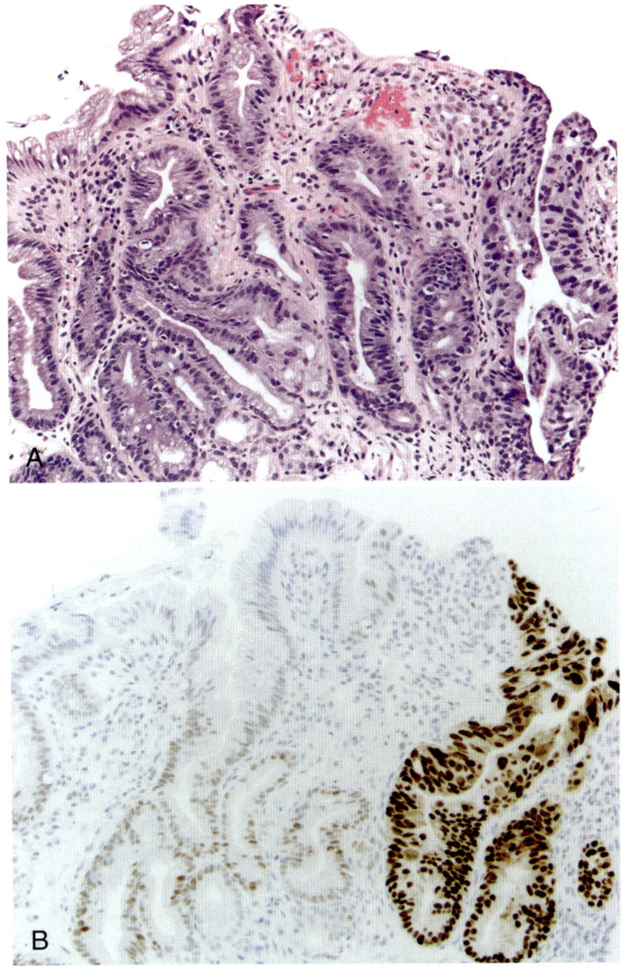

FIGURE 2.12

High-grade dysplasia in Barrett's esophagus. Abrupt transition to two crypts on the right that show marked nuclear pleomorphism with loss of polarity (**A**). The p53 immunostain shows a diffuse strong "mutant pattern" of staining restricted to the focus of dysplasia (**B**).

Barrett's Esophagus, High-Grade Dysplasia

In high-grade dysplasia (HGD), the metaplastic glands show significant glandular crowding with back-to-back arrangement and scant lamina propria between the glands. The nuclei are large and hyperchromatic with irregular nuclear membranes, clumped chromatin and prominent nucleoli and show loss of polarity (Fig. 2.12). The nuclei may become monolayered and lose stratification, which often leads to a paradoxical bland appearance and underdiagnosis of HGD as LGD. Mitoses are readily identifiable and can also be present in the surface epithelium. HGD may be present endoscopically as nodules of variable size and may surface trauma and erosion may lead to varying degrees of inflammation in the lamina propria and even in the neoplastic epithelium.

Variants of Dysplasia

Basal "Crypt" Dysplasia. As mentioned earlier, some cases may show significant atypia involving the crypt bases with a mature surface epithelium (Fig. 2.13). Aberrant p53 expression and high Ki-67 proliferation may be present in these foci, supporting a neoplastic proliferation. Whether this represents tangential sectioning of a focus of dysplasia or early neoplastic change is unclear. More than half of such cases have been reported to be associated with concurrent dysplasia or carcinoma. The natural history of these lesions in the absence of concurrent conventional dysplasia is unknown. Unless definitive features of HGD are present, preferably supported by a mutant pattern of p53 expression, these lesions are best classified as IND which leads to repeat surveillance biopsies within 6 to 12 months.

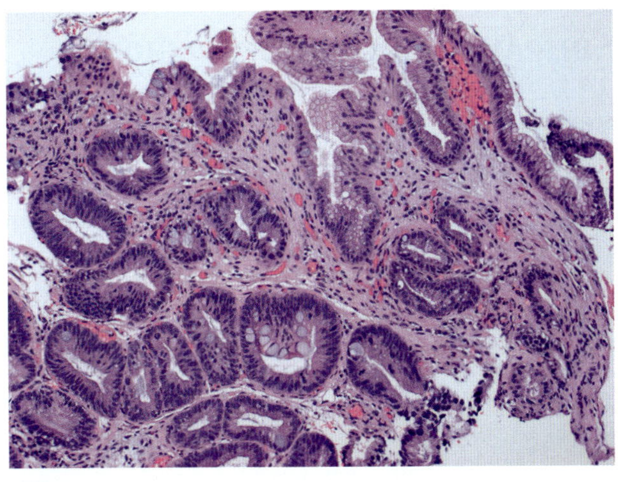

FIGURE 2.13

Basal atypia with surface maturation. Occasional examples show the epithelial changes restricted to deeper glands, sometimes as a result of tangential embedding. These biopsies are best classified as indefinite for dysplasia.

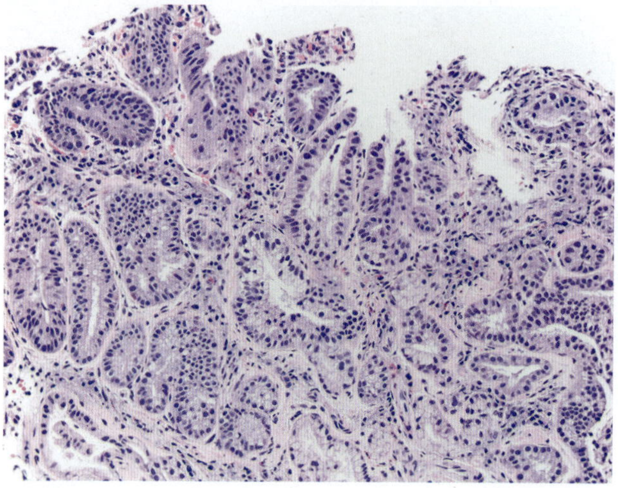

FIGURE 2.14

Foveolar type dysplasia in Barrett's esophagus is characterized by abundant pale cytoplasm that stains positively for MUC5. Nuclei are often round and monolayered, often leading to an underdiagnosis of LGD. This phenotype of dysplasia has been described variously as foveolar, gastric, and nonadenomatous in literature.

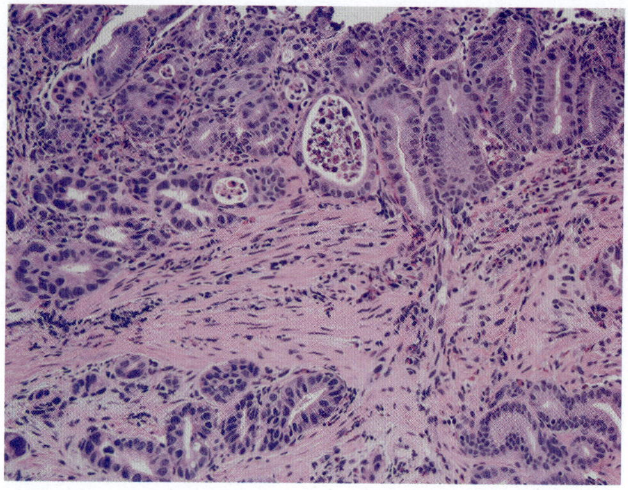

FIGURE 2.15

Intramucosal adenocarcinoma in Barrett's esophagus can be distinguished from high-grade dysplasia by the presence of anastomosing glands, sheets of neoplastic cells, single cell infiltration, intraglandular necrosis, or neoplastic glands invading into the muscularis mucosae.

Foveolar, Nonadenomatous or Gastric-Type Dysplasia. A peculiar form of dysplasia that is rich in gastric foveolar type mucin has been described variously as foveolar, nonadenomatous or gastric-type dysplasia in BE (Fig. 2.14). This accounts for approximately 6% to 8% of all dysplasia cases. It is characterized by back-to-back glands lined by a monolayer epithelium with round basally located nuclei, abundant apical cytoplasm, high nuclear-to-cytoplasmic ratio, and prominent nucleoli. Some cases may show eosinophilic instead of clear cytoplasm. There are no validated grading schemes for this pattern of dysplasia, but patients develop adenocarcinoma at rates similar to patients with high-grade conventional adenomatous dysplasia. Therefore, these lesions are best regarded as high risk and managed similar to HGD.

INTRAMUCOSAL ADENOCARCINOMA

Intramucosal adenocarcinoma is characterized by invasion of neoplastic cells into the lamina propria. This may occur more obviously but less commonly in the form of single cells infiltration or neoplastic cells floating in pools of extracellular mucin or in a more subtle but common pattern of confluent sheet-like or anastomosing glandular growth pattern, or expansile invasion by cystically dilated glands with intraluminal papillary or cribriform architecture. Intraglandular necrosis is also a helpful sign of intramucosal adenocarcinoma (Fig. 2.15). Deep infiltration into the submucosa or beyond is often associated with desmoplasia, and a clearly infiltrative growth pattern is more readily apparent in deeply invasive tumors.

Ancillary Studies

Immunohistochemistry

Various biomarkers have been examined to aid in the diagnosis of BE-related dysplasia, of which p53 is the most well-studied. Aberrant immunohistochemical staining for p53 is a useful surrogate marker of p53 mutations, but reported concordance between aberrant staining and p53 mutations is about 90%. This highlights the risk of misdiagnosis in a significant subset of cases if too much reliance is placed on p53 pattern of expression only. Whereas "wild-type" p53 staining shows scattered, weak nuclear positivity (see Fig. 2.9B), a "mutant" pattern shows confluent, "clonal" diffuse strong expression (see Fig. 2.12B) or complete loss of nuclear staining caused by truncating p53 mutations. Caution must be used when using p53 staining because a lack of a mutant pattern does not rule out dysplasia, and the presence of a mutant pattern may be seen both in LGD and HGD. Similarly, the significance of a mutant p53 staining in biopsies negative for dysplasia is uncertain and should not change the recommended surveillance interval. None of the other ancillary biomarkers reported in BE have been validated for use in clinical practice, and even routine use of p53 immunostain in classification of BE-associated dysplasia is not recommended for reasons discussed above.

Prognosis and Therapy

Guidelines for surveillance intervals have been developed by the American College of Gastroenterologists as in Table 2.2. The grade of dysplasia correlates well with

TABLE 2.2

American College of Gastroenterology Guidelines for Follow-up of Barrett's Esophagus

Dysplasia	Documentation	Follow-up
None	If adequate biopsies were obtained at index examination when diagnosis of BE was established, repeat endoscopy within 1 year not required	Endoscopy every 3–5 years
Low grade	Highest grade on repeat EGD with biopsies within 6 months. Expert review	Endoscopic eradication therapy *or* 1-year interval until two negative EGDs with biopsy
High grade	Repeat EGD with biopsies within 3 months to exclude carcinoma. Expert review	Endoscopic mucosal resection or other endoscopic eradication therapy, such as radiofrequency ablation. Surveillance every 3 months

EGD, Esophagogastroduodenoscopy.

risk of progression to invasive carcinoma, and it remains an imperfect but current gold standard for clinical decision making. Consensus diagnosis and review by an expert GI pathologist is recommended by gastroenterology society guidelines to help minimize interobserver variability and improve patient management. In the past, esophagectomy was the treatment of choice for patients with HGD and intramucosal adenocarcinoma, but this is no longer the case. In the absence of a deep invasive component (pT1b or higher) on endoscopic ultrasound, visible neoplastic lesions are removed by EMR or ESD, depending on size, followed by ablation of the remaining BE segment. Radiofrequency ablation (RFA) is the most common ablation technique currently used for eradication of early BE neoplasia. Endoscopically invisible HGD and even LGD, at some centers, is now usually treated by RFA. Interestingly, after ablation from any technique, there is a regrowth of squamous mucosa in the esophagus previously lined by the metaplastic BE segment. Postablation neoplastic recurrence typically occurs at the original site of neoplasia, commonly in the distal esophagus, and may be buried underneath the neosquamous mucosa in many cases.

ADENOCARCINOMA

Clinical Features

Esophageal adenocarcinoma is rapidly increasing in incidence in the United States and is often diagnosed at a late stage. As mentioned earlier, more than 90% of all patients with adenocarcinoma are diagnosed at the time of their first endoscopy (prevalent carcinomas) and only 5% to 10% are diagnosed during surveillance for BE (incident carcinomas). The majority of adenocarcinomas occurring in association with BE occur in white, middle-aged men, with a median age in the late fifties. The predisposing risk factors for adenocarcinoma are the same as for BE and include male gender, white race, and obesity.

Pathologic Features

Gross Findings

Esophageal adenocarcinomas are most often seen at esophagectomy as firm white mass lesions, usually involving the distal third of the esophagus (Figs. 2.16A–C). Residual Barrett's mucosa can be recognized in the background by its salmon color and "velvety appearance."

Microscopic Findings

Esophageal adenocarcinomas are composed of malignant cells with glandular differentiation. Well-recognized patterns of adenocarcinoma include tubular, papillary, mucinous, and signet-ring cell types (Figs. 2.16D–F). Some tumors may also show endocrine cells or Paneth cells or an admixed malignant squamous component. Although poorly differentiated adenocarcinomas behave more aggressively than well-differentiated ones, stage is the most important prognostic parameter. The muscularis mucosae of the esophagus tend to either thicken or duplicate, and invasion between the two muscularis mucosae should not be misinterpreted as submucosal invasion (Figs. 2.16G and H). Similarly, the thick deep muscularis mucosae should not be mistaken for muscularis propria, which has major implications for patient management.

In patients treated with preoperative chemoradiation, residual tumor cells may be rare, consisting of single or small clusters of cells associated with dense fibrosis and large pools of mucin. In some cases, acellular pools of mucin may be the only residual indication of a preexisting tumor, and this is considered complete treatment response. Grading schemes for tumor regression exist and are typically included as part of tumor synoptic reporting. The modified Ryan scheme is most commonly used and has four different tumor regression scores: 0, no viable cancer cells; 1, single or small groups of cancer cells; 2, residual cancer with evident tumor regression but more than single or small groups of cancer cells; and 3, extensive residual cancer with no evident tumor regression.

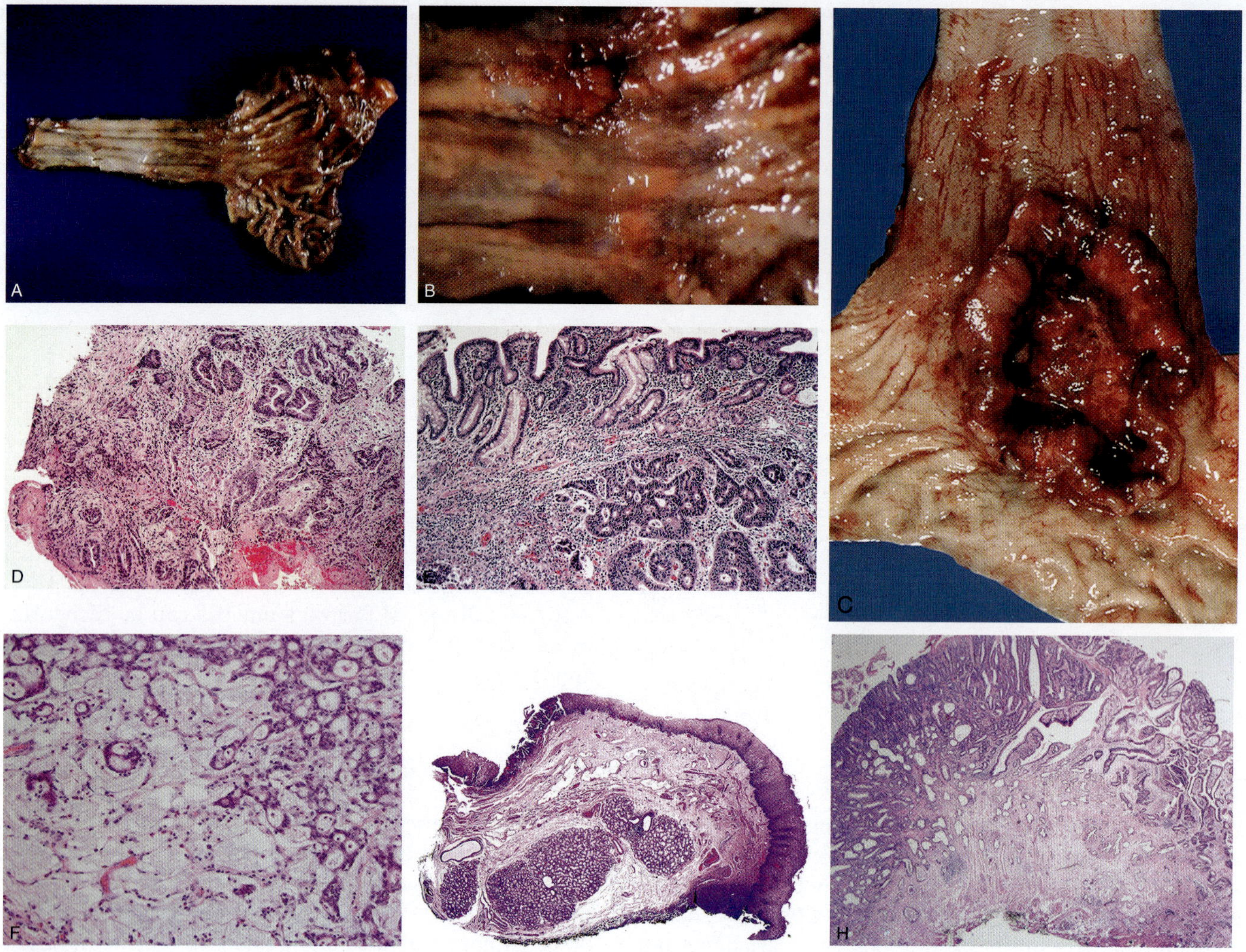

FIGURE 2.16

Esophagectomy from a patient with an early invasive adenocarcinoma (**A**). Note the columnar mucosa in the distal esophagus. A subtle nodule in the distal esophagus in another case (**B**) corresponded to an early invasive adenocarcinoma. Large bulky tumors with extensive ulceration (**C**) can be seen in patients with poor response to neoadjuvant therapy. Microscopically, esophageal adenocarcinomas show variable grades of differentiation (**D** and **E**) and may show mucinous (**F**) or signet ring cell phenotype. The phenomenon of double muscularis mucosae in Barrett's esophagus is a pitfall that may lead to misdiagnosis of submucosal invasion in endoscopic mucosal resection (EMR) or endoscopic submucosal dissection specimens. EMR specimen showing duplication of the muscularis mucosae. There are large submucosal glands at the bottom of the field, proving that the deepest portion of the sample is submucosal (**G**). EMR for T1a adenocarcinoma with invasion into (but not beyond) muscularis mucosae (**H**).

ANCILLARY STUDIES

IMMUNOHISTOCHEMISTRY

Immunohistochemical staining is not typically necessary to establish the diagnosis of esophageal adenocarcinoma but can be helpful in poorly differentiated cases to rule out squamous and neuroendocrine differentiation and to exclude metastases. Positivity for broad-spectrum cytokeratin and CK7 is typically seen, whereas positivity for CDX-2 is variable and CK20 is usually negative. Special stains for mucin are positive but may be focal in poorly differentiated cases. A subset of tumors, usually of intestinal type, demonstrate *HER2* amplification, which can be targeted for therapy. Similarly, a minority of high stage adenocarcinomas with metastatic disease are positive for PDL1, which is useful to identify patients likely to respond to anti-PD1 immunotherapy. Microsatellite instability, most often caused by sporadic methylation of MLH1, is rare in esophageal adenocarcinomas.

MOLECULAR FINDINGS

Reported molecular genetic alterations include p53 mutation and deletion; deletion of Rb, p16, and APC; overexpression of epidermal growth factor receptor (EGFR) and transforming growth factor-α; and clonal DNA aneuploidy and tetraploidy. There is no important role for Ras gene mutations. Mutations in chromatin modifier genes, such as *ARID1A*, are also reported in a small subset of tumors. Promoter methylation for numerous genes has been reported, but is of little clinical significance.

DIFFERENTIAL DIAGNOSIS

The differential diagnosis is the same as with other adenocarcinomas, including metastases and direct extension from other primary sites. The presence of adjacent BE and associated dysplasia is strong evidence of primary esophageal origin. Immunohistochemical staining may be helpful in excluding metastases. When esophageal carcinomas appear poorly differentiated or undifferentiated, the usual differential diagnosis is SCC or adenocarcinoma or a high-grade neuroendocrine carcinoma. A panel of p40/p63 in combination with CDX2, chromogranin, synaptophysin, and INSM1 can help in determining the dominant line of differentiation in most cases. Poorly differentiated neuroendocrine carcinomas may show loss of Rb protein and aberrant p53 but this finding is not lineage specific since a subset of SCC may show a similar phenotype. Undifferentiated SMARCA4 deficient carcinomas can also occur in the esophagus in a background of BE. This possibility should be considered in poorly differentiated tumors with limited keratin positivity and features reminiscent more of a lymphoma rather than carcinoma or when tumors show a rhabdoid or plasmacytoid morphology. The esophagus can also be the site of primary malignant melanoma, which can be easily diagnosed using immunostains when the diagnosis is suspected. Lymphomas involving the esophagus are very rare but primary esophageal plasmablastic lymphomas have been described in HIV positive patients. Carcinomas involving the GEJ are defined as tumors with epicenters within 2 cm from GEJ and extending into the esophagus and are staged similar to distal esophagus cancers. Tumors with epicenters in the stomach greater than 2 cm from the GEJ or those within 2 cm of the esophagogastric junction but without involvement of the GEJ are classified and staged as proximal gastric cancers.

Prognosis and Therapy

Patients with early-stage adenocarcinoma treated with EMR or ESD undergo a completion esophagectomy in the presence of deep submucosal invasion, positive deep margin of resection, or lymphovascular invasion (Fig. 2.17). For deeply invasive tumors, preoperative neoadjuvant chemotherapy and radiotherapy followed by esophagectomy is the preferred treatment. The overall 5-year survival rate is poor (~15%–20%). The few patients with a good outcome tend to be those with early lesions detected

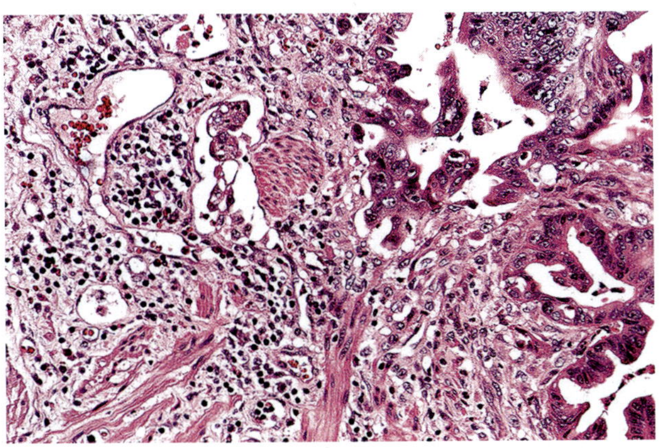

FIGURE 2.17

The presence of lymphovascular invasion in early-stage adenocarcinomas treated by endoscopic therapy is an indication for completion esophagectomy to rule out the possibility of nodal metastasis.

Esophageal Adenocarcinoma—Fact Sheet

Definition

- A carcinoma displaying varying degrees of glandular differentiation arising in the esophagus, usually in the setting of Barrett's esophagus

Incidence and Location

- The overall incidence of esophageal cancer in the United States is 2.58 cases per 100,000 persons (4.87 per 100,000 in men)
- The incidence of adenocarcinoma has increased approximately 6% per year over the past several decades
- The distal esophagus is most common site

Morbidity and Mortality

- The overall 5-year survival rate is poor (~15%–20%) because of the high stage at presentation
- Low-stage lesions have an excellent prognosis

Gender, Race, and Age Distribution

- The mean age at diagnosis is in the mid-60s with a strong white male prevalence

Clinical Features

- Dysphagia, odynophagia, and weight loss are common symptoms at presentation
- Some patients have symptomatic reflux

Esophageal Adenocarcinoma—Pathologic Features

Gross Findings

- Mass lesion typically involving the lower one-third of the esophagus
- Background Barrett's mucosa seen in most cases

Microscopic Findings

- Malignant invasive tumor with glandular differentiation
- Tubular and papillary patterns most common; signet ring cell and mucinous types less common
- Tumors show a wide spectrum of differentiation (well to poorly differentiated)
- Adjacent mucosa often shows residual Barrett's esophagus with dysplasia

Immunohistochemistry

- Not specific; often CK7+, variable CDX2
- HER2 and PDL1 expression or loss of DNA mismatch repair proteins useful in metastatic tumors to guide adjuvant therapy

Differential Diagnosis

- When poorly differentiated, squamous cell carcinoma, neuroendocrine carcinoma, SMARCA4 deficient undifferentiated carcinoma, melanoma, and lymphoma should be considered
- Can be easily differentiated by immunohistochemistry in most cases

on surveillance or those with complete response to neoadjuvant therapy. Positive lymph nodes in posttreatment resections are the worst prognostic factor in these patients. Residual or recurrent neoplastic glands may be completely buried underneath squamous mucosa after treatment with RFA (Fig. 2.18). Surveillance biopsies from the entire segment involved by BE before ablation are therefore performed routinely in these patients.

SQUAMOUS DYSPLASIA AND SQUAMOUS CELL CARCINOMA

Clinical Features

The prevalence of esophageal squamous dysplasia varies worldwide and is much more common in the East, in China and Iran. The incidence is declining in the United States. Estimates regarding the prevalence of squamous dysplasia are from higher-risk countries and range from 3% to 38%. Esophageal squamous dysplasia is a precursor to SCC and is seen adjacent to SCC in up to 90% of cases. As with adenocarcinomas, most patients with squamous carcinomas are men in their 50s. Unlike adenocarcinomas, which typically affect white men, SCC is more common among African American men.

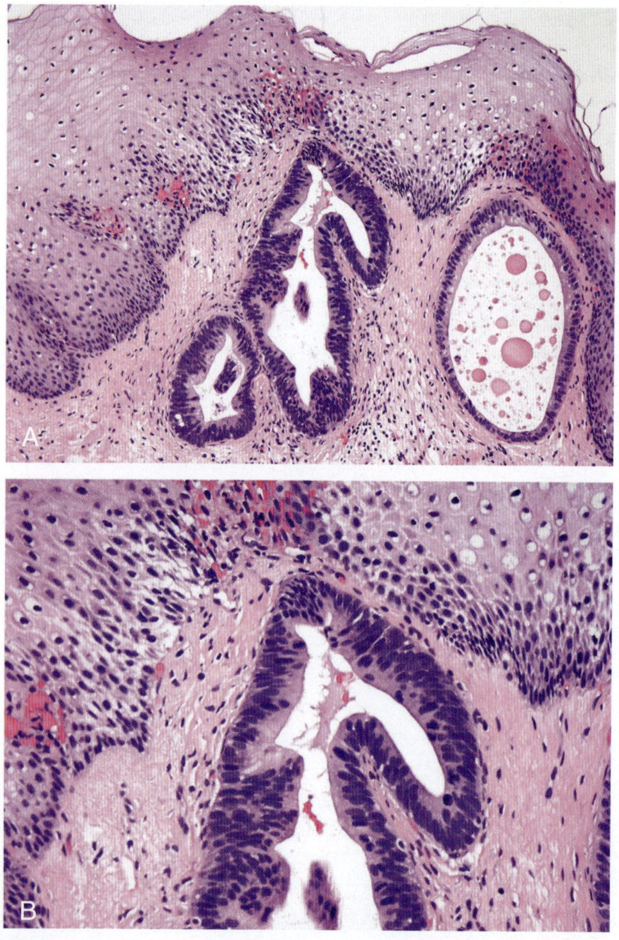

FIGURE 2.18

In patients with high-grade dysplasia or intramucosal adenocarcinoma who are treated with radiofrequency ablation, non-neoplastic metaplastic crypts or neoplastic glands may remain buried underneath squamous mucosa and are an important cause for neoplastic recurrence. (**A**). At higher magnification, the dysplastic nature of buried gland is apparent (**B**).

ESOPHAGEAL SQUAMOUS CARCINOMA—FACT SHEET

Definition

- Malignant neoplasm of the esophagus showing squamous differentiation, often with keratinization

Incidence and Location

- The incidence in US men is approximately 1.8 per 100,000 persons; it is 0.7 per 100,000 in women
- The incidence of squamous cell carcinoma is declining in the United States
- Mid- or upper esophagus involved preferentially; in contrast to adenocarcinomas that more commonly involve the distal esophagus

Morbidity and Mortality

- The overall prognosis for these tumors is poor

Gender, Race, and Age Distribution

- More common in African American men in sixth to seventh decades of life
- High tobacco and alcohol use are strong risk factors

Clinical Features

- Presenting symptoms are similar to adenocarcinoma—dysphagia, odynophagia, and weight loss

Pathologic Features

Gross Findings

Squamous dysplasia appears as foci of mucosal erythema that tends to be irregular and friable. Lugol iodine staining can be used to detect lesions that are endoscopically invisible, leaving dysplastic areas "unstained" because of decreased glycogen content. Enhanced endoscopic techniques, such as narrow-band imaging, are helpful in detecting and delineating dysplastic areas. At esophagectomy, carcinomas are firm white mass lesions of variable size that may appear exophytic or endophytic (Fig. 2.19) or present as a diffuse stricture, typically involving the middle third of the esophagus.

Microscopic Findings

Dysplasia involving esophageal squamous mucosa is morphologically similar to oropharyngeal and laryngeal squamous neoplasia and may be seen without a concurrent invasive tumor in high-risk patients undergoing screening or surveillance endoscopy. Low-grade

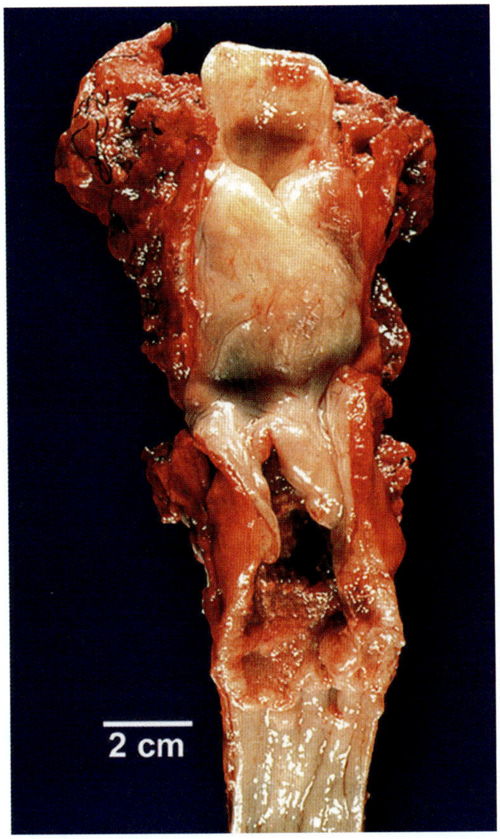

FIGURE 2.19

Squamous cell carcinoma of the esophagus. This lesion is proximal and involves the cervical esophagus. Most examples are seen in the mid-esophagus.

squamous dysplasia (Fig. 2.20A) is composed of basaloid cells with high nuclear-to-cytoplasmic ratio and typically involves the lower third of the mucosa. A greater degree of involvement by cells with similar morphologic features is diagnostic of high-grade squamous dysplasia (Fig. 2.20B). SCC of the esophagus shows a spectrum of differentiation from well-differentiated keratinizing carcinomas (Fig. 2.21A) to poorly differentiated or undifferentiated tumors (Fig. 2.21B) that can only be classified as squamous based on immunophenotypic positivity for p40/63 or the presence of adjacent high-grade squamous dysplasia. Several histologic variants of SCC exist. A prominent spindle cell component may be present, and these tumors have been variably designated as *polypoid carcinoma*, *carcinosarcoma*, and *sarcomatoid carcinoma* in the past (Fig. 2.22). *Spindle cell SCC* is the preferred designation for these tumors. Short-term survival in patients with such tumors is better than that for those with flat typical carcinomas, owing to their exophytic growth, but deeply invasive tumors have a dismal prognosis. Basaloid SCCs are characterized by solid or cribriform nests of round cells with open chromatin and scant cytoplasm (Fig. 2.23). Areas of central necrosis and peripheral palisading of nuclei may be present. Verrucous SCCs are a rare variant with an exophytic growth pattern. Histologically, these tumors

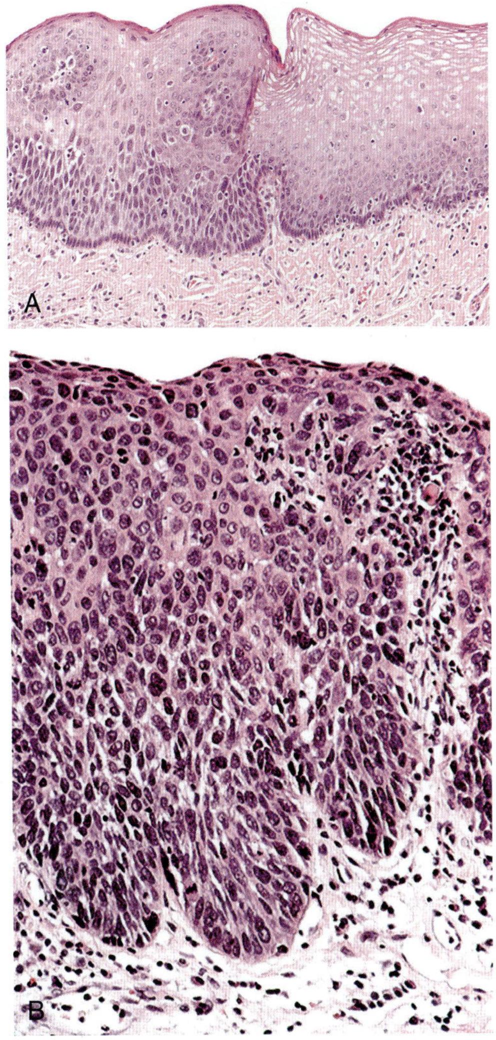

FIGURE 2.20

Squamous dysplasia may be low grade when basaloid cells with scant cytoplasm involve the lower third of the mucosa (**A**) or high grade when neoplastic cells with similar features occupy a greater thickness of the mucosa (**B**).

ESOPHAGEAL SQUAMOUS CARCINOMA—PATHOLOGIC FEATURES

Gross Findings

- Exophytic or endophytic mass or stricture involving the middle third of the esophagus

Microscopic Findings

- Carcinoma with variable grades of squamous differentiation
- Associated high-grade dysplasia or in situ carcinoma often seen
- Variants include spindle cell, basaloid, and verrucous carcinomas

Immunohistochemistry

- Positivity for CK5/6, P63, and/or P40 helpful in establishing diagnosis in poorly differentiated tumors

Differential Diagnosis

- Majority easily diagnosed on morphology; poorly differentiated tumors need confirmation by immunohistochemistry are composed of well-differentiated squamous cells with prominent acanthosis and a pushing boarder of invasion. These tumors typically grow very large before coming to clinical attention and are usually difficult to diagnose on biopsy because of their well-differentiated appearance.

- Spindle cell squamous cell carcinomas can be challenging because positivity for keratins can be focal; sampling to detect a typical invasive component or adjacent dysplasia is helpful in making the diagnosis.

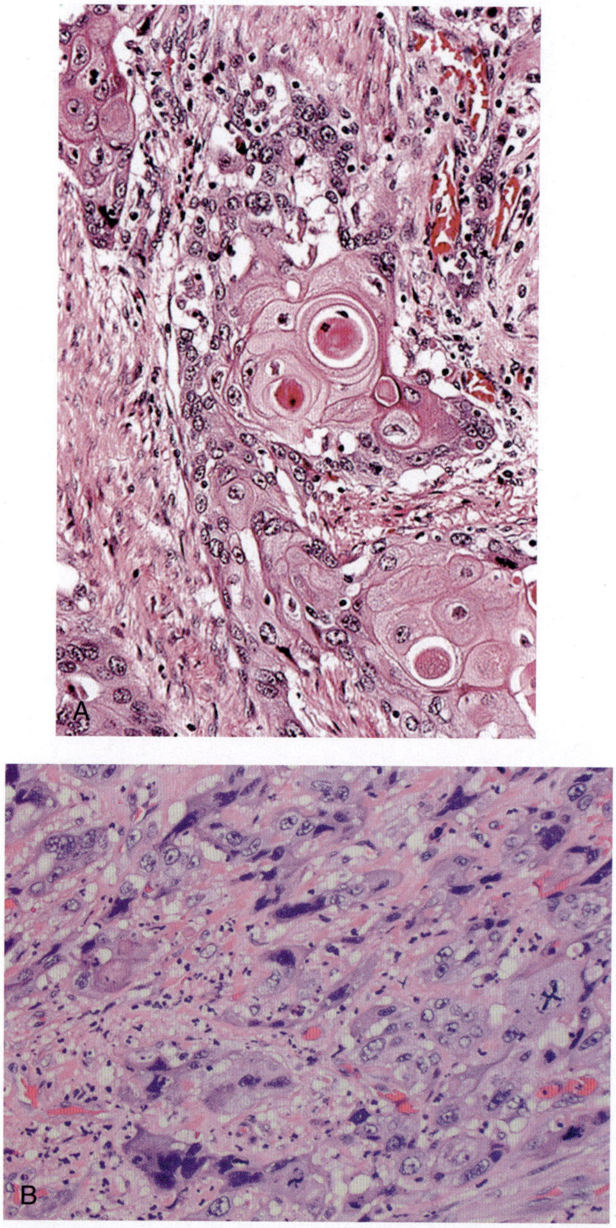

FIGURE 2.21

Typical keratinizing squamous cell carcinoma of the esophagus (**A**). Other examples may show a poorly differentiated or undifferentiated appearance (**B**) and may be recognizable as squamous only by virtue of immunohistochemical positivity for p40/63 or the presence of squamous dysplasia in the adjacent mucosa.

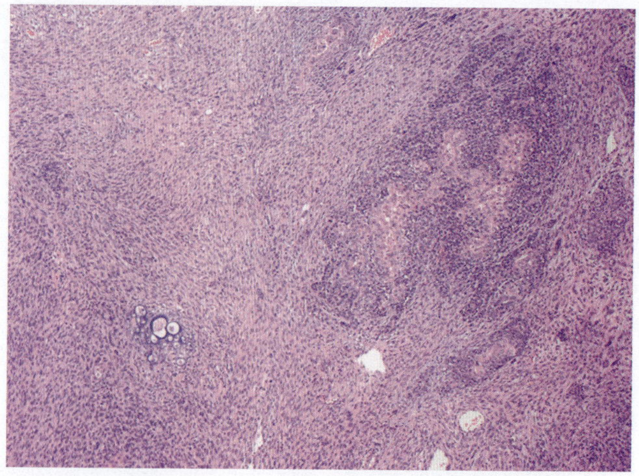

FIGURE 2.22

Spindle cell squamous cell carcinoma (SCC), also known in the literature as polypoid carcinoma or sarcomatoid carcinoma, is a SCC variant that can show undifferentiated spindle cell morphology admixed with sarcomatoid differentiation. Note the presence of malignant cartilaginous foci in this example. The presence of in situ squamous neoplasia and foci of conventional invasive SCC are helpful in establishing the diagnosis.

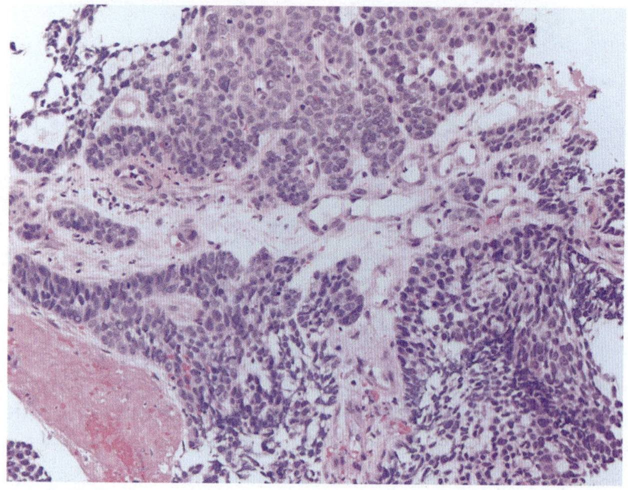

FIGURE 2.23

Basaloid squamous cell carcinoma of the esophagus may be mistaken for adenoid cystic carcinoma because of cribriform architecture and basement membrane–like material but is composed of a single population of round cells with scant cytoplasm. The tumor is present in broad nests that may show peripheral palisading and central necrosis. A myoepithelial component, as seen in adenoid cystic carcinoma, is lacking in basaloid squamous cell carcinoma.

Ancillary Studies

Immunohistochemistry

Squamous cell carcinomas are positive for CK5/6, p40, p63, and broad- spectrum keratins.

Other Studies

Reported molecular genetic abnormalities include p53 mutations and deletion; deletion of Rb and p16; amplification of EGFR; and c-*myc*, int-2/hst-1, and cyclin D1;

overexpression of EGFR and insulin-like growth factor receptor-1 has also been reported.

Differential Diagnosis

As with adenocarcinomas, the diagnosis is challenging only in poorly differentiated or undifferentiated tumors. Careful evaluation of background mucosa for BE or squamous dysplasia and a basic panel of immunostains can resolve the differential diagnosis in most cases. Primary sarcomas of the esophagus are extremely rare, and the possibility of a spindle cell SCC must be excluded before rendering such a diagnosis. Basaloid SCCs can mimic melanoma or high-grade neuroendocrine carcinomasbut this is easily resolved on immunohistochemical stains. Reactive epithelial changes are in the differential diagnosis of verrucous SCC and challenging to distinguish in a biopsy but the overall clinical context and presence of a mass lesion on endoscopy is helpful in rendering the right diagnosis.

Prognosis and Therapy

Squamous cell carcinomas are also high stage at initial presentation, and extension into periesophageal soft tissue is already present. Esophageal obstruction, extension of carcinoma into mediastinal and intrathoracic structures (tracheobronchial tree, aorta, and lung), and mediastinal lymph node metastases are frequent, but distant metastases are rare. Radiotherapy or chemotherapy is the usual treatment, sometimes with esophagectomy, which may be palliative rather than curative. Esophageal SCC has a dismal prognosis with an overall 5-year survival rate of 5% to 10%. Patients with squamous dysplasia in the absence of invasive carcinoma can be treated with endoscopic techniques such as radiofrequency ablation or mucosal resection or submucosal dissection.

UNDIFFERENTIATED CARCINOMA

Clinical Features

This tumor is rare, representing fewer than 4% of all esophageal carcinomas. It presents more commonly in men in the sixth decade of life and involves the distal esophagus and GEJ. Patients present with dysphagia and weight loss.

PATHOLOGIC FINDINGS

Gross Findings

Tumors are exophytic with a central depression or ulceration and involve the distal esophagus or GEJ.

MICROSCOPIC FINDINGS

By definition, these tumors lack squamous, glandular, and neuroendocrine differentiation. Tumors have a nested, syncytial, or sheet-like growth pattern (Fig. 2.24). The neoplastic cells reveal amphophilic to slightly eosinophilic cytoplasm and oval nuclei with vesicular chromatin. Admixed pleomorphic and rhabdoid cells are often seen.

Lymphoepithelioma-like carcinoma is considered a subtype of undifferentiated carcinoma. As opposed to those in the head and neck region, positivity for Epstein-Barr virus is not frequent.

ANCILLARY STUDIES

Immunohistochemistry

The goal of using immunostains is to exclude primary tumors with distinct differentiation (adenocarcinoma, squamous, or neuroendocrine) or involvement by other nonepithelial neoplasms such as lymphomas, melanomas, among others. SMARCA4 or INI-1 deficient undifferentiated carcinomas can also occur in the esophagus and easily diagnosed using the appropriate immunostains. SALL4 expressing undifferentiated carcinoma carry a worse prognosis compared to those which are negative.

Prognosis and Therapy

The prognosis is poor with a 1-year survival rate of approximately 25%.

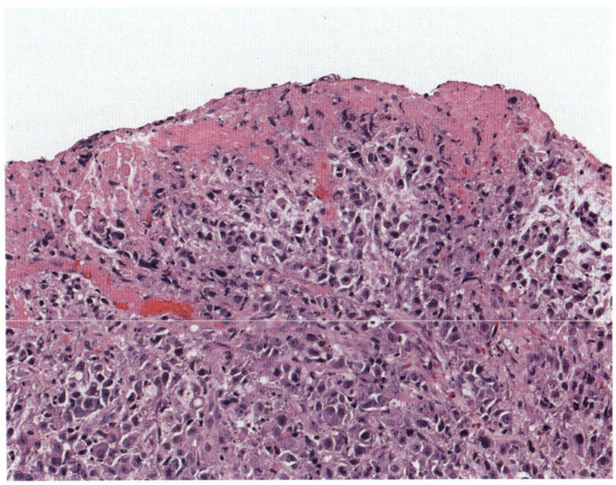

FIGURE 2.24

Undifferentiated carcinoma of the esophagus characterized by sheets of atypical cells that do not display glandular, squamous, or neuroendocrine differentiation.

UNDIFFERENTIATED CARCINOMA—FACT SHEET

Definition
- Tumors that lack glandular, squamous, or neuroendocrine differentiation

Incidence and Location
- Uncommon (<4%); usually involves the distal esophagus

Gender and Age Distribution
- More common in men in their 60s

Clinical Features
- Dysphagia and weight loss

UNDIFFERENTIATED CARCINOMA—PATHOLOGIC FEATURES

Gross Findings
- Mass forming with central depression or ulceration on endoscopy

Microscopic Findings
- Nests, syncytial, or sheet-like growth pattern
- Cell with amphophilic to eosinophilic cytoplasm and oval nuclei; rhabdoid or pleomorphic cells
- Lymphoepithelioma-like carcinoma is a subtype

Immunohistochemistry
- Lacks a characteristic staining pattern
- Stains can help exclude tumors such as squamous cell carcinoma, adenocarcinoma, or neuroendocrine neoplasms, among others; SMARCA4 and INI-1 deficient carcinomas also fall within this category

Differential Diagnosis
- Squamous cell carcinoma
- Adenocarcinoma
- Neuroendocrine carcinoma
- Melanomas
- Lymphomas
- Others

SALIVARY GLAND TYPE TUMORS

CLINICAL FEATURES

Primary tumors of the salivary glands originating from esophageal submucosal glands or ducts have also been described. These tumors are relatively rare, representing fewer than 1% of all esophageal carcinomas. Mucoepidermoid and adenoid cystic carcinomas are the most common variants and predominantly present in the seventh decade of life with a male predominance. Presenting symptoms are similar to other esophageal carcinomas and include dysphagia and weight loss.

PATHOLOGIC FEATURES

GROSS FEATURES

Mucoepidermoid carcinomas appear grossly similar to SCCs, presenting as ulcerated or infiltrative mass lesions in the midesophagus. Adenoid cystic carcinoma can present as a discrete submucosal mass or as large, polypoid or fungating mass lesions, also predominantly involving the midesophagus.

MICROSCOPIC FEATURES

Mucoepidermoid carcinomas are characterized by an intimate mixture of squamous cells, mucus secreting cells, and intermediate cells (Fig. 2.25). Squamous areas resemble SCC with intercellular bridges and keratinization. A limited in situ SCC component is present in some cases. Adenoid cystic carcinomas are composed of two cell populations: ductal epithelium and basaloid myoepithelial cells. The tumor may show cribriform, tubular, or solid growth patterns (Fig. 2.26). Areas of cribriform growth characteristically contain abundant eosinophilic basement membrane material. The tumor cells are very monomorphic and only show mild nuclear atypia. The tumor nests are sharply circumscribed unlike the streaming appearance of myoepithelial cells in benign mixed tumors.

ANCILLARY STUDIES

IMMUNOHISTOCHEMISTRY

Like SCC, mucoepidermoid carcinoma is positive for most cytokeratins and markers of squamous differentiation

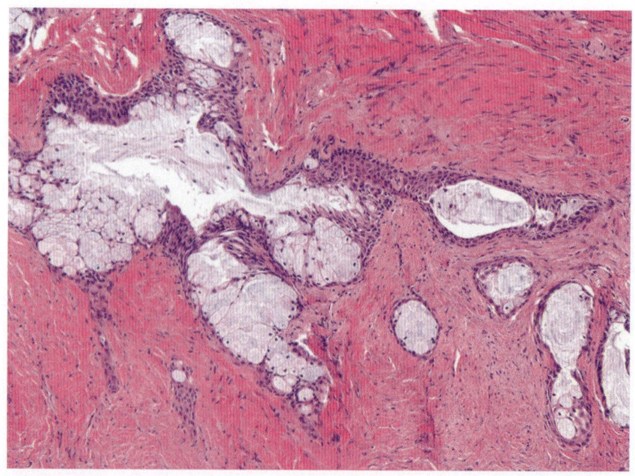

FIGURE 2.25

An example of mucoepidermoid carcinoma involving the esophagus. The tumor shows an infiltrative growth pattern in the esophageal wall and displays the typical mucoid cells admixed with intermediate and squamous cells.

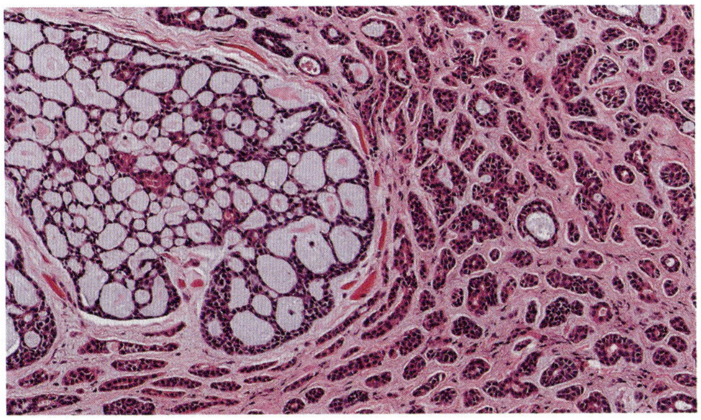

FIGURE 2.26
Adenoid cystic carcinoma in the esophagus. In this example, the two-cell population characteristic of this tumor (ductal and basal myoepithelial cells) can be appreciated on hematoxylin and eosin stain. The tumor reveals cribriform *(left)* and tubular *(right)* predominant growth patterns.

(p63, p40). In addition, mucin stains (mucicarmine, Alcian blue) highlight the mucin-secreting cells. Ductal cells of adenoid cystic carcinoma are strongly positive for cytokeratins, CEA and KIT. The basal cells may show weak keratin staining but are strongly positive for p63, S100, actin, and calponin. MYB expression can also be a helpful adjunct to diagnosis and correlates with MYB translocations seen in the majority of adenoid cystic carcinomas.

DIFFERENTIAL DIAGNOSIS

Mucoepidermoid carcinoma and adenosquamous carcinoma show extensive histologic overlap and may be difficult to distinguish. Adenosquamous carcinoma has clearly distinguishable components of adenocarcinoma and SCC, whereas in mucoepidermoid carcinoma the components are intimately admixed. Mucoepidermoid carcinoma must also be differentiated from pure SCC by identification of the mucus-secreting cells. This distinction may be difficult on biopsy samples. The main differential diagnosis for adenoid cystic carcinoma is basaloid SCC, especially if a solid growth component and basement membrane-like material is prominent. Presence of an in situ squamous component strongly favors basaloid SCC. In contrast, identification of two cell populations, histologically or immunohistochemically, supports the diagnosis of adenoid cystic carcinoma. Adenoid cystic carcinoma also typically has minimal pleomorphism and limited mitotic activity.

PROGNOSIS AND THERAPY

Treatment usually consists of surgical resection with or without chemoradiation therapy. The prognosis for patients with mucoepidermoid carcinoma is poor with

SALIVARY GLAND TYPE TUMORS OF THE ESOPHAGUS–FACT SHEET

Definition

- Primary esophageal carcinomas arising from submucosal glands or ductal epithelium of the esophagus and resembling salivary gland counterparts

Incidence and Location

- Extremely rare, representing fewer than 1% of all esophageal carcinomas
- Predominantly in the midesophagus

Morbidity and Mortality

- Mucoepidermoid carcinomas have poor prognosis
- Adenoid cystic carcinomas tend to do slightly better than squamous cell carcinomas because of the earlier stage at presentation

Gender, Age, and Race Distribution

- Middle-aged to older patients with peak incidence in the seventh decade of life
- Male predominance

Clinical Features

- Dysphagia and weight loss

SALIVARY GLAND TYPE TUMORS OF THE ESOPHAGUS–PATHOLOGIC FEATURES

Gross Findings

- Mucoepidermoid carcinomas present as ulcerated or infiltrative mass lesions in the midesophagus
- Adenoid cystic carcinomas present as submucosal lesions at early stages and progress to polypoid or fungating mass lesions

Microscopic Findings

- Mucoepidermoid carcinomas are characterized by intimate mixture of squamous cells, mucus cells, and intermediate cells
- Adenoid cystic carcinomas are characterized by two cell populations consisting of ductal cells and myoepithelial cells; typically, there are tubular and cribriform areas containing basement membrane material; solid areas mimic basaloid carcinoma

Immunohistochemistry

- Mucin stains, keratin, p63, p40 positive in mucoepidermoid carcinoma
- Keratin, KIT, and CEA positive in ductal cells of adenoid cystic carcinoma; basal myoepithelial cells are positive for p63, S100, actin, calponin; MYB positivity also helpful in diagnosis

Differential Diagnosis

- Adenosquamous carcinoma has discrete areas of adenocarcinoma and squamous cell carcinoma (SCC) rather than an intimate admixture of both components typically seen in mucoepidermoid carcinoma; intermediate cells are absent in typical adenosquamous carcinoma
- Basaloid SCC has more cytologic atypia and lacks the two cell populations of adenoid cystic carcinoma; presence of squamous dysplasia also is absent in adenoid cystic carcinoma

a 5-year survival rate of approximately 20 % to 25 %. Follow-up data for patients with adenoid cystic carcinoma are limited. In general, patients with adenoid cystic carcinoma tend to do better than patients with SCC, presenting with lower-stage disease and a lower frequency of lymph node metastases. The estimated 5-year survival rate is approximately 35 %.

NEUROENDOCRINE NEOPLASMS

Clinical Features

Well-differentiated neuroendocrine tumors are extremely uncommon lesions in the esophagus and are typically found incidentally at the time of esophagectomy for other diagnoses. Poorly differentiated (small cell and large cell) neuroendocrine carcinomas are the most common variant of neuroendocrine tumors in the esophagus but are still rare and make up fewer than 1 % of all esophageal malignancies. Like other esophageal malignancies, patients with neuroendocrine carcinomas may present with dysphagia, chest pain, weight loss, or symptoms of reflux. There is a male predominance, and the age at presentation varies greatly with most cases occurring in the sixth or seventh decade of life.

PATHOLOGIC FEATURES

Gross Findings

Neuroendocrine neoplasms are primarily found in the distal esophagus. Well-differentiated neuroendocrine tumors are usually incidental polypoid lesions. Neuroendocrine carcinomas, on the other hand, present as large ulcerated and fungating masses.

Microscopic Findings

Esophageal neuroendocrine tumors show identical histologic features, and grading is based on mitotic count and Ki-67 proliferative index, similar to other sites in the GI tract. Poorly differentiated neuroendocrine carcinomas are subclassified as small cell or large cell neuroendocrine carcinoma. Small cell variants are composed of cells with hyperchromatic, irregular nuclei, nuclear molding, and scant cytoplasm (Fig. 2.27). In contrast, large cell variants are composed of cells with moderate cytoplasm, coarse chromatin, and prominent nucleoli often growing in a nested or acinar pattern. Mixed neuroendocrine carcinomas with adenocarcinoma or SCC components do exist and are considered when at least 30 % of each tumor component is present. These tumors have been designated mixed neuroendocrine non-neuroendocrine neoplasms in the recent World Health Organization classification.

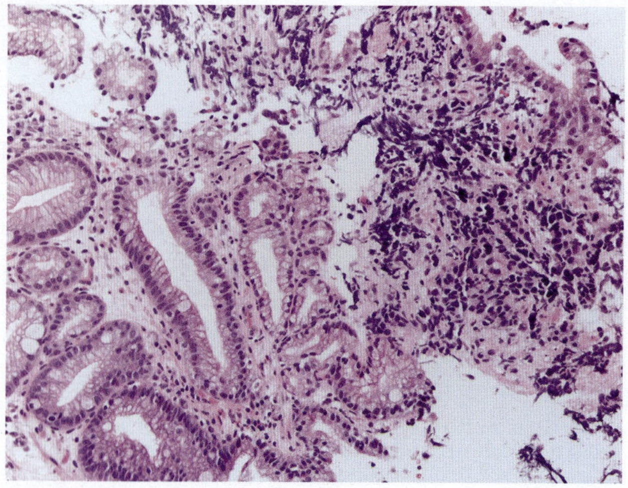

FIGURE 2.27

Small cell carcinomas of the esophagus are rare but may arise in association with both squamous cell or adenocarcinomas. The latter are often associated with a background of Barrett's esophagus, as seen in this example, with metaplastic crypts on the *left* and a poorly differentiated small cell neuroendocrine carcinoma on the *right*.

ANCILLARY STUDIES

Immunohistochemistry

Immunohistochemical stains for keratins and neuroendocrine markers, chromogranin, synaptophysin, INSM1, and CD56, and synaptophysin are positive in variable intensity and extent.

Differential Diagnosis

The main differential diagnosis for esophageal neuroendocrine carcinomas is other poorly differentiated malignancies or metastasis from another site. Positive immunohistochemical staining for neuroendocrine markers helps differentiate these tumors from other carcinomas. Discriminating metastatic neuroendocrine carcinoma is not possible on histologic grounds alone. Immunostaining for TTF-1 is not helpful in differentiating lung metastases because the majority of small cell carcinomas show positive staining regardless of primary site of origin.

Prognosis and Therapy

Follow-up data on well-differentiated neuroendocrine tumors are limited given the rarity of occurrence.

Well-differentiated neuroendocrine tumors appear benign in nature with most reported patients alive and disease free on follow-up. Poorly differentiated neuroendocrine carcinomas are aggressive tumors with nearly half of patients presenting with distant metastases at diagnosis. Treatment typically consists of neoadjuvant chemotherapy followed by esophagectomy in cases amenable to resection. However, these tumors in general show poor response to preoperative chemoradiation. The overall median survival period is approximately 14 months; patients with small cell carcinoma tend to have worse survival than those with large cell carcinoma (median, 16 months vs 22 months). Patients with localized disease have a slightly better survival (median, 28 months).

NEUROENDOCRINE NEOPLASMS OF THE ESOPHAGUS—FACT SHEET

Definition

- Neoplasms of esophagus with neuroendocrine differentiation

Incidence and Location

- Well-differentiated neuroendocrine tumors are exceedingly rare in the esophagus; poorly differentiated neuroendocrine carcinomas are more common but still account for only approximately 1% of esophageal malignancies
- Most cases are found in the distal esophagus

Morbidity and Mortality

- Well-differentiated tumors are rare but appear largely benign in nature
- Neuroendocrine carcinomas are aggressive tumors with a median survival of approximately 14 months

Gender, Race, and Age Distribution

- Most cases occur in the sixth decade of life
- Neuroendocrine carcinomas are more common in men; there is an equal distribution in men and women for well-differentiated tumors

Clinical Features

- Well-differentiated tumors are typically incidental
- Dysphagia and weight loss

NEUROENDOCRINE NEOPLASMS OF THE ESOPHAGUS—PATHOLOGIC FEATURES

Gross Findings

- Well-differentiated tumors present as incidental polypoid lesions
- Poorly differentiated neuroendocrine carcinomas appear as large, ulcerated mass lesions

Microscopic Findings

- Grading is based on mitotic count and Ki-67 proliferative index
- Well-differentiated tumors show organoid or trabecular growth and nuclei with finely granular chromatin
- Small cell neuroendocrine carcinomas show scanty cytoplasm with nuclear hyperchromasia and molding; large cell neuroendocrine carcinomas show more abundant cytoplasm and prominent nucleoli
- Admixed adenocarcinoma or squamous cell carcinoma component may be present

Immunohistochemistry

- Positive for cytokeratins, synaptophysin, chromogranin, CD56, and INSM1

Differential Diagnosis

- Immunohistochemistry can help differentiate from poorly differentiated squamous or adenocarcinoma; distinguishing metastatic neuroendocrine carcinoma from another site can only be done based on correlation with clinical or imaging findings

SECONDARY TUMORS OF THE ESOPHAGUS

CLINICAL FEATURES

Metastases to the esophagus do occur, but are rare. They are also seldom the only site of metastatic disease and hence may not be biopsied if the diagnosis is already clear based on clinical presentation. Direct extension is most common pattern of spread and typically occurs secondary to tumors arising from the larynx, hypopharynx, trachea, and stomach. The most common primary sites for secondary tumors involving the esophagus include carcinomas of the lung and breast. Metastatic malignant melanoma can also occur in the esophagus (Fig. 2.28A).

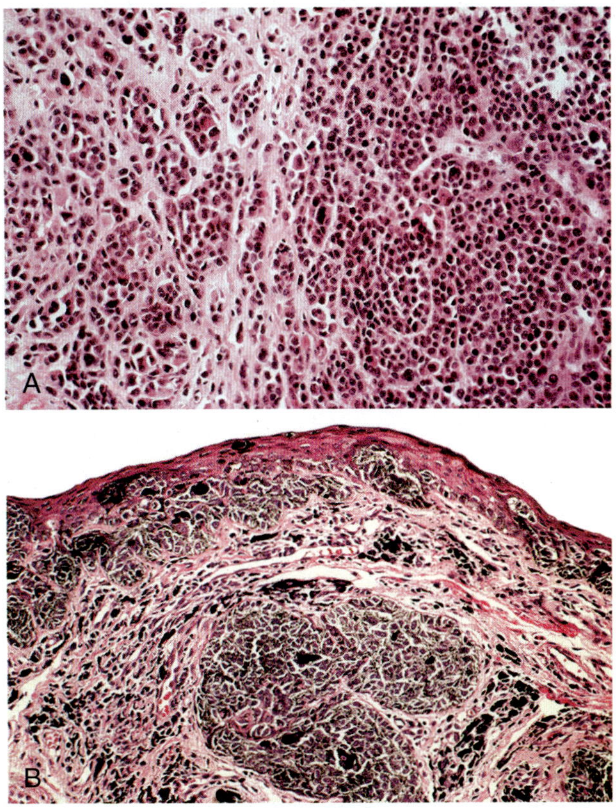

FIGURE 2.28

Malignant melanomas involving the esophagus are most often secondary tumors that display features akin to those of primary skin lesions (**A**). The presence of a junctional component (**B**) or background melanocytosis is a helpful feature that favors a primary esophageal malignant melanoma.

It should be noted that primary melanoma of the esophagus can also occur (Fig. 2.28B) but is quite rare, with fewer than 300 cases reported.

Metastases to the esophagus typically present several years after diagnosis of the primary tumor. If lesions are large and obstructive, patients may present with dysphagia, but the submucosal location of metastases often makes these lesions less likely to cause clinical symptoms. Most patients are older, presenting in the seventh or eighth decades of life.

SECONDARY TUMORS OF THE ESOPHAGUS—FACT SHEET

Definition
- Tumor metastasizing to the esophagus from another primary

Incidence and Location
- Relatively uncommon; one autopsy series reported an incidence of 6%

Morbidity and Mortality
- Varies based on underlying disease

Gender, Race, and Age Distribution
- Older individuals

Clinical Features
- Most are submucosal in location and do not cause clinical symptoms; obstructive lesions may cause dysphagia

Pathologic Features

Gross Findings

Lesions are typically submucosal with associated stricture but can present as large obstructive lesions. The midesophagus is the most common site of involvement.

Microscopic Findings

Histologic features vary based on the primary site of tumor origin. Submucosal tumor involvement with lack or mucosal extension and absence of an in situ component are clues to metastatic origin.

Secondary Tumors of the Esophagus—Pathologic Features

Gross Findings
- Submucosal mass lesion

Microscopic Findings
- Variable
- Lack of communication with mucosal surface and no in situ component

Immunohistochemistry
- TTF-1 positivity in lung metastases
- ER/PR positivity in breast metastases

Differential Diagnosis
- Primary esophageal cancer; presence of in situ component

Ancillary Studies

Immunohistochemistry

Immunohistochemistry can be useful in determining metastatic origin, and an appropriate panel can be selected based on tumor morphology and clinical history. TTF-1 positivity suggests lung origin and positivity of hormone receptors (ER/PR) can suggest breast origin. SMAD4 loss can be seen metastatic pancreatic cancer but has also been reported in primary esophageal adenocarcinomas.

Differential Diagnosis

The main differential diagnosis is primary esophageal cancer. The presence of an in situ squamous carcinoma component or BE with dysplasia in the case of adenocarcinoma strongly favors a primary esophageal tumor.

Prognosis and Therapy

The prognosis in these patients is variable owing to the heterogeneity of the underlying diseases. Reported survival has ranged from months to years after the diagnosis of esophageal metastases. Treatment is also variable with reports of resection, chemotherapy, and palliative dilation of stricturing lesions.

SUGGESTED READINGS

1. Boni A, Lisovsky M, Dal Cin P, et al. Atypical lipomatous tumor mimicking giant fibrovascular polyp of the esophagus: report of a case and critical review of the literature. *Hum Pathol*. 2013;44:1165–1170.
2. Levine MS, Bucvk JL, Pantongrag-Brown L, et al. Fibrovascular polyps of the esophagus: clinical, radiographic and pathology finding in 16 patients. *AJR Am J Roentgenol*. 1996;166:781–787.
3. Carr NJ, Bratthauer GL, Lichy JH, et al. Squamous cell papillomas of the esophagus: a study of 23 lesions for human papillomavirus by in situ hybridization and polymerase chain reaction. *Hum Pathol*. 1994;25:536–540.
4. Odze R, Antonioli D, Shocket D, et al. Esophageal squamous papillomas: a clinicopathologic study of 38 lesions and analysis for human papillomavirus by the polymerase chain reaction. *Am J Surg Pathol*. 1993;12:803–812.

5. Syrjanen K, Syrjanen S. Detection of human papillomavirus in esophageal papillomas: systemic review and meta-analysis. APMIS. 2013;121:363–374.
6. Glickman JN, Spechler SJ, Souza RF, et al. Multilayered epithelium in mucosal biopsy specimens from the gastroesophageal junction region is a histologic marker of gastroesophageal reflux disease. *Am J Surg Pathol*. 2009;33:818–825.
7. Lisovsky M, Srivastava A. Barrett esophagus: evolving concepts in diagnosis and neoplastic progression. *Surg Pathol Clin*. 2013;6(3):475–496.
8. Montgomery EA, Canto MI, Srivastava A. Evaluation and reporting of biopsies from the columnar-lined esophagus and gastro-esophageal junction (GEJ). *Ann Diagn Pathol*. 2019;39: 111–117.
9. Srivastava A, Appelman H, Goldsmith JD, et al. The use of ancillary stains in the diagnosis of Barrett esophagus and Barrett esophagus-associated dysplasia: recommendations from the Rodger C. Haggitt Gastrointestinal Pathology Society. *Am J Surg Pathol*. 2017; 41:e8–e21.
10. Shaheen NJ, Falk GQ, Iyer PG, et al. ACG clinical guideline: diagnosis and management of Barrett's esophagus. *Am J Gastroenterol*. 2016;111:30–50.
11. Spechler SJ, Sharma P, Souza RF, et al. American Gastroenterological Association medical position statement on the management of Barrett's esophagus. *Gastroenterology*. 2011;140: 1084–1091.
12. Srivastava A, Odze RD, Lauwers GY, et al. Morphologic features are useful in distinguishing Barrett esophagus from carditis with intestinal metaplasia. *Am J Surg Pathol*. 2007;31:1733–1741.
13. Brown IS, Whiteman DC, Lauwers GY. Foveolar type dysplasia in Barrett esophagus. *Mod Pathol*. 2010;23:834–843.
14. Srivastava A, Hornick JL, Li X, et al. Extent of low-grade dysplasia is a risk factor for the development of esophageal adenocarcinoma in Barrett's esophagus. *Am J Gastroenterol*. 2007;102(3): 483–493.
15. Lomo LC, Blount PL, Sanchez CA, et al. Crypt dysplasia with surface maturation; a clinical, pathologic, and molecular study of a Barrett's esophagus cohort. *Am J Surg Pathol*. 2006;30:423–435.
16. Montgomery E, Bronner MP, Goldblum JR, et al. Reproducibility of the diagnosis of Barrett esophagus: a reaffirmation. *Hum Pathol*. 2001;32:368–378.
17. Srivastava A, Golden KL, Sanchez CA, et al. High goblet cell count is inversely associated with ploidy abnormalities and risk of adenocarcinoma in Barrett's esophagus. *PLoS One*. 2015;10(7): e0133403.
18. Hur C, Miller M, Kong CY, Dowling EC, et al. Trends in esophageal adenocarcinoma incidence and mortality. Cancer. 2013;119:1149–1158.
19. Yachida S, Nakanishi Y, Shimoda T, et al. Adenosquamous carcinoma of the esophagus: clinicopathologic study of 18 cases. Oncology. 2004;66:218–225.
20. Agoston AT, Zheng Y, Bueno R, et al. Predictors of disease recurrence and survival in esophageal adenocarcinomas with complete response to neoadjuvant therapy. *Am J Surg Pathol*. 2015;39:1085–1092.
21. Agoston AT, Strauss AC, Dulai PS, et al. Predictors of treatment failure after radiofrequency ablation for intramucosal adenocarcinoma in Barrett Esophagus: a multi-institutional retrospective cohort study. *Am J Surg Pathol*. 2016;40(4): 554–562.
22. Bartel MJ, Srivastava A, Gordon S, et al. Subsquamous intestinal metaplasia is common in treatment-naïve Barrett's esophagus. *Gastrointest Endosc*. 2018;87(1):67–74.
23. Arnold M, Soerjomataram I, Ferlay J, et al. Global incidence of oesophageal cancer by histologic subtype in 2012. Gut. 2015;64: 381–387.
24. Osborn NK, Kreate RF, Trastek VF, et al. Verrucous carcinoma of the esophagus: clinicopathophysiologic features of a rare entity. *Dig Dis Sci*. 2003;48:465–474.
25. Raza MA, Mazzara PF. Sarcomatoid carcinoma of esophagus. *Arch Pathol Lab Med*. 2011;135:945–948.
26. Tayler PR, Abnet CC, Dawsy SM. Squamous dysplasia—the precursor lesion for esophageal squamous cell carcinoma. *Cancer Epidemiol Biomarkers Prev*. 2013;22 540–552.
27. Chen S, Chen Y, Yang J, et al. *Prim mucoepidermoid carcinoma esophagus*. 2011;6:1426–1431.
28. Kumagai Y, Ishiguro T, Kuwabara K, et al. Primary mucoepidermoid carcinoma of the esophagus: review of the literature. *Esophagus*. 2014;11:81–88.
29. Na YJ, Shim KN, Kang MJ, et al. Primary esophageal adenoid cystic carcinoma. *Gut Liver*. 2007;1:178–181.
30. Sawada G, Moon J, Saito A, et al. A case of adenoid cystic carcinoma of the esophagus. *Surg Case Rep*. 2015;1:119.
31. Hoang MP, Hobbs CM, Sobin LH, et al. Carcinoid tumor of the esophagus: a clinicopathologic study of four cases. *Am J Surg Pathol*. 2002;26:517–522.
32. Maru DM, Khurana H, Rahid A, et al. Retrospective study of clinicopathologic features and prognosis of high-grade neuroendocrine carcinoma of the esophagus. *Am J Surg Pathol*. 2008;32: 1404–1411.
33. Kumagai Y, Miura K, Nishida T, et al. Simultaneous resection of metastatic melanoma in the esophagus and primary cutaneous melanoma showing partial regression: report of a case. Surg Today. 2012;42:884–890.
34. Mizobuchi S, Tachimori Y, Kato H, et al. Metastatic esophageal tumors from distant primary lesions: report of three esophagectomies and study of 1835 autopsy cases. *Jpn J Clin Oncol*. 1997;27: 410–414.
35. Simchuk EJ, Low DE. Direct esophageal metastasis from a distant primary tumor is a submucosal process: a review of six cases. *Dis Esophagus*. 2001;14(3–4):247–250.

3

Non-Neoplastic Disorders of the Stomach

Sarah E. Umetsu, MD and Gregory Y. Lauwers, MD

The recognition of the central role of *Helicobacter pylori* in the development of what was once the most common form of chronic gastritis has elicited a significant interest in non-neoplastic gastric pathology. This has been paralleled by easier access to upper endoscopic examinations, which has allowed the characterization of various patterns of gastritis with defined etiologic associations.

The prevalence of *H. pylori* gastritis has significantly decreased over time because of effective antibiotic therapy and improved sanitary conditions, and reactive gastropathy has become the most common histologic diagnosis rendered in gastric biopsies in Western countries.

Numerous attempts at classifying the different types of gastritides have been made, mostly based on the acuteness or chronicity of gastric mucosal injury. This chapter does not offer a new classification but presents a review of the major clinicopathological entities, based either on the salient morphologic features or the underlying etiologies.

ACUTE EROSIVE/HEMORRHAGIC GASTRITIS ("STRESS" GASTRITIS)

Acute erosive/hemorrhagic gastritis is the result of severe and often acute mucosal injury. It is commonly associated with abrupt onset of abdominal pain and mucosal bleeding. Common causes include alcohol, steroids, nonsteroidal antiinflammatory drugs (NSAIDs), various iatrogenic injuries, and low hemodynamic state after major trauma.

The pathogenesis of acute hemorrhagic gastritis reflects an imbalance between mucosal irritants such as acid, pepsin, bile salts, NSAIDs, and other chemicals and mucoprotective mechanisms such as mucin, bicarbonates, prostaglandins, epidermal growth factors, mucosal blood flow, and the remarkable ability of gastric mucosa to reepithelialize. Various mechanisms can be at play to damage the mucosa (Box 3.1):

ACUTE EROSIVE/HEMORRHAGIC GASTRITIS (STRESS GASTRITIS)—FACT SHEET

Definition

- Direct irritant action of chemical agents such as ferrous sulfate, NSAIDs, and alcohol
- Hydrochloric acid, pepsin, and bile salts that gain entry, resulting from the disrupted mucosal barrier
- NSAIDs with their cyclo-oxygenase–inhibiting action inhibit prostaglandins, which in turn reduces bicarbonate and mucin secretions that have mucosal protective roles
- In cases of hypoperfusion-related stress ulcers, the pathogenesis is related to reduced mucosal blood flow, vasoconstriction, and reperfusion injury with release of free oxygen radicals
- Abrupt onset of abdominal pain and bleeding associated with alcohol, nonsteroidal antiinflammatory drugs, or low hemodynamic state after major trauma
- Present with multiple erosions in the gastric mucosa

Morbidity and Mortality

- Bleeding can be minimal and self-resolving or life threatening.
- Patients with comorbid conditions such as liver disease have higher morbidity and mortality rates

Clinical Features

- Abrupt onset of abdominal pain, vomiting, and gastrointestinal bleeding

Prognosis and Therapy

- Most patients have an uneventful course with full recovery within a short period
- Intravenous fluids and blood transfusion
- Stop the offending agent
- H_2 blockers, proton pump inhibitors, prostaglandin analogues
- Life-threatening hematemesis may require surgical intervention

CLINICAL FEATURES

Patients commonly present with abrupt onset of burning epigastric pain, nausea, vomiting, and gastrointestinal (GI) bleeding. The bleeding can be minimal occult bleeding, self-resolving melena, or life-threatening hematemesis. Patients with aspirin- or alcohol-induced injury usually make a quick recovery, whereas hypoperfusion-related gastritis (stress ulcers) is associated with greater morbidity and mortality. Acute erosive gastropathy is a common cause of upper GI bleeding and accounts for 6% to 34% of cases.

Acute Erosive/Hemorrhagic Gastritis (Stress Gastritis)—Pathologic Features

Gross Findings

- Superficial, round, dark erosions, few millimeters in size; frequently multiple
- The intervening mucosa is edematous and hyperemic
- Stress-related ulcers are present in the fundus and body
- Nonsteroidal antiinflammatory drug–related erosions are usually present in the antrum

Microscopic Findings

- Superficial lamina propria hemorrhage, mucosal sloughing, fibrinous exudate with neutrophils, and mucosal necrosis
- Changes limited to the mucosa
- Lack of significant lymphoplasmacytic infiltrate in lamina propria
- The healing phase is associated with regenerative epithelium with dark enlarged nuclei with prominent nucleoli

Differential Diagnosis

- Mallory-Weiss tear, peptic ulcers
- Nasogastric tube trauma
- Dysplasia in cases with marked regenerative changes

Pathologic Features

Gross Findings

The gastric erosions are multiple, 2 to 5 mm in diameter, superficial, round, and dark. The intervening mucosa is edematous and hyperemic with petechial hemorrhage.

Stress-related ulcers are mostly located in the fundus and body, whereas NSAID-related erosions are present in the antrum.

Microscopic Findings

Acute damage presents as mucosal denudation and sloughing, surface hemorrhage, or fibrin exudate with neutrophils, epithelial necrosis, and lack of significant lymphoplasmacytic infiltration in the lamina propria (Fig. 3.1). Mucosal damage ranges from gastric erosions limited to the mucosa to deep ulcers that extend beyond the submucosa. Etiologically specific changes may sometimes be seen (Figs. 3.2 to 3.4). Mucosal healing is associated with regenerative epithelial changes with enlarged hyperchromatic nuclei with prominentf nucleoli, amphophilic cytoplasm, and sometimes syncytial glandular architecture with increased mitotic activity (Figs. 3.5 and 3.6). These changes can be alarming and may be mistaken for dysplasia or adenocarcinoma. The presence of an overlying ulcer or erosion with active fibrin and neutrophilic exudate should caution against making a diagnosis of malignancy.

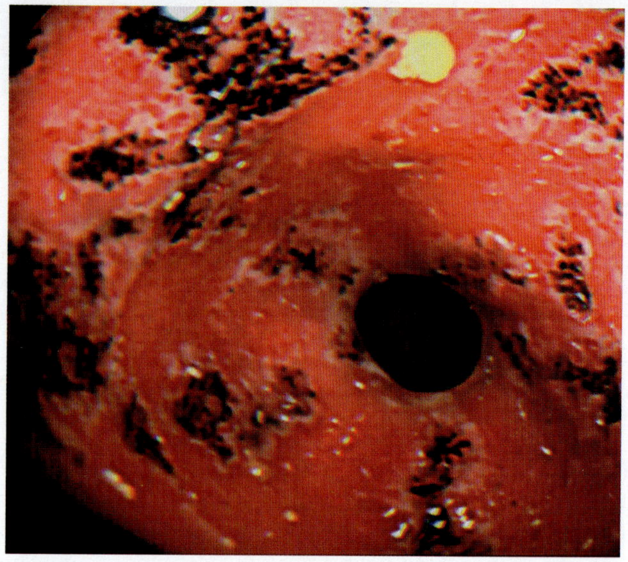

FIGURE 3.1

Endoscopic appearance of acute erosive gastritis with mucosal necrosis and hemorrhage.

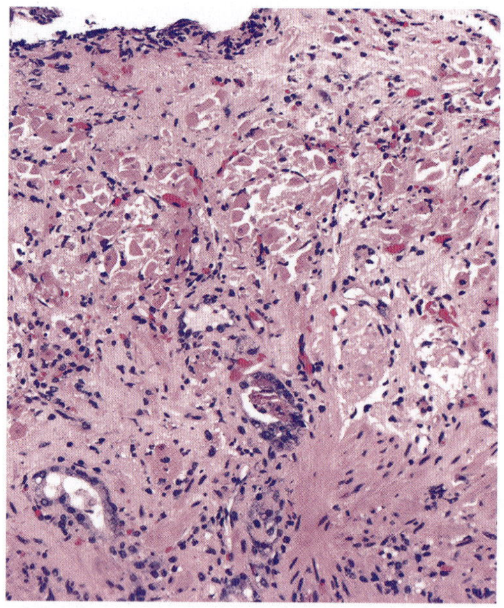

FIGURE 3.2

Acute erosive gastritis involving the gastric antrum with denuded surface mucosa covered by a band of fibrin and acute inflammatory cells. Necrotic debris is present within remnants of glandular epithelium toward the base

Differential Diagnosis

- Trauma related to nasogastric tubes presents as a very focal erosion and hemorrhage with unremarkable surrounding mucosa. The clinical scenario makes the diagnosis obvious, and these lesions are seldom biopsied.
- Severe chronic active *H. pylori* gastritis: Ulcers are associated with diffuse lymphoplasmacytic inflammation in lamina propria with variable neutrophilic

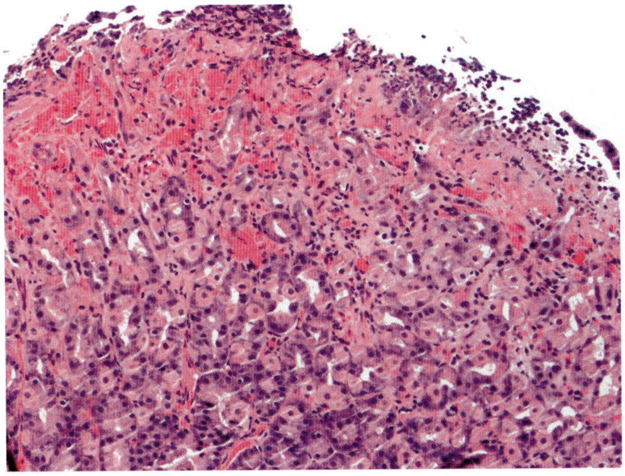

FIGURE 3.3

Erosive gastritis secondary to an alcoholic binge involving gastric corpus mucosa characterized by superficial necrosis with marked vascular congestion and fibrinopurulent exudate.

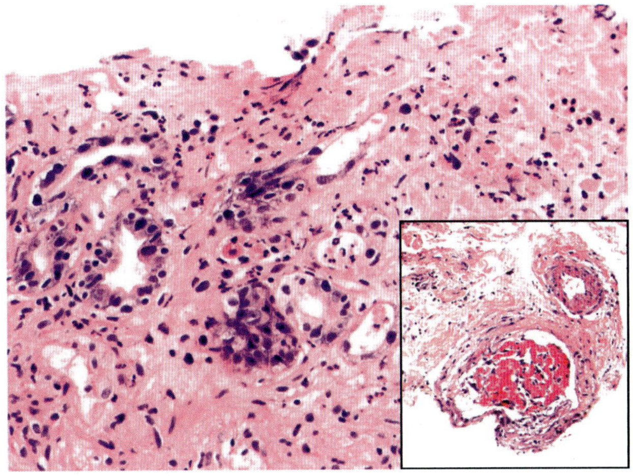

FIGURE 3.5

Erosive gastritis secondary to radiation injury may be associated with marked reactive glandular changes mimicking neoplasia and often shows vascular thrombi *(inset)*.

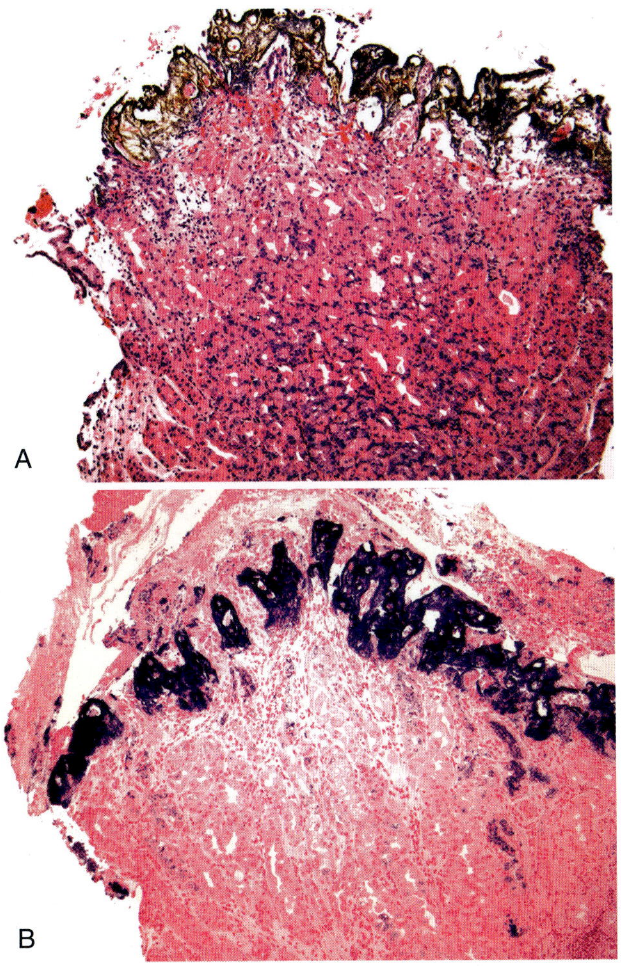

FIGURE 3.4

Brown-yellow refractile deposits (**A**) in erosive gastritis secondary to iron pills; special stain for iron (Prussian blue) is positive (**B**).

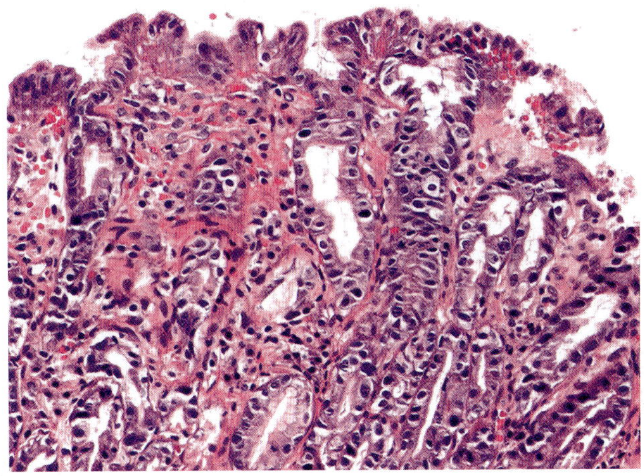

FIGURE 3.6

Healing erosive gastritis with marked regenerative epithelial changes with amphophilic cytoplasm and enlarged nuclei. There appears to be surface maturation.

infiltrate in gastric epithelium. Organisms are seen on hematoxylin and eosin (H&E) or ancillary stains.

- Dysplasia or malignancy: Regenerative epithelial change in a setting of erosion or ulcers can mimic neoplasia caused by hyperchromatic nuclei with prominent nucleoli, increased mitotic activity, and amphophilic cytoplasm. The changes are limited to epithelium adjacent to the erosion or ulcer, which cautions against a diagnosis of neoplasia.
- Chemical gastropathy: Usually associated with bile reflux, alcohol, and NSAIDs. This is histologically characterized by surface mucin depletion, foveolar hyperplasia, and smooth muscle hyperplasia in the lamina propria.

Prognosis and Therapy

Most patients make an uneventful recovery within a short time period. Depending on the hemodynamic state, management consists of supportive measures such as intravenous fluids and blood transfusion, stopping the offending agent, H_2 blockers, proton pump inhibitors (PPIs), and prostaglandin analogues. In cases of life-threatening bleeding, surgical intervention may be necessary.

REACTIVE (CHEMICAL) GASTROPATHY

Reactive gastropathy is the result of surface mucosal damage induced by bile, medications, or chemical agents. It is a histologic diagnosis characterized by surface mucin depletion, foveolar hyperplasia, regenerative epithelial changes, smooth muscle proliferation in the lamina propria, and vascular congestion of the gastric mucosa. The lamina propria does not typically show an increase in lymphoplasmacytic infiltrate. *Reactive gastropathy* is synonymous with *type C gastritis, chemical gastropathy*, and *alkaline or bile reflux gastritis*.

CLINICAL FEATURES

Reactive gastropathy is one of the most common diagnosis rendered in gastric biopsies. It is commonly asymptomatic; however, some patients report vague upper abdominal pain, nausea, and vomiting. The mean age at presentation is 66 years (range, 22–88 years), without any gender predilection. Common causes include chronic aspirin or other NSAID use and various medications (e.g., ferrous sulfate), bile reflux after gastroenterostomies, vagotomy, and pyloroplasty. In nonsurgical patients, bile reflux may be caused by an incompetent pyloric sphincter or gastric dysmotility. Other putative causes include alcohol intake and smoking.

REACTIVE (CHEMICAL) GASTROPATHY—FACT SHEET

Definition

- Surface mucosal damage characterized by mucin depletion, foveolar hyperplasia, regenerative epithelial changes, smooth muscle proliferation in the lamina propria, and vascular congestion in the absence of significant lymphoplasmacytic infiltration in the lamina propria

Morbidity and Mortality

- Often an incidental finding with no clinical implications; some cases may be associated with gastrointestinal (GI) bleeding caused by concurrent erosions or ulcers

Gender, Race, and Age

- Seen at any age but more prevalent in older adults; mean age, 66 years (range, 22–88 years)
- No gender predilection

Clinical Features

- Frequently asymptomatic; vague upper abdominal pain, nausea, vomiting, gastroduodenal ulcers, and GI bleeding can be reported
- Causes include long-term aspirin use, nonsteroidal antiinflammatory drug (NSAID) use, various iatrogenic injuries, and bile reflux after gastroenterostomies

Prognosis and Therapy

- Treatment involves proton pump inhibitors and discontinuing offending agents such as NSAIDs

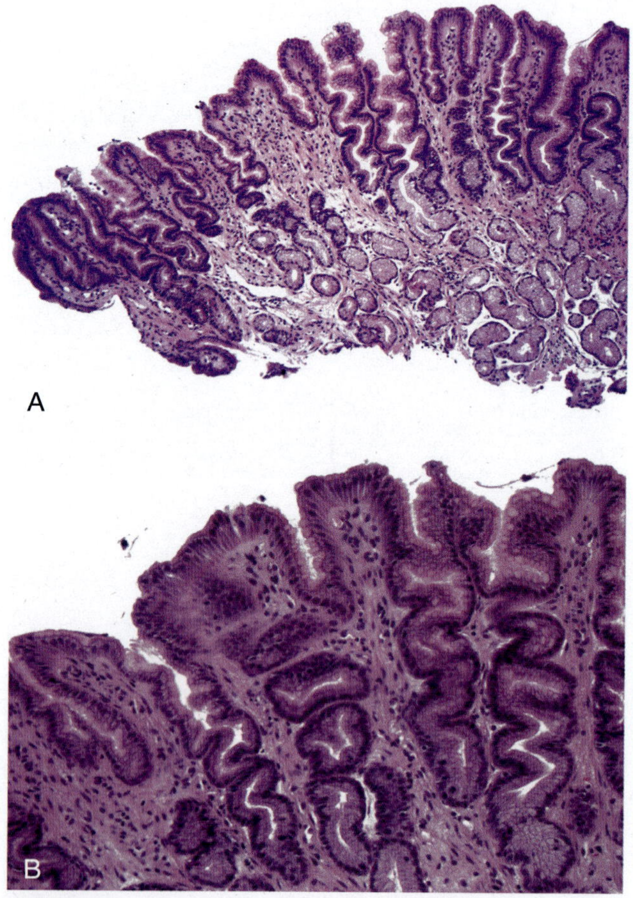

FIGURE 3.7

Reactive gastropathy involving antral mucosa and showing foveolar hyperplasia and corkscrew appearance of gastric pits (**A**). Note the mucin-depleted surface and lamina propria with smooth muscle proliferation and paucity of inflammatory cells (**B**).

PATHOLOGIC FEATURES

GROSS AND ENDOSCOPIC FINDINGS

The endoscopy may be normal or display nonspecific findings, including erythema and localized erosions. Visible gastric bile staining on endoscopic examination can be helpful in the diagnosis.

MICROSCOPIC FINDINGS

The mucosa shows marked surface mucin depletion accompanied by foveolar hyperplasia, which is characterized villiform change, elongation, and tortuosity of gastric pits with a corkscrew appearance (Fig. 3.7). The lamina propria shows smooth muscle proliferation and vascular congestion. There is typically a paucity of inflammatory cells in the lamina propria, hence the term *gastropathy* instead of *gastritis*. Focal erosions may be associated with small clusters of neutrophils and eosinophils but are restricted to the foci of injured mucosa, and diffuse lamina propria infiltrate is not seen. The changes are commonly limited to the antrum, whereas the oxyntic mucosa occasionally may occasionally show subtle reactive changes limited to the surface with separation of the surface foveolar epithelium from the glandular compartment. Reactive gastropathy may also be, at times, associated with intestinal metaplasia in cases with recurrent injury over a long period. Bile reflux gastropathy after Billroth I to II surgery with antrectomy is present in the body. Findings of histochemical or immunostains for *H. pylori* are negative.

REACTIVE (CHEMICAL) GASTROPATHY—PATHOLOGIC FEATURES

Endoscopic Findings

- Can be normal or show erythema, typically in the gastric antrum
- Visible bile reflux on endoscopic examination or erosions may also be seen

Microscopic Findings

- Changes are commonly in the antrum and prepyloric area
- Marked foveolar hyperplasia characterized by villiform change of the surface foveolae and elongation and corkscrew tortuosity of the gastric pits
- Surface mucin depletion leads to high nuclear-to-cytoplasmic ratio that may be mistaken for dysplasia
- Smooth muscle proliferation and vascular congestion in the lamina propria
- Paucity of inflammatory cells; focal erosions may be associated with neutrophils and eosinophils limited to the injured focus

Ancillary Studies

- Stains for *H. pylori* are negative

Differential Diagnosis

- Hyperplastic polyp
- Gastric antral vascular ectasia

DIFFERENTIAL DIAGNOSIS

The marked foveolar hyperplasia in chemical gastropathy may resemble hyperplastic polyps and the endoscopic appearance of a polyp or nodule is important in making this distinction. Changes similar to reactive gastropathy are also present in gastric antral vascular ectasia (GAVE), but the typical endoscopic appearance is that of a "watermelon stomach," and vascular ectasia with fibrin thrombi in lamina propria capillaries are helpful in establishing a diagnosis of GAVE.

PROGNOSIS AND THERAPY

Management involves discontinuing the offending agents, such as NSAIDs, and medical management with PPIs.

HELICOBACTER PYLORI GASTRITIS

H. pylori gastritis is a chronic infectious form of gastritis caused by spiral, flagellated gram-negative rods and characterized by a diffuse chronic active gastritis.

CLINICAL FEATURES

The prevalence of infection varies worldwide, and most people acquire infection during childhood. Transmission of infection is human to human, with poor sanitary conditions and overcrowding being risk factors. It is more prevalent in developing countries, where up to 75% of the population older than 25 years of age is infected. In developed countries, the overall prevalence is 25% to 30%, and the seroprevalence ranges from 5% to 27% in early childhood to 50% to 60% in adults older than 60 years of age. Currently, despite a decrease of infection worldwide, at least 50% of the world's population is actively infected. In the United States, African Americans, Asian Americans, and Hispanics have a higher prevalence (70%) than whites (35%).

H. pylori is a 3.5-µm-long, microaerophilic gram-negative rod with S-shaped or seagull wing appearance that appears comma or spiral shaped on routine or special stains. This organism has a tropism for gastric mucosa or gastric metaplasia in the duodenum. The pathogenesis depends on its ability to colonize gastric epithelium via adhesins such as BabA, SabA, urease and virulence factors such as Cag A, Vac A, and urease, which in turn generates cytokines such as interleukin-8 to attract neutrophils.

The majority of infected patients carry and transmit *H. pylori* without any symptoms or are mildly symptomatic. Other patients may develop moderate to severe symptoms of abdominal pain, nausea, vomiting, dyspepsia, weight

TABLE 3.1
***Helicobacter pylori* Tests**

INVASIVE TESTS		
Biopsy, special stains	Modified Giemsa, Diff-Quik, silver stains—Warthin-Starry, Genta stain.	Diff-Quik and modified Giemsa are preferred over silver stains (cost). Sensitivity is 84%–99%, and specificity is 90%–99%.
Immunostain for *Helicobacter pylori*	Especially useful in demonstrating variant forms of *H. pylori*, such as the coccoid forms (see Fig. 3.13D) that can occur in partially treated cases, patients taking antibiotics or PPIs, and resistant forms. PPI therapy can drive the organisms into the parietal cells when they become visible by immunostains.	Costly compared with special stains such as Diff-Quik; performed when the findings of special stains are questionable. Immunostain is also positive in *H. heilmannii* gastritis.
Biopsy-based rapid urease tests	Biopsy tissue is placed on urea medium, and positive test result is indicated by color change caused by an increase in pH as a result of urea breakdown into ammonia catalyzed by urease produced by all strains of *Helicobacter* organisms.	CLOtest, Hpfast, PyloriTek Sensitivity is 89%–98%, and specificity is up to 93%–98%. Sensitivity depends on organism load in the biopsy tissue and number of biopsy samples used. Less sensitive in pediatric population.
Culture	Incubation in nonselective mediums such as chocolate or blood agar for 5–7 days.	Sensitivity is 77%–92%, and specificity is 100%. Not used routinely but may gain importance in the future owing to the emergence of resistant strains.
Molecular tests	PCR-based detection of *H. pylori* using various genetic targets such as 23 S ribosome, vac A, ure A, and cag A gene.	Rarely used in clinical practice.
NONINVASIVE TESTS		
Serology	Detect IgG antibodies in serum or even whole blood to *H. pylori* antigens using ELISA.	Screening test used to detect current or past infection. Performance varies with the different commercial kits with an overall sensitivity and specificity of 88%92% and 86%–95%, respectively. Reduced sensitivity in HIV-infected individuals. Patients with *H. heilmannii* may have a negative test result to anti–*H. pylori* IgG assays. Serologic results can stay positive for a very long time, making them less useful for follow-up. Follow-up serology to test for eradication should be done only after 1 year.
Urea breath test (UBT)	Patient is given radioactively labeled urea to drink. The urease produced by *Helicobacter* organisms breaks down urea, and the labeled CO_2 is detected in the exhaled breath.	Sensitivity is 90%–100%, and specificity is 98%–100%. UBT is used as a follow-up for patients who continue to be symptomatic.
Stool antigen test	*H. pylori* antigen is detected from fecal sample by enzyme immunoassay.	Sensitivity is 89%, and specificity is 94%. Like UBT, this test can also be used to confirm eradication.

ELISA, Enzyme-linked immunosorbent assay; *IgG*, immunoglobulin G; *PCR*, polymerase chain reaction; *PPI*, proton pump inhibitor.

loss, and iron-deficiency anemia. The recognition of the *Helicobacter* organism and its association with peptic ulcer disease, gastric mucosa–associated lymphoid tissue (MALT) lymphoma, and carcinoma has revolutionized modern understanding of disease processes and influenced patient management. The World Health Organization has classified *H. pylori* as a group I human carcinogen of gastric cancer. Infected persons have a three- to sixfold greater risk of developing gastric cancer over that of uninfected persons. Australian researchers Robin Warren, a pathologist, and Barry Marshall, a gastroenterologist, became the recipients of the Nobel Prize in 2005 for this significant discovery. Noninvasive and invasive tissue-based, serologic, and stool tests for diagnosis of *H. pylori* infection have been developed and are summarized in Table 3.1.

Pathologic Features

Gross Findings

Endoscopic findings are variable and include mucosal erythema, erosions, granularity, and nodularity. Gastric and duodenal ulcers may be present in severe cases. Mucosal nodularity may be prominent in cases associated with marked lymphoid hyperplasia or MALT lymphoma. In rare instances, the mucosa may appear completely normal. For optimal evaluation, at least two mucosal biopsy specimens, one each from the antrum and body, are recommended. Sampling of a single site may reduce the test sensitivity. The Sydney system and the Operative Link for Gastritis Assessment (OLGA) staging

HELICOBACTER PYLORI GASTRITIS—FACT SHEET

Definition

- Chronic infectious form of gastritis caused by curved, flagellated gram-negative rods—*Helicobacter pylori*—and characterized by a chronic active gastritis of variable severity

Incidence and Location

- Variable prevalence across the globe
- In developing countries, up to 75% of the population older than 25 years is infected, with the prevalence reaching 80% to 90%
- In developed countries, the overall prevalence is 25%–30%; the seroprevalence ranges from 5% to 27% in early childhood and exceeds 50% in adults older than 60 years of age
- In the United States, African Americans and Hispanics have a higher prevalence than whites

Morbidity and Mortality

- Epidemiologic association with peptic ulcer disease, gastric lymphoma, and carcinoma
- Group I human carcinogen (World Health Organization)

Clinical Features

- Abdominal pain, nausea, vomiting, dyspepsia, weight loss, iron-deficiency anemia, and possibly ulcer-related bleeding in symptomatic patients

Prognosis and Therapy

- Triple therapy for 14 days consisting of either bismuth or proton pump inhibitors combined with two antibiotics such as metronidazole, clarithromycin, tetracycline, or amoxicillin
- Cure rate is greater than 95%
- Short treatment courses of 1 to 5 days may be effective with a slightly lower eradication rate

system have been proposed for systematic reporting of gastritis but are seldom followed in the West.

Microscopic Findings

H. pylori typically presents as a chronic active gastritis of variable severity. The infection can be antrum predominant or a pangastritis at initial presentation. Posttreatment cases may show persistence of infection in the gastric corpus or cardia with resolution of inflammation and lack of organisms in the distal stomach.

In involved regions, the superficial lamina propria shows a diffuse bandlike mononuclear infiltrate of lymphocytes and plasma cells along with activated lymphoid follicles with germinal centers (Fig. 3.8). The term *follicular gastritis* has been used in the past for cases with prominent lymphoid aggregates (Fig. 3.9). Various degrees of neutrophilic infiltrate, reported as evidence of activity, may be seen in the surface epithelium and gastric pits and crypt abscesses (Fig. 3.10). A pattern of lymphocytic gastritis can also be seen with

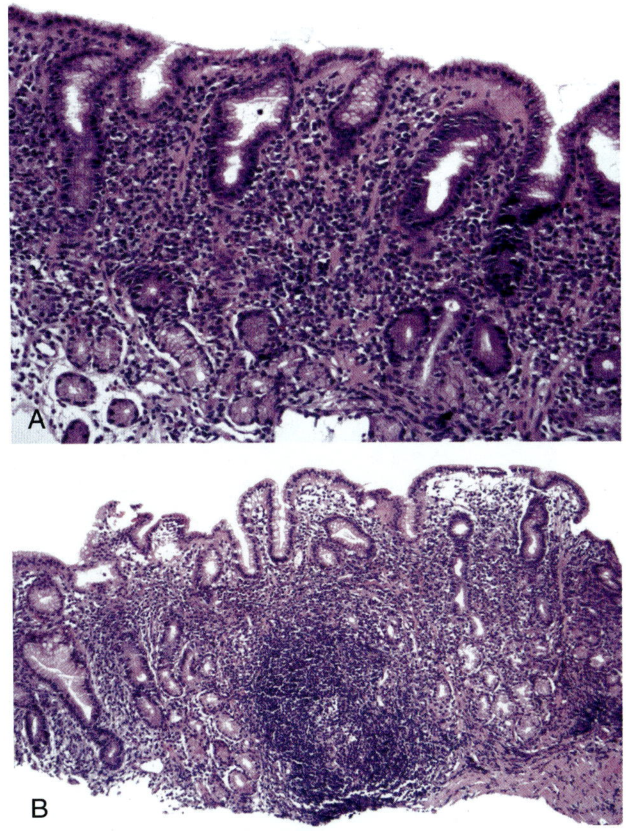

FIGURE 3.8

Chronic gastritis secondary to *Helicobacter pylori* is associated with a diffuse bandlike infiltrate of lymphocytes and plasma cells separating the surface epithelium from the glandular compartment (**A**). Lymphoid follicles with active germinal centers are often present (**B**).

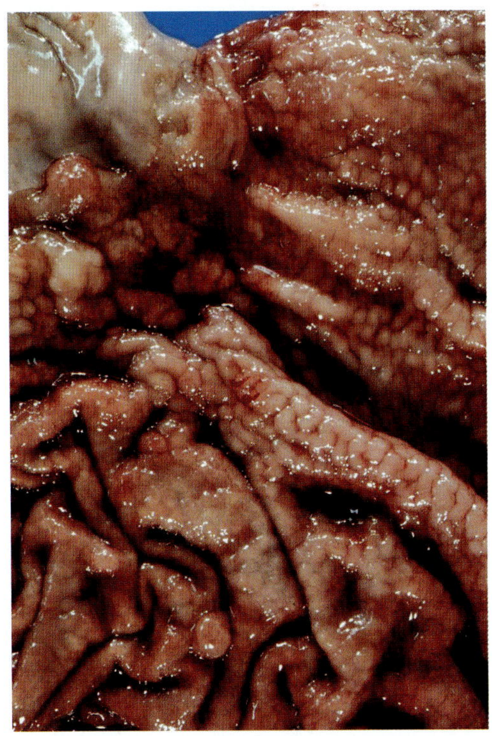

FIGURE 3.9

Gastric mucosal nodularity simulating lymphoma or carcinoma. Such a nodularity as this is often present in *Helicobacter* gastritis, caused by the florid lymphoid hyperplasia. (Courtesy of Shriram Jakate, MD, Rush Medical College, Chicago).

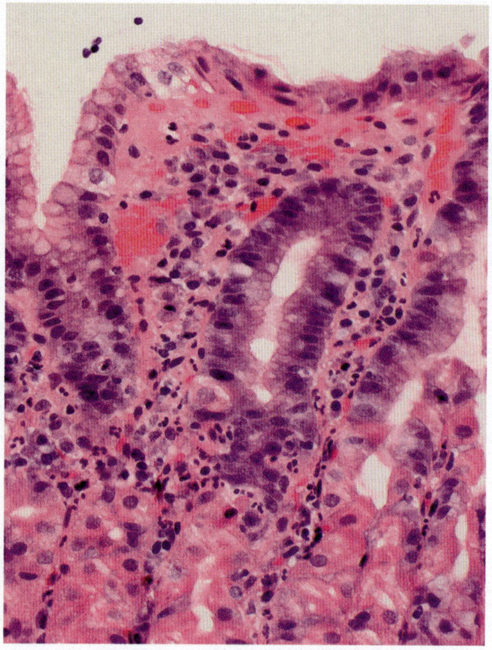

FIGURE 3.10

High-power view of *Helicobacter pylori* gastritis showing active neutrophilic inflammation infiltrating gastric pit and glandular epithelium.

H. pylori infection. Severe cases with ulcers may show regenerative foveolar hyperplasia, and intestinal metaplasia is already present in a subset of patients at first diagnosis.

The organisms appear as slightly curved seagull wing–shaped rods, clustered in the gastric mucus, adherent to the gastric surface foveolar epithelium, or deep in the gastric pits. When abundant, the organisms are easily visible on H&E, but special stains (e.g., Giemsa, silver stains) and immunohistochemistry can aid in their detection (Fig. 3.11) when the density is low or posttreatment change has transformed the typical spiral shape of the organisms into a more coccoid appearance. Table 3.2 highlights other manifestations that may be attributed to *H. pylori* infection. A pattern of chronic inactive gastritis with residual mononuclear cell infiltration in the lamina propria but without any foci of neutrophilic infiltration may be seen in biopsies obtained soon after treatment with antibiotics (Fig. 3.12). The pattern is not etiologically specific, and organisms are usually absent in posttreatment biopsies. The only way to establish the diagnosis is by correlating findings with patient history.

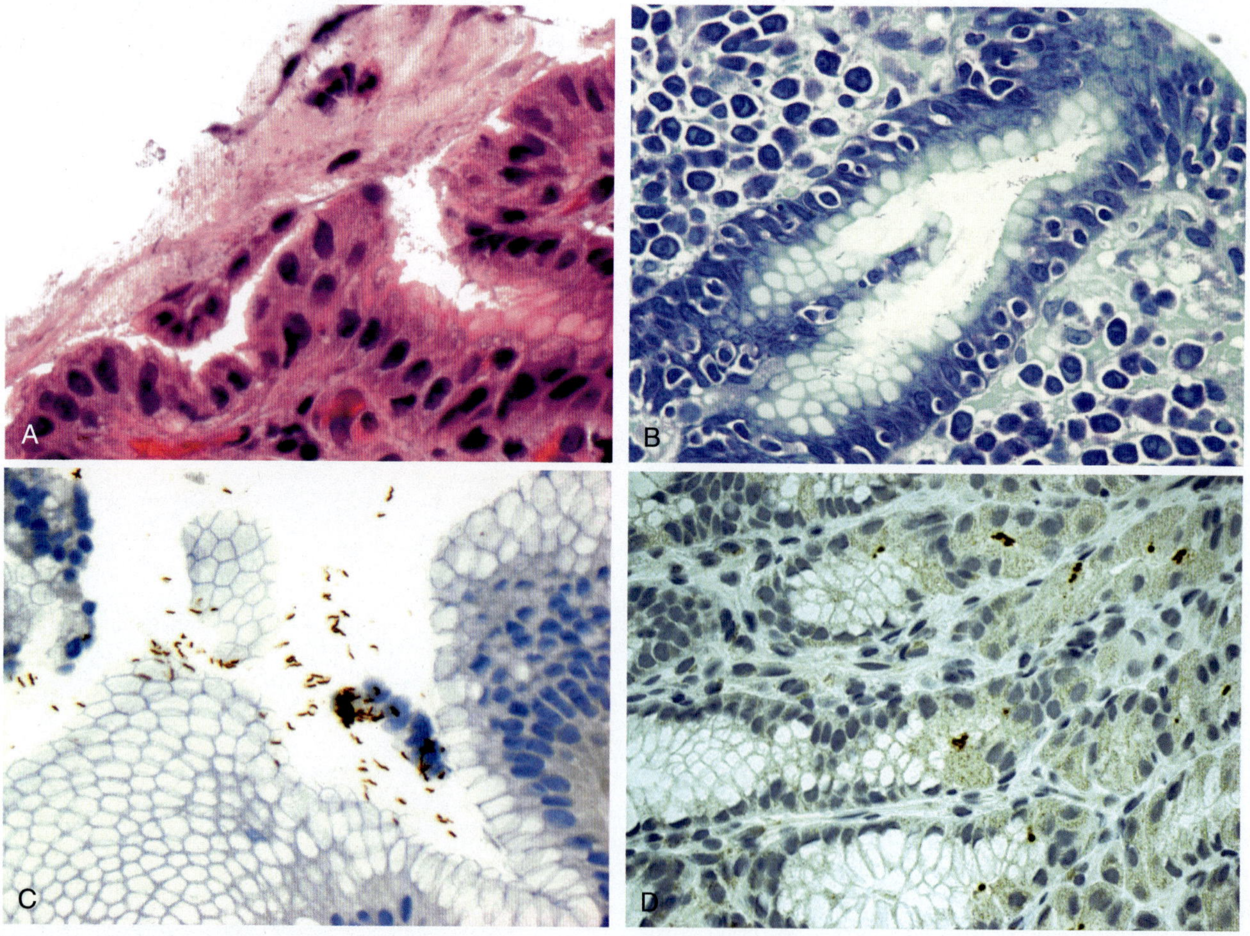

FIGURE 3.11

A, *Helicobacter pylori* organisms seen on hematoxylin and eosin stain, admixed in surface mucin. Notice the curved shapes. **B**, *Helicobacter* gastritis. Diff-Quik stain highlights the slightly curved seagull wing–shaped *H. pylori* organisms in the gastric pits lining the foveolar epithelium. **C**, Immunostain for *H. pylori* shows the organisms lining the gastric foveolae. **D**, Coccoid, deep, intracellular location of *H. pylori* is common after treatment and best visualized on immunostains.

TABLE 3.2
Histologic Manifestations Indicative of Present or Past *Helicobacter pylori* Infection

Acute *Helicobacter* gastritis	Acute manifestation at the time of initial acquisition of the infection. It almost never comes to medical attention and therefore is not biopsied. Best evidence came from Dr. Marshall himself, who drank from a Petri dish containing the organisms from the culture of a patient with *H. pylori* infection and had acute gastritis with nausea, vomiting, and halitosis.
Chronic active gastritis	Neutrophilic inflammation within the epithelium, most prominent in gastric pits accompanied by diffuse lymphoplasmacytic infiltrate in the lamina propria.
Chronic inactive gastritis	Characterized by clusters of plasma cells in the lamina propria (see Fig. 3.14); lacks active inflammation and may reflect past *Helicobacter* infection.
Lymphocytic gastritis	Lymphocytic gastritis contains prominent intraepithelial lymphocytosis.
Hyperplastic polyp	May be a marker of *H. pylori* infection in the nonpolypoid gastric mucosa in a subset of cases.
Environmental atrophic metaplastic gastritis (EMAG), multifocal atrophic gastritis, or type B gastritis	*H. pylori* is an important cause of EMAG, a precursor to gastric dysplasia and carcinoma. Characterized by gradual loss of normal glands and multifocal intestinal metaplasia, predominantly in the gastric antrum but may also present in the body and cardia. Unlike autoimmune gastritis, the gastrin level in EMAG is either low or normal. The antrum is normal in autoimmune gastritis, which is not the case in EMAG.

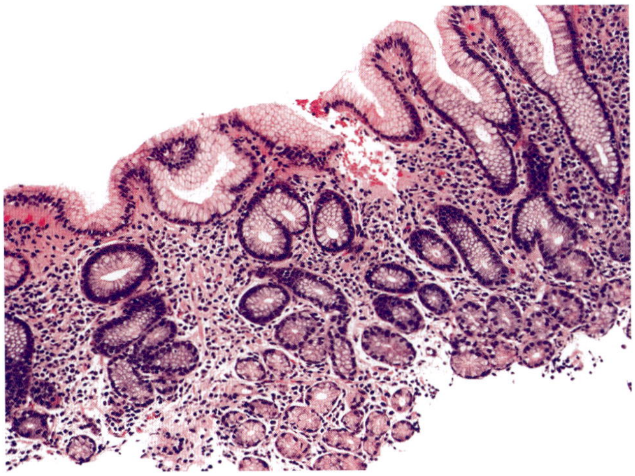

FIGURE 3.12
Chronic inactive gastritis in a patient recently treated for *Helicobacter pylori* infection. Note the lamina propria with plasma cells but without active inflammation.

Helicobacter Pylori Gastritis—Pathologic Features

Gross Findings
- Gastric mucosal erythema, erosions, granularity, and nodularity

Microscopic Findings
- For optimal evaluation, two mucosal biopsies from both the antrum and body are recommended
- Chronic active gastritis with marked lymphoplasmacytic inflammation and variable neutrophilic infiltration and prominent lymphoid aggregates
- The inflammation is predominantly in the superficial mucosa
- Active (or neutrophilic) inflammation, a marker for the presence of *Helicobacter* organisms, is prominent in the gastric pits, causing pititis
- Foveolar hyperplasia, erosion, hemorrhage, reactive epithelial changes, and in severe cases, mucosal erosion and ulceration
- Mucosal atrophy and intestinal metaplasia may be present
- *Helicobacter pylori* appear as slightly curved seagull wing–shaped rods, most prominent in the gastric mucus and the lining surface foveolar epithelium and also in gastric pits
- The organisms can be visible on hematoxylin and eosin stain, especially when numerous, but ancillary stains can be used in selected situations discussed next

Ancillary Studies
- Histochemical stains: modified Giemsa, Diff-Quik, Warthin-Starry, Genta stain, and Alcian yellow have all been used in the past
- Immunohistochemistry for *Helicobacter* is often used in current practice when:
  - Organisms are not seen on *hematoxylin and eosin* despite the presence of a chronic gastritis reminiscent of *H. pylori* infection
  - In posttreatment biopsies when the density of organisms is low and they have transformed into a coccoid appearance

Differential Diagnosis
- *Helicobacter heilmannii* gastritis
- Gastric marginal zone B-cell lymphoma
- Focally enhanced gastritis
- Autoimmune gastritis
- Non–*H. pylori* infectious gastritis

Differential Diagnosis

Helicobacter heilmannii gastritis *(Gastrospirillum hominis)* is responsible for approximately 0.3% of the cases of *Helicobacter* gastritis. It is caused by a tight spiral bacterium that is 5 to 6 μm in length, which is longer than *H. pylori* (Fig. 3.13A and 3.13B). It is also seen in cats and dogs, and the disease in humans may be a zoonotic infection. They can be seen on H&E examination easily because of their large size and are present in the gastric mucus and lumen of gastric pits without coming in close contact with the epithelium. Immunostain for *H. pylori* also stains *H. heilmannii* (Fig. 3.13C). *H. heilmannii* infection has been associated with the development of marginal zone B-cell lymphoma but not with gastric cancer.

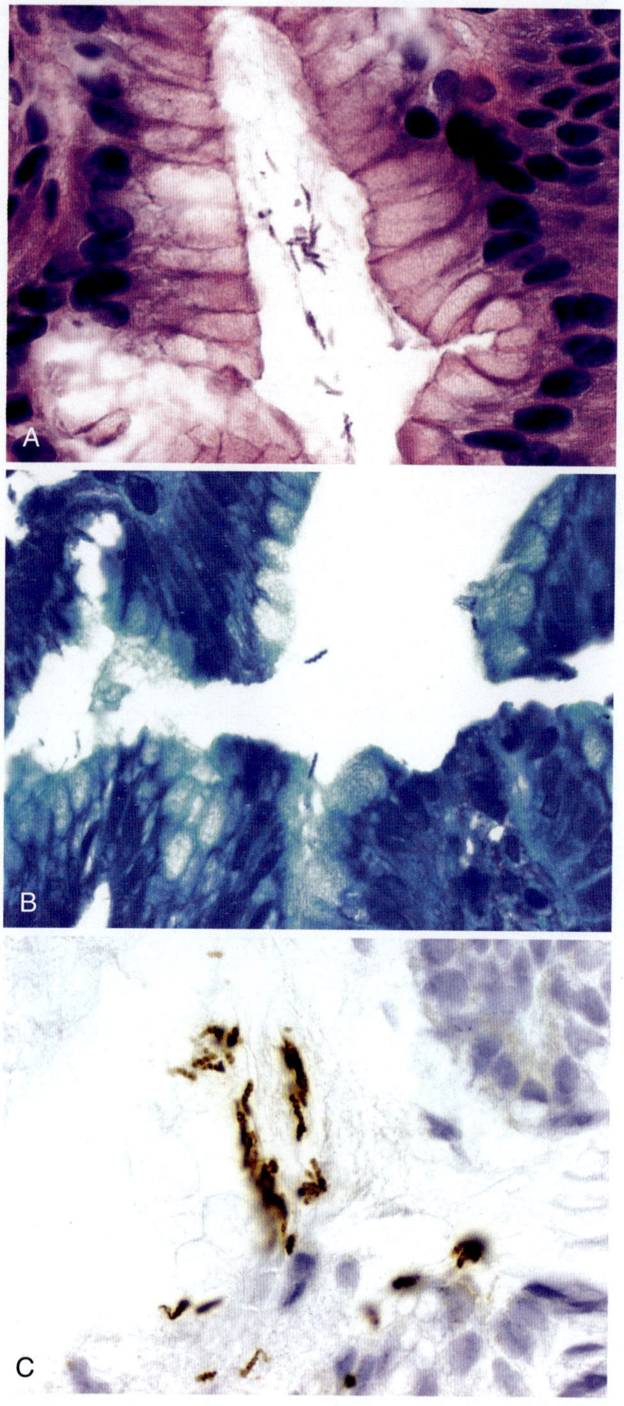

FIGURE 3.13

A, Unlike *Helicobacter pylori, Helicobacter heilmannii* organisms are longer, tightly spiraled, present in the lumen, and less tightly adherent to surface foveolar cells (hematoxylin and eosin). **B**, *H. heilmannii* in (GMS). **C**, The antibody for *H. pylori* cross reacts with *H. heilmannii and can be useful in cases with low density of the organisms.*

The florid lymphoid hyperplasia in *Helicobacter* gastritis can be mistaken for low-grade extranodal marginal zone B-cell lymphoma. However, marginal zone B-cell lymphoma is characterized by aggregates or sheets of monomorphic B cells with destructive lymphoepithelial lesions. The neoplastic lymphoid cells in marginal zone B-cell lymphoma may show aberrant coexpression of CD20 and CD43 and light chain restriction. The intraepithelial lymphocytes in *Helicobacter* gastritis are mostly CD3-positive T lymphocytes, unlike the CD20-positive neoplastic B-cells in gastric marginal zone B-cell lymphoma. A clonal population of lymphoid cells may be seen in *Helicobacter* gastritis, and a diagnosis of lymphoma should not be based on molecular studies alone (see details in Chapter 19).

Focally enhanced gastritis is typically associated with Crohn's disease, medication-induced mucosal injury, and the resolving phase of gastric erosions. The biopsy shows a localized increase in lymphoplasmacytic inflammation with neutrophilic infiltration into the epithelium and a cuff of loose histiocytic aggregates around damaged gastric pits.

Autoimmune gastritis typically involves the oxyntic mucosa and shows atrophy with marked reduction in oxyntic glands, pyloric gland and intestinal metaplasia, and enterochromaffin-like (ECL) hyperplasia. The latter feature shows a spectrum of linear to micronodular to adenomatoid hyperplasia culminating in well-differentiated neuroendocrine tumors. The presence of micronodular hyperplasia is helpful in differentiating autoimmune gastritis from *H. pylori* gastritis. Antibodies to intrinsic factor and parietal cells are diagnostic and lead to hypochlorhydria, vitamin B_{12} deficiency, and hypergastrinemia. Hypergastrinemia can also occur in *H. pylori* gastritis but not to the extent seen in autoimmune gastritis.

A variety of other bacterial, viral, fungal, and parasitic infections may rarely involve the stomach and must be excluded when the mucosa is inflamed and *Helicobacter* organisms are not identified.

PROGNOSIS AND THERAPY

In most untreated cases, the gastritis progresses to glandular atrophy (loss of specialized glandular epithelium) and intestinal metaplasia. Patients with gastric atrophy have up to a 16-fold increased risk of developing gastric neoplasia. The OLGA system arranges histologic phenotypes of gastritis along a scale of progressively increasing gastric cancer risk by scoring the extent and location of atrophy. However, this system is not typically used in daily practice. These patients are also at risk for the development of MALT extranodal marginal zone B-cell lymphoma. Antral restricted and pangastritis both increase the risk of gastric cancer, whereas antral dominant gastritis also increases risk of duodenal ulcers.

Triple therapy for 14 days consisting of either bismuth or a PPI combined with two antibiotics has been the most popular regimen, achieving up to a 95% cure rate. The recommended antibiotics are metronidazole, clarithromycin, and tetracycline or amoxicillin.

However, recent studies have shown that short treatment courses of 1 to 5 days may be equally effective with an eradication rate of 89% to 95% with better compliance, reduced cost, and fewer adverse effects.

GASTRIC PEPTIC ULCER DISEASE

Peptic ulcer disease is a clinical term used for patients with discrete ulcers in the stomach or duodenum, most often in association with *H. pylori* gastritis or NSAID use.

CLINICAL FEATURES

The incidence of gastric peptic ulcer disease has been decreasing since the 1980s. Common locations are stomach and proximal duodenum, with a mean age of 40 years and 20 years, respectively. Symptoms include severe epigastric pain exacerbated by food intake, in contrast to duodenal ulcer pain, which is relieved by food intake. In addition, vomiting, weight loss, hematemesis, melena, and gastric outlet obstruction can be caused by scarring and pyloric stenosis. Peritonitis can develop after perforation. NSAID ulcers are on the rise as the prevalence of *H. pylori* infection is declining. Certain medications, such as steroids, can also contribute to ulcer development. Other rare causes of peptic ulcers include ZES and multiple endocrine neoplasia type I (MEN-I).

PATHOLOGIC FEATURES

GROSS FINDINGS

Gastric ulcers are variably sized and usually present in the lesser curvature, round to oval in shape with a smooth base and regular, perpendicular edges (Fig. 3.14), unlike the irregular heaped-up borders of malignant ulcers.

MICROSCOPIC FINDINGS

Histologically, mucosal defects are seen extending below the muscularis mucosae with extension into the submucosa and muscularis propria in severe cases. Early ulcers are associated with fibrin, necrosis, inflammation, and granulation tissue reaction. Chronic ulcers are associated with scarring and stenosis (Fig. 3.15).

DIFFERENTIAL DIAGNOSIS

The histologic changes seen in gastric peptic ulcer disease are nonspecific. The possibility of an associated malignancy should be ruled out.

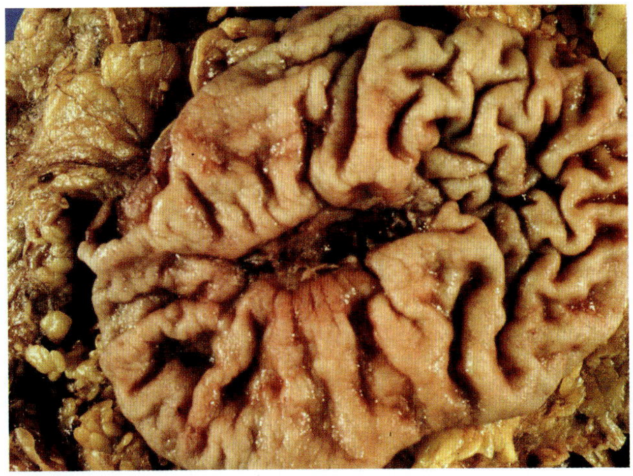

FIGURE 3.14
Benign gastric ulcer with a smooth base and regular borders.

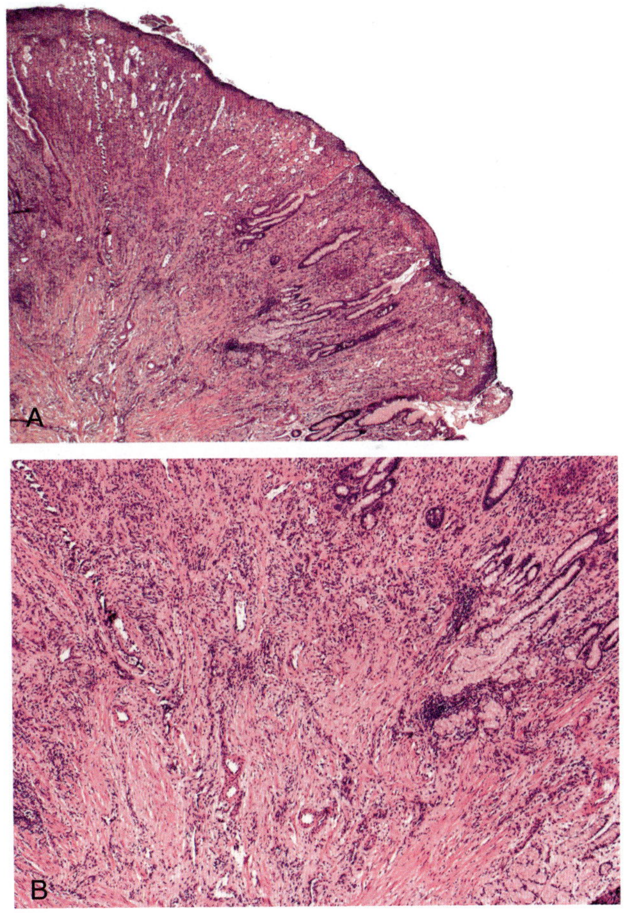

FIGURE 3.15
Gastric ulcers can be with extension below the muscularis mucosae (**A**). Chronic ulcers are characterized by fibrosis and stricture (**B**).

PROGNOSIS AND THERAPY

Eradication of *H. pylori* infection is the key to successful healing and reduces the risk of recurrence or rebleeding. Acid suppressors, especially PPIs, are used in addition to stopping intake of NSAIDs and prostaglandin analogues such as misoprostol. Discontinuing smoking and alcohol use may be helpful. Endoscopic treatment modalities such as epinephrine injection, coagulation, or clipping of bleeding sites, or in cases of perforation or severe hemorrhage, surgical management can be used in selected cases.

AUTOIMMUNE GASTRITIS

Autoimmune gastritis is an immune-mediated destruction of the oxyntic glands caused by antiparietal cell antibodies. Patients also have antibodies to intrinsic factor, and loss of oxyntic glands leads to hypochlorhydria, vitamin B_{12} deficiency, and endocrine ECL cell hyperplasia. *Type A gastritis, diffuse corporal atrophic gastritis*, and *autoimmune metaplastic atrophic gastritis* are all terms used for autoimmune gastritis in the past.

CLINICAL FEATURES

Autoimmune gastritis affects nearly 2% of the population older than 60 years old and is responsible for approximately 4% of cases of chronic gastritis. It was classically described in individuals of northern European or Scandinavian descent but is now known to be equally represented in African Americans and Latin Americans. White women in the fifth to sixth decade of life are affected three times more commonly than men. Patients may be asymptomatic or present with abdominal pain, weight loss, diarrhea, malabsorption, and neurologic complications, such as peripheral neuropathy and subacute combined degeneration of the spinal cord, related to severe vitamin B_{12} deficiency. The antiparietal cell antibodies that target H^+/K^+-ATPase proton pump are present in 60% to 85%, and anti-intrinsic factor antibodies are identified in 30% to 50% of patients (Table 3.3). Reduced gastric acid plays a role in iron deficiency in 20% to 40% of cases because gastric acid is necessary to release iron bound to proteins and to reduce ferric iron to ferrous state for absorption. Pernicious anemia is present in 15% to 25% of patients and is characterized by macrocytosis, megaloblastic anemia, pancytopenia, atrophic glossitis, low serum B_{12} concentration, and normal folate level. This is a late manifestation of autoimmune gastritis, taking 20 to 30 years to develop, and is caused by progressive loss of parietal cells, which are necessary for intrinsic factor production. Concomitant autoimmune disorders such as insulin-dependent diabetes mellitus, Hashimoto's thyroiditis, adrenal insufficiency, Graves' disease, vitiligo, or myasthenia gravis can also be seen in patients with autoimmune gastritis.

TABLE 3.3

Pertinent Laboratory Findings in Autoimmune Gastritis

Antiparietal cell antibodies	Positive (target H^+/K^+ATPase): 60%–85%
Intrinsic factor antibodies	Positive: 30%–50%
Serum gastrin	Elevated
Gastric pH	Alkaline or neutral
Vitamin B_{12} level	Reduced
Serum pepsinogen I	Reduced (loss of chief cells)
Schilling test	Positive and corrected by vitamin B_{12} injection
Helicobacter pylori serology	Usually negative
HLA haplotypes	HLA-B8, DR-3

AUTOIMMUNE GASTRITIS –FACT SHEET

Definition

- Immune-mediated chronic gastritis and loss of oxyntic glands caused by antiparietal cell and anti-intrinsic factor antibodies leading to hypochlorhydria, achlorhydria, and vitamin B_{12} deficiency

Incidence and Location

- Affects nearly 2% of people older than 60 years
- No racial predilection

Gender, Race, and Age

- Patients are usually older white women in the fifth or sixth decades of life
- Male-to-female ratio of 1 to 3

Clinical Features

- Frequently asymptomatic, but abdominal pain and discomfort, weight loss, pernicious anemia, and rarely subacute combined degeneration of spinal cord are reported
- Patients may have other immune-related disorders such as insulin-mediated diabetes mellitus, Hashimoto's thyroiditis, or adrenal insufficiency
- Serum analysis positive for antiparietal cell antibodies (~80% of patients) and anti-intrinsic factor antibodies (~30% of patients)
- Elevated serum gastrin
- Reduced B_{12}; positive Schilling test result corrected by administering intrinsic factor but is seldom performed nowadays
- *Helicobacter* serology is usually negative

Prognosis and Therapy

- 2% to 9% prevalence of gastric well-differentiated neuroendocrine tumors and a two- to threefold increase in gastric carcinomas
- Medical management includes vitamin B_{12} injections
- Management for multiple well-differentiated neuroendocrine tumors includes endoscopic polypectomies or mucosal resection, antrectomy, or rarely total gastrectomy

PATHOLOGIC FEATURES

GROSS FINDINGS

Autoimmune gastritis affects the oxyntic mucosa and spares the antrum in the vast majority of cases. On endoscopic examination, the body or fundic mucosa appears flat and congested with a prominent submucosal vascular pattern caused by mucosal atrophy. Multiple small mucosal elevations or pseudopolyps, representing preserved islands of oxyntic mucosa surrounded by flattened atrophic mucosa, may be seen. Other polypoid lesions in autoimmune gastritis include hyperplastic polyps (most common), pyloric adenomas, well-differentiated neuroendocrine tumors, and dysplastic lesions or adenocarcinoma.

Microscopic Findings

The histologic findings are limited to the oxyntic mucosa lining the gastric corpus. The antrum is normal in the vast majority of cases. The corpus mucosa shows a chronic gastritis with prominent lymphocytic and plasma cell infiltration that is more prominent in the deep aspect of lamina propria. There is a variable loss of oxyntic glands depending on stage of the disease and manifests as atrophy, pyloric gland metaplasia, and intestinal metaplasia with goblet and Paneth cells (Fig. 3.16A). Pancreatic acinar metaplasia may also be present.

The gastric atrophy leads to hypergastrinemia, which acts as a trophic signal to the ECL cells in the gastric corpus. This results in a unique hyperplasia to neoplasia continuum culminating in the development of well-differentiated neuroendocrine tumors. Linear, micronodular, adenomatoid hyperplasia and dysplastic nodular lesions have been described, but this subclassification is seldom used in daily practice other than using the presence of neuroendocrine cell hyperplasia to render a diagnosis of autoimmune gastritis. Expansile nodules greater than 0.5 mm or lesions infiltrative into the muscularis mucosa or submucosa are designated as well-differentiated neuroendocrine tumor.

An atrophic corpus in the late stages of the disease can resemble the antrum and the diagnosis can be easily missed when antrum and corpus biopsies are submitted in the same container, a common practice in many parts of the world. Immunostains for gastrin and chromogranin can aid in establishing the diagnosis. Therefore, the presence of a patchy chronic gastritis or intestinal metaplasia restricted to corpus biopsies in the setting of a negative *H. pylori* immunostain should always lead to work-up for autoimmune gastritis in gastric biopsies.

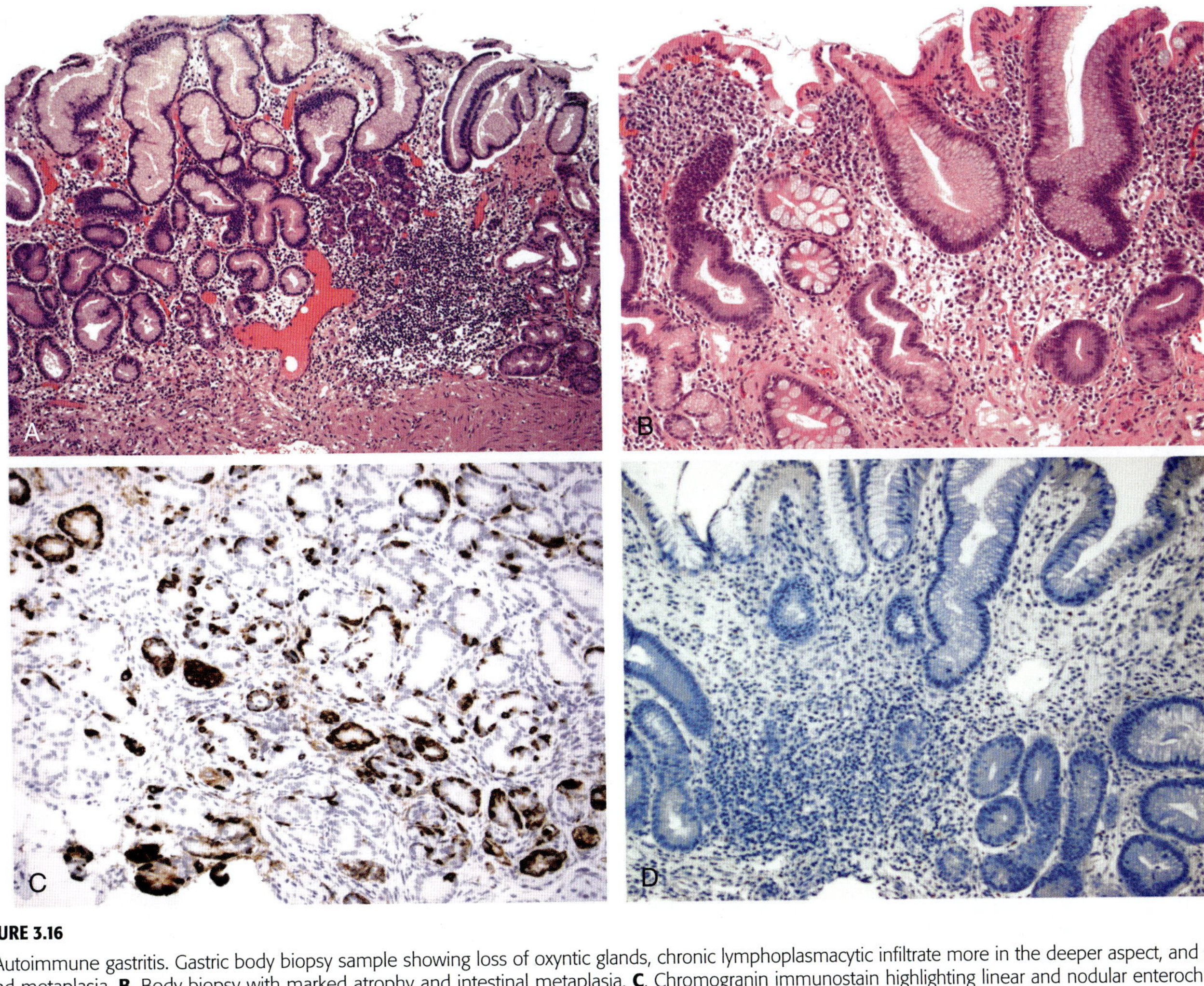

FIGURE 3.16

A, Autoimmune gastritis. Gastric body biopsy sample showing loss of oxyntic glands, chronic lymphoplasmacytic infiltrate more in the deeper aspect, and pyloric gland metaplasia. **B**, Body biopsy with marked atrophy and intestinal metaplasia. **C**, Chromogranin immunostain highlighting linear and nodular enterochromaffin-like cell hyperplasia in the body mucosa. **D**, Gastrin immunostain in the body is negative. Based on this, some observers refer to the presence of metaplastic antral type glands as *pseudopyloric metaplasia* because the glands do not produce gastrin.

The antral mucosa may show only limited changes including foveolar hyperplasia or mild chronic inflammation. Furthermore, the low-acid state created by the loss of parietal cells stimulates antral gastrin cell hyperplasia presenting as increased density of gastrin-positive G cells in the gastric pits. Extremely rare cases of an autoimmune pangastritis with antral involvement have also been reported.

Other associated findings in autoimmune gastritis include gastric hyperplastic polyps, pyloric gland adenomas, well-differentiated neuroendocrine tumors of variable size, and gastric dysplasia and adenocarcinoma.

Autoimmune Gastritis—Pathologic Features

Gross Findings

- Involves the gastric body and fundus and spares the antrum
- Effacement of rugal folds and prominent submucosal vascular pattern in gastric corpus caused by glandular atrophy

Microscopic Findings

- Chronic gastritis with prominent lamina propria lymphocytic and plasma cell infiltration, often prominent within the deep lamina propria
- Loss of specialized glandular epithelium (atrophy) in the gastric corpus
- Pyloric gland metaplasia, intestinal metaplasia, and linear or micronodular enterochromaffin-like (ECL) hyperplasia is characteristic

Immunohistochemical Features

- Gastrin and chromogranin A can be used to demonstrate ECL-cell hyperplasia when antrum and corpus biopsies are submitted together in the same container

Differential Diagnosis

- *Helicobacter pylori* gastritis
- Lymphocytic and collagenous gastritis
- Infectious gastritis, other than H. pylori
- Pernicious anemia associated with autoimmune polyglandular syndrome

Immunohistochemistry

Gastrin and chromogranin immunohistochemical stains are helpful, especially when the gastroenterologist places multiple biopsies in the same container or if the specimen site is unspecified (Fig. 3.16B–D). The neuroendocrine ECL cell hyperplasia stains positive with chromogranin but is negative for gastrin, confirming the corpus-restricted nature of the disease. The gastrin immunostain highlights normal G cells in the gastric antral fragments (Fig. 3.17). *H. pylori* immunostain is usually negative.

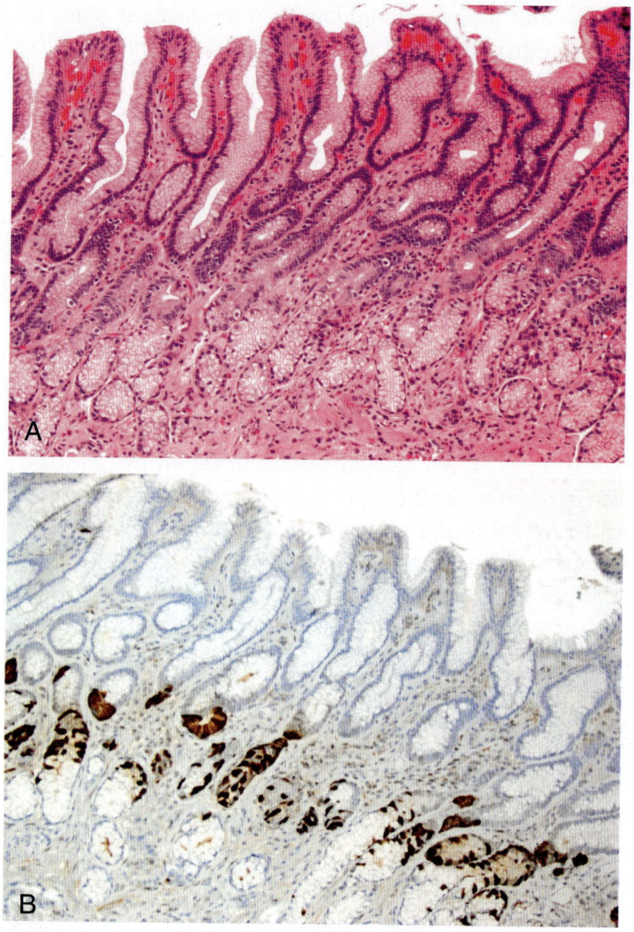

FIGURE 3.17

A, Antral biopsy specimen from an autoimmune gastritis case showing mild reactive gastropathy and lack of chronic gastritis and metaplasia. **B**, Gastrin immunostain of the antrum highlights G cells.

Differential Diagnosis

Chronic H. pylori gastritis, when associated with gastric atrophy, can mimic autoimmune gastritis (Table 3.4). Involvement of the antrum, demonstration of *H. pylori* on H&E or ancillary stains, and the lack of ECL cell hyperplasia and antiparietal and anti-intrinsic factor antibodies can help rule out the diagnosis of autoimmune gastritis.

Lymphocytic and collagenous gastritis can resemble autoimmune gastritis when restricted or predominantly involving the gastric corpus or when associated with atrophy. However, neither is associated with endocrine cell hyperplasia, and autoimmune gastritis is not associated with marked intraepithelial lymphocytosis or abnormality of subepithelial collagen. Infections other than *H. pylori*, such as Epstein-Barr virus, may cause a destructive gastritis with loss of parietal cells that mimics autoimmune gastritis. The corpus-restricted nature and the associated endocrine cell hyperplasia and lack of EBER CISH positivity in the mononuclear cells are helpful in establishing the correct diagnosis.

Pernicious anemia related to autoimmune polyglandular syndrome type I is a rare childhood disorder characterized by antibodies directed against endocrine cells that leads to a generalized loss of GI endocrine cells, including gastrin-secreting G cells. Patients have a low serum gastrin, unlike typical autoimmune gastritis, and variably present with antiparietal cell antibodies. The loss of parietal cells in the gastric corpus is a result of the low serum gastrin.

Prognosis and Therapy

Autoimmune gastritis carries a 2% to 9% prevalence of gastric well-differentiated neuroendocrine tumors that are often multiple, usually less than 1 cm in diameter, and typically have a better prognosis than their sporadic counterparts. There is also a two- to threefold increase in the risk of gastric adenocarcinoma in patients with autoimmune gastritis.

Medical therapy includes vitamin B_{12} injections and iron supplementation for those with pernicious anemia or iron-deficiency anemia, respectively. In patients with multiple well-differentiated neuroendocrine tumors, management includes endoscopic polypectomy or mucosal resection with continued surveillance. Antrectomy is reserved for selected patients with numerous lesions or rapidly enlarging lesions and causes resolution of the hypergastrinemic state and reduction in the size of tumors.

TABLE 3.4

Features of Autoimmune versus Environmental Atrophic Gastritis

	Autoimmune Gastritis	Environmental Metaplastic Atrophic Gastritis
Synonyms	Type A gastritis Diffuse corporal gastritis	Type B gastritis Diffuse antral gastritis Multifocal atrophic gastritis
Population affected	Northern European and Scandinavian descent	Worldwide
Sex	Female predominance	No sex predilection
Etiology	Immune mediated	*Helicobacter pylori* infection
H. pylori colonization	<20%	90%–100%
Affected mucosa	Oxyntic mucosa	Antrum predominantly with extension to body, multifocal
Antiparietal cell antibody	Positive	Negative
Anti-intrinsic factor antibody	Positive	Negative
Vitamin B_{12} level	Low	Normal
Serum gastrin	Very high	Normal or low

GRANULOMATOUS GASTRITIS

Granulomatous gastritis is an uncommon form of gastritis, comprising 0.27% to 0.35% of all gastritides. It encompasses a wide spectrum of diseases that lead to the development of mucosal or submucosal granulomas as the defining histologic feature. The types of granulomas vary widely from discrete nodular circumscribed collection of epithelioid histiocytes, reminiscent of sarcoidosis, to those admixed with lymphocytes, eosinophils, and even neutrophils, with or without giant cells, to others with prominent central necrosis and a lymphoid cuff similar to necrotizing granulomas seen in *Mycobacterium tuberculosis* infection. Notably, determining the underlying cause usually requires correlation with the clinical, radiologic, endoscopic, and microbiological findings and sometimes the response to treatment (Table 3.5). When a granuloma is seen on H&E examination, additional studies such as the use of polarized light to rule out presence of foreign body and special stains such as acid-fast bacilli, Gomori methenamine silver, and periodic acid–Schiff (PAS) are obligatory parts of the diagnostic assessment. A controversial diagnosis of *idiopathic granulomatous gastritis* has been reported in the literature to define patients with large and compact granulomas limited to the stomach and after exclusion of known entities such as Crohn's disease and sarcoidosis. Some authors have linked these granulomas to an inflammatory response to *H. pylori*

TABLE 3.5

Differential Diagnoses of Granulomatous Gastritis

Gastric Crohn's disease—52%
Sarcoidosis-1—21%
Foreign body granuloma-food, suture material, barium, mucin—10%
Isolated granulomatous gastritis—25%
Tumor-associated granulomas—7%
Infections (tuberculosis, histoplasmosis, schistosomiasis Whipple's disease, leprosy, syphilis)
Vasculitis-associated granulomas (Churg Strauss disease)
Helicobacter pylori gastritis

Data from Ectors NL, Dixon MF, Geboes KJ, et al. Granulomatous gastritis: a morphological and diagnostic approach. *Histopathology*. 1993;23:55–61; and Shapiro JL, Goldblum JR, Petras RE. A clinicopathologic study of 42 patients with granulomatous gastritis: is there really an "idiopathic" granulomatous gastritis? *Am J Surg Pathol*. 1996;20:462–470.

infection after reporting the disappearance of the granulomas following successful eradication of the bacteria. Other authors have found an association with vasculitis.

GASTRIC CROHN'S DISEASE

Approximately 30% to 50% of patients with Crohn's disease have upper GI manifestations. Patients with both small and large bowel involvement are more likely to have upper GI involvement. Patients are usually younger and often belong to the pediatric age group. Patients may present with symptoms of abdominal pain, nausea, and vomiting, often combined with lower GI symptoms such as chronic diarrhea and weight loss. In the West, Crohn's disease accounts for 17% to 55% of all cases with granulomatous gastritis.

Endoscopically, the mucosal appearance is quite variable and ranges from completely normal mucosa to findings that include erythema, erosions or ulcers, nodules, thickened folds (so-called bamboo stomach), and even gastric outlet stenosis. Findings are usually predominant in the antrum.

The finding of granulomas is helpful in establishing the diagnosis of Crohn's disease in the appropriate clinical setting. However, granulomas are present in only 7% to 34% of cases. Crohn's granulomas usually consist of small clusters of epithelioid histiocytes. Notably, granulomas can also be detected in apparently normal mucosa, thus emphasizing the importance of sampling.

More commonly, the gastric involvement in patients with Crohn's disease may show a spectrum of inflammatory changes that range from focally enhanced gastritis to a patchy or diffuse chronic active gastritis of variable severity (Fig. 3.18). Focally enhanced gastritis is a patchy inflammatory process composed of inflamed gastric pits surrounded by a cuff of loose lymphohistiocytic aggregates (Fig. 3.19). Focally enhanced gastritis, particularly in adults, can also be associated with drug-induced mucosal injury, graft-versus-host disease, or incompletely treated *H. pylori* gastritis.

GASTRIC SARCOIDOSIS

Sarcoidosis is a systemic granulomatous disorder that commonly affects the lungs and hilar lymph nodes. It usually affects young adults and is more common in African Americans. Gastric antral involvement can be seen in 10% of patients with systemic disease.

The gastric mucosa may be macroscopically nodular (Fig. 3.20) with ulcers, thickening, and a segmental linitis plastica–like appearance. Gastric outlet obstruction and bleeding have been reported.

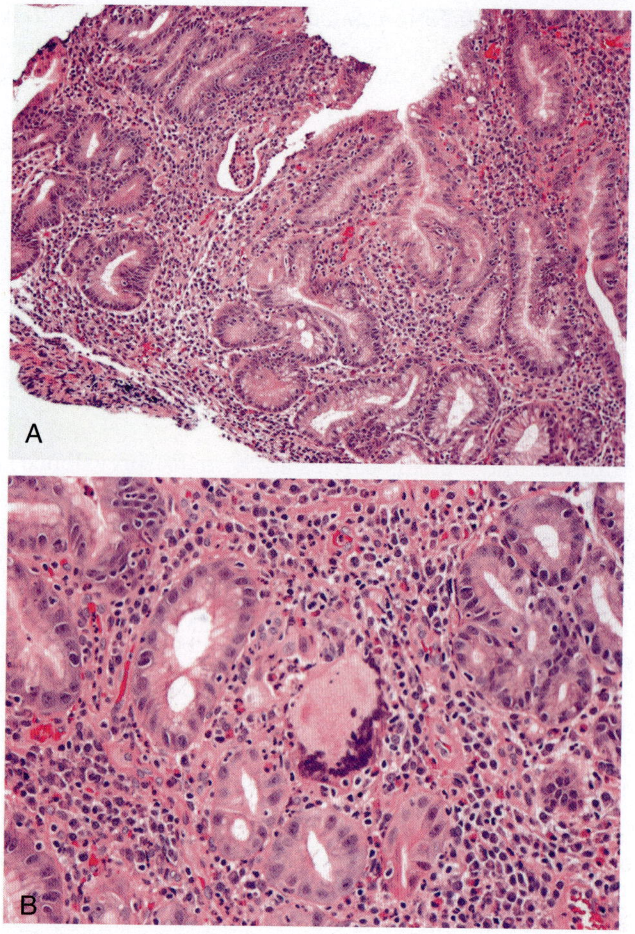

FIGURE 3.18

Gastric Crohn's showing lymphoplasmacytic infiltrate and crypt abscess (**A**) and giant cell (**B**). Immunostain for *Helicobacter pylori* was negative.

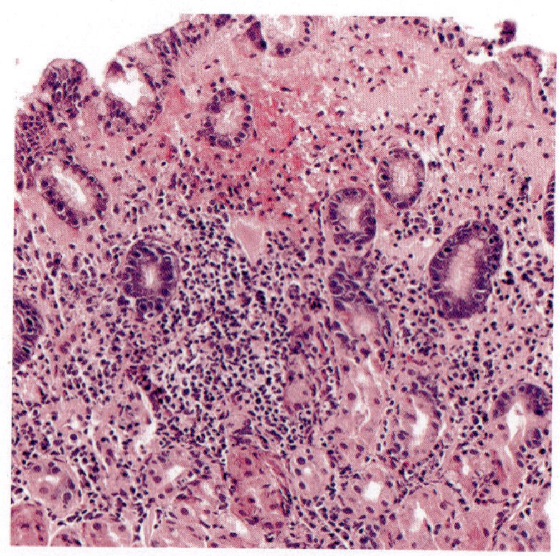

FIGURE 3.19

Focal enhancing gastritis can be a manifestation of Crohn's disease and is characterized by active inflammation surrounded by a loose cuff of lymphocytes and histiocytes.

Compact noncaseating granulomas (Figs. 3.21) are seen in gastric sarcoidosis, which is a diagnosis of exclusion and confirmed by correlation with clinical and imaging findings. Patients often respond to steroid therapy.

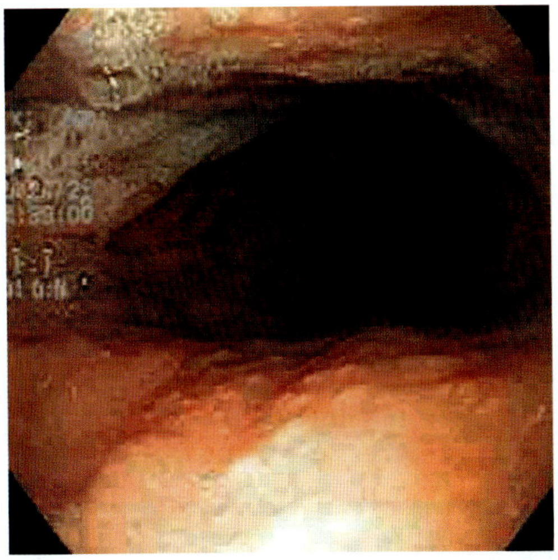

FIGURE 3.20
Gastric sarcoidosis with a nodular mucosal appearance on endoscopy.

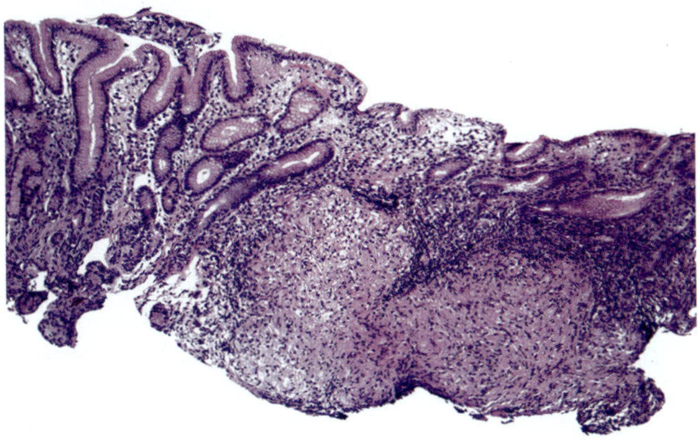

FIGURE 3.21
Antral mucosa showing noncaseating granulomas in the lamina propria in a patient with sarcoidosis.

LYMPHOCYTIC GASTRITIS

Lymphocytic gastritis is an uncommon form of chronic gastritis characterized by marked intraepithelial lymphocytosis in the gastric surface and pit epithelium; the glandular compartment is often spared. *Lymphocytic gastritis* is synonymous with *varioliform gastritis*, which refers to the endoscopic appearance and with chronic erosive verrucous gastritis.

CLINICAL FEATURES

Lymphocytic gastritis has a prevalence of 1% to 4% in upper GI endoscopies. Symptoms include dyspepsia, iron-deficiency anemia, and diarrhea. It has been seen in adults and children (age range, 1–89 years) but is more common in older adults. A slight female predominance is present. Etiologic associations are broad with approximately 38% of patients with lymphocytic gastritis having celiac disease and 29% having *H. pylori* gastritis. Other less common associations consist of Crohn's disease, human immunodeficiency virus (HIV) infection, esophageal carcinoma, and gastric lymphoma. Lymphocytic gastritis is found in 33% of patients with celiac disease who undergo gastric biopsies, and 4% of patients with *H. pylori* gastritis have lymphocytic gastritis. Patients with celiac disease with lymphocytic gastritis may also have lymphocytic colitis (38%). More recently, a lymphocytic gastritis pattern has also been shown in patients with an immune checkpoint inhibitor therapy–associated gastritis.

LYMPHOCYTIC GASTRITIS—FACT SHEET

Definition
- Chronic gastritis characterized by marked intraepithelial lymphocytosis, similar to the pattern seen in lymphocytic colitis

Incidence and Location
- 1% to 4% of all upper endoscopies
- May show diffuse involvement or be restricted to antrum or corpus mucosa

Gender, Race, and Age
- Seen across all age groups; more common in older adults
- Slight female predominance
- No racial predilection

Clinical Features
- May be asymptomatic or present with dyspepsia, iron-deficiency anemia, or diarrhea
- Common etiological associations include celiac disease (38%) and *Helicobacter pylori* infection (29%)
- Other causes include Crohn's disease, immune deficiency disorders, and drug-induced gastritis

Prognosis and Therapy
- Treatment of *H. pylori* infection leads to resolution in cases associated with this organism
- Similarly, treatment of the underlying cause, such as gluten withdrawal, leads to histologic resolution

PATHOLOGIC FEATURES

GROSS FINDINGS

The endoscopic appearance may either be normal or consist of mucosal nodules, erosions, and enlarged gastric folds resembling Ménétrier-like protein-losing gastropathy. The latter appearance can mimic neoplastic processes. The nodules may contain a central depression or erosion and are described as varioliform or aphthoid erosions.

MICROSCOPIC FINDINGS

Histologic findings include marked intraepithelial lymphocytosis predominantly involving the surface foveolar and pit epithelium; the deeper glandular compartment is frequently spared. Lymphocytic gastritis is typically characterized by the presence of greater than 25 lymphocytes per 100 epithelial cells. It has been shown that normal gastric epithelium usually harbors around 3.5 lymphocytes per 100 cells, and diseased control participants s such as patients with *Helicobacter* gastritis have 5 lymphocytes per 100 cells. The lamina propria is also expanded by lymphocytes and plasma cells (Fig. 3.22). The intraepithelial lymphocytes are recognized by their condensed, dark nuclei surrounded by a clear halo (Fig. 3.23). The foveolar pits are slightly tortuous and elongated. Patchy foci of active neutrophilic infiltration may also be present in some cases, usually close to foci of erosion, and are acceptable within the spectrum of lymphocytic gastritis.

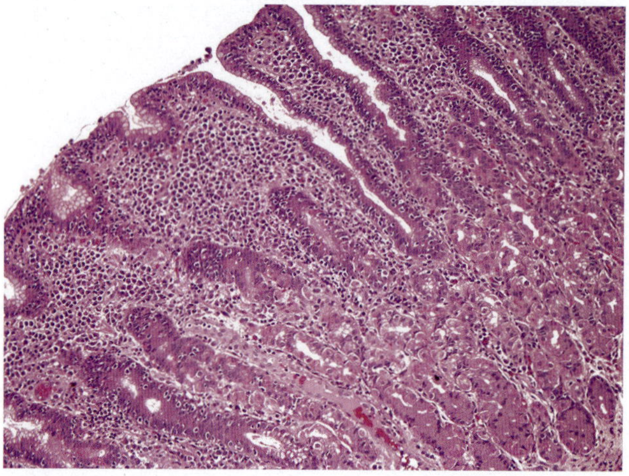

FIGURE 3.22

Lymphocytic gastritis. Oxyntic mucosa with marked increase in intraepithelial lymphocytes in the surface epithelium and gastric pits. The lamina propria is expanded by plasma cells and lymphocytes.

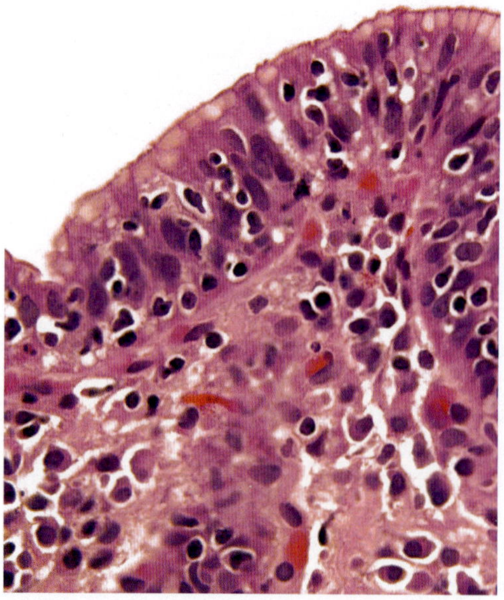

FIGURE 3.23

Lymphocytic gastritis. High-power view showing the condensed dark nuclei of intraepithelial lymphocytes surrounded by a clear halo.

Lymphocytic gastritis can involve the entire gastric mucosa or may predominantly involve the antrum or the body and fundic region. The antrum-predominant distribution is more often associated with celiac disease, whereas *H. pylori*–associated lymphocytic gastritis is more likely to involve the body or fundus. The intraepithelial lymphocytes are CD3- and CD8-positive cytotoxic/suppressor T-lymphocytes and thus easily distinguishable from CD20-positive B cells seen in lymphoepithelial lesions of extranodal marginal zone lymphoma (MALT lymphoma). Stains for *Helicobacter* organisms may be positive in a subset of cases.

Lymphocytic Gastritis—Pathologic Features

Gross Findings

- May be normal or show a nodular appearance with or without erosions or diffuse enlargement of gastric rugal folds

Microscopic Findings

- Chronic gastritis with prominent intraepithelial lymphocytes
- The lymphocytes preferentially infiltrate the surface foveolar epithelium and the superficial gastric pit epithelium while sparing the deep glandular compartment
- Patchy foci of neutrophilic infiltration may also be present in some cases, usually close to mucosal erosions, and are compatible with this diagnosis
- *Helicobacter pylori* may be present in a subset of cases

Immunohistochemical Features

- The intraepithelial lymphocytes show a CD3/CD8-positive cytotoxic/suppressor T-cell phenotype, unlike the CD20-positive B cells present in lymphoepithelial lesions of extranodal marginal zone B-cell lymphoma

Differential Diagnosis

- *H. pylori* gastritis
- Collagenous gastritis
- Extranodal marginal zone B-cell lymphoma

Differential Diagnosis

H. pylori gastritis can show foci of intraepithelial lymphocytosis, but in its typical form, it shows a chronic active gastritis with diffuse lymphoplasmacytic infiltrate and prominent neutrophilic activity. The intraepithelial lymphocytes are minimal and patchy and do not approach the 25 lymphocytes per 100 epithelial cells cut-off commonly seen in lymphocytic gastritis. Similar to colonic biopsies, whenever a diagnosis of lymphocytic gastritis is entertained, a close look at the subepithelial collagen is warranted to rule out the possibility of a collagenous gastritis.

Extranodal marginal zone lymphoma (MALT lymphoma) is characterized by significant expansion of the lamina propria by a monotonous lymphoid infiltrate composed of small- to medium-sized lymphocytes that is associated with characteristic lymphoepithelial lesions. The lymphoid population is composed of CD20 positive B cells that often show aberrant CD43 coexpression. In contrast, the lymphocytes in lymphocytic gastritis are CD3-positive mature T lymphocytes.

Prognosis and Therapy

Treatment is directed at the underlying conditions such as a gluten-free diet in patients with celiac disease or eradication of *Helicobacter* gastritis or discontinuation of the offending medication in patients with drug-induced gastritis.

INFECTIOUS GASTRITIS

The most common form of infectious gastritis is *Helicobacter* infection, which has been discussed already. Various other infectious causes, such as cytomegalovirus (CMV) and adenovirus (Figs. 3.24 and 3.25) in

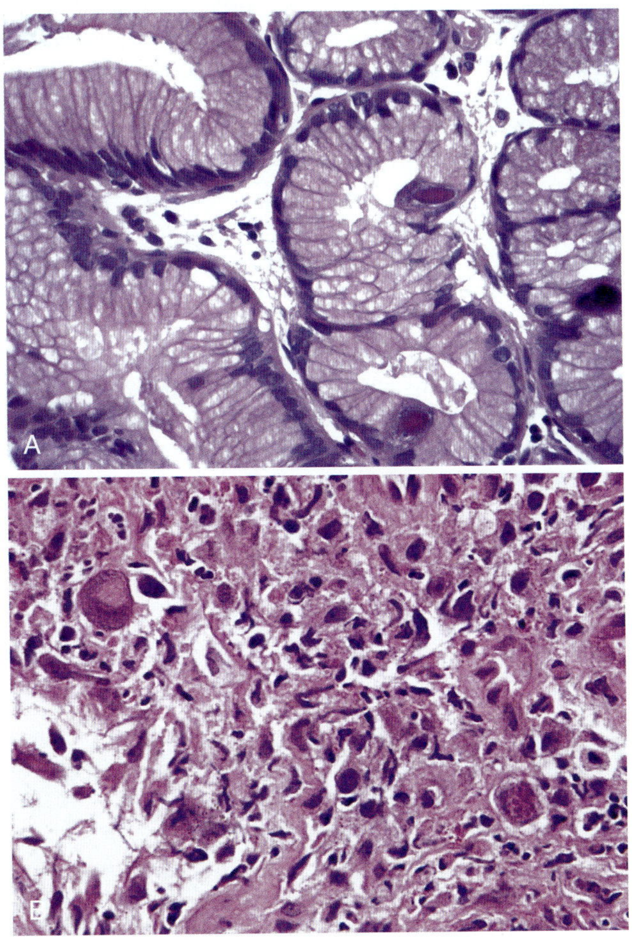

FIGURE 3.24

Gastric foveolar epithelial cells with cytomegalovirus (CMV) inclusions. Note both nuclear and cytoplasmic inclusions (**A**). Similar CMV inclusions may be seen in endothelial and stromal cells (**B**).

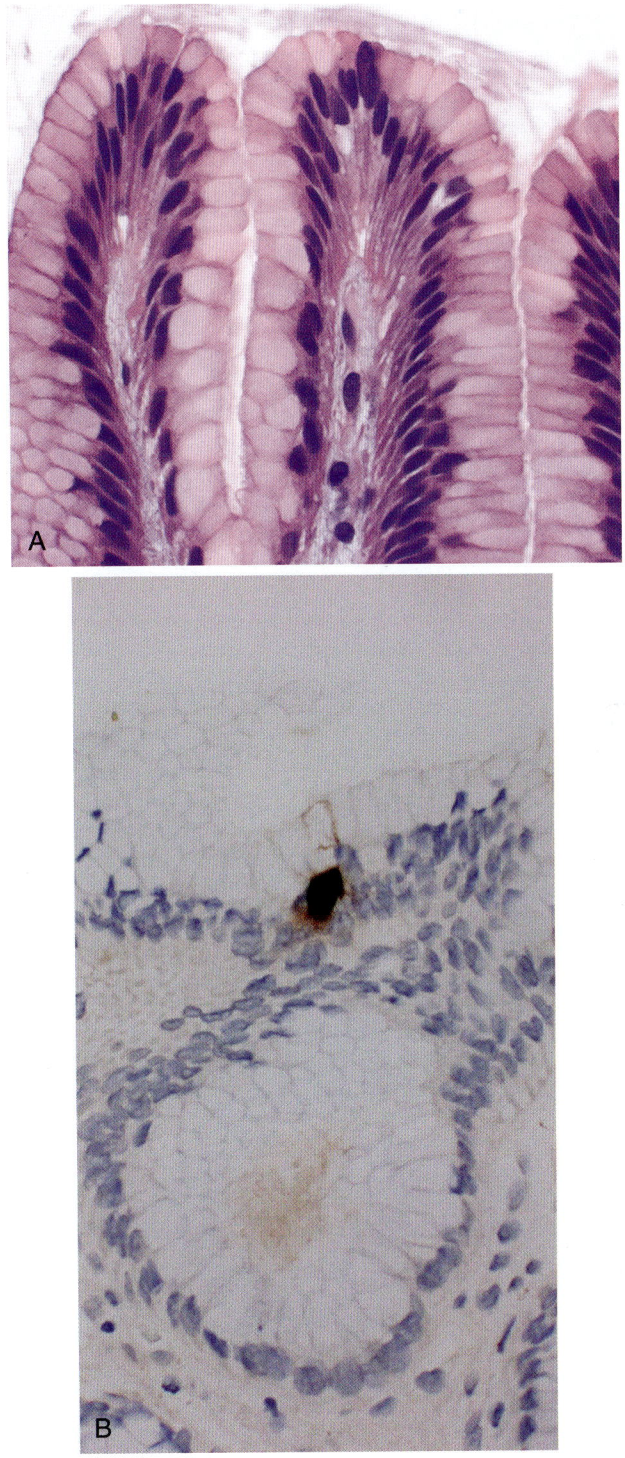

FIGURE 3.25

Smudgy nuclear inclusions in adenovirus gastritis can be easily missed (**A**). The mucosa may not be significantly inflamed because the infection typically occurs in immunocompromised patients. Immunostain for adenovirus is essential for establishing the diagnosis (**B**).

immunocompromised patients and a wide array of other bacterial, viral, fungal, and parasitic infections in the stomach have been described. The diagnostic findings in these infections are not site specific and are discussed in detail in Chapter 9 on infectious disorders of the GI tract.

EOSINOPHILIC GASTRITIS

Eosinophilic gastritis is a morphologic pattern of injury characterized by a dense eosinophilic infiltrate in the lamina propria accompanied by foci of epithelial destruction by eosinophils. The common underlying etiologic conditions associated with eosinophilic gastritis include primary eosinophilic gastroenteritis, drug-induced hypersensitivity or other allergic reactions, and parasitic infections. The discussion here is limited to gastric involvement in eosinophilic gastroenteritis, which is defined by the presence of GI symptoms, dense tissue infiltration by eosinophils, lack of extraintestinal eosinophilia, and exclusion of all other known causes of eosinophilic infiltration.

EOSINOPHILIC GASTRITIS—FACT SHEET

Definition

- Eosinophilic gastritis is a rare inflammatory condition characterized by dense eosinophilic infiltration in the lamina propria with epithelial injury

Morbidity and Mortality

- Patients may present with acute abdominal emergency and perforation
- Gastrointestinal bleeding

Gender, Race, and Age

- Patients are usually 20 to 50 years old
- Pediatric involvement in 15% to 20% of cases
- Male-to-female ratio is 1 to 1

Clinical Features

- History of allergy, asthma, food intolerance, eczema, drug sensitivities, peripheral blood eosinophilia, and increased immunoglobulin E levels
- Symptoms depend on the site and extent of eosinophilic infiltration
- Mucosal disease can present as abdominal pain, nausea, vomiting, diarrhea, weight loss, malabsorption, protein-losing enteropathy, and gastrointestinal bleeding
- Submucosal and muscularis propria involvement present in cases with obstructive symptoms
- Eosinophilic ascites with serosal involvement
- Other causes of tissue eosinophilia such as parasitic infestation, drug reaction, and hypereosinophilic syndrome should be excluded

Endoscopic and Radiologic Features

- Marked edema and thickening of the gastric folds and wall

Prognosis and Therapy

- Dramatic improvement with steroids in cases with primary eosinophilic gastroenteritis
- Surgery in obstructive or refractory cases

CLINICAL FEATURES

The diagnostic criteria for eosinophilic gastroenteritis include (1) GI symptoms; (2) histologic evidence of eosinophilic infiltration of the GI tract; (3) absence of eosinophilic infiltration in extraintestinal organs; and (4) exclusion of known causes of eosinophilia, such as healing ulcer site, parasitic infestation, and drug hypersensitivity reaction.

Eosinophilic gastroenteritis may affect all races and any age group but usually affects adults between 20 and 50 years of age. There is no sex predominance. Pediatric presentation is common with 15% to 20% of cases diagnosed in children. Any part of the GI tract from the esophagus to the rectum can be involved, and the gastric antrum is the most common site of involvement. The esophagus and small bowel are also commonly affected. Eosinophilic proctocolitis is seen most often in infants (an important cause of bloody stool) and is usually attributed to cow's milk allergy. The estimated prevalence of eosinophilic gastritis and gastroenteritis is 6.3 and 8.4 per 100,000, respectively, in some recent studies.

Eosinophilic gastroenteritis can show preferential involvement of the mucosa, muscle layer, or serosa, but this subclassification is seldom used in daily practice. Symptoms depend on the site and extent of eosinophilic infiltration. Mucosal disease can present as abdominal pain, nausea, vomiting, diarrhea, weight loss, malabsorption, protein-losing enteropathy, and anemia caused by bleeding. Patients with involvement of the submucosa and muscularis propria present with obstructive symptoms and symptoms mimicking pyloric stenosis. Thickening of the stomach may also be noted on imaging studies in cases with dominant mural involvement. Serosal involvement is characterized by eosinophilic ascites, peripheral eosinophilia, and dramatic response to steroids. Rarely, patients may present with an acute abdominal emergency and perforation necessitating emergency laparotomy.

The patients commonly present with a history of allergy (25%–50%), asthma, food intolerance (52%), eczema, drug sensitivities, peripheral blood eosinophilia (80%), and elevated serum immunoglobulin E levels. Connective tissue diseases (scleroderma, polymyositis) are also commonly described associations.

PATHOLOGIC FEATURES

GROSS FINDINGS

Gastric mucosa may be normal on endoscopic examination or reveal erosions, ulcerations, erythema, and nodularity.

Microscopic Findings

Gastric involvement in eosinophilic gastroenteritis is characterized by intense eosinophilic infiltration of the lamina propria (>20 per high-power field [hpf]), intraepithelial eosinophils, and eosinophilic crypt abscesses (Fig. 3.26). The finding of greater than 30 eosinophils/hpf in at least 5 hpf has also been proposed as diagnostic criteria. The eosinophilic infiltration is accompanied by epithelial damage, regenerative change, and marked edema. Eosinophils are the dominant cell type, and other inflammatory cells are not prominent, with the exception of an increase in mast cells. The eosinophilic infiltrate can be patchy or diffuse, and mucosal biopsies can be nondiagnostic in up to 10% of cases. The presence of clusters of eosinophils deep in the submucosa, muscularis propria, or serosa should prompt careful evaluation of clinical and histologic findings to ensure prompt diagnosis of eosinophilic gastroenteritis.

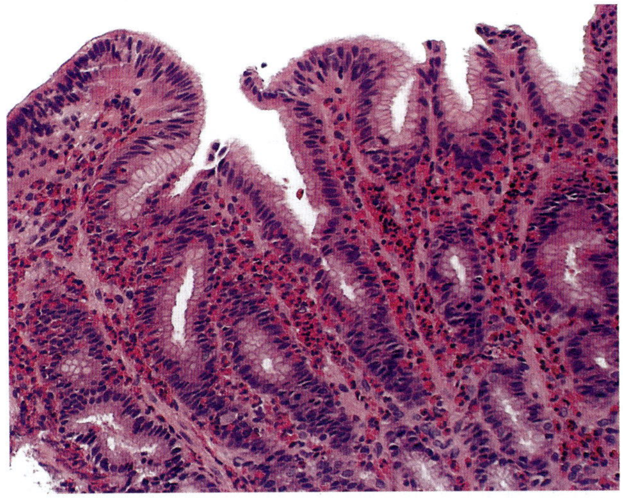

FIGURE 3.26

Intense eosinophilic infiltration in a case of eosinophilic gastritis. Notice the surface regenerative changes and glandular infiltration by eosinophils.

Eosinophilic Gastritis—Pathologic Features

Gross Findings

- Gastric mucosa may be normal or display erosions, ulcerations, erythema, and nodules

Microscopic Findings

- Gastric antral mucosa commonly involved
- Intense eosinophilic infiltration with prominent lamina propria eosinophils, eosinophilic crypt abscesses, and epithelial damage
- >20/HPF or >30/HPF in at least five fields have been proposed criteria for diagnosis
- Eosinophilic infiltrate can be patchy or diffuse, and mucosal biopsies can be nondiagnostic in up to 10%
- Involvement of deep submucosa, muscularis propria, or serosa should raise suspicion for diagnosis

Differential Diagnosis

- Infiltrate secondary to mucosal ulcers
- Parasitic infestation
- Hypereosinophilic syndrome
- Langerhans cell histiocytosis
- Systemic mastocytosis
- Drugs such as nonsteroidal antiinflammatory drugs, gold, azathioprine, carbamazepine, enalapril, and cotrimoxazole
- Eosinophils can be focally prominent in gastric Crohn's disease, gastric carcinomas, lymphomas, connective tissue disorder, and peptic ulcer disease

Differential Diagnosis

- Eosinophils can be present in the stroma whenever there is a breach of surface epithelium, allowing luminal contents to come in contract with connective tissue in the lamina propria. Healing erosions and ulcers often show lamina propria eosinophilia to varying degrees. This is seldom to a degree typical for eosinophilic gastroenteritis, and the localization adjacent to foci of ulceration is a clue to the right diagnosis.
- Parasitic infestation is associated often with intense eosinophilic infiltration surrounding parasitic ova, larvae, or nematode such as anisakiasis, *Strongyloides*, and *Ascaris*. Careful histologic examination for ova and parasites (Fig. 3.27) and stool examination are important.
- Drugs such as gold, azathioprine, carbamazepine, enalapril, and cotrimoxazole can also cause a hypersensitivity reactive, leading to tissue eosinophilia in the GI tract.
- Hypereosinophilic syndrome is a fatal disease characterized by peripheral eosinophilia (>1500/mm^3) and diffuse infiltration of eosinophils in various organs such as the myocardium, lungs, and GI tract.
- Eosinophilic infiltration is also prominent in cases of Langerhans cell histiocytosis and systemic mastocytosis, where it is recruited secondarily by the neoplastic cells. The diagnosis can easily be made by using the appropriate immunostains for Langerhans cells (CD1a and S-100) and abnormal mast cells (KIT and CD25).
- Eosinophils can be focally prominent in gastric Crohn's disease, gastric carcinomas, lymphomas, connective tissue disorder, vasculitis such as Churg-Strauss disease, and peptic ulcer disease.

Prognosis and Therapy

Patients with eosinophilic gastroenteritis show an excellent response to steroids and relapse can occur after discontinuation. Patients have also shown good response to oral sodium cromoglycate. Surgical resection may be necessary in patients with obstruction or in refractory cases.

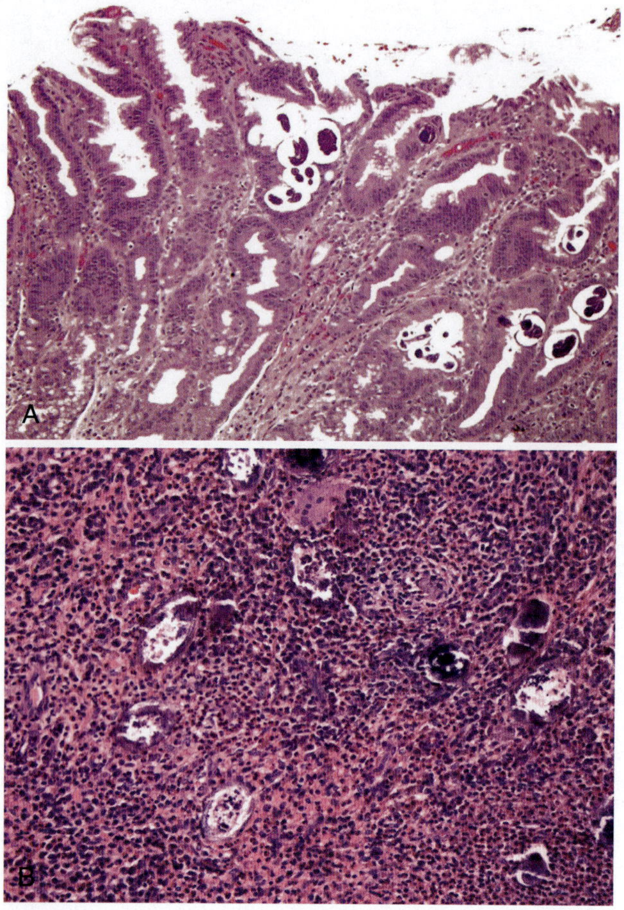

FIGURE 3.27

Eosinophilic infiltrate can be striking in parasitic infections involving the stomach. Gastric antral mucosa with cross sections of *Strongyloides stercoralis* larvae in gastric pits (**A**) and numerous schistosome eggs; some are calcified (**B**).

COLLAGENOUS GASTRITIS

Collagenous gastritis is a rare entity characterized by subepithelial collagen deposition in superficial gastric mucosa exceeding 10 μm in thickness accompanied by surface epithelial damage, increased lymphoplasmacytic inflammation of the lamina propria, and variable intraepithelial lymphocytosis.

CLINICAL FEATURES

The disease presents over a wide age range, including children and older adults, with a slight female predominance. Clinical manifestations are broad include chronic diarrhea, anorexia, nausea, vomiting, abdominal pain, weight loss, anemia, and bleeding. According to several series, patients with collagenous gastritis generally fall into two clinical groups, (1) children and young adults presenting with anemia and disease limited to the stomach with a nodular gastric mucosa on endoscopy and (2) older adult patients presenting with chronic watery diarrhea, often associated with collagenous colitis. In some patients, collagenous gastritis is associated with other inflammatory conditions, including collagenous colitis, lymphocytic colitis, celiac or collagenous sprue, inflammatory bowel disease, or autoimmune disorders, or it may be a manifestation of drug-induced gastritis, including immunotherapy-associated gastritis. The pathogenesis is unknown. Proposed mechanisms are excessive collagen deposition caused by a reparative process after chronic inflammation, collagen deposition by abnormal pericryptal fibroblasts, and leakage of plasma proteins and fibrinogen with subsequent replacement by collagen

COLLAGENOUS GASTRITIS—FACT SHEET

Definition

- Chronic gastritis characterized by subepithelial collagen deposition of more than 10 μm, surface epithelial damage, lymphoplasmacytic inflammation of the lamina propria, and variable intraepithelial lymphocytosis

Incidence

- Rare entity

Morbidity and Mortality

- Can cause chronic morbidity, including anemia, chronic diarrhea, and significant weight loss

Gender, Race, and Age

- Slight female predominance
- Seen both in children and adults over a wide age range

Clinical Features

- Symptoms include chronic watery diarrhea, weight loss, anorexia, nausea, vomiting, abdominal pain, anemia, and bleeding
- Can be associated with collagenous colitis, lymphocytic colitis, celiac sprue, collagenous sprue, lymphocytic gastritis, inflammatory bowel disease, autoimmune disorders, and drug-induced mucosal injury

Prognosis and Therapy

- Prednisone, budesonide, azathioprine, and a gluten-free diet have been shown to improve symptoms and cause weight gain
- It is important to biopsy the duodenum and colon to exclude concurrent celiac and collagenous sprue, as well as collagenous and lymphocytic colitis

PATHOLOGIC FEATURES

GROSS FINDINGS

The disease can be patchy or manifest as a pangastritis involving both the gastric antrum and body. The endoscopic appearance consists of diffuse nodularity, erythema, and erosions.

MICROSCOPIC FINDINGS

Histologic findings resemble those seen in collagenous colitis. The lamina propria is expanded by a prominent lymphoplasmacytic infiltrate accompanied by a variable

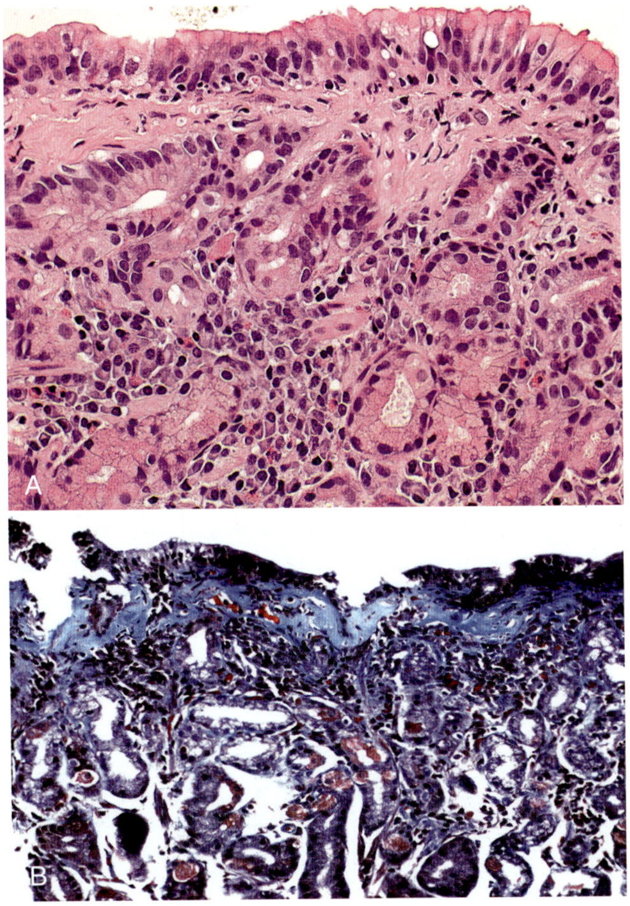

FIGURE 3.28

Collagenous gastritis with increased subepithelial deposition of collagen. The thick collagen band entraps capillaries and inflammatory cells (**A**). The subepithelial collagen thickness and irregularity can be highlighted by a trichrome stain that stains collagen blue (**B**).

COLLAGENOUS GASTRITIS—PATHOLOGIC FEATURES

Gross Findings

- The gastric antrum and/or corpus can be affected
- Endoscopy shows diffuse nodularity (common), diffuse or patchy erythema, or erosions

Microscopic Findings

- The lamina propria is expanded by lymphoplasmacytic infiltrate, and the subepithelial collagen layer is thick and frayed
- Subepithelial collagen band abnormality can be patchy, and surface epithelium can strip off
- Variable degrees of intraepithelial lymphocytosis may be present
- A prominent eosinophilic infiltrate may be present in the lamina propria
- Masson's trichrome may help to highlight the subepithelial collagen layer

Differential Diagnosis

- Autoimmune gastritis
- Lymphocytic gastritis
- Gastric amyloidosis
- Radiation gastritis

intraepithelial lymphocytosis, and the subepithelial collagen is increased in thickness and frayed in nature, often entrapping capillaries and mononuclear cells within it (Fig. 3.28A). The collagen thickness is typically greater than 10 μm, ranging from 20 to 120 μm, and the surface epithelium may strip off. The lamina propria may also show prominent eosinophils and contain foci of active gastritis. Most patients with collagenous gastritis are negative for *H. pylori* infection. Collagenous gastritis is a chronic gastritis and can show atrophy and intestinal metaplasia in some cases, mimicking autoimmune gastritis. The lack of neuroendocrine cell hyperplasia and presence of collagen abnormalities are key to making this distinction. Trichrome or Sirius red stains can help in highlighting the abnormalities of subepithelial collagen in subtle cases (Fig. 3.28B).

DIFFERENTIAL DIAGNOSIS

- Atrophy and intestinal metaplasia can be present in collagenous gastritis involving the gastric corpus, raising the possibility of autoimmune gastritis. Whereas the presence of linear and micronodular hyperplasia is a hallmark of autoimmune gastritis, subepithelial collagen layer abnormalities are diagnosis of collagenous gastritis.
- Lymphocytic gastritis is in the differential diagnosis because of increased intraepithelial lymphocytosis that may be present in collagenous gastritis cases. However, similar to interpretation of small intestine and colon biopsies, the presence of a thick or abnormal collagen layer is diagnostic of collagenous gastritis. Special stains for collagen are helpful in cases with subtle abnormalities.
- Gastric amyloidosis may mimic collagenous gastritis because the amyloid deposition may in some cases be superficial and resemble a collagen band. However, the deposit is not just limited to the superficial mucosa as in collagenous gastritis but often involves the blood vessels and may be present as stromal deposits in severe cases. Amyloid is more homogeneous in appearance compared with the fibrillary character of collagen in collagenous gastritis. The distinction is easily achieved using special stains for amyloid such as Congo red that show characteristic apple-green birefringence upon polarization.
- Lamina propria fibrosis in radiation and ischemic gastritis or scleroderma is not restricted to the subepithelial zone. Furthermore, scleroderma can involve the submucosa and muscularis propria and even subserosa. Radiation gastritis also shows hyalinized blood vessels and atypical stromal fibroblasts.

PROGNOSIS AND THERAPY

Treatment is empirical and includes budesonide, prednisone, azathioprine, 5-aminosalicylates, nutritional supplements, and even a gluten-free diet. In most instances, despite symptomatic improvement, follow-up biopsies show a persistence of collagen. Considering the frequent association with other collagenous enterocolitides, it is important to biopsy the duodenum and colon in all cases of collagenous gastritis.

GASTRIC MUCOSAL CALCINOSIS

Gastric mucosal calcinosis (GMC) is infrequently encountered in biopsies and is associated with calcium deposition in the gastric mucosa.

CLINICAL FEATURES

Gastric mucosal calcinosis is mostly seen in chronic renal failure, organ transplant patients, and patients taking aluminum-containing antacids or sucralfate. It is also seen and been classified as dystrophic when encountered in inflamed or necrotic gastric mucosa and as "metastatic" when developing in normal gastric mucosa of patients with hypercalcemia and hyperphosphatemia. Other associations include hyperparathyroidism, sarcoidosis, multiple myeloma, tumor lysis syndrome, hypervitaminosis D, hypervitaminosis A, milk-alkali syndrome, and isotretinoin use. The overall incidence of mucosal calcinosis is fewer than 0.1% of all gastric biopsies but can be as high as 14% to 60% in selected patients with transplants and chronic renal disease. A report quoted an incidence of 5% in nontransplant patients with gastric ulcers. An underlying etiology may not be apparent in some patients. Patients may present with nausea, vomiting, dyspepsia, abdominal pain, anemia, or GI bleeding.

GASTRIC MUCOSAL CALCINOSIS—FACT SHEET

Definition

- Condition characterized by gastric mucosal deposits of calcium beneath the foveolar epithelium

Incidence and Location

- Rare condition; more likely to occur in selected clinical settings
- 14% to 60% of gastric biopsies from transplant patients
- 5% of gastric biopsies from nontransplant patients with gastric ulcers

Morbidity and Mortality

- Usually seen in patients with end-stage renal failure, organ transplant recipients, patients on dialysis, and patients using aluminum-containing antacids and sucralfate

Clinical Features

- Asymptomatic or associated with nausea, vomiting, dyspepsia, abdominal pain, anemia, or bleeding

Prognosis and Treatment

- Benign outcome

PATHOLOGIC FEATURES

ENDOSCOPIC FINDINGS

Gastric mucosal calcinosis appears as small white plaques or nodules and may involve the antrum or corpus mucosa.

MICROSCOPIC FINDINGS

The gastric biopsies show basophilic extracellular deposits in the superficial aspect of the mucosa, usually beneath the foveolar epithelium, but can also be present deep in the mucosa as well (Fig. 3.29). The deposits are 50 to 500 μm in size, slightly refractile, and do not polarize. They may occasionally be rimmed by histiocytes and giant cells. Background stomach may show foveolar hyperplasia with mucin depletion and reactive epithelial changes. Despite the nomenclature

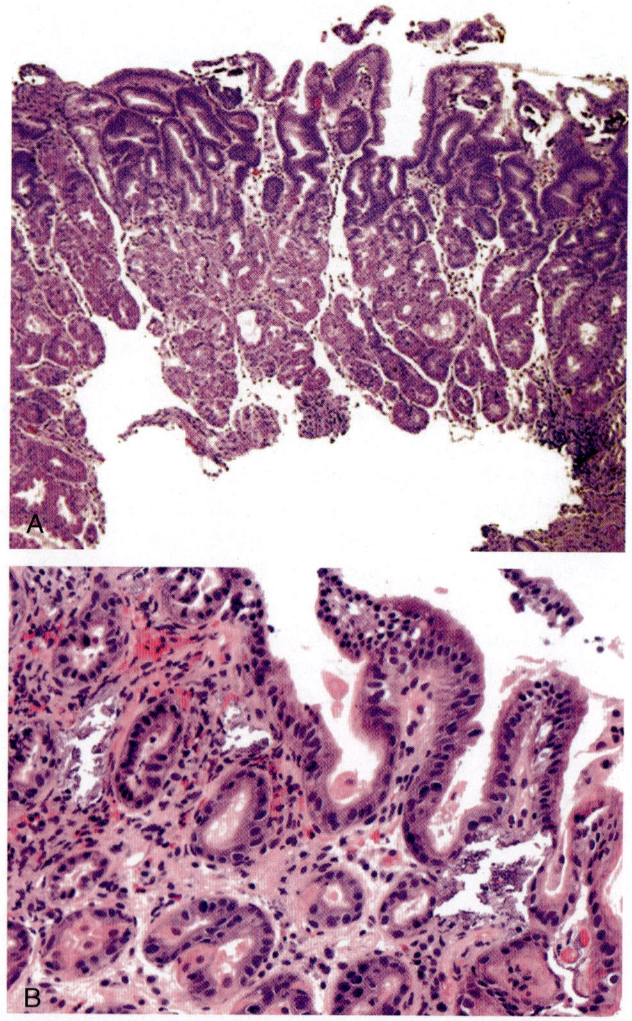

FIGURE 3.29

Gastric mucosal calcium deposits beneath the foveolar tips appear basophilic and refractile, and the surface epithelium is stripping off (**A**). Basophilic calcium deposits slightly deep in the lamina propria (**B**).

the deposits are actually composed of an admixture of calcium, aluminum, phosphorus, and chlorine, which has been demonstrated on x-ray microanalysis.

Gastric Mucosal Calcinosis—Pathologic Features

Endoscopic Findings

- Appear as white plaques or nodules

Microscopic Findings

- Basophilic, extracellular deposits located beneath the foveolar tips or deep in lamina propria
- May be rimmed by macrophages
- Slightly refractile but do not polarize
- Deposits shown to contain calcium, aluminum, phosphorus, and chlorine on x-ray microanalysis

Immunohistochemical Findings

- Variably positive with calcium stains such as Von Kossa and Alizarin red

Differential Diagnosis

- Deposit of lanthanum carbonate
- Gastric siderosis

Differential Diagnosis

The basophilic deposit of Lanthanum carbonate prescribed to lower hyperphosphatemia can vaguely mimic GMC. Furthermore, the same population is at risk. In patients with lanthanum deposition, the gastric mucosa shows a histiocyte-rich inflammatory infiltrate that is usually subepithelial in distribution. The histiocytes are filled with pale to amphophilic material that is fine or coarse in appearance. The lanthanum accumulation within the histiocytes has been found to stain positively for PAS; PAS after diastase digestion; and, in some cases, Prussian blue (Fig. 3.30). In contrast, mucosal calcinosis consists of large, extracellular, basophilic deposits that are PAS negative but Prussian blue positive.

Prognosis and Therapy

The significance of GMC is unclear. However, it is important to report the findings, given their frequent association with underlying medical conditions, such as chronic renal failure, and with history of transplantation. Calcium deposits in the stomach may also be an indicator of generalized deposition of calcium within other organs.

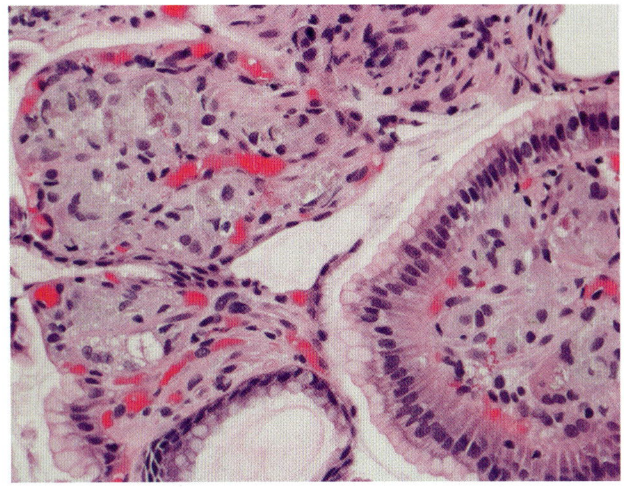

FIGURE 3.30

Lanthanum deposits in the lamina propria appear as brown-purple amorphous grungy material engulfed within large histiocytes. Deposits may be refractile and can stain positive with calcium stains. The localization within histiocytes is different from mucosal calcinosis, and the patient history is key to making the right diagnosis.

Iron Pill Gastritis

Patients prescribed oral iron therapy for anemia may develop gastric mucosal injury secondary to the medication. It is seen in about 15% of patients taking iron supplements. The changes are more frequently detected in older adult patients and particularly women.

Clinical Features

Many patients are asymptomatic, but others present with abdominal pain, nausea, and vomiting. Melena can also develop, and in extremely rare instances, recurrent ulcers may lead to stricture.

Pathologic Features

The mucosa is normal in most cases, but mucosal erythema and erosions and ulcerations can be detected. Brown-green discoloration of the mucosa may be seen in severe cases.

Microscopically, the gastric biopsy shows golden brown refractile crystalline material that is either embedded in the superficial lamina propria within macrophages and stromal elements or as a layer of encrustation on the damaged epithelium (see Fig. 3.31). It may even be seen within in vessel walls. The epithelium shows regenerative foveolar hyperplasia, but infarct-like necrosis can be observed as well. Prussian blue stain is confirmatory and highlights deposits that were not detected on H&E.

Differential Diagnosis

Exogenous deposits form the differential diagnosis, including mucosal calcinosis (see earlier), kayexalate resin crystals (nonpolarizing refractile crystals with a fish-scale appearance staining with acid fast stain), cholestyramine (PAS positive) angulated crystals, sevelamer (tree bark–shaped yellowish crystals), and colesevelam (red-brown angulated crystals). Gastric glandular siderosis (Fig. 3.31) also consists of iron deposition in gastric mucosa in patients with primary or secondary iron overload. In contrast to pill gastritis, the iron in gastric siderosis is present as granular intracytoplasmic deposits within macrophages or glandular epithelium deep in the mucosa.

Prognosis and Therapy

The symptoms decrease, and mucosal changes heal after ferrous sulfate medication is discontinued and less corrosive supplements, such as ferrous gluconate, are substituted.

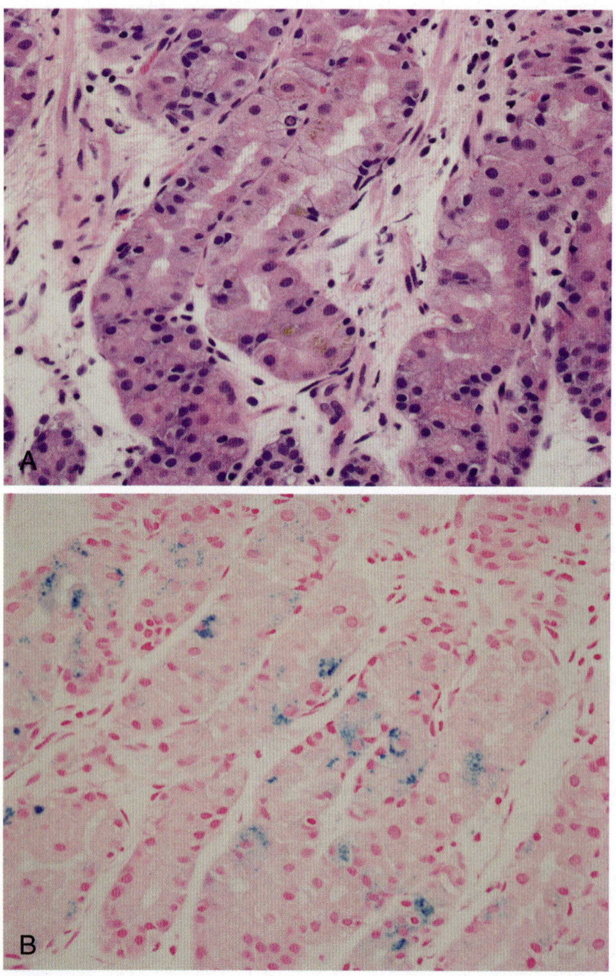

FIGURE 3.31

Iron pill gastritis with reactive epithelial changes and ill defined granular material on the mucosal surface and the lamina propria (**A**). The Iron stain highlights the deposition of ferrous sulfate (**B**).

DOXYCYCLINE GASTRITIS

Esophageal and gastric mucosal alterations can also be seen in patients taking tetracycline. The antibiotic is ulcerogenic and can sometimes produce distinctive changes in the gastric mucosa.

CLINICAL FEATURES

Some patients maybe asymptomatic, but most present with epigastric pain. The endoscopy may reveal either white-yellow plaque-like lesions or nonbleeding ulcers

Pathologic Features

The gastric biopsy shows superficial mucosal necrosis and erosion, with variable neutrophilic infiltrate and regenerative epithelial changes. Characteristic vascular degeneration of the capillaries in the superficial lamina propria is seen, consisting of eosinophilia of the vessel wall creating a ring-like deeply eosinophilic structures (Fig. 3.32). Microthrombi are noted in some of the vessels. Regenerative foveolar hyperplasia may be seen in cases associated with erosions and ulcers.

Differential Diagnosis

The differential diagnosis includes exogenous deposits such as calcium and iron discussed earlier or GAVE in cases associated with prominent foveolar hyperplasia. However, endoscopically, GAVE shows a characteristic

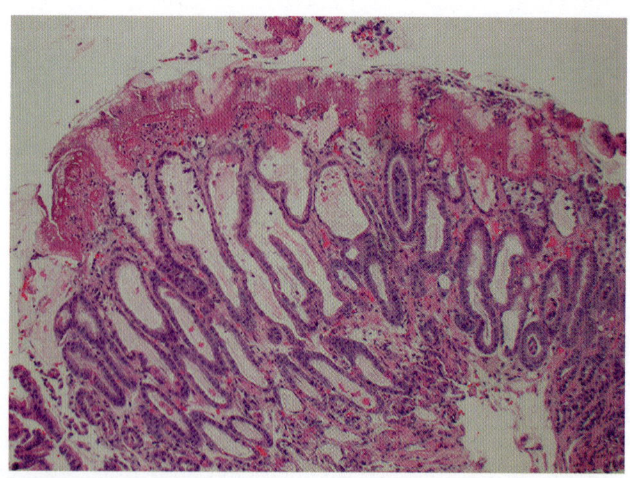

FIGURE 3.32

Acute erosive gastritis secondary to doxycycline involving antrum. The surface is completely denuded and replaced by a fibrinous exudate. The striking eosinophilic necrosis of the walls of superficial capillaries in the mucosa *(top left)* is typical of this entity.

"watermelon stomach" pattern. Reactive gastropathy, such as that caused by NSAIDs, might also be a consideration in cases with foveolar hyperplasia but lacks the characteristic vascular degenerative changes seen with doxycycline. Small vessel vasculitis is rare in the stomach, and changes in doxycycline injury are restricted to the areas of mucosal erosion and necrosis and clinical features suggestive of vasculitis are lacking.

Prognosis and Therapy

The symptoms decrease and mucosal changes heal after discontinuation of doxycycline.

MÉNÉTRIER'S DISEASE

Ménétrier's disease is a rare acquired disorder involving the gastric body characterized by diffuse gastric rugal hypertrophy, hypoproteinemia, and hypochlorhydria secondary to excessive mucosal protein loss. Synonyms include *giant hypertrophic gastritis, hypoproteinemic hypertrophic gastropathy*, and *giant mucosal rugae*.

CLINICAL FEATURES

Ménétrier's disease has been described in both adults and children (average age, fourth to sixth decades of life). It is more common in men with a male-to-female ratio of 3 to 1. CMV is associated in 70 % of affected children. In contrast, *H. pylori* has been reported in 90 % of affected adults in some series and rarely in association with herpes simplex virus infection.

The disease course is usually chronic, with an unfavorable prognosis. Patients present with hypoproteinemia resulting from nonselective protein loss across the gastric mucosal barrier and peripheral edema. Studies have shown loss of immunoglobulins, albumin, and transferrin, and acid output may be low or normal. Symptoms appear insidiously and become progressive, consisting of vomiting, abdominal pain and dyspepsia, anorexia, and peripheral edema. A thickened gastric wall with marked enlargement of gastric mucosal folds is seen on endoscopy along with a fine reticulated barium pattern resulting from mucus hypersecretion. The risk for developing carcinoma with Ménétrier's disease is debatable. It is reported that the patients have a 2 % to 15 % lifetime risk, but the exact risk is unknown, and there is no consensus on the appropriate surveillance in these patients.

The pathogenesis remains uncertain, but overexpression of transforming growth factor-α (TGF-α) has a possible role. Transgenic mice that overproduce TGF-α in the stomach have many features of Ménétrier's disease, such as foveolar hyperplasia, increased mucin content, decreased parietal cell mass, and reduced acid production.

PATHOLOGIC FEATURES

Gross Findings

Gross findings consist of massively thickened irregular "cerebriform" gastric folds (1–3 cm in thickness) with large amounts of viscous mucus and superficial erosions (Fig. 3.33). These changes are seen in the proximal stomach, although localized or diffuse cases have been reported. Localized disease of the gastric antrum, with sparing of the fundus and body, mainly manifested by polyposis has also been observed.

Microscopic Findings

Ménétrier's disease is characterized by markedly elongated and tortuous foveolae lined by mucous cells that may show cystic dilatation of the pits and massive overproliferation of the surface mucus-producing cells. The glands may also extend into the submucosa and present as gastritis cystica profunda (Fig. 3.34). A reduction or even absence of oxyntic glandular component (parietal and chief cells) is frequent. Inflammation is usually scarce or absent, although prominent eosinophilia can be observed. In a subset of cases, lymphocytic gastritis showing marked intraepithelial lymphocytosis may be seen. Other changes include a thickened and disorganized muscularis mucosae, with strands of smooth muscles extending into the lamina propria. Immunostains for CMV and *H. pylori* may be helpful.

From a practical point of view, histologic examination on conventional endoscopic biopsies usually fails to

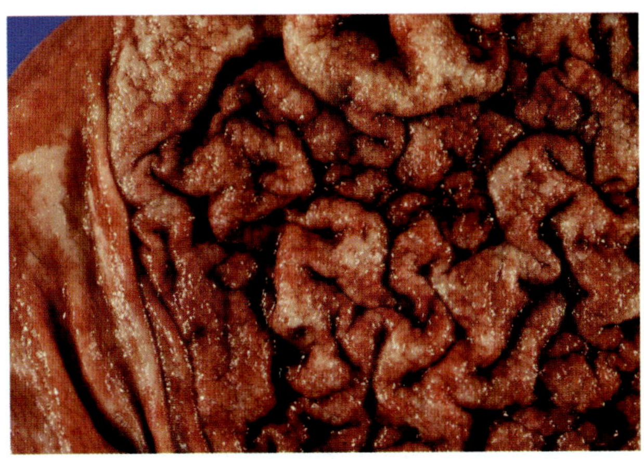

FIGURE 3.33

Ménétrier's disease. The giant mucosal hypertrophy of gastric body in Ménétrier's disease, with a cerebriform appearance. The antrum is spared. (**A**, Courtesy of Shriram Jakate, MD, Rush Medical College, Chicago).

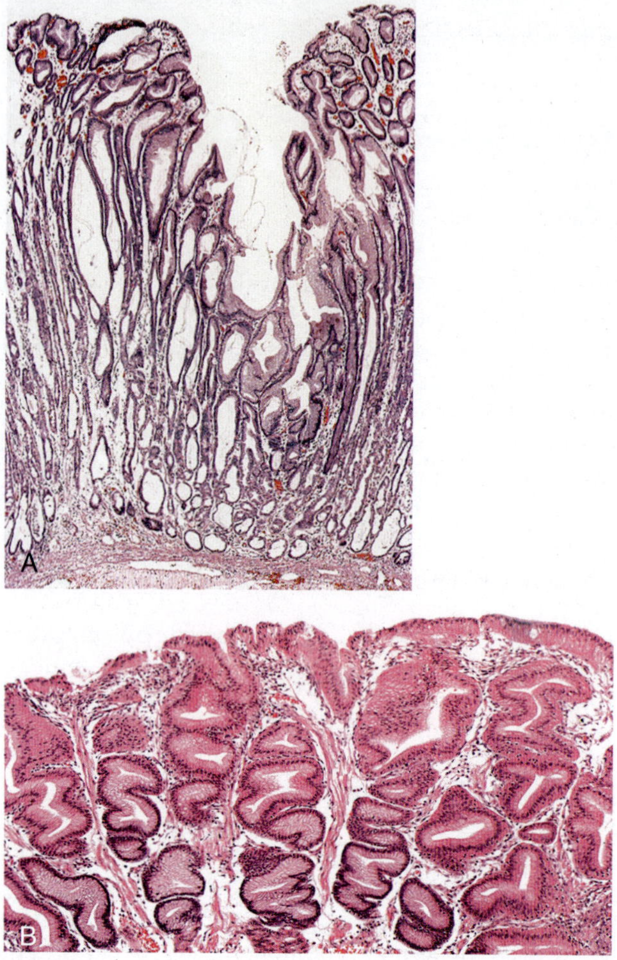

FIGURE 3.34

Low- and medium-power view of Ménétrier's disease: Marked tortuosity and elongation of gastric foveolar epithelium and cystic dilation of the deeper mucous glands (**A**). The oxyntic glands are replaced by mucous glands (**B**).

demonstrate the massive foveolar hyperplasia, and some recommend obtaining full-thickness biopsies. Because marked foveolar hyperplasia can be seen in a variety of conditions such as chemical gastropathy, hyperplastic polyps, and gastric ulcers and at the postgastroenterostomy stomal site, a diagnosis of Ménétrier's disease requires typical histologic findings in a full-thickness mucosal biopsy in conjunction with other clinical features.

Differential Diagnosis

The appearance of thick enlarged gastric folds is not specific to Ménétrier's disease and can be seen in a number of other conditions such as Zollinger-Ellison syndrome (ZES), gastric lymphoma, diffuse-type gastric cancer, *H. pylori* and CMV gastritis, granulomatous gastritis, eosinophilic gastritis, and gastric polyposis in Cronkhite-Canada syndrome. However, none of these diagnoses is associated with such a severe foveolar hyperplasia restricted to the gastric corpus.

Zollinger-Ellison syndrome shows hyperplasia of parietal and chief cells with increased acid production as a result of increased gastrin secretion caused by gastrinomas and is often associated with multiple gastric and duodenal ulcers but not with protein loss or foveolar hyperplasia.

Hyperplastic hypersecretory gastropathy is also associated with features similar to ZES, but the gastrin level is normal. Hyperplastic polyps are composed of prominent foveolae but are localized polypoid lesions and do not show the diffuse thick and enlarged gastric folds seen in Ménétrier's disease. Cronkhite-Canada syndrome involving the stomach may mimic Ménétrier's disease but is also associated with abnormalities in the colon and the gastric mucosa in Cronkhite-Canada syndrome is nodular and can also involve the antrum in contrast to the diffuse enlargement restricted to the gastric corpus seen in Ménétrier's disease.

Prognosis and Therapy

In adults, the disease course is chronic with an unfavorable prognosis. It seems reasonable to test and treat for CMV and *H. pylori* when these organisms are identified. Symptoms may improve with antibiotics, histamine H_2 blockers, anticholinergic agents that reduce gastric protein loss, corticosteroids, and octreotide (somatostatin analogue). One study reported marked improvement in symptoms such as vomiting and increased serum albumin after an experimental treatment with cetuximab, a monoclonal antibody against directed epidermal growth factor receptor. Partial or total gastrectomy is reserved for patients with severe complications such as massive bleeding and those with refractory protein loss or obstructive symptoms.

ZOLLINGER-ELLISON SYNDROME

Zollinger-Ellison syndrome is a triad consisting of hypergastrinemia caused by gastrin-secreting tumors (gastrinomas), increased acid production, and severe peptic ulcer disease.

CLINICAL FEATURES

Zollinger-Ellison syndrome has an incidence rate of 0.1 to 3 per million people in the United States and comprises 0.1% of all duodenal ulcer patients. It affects adults and children (age range, 7–90 years; average age,

50 years). Male and female patients show an equal disease distribution. ZES is characterized by gastrinomas located usually in the duodenum, pancreas, or area adjacent to the common bile duct (gastrinoma triangle). The secondary hypergastrinemia leads to persistent and massive secretion of acid and pepsin, giving rise to multiple and recurrent peptic ulcers, severe esophagitis, enteritis, epigastric pain, diarrhea, malabsorption, and weight loss. The massive acid output causes inactivation of pancreatic enzymes and bile salts, leading to malabsorption and diarrhea. An elevated fasting serum gastrin level of greater than 1000 pg/mL is virtually diagnostic of ZES.

Other clinical features include a positive secretin test result (secretin injection followed by elevation of gastrin >200 pg/mL above basal level) and basal acid output greater than 10 mEq/hr but is seldom needed now for diagnosis.

Eighty percent of patients with ZES have sporadic gastrinomas. In the remaining 20% of patients with ZES, gastrinomas are part of MEN-I syndrome. MEN-I is an autosomal dominant disorder resulting from mutations in the MEN-I gene on chromosome 11q13, which encodes for a 610–amino acid protein, menin. MEN-I is characterized by parathyroid hyperplasia, pancreatic endocrine tumors, pituitary adenomas, and adrenal adenomas.

Imaging studies such as computed tomography (CT) and magnetic resonance imaging (MRI) demonstrate markedly thickened gastric folds. Imaging studies such as somatostatin receptor scintigraphy (gastrinomas have somatostatin type 2 receptors) and endoscopic ultrasonography are sensitive modalities to localize gastrinomas and are often used along with abdominal CT and MRI for staging.

Pathologic Features

Gross Findings

Zollinger-Ellison syndrome causes massive hypertrophy of gastric rugae in the body and fundus that can range from 0.6 to 4.5 cm in thickness (Fig. 3.35). The antral mucosa is often reduced in thickness.

Microscopic Findings

The trophic effect of gastrin causes increased thickness of oxyntic mucosa in ZES (Fig. 3.36). Parietal cells show hypertrophy and hyperplasia and extend up to the foveolar neck region (Fig. 3.37). Parietal cells can also extend into the gastric antrum. Excess gastrin also causes physiologic hyperplasia of ECL cells in the gastric corpus, leading to linear and nodular ECL hyperplasia. Well-differentiated neuroendocrine tumors may be seen in up to 37% of patients with MEN-I–associated ZES. However, this is almost never seen in patients with sporadic ZES.

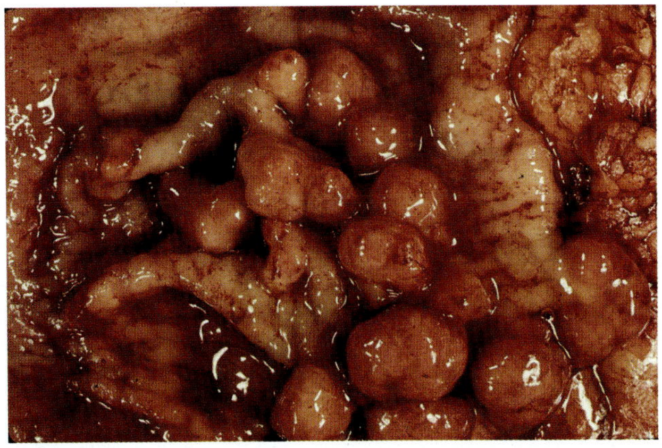

FIGURE 3.35

Zollinger-Ellison syndrome. Note the massive hypertrophy of gastric rugal folds with polypoid appearance. (Courtesy of Shriram Jakate, MD, Rush Medical College, Chicago).

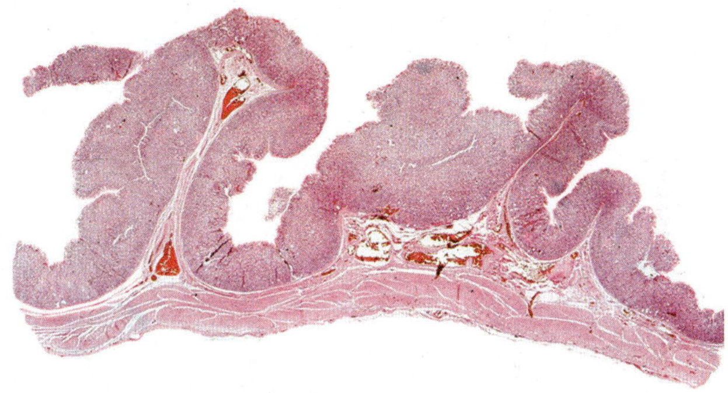

FIGURE 3.36

Low-power view shows the diffuse hyperplasia of gastric oxyntic mucosa in Zollinger-Ellison syndrome.

Gastrinomas stain for gastrin, chromogranin, and synaptophysin. ECL hyperplasia and neuroendocrine tumors stain for chromogranin and vesicular monoamine transporter, isoform 2 (VMAT-2), which regulates the intravesicular accumulation of histamine. The ECL cells are negative for gastrin, somatostatin, and serotonin.

Differential Diagnosis

Ménétrier's disease is associated with gastric rugal hypertrophy, protein-losing gastropathy, and hypochlorhydria. In contrast to ZES, acid secretion is generally reduced. Microscopically, Ménétrier's disease is associated with giant foveolar hyperplasia, and the oxyntic cells are replaced by mucous cells, whereas ZES is associated with hypergastrinemia, leading to hyperplasia of oxyntic mucosa and ECL

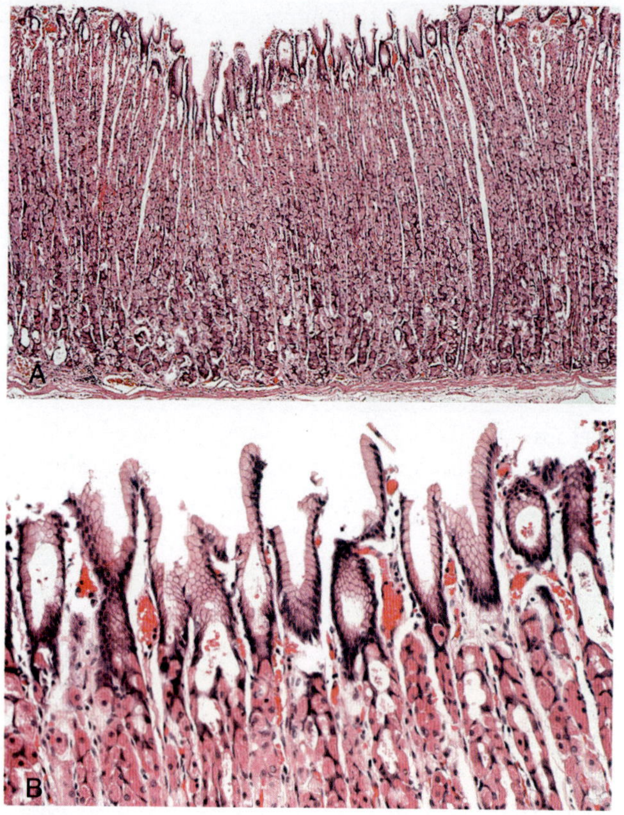

FIGURE 3.37
Zollinger-Ellison syndrome, medium-power view shows striking parietal cell hyperplasia and hypertrophy of parietal cells extending up to foveolar neck.

cells in the gastric body and fundus. Autoimmune gastritis is another important cause of hypergastrinemia. However, unlike ZES, the gastric body shows atrophy rather than hypertrophy of oxyntic glands along with hypochlorhydria or achlorhydria. The majority of patients with autoimmune gastritis have antibodies against the intrinsic factor and parietal cells. In addition, most patients present with symptoms associated with megaloblastic and iron-deficiency anemia caused by reduced vitamin B_{12} concentration and concurrent reduced iron absorption.

Chronic active *H. pylori* gastritis often results in antral G-cell hyperplasia, acid hypersecretion, and peptic ulcer disease. However, the nature of inflammatory infiltrate (superficial predominant lymphoplasmacytic inflammation with or without activity) and the presence of curved bacilli help in distinguishing it from ZES.

Prognosis and Therapy

Patients with ZES require long-term medical therapy for adequate control of gastric hypersecretion with PPIs such as omeprazole or lansoprazole. Partial or total gastrectomy may be required for intractable cases. Patients with localized well-differentiated gastrinomas without metastases are ideal candidates for surgical removal of the tumor. Patients with hepatic or distant metastases are managed with chemotherapy, hormonal therapy, or surgical debulking. Achieving surgical cure in ZES patients with MEN-I is more difficult, and patients need to be on lifelong acid suppressors. The need for family screening and screening for endocrine tumor elsewhere also is important. ZES patients who have had successful tumor resection show a 60 % to 100 % survival rate at 10 years. Patients with unresectable tumors have a 40 % survival rate at 5 years. Patients with MEN-I have better 5- and 10-year survival rates than do those with sporadic ZES

GASTRIC AMYLOIDOSIS

Amyloidosis is a group of disorders thought to be secondary to misfolding of extracellular proteins. Similar to other organs, the stomach can also be affected by amyloidosis. Gastric involvement almost always represents the systemic form of amyloidosis and is characterized by the deposition of extracellular, insoluble, β-pleated fibrillary protein sheets anywhere within the wall of the stomach. Localized form of amyloidosis is extremely rare.

CLINICAL FEATURES

Amyloidosis is classified based on the fibril precursor protein (AL, amyloid light chain; AA, amyloid; ATTR, amyloid transthyretin; Aβ2M, β2 microglobulin related) and can be present as following clinical syndromes: systemic AL amyloidosis (associated with plasma cell neoplasia), systemic AA amyloidosis (associated with infectious or inflammatory or neoplastic disorders), β2-microglobulin amyloidosis (associated with long-term renal dialysis), hereditary systemic amyloidosis (associated with autosomal dominant deposition of ATTR), and senile systemic amyloidosis (associated with wild-type transthyretin deposition). In general, the GI tract, including the stomach, is most commonly affected by systemic AL form of amyloidosis.

Patients present with nausea and vomiting, weight loss, malabsorption, gastric outlet obstruction, gastroparesis, and stasis-related change such as bacterial overgrowth and diarrhea. Amyloid deposits in the blood vessels make the vessels fragile and leaky, leading to hemorrhage. Rarely, gastric amyloidosis may present as a tumoral mass and can be mistaken for a carcinoma.

GASTRIC AMYLOIDOSIS—FACT SHEET

Definition

- Extracellular deposition of insoluble, fibrillary β-pleated amyloid protein sheets in the gastric mucosa

Morbidity and Mortality

- May be associated with fatal bleeding

Gender, Race, and Age

- Patients are usually old adults, except in hereditary cases

Clinical Features

- Hemorrhage, nausea and vomiting, weight loss, malabsorption, and diarrhea
- Gastric outlet obstruction, gastroparesis, and stasis-related changes

Prognosis and Therapy

- Depends on the type and extent of deposits as well involvement of other organs
- AL amyloidosis has the worst prognosis
- Therapy is directed at reducing the supply of precursor proteins
- Bortezomib (a proteasome inhibitor) as a single agent or in combination with dexamethasone is now considered first-line therapy for patients with AL amyloidosis

Pathologic Features

Gross Findings

Endoscopic appearance consists of mucosal erosions, ulcers, thickened folds, and less commonly, a localized mass (Fig. 3.38). Resection specimens with massive amyloid deposition have thick and rigid walls with a waxy appearance.

Microscopic Findings

The distribution of amyloid can be patchy or diffuse. On H&E section, amyloid deposits appear as dense, homogenous, acellular, eosinophilic extracellular deposits within the lamina propria, submucosa, muscularis propria, nerve trunks, and vessel walls (Fig. 3.39). Amyloid deposits often show "cracking" with slit-like spaces as a result of tissue processing artifact. In biopsy specimens, amyloid is often present within the lamina propria as irregularly distributed deposits, which may have a globular appearance. If the specimen contains superficial submucosa, these deposits are visible in the perivascular region as well as within the vessel wall.

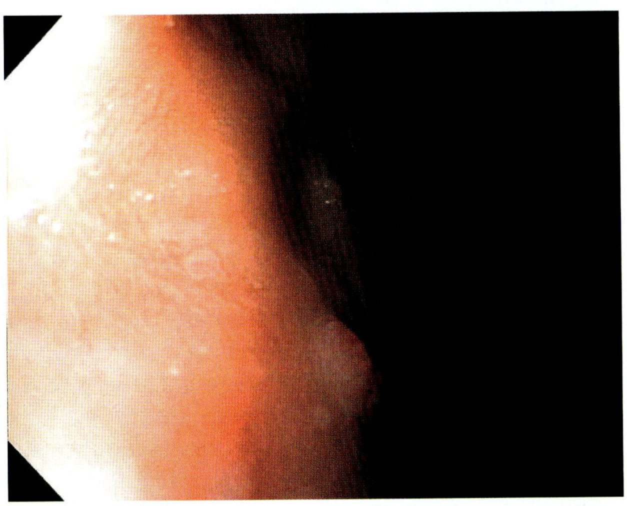

FIGURE 3.38

Endoscopic appearance of gastric amyloidosis with thick, vaguely nodular mucosa. (Courtesy of Shriram Jakate, MD, Rush Medical College, Chicago).

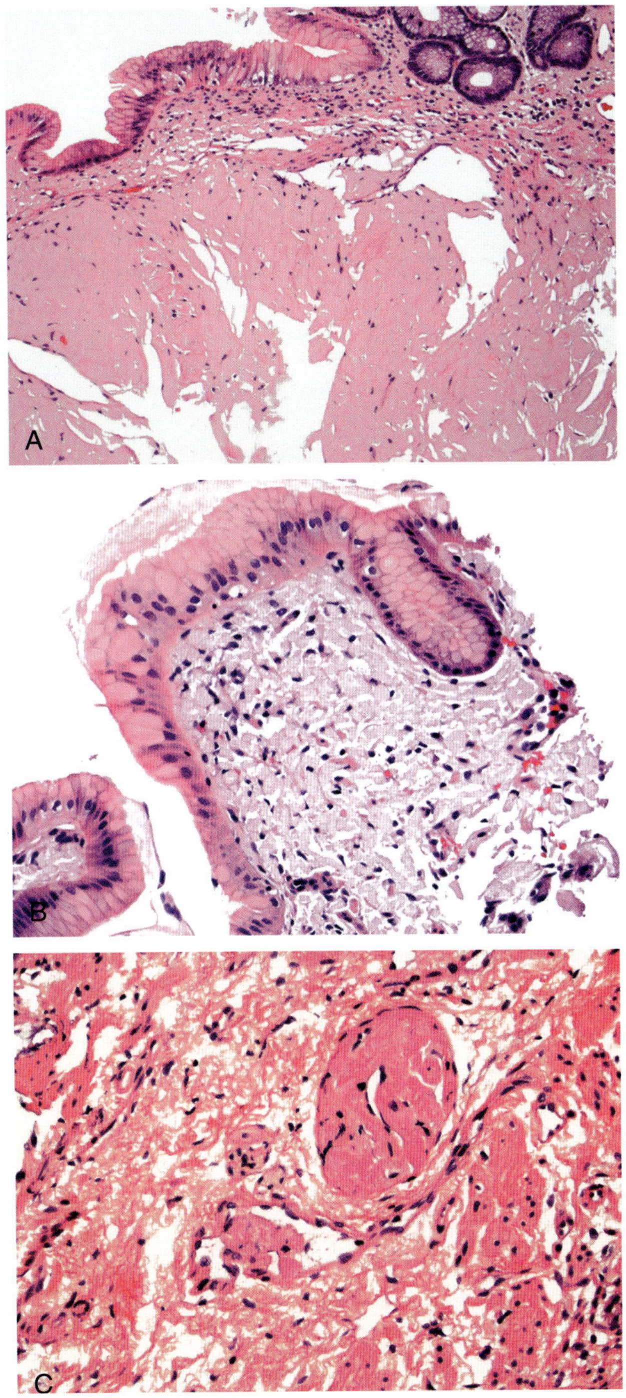

FIGURE 3.39

A, Gastric amyloid, consisting of eosinophilic, acellular deposits with cracking artifact appearing as a tumoral mass. **B**, Notice the globular amyloid deposits beneath the foveolar epithelium. **C**, Vascular amyloid deposits.

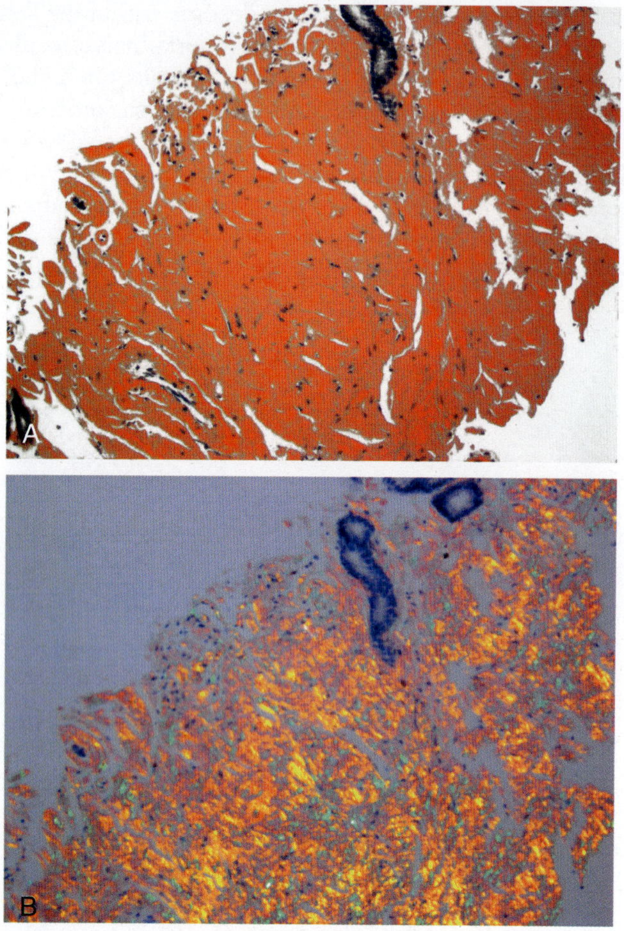

FIGURE 3.40
The amyloid appears brick red using standard illumination light (**A**) and, with polarization (**B**), showing bright-green birefringence.

A Congo red stain shows bright orange positivity in areas of amyloid deposition with a characteristic apple-green birefringence on polarized microscopy (Fig. 3.40). Immunostains may be used to classify the type of amyloid, which is helpful with patient management.

Gastric Amyloid—Pathologic Features

Gross Findings

- Mucosal erosions, ulcers, thickened folds, tumoral mass
- Thick and rigid walls with waxy appearance

Microscopic Findings

- Dense, homogenous, acellular, eosinophilic extracellular deposits in the lamina propria, submucosa, muscularis propria, nerve trunks, and vascular wall
- Nonbranching fibrils 7.5 to 10 nm in diameter on ultrastructural examination
- Congo red—characteristic apple-green birefringence on polarized light
- Thioflavin T—fluorescent dye
- Immunostains can be used to subclassify type of amyloid

Differential Diagnosis

- Vascular arteriosclerosis
- Systemic sclerosis
- Ischemic gastritis, radiation gastritis, and other causes of lamina propria fibrosis

Differential Diagnosis

Arteriosclerosis of vessels with hyalinization may be mistaken for amyloid deposits. Masson's trichrome stains the sclerosis blue, and Congo red stain is negative. Connective tissue disorder such as scleroderma, resulting in fibrosis of muscularis and submucosa, which may be mistaken for amyloid but are seldom biopsied. Masson's trichrome stains the collagen blue, and Congo red is negative. Ischemic gastritis is associated with hemorrhage, unlike amyloidosis, and radiation gastritis and other causes of lamina propria fibrosis are associated with increased collagen in the lamina propria that is easily distinguished from amyloid deposits

Prognosis and Therapy

Prognosis depends on the type, extent, and severity of amyloid deposit; organs involved; and severity of the underlying disease. Microscopic focal deposits in older adults may be of no clinical significance, but widespread deposition can be a progressive and even fatal disease. Therapy is mostly directed at reducing the supply of precursor proteins, correcting bleeding problems, and enhancing motility. Liver transplantation is curative in hereditary transthyretin amyloidosis because the mutated transthyretin is produced by the liver.

GASTRIC ANTRAL VASCULAR ECTASIA ("WATERMELON STOMACH")

Gastric antral vascular ectasia is an uncommon cause of acute or chronic occult GI bleeding that is characterized endoscopically by linear vascular stripes in the gastric antrum.

CLINICAL FEATURES

Gastric antral vascular ectasia is an uncommon condition that is increasingly recognized as a cause of acute or chronic GI blood loss leading to iron-deficiency anemia. The anemia can be severe and refractory to iron replacement therapy and may require blood transfusions. GAVE primarily affects women (76%), with a mean age of 69 years (range, 42–89 years). Clinical presentations include iron-deficiency anemia (88%), heme-positive stool (42%), melena (15%), and rarely hematemesis (3%) and hematochezia (1%). GAVE is commonly associated with autoimmune and connective tissue disorders such as Raynaud's phenomenon, sclerodactyly, autoimmune gastritis, hypothyroidism, primary biliary cirrhosis, autoimmune liver disease, and diabetes mellitus. Other associations include cirrhosis, chronic renal failure, and cardiovascular disease. The pathogenesis is unknown. It has been proposed that traumatic gastric peristalsis and subsequent prolapse of antral mucosa through the pylorus may cause vascular ectasia. Humoral factors such as hypergastrinemia, proliferation of neuroendocrine cells secreting vasoactive intestinal polypeptide (VIP), and 5-hydroxy tryptamine (serotonin) have also been speculated.

GASTRIC ANTRAL VASCULAR ECTASIA ("WATERMELON STOMACH")—FACT SHEET

Definition

- Uncommon cause of acute or chronic gastric bleeding characterized endoscopically by linear vascular stripes in the gastric antrum

Morbidity and Mortality

- Related mainly to gastrointestinal blood loss
- May give rise to severe anemia refractory to iron replacement therapy, requiring blood transfusions

Gender, Race, and Age

- Female predominance (76% are women)
- Mean age 69 years (range, 42–89 years)

Clinical Features

- Iron-deficiency anemia (88%), heme-positive stool (42%), melena (15%), and rarely hematemesis (3%) and hematochezia (1%)
- Commonly associated with autoimmune and connective tissue disorders such as Raynaud's phenomenon, sclerodactyly, autoimmune gastritis, hypothyroidism, primary biliary cirrhosis, autoimmune liver disease, and diabetes mellitus
- Other associations include cirrhosis, chronic renal failure, after bone marrow transplantation, and cardiovascular disease

Prognosis and Therapy

- Treatment is dictated by the rate of blood loss
- Conservative management includes iron supplement or blood transfusion, which may be insufficient
- Various endoscopic treatment modalities include laser, heater probe therapy, bipolar electrocautery, and injection sclerotherapy
- Surgical antrectomy offers definitive therapy but carries a mortality rate of 7.4%

PATHOLOGIC FEATURES

GROSS FINDINGS

The phrase "watermelon stomach" describes the characteristic endoscopic appearance of GAVE consisting of parallel, intensely red vascular stripes situated at the crests of mucosal folds traversing the gastric antrum and converging on the pylorus (Fig. 3.41). A surgical resection specimen can show a thickened antral wall with prominent submucosal vessels running in a longitudinal direction toward the pylorus.

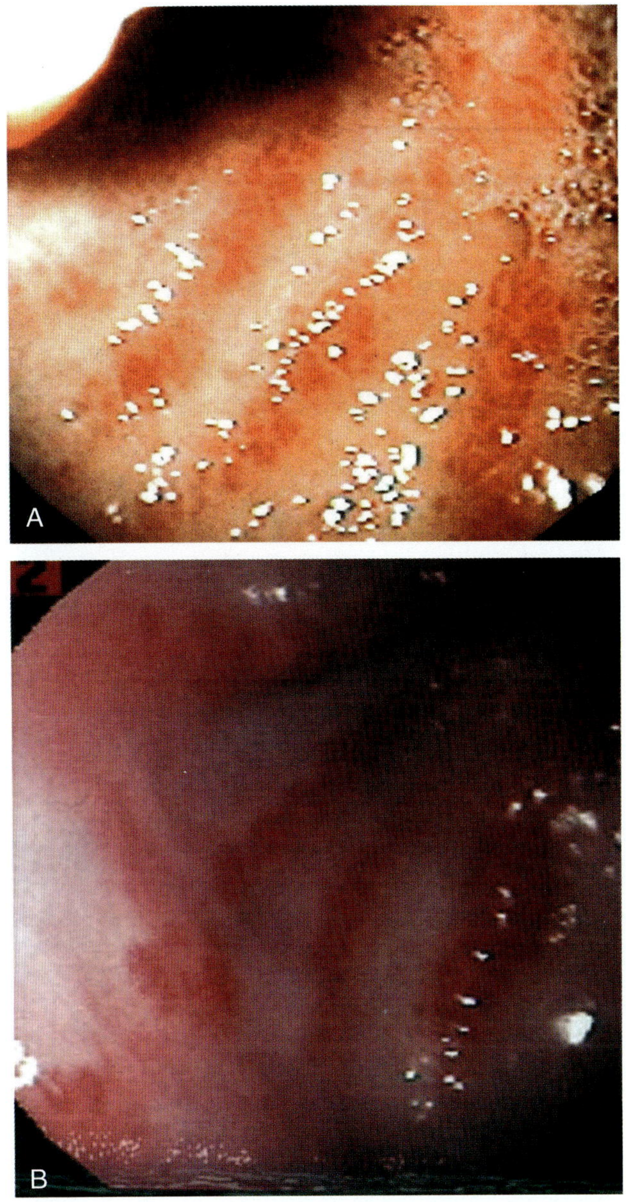

FIGURE 3.41

Characteristic endoscopic appearance of gastric antral vascular ectasia. Note the parallel, intensely red vascular stripes resembling watermelon, in two separate patients (**A** and **B**). (A, Courtesy of Shriram Jakate, MD, Rush Medical College, Chicago).

MICROSCOPIC FINDINGS

The histologic appearance consists of foveolar hyperplasia, dilated mucosal capillaries with fibrin thrombi, and fibromuscular hyperplasia of lamina propria with minimal or absent inflammation. The presence of fibrin thrombi is important for diagnosis (Fig. 3.42). In subtle cases, CD61 stain can highlight thrombi within capillaries to support the diagnosis. The submucosal vessels are also dilated and tortuous. The foveolar epithelium may show reactive

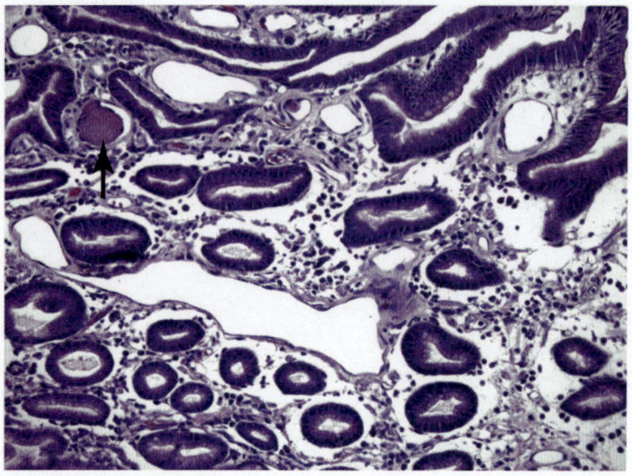

FIGURE 3.42

Gastric antral vascular ectasia. Antral biopsy shows foveolar hyperplasia, dilated mucosal capillaries with fibrin thrombi, the fibrin thrombi *(arrows)*, which are helpful for diagnosis.

epithelial changes consisting of mucin loss and preserved nuclear-to-cytoplasmic ratio. The gastric body may show atrophic gastritis with intestinal metaplasia. The gastric cardia can also be involved in a subset of cases.

Gastric Antral Vascular Ectasia ("Watermelon Stomach")—Pathologic Features

Gross Findings

- Predominantly located in the antrum; may also involve the cardia
- Endoscopic appearance consisting of intense red, linear, vascular stripes situated at the crests of mucosal folds traversing the gastric antrum and converging on the pylorus
- Resection specimen shows thickened antral wall with dilated and tortuous submucosal vessels

Microscopic Findings

- Dilated mucosal capillaries with characteristic fibrin thrombi (CD61 positive) and fibromuscular hyperplasia of lamina propria with minimal or absent inflammation
- The submucosal vessels may also be dilated and tortuous
- Minimal or no inflammation in the lamina propria

Differential Diagnosis

- Portal hypertensive gastropathy

Differential Diagnosis

The distinction between GAVE and *portal hypertensive gastropathy* (PHG) is summarized in Table 3.6. PHG involves the gastric corpus, usually spares the antrum, and is seen in patients with cirrhosis and portal hypertension. The gastric corpus mucosa shows distended capillaries but may be completely normal because the shunts may involve the larger submucosal vessels. Endoscopy in PHG shows a characteristic "snake-skin" appearance unlike the watermelon appearance seen in GAVE. It is important to emphasize that GAVE may be present in a subset of patients with cirrhosis, and severe PHG may also involve the antrum. The distinction is important because GAVE is a localized disorder that can be treated with endoscopic therapy, but PHG is a systemic condition that requires medical or surgical intervention to lower portal pressures in patients with varices.

TABLE 3.6

Comparison of Distinction between Gastric Antral Vascular Ectasia and Portal Hypertensive Gastropathy

	Gastric Antral Vascular Ectasia	Portal Hypertensive Gastropathy
Location	Predominantly antrum	Predominantly body
Endoscopic appearance	Linear red stripes resembling a watermelon	Diffuse mosaic vascular pattern, cherry-red spots, scarlatina rash
Endoscopic ultrasound	Thin atrophic gastric wall with thickening limited to antral region	Diffusely thickened gastric wall with dilated veins
Characteristic histology	Dilated mucosal capillaries with thrombi	Vascular ectasia, perivascular stromal thickening
Associated conditions	AutoiDmmune and connective tissue diseases, also cirrhosis	Cirrhosis with portal hypertension
Management	Endoscopic laser therapy, antrectomy	Portal decompression, shunting

Prognosis and Therapy

Treatment is based mainly on the rate of blood loss. Conservative management with iron supplement or blood transfusion may be insufficient. Various endoscopic modalities are available and include laser, heater probe therapy, bipolar electrocautery, and injection sclerotherapy. Excellent results have been shown with laser therapy. Surgical antrectomy offers definitive therapy but carries a mortality rate of 7.4%.

PORTAL HYPERTENSIVE GASTROPATHY

The term *portal hypertensive gastropathy* is used to describe the vascular manifestations of portal hypertension in the stomach characterized by a mosaic mucosal appearance ("snake skin") with or without red spots on endoscopy.

CLINICAL FEATURES

Portal hypertensive gastropathy is seen in patients with cirrhotic or noncirrhotic portal hypertension. Patients usually present with mild bleeding, and unlike GAVE, anemia or transfusion requirement is less common. The stomach is most often involved, but the small intestine and colon can also show manifestations of portal hypertension (portal hypertensive intestinal vasculopathy, portal colopathy). PHG can affect adults and children, and a male predominance is present. The pathogenesis of PHG is thought to be hemodynamic alterations and increased splenic circulation resulting in increased gastric mucosal blood flow caused by portal hypertension. Patients who have undergone sclerotherapy or banding for their esophageal varices are at higher risk of developing PHG.

PORTAL HYPERTENSIVE GASTROPATHY—FACT SHEET

Definition

- Vascular manifestations of portal hypertension in the stomach consisting of a mosaic mucosal pattern ("snake-skin" appearance) with or without red spots on endoscopy

Morbidity and Mortality

- Morbidity is related to the low-volume blood loss
- Not a significant cause of mortality

Gender, Race, and Age

- Male predominance

Clinical Features

- Seen in patients with cirrhotic or noncirrhotic portal hypertension
- Mild bleeding
- Patients who have undergone sclerotherapy or banding for their esophageal varices are at higher risk of developing portal hypertensive gastropathy

Prognosis and Therapy

- Transjugular intrahepatic portosystemic shunt and shunt surgery
- Nonselective β-blockers such as propranolol

PATHOLOGIC FEATURES

GROSS FINDINGS

Portal hypertensive gastropathy typically involves the proximal stomach (an important distinction from GAVE). The endoscopic appearance ranges from diffuse fine pink speckling or "scarlatina" rash with a mosaic pattern resembling snake skin (Fig. 3.43) to severe gastropathy with cherry-red spots and diffuse hemorrhagic gastropathy.

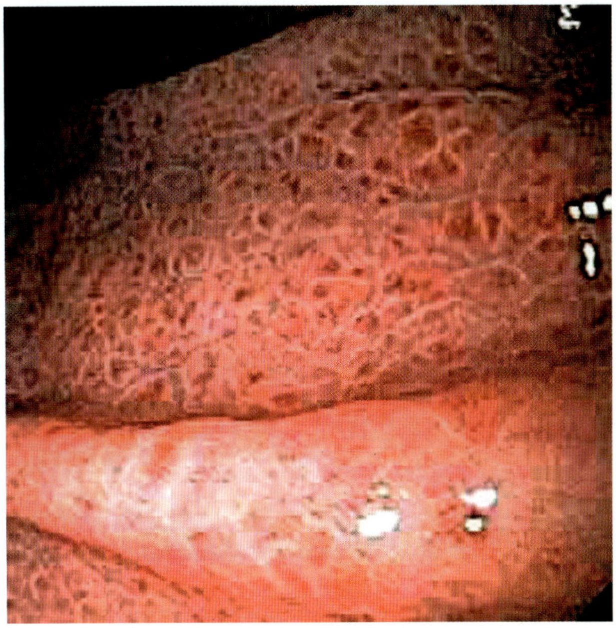

FIGURE 3.43
"Mosaic" or snake-skin appearance of the gastric body mucosa in a patient with portal hypertensive gastropathy.

MICROSCOPIC FINDINGS

The histologic findings consist of marked congestive vasculopathy with dilated mucosal capillaries and venules (Figs. 3.44 and 3.45), but the mucosa may also be completely normal and changes confined to larger submucosal vessels. The submucosal veins show marked congestion, intimal thickening, and tortuosity. The ectatic vessels are accompanied by perivascular stromal fibrosis, lamina propria edema, and scant or absent inflammation. Fibrin thrombi are absent.

For these reasons, mucosal biopsies often have low yield given the predominantly submucosal vascular abnormalities, and endoscopists are reluctant to get deeper biopsies given the coagulation abnormalities in these cirrhotic patients.

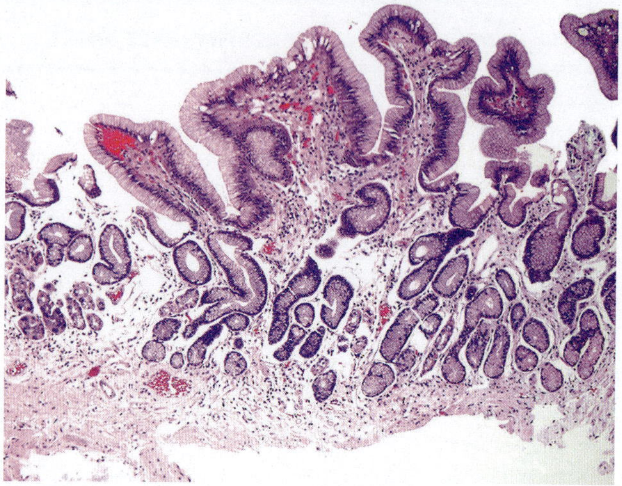

FIGURE 3.44

Gastric mucosal biopsy in a portal hypertensive gastropathy with dilated mucosal capillaries and congestion. Note the absence of fibrin thrombi.

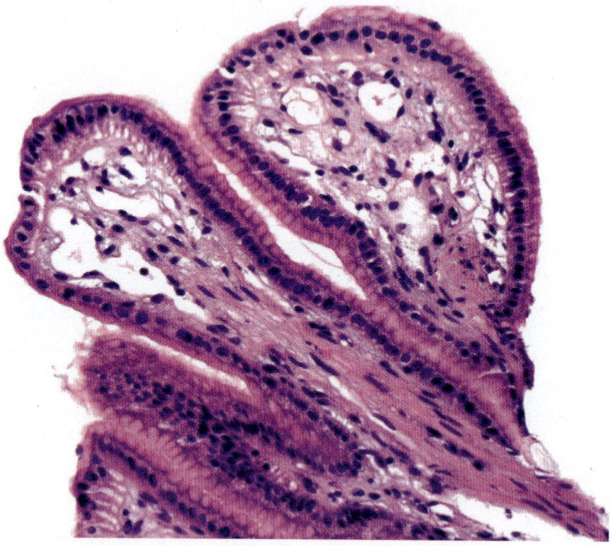

FIGURE 3.45

High-power view showing prominent and dilated mucosal capillaries in *portal hypertensive gastropathy.*

Differential Diagnosis

The differential diagnosis is typically with GAVE which is discussed in the section earlier and summarized in Table 3.6.

Prognosis and Therapy

Portal decompression procedures such as transjugular intrahepatic portosystemic shunt and shunt surgery are effective in resolving the gastropathy and bleeding. Nonselective β-blockers such as propranolol have shown promise in preventing bleeding.

Portal Hypertensive Gastropathy—Pathologic Features

Gross Findings

- Portal hypertensive gastropathy involves the fundus and body; may also involve the antrum in some cases
- Endoscopic appearance ranges from diffuse fine pink speckling or "scarlatina" rash with a mosaic pattern resembling "snake-skin" to severe gastropathy with cherry-red spots and diffuse hemorrhagic gastropathy

Microscopic Findings

- Marked congestive vasculopathy with dilated mucosal capillaries and venules
- Changes are more prominent in submucosal veins, which show marked congestion, intimal thickening, and tortuosity
- Fibrin thrombi are absent
- Mucosal biopsies often have low yield

Differential Diagnosis

- Gastric antral vascular ectasia

DIEULAFOY'S LESION (CALIBER PERSISTENT ARTERY)

Dieulafoy's lesion is an uncommon cause of recurrent and often massive upper GI bleeding. It presents as a small mucosal defect overlying an artery of persistent large caliber in the mucosa.

CLINICAL FEATURES

Dieulafoy's lesion typically presents as recurrent, often massive upper GI bleeding without preceding symptoms. Patients develop hematemesis, melena, and anemia frequently needing red cell transfusions. Symptoms such as abdominal pain, anorexia, and dyspepsia are not common. History of NSAID use, peptic ulcer, and alcohol abuse is notably absent.

The lesion is usually found in the proximal fundus within 6 cm of the gastroesophageal junction, along the lesser curvature. Apart from stomach, other sites such as the duodenum, jejunum, large intestine, and rectum can be involved. It is slightly more common in boys and men (male-to-female ratio, 2 to 1), with a median age of 54 years (range, 16–91 years).

Pathologic Features

Gross Findings

The endoscopic appearance consists of a 2- to 5-mm mucosal defect with a protruding vessel. The mucosa may

DIEULAFOY'S LESION (CALIBER PERSISTENT ARTERY)—FACT SHEET

Definition

- Dieulafoy's lesion is an uncommon cause of upper gastrointestinal (GI) bleeding consisting of a small mucosal defect overlying an artery of persistent large caliber in the mucosa

Incidence and Location

- The incidence as a cause of GI bleeding varies from 0.3% to 6.7%
- Typically located in the proximal fundus within 6 cm of the gastroesophageal junction, along the lesser curvature
- Extra gastric lesions are uncommon, but rarely, the duodenum, jejunum, large intestine, and rectum can also be involved

Morbidity and Mortality

- Modern endoscopic therapeutic modalities have reduced morbidity and mortality rates

Gender, Race, and Age

- Slightly more common in males, with a male-to-female ratio of 2 to 1
- Median age, 54 years; range, 16 to 91 years

Clinical Features

- Presents as recurrent, often massive upper GI bleeding without preceding symptoms
- Symptoms include hematemesis, melena, and anemia frequently needing red cell transfusions
- Abdominal pain, anorexia, and dyspepsia are uncommon
- History of nonsteroidal antiinflammatory drug use, peptic ulcer, or alcohol abuse is notably absent
- Almost 80% of the lesions are identified by endoscopy, sometimes requiring multiple endoscopies
- Angiography and endoscopic ultrasonography are useful to identify lesions not detected by white-light endoscopy

Prognosis and Therapy

- Endoscopic therapeutic modalities are the first line of treatment, including electrocoagulation, hemoclipping, banding, epinephrine injection, and injection sclerotherapy
- Recurrent bleeding may warrant surgical therapy, which includes gastrotomy with ligation of the responsible vessel and proximal gastric resection

look normal between bleeding episodes. This diagnosis should be seriously considered when a patient presents with massive GI bleeding without an endoscopically identifiable source of bleeding because this lesion may be difficult to visualize because of its proximal fundic location.

MICROSCOPIC FINDINGS

The characteristic histology on resection consists of a large-caliber muscular artery with a tortuous course through the submucosa, focally extending to the mucosa and communicating with the gastric lumen. The vessel may show partial disruption, with the overlying mucosa showing erosion, hemorrhage, and blood clots. There is no evidence of deep ulceration or disruption of the muscularis propria. Arteriosclerosis, calcification, aneurysmal dilation, and vasculitis are absent, and the surrounding gastric mucosa is essentially normal.

DIEULAFOY'S LESION (CALIBER PERSISTENT ARTERY)—PATHOLOGIC FEATURES

Gross Findings

- The endoscopic appearance consists of a 2- to 5-mm mucosal defect with a protruding vessel

Microscopic Findings

- Histology consists of a large-caliber muscular artery with a tortuous course through the submucosa focally extending to the mucosa and into the gastric lumen
- The large-caliber vessel may show partial disruption with the overlying mucosa showing erosion, hemorrhage, and blood clots; arteriosclerosis, calcification, aneurysmal dilation, and vasculitis are not observed. The surrounding gastric mucosa is essentially normal

Differential Diagnosis

- Other causes of bleeding, such as Mallory Weiss tear, peptic ulcer disease, angiodysplasia, chemical gastropathy, and gastric antral vascular ectasia, need to be ruled out

DIFFERENTIAL DIAGNOSIS

Other causes of bleeding such as Mallory-Weiss tear, peptic ulcer disease, angiodysplasia, chemical gastropathy, and GAVE need to be ruled out, at least clinically.

PROGNOSIS AND THERAPY

Once associated with a high mortality rate, endoscopic therapeutic modalities have reduced mortality rates considerably provided that the lesion is identified and treated early. Therapeutic interventions consist of electrocoagulation, hemoclipping, banding, epinephrine injection, and injection sclerotherapy. Recurrent bleeding may warrant surgical therapy, which includes gastrotomy with ligation of the responsible vessel or proximal gastric resection.

SUGGESTED READINGS

1. Dixon MF, Genta RM, Yardley JH, et al. Classification and grading of gastritis. The updated Sydney System. International Workshop on the Histopathology of Gastritis, Houston 1994. *Am J Surg Pathol*. 1996;20(10):1161–1181.
2. Rugge M, Correa P, Di Mario F, et al. OLGA staging for gastritis: a tutorial. *Dig Liver Dis*. 2008;40(8):650–658.
3. Srivastava A, Lauwers GY. Pathology of non-infective gastritis. *Histopathology*. 2007;50(1):15–29.
4. El-Zimaity H, Choi WT, Lauwers GY, et al. The differential diagnosis of *Helicobacter pylori* negative gastritis. *Virchows Arch*. 2018;473(5):533–550.

5. Sugawa C, Lucas CE. Caustic injury of the upper gastrointestinal tract in adults: a clinical and endoscopic study. *Surgery*. 1989;106:802–806. Discussion 806–807.
6. Chamberlain CE. Acute hemorrhagic gastritis. *Gastroenterol. Clin. North Am*. 1993;22:843–873.
7. Dixon MF, O'Connor HJ, Axon AT, et al. Reflux gastritis: distinct histopathological entity? *J Clin Pathol*. 1986;39:524–530.
8. Quinn CM, Bjarnason I, Price AB. Gastritis in patients on non- steroidal anti-inflammatory drugs. *Histopathology*. 1993;23:341–348.
9. Abraham SC, Yardley JH, Wu TT. Erosive injury to the upper gastrointestinal tract in patients receiving iron medication: an underrecognized entity. *Am J Surg Pathol*. 1999;23:1241–1247.
10. Marginean EC, Bennick M, Cyczk J, et al. Gastric siderosis: patterns and significance. *Am J Surg Pathol*. 2006;30:514–520.
11. Greenson JK, Trinidad SB, Pfeil SA, et al. Gastric mucosal calcinosis. Calcified aluminum phosphate deposits secondary to aluminum-containing antacids or sucralfate therapy in organ transplant patients. *Am J Surg Pathol*. 1993;17:45–50.
12. Abraham SC, Bhagavan BS, Lee LA, et al. Upper gastrointestinal tract injury in patients receiving kayexalate (sodium polystyrene sulfonate) in sorbitol: clinical, endoscopic, and histopathologic findings. *Am J Surg Pathol*. 2001;25:637–644.
13. Torbenson M, Abraham SC, Boitnott J, et al. Autoimmune gastritis: distinct histological and immunohistochemical findings before complete loss of oxyntic glands. *Mod Pathol*. 2002;15:102–109.
14. Jevremovic D, Torbenson M, Murray JA, et al. Atrophic autoimmune pangastritis: a distinctive form of antral and fundic gastritis associated with systemic auto-immune disease. *Am J Surg Pathol*. 2006;30(11):1412–1419.
15. Wright CL, Riddell RH. Histology of the stomach and duodenum in Crohn's disease. *Am J Surg Pathol*. 1998;22:383–390.
16. Oberhuber G, Puspok A, Oesterreicher C, et al. Focally enhanced gastritis: a frequent type of gastritis in patients with Crohn's disease. *Gastroenterology*. 1997;112:698–706.
17. Ectors NL, Dixon MF, Geboes KJ, et al. Granulomatous gastritis: a morphological and diagnostic approach. *Histopathology*. 1993;23:55–61.
18. Fireman Z, Sternberg A, Yarchovsky Y, et al. Multiple antral ulcers in gastric sarcoid. *J Clin Gastroenterol*. 1997;24:97–99.
19. Croxon S, Chen K, Davidson AR. Sarcoidosis of the stomach. *Digestion*. 1987;38:193–196.
20. Haot J, Hamichi L, Wallez L, et al. Lymphocytic gastritis: a newly described entity: a retrospective endoscopic and histological study. *Gut*. 1988;29:1258–1264.
21. Wu TT, Hamilton SR. Lymphocytic gastritis: association with etiology and topology. *Am J Surg Pathol*. 1999;23:153–158.
22. Haot J, Bogomoletz WV, Jouret A, et al. Menetrier's disease with lymphocytic gastritis: an unusual association with possible pathogenic implications. *Hum Pathol*. 1991;22:379–386.
23. Wolfsen HC, Carpenter HA, Talley NJ. Menetrier's disease: a form of hypertrophic gastropathy or gastritis? *Gastroenterology*. 1993;104:1310–1319.
24. Lagorce-Pages C, Fabiani B, Bouvier R, et al. Collagenous gastritis: a report of six cases. *Am J Surg Pathol*. 2001;25:1174–1179.
25. Pulimood AB, Ramakrishna BS, Mathan MM. Collagenous gastritis and collagenous colitis: a report with sequential histo-logical and ultrastructural findings. *Gut*. 1999;44:881–885.
26. Goldman H, Proujansky R. Allergic proctitis and gastroenteritis in children. Clinical and mucosal biopsy features in 53 cases. *Am J Surg Pathol*. 1986;10:75–86.
27. Talley NJ, Shorter RG, Phillips SF, et al. Eosinophilic gastroenteritis: a clinicopathological study of patients with disease of the mucosa, muscle layer, and subserosal tissues. *Gut*. 1990;31:54–58.
28. Primignani M, Carpinelli L, Preatoni P, et al. Natural history of portal hypertensive gastropathy in patients with liver cirrhosis. The New Italian Endoscopic Club for the study and treatment of esophageal varices (NIEC). *Gastroenterology*. 2000;119:181–187.
29. Carpinelli L, Primignani M, Preatoni P, et al. Portal hypertensive gastropathy: reproducibility of a classification, prevalence of elementary lesions, sensitivity and specificity in the diagnosis of cirrhosis of the liver. A NIEC multicentre study. New Italian Endoscopic Club. *Ital J Gastroenterol Hepatol*. 1997;29:533–540.
30. Viggiano TR, Gostout CJ. Portal hypertensive intestinal vasculopathy: a review of the clinical, endoscopic, and histopathologic features. *Am J Gastroenterol*. 1992;87:944–954.
31. Jabbari M, Cherry R, Lough JO, et al. Gastric antral vascular ectasia: the watermelon stomach. *Gastroenterology*. 1984;87:1165–1170.
32. Payen JL, Cales P, Voigt JJ, et al. Severe portal hypertensive gastropathy and antral vascular ectasia are distinct entities in patients with cirrhosis. *Gastroenterology*. 1995;108:138–144.
33. Hoda RS, Sanyal S, Abraham JL, et al. Lanthanum deposition from oral lanthanum carbonate in the upper gastrointestinal tract. *Histopathology*. 2017;70(7):1072–1078.
34. Xiao SY, Zhao L, Hart J, et al. Doxycycline-induced gastric and esophageal mucosal injuries with vascular degeneration. *Am J Surg Pathol*. 2013;37(7):1115–1116.
35. Ebert EC, Nagar M. Gastrointestinal manifestations of amyloidosis. *Am J Gastroenterol*. 2008;103(3):776–787.
36. Said SM, Grogg KL, Smyrk TC. Gastric amyloidosis: clinicopathological correlations in 79 cases from a single institution. *Hum Pathol*. 2015;46(4):491–498.

4

Epithelial Polyps and Neoplasms of the Stomach

Bence Kővari, MD, PhD, Kwun Wah Wen, MD, PhD and Gregory Y. Lauwers, MD, PhD

Gastric carcinoma is the second most common gastrointestinal (GI) cancer worldwide, only behind colorectal carcinoma, with more than 1 million cases diagnosed annually. With the increasing use of endoscopy, the diagnosis of early gastric cancer is more frequent, and previously rare or unrecognized preneoplastic lesions have been described and better characterized. Diagnosis of gastric neoplasms and preneoplastic conditions has clinical management implications that impact surveillance or resection and sometimes screening of other organs and family members for inheritable syndromes.

GASTRIC POLYPS

Gastric polyps have many subtypes, all with characteristic endoscopic appearance, topography, and predisposing conditions, such as proton pump inhibitor (PPI) therapy, autoimmune gastritis, or polyposis syndromes. Assessment of the background antral and oxyntic mucosa is essential for the accurate evaluation of gastric polyps.

FUNDIC GLAND POLYPS

Fundic gland polyps (FGPs) are the most commonly diagnosed gastric polyps, comprising 77% of all polyps. These benign epithelial lesions are found in the gastric body and fundus and are characterized oxyntic gland proliferation with luminal dilation and various degrees of parietal cell hyperplasia and hypertrophy.

Clinical Features

Fundic gland polyps occur in two common settings, sporadic and syndromic. In the sporadic setting, the polyps are most commonly detected in the fourth to sixth decade of life. However, in syndromic cases, the polyps occur in younger individuals in the second or third decade. They can be seen even in children and show an equal sex distribution. Patients are mostly asymptomatic or may present with mild abdominal pain, dyspepsia, or reflux.

The increased prevalence noted over the past 2 decades is attributed to the decreasing *Helicobacter pylori* infection and widespread use of PPIs. In fact, FGPs have an inverse correlation with *H. pylori* infection and atrophy. Long-term PPI use is associated with a fourfold risk of developing FGPs. Moreover, complete regression of some FGPs has been shown on cessation of the PPI therapy.

Fundic gland polyps are present in 0.8% to 1.9% of all patients undergoing gastroscopy. Among the syndromic conditions, they are most commonly found in patients with familial adenomatous polyposis (FAP) followed by gastric adenocarcinoma and proximal polyposis of stomach (GAPPS) and rarely in those with *MUTYH*-associated polyposis (MAP). FGP is diagnosed in 26% to 84% of patients with FAP.

Pathologic Features

Gross Findings

Fundic gland polyps are present exclusively in the body or fundus. In the syndromic setting, these polyps

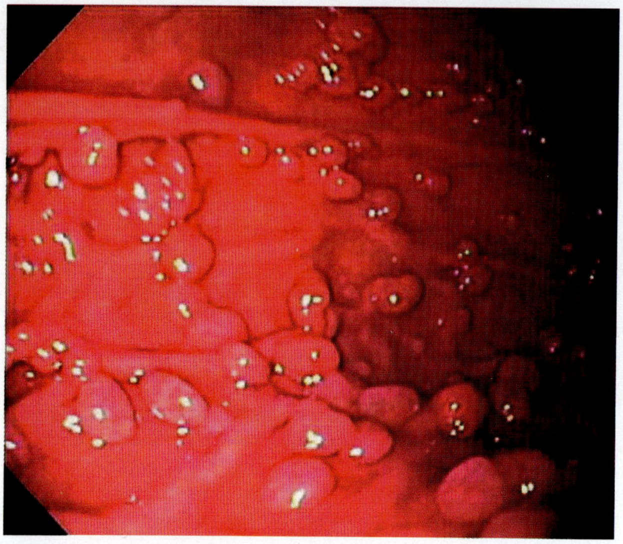

FIGURE 4.1

Endoscopic appearance of fundic gland polyps. In this patient with familial adenomatous polyposis, the fundic mucosa is studded by hundreds of small sessile polyps.

often carpet the oxyntic mucosa. They are soft, sessile, and hemispherical, with a smooth and translucent appearance (Fig. 4.1). FGPs are small, ranging from 1 to 7 mm in size. Because of their small size, these polyps are often hidden by gastric rugal folds and become visible when the stomach is fully distended. They are usually identical in color to the surrounding gastric mucosa. The nonpolypoid gastric mucosa is typically normal.

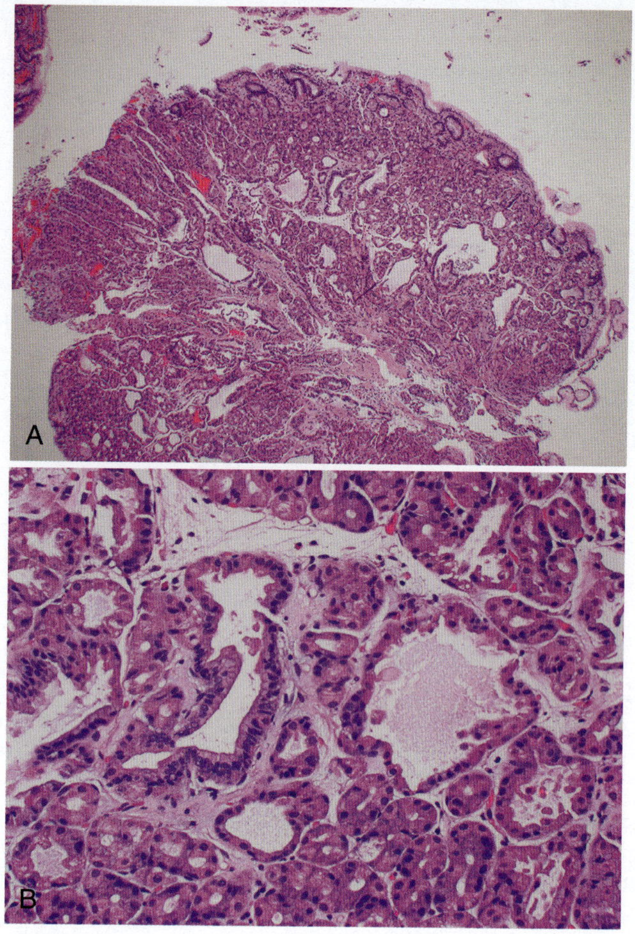

FIGURE 4.2

Fundic gland polyps with cystically dilated fundic glands (**A**) lined by parietal and chief cells (**B**).

Microscopic Findings

Fundic gland polyps consist of proliferation of oxyntic glands with cystic dilation. The proliferating glands are formed predominantly by parietal cells, but chief cells and mucous neck cells may also be present (Fig. 4.2). The morphology of FGPs is slightly different according to the etiologic background of the polyp. PPI therapy–induced lesions are characterized by the presence of more prominent parietal cell hyperplasia, increased diameter of dilated oxyntic glands, and elongation of surface foveolar epithelium. FAP-associated lesions tend to show smaller microcysts lined by pure fundic epithelium with limited parietal cell and surface foveolar hyperplasia. FGPs in patients with GAPPS tend to be generally large, but the microcysts are smaller than PPI-related lesions and are lined by a mixture of fundic and foveolar type cells. The characteristic inverted foveolar epithelium in this setting is designated as *hyperproliferative aberrant pits*. The lamina propria lacks inflammation and is mildly edematous. There may be slight hyperplasia of the surface foveolar epithelium with shallow to absent pits.

In 25% to 46% of FGPs in FAP and fewer than 1% of sporadic FGPs, low-grade epithelial dysplasia characterized by nuclear hyperchromasia, enlargement, mild pseudostratification, and loss of mucin (Fig. 4.3) may be present. The dysplasia in FGPs is usually of the foveolar type. High-grade dysplasia or adenocarcinoma are uncommon in patients with FAP. In contrast, low- and high-grade dysplasia as well as adenocarcinoma can be seen in patients with GAPPS.

Molecular Studies

Studies have revealed molecular abnormalities in FGPs, suggesting they are neoplastic lesions. FGPs associated with FAP and even sporadic FGPs with dysplasia harbor somatic *APC* gene alterations in 50% of cases. Sporadic FGPs show activating *β-catenin* mutations in

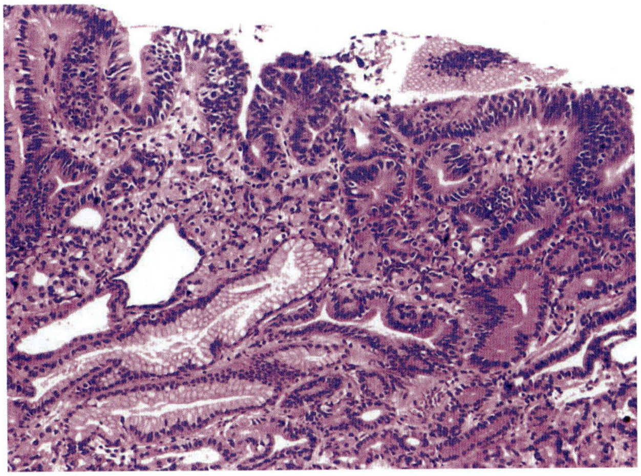

FIGURE 4.3
Low-grade surface epithelial dysplasia with hyperchromatic and pseudostratified nuclei in a sporadic fundic gland polyp.

up to 90% of cases. In the setting of MAP, the changes are driven by biallelic mutations in *MUTYH*. Recently, point mutations in the YY1 binding site of the *APC* promoter 1B were reported in several patients with GAPPS.

Differential Diagnosis

Biopsies of oxyntic mucosa from patients on PPI therapy can show hypertrophic parietal cells with apical cytoplasmic protrusions and dilated glands. The low-acid environment created by the H+/K+-ATPase inhibiting action of the PPIs causes gastrin stimulation, which in turn has a trophic effect on parietal cells, resulting in dilated intracytoplasmic canaliculi caused by the inspissated hydrogen ion. FGPs, on the other hand, show fundic gland cysts with flattened oxyntic lining. Compensatory hyperplastic parietal cells in remnant oxyntic mucosal islands of patients with autoimmune gastritis may mimic hyperplastic features reminiscent to the effect of PPI therapy. This phenomenon can lead to the development of endoscopic pseudopolyposis when the remnant nonatrophic mucosal patches appear polypoid between the depressed atrophic areas.

Oxyntic gland adenomas (OGAs) are also composed of proliferating fundic or oxyntic gland but display unmistakable neoplastic features, including an irregular tubular growth pattern and usually mild but obvious cytologic atypia. Hyperplastic polyps are also common polypoid lesions involving the stomach but are composed entirely of mucous neck cells. Parietal cells and chief cells are not part of the polyp lining epithelium in hyperplastic polyps

Prognosis and Therapy

Sporadic- and FAP-associated low-grade dysplastic FGPs have a low progression rate to high-grade dysplasia or adenocarcinoma. Conversely, GAPPS-associated FGPs have a higher risk of progression. The diagnosis of FGPs virtually never requires surgical resection, but endoscopic mucosal resection may be considered in large dysplastic FGPs. Upper endoscopic surveillance in patients with FAP is warranted to monitor the 300-fold risk for duodenal adenocarcinoma, but the question whether dysplastic FGPs deserve follow-up surveillance remains controversial.

FUNDIC GLAND POLYPS—FACT SHEET

Definition

- Benign epithelial polyps developing in oxyntic mucosa and composed of disordered proliferation and dilation of fundic glands with variable degrees of foveolar hyperplasia

Incidence

- Commonest gastric polyps (0.8%–1.9% of patients undergoing gastroscopy)
- Prevalence ranges from 26% to 84% in patients with familial adenomatous polyposis, the most common causative syndrome
- Patients with gastric adenocarcinoma and proximal polyposis (GAPPS), a recently described autosomal dominant inherited syndrome, present with multiple (30–100), usually small, fundic gland polyps (FGPs). Dysplasia and early adenocarcinoma may be present in these patients
- FGPs can also be detected in about 10% of patients with *MUTYH*-associated polyposis, frequently in association with adenomas

Morbidity and Mortality

- Benign with limited malignant potential in the sporadic setting
- Dysplasia and carcinoma develop more commonly in the syndromic setting

Gender, Race, and Age

- Patients are 40 to 69 years of age (average, 57 years)
- FGPs in FAP occur in younger individuals in their 20s and 30s
- FGPs in children are extremely rare and warrant a search for FAP

Clinical Features

- Most are asymptomatic

Prognosis and Therapy

- Malignant potential is limited in sporadic cases (incidence of dysplasia, ~1%)
- In FAP, dysplasia occurs with a reported prevalence of 25% to 46% and correlates with increased severity of duodenal polyposis, larger polyp size, and the presence of antral gastritis
- Low- and high-grade dysplasia and early adenocarcinoma are detected in GAPPS-associated FGPs

Fundic Gland Polyps—Pathologic Features

Gross Findings

- Present exclusively in the body or fundus
- Often multiple, occurring in clusters
- Soft, sessile, hemispherical, with a smooth and translucent appearance
- Small (1–7 mm in size), identical in color to the surrounding gastric mucosa
- Normal surrounding gastric mucosa

Microscopic Findings

- Disarrayed proliferation of oxyntic mucosa with cystically dilated fundic glands lined mostly by parietal cells; less often by chief cells and mucous neck cells
- Minimal or absent inflammation
- Fundic gland polyps (FGPs) may contain foveolar low-grade dysplasia characterized by hyperchromasia, nuclear enlargement, pseudostratification, and loss of mucin

Molecular Features

- Sporadic FGPs: β-catenin mutations, 90%
- Familial adenomatous polyposis: somatic *APC* gene mutation
- Gastric adenocarcinoma and proximal polyposis of stomach: point mutation in the binding site of the *APC* promoter 1B
- In *MUTYH*-associated polyposis, the alteration is a biallelic mutation of the *MUTYH* gene

Differential Diagnosis

- Proton pump inhibitor effect with prominent parietal cell hyperplasia
- Oxyntic gland pseudopolyps in autoimmune gastritis
- Oxyntic gland (chief cell) adenoma
- Hyperplastic polyps

GASTRIC HYPERPLASTIC POLYPS

Hyperplastic polyps are the second most common type of gastric epithelial polyps and are composed of elongated and tortuous foveolar epithelium. Given the strong association with background gastritis, hyperplastic polyps are believed to represent a regenerative response to mucosal injuries. In the past, these polyps were often referred to as *regenerative polyps* or *hyperplasiogenous polyps*.

Clinical Features

Hyperplastic polyps have a prevalence rate of approximately 1% to 2% at endoscopic examination in the adult population and represent about 20% of all gastric polyps. The prevalence of hyperplastic polyps has significantly decreased over the past 20 years because of the declining rate of *H. pylori* infection.

Hyperplastic polyps are antral predominant (60%). They are usually single but can be multiple in 20% of cases. The term *hyperplastic polyposis* is used to denote greater than 50 hyperplastic polyps in the stomach. A slight female predominance may be seen (male-to-female ratio, 1 to 2.4), and adults in the sixth and seventh decades of life are commonly affected. Hyperplastic polyps are the most common polyps in pediatric patients, accounting for 42% of gastric polyps in children.

Most (especially small) polyps are incidental findings during endoscopy performed for other reasons. Symptoms sometimes associated with large hyperplastic polyps include bleeding, abdominal pain, anemia, nausea, and vomiting. Large pedunculated polyps in the pyloric region may produce gastric outlet obstruction. Gastric hyperplastic polyps are frequently associated with abnormalities in the surrounding nonpolypoid mucosa in up to 85% of cases. These changes include *H. pylori* gastritis (25%), chemical gastropathy (21%), autoimmune gastritis (12%), intestinal metaplasia (37%), dysplasia (2%), and synchronous or metachronous carcinoma (6%). Other common etiological associations include partial gastrectomies for ulcers, postlaser therapy for gastric antral vascular ectasia, and cytomegalovirus gastritis. An increased prevalence of hyperplastic polyps has also been reported in the transplant setting.

Finally, a rare family pedigree with hyperplastic polyposis and increased incidence of poorly cohesive gastric carcinoma has been reported and associated with *KRAS* point mutation at codon 12. In recent studies on small cohorts, no pathogenic mutations were detected in small hyperplastic polyps without dysplasia; however, *TP53* gene mutations were the most common alteration in hyperplastic polyps with dysplasia. Large hyperplastic polyps may show loss of MGMT expression or *APC*, *CTNNB1* (beta-catenin), *KRAS*, or *BRAF* mutations.

Pathologic Features

Gross Findings

Most hyperplastic polyps are smaller than 1 cm, but they can sometimes grow up to 12 cm in size and be mistaken for a carcinoma. They are usually broad based or sessile but can also be pedunculated. The polyps have a smooth, lobulated, and glistening surface, often containing areas of erosion (Fig. 4.4).

Microscopic Findings

The polyps are composed of hyperplastic, elongated, and tortuous gastric foveolae (Fig. 4.5) with outpouchings, papillary infoldings, or cystic dilation. The foveolar cells may become hypertrophic and reminiscent of goblet cells because of accumulation of abundant cytoplasmic mucin. Scattered single hyperplastic foveolar cells created by the damage and disintegration of such foveolar epithelium

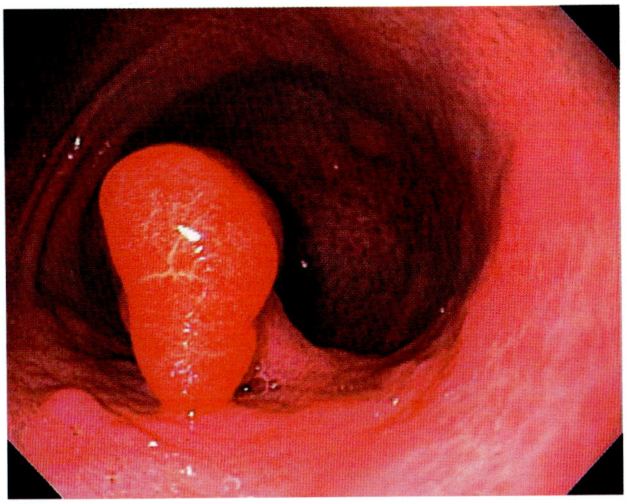

FIGURE 4.4

Single smooth and hyperemic pedunculated gastric hyperplastic polyp. (Courtesy of Shriram Jakate, MD, Rush Medical College, Chicago.)

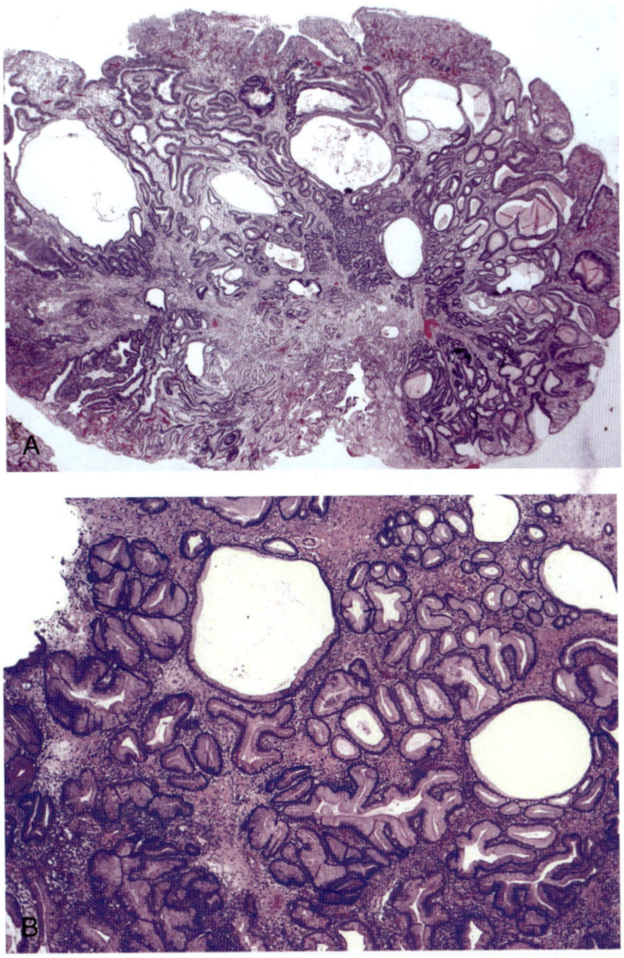

FIGURE 4.5

Dilated, tortuous gastric foveolar epithelium (**A**) in a gastric hyperplastic polyp with frequent outpouchings and edematous and inflamed stroma (**B**).

should not be mistaken for signet ring cells. The stroma is edematous, causing separation of glands, and contains variable numbers of inflammatory cells such as lymphocytes, plasma cells, eosinophils, and even lymphoid aggregates. A subset of larger polyps contain prominent vessels and wisps of smooth muscle bundles extending from muscularis mucosae into the lamina propria of the polyp, a phenomenon most likely caused by mucosal prolapse. Areas with erosion may show regenerative changes with depleted mucin, hyperchromatic nuclei, and visible nucleoli that should not be mistaken for dysplasia.

Hyperplastic polyps may contain foci of intestinal metaplasia (16%), dysplasia (4%), and rarely malignant transformation (0.6%). Dysplastic foci are characterized by lack of surface maturation, pseudostratified epithelium with enlarged hyperchromatic nuclei, and increased mitotic figures. High-grade dysplasia is characterized by loss of polarity, marked cytologic atypia, and architectural abnormalities such as cribriform glands. Size appears to be the biggest risk factor with most lesions harboring dysplasia or carcinoma measuring 2 cm or more.

Differential Diagnosis

Focal foveolar hyperplasia or polypoid foveolar hyperplasia is often seen adjacent to ulcers, and small sessile excrescences with elongated superficial gastric foveolae occur as part of chemical gastropathy. Gastritis cystica glandularis usually develops in patients after Billroth gastrectomies or near stomal sites and shows marked foveolar hyperplasia. The hallmark of these lesions is the cystically dilated glands misplaced in the submucosa and muscularis propria. Mucosal prolapse polyps can show foveolar hyperplasia but also contain a prominent glandular component and smooth muscle proliferation in the lamina propria. Hyperplastic and hamartomatous polyps are both composed of proliferating foveolar epithelium and can be indistinguishable, especially when only superficial pinch biopsies are available. Some histologic features are suggestive of hamartomas, but the correct diagnosis often cannot be reached without proper clinical correlation. Peutz-Jeghers polyps may present with characteristic arborizing bundles of smooth muscle that cause mucosal splitting, along with other clinical stigmata characteristic of the syndrome. Juvenile polyps contain prominent cystic glands, often filled with neutrophils in a distinctive abundant, edematous, and inflamed stroma. These polyps are more common in children and have a smooth rounded surface that is frequently eroded. Gastric polyps in PTEN hamartoma tumor syndrome (e.g., Cowden's disease) show great phenotypic diversity and may resemble hyperplastic or juvenile polyps. However, peculiar stromal changes (fibrosis, lipomatosis, ganglion cells) and the presence of multiple different histologic types of polyps (e.g., intramucosal lipomas and ganglioneuromas), simultaneous esophageal glycogenic acanthosis, or extra-GI manifestations help in establishing the diagnosis. Endoscopically, diffuse mucosal hyperplasia is encountered in diseases that may clinically present with protein-losing gastropathy. Ménétrier's disease involves the gastric body with dramatic foveolar hyperplasia and concurrent oxyntic gland atrophy. Cronkhite-Canada syndrome also causes diffuse mucosal involvement by confluent polyposis containing marked lamina propria edema. Abnormal skin pigmentation and nail dystrophy are helpful in establishing the diagnosis.

Prognosis and Therapy

Hyperplastic polyps are benign lesions, and although small lesions seem to be truly regenerative, large polyps that harbor clonal mutations and could be regarded as neoplastic. On follow-up, approximately 70 % of polyps are stable, and 30 % polyps increase or decrease in size. Complete regression has been noted after *H. pylori* eradication. Polyps larger than 1 cm in size may recur after endoscopic resection in roughly half of the cases, and neoplastic transformation may occur in 10.4 %. Polyps larger than 25 mm and harboring intestinal metaplasia are associated with an increased risk of neoplastic transformation. The risk of adenocarcinoma is about 0.7 % to 2.2 %. These carcinomas are mostly intramucosal and carry a good prognosis; complete removal of the lesion is recommended. The risk of metachronous or synchronous epithelial dysplasia or adenocarcinoma elsewhere in the stomach is also increased.

GASTRIC HYPERPLASTIC POLYPS—FACT SHEET

Definition

- Epithelial polyps composed of elongated, dilated, branched, and tortuous foveolar epithelium and edematous stroma containing inflammatory cells

Incidence and Location

- Represent approximately 20% of stomach polyps
- Most are located in the antrum (60%)

Morbidity and Mortality

- Large polyps may cause bleeding and gastric outlet obstruction
- Dysplasia and adenocarcinoma develop in 10% of large hyperplastic polyps (particularly those >2.5 cm in size)

Gender, Race, and Age

- Slight female predominance (male-to-female ratio, 1 to 2.4)
- Adults in their sixth to seventh decades of life are commonly affected

Clinical Features

- Smaller polyps are often incidental findings during surveillance
- Patients can present with bleeding, iron-deficiency anemia, abdominal pain, and dyspepsia
- Patients with large prepyloric polyps can present with gastric outlet obstruction

Prognosis and Therapy

- The majority of hyperplastic polyps (especially small ones) are benign
- Treatment includes snare polypectomy, endoscopic mucosal resection, and treating associated conditions such as *Helicobacter* gastritis
- Large polyps (>1 cm) may recur after endoscopic resection in 50% of the cases
- Associated carcinomas are mostly intramucosal and carry a good prognosis

Gastric Hyperplastic Polyps—Pathologic Features

Gross Findings

- Range in size from a few millimeters up to 12 cm (average, 1 cm)
- Have a smooth, lobulated, and glistening surface, often with areas of erosion
- Usually sessile; can be pedunculated
- Multiple in 20% of cases

Microscopic Findings

- Dilated, elongated, branched, and tortuous foveolar epithelium
- Edematous and inflamed stroma
- Regenerative foci can mimic dysplasia because of depleted mucin, hyperchromatic nuclei, and prominent nucleoli
- May contain foci of intestinal metaplasia, dysplasia, or invasive carcinoma. Risk of neoplasia is greater in large lesions
- Often associated with mucosal pathology in the surrounding mucosa

Histochemistry and Immunohistochemistry

- Stains for highlighting *Helicobacter pylori* useful in polyps with inflamed epithelium or stroma
- Increased and surface Ki-67 staining and overexpression of p53 staining may aid in confirming a hematoxylin and eosin–based impression of dysplasia in difficult cases

Differential Diagnosis

- Focal foveolar hyperplasia or polypoid foveolar hyperplasia
- Mucosal prolapse polyps
- Gastritis cystica glandularis
- Peutz-Jeghers polyp
- Juvenile polyp
- Cronkhite-Canada syndrome
- Ménétrier's disease

GASTRITIS CYSTICA POLYPOSA

Gastritis cystica polyposa is characterized by cystically dilated glands misplaced within the submucosa, forming polypoid lesions near postgastroenterostomy anastomoses and stomas. *Gastritis cystica polyposa* is synonymous with *gastritis cystica profunda, gastritis cystica superficialis, gastric cystic polyposis, polypoid mucosal prolapse, stromal polypoid hypertrophic gastritis*, and *polypoid cystic gastritis*. Although a non-neoplastic lesion, it is discussed in this section because it can mimic an invasive adenocarcinoma on endoscopy, and a subset may undergo neoplastic transformation.

Clinical Features

This rare entity is similar to mucosal prolapse lesions elsewhere in the GI tract, such as solitary rectal ulcer, colitis cystica profunda, and prolapse at colostomy and ileostomy sites. Gastritis cystica polyposa presents near gastroenterostomy stomal sites 3 to 40 years after surgery, typically in men in their 70s who have history of Billroth I and II procedures.

Clinically, the patients are frequently suspected of having stump carcinoma or an adenoma. Computed tomography examination can demonstrate multiple exophytic masses around gastric stomal or anastomotic sites. Anastomotic site changes, including mechanical or ischemic injury, mucosal prolapse, and bile reflux, are thought to play a role in the pathogenesis. Unlike the benign rectal mucosal prolapse lesions, gastritis cystica polyposa can be associated with dysplasia and gastric stump carcinoma.

Gross Findings

Gastritis cystica polyposa presents as single or multiple, soft, sessile 1- to 3-cm polyps or confluent, circumferential masses around gastric stomal or anastomotic sites. The mucosa overlying the polyp is usually smooth and resembles the surrounding gastric mucosa or may be red. Cut sections show thickened gastric wall containing numerous cystic structures.

Microscopic Findings

Histologic features include foveolar hyperplasia, regenerative surface epithelial changes, and cystically dilated pyloric-type glands in the mucosa, the submucosa, and even the muscularis propria (Fig. 4.6). Depending on the location of the cystic glands, these lesions can also be termed *gastritis cystica superficialis* or *gastritis cystica profunda*. The lamina propria and submucosa contain increased chronic inflammation, fibrosis, and scarring and often display thickened and splayed muscle bundles. Biopsy of the gastric remnant shows reduced oxyntic glands owing to the lack of gastrin caused by antrectomy, lamina propria edema, and chronic inflammation. There may be intestinal metaplasia or dysplasia.

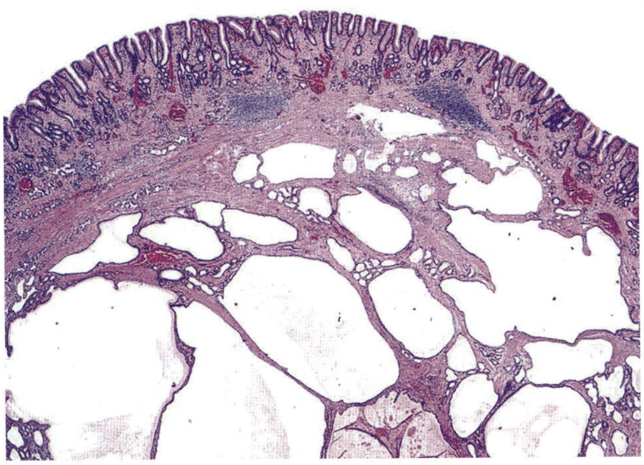

FIGURE 4.6

Gastritis cystica profunda showing cystically dilated glands extending into the submucosa. The overlying mucosa shows atrophic changes. (Courtesy of Richard Lash, MD, Caris Diagnostics, Irving)

Differential Diagnosis

The presence of epithelial elements deep in the submucosa or even muscularis propria in gastritis cystica profunda can be mistaken for invasive adenocarcinoma. Unlike in carcinomas, these cystic glands lack pleomorphism and desmoplastic stroma and are often surrounded by lamina propria or smooth muscle bundles.

Prognosis and Therapy

Although benign, gastritis cystica polyposa can be associated with dysplasia and stump carcinoma. Thus, regular follow-up is important.

Gastritis Cystica Polyposa—Pathologic Features

Gross Findings

- Single or multiple, soft, sessile 1- to 3-cm polyps around gastric stomal or anastomotic sites
- Cut sections show thickened gastric wall containing numerous cystic glands

Microscopic Findings

- Foveolar hyperplasia, regenerative surface epithelial changes, cystically dilated pyloric-type glands surrounded by lamina propria in the mucosa, submucosa, and even muscularis propria
- Lamina propria and submucosa display scarring, fibrosis, and thickened and splayed muscle bundles
- Gastric remnant shows reduced oxyntic glands, edema, and chronic inflammation

Differential Diagnosis

- Invasive adenocarcinoma

PANCREATIC HETEROTOPIA

Pancreatic heterotopia is the presence of pancreatic tissue outside the normal pancreas with no vascular or ductal continuity with the organ. It is synonymous with *pancreatic rest* and *ectopic pancreas*. It is believed to originate during embryologic development from duodenal invaginations that persist in the GI wall.

Clinical Features

Pancreatic heterotopia is an uncommon lesion, detected in 0.5% to 13% of autopsies, the majority of which are seen in the stomach (30%) followed by the duodenum, jejunum, and Meckel's diverticulum. Less common sites include the lungs, gallbladder, mediastinum, mesentery, esophagus, bile ducts, and umbilical cord. It can affect adult and pediatric patients, and the average age is 45 years with a slight male predominance. Most patients are not symptomatic, but abdominal pain, epigastric discomfort, nausea, vomiting, and bleeding can develop.

Large prepyloric lesions may present with gastric outlet obstruction. Rarely, the heterotopic tissue may develop pancreatitis, pancreatic cysts, neuroendocrine (islet cell) tumor, or even ductal adenocarcinoma.

Pathologic Features

Gross and Endoscopic Findings

Pancreatic heterotopias present as usually solitary, 0.2- to 5-cm nodules of the antrum or prepyloric area. Endoscopic appearance consists of a smooth surfaced, hemispherical, intramural nodule with normal or eroded overlying mucosa and a central dimple that represents the draining pancreatic duct. On cut section, the lesion is well demarcated, located in the submucosa or muscularis propria, yellowish, and lobulated, resembling normal pancreas.

Microscopic Findings

The heterotopic pancreas (Fig. 4.7) may contain varying proportions of acinar, ductal, and islet cell components and can be divided into four types: type I, total heterotopia (all cell types, most common variant); type II, canalicular heterotopia (ducts only); type III, exocrine heterotopia (acinar cells only); and type IV, endocrine heterotopia (islets only, rare).

Because the usually submucosal location, superficial biopsies may not be diagnostic. Thus, deeper biopsies or endoscopic removal are important for a definite diagnosis.

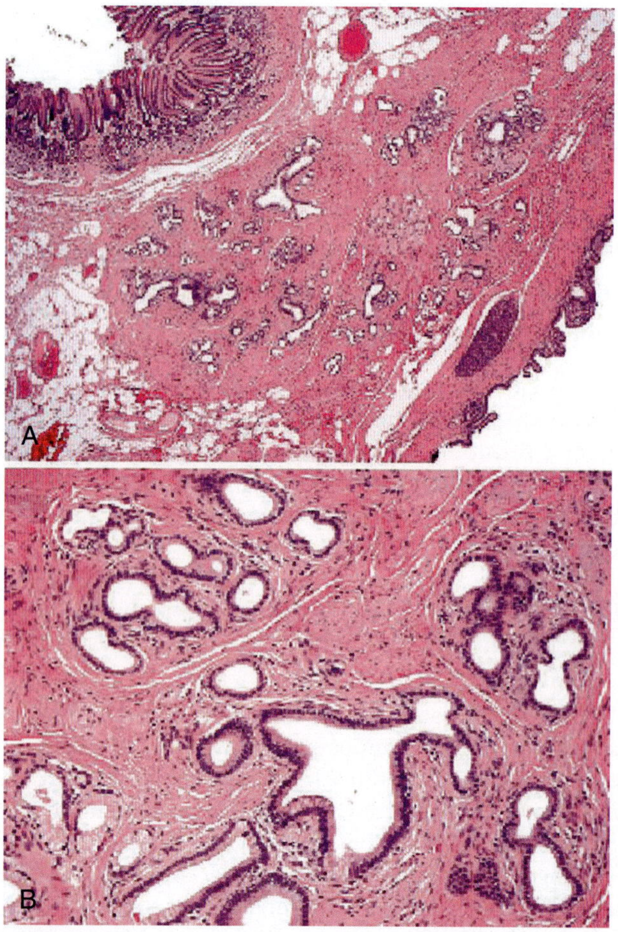

FIGURE 4.7

Heterotopic pancreatic tissue usually manifests as an intramural lesion (**A**) and is composed of pancreatic ducts and rare acini showing a lobulocentric distribution interspersed among smooth muscle bundles (**B**).

Pancreatic Heterotopia—Pathologic Features

Gross Findings

- Usually solitary, antral or prepyloric, dome-shaped polypoid nodules
- Covered by smooth normal or ulcerated mucosa with a central umbilication
- Cut sections show a well-demarcated tan-yellow and often lobulated intramural mass, resembling normal pancreatic parenchyma

Microscopic Findings

- The heterotopic tissue contains admixture of pancreatic acini, ducts, and islets in varying proportions
- Superficial biopsies may not be diagnostic because of the submucosal location, thus necessitating deeper sampling

Immunohistochemical Features

- Most cases are easily diagnosed based on the hematoxylin and eosin stain
- Endocrine or islet cell stain with chromogranin A and synaptophysin
- Pancreas exocrine markers mark the acinar cells

Differential Diagnosis

- Invasive well-differentiated adenocarcinoma
- Gastritis cystica profunda
- Neuroendocrine tumor

Differential Diagnosis

The submucosal location of the lesion brings about an endoscopic differential of GI stromal tumors, lipomas, and leiomyomas, which is easily resolved on histologic examination. Invasive adenocarcinoma is an important microscopic differential diagnosis considering that most pancreatic heterotopias arise in deep submucosa or muscularis and can be misinterpreted, especially during frozen sections. The key to the correct diagnosis is the lobulated arrangement of acinar and duct structure (like in normal pancreas) and the lack of malignant cytoarchitectural features and desmoplasia. Gastritis cystica profunda occurs in stomal or anastomotic sites and consists of surface foveolar hyperplasia with prominent features of mucosal prolapse, cystically dilated mucous glands located in the submucosa and muscularis propria. The finding of acinar and islet tissue in pancreatic heterotopias is especially helpful in excluding this possibility. Pure endocrine heterotopia (the rarest among the pancreatic heterotopias) may present a diagnostic challenge with neuroendocrine tumors (NETs). Endocrine heterotopias present as microscopic nests scattered in the submucosa and muscularis and are not associated with any stromal response. NETs present as mass lesions with the tumor cells arranged as trabeculae, tubules, and rosettes.

PROGNOSIS AND THERAPY

Pancreatic heterotopias are benign non-neoplastic lesions, and reports of islet cell tumors or ductal adenocarcinomas developing in the heterotopic tissue are extremely rare. Symptomatic superficial lesions are effectively treated by endoscopic resections. Deeper lesions may require wedge resection by laparoscopy.

GASTRIC MUCOSAL XANTHOMA

Gastric xanthomas consist of loose collections of lipid-laden macrophages in the lamina propria.

CLINICAL FEATURES

The stomach is a common site for these lesions, which also occur rarely in the esophagus, small intestine, and colon. Gastric xanthomas present as sessile, single, or multiple, 1- to 5-mm, yellowish-white mucosal nodules or plaques. They tend to be more common in the antrum, especially the prepyloric area, lesser curvature, and adjacent to gastric stoma. Adults in their 60s are commonly affected with a three to one male predominance. Notably, gastric xanthomas usually do not show any relation to skin xanthelasmas or hyperlipidemia but have been associated with bile reflux, and some studies have implied an underlying dyslipidemia. Endoscopic studies have shown an incidence ranging from 0.3% to 7%. They can be seen in association with *H. pylori* gastritis, bile reflux, chemical gastropathy, gastric ulcers, after gastroenterostomies (Billroth), chronic atrophic gastritis, and carcinomas. The frequent association with various pathologies suggests that it represents a reparative response to a wide array of mucosal injuries.

PATHOLOGIC FEATURES

GROSS AND ENDOSCOPIC FINDINGS

These are small, sessile, yellowish-white nodules or plaques, usually multiple, and 1 to 5 mm in size (Fig. 4.8).

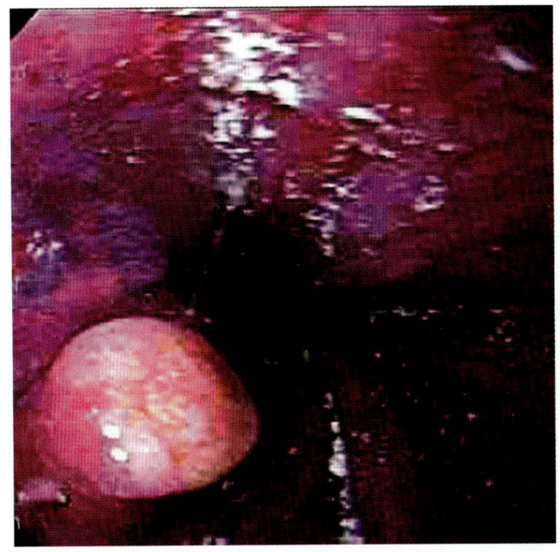

FIGURE 4.8

The typical endoscopic appearance of a gastric xanthoma. It usually consists of a small, sessile yellowish nodule or plaque. (Courtesy of Shriram Jakate, MD, Rush Medical College, Chicago.)

MICROSCOPIC FINDINGS

Gastric xanthomas consist of a loose cluster of lipid-laden macrophages in the lamina propria. The macrophages show abundant foamy cytoplasm containing cholesterol and neutral fats with central bland nondescript nuclei (Figs. 4.9A and B). The surrounding gastric mucosa may show chemical or bile reflux gastropathy, chronic gastritis with intestinal metaplasia, or *Helicobacter* gastritis.

ANCILLARY STUDIES

HISTOCHEMISTRY AND IMMUNOHISTOCHEMISTRY

Sudan Black and oil red O can demonstrate intracytoplasmic lipid, and CD68 (see Fig. 4.9B) stains the macrophages. Periodic acid–Schiff (PAS; see Fig. 4.9C), mucicarmine, cytokeratins, and S-100 stains are all negative.

DIFFERENTIAL DIAGNOSIS

The differential diagnosis is broad and includes inflammatory and infiltrative disorders involving the lamina propria. Signet ring cell carcinoma contains cytoplasmic mucin vacuoles, hyperchromatic eccentrically placed atypical nuclei, and frequent mitoses and shows positive staining with cytokeratins and mucin stains. Granular cell tumor is composed of clusters of polygonal cells with abundant eosinophilic granular cytoplasm, centrally placed nuclei, that are positive for S-100 and CD68. Clear cell NETs can grossly resemble xanthomas, appearing as yellow nodules. Positivity for chromogranin-A and synaptophysin by immunohistochemistry are diagnostic for NETs. Metastatic clear cell renal cell carcinoma

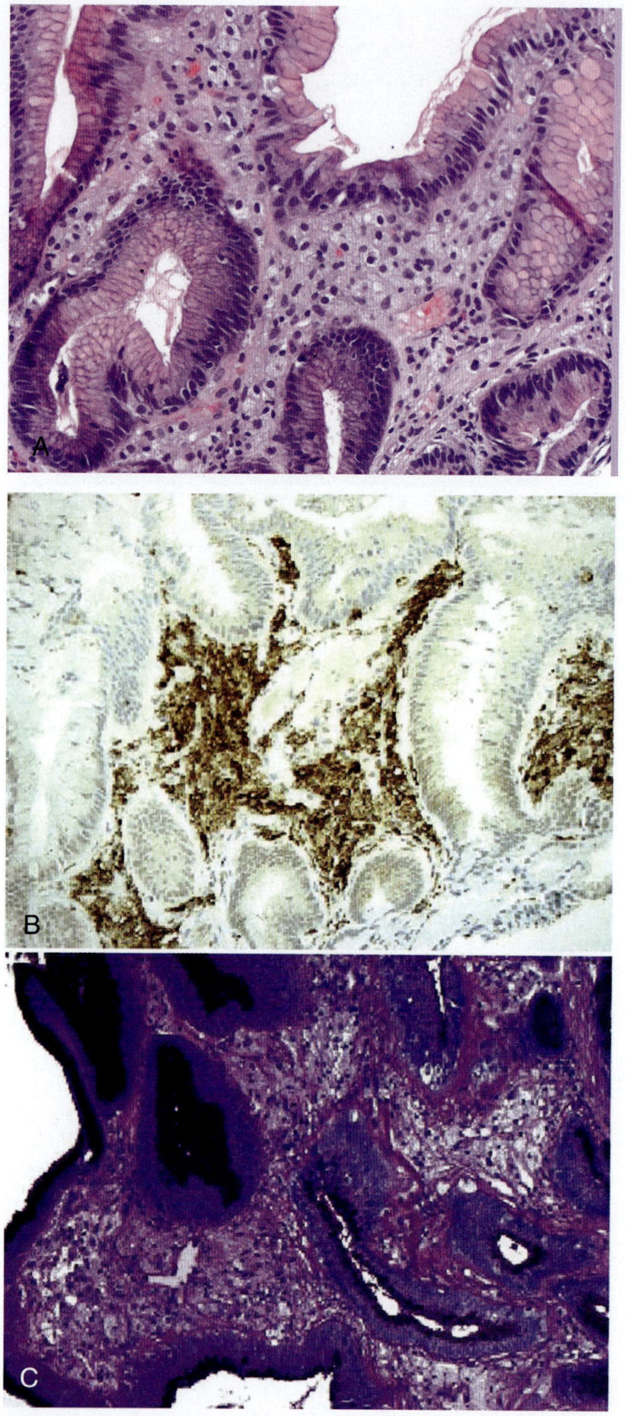

FIGURE 4.9

Gastric xanthoma in a patient who had undergone Billroth surgery and presented with bile reflux gastropathy (**A**). Note the collection of foamy lipid-laden macrophages in the lamina propria. Special studies in gastric xanthoma with strongly positive CD68 in the gastric xanthoma cells (**B**), but the result on periodic acid–Schiff stain is negative owing to the lipid content (**C**).

is positive for PAX8, CA-IX, and low-molecular-weight keratins. *Mycobacterium avium-intracellulare* infections occur in immunosuppressed patients (e.g., those with AIDS) and are characterized by the accumulation of foamy macrophages containing abundant bacilli, which are intensely positive on an acid-fast stain. Malakoplakia is a xanthogranulomatous reaction to gram-negative bacterial infections such as *Escherichia coli* and can rarely involve the stomach. Characteristic Michaelis-Guttman bodies that stain with calcium stains such as Von Kossa are diagnostic. Whipple disease can also show foamy macrophages stuffed with bacillary forms of *Tropheryma whipplei* and show positive staining with PAS (intensely positive).

Prognosis and Therapy

Benign lesions that may regress with time. If needed, therapy is directed at the associated gastric pathology.

Gastric Xanthomas (Xanthelasmas)—Pathologic Features

Gross Findings

- Small, sessile, single or multiple yellowish white nodules
- 1 to 5 mm in size

Microscopic Findings

- Lipid-laden macrophages in the lamina propria
- Macrophages contain foamy cytoplasm with centrally placed bland nuclei
- No increase in mitoses

Immunohistochemistry

- Positive for Sudan black, oil red O, and CD68
- Negative for mucicarmine, periodic acid–Schiff, cytokeratins, and S-100

Differential Diagnosis

- Signet ring cell carcinoma
- Granular cell tumor
- Neuroendocrine tumor with clear cell phenotype
- Metastatic clear cell carcinoma (e.g., renal cell carcinoma)
- Epithelioid gastrointestinal stromal tumor
- *Mycobacterium avium-intracellulare* infection
- Malakoplakia
- Whipple disease

GASTRIC CARCINOMAS, NEUROENDOCRINE TUMORS, AND THEIR PRECURSOR LESIONS

Gastric carcinomas usually develop from precursor lesions, which can be broadly classified into gastric epithelial dysplasia (GED) (flat [endoscopically invisible] lesions) and gastric adenoma (raised or polypoid visible lesions). The role of the endoscopist and pathologist is to enable early detection, diagnosis, and complete resection of precursor lesions to prevent the development of invasive carcinoma. Adenocarcinomas are the most common type of gastric malignancies, and these are divided into intestinal and diffuse subtypes in the Lauren classification. Alternatively, the 2019 World Health Organization (WHO) classification subdivides gastric carcinoma into tubular, papillary, mucinous, poorly cohesive carcinoma, mixed adenocarcinoma, and other rare histologic subtypes.

The diagnosis and grading of gastric epithelial neoplasms have historically differed between Japanese and Western pathologists. A consensus approach led to the Vienna classification of GI epithelial neoplasia. This classification divided neoplastic lesions into the following categories: (1) negative for dysplasia, (2) indefinite for dysplasia, (3) noninvasive low-grade dysplasia, (4) noninvasive high-grade dysplasia (including carcinoma in situ), and (5) invasive carcinoma (including both intramucosal carcinoma and submucosal invasive carcinoma).

GASTRIC EPITHELIAL DYSPLASIA AND GASTRIC ADENOMAS

Clinical Features

It is widely recognized that GED and gastric adenomas are precancerous lesions that can progress to gastric carcinoma. In contrast to GED, which is endoscopically flat or invisible lesions, gastric adenomas are polypoid growths of dysplastic epithelium that project above the surrounding mucosa. GED is associated with 40% to 100% of early gastric cancers and 5% to 80% of advanced carcinomas. In addition, approximately 60% of gastric cancers are discovered after a diagnosis of dysplasia.

The incidence of GED or gastric adenoma increases with age and peaks after the seventh decade of life. The male-to-female ratio is approximately 2 to 1. Most lesions are found incidentally at the time of endoscopy, primarily in the antrum. Whereas Western populations demonstrate a low prevalence of GED (0.7%–3.7%), it can be as high as 20% in high-risk areas such as Japan and Eastern Europe. A common cause is *H. pylori* gastritis, and other risk factors for the development of GED include autoimmune gastritis and polyposis syndromes. Gastric adenomas follow fundic gland and hyperplastic polyps in overall incidence, accounting for approximately 7% to 10% of gastric polyps in North America.

Half of all cases of low-grade GED, diagnosed by either biopsy or resection, may regress. This observation raises the possibility that many lesions diagnosed as low-grade dysplasia may instead be misdiagnosed atypical reactive lesions. In fact, only approximately 3% of patients with low-grade GED (in a Western population) progress to adenocarcinoma within 5 years. Conversely, about 30% to 60% of those with high-grade dysplasia progress to adenocarcinoma. However, more than 80% to 90% of high-grade dysplasia transform into adenocarcinoma within the first year of follow-up, suggesting that these are cases of prevalent invasive adenocarcinomas that were missed because of undersampling at the first endoscopy. Excluding cases that progress within the first year of follow up, only approximately 5% of high-grade lesions transform into cancer within five years.

GASTRIC DYSPLASIA AND ADENOMA—FACT SHEET

Definition

- Noninvasive neoplastic epithelial proliferation with variable risk of malignant transformation into an invasive adenocarcinoma

Incidence and Location

- Incidence varies (0.3%–20%) with geography; higher in countries endemic for gastric cancer
- Associated with 40% to 100% of early gastric cancers and 5% to 80% of advanced carcinomas
- Antral location common; adenomas account for 7% to 10% of all gastric polyps

Morbidity and Mortality

- Half of all cases of low-grade gastric epithelial dysplasia (GED), diagnosed by either biopsy or resection, may regress
- 3% of low-grade GED cases progress to carcinoma in 5 years in contrast to 30% to 60% of high-grade GED cases

Gender, Race, and Age

- Increasing incidence with age; more common in the Far East and Eastern Europe
- Male-to-female ratio is 2 to 1

Clinical Features

- GED is a flat, endoscopically invisible lesion incidentally picked up on a random biopsy
- Gastric adenomas are raised endoscopically visible lesions of variable size that can often be completely excised on endoscopy
- Variable risk of progression to adenocarcinoma (depending on grade of lesion)

Prognosis and Therapy

- Systematic biopsies to rule out concurrent carcinoma in patients with GED
- Complete resection of gastric adenomas by endoscopy after excluding the possibility of underlying invasive carcinoma on endoscopic ultrasound
- Large lesions and those associated with deep submucosal invasion or evidence of locoregional spread on imaging are treated with surgical resection

Gastric Dysplasia and Adenomas—Pathologic Features

Gross Findings

- Most common in the antrum
- Range in size from a few millimeters to several centimeters
- Gastric epithelial dysplasia: endoscopically poorly recognizable, mucosal irregularity, and erythematous changes can be seen
- Gastric adenoma: pedunculated or sessile polypoid lesion; cannot be reliably distinguished from benign polyps by endoscopy

Microscopic Findings

- Divided into intestinal type and gastric (foveolar) type
- Intestinal type defined by presence of goblet cells or Paneth cells; mostly tubular, less frequently tubulovillous or villous architecture; pseudostratified columnar epithelium with overlapping, elongated, pencil-shaped nuclei
- Gastric-type composed of foveolar epithelial cells with apical mucin cap; small round to oval, basally oriented nuclei, without marked stratification
- High-grade dysplasia associated with back-to-back glands with loss of intervening stroma, complex (e.g., cribriform) architecture, and complete loss of nuclear polarity
- Background mucosa often shows chronic atrophic gastritis and intestinal metaplasia

Genetics

- Associated with genetic alterations of *APC*, *KRAS*, *TP53*, and microsatellite instability
- *TP53*-mutated gastric dysplasia may represent a subtype with an increased risk for progression into adenocarcinoma

Differential Diagnosis

- Gastric adenoma indistinguishable endoscopically from other gastric polyps
- Gastric adenoma and gastric epithelial dysplasia need to be distinguished microscopically from reactive epithelial changes and intramucosal adenocarcinoma

PATHOLOGIC FEATURES

GROSS FINDINGS

Gastric dysplastic lesions occur throughout the stomach with the antrum being the most common location. GEDs are endoscopically flat or invisible lesions, also referred to as flat dysplasia. These lesions are often grossly unremarkable or virtually invisible by standard endoscopy, although sometimes they may appear as irregular, erythematous patches. Gastric adenomas are localized polypoid growths of dysplastic epithelium that by definition project above the surrounding gastric mucosa. They range in size from a few millimeters to several centimeters and may be sessile or pedunculated.

MICROSCOPIC FINDINGS

Gastric dysplastic lesions are divided histologically into intestinal and foveolar types based on the type of glandular epithelium. Intestinal-type adenomas are more prevalent than the gastric foveolar-type adenoma and often arise in a background of intestinalized and atrophic gastric mucosa. Intestinal-type lesions resemble conventional colonic adenoma and are defined by the presence of cells specific to intestinal differentiation as absorptive cells with brush border, goblet cells, or Paneth cells (Fig. 4.10). Mostly, these cells form a tubular growth pattern. Tubulovillous or villous architecture is less frequent. The pseudostratified columnar epithelium shows overlapping, elongated, and pencil-shaped nuclei. Foveolar-type dysplasia is composed of gastric foveolar epithelial cells containing neutral mucin forming an apical mucin cap (Fig. 4.11). The epithelial lining is characteristically nonstratified, with basally oriented, round to oval, small nuclei. Both foveolar and intestinal types of gastric dysplasia show epithelial and nuclear changes ranging from low to high grade. Whether the foveolar or intestinal type has a higher likelihood to harbor high-grade dysplasia or adenocarcinoma remains controversial.

Low-grade dysplastic epithelial changes include mild to moderate architectural irregularity with mild nuclear enlargement, hyperchromasia, pleomorphism, and increased mitotic activity. In high-grade dysplasia, the architecture becomes increasingly complex and crowded

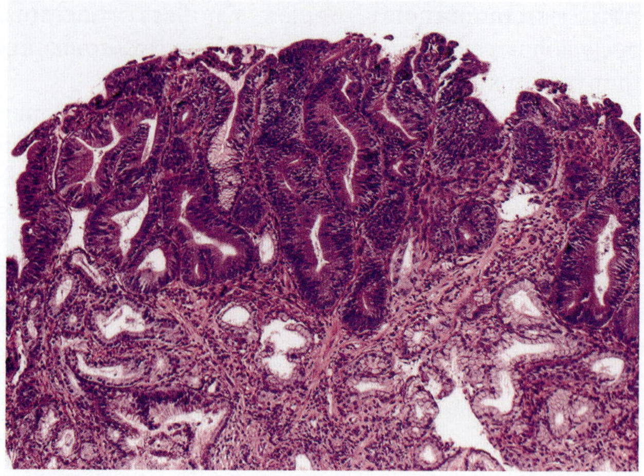

FIGURE 4.10

Low-grade intestinal type dysplasia with nuclear enlargement and elongation, nuclear crowding, and pseudostratification. Overall, the architecture is only moderately distorted.

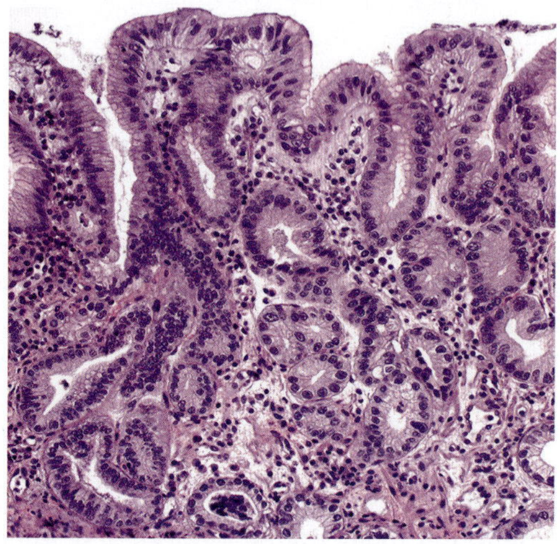

FIGURE 4.11

Low-power view of a foveolar-type adenoma with high grade-dysplasia.

with irregular branching, budding, a loss of intervening stroma, and back-to-back and cribriform architecture. Intraluminal necrotic material may be seen. Cytologically, the nuclei show more severe atypia with enlarged, hyperchromatic, vesicular nuclei and prominent nucleoli. There is also complete loss of nuclear polarity with the nuclei reaching the luminal surface of the epithelium and showing a rounded form. When an early infiltrating carcinoma confined to the lamina propria is identified within GED (i.e., laterally fusing gland manifesting in a lacy or overtly cribriform pattern), it is termed *intramucosal adenocarcinoma* (Fig. 4.12).

Molecular Studies

Gastric dysplasias may harbor molecular alterations in the *APC*, *KRAS*, *ERBB3*, and *TP53* genes and can also show mismatch repair (MMR) gene inactivation similar to that described for colon cancer. However, although the colon demonstrates a well-characterized adenoma–carcinoma sequence of molecular genetic events, the progression pathway is not fully elucidated in the stomach. For example, alterations in the *APC* gene are frequently seen in gastric adenomas but rarely in gastric adenocarcinomas. Instead, multiple studies have published data suggesting that the presence of *APC* mutation in gastric dysplasia may be the sign of an indolent lesion that infrequently progresses into adenocarcinoma, and dysplasia with *TP53* alterations could be a subtype more prone for malignant transformation.

Differential Diagnosis

Endoscopically, all polyp types can enter into the differential diagnosis of gastric adenoma. Histologically, they should also be differentiated from dysplastic foci developing in other polyps (e.g., hyperplastic polyps or FAP associated FGPs). The main differential diagnosis of GED is reactive epithelial change. Of note, in a single study of epithelial dysplasia of the stomach, half of the cases considered to be dysplastic by general surgical pathologists were diagnosed as non-neoplastic by GI pathologists. Thus, when a definitive diagnosis of dysplasia cannot be rendered, the use of the term *indefinite for dysplasia* is encouraged. As in other organs, interobserver variation is diminished as the severity of the lesions increases. In differentiating low-grade dysplasia from reactive changes, it is important to note both the cytologic and architectural features of these lesions. In reactive changes, the cells are frequently cuboidal and appear immature with basophilic cytoplasm secondary to reduced mucus secretion. The regenerative nuclei are often large, vesicular, and at times pleomorphic with smooth nuclear contours and red conspicuous nucleoli. Architecturally, normal epithelial architecture is retained in reactive proliferations with basally localized nuclei and only mild pseudostratification (Fig. 4.13). Mitotic figures, when present, are confined to the basal aspects of the glands. Finally, the transition of the epithelium from the basal portion of the glands to the luminal surface shows surface maturation, which is helpful in diagnosis of reactive change. The presence of active inflammation or granulation tissue-like stroma is in favor of regenerative atypia, and one should be wary of diagnosing neoplasia in this setting unless the changes are prominent enough or not proportionate to the degree of inflammation. Conversely, abrupt transition of the atypical into evidently non-neoplastic epithelium is a sign of neoplasia, although the border of metaplastic and native epithelium can also show this phenomenon.

Prognosis and Therapy

Although it is frequently quoted that 50% of low-grade GED regress, it is likely that some of these in fact represent misdiagnosed reactive or regenerative epithelial change. Nevertheless, the importance of early

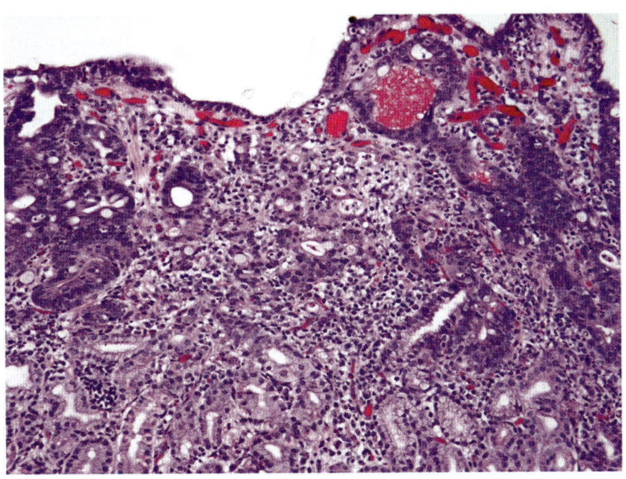

FIGURE 4.12
Example of intramucosal carcinoma. The neoplasm is characterized by syncytial growth pattern with fused glands and single cells in lamina propria.

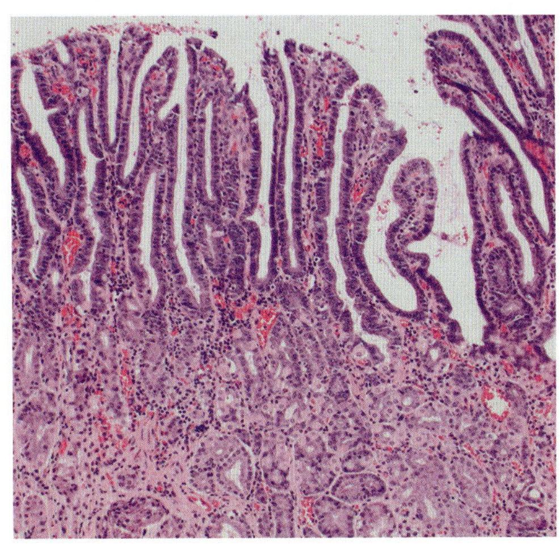

FIGURE 4.13
Reactive epithelial changes simulating epithelial dysplasia. The reactive changes include nuclear hyperchromasia and enlargement. Nuclear pseudostratification, crowding, and elongation are lacking.

detection is emphasized by the fact that more than half of gastric cancers are discovered after a diagnosis of dysplasia. Among all low-grade dysplasia, 20% to 30% of cases persist without progression, and an additional 3% of cases progress to carcinoma within a 5-year period. A meta-analysis showed that a biopsy diagnosis of low-grade gastric dysplasia was upgraded after endoscopic resection to high-grade dysplasia or cancer in 17% and 7% of the cases, respectively. In a large population-based study, 30% of high-grade dysplasia progressed to infiltrating carcinoma during a 5 year follow-up, including cases "transforming" in the first year. However, two similar studies have found that only about 5% of high-grade lesions progress on follow up when cases detected within the first year of surveillance are excluded. Recent guidelines for the management of gastric dysplasia published by the British Society of Gastroenterology recommend en bloc endoscopic resection of visible gastric dysplasia and early cancer. The same guidelines recommend that patients with nonvisible dysplasia should undergo a second endoscopy and extensive biopsy sampling. If persistent nonvisible low-grade dysplasia is detected, endoscopy should be repeated annually thereafter. In patients with nonvisible, high-grade dysplasia, 6-month interval surveillance endoscopies are advised.

PYLORIC GLAND ADENOMA

Clinical Features

Pyloric gland adenomas represent an uncommon neoplastic polyp. They usually arise in patients with autoimmune gastritis but are also detected in the setting of FAP, Lynch syndrome, and juvenile polyposis syndrome. A retrospective study, excluding FGPs, observed that pyloric gland adenomas represented up to 2.7% of all gastric polyps. Pyloric gland adenomas were associated with adenocarcinoma in one-third of the cases in one series. There is a female predominance (52%), and the mean age at diagnosis is in the seventh decade. The genetics of pyloric gland adenoma has recently been described. Activating *GNAS* mutations are found in about 50% of cases and are often associated with *KRAS* mutations.

Pathologic Features

Gross Findings

Gastric pyloric gland adenomas are polypoid lesions, although recently an inverted gross presentation was also described. They have a mean size of about 2 cm and are most often located in the gastric body. Whereas in the nonpolypoid mucosa, atrophic corpus gastritis can be recognized in patients with autoimmune gastritis, multiple FGPs can be noted studding the oxyntic mucosa in patients with FAP.

Microscopic Findings

Pyloric gland adenoma includes tubular glands composed of cuboidal or columnar cells (Figs. 4.14A–C). The cytoplasm is ground glass and either eosinophilic or amphophilic. In contrast to foveolar adenomas, pyloric gland adenomas do not have a mucin cap. Most examples show low-grade dysplasia with cells that are typically cytologically bland: cytoplasm is abundant, and nuclei are basally located and relatively uniform. In high-grade lesions, the architecture becomes more complex and crowded with pseudostratified, hyperchromatic, and markedly pleomorphic nuclei and prominent nucleoli with loss of nuclear polarity (Fig. 4.14D). The background mucosa may show variable degree of gastritis, which is most frequently autoimmune in origin (33.9%). Association with *H. pylori* (41.5%) gastritis or chemical gastropathy (20.8%) has also been reported.

Immunohistochemical studies have demonstrated that pyloric gland adenomas typically show diffuse MUC6 expression and variable MUC5AC positivity, the latter either limited to the surface or intermixed. This pattern of expression is in contrast to gastric foveolar–type gastric adenomas, which predominantly express MUC5AC and limited MUC6 staining.

Differential Diagnosis

The main differential diagnoses for pyloric gland adenomas include gastric foveolar and intestinal-type adenomas and OGA. Pyloric gland adenomas are difficult to distinguish from low-grade foveolar adenomas because pale cytoplasm and bland cytologic appearance is present in both lesions. Histologic features in favor of pyloric gland adenoma are the pale, ground-glass quality of the entire cytoplasm versus a well-formed apical mucin cap, the lack of neutral mucin on PAS stain, and the presence of MUC6 expression. OGA can be excluded on the basis of parietal and chief cell differentiation that is diagnostic of this lesion.

Prognosis and Therapy

Complete excision and careful evaluation of the lesion and the surrounding nonlesional mucosa are needed because of the association with adenocarcinoma.

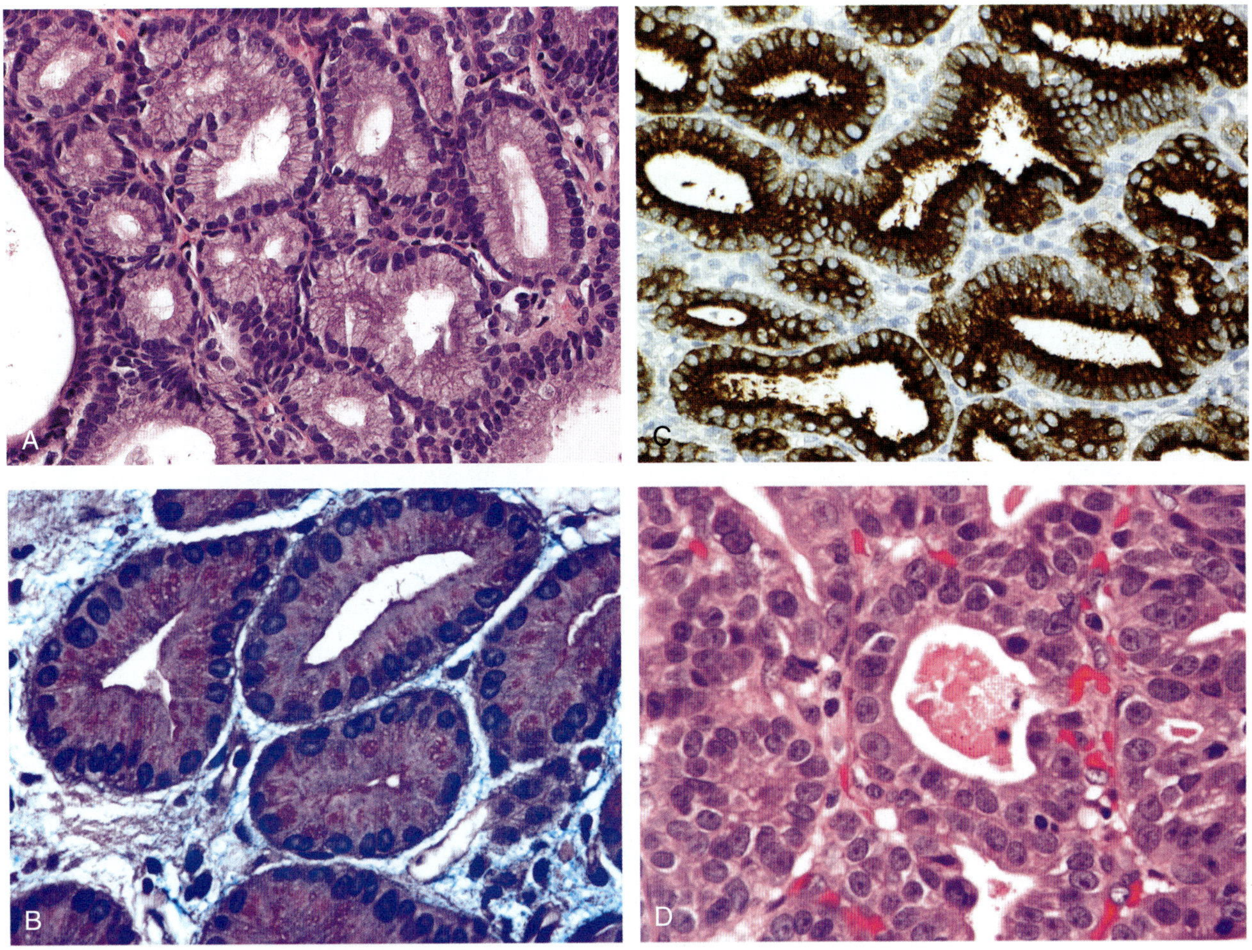

FIGURE 4.14
Pyloric gland adenoma composed of tightly packed glands lined by composed columnar cells with amphophilic cytoplasm (**A**). Note the lack of apical mucin cap using periodic acid–Schiff stain (**B**). MUC6 immunohistochemistry may help in supporting the diagnosis (**C**). A subset of cases may be associated with high-grade dysplasia (**D**) or carcinoma.

PYLORIC GLAND ADENOMA—FACT SHEET

Definition

- Neoplastic epithelial proliferation that shows pyloric gland type differentiation

Incidence and Location

- Uncommon lesions; 2.7% of all gastric polyps (excluding fundic gland polyps)
- Most often located in the gastric corpus

Morbidity and Mortality

- Most cases show low-grade dysplasia
- One-third may be associated with adenocarcinoma (usually large lesions)

Gender, Race, and Age

- Slight female predominance
- Typically present in seventh decade of life

Clinical Features

- Common associations include autoimmune gastritis, familial adenomatous polyposis, Lynch syndrome, and juvenile polyposis
- *Helicobacter pylori* gastritis and chemical gastropathy may be present in background mucosa
- No abnormality is detected in background mucosa in a subset of cases

Prognosis and Therapy

- Complete resection after excluding possibility of underlying invasive carcinoma on endoscopic ultrasound in larger lesions
- Proper evaluation of background mucosa to determine risk of metachronous lesions and need for surveillance

PYLORIC GLAND ADENOMA—PATHOLOGIC FEATURES

Gross Features

- Predominantly in the body and fundus
- Cannot be reliably distinguished from benign gastric polyps endoscopically

Microscopic Features

- Background mucosa often with autoimmune gastritis (atrophy and intestinal metaplasia)

- Amphophilic to eosinophilic cytoplasm with a ground-glass quality
- Low-grade dysplasia with well-organized glands of bland, nonpleomorphic, basally located nuclei
- High-grade dysplasia with crowding of glands, cribriform glands, nuclear stratification, cytologic atypia, and loss of nuclear polarity

Genetics

- Activating *GNAS* mutations, often associated with *KRAS* mutations

Differential Diagnosis

- Gastric foveolar or intestinal-type adenoma
- Oxyntic gland adenoma
- Hyperplastic polyp

OXYNTIC GLAND ADENOMA

CLINICAL FEATURES

Oxyntic gland adenomas are rare lesions that develop exclusively in the oxyntic mucosa and are composed primarily of chief cells with variable numbers of parietal and mucous neck cells. OGAs form the benign end of the oxyntic gland neoplasia spectrum with gastric adenocarcinomas of fundic gland type representing the malignant counterpart.

PATHOLOGIC FEATURES

GROSS FINDINGS

The polyps range in size from 4 to 20 mm, with an equal gender distribution and an average age at presentation of 65 years. The lesions are located in the gastric body or fundus and can either be depressed or elevated.

MICROSCOPIC FINDINGS

Oxyntic gland adenomas are composed of chief cells, parietal cells, and mucous neck cells that line closely packed tubules and anastomosing cords that can mimic a NET (Fig. 4.15). Most frequently, OGAs show a chief cell predominant pattern, but a balanced admixture of chief and parietal cells resembling normal fundic glands and a mucous neck cell–dominated form have also been recognized. Nuclear atypia, increased mitotic activity, necrosis, desmoplasia, perineural, and lymphovascular invasion are typically absent. The tumor can show "pseudoinvasion," but rare cases of true deep submucosal invasion and lymph node metastasis have also been reported. The surrounding nonlesional oxyntic gastric mucosa is usually normal.

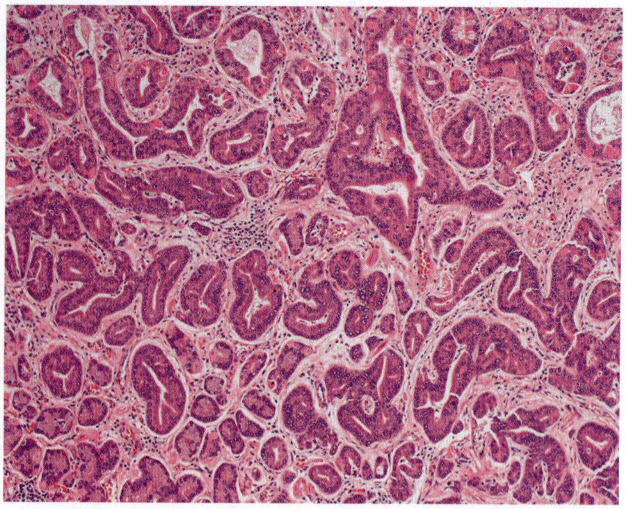

FIGURE 4.15
Oxyntic gland adenoma displaying irregularly anastomosing tubules and glands lined by bland chief and parietal cells.

ANCILLARY STUDIES

Gastric immunophenotypic markers MUC5AC and MUC6 are usually positive. Pepsinogen-I and H+/K+-ATPase immunohistochemistry may be used to highlight chief cells and parietal cells, respectively.

MOLECULAR STUDIES

Similar to pyloric adenoma, activating *GNAS* mutations associated with *KRAS* mutations are recognized in these polyps.

DIFFERENTIAL DIAGNOSIS

Pyloric gland adenoma represents the main differential diagnosis. Helpful histologic features are the cytoplasmic basophilia of chief cells and the identification of plump, intensely eosinophilic parietal cells with central bland nuclei.

PROGNOSIS AND THERAPY

Assessing the presence of submucosal invasion and predicting the biological behavior of oxyntic gland neoplasms can be difficult. Only limited data are available on the follow-up of these lesions. However, in the largest series available to date, no evidence of recurrence or metastasis was documented. OGAs limited to the mucosa pursue a benign course and can be managed by endoscopic resection. Lesions with atypical cytoarchitectural features and submucosal invasion have a low malignant potential, rarely with lymphovascular invasion, and can be diagnosed as "adenocarcinoma of fundic gland mucosa type."

OXYNTIC GLAND ADENOMA—PATHOLOGIC FEATURES

Gross Features

- Exclusively in the body and fundus
- May be elevated or depressed lesions; variable size

Microscopic Features

- Closely packed tubules and cords that can mimic a neuroendocrine tumor
- Lining epithelium composed predominantly of chief cells with variable number of parietal cells and mucous cells
- Nuclear atypia is minimal
- A minor subset of cases may show submucosal invasion, and lymphovascular invasion is reported in extremely rare cases ("adenocarcinoma of fundic gland mucosa type")

Genetics

- Activating *GNAS* mutations, often associated with *KRAS* mutations, similar to pyloric gland adenomas

Differential Diagnosis

- Pyloric gland adenoma

GASTRIC ADENOCARCINOMA

CLINICAL FEATURES

Gastric cancer is the fifth most common cancer worldwide and is a leading cause of cancer-related deaths. Overall, gastric cancer rates are higher in lower socioeconomic groups. The incidence of gastric cancer also shows geographical differences, with the lowest rates found in North America, Northern Europe, and Africa and the highest rates found in Korea, Japan, Costa Rica, East Asia, and Eastern Europe. Gastric cancer peaks in the seventh decade of life and affects men twice as often as women. Over the past decades, the rate of gastric cancer has been declining in older patients; however, the number of early onset carcinomas is increasing in North America.

There is also a difference between the epidemiologic trends of proximal and distal gastric cancers. Whereas the incidence of cancers arising from the gastroesophageal junction (GEJ) and the gastric cardia have been increasing, the number of distal carcinomas has been declining. These trends suggest that proximal gastric cancers may have a distinct pathogenesis and may be more closely related to esophageal adenocarcinomas. Because of this, the eighth edition of the tumor, node, metastasis (TNM) staging uses the following modification from prior editions: "Cancers involving the GEJ that have their epicenter within the proximal 2 cm of the cardia are to be staged as esophageal cancers. Cancers whose epicenter is more than 2 cm distal from the GEJ, even if the GEJ is involved, will be staged using the stomach cancer TNM and stage groupings."

GASTRIC CANCER RISK FACTORS

Several environmental risk factors have been associated with the development of gastric cancer. Whereas diets rich in nitrites, nitrates, salt, smoked foods, and complex carbohydrates are linked to increased gastric cancer risks, consumption of fresh fruits and vegetables is associated with reduced cancer risks. Cigarette smoking is also associated with a two- to threefold increased risk of gastric cancer.

Gastric carcinoma has a weak association with chronic atrophic gastritis and intestinal metaplasia. Several studies have shown an association between incomplete type of intestinal metaplasia and increased risk of gastric carcinoma; however, screening for the presence of this subtype is not a reliable tool in the absence of endoscopic mapping to determine the extent of metaplasia. Gastric carcinomas of the intestinal type have a greater association with intestinal metaplasia than do the poorly cohesive (i.e., diffuse) type.

H. pylori infection is now a well-established cause of both intestinal and poorly cohesive (i.e., diffuse) types of gastric carcinomas. The risk of gastric cancer is significantly increased if the *H. pylori* infection is acquired in childhood or is present for longer than 10 years. The relative risk of developing gastric adenocarcinoma because of chronic infection with *H. pylori* has been reported to be 5.9 times higher. Furthermore, *H. pylori* eradication at the time of localized gastric cancer resection decreases recurrence and the future risk of metachronous gastric cancer.

H. pylori is a heterogeneous group of strains with various factors associated with colonization and pathogenicity. Strains that produce the CagA protein induce a greater degree of inflammation and are associated with a higher risk of cancer. In the West, *H. pylori* strains expressing the vacA s1, m1, i1, or d1 genotypes have also been variably associated with an increased risk of gastric cancer.

Finally, the host response to *H. pylori* specific to the population infected is also important, as demonstrated by differing individual susceptibilities to gastric atrophy and carcinoma. Proinflammatory polymorphisms of the interleukin (IL)-1β gene (initiating and amplifying the inflammatory response) and the IL-1 receptor antagonist gene (an inflammatory cytokine that competitively binds to IL-1 receptors and modulates the potentially damaging effects of IL-1) are associated with individual or familial susceptibility to *H. pylori*–related carcinogenesis.

Other factors that increase the risk of gastric cancer include a history of prior gastrectomy, autoimmune gastritis, obesity, and Ménétrier's disease. Although the vast majority of gastric cancers occur sporadically, syndromic associations are also well recognized. Patients with FAP, gastric adenocarcinoma and proximal polyposis of the stomach, MAP, Lynch syndrome, Peutz-Jeghers syndrome, juvenile polyposis syndrome, Li-Fraumeni syndrome, and *BRCA2* mutations all have increased risk of developing gastric cancer. In addition, *CDH1* mutations affecting the adhesion molecule E-cadherin have been associated with autosomal dominant hereditary diffuse gastric cancer (HDGC).

Pathologic Features

Gross Findings

The majority of gastric carcinomas are located in the pylorus and antrum (50%–60%) followed by the cardia (25%) and the body or fundus (15%–25%). Advanced cancers of the intestinal type commonly appear as polypoid, fungating masses with surface ulceration. In contrast, poorly cohesive (diffuse-type) cancers usually appear as deep infiltrating or depressed cancers with no obvious mass present in the mucosa. Linitis plastica is a rare lesion in which the majority of the stomach wall is infiltrated by diffuse-type cancer, conferring a thick, firm, leathery appearance to the stomach.

Early gastric cancers are defined as those confined to the mucosa or submucosa regardless of lymph node status and are often incidental findings. The Japanese Gastroenterological Endoscopic Society devised an endoscopic classification for early gastric cancers, which aids in the detection of early subtle cancers. This scheme has a good correlation with the microscopic phenotype and was later adopted in the Paris classification of GI superficial neoplastic lesions. Most polypoid lesions have a tubular phenotype, but flat and ulcerated lesions are more commonly poorly cohesive.

Microscopic Findings

The overwhelming majority (95%) of malignant gastric cancers are adenocarcinomas. The 2019 WHO classification subdivides gastric carcinoma into the following subtypes: tubular; papillary; mucinous (Fig. 4.16); poorly cohesive carcinoma, including signet ring cell carcinoma and other subsets (Fig. 4.17); mixed adenocarcinoma; and other rare histologic subtypes (including gastric adenocarcinoma with lymphoid stroma [Fig. 4.18] hepatoid and micropapillary adenocarcinoma, and gastric adenocarcinoma of fundic-gland type; Table 4.1). The historic Lauren scheme separates gastric adenocarcinomas into intestinal and diffuse subtypes. The intestinal type generally corresponds to the tubular, papillary, and mucinous WHO categories and resembles colorectal adenocarcinoma. It is characterized by well-formed glands lined by columnar epithelium, often with a luminal brush border. In some cases, interspersed neuroendocrine cells can be detected. Intraluminal mucin is often present, but intracytoplasmic mucin droplets are restricted to goblet cells. Diffuse-type adenocarcinoma corresponds to the poorly

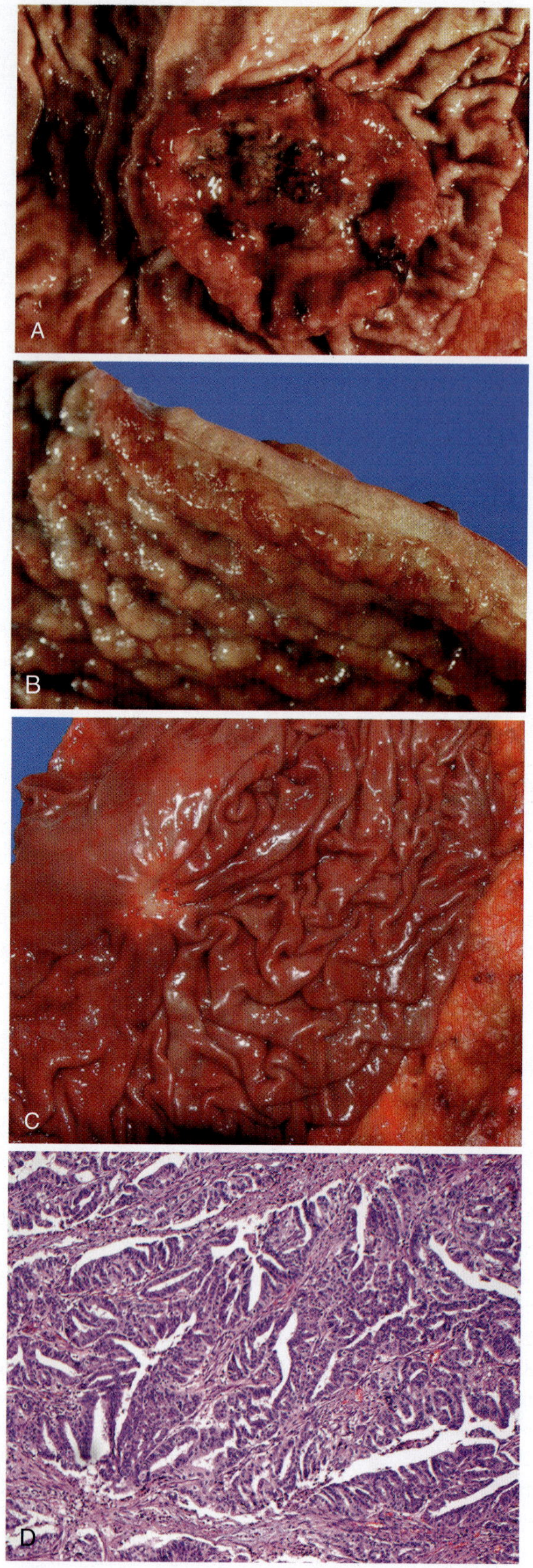

FIGURE 4.16

Gross appearances of gastric carcinoma. **A**, Intestinal-type adenocarcinoma with a large, exophytic, polypoid mass. **B**, Linitis plastica with markedly thickened, firm, and fibrotic gastric wall without a discrete mass. **C**, Early gastric cancer with a small area of mucosal ulceration. **D**, On microscopy, intestinal type tumors are mostly tubular adenocarcinomas characteristically composed of neoplastic tubules with an infiltrative growth pattern and show variable grade of differentiation.

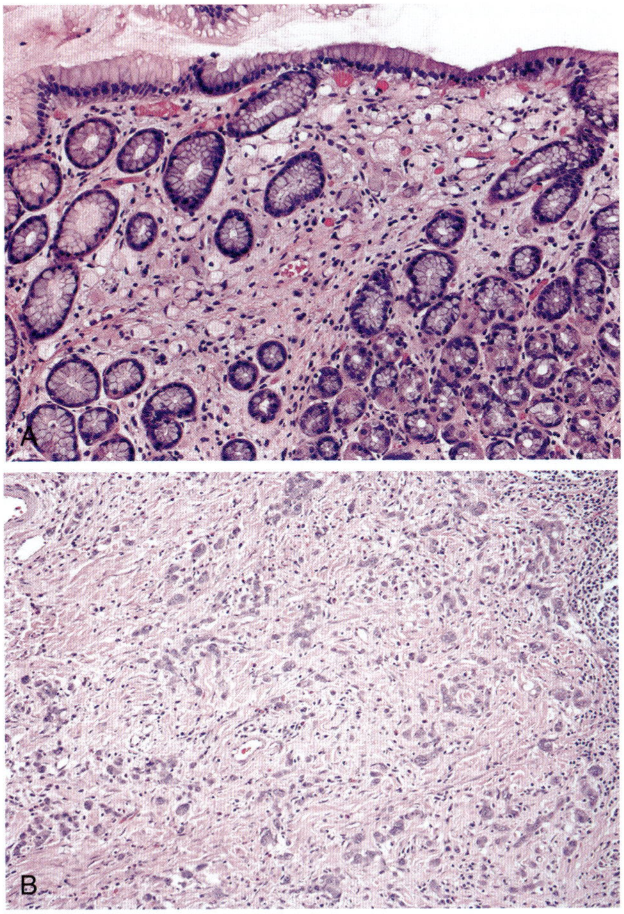

FIGURE 4.17

Poorly cohesive carcinomas. The neoplasm is composed of single cells and cells forming small aggregates some with various cytologic features. These tumors may show a signet ring cell morphology (**A**) or a small cell undifferentiated phenotype with scant cytoplasm (**B**). Metastatic breast cancer should be excluded before rendering a diagnosis of diffuse-type gastric cancer in these cases.

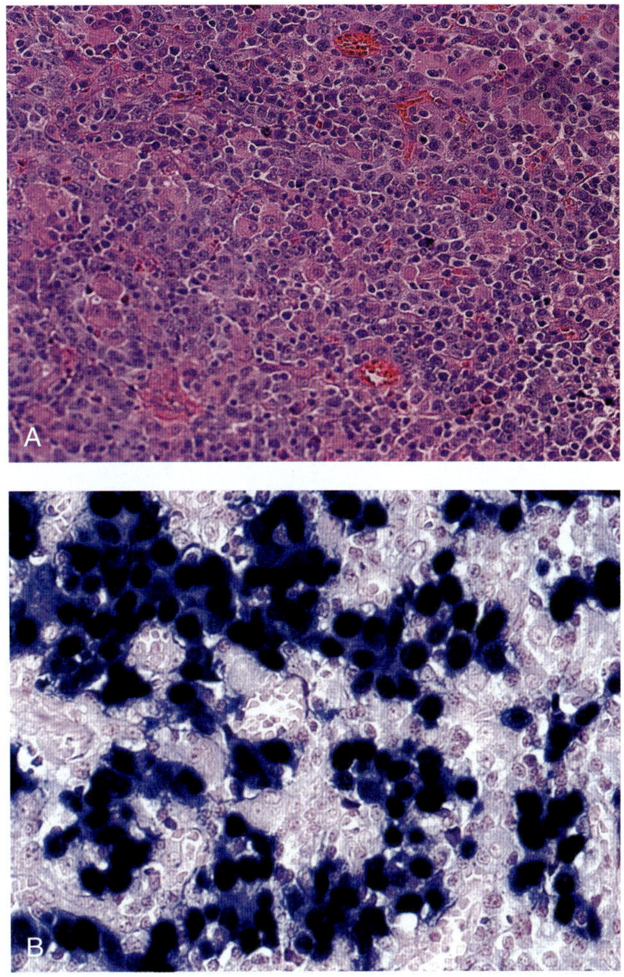

FIGURE 4.18

Example of gastric carcinoma with lymphoid stroma characterized by irregular sheets of epithelial cells embedded within a dense lymphocytic infiltrate (**A**). EBER ISH in situ hybridization confirms the diagnosis (**B**).

cohesive WHO category and is composed of individual cells or poorly formed nests growing in an infiltrative pattern. The amount of intracytoplasmic mucin present in these cells is highly variable. Sometimes these cells have abundant intracytoplasmic mucin pushing the nucleus to the periphery, leading to a signet ring appearance, hence the term *poorly cohesive carcinoma–signet ring cell type*. In other cases, including histiocytic, plasmacytoid, and pleiomorphic variants, mucin may be inconspicuous. Such tumors are designated as poorly cohesive carcinoma not otherwise specified. One rare presentation of diffuse-type gastric adenocarcinoma occurs in the setting of hereditarty diffuse gastric cancer (HDGC). In one-third of these families, a germline E-cadherin mutation can be detected. These patients may present with invasive carcinoma during their teenage years. Although this presentation is rare, examination of the histologic precursors of this hereditary carcinoma is instructive for reviewing the various morphologic variants of signet ring cell carcinomas (Fig. 4.19). Some gastric adenocarcinomas show features of both intestinal and diffuse types; these are classified as mixed types. It is important to note that the terms *intestinal* and *diffuse* are not synonymous with *well-* and *poorly differentiated carcinomas*.

Gastric carcinoma with lymphoid stroma usually develops in the proximal stomach or in the gastric stump after partial gastrectomy. Typically, these tumors present a well-demarcated pushing margin and are composed of irregular sheets, trabeculae, and ill-defined tubules, resulting in a lace-like pattern embedded in a dense lymphocytic infiltrate that may mimic a lymphoma (see Fig. 4.18). Epstein-Barr virus (EBV) can be detected in 22% to 100% of these tumors; furthermore, the infection likely occurs early because EBV can also be found in adjacent dysplasia. Two other histologic variants of EBV-associated gastric cancers have been recognized: tubular carcinomas with prominent lymphoid follicles (i.e., "carcinoma with Crohn's disease-like lymphoid reaction") and conventional-type adenocarcinomas with scant lymphocytic infiltrate. Global CpG island hypermethylation with epigenetic silencing of tumor

TABLE 4.1

Examples of Rare Variants of Gastric Adenocarcinomas and Their Characteristics

Type	Histology	Other Characteristics
Hepatoid or AFP-producing adenocarcinoma	• Hepatoid adenocarcinoma with large polygonal eosinophilic cells • Well-differentiated tubular-papillary lesions with clear cytoplasm • Yolk-sac tumor-like carcinoma	• AFP can be detected immunohistochemistry and in the serum • Bile and PAS(+) and diastase-resistant intracytoplasmic eosinophilic globules can be detected in the hepatoid cells
Adenosquamous carcinoma	• Squamous component >25% of the tumor	• Usually diagnosed at an advanced stage
Squamous cell carcinoma	• Carcinoma with uniform squamous cell differentiation and sometimes keratin pearls	• Usually diagnosed at an advanced stage

AFP, Alpha-fetoprotein; *PAS*, period acid–Schiff.

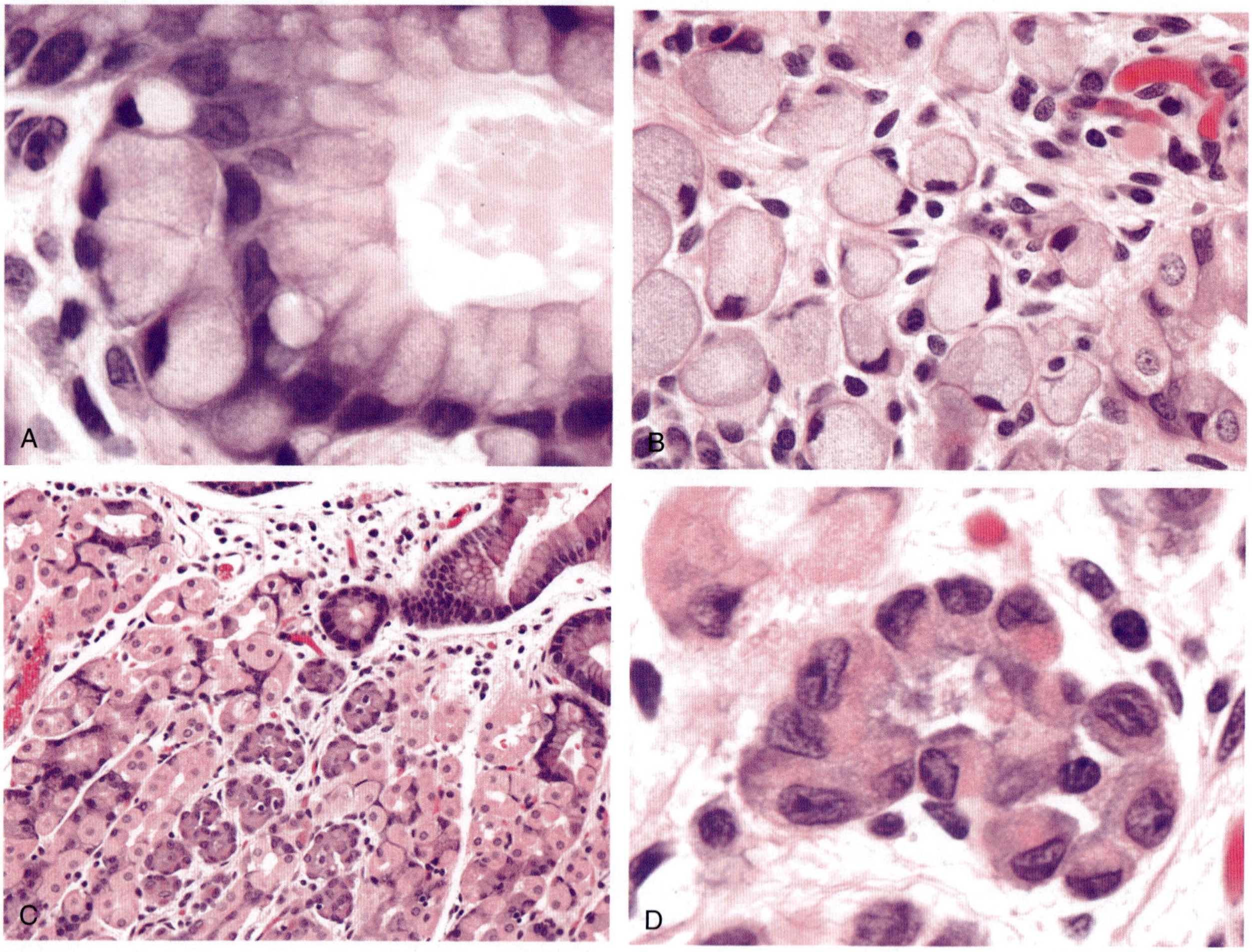

FIGURE 4.19

In situ signet ring cells (**A**) in a prophylactic gastrectomy in a patient with hereditary diffuse gastric cancer syndrome that also showed foci of superficial invasion into the lamina propria (**B**). Subtle replacement of a gland with neoplastic cells (**C**) with higher magnification of the tumor cells (**D**).

suppressor genes is a unique feature of this variant and is considered to be crucial for its carcinogenesis. Another subset of gastric carcinoma with lymphoid stroma has been associated with microsatellite instability and MMR protein deficiency but shows a distinct transcriptomic profile. The prognosis of these carcinomas is better than that of typical adenocarcinomas.

Ancillary Studies

Gastric adenocarcinomas are cytokeratin, epithelial membrane antigen (EMA), and carcinoembryonic antigen positive. CK7/CK20 profiles vary considerably with the majority being CK7 positive and CK20 negative. The testing for HER2 as a predictive biomarker of anti-HER2 therapy for unresectable and metastatic gastric cancer is well established. Primary testing by immunohistochemistry should be followed by in situ hybridization (ISH) in equivocal cases.

Given the superior prognosis, a diagnosis of gastric carcinoma with lymphoid stroma should prompt testing for the presence of EBV by EBER ISH and MMR protein deficiency by immunohistochemistry. Although not recommended by the WHO, immunophenotyping using p53, MMR proteins, E-cadherin, and EBER ISH can be used as a surrogate technique to determine the recently reported molecular subtypes of gastric cancer and may have clinical relevance in the future.

Molecular Pathology

Gastric adenocarcinomas also show marked heterogeneity at the molecular level.

The Cancer Genome Atlas performed a comprehensive analysis and identified four major molecular subtypes of gastric cancer:

1. *Genetically stable gastric cancers*, which represent about 20% of the cases. These tumors are usually aneuploid and diagnosed at an earlier age. *CDH1* somatic mutations are present in about 37% of the cases. Inactivating mutations of *ARID1A* are also noted within this group, and mutations of *RHOA* are common as well.
2. *Chromosomally unstable gastric cancers*, which represent about 50% of all gastric cancers. A large proportion (70%) of these cancers harbor *TP53* mutations.
3. *Microsatellite unstable gastric cancers* represent about 20% of the cases and are characterized by hypermethylation, including of the *MLH1* promoter region, and high rates of mutation in *KRAS*, *ALK*, *ARID1A*, and the PI3K-PTEN-mTOR pathway. These cancers tend to occur in women of older age, arise in the antrum, and have an intestinal phenotype.
4. *Gastric cancers with EBV infection*, which constitute about 10% of gastric cancers and tend to affect males. These lesions have a lower frequency of lymph node metastasis and a lower mortality rate. EBV-positive tumors also show a high CpG island methylator phenotype. Characteristics of these tumors include *CDKN2A* promoter hypermethylation and nonsilent mutations of *PIK3CA* in 80% of the cases.

Differential Diagnosis

Because of the frequently bland cytological features, poorly cohesive carcinoma can often be mistaken for a variety of benign processes, including lymphoid infiltrate in chronic gastritis, foamy macrophages, or reactive endothelial cells seen in granulation tissue. Furthermore, cells of damaged and detached foveolar epithelium can mimic signet ring cells. It may also mimic lymphoma because of its diffuse growth pattern and round, plasmacytoid cell outlines. Therefore, pathologists should always be alert when evaluating gastric biopsies and keep this possibility in mind. Stains for cytokeratin, EMA, and mucin can highlight the discohesive and infiltrating neoplastic cells and help in diagnosis in some cases. Other cancers with discohesive cells may spread to the stomach and mimic primary poorly cohesive carcinoma. The most common one is invasive lobular carcinoma of the breast. Therefore, one should always consider the possibility of a metastasis and have a low threshold to order immunohistochemical work-up to avoid this diagnostic pitfall, especially in female patients with normal background mucosa.

Prognosis and Therapy

Gastric adenocarcinoma has an overall poor prognosis with 5-year survival rates of 10% to 30%. The best predictor of prognosis is the pathologic stage, which includes the depth of invasion, the extent of nodal involvement, and the presence or absence of distant metastasis. Poor prognostic indicators include older age, proximal tumor location, and venous or lymphatic invasion. Surgical resection remains the standard of care, but patients with proximal cardia tumors with GEJ involvement are often treated with neoadjuvant therapy. More than 50% of patients present with unresectable metastatic or locally advanced disease. In these cases, palliative treatments include palliative surgery, radiation, or endoscopic procedures to alleviate obstruction. Testing for HER2 overexpression or amplification is well established in routine practice now. Immunotherapy may be indicated in cases with PDL1 expression or deficient staining for MMR proteins on immunohistochemistry.

GASTRIC ADENOCARCINOMA—FACT SHEET

Definition

- Malignant gastric epithelial neoplasm with wide array of morphological patterns and varying grades of histologic differentiation

Incidence and Location

- Fifth most common cancer worldwide
- Higher incidence in parts of the world endemic for *Helicobacter pylori*
- Incidence of distal gastric cancer declining; proximal gastric cancer and diffuse-type gastric cancer incidence is increasing in the United States
- Antrum or pylorus is commonest location followed by cardia and gastric body

Morbidity and Mortality

- Good prognosis for early gastric cancer confined to mucosa and submucosa
- Advanced-stage tumors have a poor outcome (5-year survival rate is only 10%–30%)

Gender, Race, and Age

- Men affected twice as often as women; peak incidence in the seventh decade of life
- High incidence in Far East and Eastern Europe

Clinical Features

- Can be sporadic or syndromic (e.g., germline *CDH1* mutation)
- Increased risk in patients with *H. pylori* gastritis and autoimmune gastritis, which is related to mucosal atrophy and intestinal metaplasia
- Abdominal pain or discomfort and unintentional weight loss are common presenting symptoms
- Lesions may be polypoid, flat, or depressed on endoscopic or gross examination

Prognosis and Therapy

- Complete resection after excluding possibility of underlying invasive carcinoma on endoscopic ultrasound in larger lesions
- Proper evaluation of background mucosa to determine risk of metachronous lesions and need for surveillance

Gastric Adenocarcinoma—Pathologic Features

Gross Features

- May be exophytic, flat, or ulcerated
- Linitis plastica corresponds to broad area of gastric wall thickening, typically in diffuse-type gastric cancer

Microscopic Features

- Classified as intestinal type or diffuse type (Lauren classification)
- Intestinal type: well-formed glands lined by columnar to cuboidal epithelial cells
- Diffuse type: individual or poorly formed nests of cells growing in an infiltrative pattern
- Diffuse type (poorly cohesive type in World Health Organization classification) may show signet ring cells, plasmacytoid or histiocytoid cells and mimic lymphoma
- Intestinal-type tumors are often associated with *Helicobacter pylori* or autoimmune gastritis in the background mucosa
- Metastatic breast (lobular) carcinoma can mimic diffuse-type gastric cancer and should be excluded in female patients
- Prominent lymphoid infiltrate may be present in tumors that are microsatellite instability (MSI) high or associated with Epstein-Barr virus (EBV) infection

Molecular Pathology

- Four subtypes of sporadic gastric adenocarcinoma have been recognized:
  1. Genetically stable (~20%) and corresponding to diffuse-type gastric cancer
  2. Chromosomally unstable (50%) and showing *TP53* mutations
  3. Microsatellite unstable (20%) that are deficient in mismatch repair protein expression on immunohistochemistry or show MSI
  4. Gastric cancers with EBV infection (10%)

Immunohistochemical Findings

- Variable CK7/CK20 profile (most common CK7+/CK20-)
- Carcinoembryonic antigen positive

Differential Diagnosis

- Lymphoma (for diffuse type)
- Metastatic carcinoma (especially invasive lobular carcinomas of the breast)
- Gastritis cystica polyposa

TABLE 4.2

Gastric Cancer–Predisposing Polyposis and Nonpolyposis Syndromes with Characteristic Molecular Features

Syndrome	Genes	Gastric Cancer Risk (%)
Hereditary diffuse gastric cancer syndrome	*CDH1*	56–70
Gastric adenocarcinoma and proximal polyposis syndrome	*APC (promoter 1B)*	Not determined
Lynch syndrome	*MLH1, MSH2, MSH6, PMS2*	2–30
Peutz-Jeghers syndrome	*STK11*	29
Juvenile polyposis	*SMAD4, BMPR1A*	21
Hereditary breast and ovarian cancer syndrome	*BRCA1, BRCA2*	5.5, 2.6
Li-Fraumeni syndrome	*TP53*	3.1–4.9
Familial adenomatous polyposis	*APC*	2.1–4.2
MUTYH-associated polyposis	*MUTYH (MYH)*	Very low

Modified from Setia N, Clark JW, Duda DG, et al. Familial gastric cancers. *Oncologist*. 2015;20:1365–1377.

Syndromic Gastric Cancers

The majority of gastric carcinomas are sporadic; however, approximately 10% show familial clustering, and a hereditary gene defect is recognized in 1% to 3% of cases.

Syndromic gastric cancer (Table 4.2) includes HDGC syndrome (see Fig. 4.19), FAP, GAPPS, Lynch syndrome, Peutz-Jeghers syndrome, juvenile polyposis syndrome, hereditary breast and ovarian cancer syndrome, Li-Fraumeni syndrome, FAP, and MAP.

Heterozygous mutation in the tumor suppressor gene *CDH1*, which encodes for the calcium-dependent adhesion protein E-cadherin, is found in HDGC syndrome. Carcinomas start to develop when the second allele is inactivated by hypermethylation of the promoter, intragenic deletions, or somatic mutations of *CDH1*. In addition, germline mutations in *CTNNA1* gene have also been reported. The inactivation of *CDH1* leads to absent or decreased E-cadherin protein expression by immunohistochemistry on neoplastic cells. Because of the high lifetime risk of gastric carcinoma (70%) in male carriers, endoscopic surveillance biopsies to evaluate for microscopic carcinoma and/or prophylactic gastrectomy are often recommended for carriers of *CDH1* truncating mutations.

GASTRIC SECONDARY TUMORS

Metastases to the stomach are reported in 5.4% of patients with cancer. One-third of endoscopically detected secondary tumors in the GI tract are found in the stomach. Malignant melanoma, breast (especially lobular carcinoma), pulmonary, and renal cell carcinomas represent the most common metastatic tumors involving the stomach. Finally, reports of pancreaticobiliary tract, gynecologic primaries (ovary, uterus), hepatocellular carcinoma, bladder, colon, prostate, testis, head and neck, and bone and soft tissue primary tumors have also been reported.

CLINICAL FEATURES

Abdominal pain, nausea, and vomiting are common symptoms. Guaiac-positive stools or upper GI bleeding can also be initial manifestations of the disease. Gastric metastases are usually indicative of advanced disease with a reported overall survival of less than 1 year. In many patients, the diagnosis is straightforward because a history of primary neoplasm is already known. Furthermore, in many cases, additional synchronous sites of metastatic disease are recognized. Only in rare cases is gastric metastasis the initial manifestation of an occult malignancy.

PATHOLOGIC FEATURES

GROSS FINDINGS

Metastatic tumors to the stomach are often nonspecific and may mimic a primary gastric malignancy. Only rarely, subtle findings such as multiple, small black spots may be noted indicative of a metastatic malignant melanoma. Furthermore, the metastases may be submucosal with a smooth overlying mucosa, or they can present as a diffuse infiltration mimicking linitis plastica.

MICROSCOPIC FINDINGS

The morphologic features are specific to the primary sites of origin because in many cases, they may overlap with features of primary gastric carcinoma. The availability of clinical history and radiologic reports and review of previous material are important in making a definitive diagnosis. Ancillary immunohistochemical studies have a vital role to play in the differential diagnosis, especially in the absence of sufficient clinical information or in the case of poorly differentiated neoplasms. Metastasis to the stomach is reported in 5.9% to 11.6% of patients with breast carcinomas. In nearly half of the cases, the gastric metastases are diagnosed at least 3 years after the primary diagnosis. Invasive lobular carcinoma is the source of the majority (70%–75%) of cases, and the distinction with diffuse-type gastric cancer can be difficult because both tumors show single cell infiltration and cytoplasmic lumen formation (Fig. 4.20). Furthermore, only a minor subset of metastases presents as localized lesions, and more than half of the cases show diffuse infiltration of the gastric wall. The use of immunohistochemistry is essential, with estrogen receptor (ER), progesterone receptor (PR), gross cystic disease fluid protein 15 (GCDFP-15), GATA binding protein 3 (GATA3), and mammaglobin expression favoring a breast primary. Strong CDX2 labeling favors a gastric primary but is seldom seen in diffuse-type gastritis cancer, which is the main differential diagnosis. Metastasis to the stomach is also reported in 2.4% to 6.8% of patients with lung carcinoma, and most cases are recognized within 1 year after the diagnosis of the primary malignancy. Metastasis from a pulmonary primary is more frequently diagnosed in the autopsy setting and less commonly by endoscopic

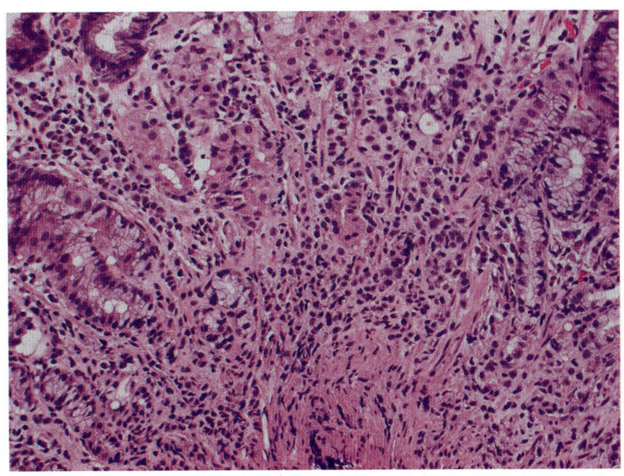

FIGURE 4.20

Lobular breast carcinoma metastatic to the stomach showing infiltrating single cell mimicking a poorly cohesive carcinoma. Immunohistochemical stains are helpful to confirm the diagnosis of metastatic breast carcinoma.

biopsy, presumably because of the dismal prognosis of advanced lung cancer. The detection of dysplasia in the gastric mucosa is the most definitive way of establishing the diagnosis of a gastric primary and to exclude a metastatic adenocarcinoma. Ancillary studies may be helpful as well because nearly 75% of pulmonary adenocarcinomas are positive for thyroid transcription factor 1 (TTF-1). However, CDX-2 or CK20, both markers of gastric adenocarcinomas, are also frequently expressed in the mucinous, colloid, and enteric subtypes of pulmonary adenocarcinomas. To differentiate a pulmonary neuroendocrine carcinoma (NEC) from a rare gastric primary, one has to rely on clinical investigation because the morphology is similar, and the expression of TTF-1 is not helpful because more than 10% of primary gastric NECs are positive.

Malignant melanoma metastasizes to the stomach in approximately 20% to 25% of patients and may be detected synchronously at the time of diagnosis of the primary lesion or years later as a recurrence. The microscopic features are similar to those seen in cutaneous lesions with diffuse and strong immunoreactivity for S-100, SOX10, HMB-45, and MART-1.

NEUROENDOCRINE NEOPLASMS

Neuroendocrine neoplasms (NENs) have prognoses that span from indolent to very aggressive. The 2019 edition of the WHO classification of digestive tumors divides NENs into well-differentiated neoplasms also known as NETs and poorly differentiated neoplasms also known as NECs based on their distinctive histomorphology. This new classification also uses a three-tier grading scheme for NETs, according to the mitotic count and Ki-67 proliferation index:

Grade 1: less than 2/10 hpf mitosis or less than 3% Ki-67 index
Grade 2: 2 to 20/10 hpf mitosis or 3% to 20% Ki-67 index
Grade 3: greater than 20/10 hpf mitosis or greater than 20% Ki-67 index

A rare subset of well-differentiated NENs may also be grade 3 based on mitotic activity or proliferative index. Neoplasms with a mixture of distinct non-neuroendocrine and neuroendocrine components (the latter should constitute >30% of the lesion) should be designated as mixed neuroendocrine–non-neuroendocrine neoplasm (MiNENs). The category of mixed adenoneuroendocrine carcinoma (MANEC) with adenocarcinoma and poorly differentiated NEC component is now considered a subtype of MiNEN because it was recognized that in rare cases, the exocrine component of mixed tumors can be benign, but the neuroendocrine component can be well-differentiated, designated as mixed adenoma neuroendocrine tumor (MANET). Other rare variants with a non-neuroendocrine component other than adenocarcinoma (e.g., acinar cell differentiation) have also been reported.

Neuroendocrine Tumors

Gastric NETs are uncommon neoplasms usually detected in middle-aged adults. These lesions represent fewer than 2% of all gastric malignancies and about 9% of all GI NETs. A rise in incidence, possibly related to a greater use of endoscopy, has been recently recognized. The clinical history and the microscopic appearance of the background gastric mucosa is helpful in determining the site-specific subtype and the expected prognosis.

Clinical Features

The WHO classification of gastric NETs recognizes three types divided primarily according to their underlying pathogenesis related to presence or absence of hypergastrinemia and autoimmune gastritis. In type I NETs, the hypergastrinemia is caused by chronic atrophic gastritis of the corpus caused by autoimmune gastritis and the attendant hypochlorhydria. In type II NETs, the hypergastrinemia is caused by Zollinger-Ellison syndrome (ZES), and the tumors nearly always arise in the context of multiple endocrine neoplasia type I (rather than a sporadic gastrinoma) and are accompanied by hyperchlorhydria. They represent 80% to 90% and 5% of all gastric NETs, respectively, and are typically small, multifocal, slow growing, and asymptomatic. Tumors smaller than 1 cm in diameter that are confined to the mucosa and submucosa and show no angioinvasion on microscopy rarely metastasize. Type III NETs, which represent 10% to 15% of all gastric NETs, are fundamentally different because they are sporadic, usually solitary, and larger neoplasms that do not arise within the context of hypergastrinemia or endocrine cell hyperplasia. These tumors tend to be located in the prepyloric region, and their outcome is usually more guarded because they may present with hemorrhage, obstruction, or metastasis. These lesions are more likely to spread, usually to regional lymph nodes and to the liver.

Neuroendocrine carcinomas are highly aggressive neoplasm that account for 6% to 20% of gastric NENs. Most cases arise de novo, and there are only few examples of progression from NET (G1 and G2) to high-grade (G3) NEC. Cases with paraneoplastic syndromes are rare.

Pathologic Findings

Gross and Endoscopic Findings

Type I and II gastric NETs are usually multifocal, small, (<1 cm) polypoid, firm, well-circumscribed elevations in the corpus and fundus. Whereas the background corpus mucosa typically shows chronic atrophic changes in type I enterochromaffin-like cell NETs (related to autoimmune gastritis), in type II, it may be hypertrophic with prominent rugae, reflecting parietal cell hyperplasia that is typical of the ZES. Type III NETs tend to be solitary and larger (>2 cm in diameter) and can show central umbilication with focal superficial erosion and hemorrhage. The background mucosa is usually normal in type III NETs

Neuroendocrine carcinomas usually form a large fungating mass indistinguishable from typical adenocarcinomas. Larger tumors may present with central umbilication and ulceration. Most cases are deeply infiltrating and frequently present with nodal and hepatic metastases at the time of initial diagnosis.

Microscopic Findings

Type I and II NETs are composed of ECL cells and usually show a mixture of growth patterns with nests, ribbon-like trabeculae, and rosettes, but sometimes acinar structures can also be seen. They are composed of small, uniform, polygonal or cuboidal cells with lightly eosinophilic, finely granular cytoplasm; regular, round, or oval nuclei; minimal nuclear pleomorphism; and a characteristic stippled ("salt and pepper") chromatin (Fig. 4.21). Type I and II gastric NETs usually display low mitotic activity (<2/10 hpf) and Ki-67 index (≤2 %) and usually fall under the grade 1 category. Invasion into the submucosa is common but deeper infiltration and lymphovascular invasion is rarely seen.

Type III NETs can be composed of serotonin-producing enterochromaffin cells and may display a higher degree of nuclear pleomorphism, hyperchromasia, prominent nucleoli, or necrosis. With the increasing size, the risk of vascular or muscularis propria invasion, cytologic atypia, and mitotic activity also increases. Finally, the proliferative activity typically qualifies as grade 2 in these tumors.

Gastric NECs are by definition poorly differentiated grade 3 NENs and classified into small cell NEC (SCNEC) and large cell NEC (LCNEC) analogous to their pulmonary counterparts. SCNEC forms sheets of densely packed small round to ovoid tumor cells with finely granular chromatin. LCNECs are composed of solid nests with large tumor cells that have abundant cytoplasm and prominent nucleoli (Fig. 4.22). Although SCLCs only occasionally show features of neuroendocrine growth pattern, LCNECs frequently contain rosettes or show peripheral palisading and organoid nesting. Both types are characterized by an infiltrative growth pattern and multifocal necrosis. Although the diagnosis of NECs is now based on the histomorphology and not the proliferative activity a high mitotic rate (>20 mitoses/hpf) and a Ki-67 labeling index of greater than 20 % (typically >75 %) are usually observed. Lymphovascular invasion is commonly reported in these lesions.

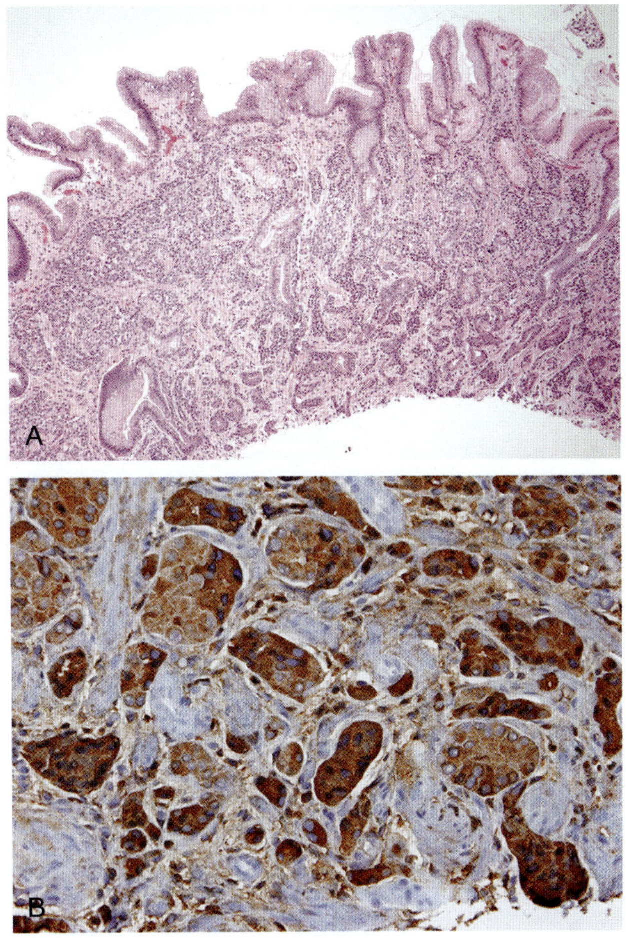

FIGURE 4.21

Type I neuroendocrine tumors characterized by enlarging nests of small, uniform, cuboidal cells with lightly eosinophilic cytoplasm and regular, round nuclei and minimal nuclear pleomorphism (**A**). The neoplasm is highlighted by synaptophysin immunohistochemistry (**B**).

Precursor Lesions

The background oxyntic mucosa of patients with type I NET shows features of autoimmune gastritis with atrophy, pseudopyloric, intestinal, and pancreatic acinar metaplasia. In type II NETs, the corpus-fundus mucosa often shows a marked hypertrophy of the oxyntic glands with hyperplasia of parietal cells, which is typical of ZES. Whereas in both type I and II NETs, striking proliferation of small, cuboidal, histamine-producing ECL cells can be detected, hyperplasia of gastrin-producing G-cells is only associated with type I tumors. The ECL cell hyperplasia can appear in three patterns representing stages of disease progression: (1) the mildest diffuse scattered

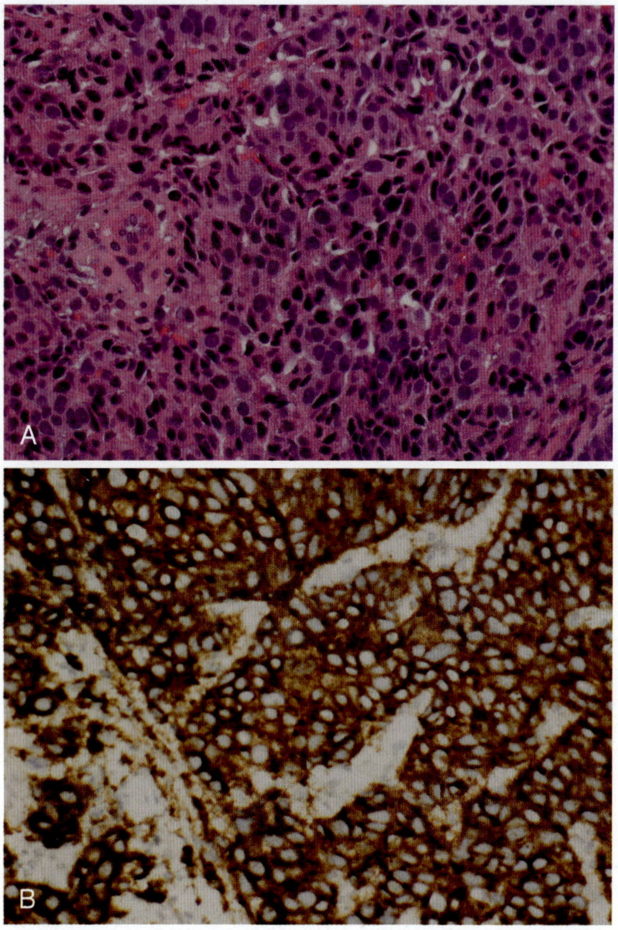

FIGURE 4.22

Neuroendocrine carcinoma characterized by infiltrative sheets of anaplastic round cells (**A**). The carcinoma is positive for general neuroendocrine markers, including synaptophysin (**B**).

ECL cell hyperplasia, (2) the moderate linear hyperplasia (forming chains of more than five contiguous cells), and (3) the advanced nodular hyperplasia with small cell nests which may extend into the lamina propria and/or muscularis mucosae. The fusion of at least five micronodules or the aggregates of nodules measuring greater than 150 microns in greatest dimension is designated as ECL cell dysplasia by some authors. The diagnosis of NET can be used for ECL cell aggregates exceeding 0.5 mm in diameter or those invading the submucosa. Type III NETs are not known to be associated with any underlying disease or specific mucosal changes.

Ancillary Studies

The diagnosis of gastric NETs can be confirmed by immunohistochemistry for neuroendocrine markers such as chromogranin A, synaptophysin, or insulinoma-associated protein 1 (INSM1). Vesicular monoamine transporter type II is a specific marker of ECL cells but is only rarely used in routine histopathology because the recognition of autoimmune gastritis in the background mucosa is a sufficient surrogate tool to recognize the ECL cell nature. Immunohistochemical detection of specific peptide hormones that may be expressed by the tumor does not have any clinical implication.

Neuroendocrine carcinomas are reactive for general neuroendocrine markers, including chromogranin A, synaptophysin, and INSM1. TTF-1 expression is present in more than 10% of primary gastric NECs and should not be regarded as evidence for metastatic disease of a pulmonary origin.

Differential Diagnosis

The main differential diagnosis of gastric NETs is with glomus tumors. Glomus tumors are composed of small, round cells with centrally placed hyperchromatic nuclei and thus show considerable overlap with NETs, including rare cases with patchy synaptophysin positivity. However, glomus tumor cells have lumpy, coarse chromatin. In addition, these cells have a pale eosinophilic to clear cytoplasm instead of the amphophilic cytoplasm of NETs, usually surround blood vessels, and are positive for myoid markers on immunohistochemistry.

The main differential diagnosis of NEC is with a poorly differentiated adenocarcinoma and malignant lymphoma. Appropriate use of immunohistochemistry allows the diagnosis in most cases. Furthermore, it is important to recall that whereas LCNEC presents frequently with organoid, trabecular pattern, the cells have a prominent eosinophilic cytoplasm, coarse nuclear chromatin, and numerous nucleoli. Infrequently, NENs may show a morphology overlapping between NEC and grade 3 NET. Given that genetic alterations in *TP53* and *RB1* are more frequent in NECs than in NETs, identification of such mutations or immunohistochemical detection of aberrant p53 and retinoblastoma expression s can help in the differential diagnosis of these neoplasms.

Prognosis and Therapy

In general, gastric NETs have a relatively good prognosis compared with adenocarcinomas. The 5-year survival rates of localized tumor versus regional spread versus distant spread are 73% versus 65% versus 25%, respectively. Type I NETs have the best 5-year survival rate of practically 100%, yet about 3% of these patients develop lymph node or liver metastases. Not surprisingly, type III tumors have the worst prognosis. It is estimated that patients with these lesions have a 5-year survival rate of 50% with half of the patients developing lymph node or liver metastases. Type II NETs have a prognosis between types I and III. It is important to note that although a worse prognosis may depend on the NET type, the most important and worst prognostic factor for all NETs is a tumor size of greater than 2 cm. Low-grade NETs can be managed conservatively because they may regress with long-acting somatostatin analogues or may be completely removed by endoscopic excision, with subsequent endoscopic follow-up. In the few cases of type I NETs with numerous polyps, antrectomy to remove the trophic stimulus from antral G cells may be indicated. Only patients with large or numerous tumors or dominant grade 2 tumors should be considered for surgery.

Patients with localized NEC should be considered for resection that should include adequate regional lymph node staging. In addition, intensive chemotherapy, with or without surgery, is recommended for patients with gastric NEC at any stage. Chemotherapy is not standardized, and various mainly platinum-based protocols, including cisplatin, etoposide, cyclophosphamide, and doxorubicin are used. The distinction between NEC and grade 3 well-differentiated NET has prognostic significance, but both groups are treated in a similar fashion with platinum-based chemotherapy.

GASTRIC NEUROENDOCRINE NEOPLASMS—FACT SHEET

Definition

- Neoplastic endocrine proliferations that span a spectrum from benign indolent tumors to highly aggressive tumors with dismal prognosis

Incidence and Location

- Rare and make up 0.1% to 0.6% of all gastric neoplasms and 7% to 8% of all neuroendocrine tumors (NETs)
- Increasing incidence may be related to greater access to upper endoscopy and higher detection
- NETs in autoimmune gastritis and Zollinger-Ellison syndrome (ZES) typically involve the corpus; sporadic type III tumors are usually present in the antrum

Morbidity and Mortality

- Type I tumors are the most indolent, and type III carry the worst prognosis among NETs with type II somewhere in the middle
- Neuroendocrine carcinomas (NECs) are highly aggressive tumors with a dismal prognosis

Gender, Race, and Age

- Type I tumors more frequent in women because of greater prevalence of autoimmune gastritis
- Median age of patients is around 60 years

Clinical Features

- Common predisposing conditions include autoimmune gastritis and ZES in the setting of multiple endocrine neoplasia type I; type III NETs are sporadic tumors with normal background mucosa
- NECs present as large bulky tumors with ulceration that mimic conventional carcinoma

Prognosis and Therapy

- Complete excision on endoscopy and surveillance for small NETs; surgical resection for large or deeply infiltrating or multicentric tumors; chemotherapy with or without surgery for grade 3 NETs and NEC
- NECs are aggressive tumors with a poor prognosis

GASTRIC NEUROENDOCRINE NEOPLASMS—PATHOLOGIC FEATURES

Gross Findings

- Neuroendocrine tumors (NETs)are small, well-circumscribed submucosal lesions
- Larger tumors can show central umbilication
- Type I and II NETs are small, often multiple, and are located in the corpus fundus
- Type III tumors tend to be larger, solitary, and located in the prepyloric region
- NECs are deeply infiltrative and frequently ulcerated, grossly indistinguishable from adenocarcinomas

Microscopic Findings

- NETs: ribbon-like trabecular, nesting, or acinar growth patterns; uniform small round cells with salt-and-pepper chromatin
- Grading of NETs is based on the mitotic count and Ki-67 proliferation index
- Gastric NETs are subcategorized based on their underlying pathogenesis
- Type I NETs are associated with features of autoimmune gastritis and have an excellent prognosis
- Type II NETs are associated with features of Zollinger-Ellison syndrome and have an intermediate prognosis
- Type III NETs are not associated with other mucosal changes and have a poor prognosis
- NECs: Subclassified into small cell NEC and large cell NEC similar to the pulmonary equivalents
- Neoplasms with a mixture of distinct non-neuroendocrine and neuroendocrine components (>30% of the lesion) are designated as mixed neuroendocrine–non-neuroendocrine neoplasm, including mixed adenoneuroendocrine carcinomas and other rare variants

Immunohistochemical Features

- Positive immunoreactivity with synaptophysin, chromogranin A, or INSM1
- Thyroid transcription factor 1 may be positive in a subset of primary gastric NECs
- Positive immunoreactivity to pancytokeratin markers (frequently dotlike)

Differential Diagnosis

- Glomus tumors
- Metastatic NET
- Poorly differentiated adenocarcinoma
- Lymphoma

SUGGESTED READINGS

1. Carmack SW, Genta RM, Schuler CM, et al. The current spectrum of gastric polyps: a 1-year national study of over 120,000 patients. *Am J Gastroenterol*. 2009;104(6):1524–1532.
2. Abraham SC, Nobukawa B, Giardiello FM, et al. Fundic gland polyps in familial adenomatous polyposis: neoplasms with frequent somatic adenomatous polyposis coli gene alterations. *Am J Pathol*. 2000;157(3):747–754.
3. de Boer WB, Ee H, Kumarasinghe MP. Neoplastic lesions of gastric adenocarcinoma and proximal polyposis syndrome (GAPPS) are gastric phenotype. *Am J Surg Pathol*. 2018;42(1):1–8.
4. Fukuda M, Ishigaki H, Sugimoto M, et al. Histological analysis of fundic gland polyps secondary to PPI therapy. *Histopathology*. 2019;75(4):537–545.
5. Arnason T, Liang WY, Alfaro E, et al. Morphology and natural history of familial adenomatous polyposis-associated dysplastic fundic gland polyps. *Histopathology*. 2014;65(3):353–362.

6. Abraham SC, Nobukawa B, Giardiello FM, et al. Sporadic fundic gland polyps: common gastric polyps arising through activating mutations in the beta-catenin gene. *Am J Pathol.* 2001;158(3):1005–1010.
7. Gonzalez-Obeso E, Fujita H, Deshpande V, et al. Gastric hyperplastic polyps: a heterogeneous clinicopathologic group including a distinct subset best categorized as mucosal prolapse polyp. *Am J Surg Pathol.* 2011;35(5):670–677.
8. Hattori T. Morphological range of hyperplastic polyps and carcinomas arising in hyperplastic polyps of the stomach. *J Clin Pathol.* 1985;38(6):622–630.
9. Takayama Y, Ono Y, Mizukami Y, et al. Comparative genome-wide analysis of gastric adenocarcinomas with hyperplastic polyp components. *Virchows Arch.* 2019;475(3):383–389.
10. Salomao M, Luna AM, Sepulveda JL, et al. Mutational analysis by next generation sequencing of gastric type dysplasia occurring in hyperplastic polyps of the stomach: mutations in gastric hyperplastic polyps. *Exp Mol Pathol.* 2015;99(3):468–473.
11. Franzin G, Novelli P. Gastritis cystica profunda. *Histopathology.* 1981;5:535–547.
12. Rezvani M, Menias C, Sandrasegaran K, et al. Heterotopic pancreas: histopathologic features, imaging findings, and complications. *Radiographics.* 2017;37(2):484–499.
13. Chandan VS, Wang W. Pancreatic heterotopia in the gastric antrum. *Arch Pathol Lab Med.* 2004;128:111–112.
14. Coates AG, Nostrant TT, Wilson JA, et al. Gastric xanthomatosis and cholestasis. A causal relationship. *Dig Dis Sci.* 1986;31:925–928.
15. Luk IS, Bhuta S, Lewin KJ. Clear cell carcinoid tumor of stomach. A variant mimicking gastric xanthelasma. *Arch Pathol Lab Med.* 1997;121:1100–1103.
16. Oviedo J, Swan N, Farraye FA. Gastric xanthomas. *Am J Gastroenterol.* 2001;96:3216–3218.
17. Banks M, Graham D, Jansen M, et al. British Society of Gastroenterology guidelines on the diagnosis and management of patients at risk of gastric adenocarcinoma. *Gut.* 2019;68 (9):1545–1575.
18. Abraham SC, Montgomery EA, Singh VK, et al. Gastric adenomas: intestinal-type and gastric-type adenomas differ in the risk of adenocarcinoma and presence of background mucosal pathology. *Am J Surg Pathol.* 2002;26(10):1276–1285.
19. Park DY, Srivastava A, Kim GH, et al. Adenomatous and foveolar gastric dysplasia: distinct patterns of mucin expression and background intestinal metaplasia. *Am J Surg Pathol.* 2008;32(4):524–533.
20. Valente P, Garrido M, Gullo I, et al. Epithelial dysplasia of the stomach with gastric immunophenotype shows features of biological aggressiveness. *Gastric Cancer.* 2015;18(4):720–728.
21. Abraham SC, Park SJ, Lee JH, et al. Genetic alterations in gastric adenomas of intestinal and foveolar phenotypes. *Mod Pathol.* 2003;16(8):786–795.
22. Rokutan H, Abe H, Nakamura H, et al. Initial and crucial genetic events in intestinal-type gastric intramucosal neoplasia. *J Pathol.* 2019;247(4):494–504.
23. Lee JH, Abraham SC, Kim HS, et al. Inverse relationship between APC gene mutation in gastric adenomas and development of adenocarcinoma. *Am J Pathol.* 2002;161(2):611–618.
24. Vieth M, Kushima R, Borchard F, et al. Pyloric gland adenoma: a clinico-pathological analysis of 90 cases. *Virchows Arch.* 2003;442(4):317–321.
25. Hackeng WM, Montgomery EA, Giardiello FM, et al. Morphology and genetics of pyloric gland adenomas in familial adenomatous polyposis. *Histopathology.* 2017;70(4):549–557.
26. Matsubara A, Sekine S, Kushima R, et al. Frequent GNAS and KRAS mutations in pyloric gland adenoma of the stomach and duodenum. *J Pathol.* 2013;229(4):579–587.
27. Choi WT, Brown I, Ushiku T, et al. Gastric pyloric gland adenoma: a multicentre clinicopathological study of 67 cases. *Histopathology.* 2018;72(6):1007–1014.
28. Hashimoto T, Ogawa R, Matsubara A, et al. Familial adenomatous polyposis-associated and sporadic pyloric gland adenomas of the upper gastrointestinal tract share common genetic features. *Histopathology.* 2015;67(5):689–698.
29. Ma C, Giardiello FM, Montgomery EA. Upper tract juvenile polyps in juvenile polyposis patients: dysplasia and malignancy are associated with foveolar, intestinal, and pyloric differentiation. *Am J Surg Pathol.* 2014;38(12):1618–1626.
30. Kushima R, Vieth M, Borchard F, et al. Gastric-type well-differentiated adenocarcinoma and pyloric gland adenoma of the stomach. *Gastric Cancer.* 2006;9(3):177–184.
31. Ushiku T, Kunita A, Kuroda R, et al. Oxyntic gland neoplasm of the stomach: expanding the spectrum and proposal of terminology. *Mod Pathol.* 2020;33(2):206–216.
32. Singhi AD, Lazenby AJ, Montgomery EA. Gastric adenocarcinoma with chief cell differentiation: a proposal for reclassification as oxyntic gland polyp/adenoma. *Am J Surg Pathol.* 2012;36(7):1030–1035.
33. Hidaka Y, Mitomi H, Saito T, et al. Alteration in the Wnt/β-catenin signaling pathway in gastric neoplasias of fundic gland (chief cell predominant) type. *Hum Pathol.* 2013;44(11):2438–2448.
34. Nomura R, Saito T, Mitomi H, et al. GNAS mutation as an alternative mechanism of activation of the Wnt/β-catenin signaling pathway in gastric adenocarcinoma of the fundic gland type. *Hum Pathol.* 2014;45(12):2488–2496.
35. Fukase K, Kato M, Kikuchi S, et al. Effect of eradication of Helicobacter pylori on incidence of metachronous gastric carcinoma after endoscopic resection of early gastric cancer: an open-label, randomised controlled trial. *Lancet.* 2008;372 (9636):392–397.
36. Lauren P. The two histological main types of gastric carcinoma: diffuse and so called intestinal type. An attempt at a histo-clinical classification. *Acta Pathol Microbiol Scand.* 1965;64:31–39.
37. Odze RD, Montgomery EA, Wang H, et al. Gastric carcinomas. In: Robert Odze RD, Montgomery EA, Wang H, eds. *Tumors of the Esophagus and Stomach (AFIP Atlas of Tumor Pathology, Series 4).* : American Registry of Pathology; 2019:199–280.
38. Setia N, Clark JW, Duda DG, et al. Familial gastric cancers. *Oncologist.* 2015;20:1365–1377.
39. van der Post RS, Vogelaar IP, Carneiro F, et al. Hereditary diffuse gastric cancer: updated clinical guidelines with an emphasis on germline CDH1 mutation carriers. *J Med Genet.* 2015;52:361–374.
40. Bass AJ, Thorsson V, Shmulevich I, et al. Cancer Genome Atlas Research Network. Comprehensive molecular characterization of gastric adenocarcinoma. *Nature.* 2014;513(7517):202–209.
41. Setia N, Agoston AT, Han HS, et al. A protein and mRNA expression-based classification of gastric cancer. *Mod Pathol.* 2016;29(7):772–784.
42. Gilg MM, Gröchenig HP, Schlemmer A, et al. Secondary tumors of the GI tract: origin, histology, and endoscopic findings. *Gastrointest Endosc.* 2018;88(1):151–158. e1.
43. El-Hage A, Ruel C, Afif W, et al. Metastatic pattern of invasive lobular carcinoma of the breast-Emphasis on gastric metastases. *J Surg Oncol.* 2016;114(5):543–547.
44. Oda Kondo H, Yamao T, et al. Metastatic tumors to the stomach: analysis of 54 patients diagnosed at endoscopy and 347 autopsy cases. *Endoscopy.* 2001;33(6):507–510.
45. Rindi G, Klimstra DS, Abedi-Ardekani B, et al. A common classification framework for neuroendocrine neoplasms: an International Agency for Research on Cancer (IARC) and World Health Organization (WHO) expert consensus proposal. *Mod Pathol.* 2018;31(12):1770–1786.
46. Nishikura K, Watanabe H, Iwafuchi M, et al. Carcinogenesis of gastric endocrine cell carcinoma: analysis of histopathology and p53 gene alteration. *Gastric Cancer.* 2003;6(4):203–209.
47. Srivastava A, Hornick JL. Immunohistochemical staining for CDX-2, PDX-1, NESP-55, and TTF-1 can help distinguish gastrointestinal carcinoid tumors from pancreatic endocrine and pulmonary carcinoid tumors. *Am J Surg Pathol.* 2009;33:626–632.
48. Thomas RM, Baybick JH, Elsayed AM, et al. Gastric carcinoids. An immunohistochemical and clinicopathologic study of 104 patients. *Cancer.* 1994;73:2053–2058.

5

Non-Neoplastic and Inflammatory Disorders of the Small Bowel

Scott Robertson, MD, PhD and Deepa T. Patil, MD

PATTERNS OF SMALL BOWEL DISORDERS

The most common indication for histologic assessment of small bowel mucosa is to evaluate for a malabsorption disorder. Although the spectrum of small intestinal diseases that can result in symptoms of malabsorption can seem daunting at first, most diseases produce histologic findings that fall into a limited number of injury patterns. A pattern-based approach is useful because, in practice, it is often difficult, if not impossible, for the pathologist to diagnose a specific cause. Furthermore, lack of available clinical history can add to this challenge. The small bowel disorders presented here mostly fall into one of two major patterns of injury based on assessment of the architecture at low magnification: the flattened villi pattern and the intact villi pattern (Table 5.1). Small bowel mucosa with intact villi pattern can be further subdivided based on the nature of the inflammatory infiltrate into neutrophilic inflammation, eosinophilic inflammation, lymphoplasmacytic inflammation, and disorders with minimal or no inflammation. Lastly, some disorders can alter the lamina propria and result in villous blunting without significant inflammation. These include infectious enteritis caused by Whipple disease, *Mycobacterium avium-intracellulare* infection, and histoplasmosis and conditions that alter the lacteals, including primary and secondary lymphangiectasia.

Flattened Villi Pattern

The flattened villi pattern of injury has also been called the malabsorption pattern and is characterized by villous blunting, crypt hyperplasia with or without significant intraepithelial lymphocytosis, and expansion of the lamina propria by lymphocytes and plasma cells. The prototypical malabsorption disorder is celiac disease (CD), but a number of other disorders can produce similar histologic findings, including peptic injury, tropical sprue, collagenous sprue, nongluten protein sensitivity, small intestinal bacterial overgrowth (SIBO), autoimmune enteropathy, common variable immunodeficiency (CVID), and drug-related sprue-like enteropathy, among others.

Intact Villi Pattern

Several conditions result in small bowel mucosal injury without altering the villous architecture. These may or may not be accompanied by prominent inflammation and can be further categorized based on the inflammatory component into conditions with neutrophilic inflammation, eosinophilic inflammation, lymphoplasmacytic inflammation, and disorders with minimal or no inflammation.

Intact Villi with Neutrophilic Inflammation

The characteristic feature of this pattern is the presence of neutrophilic inflammation within the epithelium. In most cases, the lamina propria is also expanded by a mixed inflammatory cell infiltrate composed of neutrophils, eosinophils, lymphocytes, and plasma cells. The epithelium shows regenerative epithelial changes in the form of reactive mucin loss and slight nuclear hyperchromasia, with preservation of the nucleus-to-cytoplasmic ratio. The potential causes are drug injury (especially nonsteroidal antiinflammatory drugs [NSAIDs]), infections (including *Helicobacter pylori*), peptic injury, inflammatory bowel disease (IBD), Zollinger-Ellison syndrome (ZES), and early ischemia.

Intact Villi with Eosinophilic Inflammation

This pattern is characterized by excessive number of eosinophils in the mucosa along with eosinophil-mediated epithelial injury in the form of cryptitis or crypt abscesses. Similar to the rest of the gastrointestinal (GI) tract, increased eosinophils can be associated with idiopathic eosinophilic enteritis, parasitic infection, allergies, drug- or medication-induced injury, connective tissue disease,

TABLE 5.1

Patterns of Small Intestinal Injury and Differential Diagnosis

FLATTENED VILLI PATTERN (WITH OR WITHOUT INTRAEPITHELIAL LYMPHOCYTOSIS)
- Celiac disease
- Peptic injury
- Medications
- Tropical sprue
- Nongluten protein sensitivity
- Small intestinal bacterial overgrowth
- Collagenous sprue
- Common variable immunodeficiency
- Autoimmune enteropathy

INTACT VILLI WITH NEUTROPHILIC INFLAMMATION
- Peptic ulcer disease
- Infection
- Medications
- Inflammatory bowel disease
- Zollinger-Ellison syndrome
- Radiation injury
- Vasculitis
- Ischemia

INTACT VILLI WITH EOSINOPHILIC INFLAMMATION
- Idiopathic eosinophilic enteritis
- Medications
- Allergy
- Parasite infection
- Inflammatory bowel disease
- Connective tissue disorder
- Vasculitis
- Systemic mastocytosis
- Langerhans cell histiocytosis

INTACT VILLI WITH LYMPHOPLASMACYTIC INFLAMMATION
- Celiac disease
- Inflammatory bowel disease
- Medications (especially NSAIDs)

INTACT VILLI WITH PAUCICELLULAR INFLAMMATION
- Infections: giardiasis, CMV
- Radiation injury
- Amyloidosis
- Chemotherapy agents
- Graft-versus-host disease
- Transplant rejection
- Medications (e.g., MMF)
- Inflammatory bowel disease
- Medications (especially NSAIDs)

CMV, Cytomegalovirus; *MMF*, mycophenolate mofetil; *NSAID*, nonsteroidal antiinflammatory drug.

vasculitis, systemic mastocytosis, and Langerhans cell histiocytosis (LCH).

Intact Villi with Lymphoplasmacytic Inflammation

This pattern of injury is characterized by expansion of the lamina propria by lymphocytes and plasma cells. The possible causes of this pattern of injury include CD, IBD, and drug- or medication-related injury (especially NSAIDs).

Intact Villi with Paucicellular Inflammation

Some conditions are associated with intact villous architecture and minimal or no inflammation. These disorders include certain infections, such as giardiasis, cytomegalovirus (CMV), radiation injury, amyloidosis, chemotherapeutic agents, drugs or medications (especially mycophenolate mofetil [MMF]), graft-versus-host disease (GVHD), and transplant rejection.

Applying the Pattern-Based Approach

Identifying the two major patterns of small bowel injury (flat villi and intact villi) is helpful in generating a differential diagnosis and determining the cause of mucosal injury. However, the patterns are not etiologically specific. For instance, many conditions can manifest with flattened villi pattern of injury. Furthermore, one specific etiology may result in a variety of patterns of injury. For instance, NSAID-related injury can manifest with all major patterns of injury. It is therefore important to identify the pattern of injury and provide a comment enlisting all the potential etiologies that may contribute to injury. The sections in this chapter have been organized based on causes of small bowel injury.

MALABSORPTION DISORDERS

The term *malabsorption* is broadly used to describe any type or degree of dysfunction in the uptake of substances that are normally retained or absorbed by the small intestine. Malabsorption can result from a multitude of causes, which can be broadly categorized into disorders of inadequate digestion (pancreatic disorders, disorders of decreased intestinal bile salt concentration), endocrine or metabolic disorders (diabetes mellitus, thyroid dysfunction, ZES), biochemical or genetic diseases (CD, disaccharidase deficiency, abetalipoproteinemia, hypogammaglobulinemia), mucosal disorders (infections, immunologic conditions, infiltrative disorders), and postmucosal disorders (lymphatic obstruction, cardiac failure, vascular obstruction). Conditions that affect the small bowel mucosa may drastically reduce the amount of villous surface area, preventing adequate uptake of nutrients. Microscopically, malabsorption disorders often show villous blunting, crypt hyperplasia, and intraepithelial lymphocytosis—*the flattened villi pattern of injury*. Having said that, some malabsorption disorders have no specific pathologic findings (e.g., disaccharidase deficiency, transporter defects), and lack of inadequate nutrient uptake is not caused by global surface area loss but by defects in specific protein function.

CELIAC DISEASE

Clinical Features

Once considered to be a rare childhood disorder, CD (also known as gluten-sensitive enteropathy or celiac sprue) is a chronic immune-mediated disorder induced by dietary exposure to gluten in genetically predisposed individuals. Confirmation of a diagnosis also requires prompt improvement of clinical symptoms and mucosal pathology after withdrawal of dietary gluten.

Celiac disease occurs both in adults and children with a female predominance (female-to-male ratio, 2–3 to 1). It is estimated to affect between 0.5% and 1% of individuals in both Europe and the United States. The peak age of incidence is the third to fourth decades of life. However, up to 20% of individuals may be diagnosed after 60 years of age.

The classification and diagnosis of CD are based on GI manifestations; however, patients with extraintestinal complications are increasingly being recognized (Table 5.2). The clinical presentation of CD ranges from asymptomatic to severe malnutrition. CD may be divided into four clinical subtypes, two symptomatic types and two asymptomatic types. In the classic symptomatic subtype, patients present with chronic diarrhea, abdominal distension, and pain. In the atypical symptomatic subtype, GI symptoms may be less pronounced to absent. Instead, extraintestinal features such as anemia, short stature, neurologic symptoms, dermatitis herpetiformis, delayed puberty, osteoporosis, infertility, vitamin and protein deficiencies, and elevated liver enzyme levels are predominant. Some patients have asymptomatic or silent CD; they lack classic or atypical symptoms but have unequivocal villous atrophy found incidentally for other reasons or after serologic screening. Finally, latent CD is defined by a positive serology but lack of villous atrophy on initial biopsies. Individuals are asymptomatic but may develop symptoms, histologic changes, or both.

TABLE 5.2

Extraintestinal Disorders Associated with Celiac Disease

Endocrine disorders
Type 1 diabetes mellitus
Autoimmune thyroid disorders
Addison's disease
Reproductive disorders (infertility, miscarriages)
Osteoporosis
Alopecia areata
Neurologic disorders
Cerebellar ataxia
Neuropathy
Epilepsy
Migraines
Cardiac disorders
Idiopathic dilated cardiomyopathy
Autoimmune myocarditis
Hepatic disorders
Primary biliary cirrhosis
Autoimmune hepatitis
Autoimmune cholangitis
Other
Dermatitis herpetiformis
Anemia
Selective immunoglobulin A deficiency
Sjögren syndrome
Juvenile chronic arthritis
Turner syndrome
Down syndrome
Dental enamel defects

High-risk groups to be screened for CD are those with other autoimmune disorders such as type 1 diabetes mellitus and autoimmune thyroiditis, a family history of CD, selective immunoglobulin (Ig) A deficiency, or dermatitis herpetiformis. CD is also more common in certain pediatric populations, including those with Down syndrome, in whom the frequency of CD is as high as 10%. In this group, CD is usually not detected on the basis of GI symptoms.

Celiac disease is a clinicopathologic diagnosis that is most often based on positive serology and specific histologic findings. Antitissue transglutaminase (anti-tTG) antibodies are both highly sensitive (90%–98%) and specific (95%–97%) for CD. Antiendomysial (EMA) antibodies are specific (97%–100%) but have slightly inferior sensitivity (85%–98%). Antigliadin antibody testing should no longer be used because of its low positive predictive value. A diagnosis of CD may be made if both tissue biopsy and serologic testing are consistent with CD. CD may be excluded if results of both are negative.

Sometimes there is discordance between the histologic and serologic findings, which may occur for a number of reasons. First, IgA deficiency is more common in individuals with CD than in the general population. Because tTG and EMA serologic tests are based on IgA, they may be falsely negative in patients with IgA deficiency. Total IgA can be measured to identify these patients, and IgG-based assays, particularly deamidated gliadin peptide or IgG-tTG, may be used in these situations. Second, the flattened villi pattern of injury is not specific for CD. Consideration of an alternative cause (e.g., SIBO, tropical sprue, drug-associated enteropathy) should be explored in patients with negative celiac serologies. Sometimes HLA genotyping is useful from excluding the possibility of CD. HLA-DQ2 or HLA-DQ8 is present in almost all cases of CD. Negative testing for these alleles virtually eliminates the possibility of CD. Human leukocyte antigen (HLA) typing is particularly useful in patients who may have initiated a gluten-free diet (GFD) before proper diagnostic work-up. This complicates diagnosis because both serologic and histologic abnormalities may normalize with GFD. HLA genotyping can be used to rule out CD in a subset of these patients.

In patients who test positive for HLA-DQ2 or HLA-DQ8, a gluten challenge can be performed, in which biopsy and serologic analysis takes place after gluten has been reintroduced for a period time. In patients with CD, gluten challenge should elicit typical serologic and histologic features. However, some patients may experience a return of their symptoms (e.g., abdominal pain, bloating) but without serologic or histologic evidence of CD. An alternate diagnosis should be considered in these patients, such as IgE-mediated wheat allergy or nonceliac gluten sensitivity.

PATHOGENESIS

The pathogenesis of CD is related to a combination of environmental, genetic, and immunologic features and can be viewed as both luminal events and cellular events leading to the activation of immune cells and ensuing tissue damage. Enteric exposures to certain glutamine-rich proteins in the dietary grains wheat, rye, and barley are essential for the development of CD. The actual proteins that trigger the disease are the gliadins in wheat, the hordeins in barley, and the secalins in rye. In CD, many of these peptides are poorly digested by the intestinal tract proteases and traverse through the epithelium into the lamina propria as intact molecules. tTG is a multifunctional enzyme that is essential for the pathogenesis of CD. tTG has two essential functions, deamidation of glutamine to glutamic acid and cross-linking glutamine and lysine residues. After absorption, intact peptides are deamidated by tTG, converting the abundant glutamine residues to glutamic acid, thus rendering them negatively charged. The negatively charged peptides are more efficiently bound to HLA-DQ2 or HLA-DQ8 receptors on the surface of the antigen presenting cells. Intestinal DQ2- or DQ8-restricted CD4+ T cells then recognize the deaminated gliadin peptides and elicit a cytokine-mediated inflammatory response. Importantly, tTG also forms complexes with gliadin, mediated by its glutamine-lysine cross-linking function. In an environment already primed by gliadin peptide presentation on DQ2/8T cells, tTG–gliadin complexes serve as neoepitopes that stimulate the formation of anti-tTG autoantibodies.

Finally, it was recently discovered that infection with certain viruses can trigger immunopathologic responses to dietary gluten. Specifically, infection with reovirus, which is nonvirulent and otherwise nonpathogenic, can trigger certain events critical for CD pathogenesis. In mouse models, reovirus infection represses regulatory T-cell (T_{reg}) conversion and promotes T helper-1 (T_H1) immunity to dietary antigen. Reovirus infection also breaks oral tolerance to gluten and promotes activation of transglutaminase 2. In humans, patients with CD were much more likely to have circulating antibodies against reovirus than normal control participants, suggesting a link between CD and prior reovirus infection. It remains to be seen if other infectious agents can elicit similar immunologic derangements.

GENETIC

The major genetic risk factors for CD are the HLA class II genes *HLA-DQ2* and *HLA-DQ8*. Approximately 95 % of all patients with CD have a DQ2 heterodimer, and almost all remaining patients with CD have a DQ8 heterodimer. Gene dosage correlates with the risk for developing CD, with patients homozygous for DQ2 carrying the greatest risk. CD is concordant in 70 % to 80 % of monozygotic twins, 30 % to 40 % of HLA-identical siblings, and fewer than 20 % of dizygotic twins, a rate similar to that for all first-degree relatives. However, recent linkage studies suggest that non-HLA disease-associated genes may also play a role.

CELIAC DISEASE—FACT SHEET

Definition

- A multisystem autoimmune disorder caused by an immune response to dietary gluten and related proteins

Incidence

- 1% of the US population
- 1 in 133 patients with no risk factors
- 1 in 29 patients with at least one first-degree relative with celiac disease (CD)

Morbidity and Mortality

- 20-fold higher risk for enteropathy-associated T-cell lymphoma
- 30-fold higher risk for small intestinal adenocarcinoma
- Two- to fourfold higher risk for oropharyngeal and esophageal carcinoma

Gender, Race, and Age Distribution

- Wide age range: children and adults
- Common in Northern Europeans; rare in Southeast Asians and Middle East

Clinical Features

- Variable: ranges from asymptomatic to severe malnutrition
- Most common presentation is weight loss, abdominal pain, and diarrhea
- Extraintestinal manifestations include infertility, osteoporosis, dermatitis herpetiformis, and various neuropathies

Prognosis and Therapy

- Complete resolution of mucosal injury with a strict gluten-free diet (GFD)
- Refractory CD refers to patients on GFD for a period of 1 year or longer without resolution of symptoms
- Type II refractory CD is commonly associated with a clonal T-cell population and is at high risk for developing enteropathy-associated T-cell lymphoma

Pathologic Features

Gross Findings

If the mucosal biopsy specimen is examined under a dissecting microscope (which is seldom done), delicate villi are found to be attenuated or even absent. Endoscopically, a reduction in folds, scalloping, a mosaic pattern, or nodular mucosa may be seen (Fig. 5.1).

Microscopic Findings

Histologic abnormalities in the duodenum may be patchy. Current guidelines from the American College of Gastroenterology (ACG) recommend multiple biopsies of the duodenum, with one or two biopsies from the bulb and at least four biopsies from the distal duodenum. CD produces the flattened villi pattern of injury—intraepithelial lymphocytosis, villous blunting, and crypt hyperplasia (Figs. 5.2 and 5.3). The earliest change in CD is the presence of increased intraepithelial lymphocytes (IELs), most conspicuously within the villous tips, with intact villous architecture (Fig. 5.4). With persistent disease, epithelial damage ensues with reactive mucin loss. The lamina propria is expanded by lymphocytes and plasma cells, thus contributing to partial or complete villous blunting. Villous blunting is accompanied by crypt hyperplasia. Active inflammation is occasionally seen but is generally not prominent. Marked neutrophilic epithelial injury should suggest an additional or alternative cause, such as peptic duodenitis, NSAID injury, infection, or Crohn's disease.

Duodenal biopsies exhibiting all the features of CD—increased IELs, villous blunting, crypt hyperplasia—are easy to recognize. However, changes of early CD can be quite subtle and include intact villous and crypt architecture with increased IELs. The increase in IELs is sometimes obvious, but in some cases, an objective

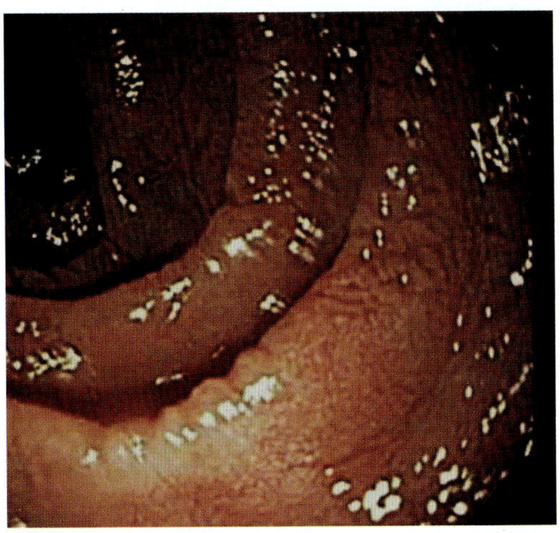

FIGURE 5.1

Endoscopic appearance of celiac disease. The duodenal mucosa shows characteristic scalloping with reduction in the mucosal folds.

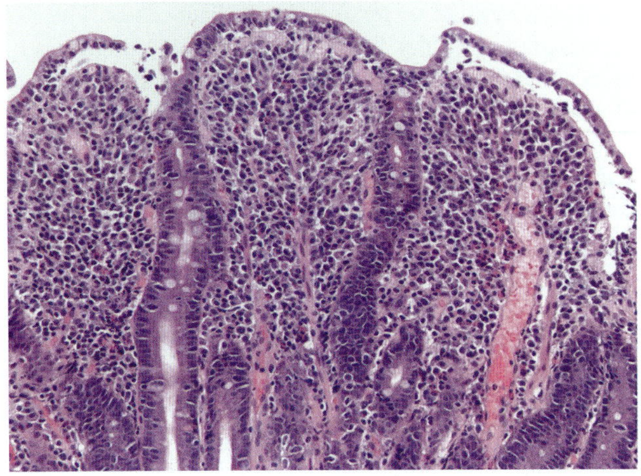

FIGURE 5.2

Celiac disease. The duodenal biopsy shows marked villous blunting with expansion of the lamina propria by lymphocytes and plasma cells along with crypt hyperplasia.

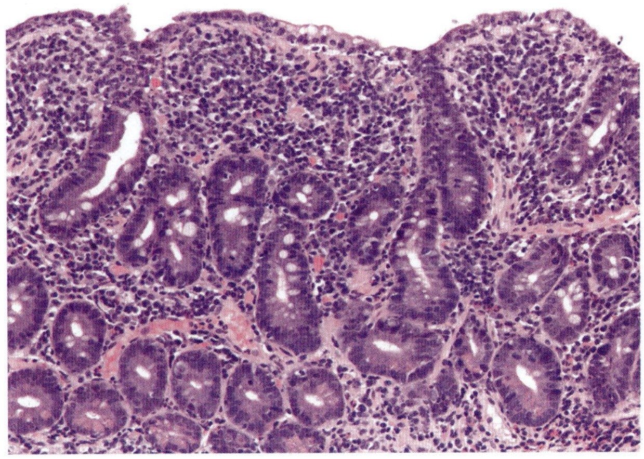

FIGURE 5.3

Higher magnification of duodenal biopsy with celiac disease showing marked expansion of the lamina propria by lymphocytes and plasma cells. There is crypt as well as surface intraepithelial lymphocytosis.

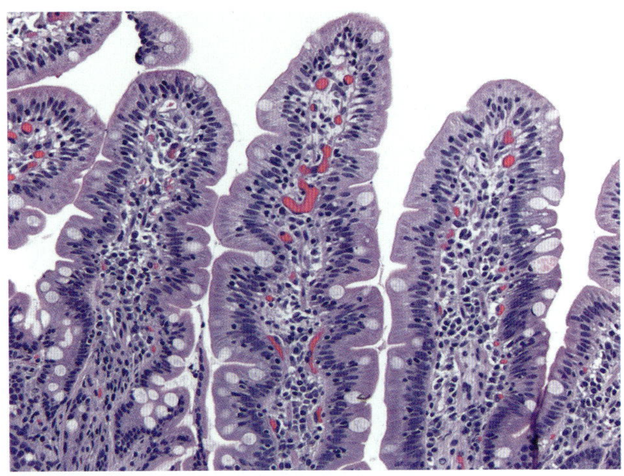

FIGURE 5.4

Early celiac disease. The duodenal biopsy shows preservation of the villous architecture with intraepithelial lymphocytes within the villous tips.

measure is needed to resolve borderline cases. The normal range of IELs has been reported as 11 to 23 per 100 enterocytes. According to ACG guidelines, more than 25 IELs per 100 enterocytes is abnormal. One rapid method to determine this number is to evaluate 5 villous tips, counting the number of lymphocytes present within the distal-most 20 enterocytes. The final values can be expressed as IEL per 100 enterocytes. When possible, evaluate only well-oriented villi that are anchored by intact muscularis mucosae because tangentially sectioned lateral aspects of the villi may result in overestimation and inaccurate estimation of the lymphocyte count. A CD3 immunostain can also be used to highlight IELs. However, the utility of this approach has not been established or validated for clinical practice. Some studies have shown that CD3 immunohistochemistry (IHC) does not improve detection of CD in cases in which the hematoxylin and eosin–stained sections are normal.

Upon initiation of a GFD, patients often report a marked improvement in clinical symptoms. Microscopically, intestinal biopsies show diminished surface epithelial injury, a reduced number of IELs, and partial to complete resolution of villous architectural abnormalities. However, in some cases, despite resolution of clinical symptoms and normal serology, the inflammatory component may persist for up to a period of 1 to 2 years after GFD. If patients consume gluten-containing products, there is a rapid return of all lesions, and malabsorption ensues.

Celiac Disease—Pathologic Features

Gross Findings

- Attenuated to absent villi (as seen under a dissecting microscope)
- Scalloping or mosaic appearance of the mucosa

Microscopic Findings

- Variable degrees of villous blunting
- Intraepithelial lymphocytosis, most prominent on villous tips (>25 IELs per 100 enterocytes)
- Crypt hyperplasia

Differential Diagnosis

- Bacterial overgrowth
- Infection
- Tropical sprue
- Nongluten protein sensitivity
- Crohn's disease
- Protein intolerance
- Autoimmune enteropathy
- Medications (nonsteroidal antiinflammatory drugs, olmesartan)

Differential Diagnosis

The flattened villi pattern of injury is not specific for CD, and therefore, a diagnosis of CD can only be confirmed with the knowledge of positive celiac serologies. Without this information, the pathologist must be descriptive in the report by stating the pattern of injury (e.g., duodenal mucosa with villous blunting and increased IELs) and providing a comment with the differential diagnosis. In biopsies showing well-developed features of the flattened villi pattern of injury, the differential diagnosis includes infection, protein intolerance, tropical sprue, nongluten protein sensitivity, bacterial overgrowth, Crohn's disease, CVID, autoimmune enteropathy (AIE), and medication injury (particularly from NSAIDs and olmesartan). In biopsies with increased IELs and normal villous and crypt architecture, the differential diagnosis is slightly different and includes viral infections, *H. pylori* infection, NSAID injury, peptic injury, tropical sprue, nongluten protein sensitivity, bacterial overgrowth, Crohn's disease, and AIE.

Prognosis and Therapy

A lifelong adherence to a GFD is the mainstay of safe and effective treatment of patients with CD. Commonly substituted grains in the GFD include rice, corn, quinoa, and buckwheat. Serologic testing may be used to check the effectiveness of a GFD. Patients whose disease does not respond to dietary therapy should undergo a systematic evaluation, including review of the patient's diet by an expert dietician.

Patients with CD have more than a 30-fold increased risk for small bowel adenocarcinoma compared with the general population, and 13% of patients with a small bowel adenocarcinoma have underlying CD. Other malignancies potentially associated with CD include enteropathy-associated T-cell lymphoma (EATL), papillary thyroid carcinoma, and malignant melanoma.

NONRESPONSIVE OR REFRACTORY CELIAC DISEASE

Nonresponsive CD is defined as persistent symptoms, signs, or laboratory abnormalities despite 6 to 12 months of gluten avoidance. It is common, occurring in 7% to 30% of patients. The most common cause is inadvertent gluten ingestion. Other causes include SIBO, other food intolerances, irritable bowel disease, pancreatic insufficiency, and microscopic colitis. In patients with nonresponsive CD, the diagnosis of CD should be reconfirmed, and the patient's diet should be closely examined to rule out inadvertent gluten ingestion. Additional studies, including upper and lower endoscopy, may also be indicated to exclude other diseases in the differential diagnosis.

If there are persistent signs and symptoms after 12 months on a strict GFD and if alternative disorders have been ruled out, the diagnosis of refractory celiac disease (RCD) is appropriate. RCD is rare (1%–2% of patients with CD) and can be subdivided into two types based on the immunophenotype of the lymphocyte population. In type I RCD, the infiltrating lymphocytes are morphologically and immunophenotypically similar to those seen in untreated CD. Patients with type I RCD usually respond to immunosuppressive regimens and are at low risk for progression to lymphoma. In type II RCD, the lymphocytes display an abnormal immunoprofile, lacking one or more normal T-cell markers (CD3, CD4, and CD8). Furthermore, monoclonal or oligoclonal T-cell receptor rearrangements can be detected. Having said that, a recent study has shown clonal T-cell populations even in typical patients with CD. Thus, the utility of TCR gene-rearrangement studies in this setting is somewhat limited. Given these findings, some consider RCD II to be a form of in situ T-cell lymphoma, and there is a much higher risk of progression to malignancy compared with RCD I. Patients with RCD II are often refractory to steroid therapy. Optimal treatment is unclear, but a variety of immunomodulatory and chemotherapeutic agents have been used.

Enteropathy-associated T-cell lymphoma is a high-grade T-cell non-Hodgkin's lymphoma of the upper small intestine. This rare T-cell disorder is 20 times more common in patients with CD. Two types of EATL are recognized and have slightly different clinical and pathologic features, though both are very aggressive. Type I EATL is closely associated with CD. Type II EATL is less common and is not associated with CD. Pathologically, type I EATL most commonly involves the jejunum or ileum. Plaques, nodules, or strictures can be seen grossly. Microscopically, there is a dense, diffuse proliferation of atypical medium to large lymphoid cells, usually in a background of mixed inflammatory cells (Fig. 5.5). Immunohistochemically, the neoplastic cells usually express CD45 and cytoplasmic CD3 while lacking other T-cell markers, including CD4, CD5, and CD8. CD30 expression is present in some cases. The neoplastic cells have a cytotoxic T-cell phenotype with expression of TIA-1, granzyme B, and perforin. Type II EATL usually involves the jejunum, but in contrast to type I EATL, it may also involve the stomach or colon. Microscopically, EATL type II is composed of a more monotonous population of smaller cells, and there are fewer admixed non-neoplastic inflammatory cells. Immunohistochemically, type II EATL is similar to type I but more often expresses CD8 but less often expresses CD30 (see Chapter 19 for additional details). The prognosis is similarly poor for both types; the 5-year survival rate is approximately 10%. About half of patients require laparotomy for complications of hemorrhage, perforation, or obstruction.

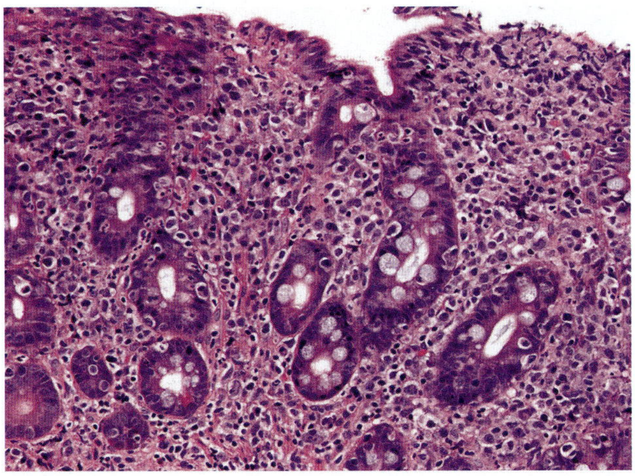

FIGURE 5.5

Enteropathy-associated T-cell lymphoma. The duodenal biopsy shows marked villous blunting with expansion of the lamina propria by a monomorphic population of atypical medium to large lymphoid cells.

COLLAGENOUS SPRUE

Collagenous sprue, also known as collagenous enteritis, is a rare but severe form of malabsorption disorder. Given the limited number of small case series reported in the literature, the nature of collagenous sprue and its relationship to other malabsorption disorder are unclear. Initially, collagenous sprue was thought to represent an uncommon variant of CD, enriched in patients who have refractory disease. However, it is now clear that a proportion of cases occur in patients with no other evidence of CD (based on serology, genetics, or response to a GFD). Therefore, collagenous sprue seems to represent an unusual, nonspecific injury pattern associated with a variety of pathogenic mechanisms. Beyond its association with CD, collagenous sprue has also been reported in the context of collagenous gastritis, microscopic colitis, and olmesartan-induced injury. It is most common in middle-age to older women, and, unlike collagenous gastritis, it is rare in children.

Histologically, the key feature is a thick subepithelial collagen layer (Fig. 5.6). The required thickness of the collagen layer is not well defined, but some reports use greater than 12 µm as a cut-off. Similar to collagenous colitis, there are entrapment of capillaries and irregular extension of the collagen layer into the lamina propria. The background mucosa shows villous atrophy. However, in contrast to CD, the crypts are typically atrophic rather than hyperplastic. The degree of intraepithelial lymphocytosis can be variable.

Early descriptions of this entity indicated that patients usually have a poor prognosis. However, more recent studies have revealed that the clinical outcome can be quite heterogeneous. GFD is sufficient treatment for some patients, though about half are refractory to GFD, in which case immunosuppressive or chemotherapeutic agents are needed. Some patients die of intractable disease.

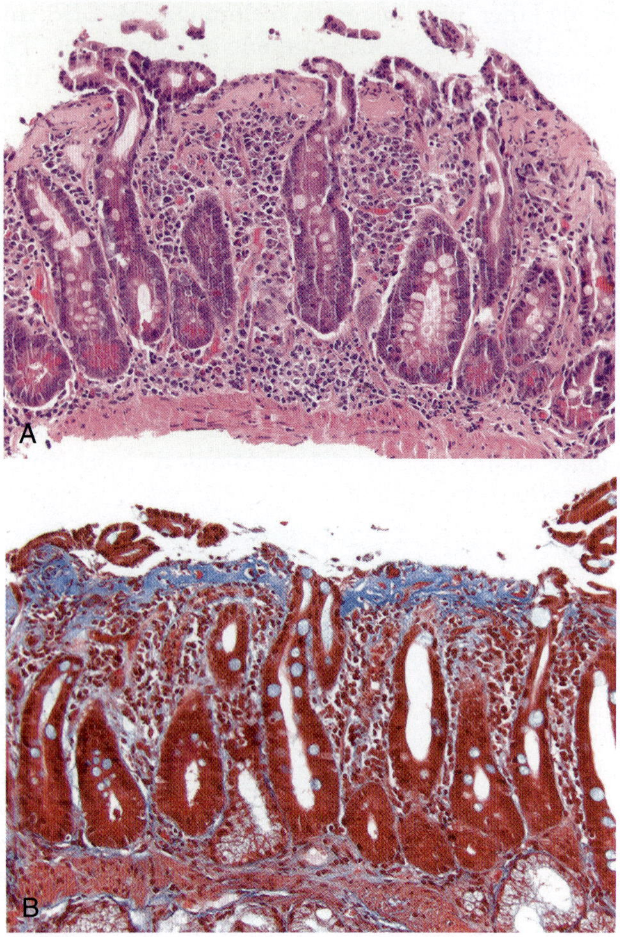

FIGURE 5.6

Collagenous sprue. **A**, Duodenal mucosa shows villous blunting and expansion of the lamina propria by lymphocytes and plasma cells. A thick collagen layer is present beneath the epithelium. It has an irregular contour and entraps capillaries as well as stromal and inflammatory cells. In addition, there is intraepithelial lymphocytosis. **B**, A trichrome stain highlights the collagen layer.

TROPICAL SPRUE

Tropical sprue (also known as postinfective tropical malabsorption) is a rare disorder that mimics several aspects of CD. It is an intestinal malabsorption of unknown etiology that occurs among residents in or visitors to the tropics. No single causative agent has been identified to account for tropical sprue. However, the following evidence favors an infectious cause: infection often initiates and sustains tropical sprue, tropical sprue occurs in specific geographic areas (West Indies and the Indian subcontinent) where enteric infections are common, tropical sprue is endemic in some areas, and recovery from tropical sprue with antibiotics is usually rapid and dramatic. Protozoan infections such as with *Cyclospora* have been suggested to play a role.

Gross findings are not well described but may include an abnormal villous pattern. Microscopically, tropical sprue produces a marked increase in IELs. The villous architecture of the mucosa is typically preserved in tropical sprue and a completely flat mucosa—like that seen in patients with CD—is never seen. Intraepithelial lymphocytosis is very prominent in tropical sprue and is seen in both the villi and crypts. In addition, there may be a significant increase in the number of lamina propria eosinophils. Finally, unlike CD, in which mucosal changes are greatest in the proximal small bowel, the lesions are similar throughout the entire small bowel in tropical sprue. Mechanistically, this fits with the resulting secondary vitamin B_{12} and folate deficiency states that are commonly a consequence of tropical sprue. In fact, vitamin B_{12} and folate deficiency may produce megaloblastic changes in the epithelium with enlarged nuclei and reduced mitotic activity.

After the diagnosis is made, tropical sprue is eminently treatable with antibiotics; a 3-month course of doxycycline is generally sufficient. Folic acid vitamin B_{12} supplementations are also useful to correct nutritional deficiencies. Unfortunately, given the rarity of the disorder, this diagnosis is often not considered either clinically or pathologically.

PEPTIC DUODENAL DISEASE

Clinical Features

Peptic duodenitis and peptic ulcer disease (PUD) represent a continuum of the same disease process, namely damage to the duodenal mucosa caused by exposure to excessive gastric acid. It is estimated to affect up to 10% of the Western population. Peptic disease is more common among men who are older than 40 years. Patients often present with burning epigastric pain relieved by eating. In severe cases, the pain may be constant and accompanied by nausea and vomiting.

Chronic infection with *H. pylori* is highly correlated with peptic disease of the duodenum and is associated with more than 80% of peptic ulcers. Mechanistically, this occurs with antrum-predominant *H. pylori* infection, which stimulates gastrin secretion, and in turn, increases acid production. Furthermore, peptic injury often results in gastric foveolar metaplasia, which can become secondarily colonized with *H. pylori*, further contributing to mucosal injury. Gastric foveolar metaplasia may represent an adaptation to chronic exposure to hyperacidity. Other factors, such as smoking, NSAIDs, renal insufficiency, or duodenal dysmotility, compromise mucosal defense mechanism and allow prolonged contact with gastric acid, resulting in peptic injury.

Patients with multiple duodenal ulcers represent the most severe form of the disease; multiple duodenal or jejunal ulcers should raise concern for ZES. In the absence of ZES, refractory ulcers may be seen in patients with chronic NSAID use, gastric outlet obstruction or duodenal stenosis, or those with a history of gastric bypass procedure.

Pathologic Features

Gross Findings

Peptic duodenitis is most commonly seen in the duodenal bulb. The endoscopic appearance varies from simple erythema to friability, erosions, and nodularity of the mucosa (Fig. 5.7). Nodularity and polypoid lesions most often correspond to Brunner's gland hyperplasia or prominent foveolar hyperplasia. In PUD, the ulcers are usually circular and rarely exceed 3 cm in diameter. They are typically located along the posterior wall of the duodenal bulb and are more likely to present with perforation and massive hemorrhage because of their proximity to pancreaticoduodenal and gastroduodenal arteries.

Microscopic Findings

In general, peptic duodenal disease shows the intact villi with a neutrophilic inflammation pattern of injury. There are expansion of the lamina propria by neutrophils and neutrophil-mediated epithelial injury (Fig. 5.8). There are an accompanying increase in lamina propria plasma cells, reactive epithelial changes (mucin loss, nuclear hyperchromasia), gastric foveolar metaplasia (Fig. 5.9) and Brunner's gland hyperplasia. In some instances, the Brunner's glands may extend from the submucosa into the basal aspect of the mucosa. In severe cases, villous blunting can be present as well—a feature more in keeping with the flattened villi pattern of injury. Severe peptic injury leads to ulceration (PUD).

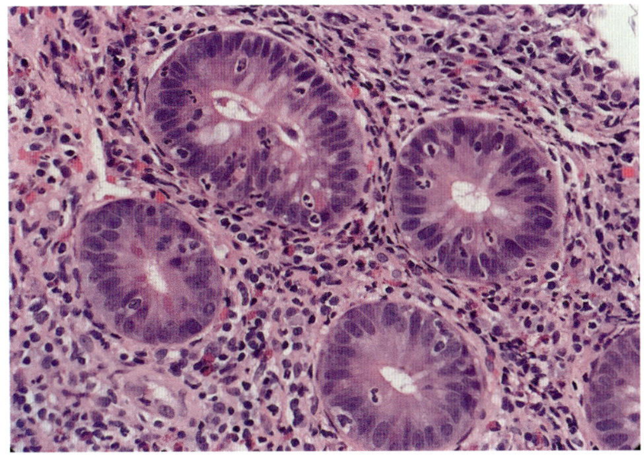

FIGURE 5.8

Peptic duodenitis. The duodenal biopsy shows expansion of the lamina propria by a mixed inflammatory cell infiltrate that is predominantly composed of neutrophils. In addition, there is neutrophilic cryptitis.

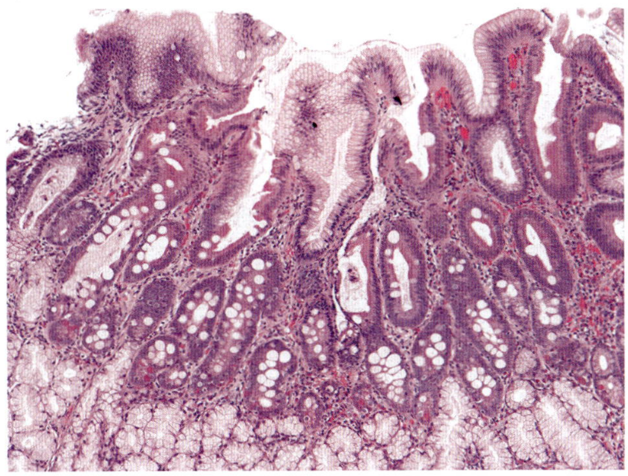

FIGURE 5.9

Peptic duodenitis. Duodenal biopsy shows gastric surface foveolar metaplasia as well as extension of Brunner's gland within the lamina propria.

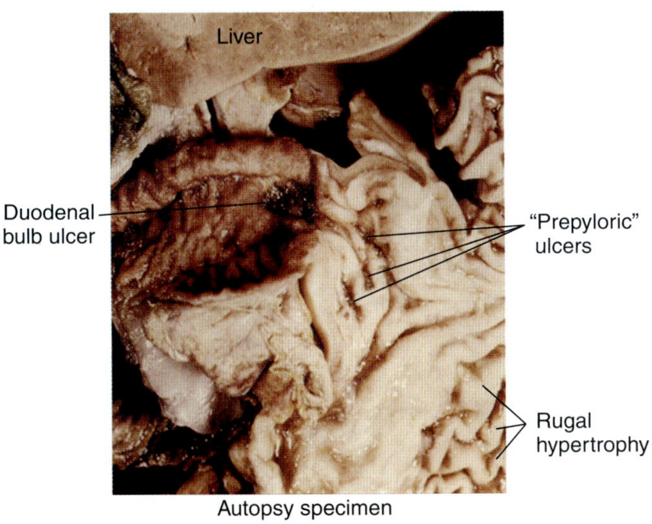

FIGURE 5.7

Peptic duodenal ulcer. The specimen shows an acute duodenal ulcer within the duodenal bulb. Several small acute ulcers are also present in the prepyloric region.

Ancillary Studies

Ancillary stains are not generally used for diagnosis of peptic disease but may be used to highlight a few interesting features. Gastric foveolar metaplasia can be highlighted by a combination periodic acid–Schiff (PAS) and Alcian blue (AB) stain that highlights the presence of neutral mucin characteristic of the gastric foveolar metaplasia (Fig. 5.10). *H. pylori* may colonize areas of metaplastic gastric epithelium because these cells express the same surface receptors as the native gastric epithelium. The organisms may be highlighted by special stains such as IHC, Giemsa, or Diff-Quik (Fig. 5.11). However, evaluation of the gastric mucosa, when provided, is a preferred method to detect *H. pylori* infection.

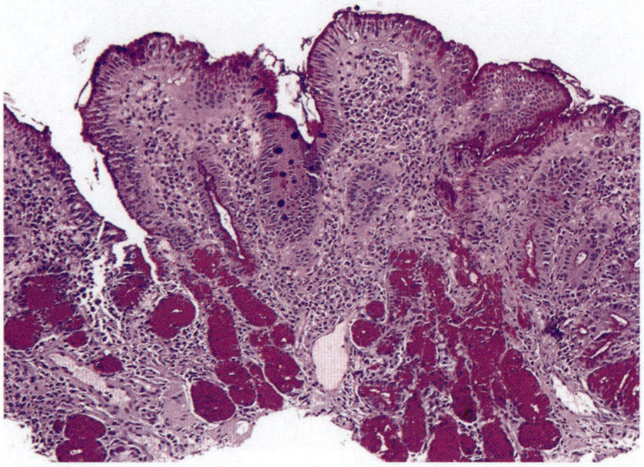

FIGURE 5.10

Peptic duodenitis. The periodic acid–Schiff stain highlights the neutral mucin present within the gastric foveolar metaplastic epithelium and the intramucosal Brunner's glands. The only residual Alcian blue–positive epithelium consists of scattered goblet cells, which represent intestinal-type mucin.

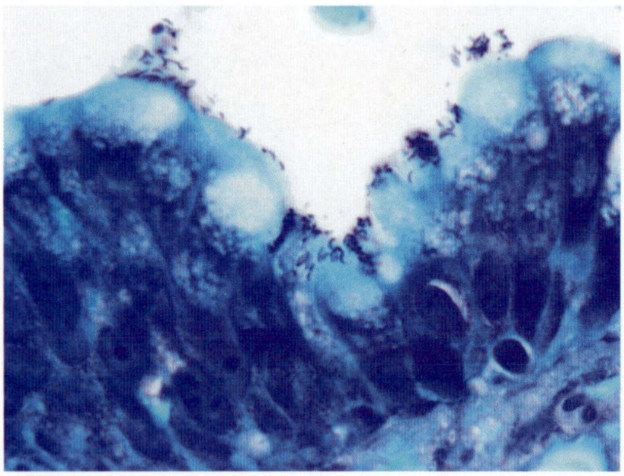

FIGURE 5.11

Peptic duodenitis with *Helicobacter pylori* organisms (Diff-Quik stain). There is gastric surface foveolar metaplasia with *H. pylori* organisms.

Differential Diagnosis

Peptic duodenal disease typically shows a neutrophilic pattern of inflammation, and other causes that produce this pattern of injury include drug or medication injury (particularly from NSAIDs), infections (other than from *H. pylori*), and IBD. Occasionally, there are specific clues to distinguish between these possibilities. For example, crypt distortion and granuloma formation in conjunction with involvement of the rest of the GI tract would be highly suspicious for Crohn's disease. Some infectious causes, including CMV and adenovirus, can be detected microscopically.

Although gastric foveolar metaplasia is a common feature of peptic duodenal disease, "lipid hang-up" is a common mimic. It results from physiologically normal vacuolization of the enterocyte cytoplasm resulting from a recent fatty meal (Fig. 5.12). Compared with gastric foveolar metaplasia, which is PAS positive, these vacuoles are PAS–AB negative and are only localized to the tips of the villi. A similar

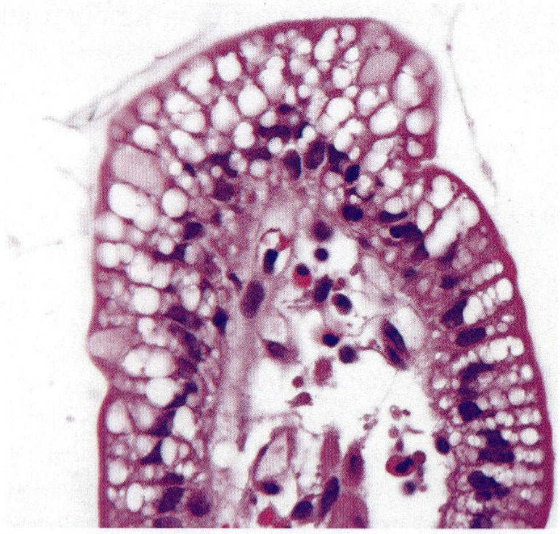

FIGURE 5.12

"Lipid hang-up." Duodenal biopsy showing vacuolization of the enterocyte epithelium. These are physiologically normal enterocytes that retain lipid after a meal.

finding is seen in abetalipoproteinemia; however, the vacuolization affects the tips as well as the lateral aspect of the villi. Gastric heterotopia may also be included in the differential diagnosis with peptic duodenitis resulting from the prominent gastric foveolar epithelium. However, unlike peptic duodenitis, gastric heterotopia can be recognized by normal-appearing oxyntic glands in association with the surface gastric mucinous epithelium. Finally, chronic peptic injury can also cause villous blunting with a variable degree of intraepithelial lymphocytosis. Therefore, these findings should prompt consideration of other disorders that produce the flattened villi pattern of injury (e.g., CD).

Finally, although marked histologic abnormalities are highly correlated with *H. pylori* infection, many duodenal biopsies show mild changes, with increased lymphoplasmacytic inflammation in the lamina propria, gastric foveolar cell metaplasia, and reactive epithelial changes (hyperchromasia and apical mucin attenuation). Neutrophils may or may not be present. If a concurrent stomach biopsy shows no suggestion of *H. pylori* infection, it is unclear what diagnosis is most appropriate. Various terms are commonly used, including *peptic duodenitis* and *peptic duodenopathy*. However, in the absence of *H. pylori*, there is little evidence that these changes are caused by stomach acid or any other "peptic" etiology. Therefore, when these cases are encountered, it is probably best to be descriptive and simply list the specific histologic abnormalities that are present.

Prognosis and Therapy

The eradication of *H. pylori* and the use of acid-suppressive therapies improve symptoms in most patients with peptic duodenitis. Medical therapy is mainly intended to reduce gastric acid by small meals, antacids, and histamine-2 (H_2) blockers. Patients should avoid substances that promote gastric acid secretion, such as alcohol.

Aspirin and other NSAIDs should also be avoided because they inhibit mucosal defenses.

Bleeding ulcers are estimated to be responsible for up to 50% of all cases of acute hemorrhage from the upper GI tract. Up to 5% of patients may have bleeding that is brisk enough to cause hematochezia. Even if initially controlled, rebleeding can affect up to one-third of patients, most commonly patients in the seventh decade of life or beyond or those with a visible vessel in the ulcer base. Refractory ulcers heal slowly or follow a relapsing and remitting course. Scarring of duodenal ulcers may lead to duodenal stricturing and obstruction.

Free perforation of a duodenal ulcer into the peritoneal cavity can be a catastrophic, life-threatening event. Most patients with this complication are older adults, and the perforations are associated with NSAID use in up to half of cases. However, in patients younger than 75 years, smoking may be a stronger risk factor for perforation than NSAIDs.

PEPTIC DUODENAL DISEASE—FACT SHEET

Definition

- Damage to the duodenal mucosa resulting from exposure to excess gastric acid

Incidence

- Common; up to 10% of population in Western countries

Morbidity and Mortality

- Severe disease can cause perforation or life-threatening bleeding

Gender, Race, and Age Distribution

- More common among men who are older than 40 years

Clinical Features

- 70% of patients are asymptomatic
- Dyspepsia is most common symptom, classically 2 to 5 hours after a meal
- In severe cases, bleeding and perforation may occur

Prognosis and Therapy

- Antisecretory therapy to reduce acid production
- *Helicobacter pylori* eradication if *H. pylori* is present
- Prognosis usually favorable, though life-threatening ulcer perforation is possible
- Surgical therapy occasionally indicated for refractory ulcers

PEPTIC DUODENAL DISEASE—PATHOLOGIC FEATURES

Gross Findings

- Circular ulcers in the duodenum, most commonly involving the duodenal bulb
- Nodularity or polypoid areas may represent Brunner's gland hyperplasia

Microscopic Findings

- Neutrophilic inflammation (both in the lamina propria and epithelium)
- Increase plasmacytic inflammation
- Gastric foveolar metaplasia
- Brunner's gland hyperplasia
- Reactive epithelial changes (apical mucin loss, hyperchromasia)
- Villous blunting is variable

Differential Diagnosis

- Nonsteroidal antiinflammatory drug injury
- Infection
- Inflammatory bowel disease
- Malabsorptive disorders (if villous blunting is prominent)

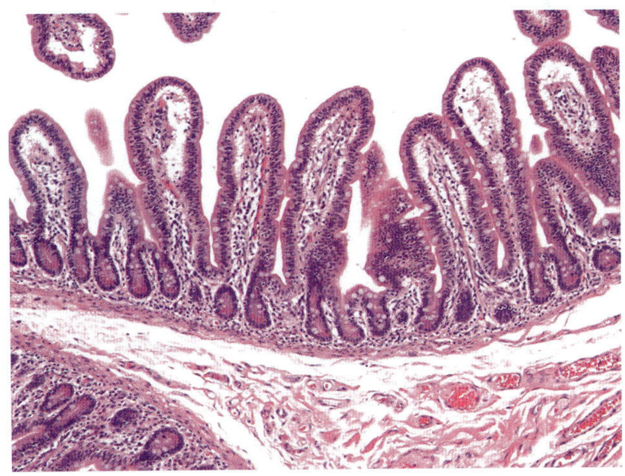

FIGURE 5.13

Bacterial overgrowth. Small intestinal mucosa with intact callous architecture and increased intraepithelial lymphocytes. The lamina propria is only slightly expanded by chronic inflammatory cells.

SMALL INTESTINAL BACTERIAL OVERGROWTH

Bacterial overgrowth is another cause of small intestinal malabsorption. Although the causes of bacterial overgrowth are numerous, most result in intestinal stasis; thus, these disorders are also known as stasis syndrome. Causes of stasis in the small bowel include motor or neural disorders that affect intestinal motility such as diabetic neuropathy and scleroderma, as well as structural lesions, such as diverticula and surgical anastomoses. Certain drugs may also slow intestinal motility (e.g., narcotics and benzodiazepines). Stasis allows accumulation of anaerobic bacteria that deconjugate bile salts, deplete vitamin B_{12}, and damage surface epithelium. Patients may experience bloating, abdominal pain, diarrhea, dyspepsia, or weight loss, though some patients are asymptomatic. The pathologic features can be quite variable. There is often mild to moderate villous blunting, but complete villous blunting is uncommon. IELs are also increased but typically not to the degree that is seen in CD (Fig. 5.13). The gold-standard test for SIBO involves aspiration of small intestinal fluid and demonstration of greater than 10^5 colony forming units per milliliter of fluid. A carbohydrate-based breath test can also be used, which is simple and noninvasive. Breath tests are based on the principle that a test dose of carbohydrate will be metabolized by bacterial flora, and certain metabolites can be detected in the breath.

The two main goals of SIBO treatment are to correct the underlying disease process, if possible, and to decrease bacterial load. Antibiotics reduce the bacterial burden, which leads to symptomatic improvement. Dietary changes may also be helpful to provide nutrients that are quickly absorbed and less metabolized by bacteria, such as a high-fat, low-carbohydrate diet. Finally, prokinetic agents (e.g., metoclopramide) may be useful, though their benefit is not well-established.

NONSTEROIDAL ANTIINFLAMMATORY DRUG–ASSOCIATED INJURY

Clinical Features

Nonsteroidal antiinflammatory drugs are a widely prescribed class of medication and can cause injury throughout the GI tract in those consuming the medication. NSAID injury occurs via both local and systemic mechanisms. Locally, NSAIDs may pass directly into epithelial cells and become ionized and trapped within. Inside the cell, these compounds can disrupt oxidative phosphorylation and deplete adenosine triphosphate stores. Systemically, NSAIDs nonselectively inhibit cyclooxygenase isoenzymes and suppresses prostaglandin synthesis. Certain prostaglandins downregulated by NSAIDs are important for maintaining several aspects of mucosal protection, including supporting mucin production, mucosal blood flow, and bicarbonate secretion. Thus, although ulceration is relatively common, chronic use can cause fibrosis, stricture, perforation, and formation of mucosal diaphragms—so-called *diaphragm disease*.

NONSTEROIDAL ANTIINFLAMMATORY DRUG–ASSOCIATED SMALL BOWEL LESIONS—FACT SHEET

Definition

- Ulcers, strictures, and mucosal diaphragms associated with nonsteroidal antiinflammatory drug (NSAID) use

Incidence

- Overall unknown
- Ulcers are most common, strictures less so, and "diaphragm disease" is rare

Morbidity and Mortality

- Data from 1997 showed 107,000 hospitalizations and 16,500 deaths resulting from NSAID consumption in the United States alone (data are not specific to the gastrointestinal [GI] tract)
- The incidence of GI perforations, symptomatic gastroduodenal ulcers, and upper GI bleeding in persons known to be taking NSAIDs is about 3% over 2 years
- A minority of these patients die of these complications

Pathologic Features

Gross Findings

Most commonly, NSAIDs injury consists of localized erosions and ulcers. More rarely, NSAID may cause chronic damage that includes varying degrees of mucosal and submucosal fibrosis, ultimately broadening and forming flat strictures. There may also be mucosal membranes that divide the lumen of the small intestine into compartments, and this appearance is termed *diaphragm disease*.

Microscopic Findings

Typically, NSAID damage shows the intact villi with neutrophilic inflammation pattern of injury, with expansion of the lamina propria by neutrophils. Epithelial injury is usually present and may be associated with erosion or ulcer surrounded by reactive epithelial changes. NSAID injury may also take the form of prominent mucosal eosinophilia, presumably via a hypersensitivity mechanism (Fig. 5.14). In resection specimens, these changes are patchy in distribution with multifocal superficial ulcers.

In chronic NSAID injury, there are villous blunting and crypt hyperplasia—features of the flattened villi pattern of injury. In other cases, crypt distortion and pyloric gland metaplasia are often present. With ongoing injury, there are thickening of the muscularis mucosae and a disorganized proliferation of smooth muscle fibers, nerves, and vessels within the submucosa. These findings indicate reparative changes that are most prominent in areas with stricture formation.

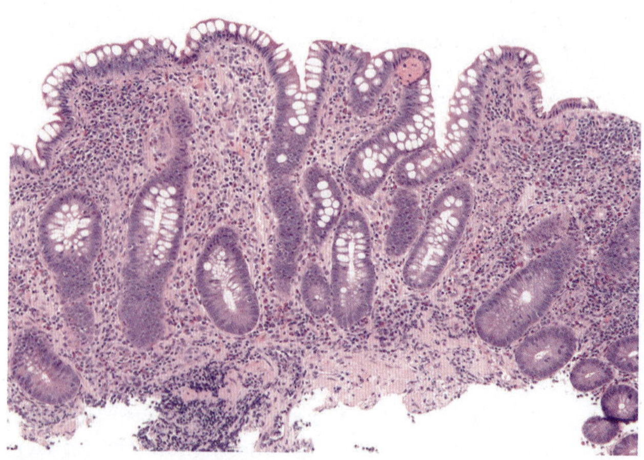

FIGURE 5.14

Nonsteroidal antiinflammatory drug (NSAID)–associated injury. The duodenal biopsy from a patient with history of NSAID use shows distortion of the villous and crypt architecture with expansion of lamina propria by eosinophils, lymphocytes, and plasma cells.

It has been suggested that ischemia, inflammation, and repeated mucosal injury contribute to these pathologic changes.

Rarely, chronic injury can lead to *diaphragm disease*. The pathogenesis of this phenomenon is not well understood but likely involves repeated cycles of injury and repair. There may be superficial annular or longitudinal ulcers. The submucosa is widened, creating annular constriction of the lumen, and it is replaced by disorganized fascicles of smooth muscles (i.e., muscularization of the submucosa), bundles of unmyelinated nerve fibers with scattered ganglion cells, and numerous blood vessels. These changes may extend to the serosa.

Nonsteroidal antiinflammatory drugs can produce any major patterns of small intestinal injury that includes neutrophilic inflammation, eosinophilic inflammation, the flattened villi pattern, and the architectural distortion pattern. Again, NSAID injury can also produce lesions with a paucity of chronic inflammation, which is a relatively distinct feature. Overall, the diagnosis of NSAID injury always requires correlation with clinical findings and exclusion of other causes.

Nonsteroidal Antiinflammatory Drug–Associated Small Bowel Lesions—Pathologic Features

Gross Findings

- Perforations and ulcers associated with nonsteroidal antiinflammatory drugs (NSAIDs) do not have a specific appearance, nor do the strictures of the small bowel
- *Diaphragm disease* has a relatively unique pattern, consisting of mucosal membranes separating segments of the small bowel

Microscopic Findings

- Intact villi with numerous neutrophils within the lamina propria along with neutrophilic epithelial injury; occasionally mucosal eosinophilia
- Erosions and superficial ulcers may be present
- Chronic NSAID injury shows crypt architectural distortion, pyloric gland metaplasia, thickening of muscularis mucosae, submucosal fibrosis, and proliferation of nerves, vessels, and smooth muscle
- Chronic NSAID injury may present as villous blunting with or without intraepithelial lymphocytosis
- In patients with *diaphragm disease*, the submucosa is widened, creating annular constriction of the lumen, and is replaced by disorganized fascicles of smooth muscles (i.e., muscularization of the submucosa), bundles of unmyelinated nerve fibers with scattered ganglion cells, and numerous blood vessels

Differential Diagnosis

- Peptic duodenal disease
- Infection
- Ischemia
- Inflammatory bowel disease
- Behçet's disease
- Malabsorption disorders (if villous blunting is prominent or IELs are increased)

Differential Diagnosis

Because NSAIDs injury can produce each of the major patterns of small intestinal injury, the differential diagnosis depends on which pattern is present. The neutrophilic inflammation pattern is most common, the differential diagnosis for which includes *H. pylori* infection, Crohn's disease, and reactive duodenopathy. In patients with chronic NSAID use, chronic ischemia, Crohn's disease, and Behçet's disease are in the differential diagnosis. Clinical findings are key in distinguishing NSAID injury from Behçet's disease. Behçet's syndrome is characterized by lymphocytic vasculitis that affects veins and less commonly the arteries. Crohn's disease is distinguished from NSAID injury by the presence of deep fissuring ulcers, transmural lymphoid aggregates, and granulomas. Chronic ischemia is a close mimic and requires assessment of mesenteric vessels. When villous blunting is a prominent feature, it should prompt consideration of other malabsorptive disorders. Ultimately, as with any other medication, confirmation of causal association requires correlation with history of drug intake and resolution of symptoms after discontinuation of the drug.

Prognosis and Therapy

The prognosis is excellent for patients with NSAID ulcers if the medication is discontinued. For patients requiring resections owing to strictures or *diaphragm disease*, the prognosis is good, and the risks are typically those associated with the surgical procedure itself.

OLMESARTAN-ASSOCIATED SPRUE-LIKE ENTEROPATHY

Olmesartan is an antihypertensive drug and a member of the angiotensin receptor blocker (ARB) family of compounds. Recently, this drug has shown to cause a sprue-like enteropathy in some patients who have negative celiac serologies. Patients typically present with diarrhea and weight loss. The length of time between olmesartan use and onset of symptoms is highly variable and ranges from a few weeks to 10 years. Histologically, olmesartan enteropathy may mimic all of the features of CD, with most cases showing villous blunting and increased IELs. Nearly one-third of cases also show features of collagenous sprue (Fig. 5.15). Finally, these patients often have concomitant collagenous or lymphocytic gastritis or colitis. Symptoms quickly resolve with cessation of drug. Other members of the ARB family result in a similar sprue-like

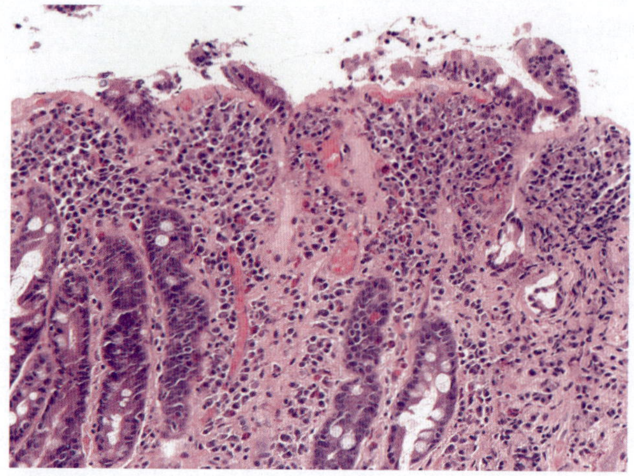

FIGURE 5.15

Olmesartan-associated sprue-like enteropathy. The duodenal biopsy shows villous blunting, intraepithelial lymphocytosis, and crypt hyperplasia along with thickening of the subepithelial collagen layer similar to collagenous sprue.

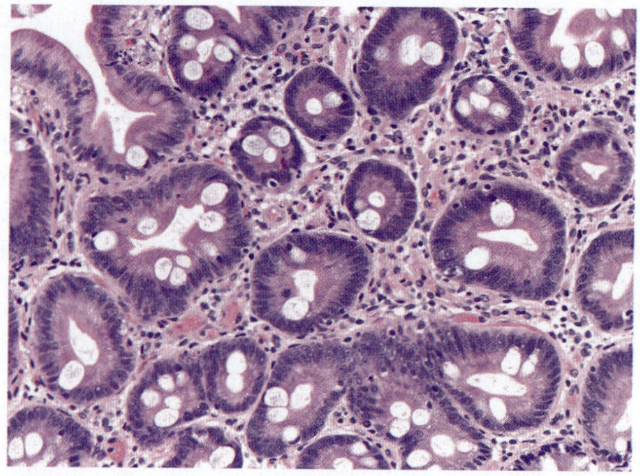

FIGURE 5.16

Common variable immunodeficiency. The duodenal biopsy shows preserved architecture without any plasma cells in the lamina propria.

enteropathy. In general, it is prudent to consider ARB-induced mucosal injury in a patient with celiac-seronegative enteropathy.

COMMON VARIABLE IMMUNODEFICIENCY

Clinical Features

Common variable immunodeficiency is the second most common primary immunodeficiency syndrome (the first being select IgA deficiency). Patients may present at any age with heterogeneous symptoms, including recurrent infections, various autoimmune diseases, GI complaints, and lymphoma. Consistent with its variable presentation, CVID actually represents a group of diseases likely caused by a variety of different gene defects but ultimately leading to immunoglobulin deficiency. Known gene defects account for only 10% of cases (mutations in inducible T-cell costimulator [*ICOS*], calcium-modulating cyclophilin ligand interactor [*TACI*], CD19, CD20, CD21, CD80, and B-cell activating factor receptor [*BAFFR*]). Nearly 80% of cases are sporadic in nature. CVID is primarily a disorder of B-cell differentiation, though T-cell dysfunction is also present in about 40% of cases.

CVID is occasionally diagnosed in childhood, but most patients are diagnosed between the ages of 20 and 45 years. CVID is diagnosed by demonstrating low immunoglobulin levels. IgG is most commonly depleted, but IgA and IgM levels may be low as well. A poor or absent response to vaccination can also be evidence of underlying CVID. Finally, CVID is a diagnosis of exclusion and can only be made when a more specific immunodeficiency disorder is ruled out.

Pathologic Features

Gross Findings

In most cases, the mucosa is grossly unremarkable.

Microscopic Findings

Common variable immunodeficiency has variable histologic findings but is most consistent with the flattened villi pattern of injury with villous blunting and intraepithelial lymphocytosis. Prominent lymphoid aggregates, increased crypt apoptosis, and granulomas are occasionally identified. A feature specific for CVID is the pronounced paucity or even absence of plasma cells, which results from defects in B-cell maturation (Fig. 5.16). However, about one-third of cases have relatively normal numbers, though, in these cases, the plasma cells are functionally abnormal. Given the susceptibility to infection, the histologic picture may be dominated by features caused by a specific infection, such as *Giardia* or CMV. Finally, CVID is often not clinically suspected, and the absence of plasma cells is subtle. Therefore, it is prudent to verify the presence of plasma cells in at least one specimen from every case regardless of indication or histologic picture.

Differential Diagnosis

Histologically, the differential diagnosis includes other diseases that produce the flattened villi pattern of injury, particularly CD. In fact, many patients ultimately diagnosed with CVID carry a prior, incorrect, diagnosis of CD. For the pathologist, the best feature to separate the two entities is the lack of plasma cells. Granulomas and prominent apoptosis are present in a minority of cases and should prompt consideration of Crohn's disease and AIE, respectively. Ultimately, the diagnosis of CVID must be confirmed by demonstrating low serum immunoglobulin levels.

Prognosis and Therapy

Therapy for most patients consists of mitigating the risk of infectious disease. The mainstay of treatment for CVID is IgG replacement, which reduces the incidence of recurrent infections and has been shown to reduce antibiotic use and decrease hospitalizations. With respect to vaccinations, certain live vaccines are contraindicated. Patients should receive killed or inactivated vaccines, although patients may only mount a partial response.

Beyond infection, patients with CVID are also at risk for autoimmune disease, chronic lung disease, granulomatous disease, and malignancy (specifically lymphoma and gastric cancer). Therapy for these patients is tailored to the specific coexisting disease. The prognosis in CVID greatly improved after the introduction of IgG therapy, before which death from bacterial infection was common. Currently, the prognosis is driven mostly by the presence of coexisting disease. Patients most commonly die of chronic lung disease or malignancy.

Common Variable Immunodeficiency—Fact Sheet

Definition

- Immunodeficiency disorder characterized by low circulating immunoglobulins

Incidence

- 1 in 25,000
- Most commonly diagnosed between ages 20 and 45 years

Morbidity and Mortality

- Rate of infections greatly reduced with IgG therapy
- Long-term prognosis driven by coexisting disease (lung disease, autoimmune disease, malignancy)

Clinical Features

- Recurrent infections (most commonly upper respiratory, lower respiratory, and gastrointestinal)
- Autoimmune disease
- Chronic lung disease
- Malignancy

Common Variable Immunodeficiency—Pathologic Features

Gross Findings

- No characteristic gross findings

Microscopic Findings

- Villous blunting
- Intraepithelial lymphocytosis
- Prominent lymphoid aggregates
- Decreased plasma cells
- Granulomas

Differential Diagnosis

- Celiac disease
- Autoimmune enteropathy
- Crohn's disease

Autoimmune Enteropathy

Clinical Features

AIE is a rare disease that typically presents with chronic diarrhea in the first few months of life. Although more common in children, AIE may be seen in adults as well. In AIE, the immune system attacks the intestinal mucosa, leading to severe malabsorption symptoms. Patients usually generate a variety of autoantibodies against self-antigens in different organs, including the pancreas, small intestine, and thyroid. Therefore, in addition to AIE, other autoimmune diseases such as diabetes mellitus, thyroiditis, or hemolytic anemia may also be seen in these patients. Patients with AIE present with severe and persistent inflammatory diarrhea, abdominal pain, weight loss, and malnutrition. Weight loss and malnutrition can be so severe that parenteral nutrition is often required. The symptoms are unresponsive to dietary restriction.

Circulating gut epithelial cell autoantibodies, such as anti–goblet cell or antienterocyte antibodies, are often present in AIE patients. The correlation between the presence of these antibodies and AIE pathogenesis is somewhat unclear; therefore, the diagnostic utility of gut autoantibodies is also a matter of debate. The presence of anti–goblet cell antibodies correlates with absence of goblet cells only in some patients. Furthermore, although almost all patients with AIE have detectable gut autoantibodies, they are not entirely specific for AIE. These antibodies can also be detected in patients with other enteropathies, including CD, IBD, and irritable bowel syndrome.

AIE is known to be part of two inherited syndromes. Immunodysregulation, polyendocrinopathy, enteropathy, and X-linked inheritance (IPEX) syndrome is a particular form of AIE seen in male infants caused by mutations in *FOXP3* gene on the X chromosome. The other inherited syndromic association is autoimmune polyendocrinopathy, mucocutaneous candidiasis, and ectodermal dystrophy (APECED) syndrome, also known as autoimmune polyendocrine syndrome type 1 (APS-1). Defects in the transcription factor autoimmune regulator *(AIRE)* underlie this syndrome. Patients present with *Candida* infections and later develop hypoparathyroidism, Addison's disease, and possibly autoimmune gastritis, autoimmune hepatitis, type 1 diabetes, gonadal dysfunction, and hair and nail loss.

AUTOIMMUNE ENTEROPATHY—FACT SHEET

Definition

- Gastrointestinal mucosal damage caused by antienterocyte or anti–goblet cell antibodies

Incidence

- 25% of infants with intractable diarrhea
- Rare in adults

Morbidity and Mortality

- Failure to thrive

Clinical Features

- Protracted hypersecretory diarrhea
- Weight loss
- Malnutrition

Prognosis

- High mortality rate (~30%) for immunodysregulation, polyendocrinopathy, enteropathy, and X-linked inheritance (IPEX)

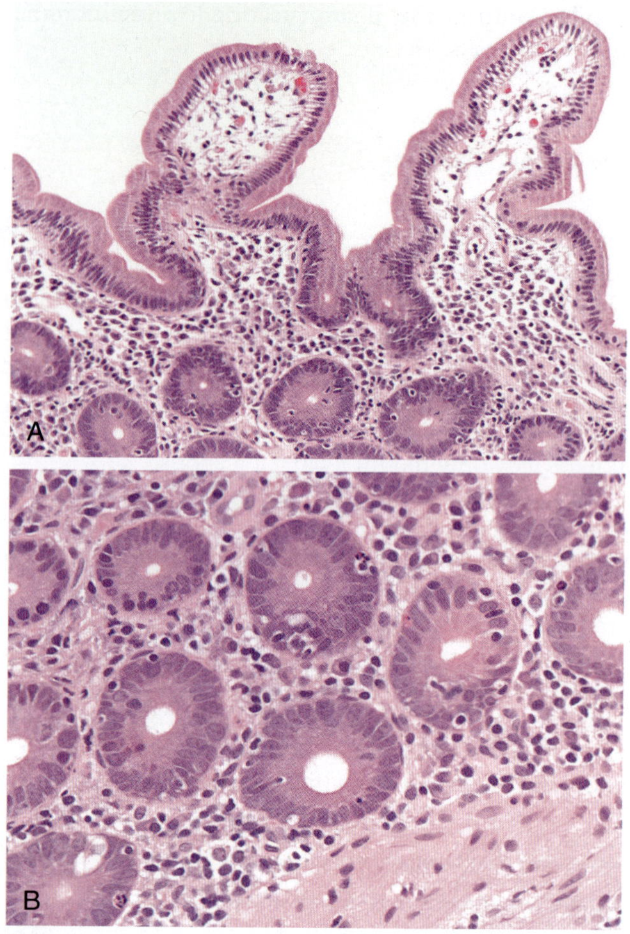

FIGURE 5.17

Autoimmune enteropathy. **A**, Duodenal mucosa shows normal villous architecture. Even at low magnification, one can see lack of goblet cells and Paneth cells within this biopsy. **B**, The crypts characteristically show increased apoptotic activity. Note the lack of Paneth cells. The crypts show more prominent intraepithelial lymphocytosis compared with the surface epithelium.

PATHOLOGIC FEATURES

GROSS FINDINGS

Endoscopic findings include loss of the normal mucosal folds with ulceration and hyperemia. The entire GI tract can be involved, though the most severe disease is often seen in the small bowel.

MICROSCOPIC FINDINGS

AIE has variable histology but falls best into the flattened villi pattern of injury with villous blunting as a constant feature. Most cases show a relatively specific pattern of additional features, with crypt lymphocytosis (more than those present within the villous tips), increased crypt apoptosis, and a prominence of mononuclear inflammatory cells in the lamina propria. Additionally, some cases lack goblet cells, Paneth cells, enteroendocrine cells, and brush border (Fig. 5.17). However, a significant proportion of cases, 20% to 50%, have histology indistinguishable from that of CD. These cases lack significant crypt apoptosis and have surface intraepithelial lymphocytosis rather than deep crypt lymphocytosis.

Finally, the absence of goblet cells, Paneth cells, and enteroendocrine cells can easily go unnoticed,

AUTOIMMUNE ENTEROPATHY—PATHOLOGIC FEATURES

Gross Findings

- Villous atrophy
- Mucosal erythema

Microscopic Findings

- Villous blunting and crypt hyperplasia
- Most cases have increased intraepithelial lymphocytosis in crypts greater than villous tips
- Increased crypt apoptosis
- Absent goblet cells, Paneth cells, brush border, or enteroendocrine cells
- Increased mononuclear inflammation of the lamina propria

Differential Diagnosis

- Celiac disease
- Common variable immunodeficiency
- Microvillus inclusion disease
- Congenital tufting enteropathy
- Enteroendocrine cell dysgenesis

especially when the histologic picture dominated by villous blunting. Therefore, it is important to verify the presence of these cell types in any abnormal small intestinal mucosa.

Differential Diagnosis

AIE is commonly considered in infants with intractable diarrhea when common illnesses, such as infections and food sensitive enteropathies, have been excluded. CD is the most common mimic. Presence of crypt apoptosis, crypt lymphocytosis more than villous tip lymphocytosis, and lack of goblet cells, Paneth cells, or enteroendocrine cells favor AIE compared with CD. Serologic tests (circulating gut epithelial cell antibodies, celiac serologies) should be performed to help this distinction. Some patients may receive an initial diagnosis of CD, but AIE should be considered if symptoms persist on a gluten-free diet.

Common variable immunodeficiency can also be associated with crypt apoptosis. However, paucity of plasma cells should raise the possibility of CVID and prompt serum immunoglobulin quantification studies. In the absence of significant inflammation, congenital enteropathies should be considered, including microvillus inclusion disease (MVID) and congenital tufting enteropathy. Lack of enteroendocrine cells should raise the possibility of enteroendocrine cell dysgenesis (see later). Although these disorders may show some features overlapping with AIE, they are not inflammatory disorders by nature, thus allowing distinction from AIE.

Prognosis and Therapy

The mainstay of treatment for AIE is immunosuppressive therapy. In infancy, nutritional support and adequate hydration are also needed to ensure optimal growth and development. Most patients respond well to this treatment with a high survival rate. Restoration of goblet and Paneth cells is observed in some patients after treatment. However, patients with IPEX syndrome usually have a poor response to therapy, show a high mortality rate, and require hematopoietic cell transplantation as a definitive form of therapy.

MICROVILLUS INCLUSION DISEASE

Microvillus inclusion disease (also known as Davidson's disease, familial microvillus atrophy, congenital microvillus atrophy, or intestinal microvillus dystrophy) is a rare congenital malabsorption disorder caused by defective organelle transport. It is inherited in an autosomal recessive pattern and results in mutations in *MYO5B*, which codes for myosin-Vb. Myosin-Vb participates in organelle transport and endosome recycling. Infants present with intractable diarrhea, severe malabsorption, and negative stool cultures.

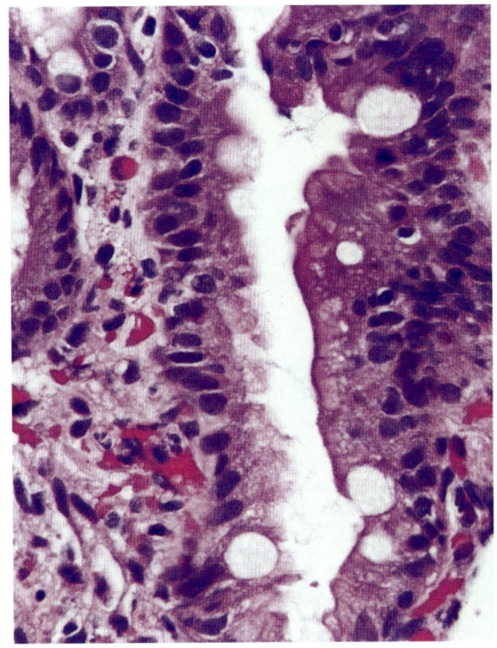

FIGURE 5.18

Microvillus inclusion disease. The duodenal biopsy shows complete loss of the brush border and apical vacuolization on the left half of the image. The section of enterocytes on the right have an intact brush border but do have early apical vacuolization.

Duodenal biopsy shows moderate to diffuse villous blunting without significant inflammatory activity or intraepithelial lymphocytosis. Because of increased crypt cell apoptosis, either crypt hypoplasia or hyperplasia can be found. The most characteristic finding of MVID is a bubbly or vacuolated appearance of the apical enterocyte cytoplasm with extensive or patchy absence of the brush border (Fig. 5.18). Definitive diagnosis requires ancillary stains or methods. PAS is a useful ancillary stain that highlights brush border. In MVID, there are disruption of the normal brush border and misplacement of brush border within the enterocyte cytoplasm, resulting in the formation of cytoplasmic inclusions (Fig. 5.19A). The diagnosis, however, should be confirmed with a more specific method. In the past, electron microscopy (EM) was required for this purpose. EM characteristically shows reduced or complete absence of microvilli on the surface of the enterocytes and vacuoles filled with microvilli (Fig. 5.19B). In addition, these cells show intracytoplasmic inclusions lined by neatly arranged brush border microvilli. The crypt epithelial cells show increased secretory granules. More recently, IHC for villin has been shown to produce a highly characteristic staining pattern in MVID. The differential diagnosis includes other diseases that cause intractable diarrhea in infancy (e.g., congenital tufting enteropathy,

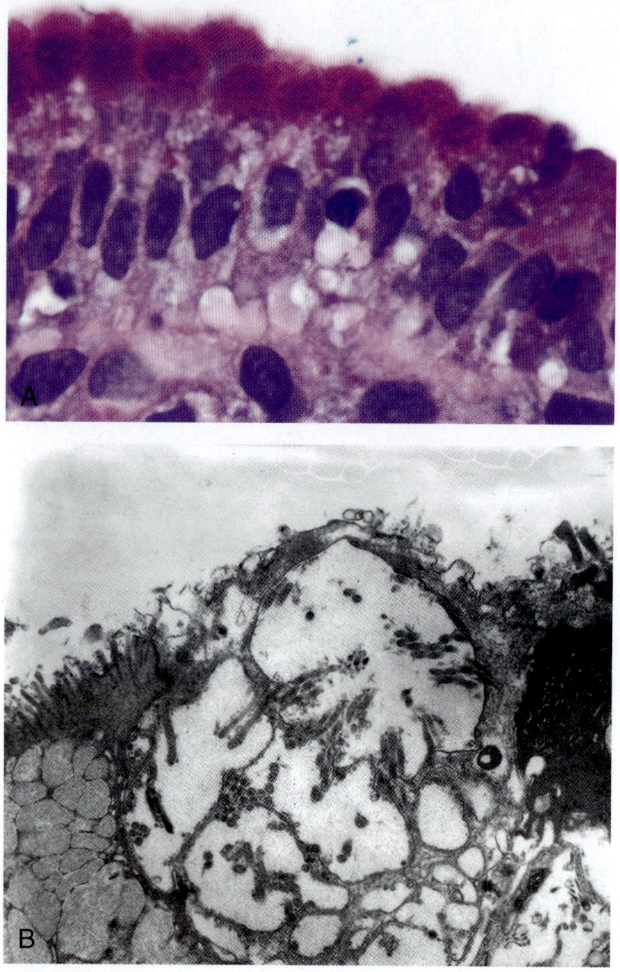

FIGURE 5.19

Microvillus inclusion disease. **A**, Duodenal biopsy stained with Alcian blue–periodic acid–Schiff highlight the alcianophilic apical vacuoles. Notice the complete absence of normal brush border. **B**, Electron microscopy shows enterocytes containing vacuoles filled with microvilli. The overlying and adjacent surface has abnormal villi.

enteroendocrine cell deficiency, AIE), though the biopsy findings are sufficient to discriminate between these possibilities. The disease is life threatening and requires lifelong total parenteral nutrition (TPN) or small bowel transplantation.

CONGENITAL TUFTING ENTEROPATHY (INTESTINAL DYSPLASIA)

Congenital tufting enteropathy is inherited in an autosomal recessive pattern and is most prevalent among individuals of Arabic origin. Clinical presentation is similar to MVID. Infants present with intractable watery diarrhea in the neonatal period. Mutations of epithelial cellular adhesion molecule (EpCAM), a cell adhesion-receptor, and *SPINT2*, a serine protease inhibitor, have been implicated in this condition.

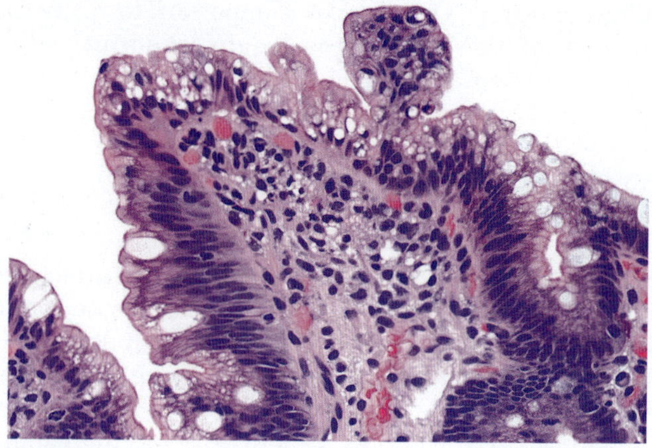

FIGURE 5.20

Congenital tufting enteropathy. The duodenal biopsy shows disorganization of the surface epithelium. These surface enterocytes show formation of clusters or tufts of cells.

The small intestinal mucosa shows severe villous atrophy. However, there is no significant increase in lamina propria inflammatory cells, and intraepithelial lymphocytosis is absent. Characteristically, the superficial epithelium shows disorganization of the surface enterocytes, forming "tufts" (Fig. 5.20). In contrast to MVID, the brush border is normal. Epithelial abnormalities can vary over time and may be extremely subtle at presentation. Immunostaining is helpful to make the diagnosis because patients with *EpCAM* mutations have decreased or absent expression of EpCAM, the target of the MOC31 antibody.

Although tufting enteropathy mimics other entities that cause intractable diarrhea of infancy, lack of EpCAM staining is helpful in confirming the diagnosis of tufting enteropathy. In most cases, the condition is life threatening and requires TPN or small bowel transplantation. However, there is a subset of patients with variant *EpCAM* mutations that have a more "benign" clinical course. Some patients in this category can eventually be weaned from TPN.

ENTEROENDOCRINE CELL DYSGENESIS

Enteroendocrine cell dysgenesis is an autosomal recessive disorder caused by mutations in *NEUROG3*, leading to an absence of intestinal enteroendocrine cells. Patients have diarrhea and profound malabsorption of all nutrients from birth. The hallmark histologic feature is an absence of enteroendocrine cells in the small bowel and colon. Otherwise, the histologic changes are minimal, often showing only mild villous atrophy, if any. The differential diagnosis includes other causes of intractable diarrhea of infancy.

Although the absence of enteroendocrine cells is highly suggestive of enteroendocrine cell dysgenesis, some cases of AIE can show absence of these cells as well. However, the histologic background should allow separation of these entities because AIE is typically associated with intraepithelial lymphocytosis, increased crypt apoptosis, and loss of goblet and Paneth cells (see section on AIE). Patients with enteroendocrine cell dysgenesis require lifelong TPN or small intestinal transplantation.

ABETALIPOPROTEINEMIA

Abetalipoproteinemia (also known as Bassen-Kornzweig disease) is a disorder caused by mutations in microsomal triglyceride transfer protein (MTTP) and is inherited in an autosomal recessive pattern. MTTP is essential for the formation of apo B–containing lipoproteins including chylomicrons, low-density lipoprotein, and very-low-density lipoprotein. Because this disorder leads to an inability to package lipids such as chylomicrons, it manifests with symptoms of fat malabsorption disorder and deficiency of fat-soluble vitamins. Patients typically present in early childhood with abdominal distension, steatorrhea, and failure to thrive. Mental retardation, neuropathic changes, and coagulopathy occur as the disease progresses. Small bowel biopsies show prominent and diffuse vacuolization of the enterocytes. This histologic feature may mimic the much more commonly-encountered phenomenon "lipid hang-up" caused by postprandial lipid accumulation. However, the changes in abetalipoproteinemia are much more florid and not restricted to the villous tips. The villous architecture is preserved, and usually there is no significant epithelial injury. Liver biopsy may reveal steatosis. The diagnosis is not solely a pathologic diagnosis, and affected patients have characteristic abnormalities in hematologic and lipid profiles. Treatment consists of strict adherence to a low-fat diet and supplementation with essential fatty acids and high doses of fat-soluble vitamins. Outcome is variable, but early diagnosis and strict compliance with diet can prevent disease progression.

SMALL INTESTINAL INFLAMMATORY BOWEL DISEASE

Traditionally, IBD of the small intestine was considered to be the exclusive domain of Crohn's disease. We now appreciate that this dichotomy is not entirely accurate because there are reports of the upper GI tract involvement in patients with ulcerative colitis (UC) as well. In this chapter, only Crohn's disease is discussed. UC is presented in Chapter 10.

CROHN'S DISEASE

CLINICAL FEATURES

Burrill Crohn published his seminal work on this entity in 1932, describing "regional ileitis," as a stricturing, fistulizing, inflammatory disease of the ileum. Crohn's disease is most prevalent in Western countries with an annual incidence of approximately 10 per 100,000. The cause of Crohn's disease is unknown but is thought to be an abnormal response to gut flora in a genetically susceptible individual. Crohn's disease has a strong genetic component with a concordance rate of 50% in monozygotic twin studies. Numerous susceptibility loci have been linked to the pathogenesis of Crohn's disease. One of the earliest genes identified was *IBD1*, which encodes the NOD2 protein (also known as CARD15). NOD2 activates nuclear factor κB (NF-κB) in response to fragments of the bacterial cell wall. In one study, *NOD2* mutations were found in 42% of children with early-onset Crohn's disease. Other susceptibility loci encode proteins involved in cell autophagy, adaptive immunity, and epithelial function and underscore the importance of these functions in the pathogenesis of Crohn's disease. Furthermore, various clinical features of Crohn's disease show heritable patterns and concordance within family members such as similar disease location (ileal vs ileocolonic) and type (stenotic, fistulizing).

Crohn's disease may involve any portion of the tubular GI tract. The Montreal classification is commonly used to classify the disease and incorporates age at disease onset, principal anatomic location, and clinical behavior (Table 5.3). Most patients have small intestinal disease (80%) usually in the distal ileum, with one-third having ileal disease exclusively. The terminal ileum is the most commonly affected location. In contrast, duodenal involvement is much more uncommon (1%–7%).

TABLE 5.3
Montreal Classification of Crohn's Disease

AGE AT DIAGNOSIS
- A1: younger than 16 years
- A2: between 17 and 40 years
- A3: older than 40 years

LOCATION
- L1: ileal
- L2: colonic
- L3: ileocolonic
- L4: isolated upper tract disease

BEHAVIOR
- B1: nonstricturing, nonpenetrating
- B2: stricturing
- B3: penetrating
- p: perianal disease

About 50% of patients show involvement of both the small bowel and colon (usually localized to ileocolonic region). In patients with involvement of both the small bowel and colon, the rectum is normal in about half of cases; this is a striking contrast to UC, in which the rectum is nearly always involved. A minority of patients have isolated colonic Crohn's disease (20%). Among these patients, about 50% have right-sided colitis, 40% have left-sided colitis, and 6% have pancolonic involvement. About one-third of patients have perianal disease, a feature that is highly specific for Crohn's disease over UC.

Most patients with Crohn's disease present with a variety of symptoms, including diarrhea, steatorrhea, chronic abdominal pain, perianal disease, oral ulcers, and malabsorption symptoms (weight loss, fatigue, anemia). Patients with the stenotic form of Crohn's disease present with symptoms of intestinal obstruction.

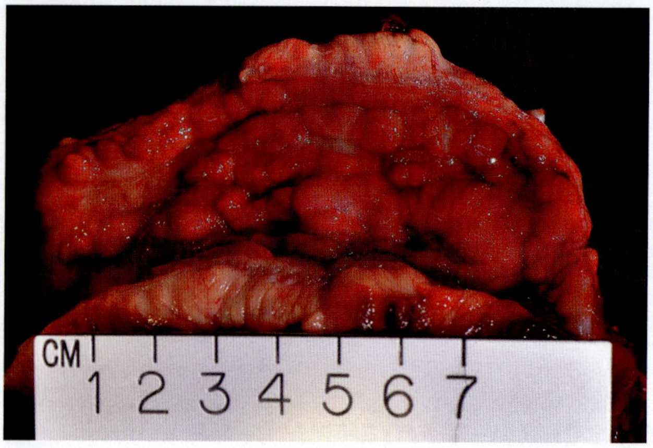

FIGURE 5.21

Crohn's disease. The small bowel resection specimen shows a segment of stenotic bowel with longitudinal, fissuring ulcers, and cobblestone appearance of the mucosa.

PATHOLOGIC FEATURES

GROSS FINDINGS

Crohn's disease has a number of distinct gross findings. Fat wrapping, or creeping fat, is characteristic of Crohn's disease and is characterized by overgrowth of mesenteric fat around the serosal surface of the bowel. There may be adhesions or fistula formation between the involved bowel and any nearby organs. Fat wrapping, adhesion formation, and fistula formation are related to the deep, transmural inflammatory activity that is characteristic of Crohn's disease. The bowel is typically fibrotic and stiff, forming "hose-like" segments that do not lie flat on the grossing bench. This stiffness is caused by a combination of submucosal fibrosis, obliterative muscularization of the submucosa, and hypertrophy of the muscularis propria. These factors also contribute to luminal stenosis that becomes evident after opening the specimen.

Aphthous ulcers are the earliest mucosal lesions found in Crohn's disease. These are pinpoint erosions often found in the distal terminal ileum and are a useful endoscopic clue for Crohn's disease. As the disease becomes more extensive, the mucosa shows characteristic fissuring, forming "bear claw" ulcers that surround intact mucosa. At this stage, mucosa often shows a "cobblestone" appearance that results from extensive anastomosing ulcers delimiting small patches of intact mucosa (Fig. 5.21).

MICROSCOPIC FINDINGS

The microscopic features of Crohn's disease can be divided into mucosal and mural findings; the latter are considered to be more pathognomonic of Crohn's disease and can only be assessed on resection specimens. Early in the disease process, the classic aphthous ulcer corresponds to a zone of active inflammation with superficial erosion, typically overlying a lymphoid aggregate. As the disease becomes more severe, these erosions may grow into "fissuring ulcers," which are penetrating ulcers that extend into the submucosa or muscularis propria.

The accompanying mucosal findings include variable degree of chronic mucosal injury with or without activity (Fig. 5.22A). Features of chronic mucosal injury include crypt or villous architectural distortion, basal lymphoplasmacytosis, basal lymphoid aggregates, and pyloric gland metaplasia (Fig. 5.22B). Activity typically consists of neutrophil- (or eosinophil-) mediated epithelial injury in the form of cryptitis and crypt abscesses. Thickening of muscularis mucosae is often present and is best assessed on resection specimens. Overall, this combination of features falls into the "chronic mucosal injury" of injury as outlined in the introduction section of this chapter. In segments of small bowel wall affected by Crohn's disease, the submucosa may show fibrosis along with obliterative muscularization. Deep fissuring ulcers usually extend into the submucosa and superficial muscularis propria. The bowel wall is characterized by transmural inflammation in the form of transmural lymphoid aggregates as well as lymphoid aggregates at the junction of muscularis propria and serosa (Fig. 5.22C). Other findings include neural hyperplasia and lymphocytic plexitis. Mural fibrosis, serositis, and adhesions are common in areas of fistula formation.

Nearly 50% to 60% of patients with Crohn's disease show granulomas in resection specimens. They are typically noncaseating and often poorly formed and perivascular in distribution (Fig. 5.22D). These granulomas need to be distinguished from crypt rupture–related granulomas, which are more common in UC. One-third of patients with Crohn's disease do not form granulomas, so the absence of granulomas does not necessarily exclude a diagnosis of Crohn's disease, especially in

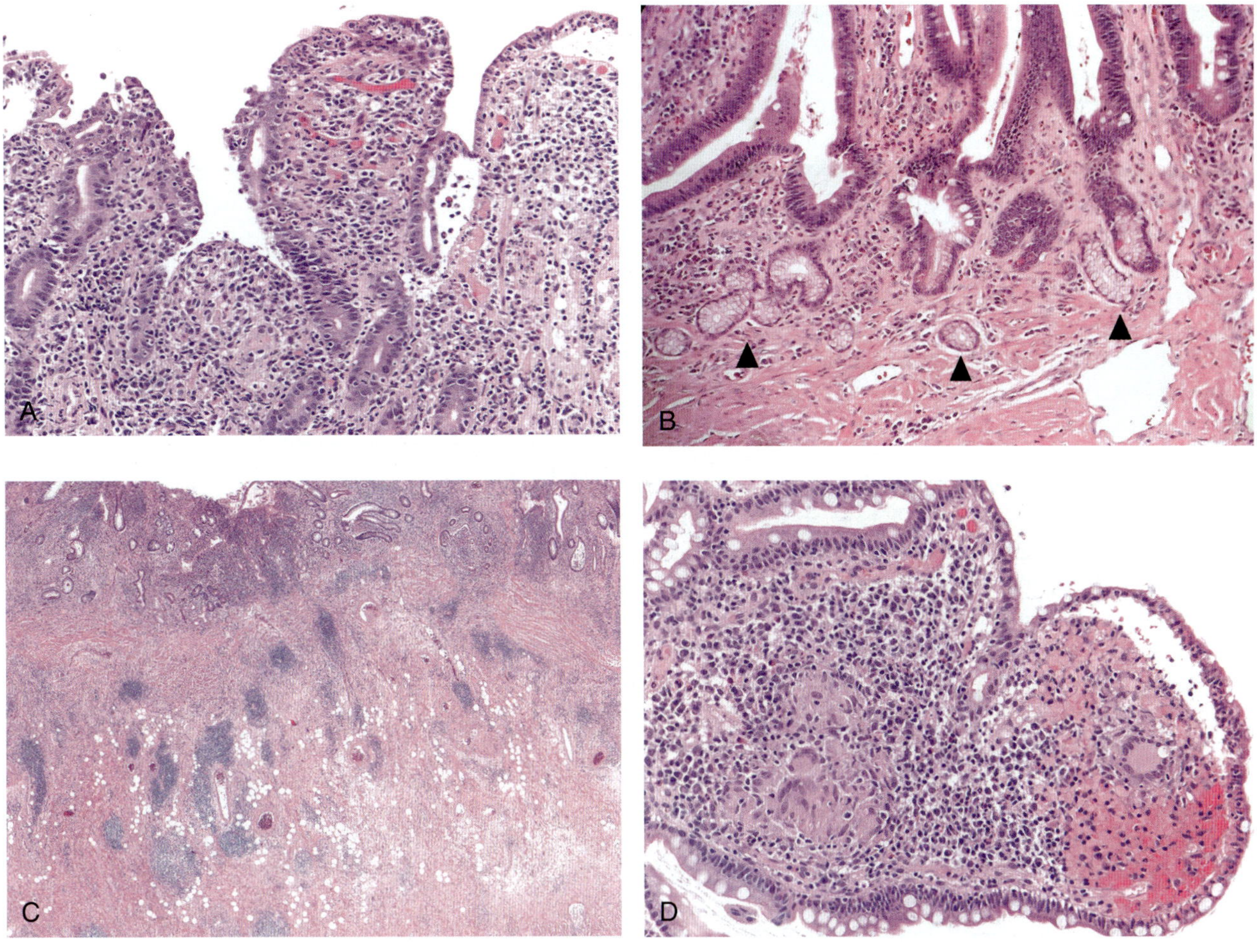

FIGURE 5.22

Crohn's disease. **A**, The duodenal mucosa shows villous blunting and crypt architectural distortion. The lamina propria is expanded by mixed inflammatory cell infiltrate, and there is prominent neutrophilic epithelial injury with erosion **B**, Pyloric gland metaplasia in a patient with Crohn's disease. This finding indicates chronic or prior mucosal injury and may be seen in conditions other than Crohn's disease, such as nonsteroidal antiinflammatory drug–related chronic small bowel injury (The black triangles are arrow heads). **C**, Small bowel resection specimen of Crohn's disease showing chronic active enteritis with mucosal erosion and characteristic transmural lymphoid aggregates with mural fibrosis. **D**, Duodenal mucosa with granulomas in a patient with Crohn's disease.

biopsy material, in which only a small sample of the mucosa is evaluated. In keeping with the transmural nature of Crohn's disease, granulomas may be seen in any layer of the bowel wall, including within and deep to the muscularis propria. Granulomas are often present within regional lymph nodes and can occasionally be seen within lymphatic spaces as well. In cases in which granulomas are far too numerous or show necrosis ("atypical" granulomas), special stains should be performed to exclude an infectious cause.

Differential Diagnosis

In biopsy specimens, the differential diagnosis for architectural distortion pattern of injury (with or without activity) includes infections, drug injury, ischemia, and IBD. However, given that the pathognomonic findings of Crohn's disease are transmural, a definitive diagnosis of Crohn's disease cannot be made on the basis of mucosal biopsy specimens. In the early phases of Crohn's disease, the biopsy may only show activity without features of chronic mucosal injury. In these cases, the differential diagnosis primarily involves infections and drug- or medication-related injury (especially NSAIDs) and less likely ischemia. When features of chronic mucosal injury (crypt and villous distortion, pyloric gland metaplasia, diffuse lymphoplasmacytosis) are present, IBD is more likely.

The differential diagnosis of granulomas includes infection (e.g., mycobacterium, fungus, *Yersinia* spp.) and sarcoidosis. A rare cause of granulomas is chronic granulomatous disease (CGD), a form of inherited immunodeficiency. CGD patients are typically infants or children with recurrent infections. Besides granulomas, the intestinal lamina propria also shows characteristic pigmented macrophages, which contain a yellow-brown lipofuscin-like pigment.

A rare mimic of Crohn's disease is Behçet's disease, a vasculitis that occurs primarily in Asians and is rare in Western countries. Behçet's disease is a systemic disorder consisting of oral ulceration plus two of the following: recurrent genital ulcers, eye lesions, skin lesions, and a positive pathergy test result (an abnormal response to minor skin injury). Patients may experience symptoms similar to Crohn's disease. In the GI tract, Behçet's disease most frequently involves the terminal ileum and may produce ulcerated lesions histologically identical to those seen in Crohn's disease. In contrast to Crohn's disease, examination of the submucosa should reveal small-vessel phlebitis (larger vessels are typically unaffected). Furthermore, strictures and fistulas are not features of Behçet's disease, and other clinical findings are usually sufficient to distinguish between these entities.

In small bowel resection specimens, the differential diagnosis for Crohn's disease includes drug-induced injury (especially NSAIDs), chronic ischemia, chronic infection, and Behçet's disease. NSAID-induced injury usually occurs in older patients with a history of NSAID intake for chronic pain. Similar to Crohn's disease, the mucosa shows chronic enteritis (with or without activity) and submucosal or mural fibrosis in a segmental distribution. However, transmural lymphoid aggregates are usually not seen in NSAID-related enteritis. Chronic NSAID injury can show characteristic mucosal and submucosal widening, creating annular constriction of the lumen ("diaphragm disease") that may mimic stenotic Crohn's disease, the results of repeated cycles of mucosal injury and repair. Ultimately, confirming NSAID-related injury is difficult because it requires a detailed examination of the patient's clinical history, specifically the timing and dosage of the suspected drug.

Often, the differential diagnosis is primarily between UC and Crohn's disease. The distribution of the disease is important to consider as Crohn's disease can affect any portion of the GI tract, often in a discontinuous fashion with intervening areas of normal mucosa (i.e., "skip lesions"). In contrast, UC typically extends proximally from the rectum in a continuous fashion, generally sparing the small bowel.

Small bowel involvement can be seen in some patients with UC (see Chapter 10). This is believed to be caused by reflux of colonic contents through the damaged ileocecal valve and was termed "backwash ileitis." A recent critical review of the literature by Patil and Odze[1] related to "backwash ileitis" suggests that the originally proposed theory of this condition, which has never been proven experimentally and was postulated during a time when little was known regarding the pathologic manifestation of Crohn's disease in the GI tract, including the colon, or the variability of involvement of the upper GI tract in Crohn's disease or UC, may be entirely false. Interestingly, most, if not all, contemporary studies of presumed "backwash ileitis" reveal data that are not compatible with the proposed mechanism of action of backwash ileitis. The more likely possibility is that ileitis in UC may simply represent a primary manifestation of UC in this portion of the GI tract, and this is a theory that needs to be tested further in future.

CROHN'S DISEASE—FACT SHEET

Definition

- Chronic multifocal relapsing and remitting inflammatory disease of unknown cause
- May affect any portion of the gastrointestinal tract (mouth to anus)

Incidence. Prevalence and Location

- Incidence: approximately 1 to 10 per 100,000
- Prevalence: 10 to 200 per 100,000
- Higher incidence in North Americans and Northern Europeans

Gender, Race, and Age Distribution

- Males and females equally affected
- Higher incidence in North Americans and Northern Europeans
- Higher incidence in Ashkenazi Jews
- Major peak at 20 to 30 years of age
- Minor peak at 60 to 70 years of age

Clinical Features

- Cramping pain, nonbloody diarrhea, fever, malaise, and anorexia
- Fistulas, stenosis
- Hemorrhage and hematochezia uncommon
- Anal and perianal fissures and fistulas
- Inflammatory involvement can occur in joints, eyes, liver, and skin

Prognosis and Therapy

- Cure: none
- Low mortality, high morbidity
- Medical treatment: 5-aminosalicylate, sulfasalazine, oral steroids, antibiotics, infliximab
- Surgical management for obstruction or medically refractory disease
- Increased risk of dysplasia and adenocarcinoma
- Ileal pouch anal anastomosis procedure is contraindicated

GRAFT-VERSUS-HOST DISEASE

CLINICAL FEATURES

Graft-versus-host disease is one of the most common complications after hematopoietic stem cell transplantation (HSCT). It occurs when donor immune cells react against recipient tissues that are not recognized as

Crohn's Disiease—Pathologic Features

Gross Findings

- Patchy involvement
- Firm, thickened, and pipe-like bowel
- Interloop adhesions
- Aphthous erosions
- Longitudinal ulcers
- Cobblestoning
- Inflammatory polyps
- Fistulas

Microscopic Findings

- Aphthous or fissuring ulcers
- Granulomas (noncaseating, frequently poorly formed)
- Chronic enteritis with or without activity, crypt and villous distortion, basal lymphoplasmacytosis, expansion of the lamina propria by lymphocytes and plasma cells, and pyloric gland metaplasia
- Submucosal fibrosis
- Transmural lymphoid aggregates
- Neural hyperplasia and lymphocytic plexitis

Differential Diagnosis

- Infectious enteritis (especially *Yersinia* spp.)
- Medication-associated colitis (especially nonsteroidal antiinflammatory drugs)
- Ileal involvement in ulcerative colitis
- Ischemia
- Behçet's disease
- If granulomas present: sarcoidosis, chronic granulomatous disease, infections (e.g., *Yersinia* spp., mycobacteria, fungus)

"self." GVHD has classically been divided into acute and chronic forms, which vary in timing, patient symptoms, end-organ involvement, treatment, and prognosis. Historically, acute GVHD was diagnosed within the first 100 days after HSCT; disease after this point was considered chronic GVHD. However, now it is recognized that acute GVHD may occur after 100 days, and features of chronic GVHD may start to appear prior to 100 days.

Acute GVHD most often occurs 2 to 3 weeks after HSCT and occurs in 40 % to 50 % of patients. The principal targets are the tubular GI tract, the liver, and the skin. GI symptoms include crampy abdominal pain, diarrhea, nausea, and vomiting. Acute GVHD of the GI tract is graded clinically according to volume of diarrhea. There are additional clinical grading criteria for skin and liver involvement.

With respect to chronic GVHD, it is unclear if it represents a late manifestation of acute GVHD or if it is a separate manifestation of immunologic injury. Acute GVHD is a risk factor for the later development of chronic GVHD. In contrast to acute GVHD, chronic GVHD more resemble autoimmune or immunologic disorders such as Sjögren syndrome, scleroderma, primary biliary cholangitis, and bronchiolitis obliterans. Whereas acute GVHD principally involves the tubular GI tract, liver, and skin, chronic GVHD can also affect the lungs, eyes, muscles, connective tissue, joints, and nails. According to the National Institutes of Health (NIH) consensus development project, feature of chronic GVHD can be divided into "diagnostic features" and "distinctive features." Diagnostic features, when present, are sufficient for the diagnosis of chronic GVHD without need for further investigation. Distinctive features, although suggestive of chronic GVHD, require additional studies, such as biopsy or laboratory testing, to verify the diagnosis. In the GI tract, the only diagnostic feature of chronic GVHD is the presence of esophageal webs, provided they were not present before HCST.

Gastrointestinal GVHD—Fact Sheet

Definition

- Gastrointestinal mucosal damage caused by the engraftment of donor T lymphocytes

Incidence

- 10% to 40% of patients with allogeneic hematopoietic stem cell transplant
- Up to 13% of patients with autologous hematopoietic stem cell transplant
- Fewer than 1% of patients with solid organ transplant

Morbidity and Mortality

- Responsible for approximately 50% of transplant-related deaths

Clinical Features

- Diarrhea
- Crampy abdominal pain
- Nausea and vomiting

Prognosis

- Fewer than 50% of patients achieve a complete resolution after treatment
- Transplant-related mortality for nonresponders is 49% to 75%

PATHOLOGIC FEATURES

Gross Findings

The gross endoscopic appearance of GVHD can be variable. In most cases, the mucosa may either appear normal or show edema with or without erythema. In severe cases, ulcer, nodularity, friability, diffuse bleeding, or mucosal sloughing can be seen. Although the entire GI tract can be involved, the involvement is usually patchy. Esophageal webs are a diagnostic feature of chronic GVHD.

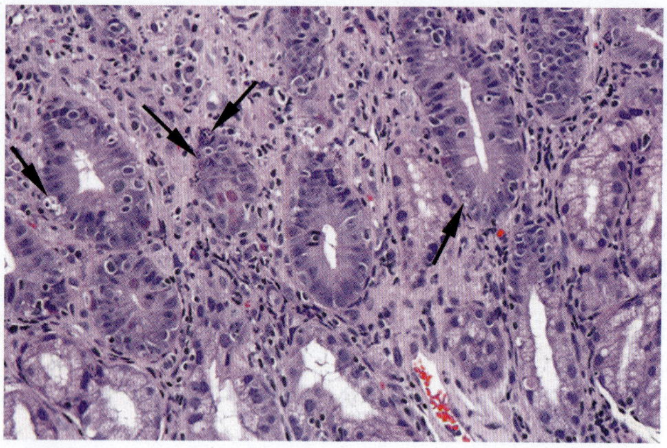

FIGURE 5.23

Graft-versus-host disease (GVHD). The duodenal biopsy shows prominent apoptotic activity within the crypts. Epithelial cell apoptosis is a key histologic feature of GVHD (black arrows).

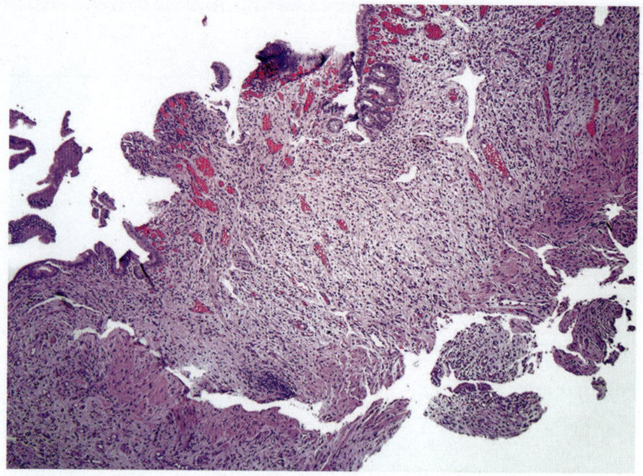

FIGURE 5.24

Grade 4 graft-versus-host disease in a duodenal biopsy. There are extensive crypt loss, mucosal denudation, and granulation tissue formation.

TABLE 5.4

Graft-versus-Host Disease Guidelines: 2014 National Institutes of Health Pathology Working Group: Recommendations for Final Diagnosis Categories.

NOT GVHD
- No evidence for GVHD

POSSIBLE GVHD
- Evidence of GVHD but other possible explanations (e.g., CMV, possible drug reaction)

LIKELY GVHD
- Clear evidence of GVHD without a competing cause of injury
- Clear evidence of GVHD with mitigating factors
- GVHD is most likely diagnosis, but relevant clinical information is limited
- GVHD is validated by sequential biopsy or by absence of a competing diagnosis

Microscopic Findings

Crypt apoptosis is the histologic hallmark of GVHD. It is prominent in the deep aspects of the crypts (Fig. 5.23). Early changes consist only of apoptotic activity. With progressive injury, apoptosis is accompanied by crypt dropout, neutrophilic epithelial injury, crypt abscesses, villous blunting, and ulceration. Paneth cell loss may occur and is associated with poor prognosis. Small clusters of enteroneuroendocrine cells may be present at the bases of crypts because these cells are much more resistant to immunologic injury.

The 2014 report from the NIH consensus project on GVHD recommended three diagnostic categories for GVHD: not GVHD, possible GVHD, and likely GVHD (Table 5.4). "Not GVHD" is appropriate when there is no evidence of GVHD. If there is some evidence of GVHD but there are other possible explanations (CMV coinfection, possibility of drug reaction such as MMF-induced injury), a diagnosis of "possible GVHD" is recommended. Finally, "likely GVHD" is appropriate when there is clear evidence of GVHD without a competing cause of injury or mitigating factors. The minimal criteria for diagnosis of GVHD are not well established, but the NIH consensus document recommends the presence of greater than one apoptotic body per fragment of the biopsy specimen is sufficient for a diagnosis of GVHD.

Graft-versus-host disease grading is still performed in many centers because it provides some quantification of mucosal injury, but it is unclear if pathologic grading offers much additional value over clinical grading alone. Various grading schemes exist, but a system modified by Lerner is most commonly used in daily practice: grade 1, isolated apoptotic bodies; grade 2, loss or damage of individual crypts; grade 3, loss of two or more contiguous crypts; and grade 4, extensive crypt loss or denudation (Fig. 5.24).

GASTROINTESTINAL GRAFT-VERSUS-HOST DISEASE—PATHOLOGIC FEATURES

Gross Findings
- Mucosal edema and erythema
- Ulcer, nodularity, friability
- Diffuse bleeding
- Mucosal sloughing

Microscopic Findings
- Crypt apoptosis
- Crypt dropout
- Crypt abscesses
- Ulcer
- Neuroendocrine cell clusters

Differential Diagnosis
- Cytomegalovirus infection
- Cryptosporidium infection
- Toxicity from conditioning regimen
- Mycophenolate mofetil-induced injury

When grade of GVHD is reported, the highest grade should be reported per anatomic segment of involvement.

Differential Diagnosis

Infections and drug toxicities can mimic GI GVHD in patients who have received HSCT. Because treatments for these conditions are very different compared with GVHD, differentiation of GI GVHD from its mimics is critical.

Cytomegalovirus infection is a frequent complication of HCST, and CMV enteritis may occur concomitantly with GI GVHD. They also share a similar key finding: increased crypt apoptosis. However, CMV enteritis is often associated with neutrophilic cryptitis and crypt abscesses. Sometimes nuclear inclusions in CMV enteritis maybe very sparse, and an immunohistochemical stain may be needed to demonstrate the inclusions. Infection with cryptosporidium can also cause crypt apoptosis. These organisms appear as basophilic, round, predominantly extracellular organisms located along the microvillous brush board (see Chapter 9 for additional details).

Early GVHD must be differentiated from toxicity due to the pretransplant conditioning regimen. The conditioning regimen may result in changes nearly indistinguishable from GVHD, with increased apoptosis, mitotic activity, and regenerative epithelial changes. However, the histologic changes caused by conditioning regimen usually resolve within 20 days after transplantation. Severe mucosal injury, such as ulcers, is unusual with conditioning regimen (even at day 20), and thus is more likely to represent GVHD.

Mycophenolate mofetil is a common immunosuppressive drug used in transplant patients (see Chapter 10 for details). In the ileum and colon, MMF may produce a variety of injury patterns such as those mimicking GVHD (increased apoptosis), acute self-limited or infectious colitis (cryptitis, crypt abscesses), and IBD (architectural distortion, crypt loss, Paneth cell metaplasia). The distinction between MMF toxicity and GVHD is particularly challenging, though some histologic features can suggest one process over the other. Whereas significant eosinophilia (>15 per 10 hpf) is more common in MMF toxicity, apoptotic crypt abscesses and neuroendocrine cell aggregates are more suggestive of GVHD. Finally, clinical information regarding the dosage of MMF is helpful to confirm MMF toxicity.

Prognosis and Therapy

For acute GVHD, steroids are the first-line treatment. For patients who do not respond to initial therapy, second-line options include MMF, tacrolimus, antithymocyte globulin, cyclosporine, photophoresis, sirolimus, and pentostatin. About 40% of patients achieve complete resolution with initial therapy. In patients requiring second-line therapy, there are a lower likelihood of complete resolution and an increased incidence of recurrent episodes of GVHD. Patients with no response have a mortality rate as high as 75%.

Chronic GVHD is the single most important determinant of long-term outcome in HSCT patients. It occurs in 50% of long-term survivors of HLA-identical sibling transplants. Mortality rate varies with severity of disease, which can be graded based on the revised 2014 NIH consensus guidelines. Mild disease involves two or fewer organs or sites with no clinically significant functional impairment (97% 2-year survival rate). Moderate disease involves three or more organs or sites with no clinically significant functional impairment or at least one organ or site with clinically significant functional impairment but no major disability (86% 2-year survival rate). Severe disease involves major disability caused by chronic GVHD (62% 2-year survival rate). The mainstay of treatment is steroids. Unfortunately, there is a 50% failure rate of front-line steroid treatment. Given the poorly understood nature of this disease, specific agents for the treatment of patients with chronic GVHD do not yet exist.

EOSINOPHILIC GASTROENTERITIS

Clinical Features

Eosinophilia in the small bowel can be seen in isolation (eosinophilic enteritis) or as part of eosinophilic gastroenteritis (EGE), which includes eosinophilic esophagitis, eosinophilic gastritis, and eosinophilic colitis. EGE is a poorly characterized clinicopathologic entity. The incidence rate in the United States is estimated to be 22 to 28 per 100,000 persons. It can occur at any age but presents most often in the third through fifth decades of life. An allergic component is suspected because some patients improve with dietary modifications.

One early description of EGE classified it into three forms, depending on the bowel layer involved: mucosal, mural, and serosal. Patients with mucosal-predominant disease present with diarrhea, hemorrhage, and protein-losing enteropathy. Patients with mural disease present with abdominal pain, intestinal obstruction, nausea, and vomiting, and those with serosal involvement may additionally develop ascites, which is rich in eosinophils. Mucosal disease is the most common form (50% of cases); the serosal EGE is much less common.

The laboratory findings in patients with EGE include a peripheral blood eosinophilia but are normal in 20%

of patients. Serum IgE is commonly elevated. Mucosal EGE may cause iron deficiency, prolonged prothrombin time, and hypoalbuminemia caused by malabsorption.

PATHOLOGIC FEATURES

Gross Findings

Mucosal EGE may show erosions or ulcers. In cases with mural disease, the bowel wall shows thickening and induration.

Microscopic Findings

In the mucosal form of EGE, there are sheets of eosinophils within the lamina propria. Eosinophils may be intact or degranulated. Features of epithelial injury, such as eosinophilic cryptitis, eosinophilic crypts abscesses, erosions, and ulceration, are usually present. Because the disease can show patchy distribution, the findings can vary between biopsy samples and within each biopsy fragment.

The mural form is characterized by eosinophilic infiltration and edema of the submucosa and muscularis propria (Fig. 5.25). In the serosal form, the eosinophils are limited to the serosa and subserosa. In the absence of mucosal disease, a diagnosis of EGE can be difficult to establish. Serosal disease can be detected with ascitic fluid analysis, but mural disease may require full-thickness biopsy or resection. In these cases, a high degree of suspicion is required.

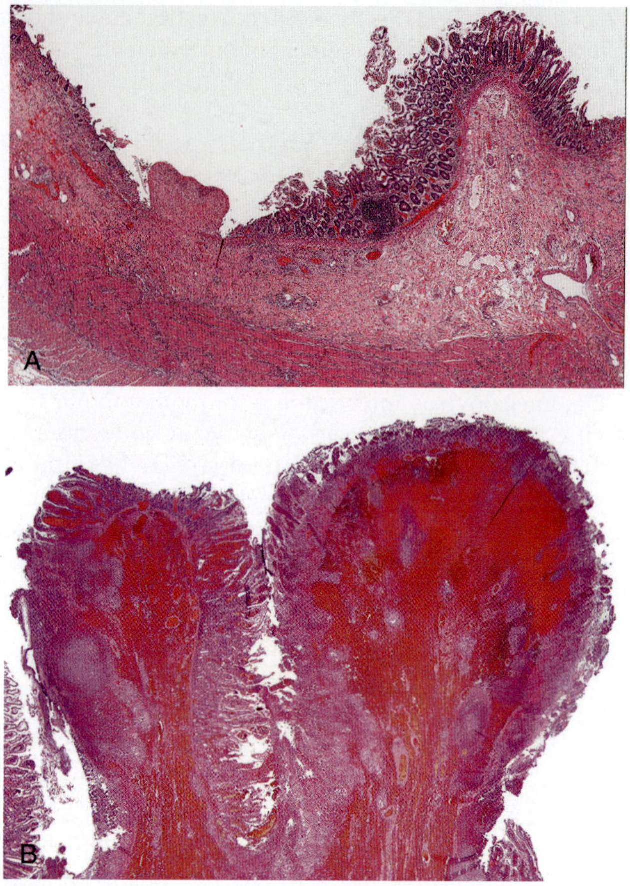

FIGURE 5.25

Eosinophilic enteritis, mural form. **A**, Segment of small bowel with ulcer and submucosal fibrosis. **B**, The bowel wall shows sheets of eosinophils with the muscularis propria.

Differential Diagnosis

Mucosal eosinophilia can be seen in the context of a variety of other diseases. In particular, increased eosinophilia can be seen in the context of hypersensitivity reactions, including allergies and hypersensitivity to drugs or medications, IBD, parasitic infection, connective tissue disorders, and vasculitis. Systemic mastocytosis also lead to mucosal eosinophilia because mast cells appear to attract eosinophils. However, mast cells can be rather inconspicuous, and the increase in eosinophils may be the most eye-catching feature at first glance. Finally, LCH is usually rich in eosinophils, though LCH is usually an endoscopically discrete lesion.

The histologic characteristic of this disorder is simple—a marked increase the number of eosinophils. Unfortunately, the normal range of eosinophils in the small bowel mucosa is quite broad, and rigorous quantitative criteria for establishing this diagnosis do not exist. Some of the proposed criteria include greater than 21 eosinophils/hpf as the cut-off. In the pediatric population, the peak numbers of eosinophils per hpf were reported as 26/hpf for duodenum and 28/hpf for the ileum in one study and 52/hpf for the duodenum and 68/hpf for the ileum in another study. Although prototypical cases show a conspicuous increase in eosinophils, often in sheets, the pathologists often encounter cases with borderline findings. In these cases, the report can be descriptive (e.g., "small bowel mucosa with increased intramucosal eosinophils"), and the comment can include a differential diagnosis of intramucosal eosinophilia. A few additional factors suggest a truly pathologic process. These include evidence of epithelial injury (e.g., eosinophilic crypt abscesses or cryptitis), the presence of eosinophils in the muscularis propria or submucosa, and eosinophilia in more than one site or organ.

Prognosis and Therapy

Patients are initially managed with dietary modification, which includes eliminating the most common food allergens (milk, eggs, wheat, soy, peanuts, tree nuts, and seafood). Alternatively, patients may be administered an elemental diet, consisting of amino acids, fat, and sugars, which contains no allergens. If necessary, oral prednisone may be necessary to manage symptoms. Surgical management is uncommon but occasionally indicated if obstruction occurs. The natural history of EGE is not well defined. Some patients remit spontaneously without treatment, and many respond completely to the initial form of treatment. Patients who experience relapses after initial therapy may require long-term treatment.

EOSINOPHILIC GASTROENTERITIS—FACT SHEET

Definition

- Idiopathic inflammatory disorder characterized by eosinophil-mediated injury

Incidence

- Approximately 22 to 28 per 100,000
- Most commonly presents in the third to fifth decades of life

Morbidity and Mortality

- Not life threatening
- Morbidity associated with obstruction and symptoms

Clinical Features

- Mucosal disease (gastrointestinal bleeding, diarrhea, protein-losing enteropathy)
- Mural disease (abdominal pain, nausea, vomiting)
- Subserosal disease (abdominal pain, nausea, vomiting, ascites)

Prognosis and Therapy

- Oral steroids
- Surgical management for obstruction is occasionally needed
- Natural history is largely unknown
- Some patients have spontaneous remission
- Some patients have a recurring or continuous course

EOSINOPHILIC GASTROENTERITIS—PATHOLOGIC FEATURES

Gross Findings

- Ulceration (mucosal disease)
- Thickening and induration of the bowel wall (mural disease)

Microscopic Findings

- Marked mucosal, mural, or serosal eosinophilia
- Epithelial injury (eosinophilic cryptitis, eosinophilic crypt abscesses)
- Erosion and ulceration in mucosal disease

Differential Diagnosis

- Allergy
- Drug reaction
- Parasite infection
- Inflammatory bowel disease
- Vasculitis
- Systemic mastocytosis
- Langerhans cell histiocytosis

ISCHEMIC OR HEMORRHAGIC ENTERITIS

CLINICAL FEATURES

Ischemic or hemorrhagic enteritis results from multiple causes that compromise the vascular supply of the small bowel. Depending on the clinical manifestation and onset of symptoms, intestinal ischemia is classified into acute versus chronic mesenteric ischemia. Patients with acute mesenteric ischemia present with sudden-onset abdominal pain that lasts for more than 2 to 3 hours. In contrast, chronic mesenteric ischemia ("intestinal angina") is characterized by postprandial abdominal pain and chronic weight loss caused by malabsorption. Intestinal ischemia results from occlusive or nonocclusive causes of vascular compromise. Occlusive causes include vascular thrombi, emboli, hypovolemia-induced vasoconstriction, extrinsic compression caused by tumors, adhesion, strictures, strangulation, and volvulus, among others. Patients at risk include those with a history of previous arterial emboli, vasculitis, deep vein thromboses, chronic postprandial pain, and hypercoagulable states (protein C and S deficiencies, antithrombin III deficiency, and activated protein C resistance, among others). In younger patients, use of oral contraceptives, polyarteritis nodosa, Henoch-Schönlein purpura, and other causes of systemic vasculitis can result in mesenteric ischemia.

Nonocclusive ischemic enteritis is caused by arterial hypoperfusion, often leading to spasm of the superior mesenteric artery. Patients are often critically ill with severe preexisting cardiovascular disease. Specific risks include heart failure or cardiogenic shock, septic shock, peripheral artery disease, aortic insufficiency, cardiac arrhythmias, and vasoconstrictive drugs or medications (e.g., alpha-adrenergics, digoxin, cocaine).

Ischemic enteritis has a poor prognosis, and mortality rates in large studies range from 30% to 65%. Diagnosis before intestinal infarction is the key factor to improve these poor results. Relief of persistent vasoconstriction, which is the cause of nonocclusive mesenteric ischemia and occurs in association with occlusive forms of ischemia, is another important factor.

Radiologic studies are important for diagnosis. Plain films are insensitive for ischemic enteritis but are useful to rule out other causes of abdominal pain (e.g., perforation). Abdominal computed tomography (CT) with intravenous contrast is the most widely used study with a sensitivity of 93% and specificity of 96% for the detection of acute mesenteric ischemia. If the CT scan is inconclusive, arteriography can be used, which is considered the gold-standard diagnosis.

ISCHEMIC OR HEMORRHAGIC ENTERITIS—FACT SHEET

Definition

- Injury to the bowel caused by insufficient blood flow

Prevalence

- Acute mesenteric ischemia accounts for 0.1% of all hospital admissions

Morbidity and Mortality

- High mortality for acute ischemic disease (30%–65%)

Gender, Race, and Age Distribution

- Risk factors overlap those for vascular diseases
- Age older than 50 years
- Nonocclusive ischemic enteritis associated with heart failure or cardiogenic shock, septic shock, cardiac arrhythmias, peripheral vascular disease, aortic insufficiency, and vasoconstrictive drugs or medications
- Occlusive ischemic enteritis associated with arterial emboli, vasculitis, deep vein thromboses, hypercoagulable states, stricture, volvulus, and strangulation
- Oral contraceptive use, polyarteritis nodosa, Henoch-Schönlein purpura, and other causes of systemic vasculitis in younger patients

Clinical Features

- Acute mesenteric ischemia: severe abdominal pain that persists for more than 2 or 3 hours
- Chronic mesenteric ischemia ("intestinal angina"): postprandial abdominal pain

Prognosis and Therapy

- Poor prognosis for acute ischemia (70% mortality rate)
- Treatment includes anticoagulation and efforts to revascularize the affected segment; chronic ischemia is treated by angioplasty or revascularization procedures
- When bowel wall necrosis and peritonitis have ensued, the necrotic segment must be excised as promptly as possible

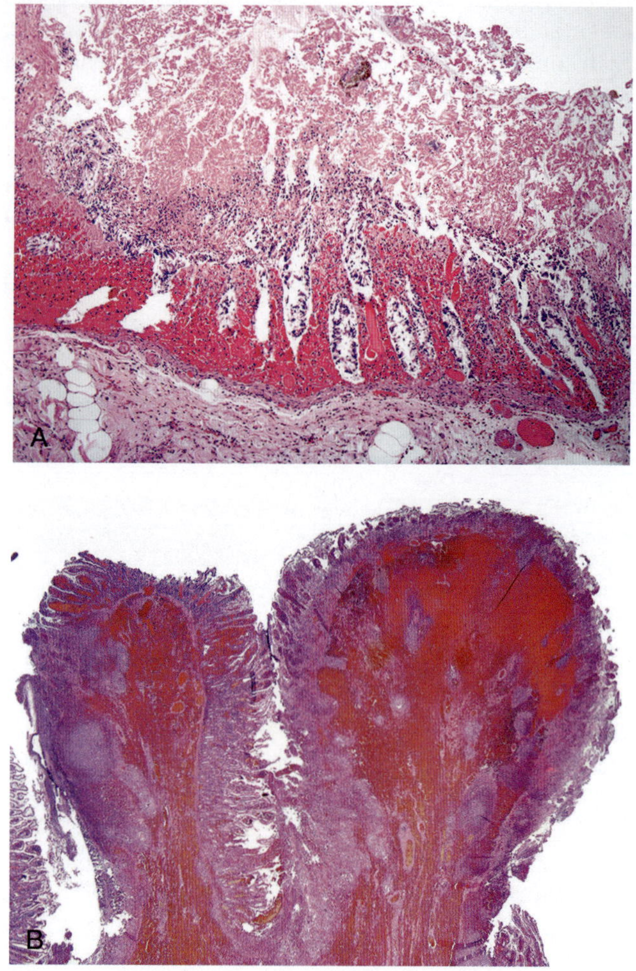

FIGURE 5.26

Ischemic or hemorrhagic enteritis. **A**, Early acute ischemia characterized by enterocyte necrosis with luminal fibrinopurulent debris *(top)* and extensive lamina propria hemorrhage. **B**, Late ischemia with extensive submucosal hemorrhage.

Pathologic Features

Gross Findings

Bowel affected by acute mesenteric ischemia appears hemorrhagic. If gangrenous changes have ensued, bowel wall may be dilated. The mucosa surface shows features of congestion, erosion, ulceration, and pseudomembrane formation. Perforation may be present in some cases. If there is pneumatosis, the segment of bowel wall may be crepitant. In long-standing cases of mesenteric ischemia, there may be evidence of stricture formation.

Microscopic Findings

In early acute ischemia, the tips of the villi appear hyperemic and show mucin loss in the surface epithelium. With progressive ischemia, there are lamina propria congestion with hyalinization and an atrophic or "withered" appearance of the residual crypts (Fig. 5.26A). Submucosa and muscularis propria are only affected in cases of severe ischemia and may appear hemorrhagic (Fig. 5.26B). Hemorrhage tends to be more pronounced in cases caused by stricture, volvulus, or strangulation. There may be prominent submucosal edema. In cases with transmural necrosis, there is often a prominent serosal fibroinflammatory response. Mesenteric blood vessels should be sampled to evaluate for possible causes. These may show evidence of vasculitis or thrombi. The presence of thrombi within a necrotic segment of bowel usually represents a secondary phenomenon and should not be considered as the cause of the ischemic episode.

In chronic ischemic enteritis, the lamina propria may show marked hyalinization. There is crypt architectural distortion with or without pyloric gland metaplasia. Neutrophilic epithelial injury is usually not seen. The bowel wall shows submucosal as well as muscular propria fibrosis. This is usually prominent in areas with stricture formation.

Ischemic or Hemorrhagic Enteritis—Pathologic Features

Gross Findings

- Acute ischemic disease: mucosal erosion, hemorrhage, ulceration, and necrosis, with or without perforation and peritonitis
- Chronic ischemia: strictures

Microscopic Findings

- Acute: mucin loss, crypt withering, lamina propria hyalinization and congestion, submucosal edema
- Chronic: architectural distortion, pyloric gland metaplasia, lamina propria hyalinization, fibrosis of the submucosa and muscularis propria

Differential Diagnosis

- Crohn's disease
- Nonsteroidal antiinflammatory drug injury

Differential Diagnosis

With features of acute ischemia (mucin loss, crypt withering lamina propria hyalinization, congestion) the differential diagnosis primarily includes a drug or medication injury. In particular, NSAIDs can produce findings that closely mimic those of ischemia. The overall clinical presentation as well as history of NSAID use is most useful in differentiating these possibilities.

With features of chronic ischemia (architectural distortion, pyloric gland metaplasia), the differential diagnosis includes IBD (typically Crohn's disease). On resected material, strictures may be seen in both diseases, but the presence of transmural inflammation away from deep ulcers, granulomas, and anal or perianal disease favors Crohn's disease over NSAID-related injury. Finally, because of the prominent lamina propria hyalinization and reactive epithelial changes, radiation enteritis is in the differential diagnosis of chronic ischemia. However, radiation injury is usually associated with either epithelial or stromal "atypia" and usually occurs only in patients who have received radiation therapy for pelvic cancers.

Prognosis and Therapy

The prognosis of acute mesenteric ischemia is poor because it is often difficult to recognize clinically. If recognized early, surgical revascularization, intraarterial perfusion with a thrombolytic agent, intraarterial infusion of vasodilators, and simple systemic anticoagulation are choices of therapy. In severe cases, surgical resection of the affected segment is the best treatment. In cases of chronic mesenteric ischemia, if a surgical revascularization is performed, success rates and recurrence rates for surgical revascularization range from 59% to 100% and 0% to 26.5%, respectively.

Infectious Enteritis

The majority of infectious agents that affect the colon can also affect the small bowel. These are addressed in Chapter 9. In particular, *Yersinia* spp., viral agents, and histoplasmosis are found in the small bowel and may mimic Crohn's disease. The most common infectious pathogens affecting the small bowel are Whipple disease and *Giardia, Cystoisospora*, and *Microsporidia* infections. In particular, Whipple disease and *M. avium-intracellulare* can expand the lamina propria and cause villous blunting without significant intraepithelial lymphocytosis.

Primary Lymphangiectasia

Clinical Features

Primary intestinal lymphangiectasia is a rare digestive disorder characterized by dilated lymphatic channels. Most patients are diagnosed before the age of 3 years and present with signs of growth retardation. GI symptoms include diarrhea, vomiting, abdominal pain, and steatorrhea. If large segments of the gut are involved, secondary edema resulting from protein-losing enteropathy and malabsorption may occur. The edema is usually generalized, but asymmetric edema is common. Lymphangiectasia also has a few characteristic radiologic and shows thickening of the bowel wall, hypodense streaks in the bowel (which represent dilated lymphatic channels), and the so-called "halo sign," which consists of distinct "rings" seen on CT scan.

Pathologic Features

Gross Findings

The mucosa show white spots or nodules, and the background mucosa may be nodular.

PRIMARY INTESTINAL LYMPHANGIECTASIA (WALDMANN'S DISEASE)—FACT SHEET

Definition

- Rare digestive disorder characterized by abnormally enlarged (dilated) lymph vessels supplying the lamina propria of the small intestine

Incidence

- Unknown

Morbidity and Mortality

- Growth retardation common
- Reduced life span
- Poor prognosis associated with delay in diagnosis

Gender, Race, and Age Distribution

- Presents in infancy
- No gender or racial predilection

Clinical Features

- Edema and nonbloody diarrhea
- Edema in primary intestinal lymphangiectasia is usually bilateral
- Secondary types often manifest as unilateral edema, which is caused by various neoplastic, infiltrative, and inflammatory lesions affecting one side of the body
- Steatorrhea, malabsorption, lymphocytopenia, and hypogammaglobulinemia
- Chylous ascites and chylous pleural effusions

Prognosis and Therapy

- The long-term course is variable
- Slow progression with intermittent clinical remissions
- Treatment includes a high-protein, low-fat diet fortified with medium-chain triglycerides; octreotides have been reported to decrease intestinal protein losses

MICROSCOPIC FINDINGS

Biopsy samples usually show multiple dilated lacteals within the tips of the villi as well as within the lamina propria. There is usually no accompanying inflammation or epithelial injury (Fig. 5.27).

PRIMARY INTESTINAL LYMPHANGIECTASIA (WALDMANN DISEASE)—PATHOLOGIC FEATURES

Gross Findings

- Numerous white spots at endoscopy

Microscopic Findings

- Many dilated lacteals with no inflammatory process

Differential Diagnosis

- Cardiac disease (congestive heart failure, constrictive cardiomyopathy)
- Local obstruction (malrotation, stricture, infection, infiltrating neoplasm, sarcoidosis, Crohn's disease, radiation therapy)

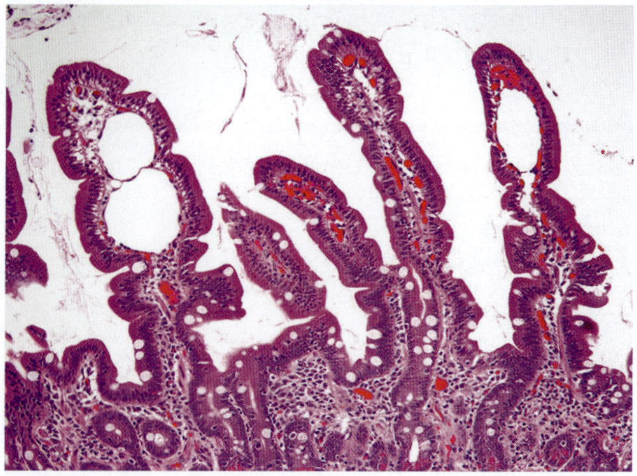

FIGURE 5.27

Primary intestinal lymphangiectasia. Duodenal biopsy shows dilated lymphatics within the villi. In the appropriate endoscopic and clinical setting, this is diagnostic of primary lymphangiectasia.

DIFFERENTIAL DIAGNOSIS

The bowel lymphatics can become dilated in other conditions resulting in "secondary lymphangiectasia." This may result from cardiac disease caused by congestive heart failure or constrictive cardiomyopathy. Alternatively, there can be a local obstruction of lymphatics caused by mechanical abnormalities (e.g., malrotation, stricture), infection (e.g., Tuberculosis), infiltrating neoplasm, sarcoidosis, or Crohn's disease or after radiation therapy. Usually, the age of the patient and overall clinical context are sufficient to distinguish between primary and secondary lymphangiectasia.

PROGNOSIS AND THERAPY

The long-term course is variable, but the disease usually shows an indolent course, with intermittent clinical remissions. The medical treatment includes high-protein, low-fat diet along with medium-chain triglycerides. Octreotides have been reported to decrease intestinal protein loss.

INCIDENTAL PIGMENTATION

Mucosal pigmentation within the small bowel may occur as an incidental finding, with no clinical significance. There are two pigments that are relatively restricted to the small intestine. The first, pseudomelanosis duodeni, as the name suggests, is typically found in the duodenum, though is occasionally detected in the stomach as well. The pigment is not melanin, nor does it have any relationship to melanocytes. In fact, the pigment is usually composed mostly of iron in combination with calcium, magnesium, aluminum, potassium, silica, and sulfur. This brown-black pigment is most commonly found within the macrophages in the tips of the villi (Fig. 5.28). An iron stain can be helpful in highlighting this pigment; however, it can be negative in about 25% of cases. Pseudomelanosis duodeni has been linked to a number of disease states, including GI bleeding, renal failure, diabetes, and hypertension as well as iron supplement intake.

The second pigment, titanium, is unique to the terminal ileum and accumulates within the Peyer's patches. This pigment is also present within macrophages and has a distinct speckled and black to brown appearance (Fig. 5.29). Titanium, specifically titanium dioxide, is a component of a number of food and hygiene products. It provides texture to food items and can be found in chocolate products and candies. It is a component of toothpaste because of its abrasive and whitening properties.

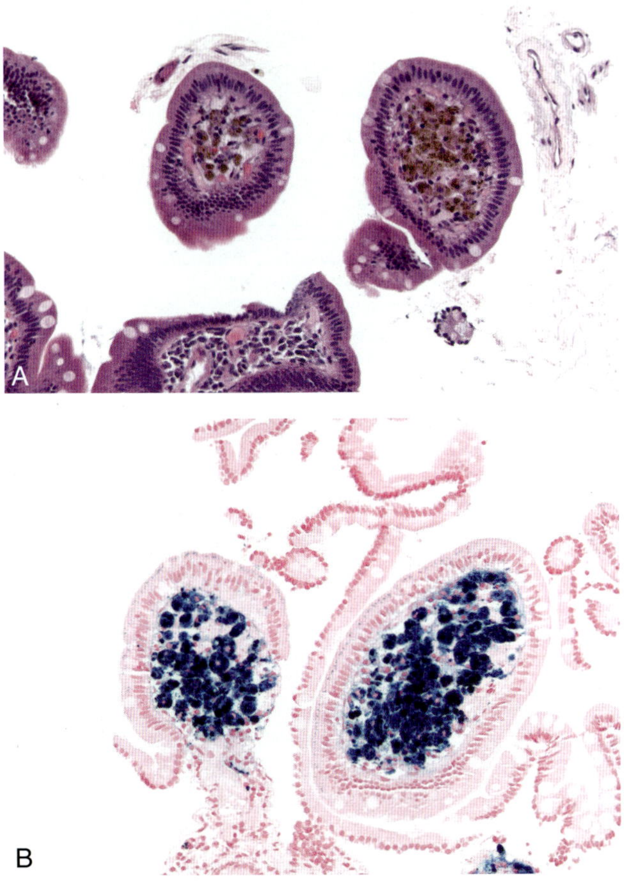

FIGURE 5.28

Pseudomelanosis duodeni. **A**, Duodenal biopsy shows brown-black pigment within macrophages that expand the lamina propria. **B**, An iron stain highlights the material in most cases.

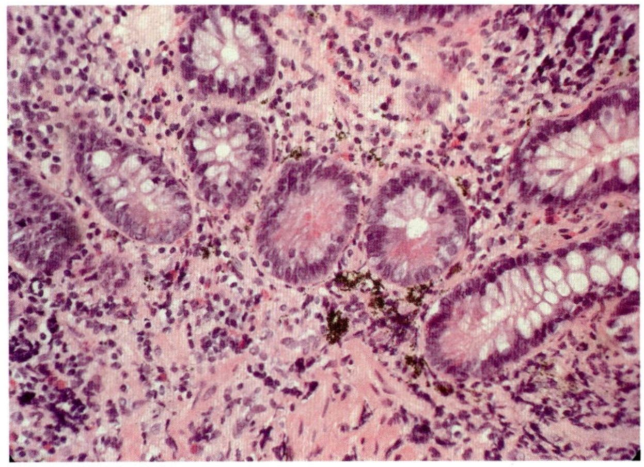

FIGURE 5.29

Titanium pigment in terminal ileum. Dark brown or black pigment within macrophages in terminal ileum Peyer's patches. This material originates from food additives.

REFERENCES

1. Patil DT, Odze RO Backwash is hogwash: The clinical significance of Ileitis in ulcerative colitis. *Am J Gastroenterol*. 2017;112(8):1211.

SUGGESTED READINGS

Nonsteroidal Antiinflammatory Drug–Associated Injury

1. Frezza M, Gorji N, Melato M. The histopathology of non-steroidal anti-inflammatory drug induced gastroduodenal damage: correlation with *Helicobacter pylori*, ulcers, and haemorrhagic events. *J Clin Pathol*. 2001;54(7):521–525.
2. Lang J, Price AB, Levi AJ, et al. Diaphragm disease: pathology of disease of the small intestine induced by non-steroidal anti-inflammatory drugs. *J Clin Pathol*. 1988;41(5):516–526.
3. Chung SH, Jo Y, Ryu SR, et al. Diaphragm disease compared with cryptogenic multifocal ulcerous stenosing enteritis. *World J Gastroenterol*. 2011;17(23):2873–2876.

Celiac Disease

4. Weir DC, Glickman JN, Roiff T, et al. Variability of histopathological changes in childhood celiac disease. *Am J Gastroenterol*. 2010;105(1):207–212.
5. Hudacko R, Kathy Zhou X, Yantiss R. Immunohistochemical stains for CD3 and CD8 do not improve detection of gluten-sensitive enteropathy in duodenal biopsies. *Mod Pathol*. 2013;26(9):1241–1245.
6. Rubio-tapia A, Hill ID, Kelly CP, et al. ACG clinical guidelines: diagnosis and management of celiac disease. *Am J Gastroenterol*. 2013;108(5):656–676.
7. Maki M, Mustalahti K, Kokkonen J, et al. Prevalence of celiac disease among children in Finland. *N Engl J Med*. 2003;348(25):2517–2524.
8. Goldstein NS, Underhill J. Morphologic features suggestive of gluten sensitivity in architecturally normal duodenal biopsy specimens. *Am J Clin Pathol*. 2001;116(1):63–71.
9. Dickey W, Hughes D. Prevalence of celiac disease and its endoscopic markers among patients having routine upper gastrointestinal endoscopy. *Am J Gastroenterol*. 1999;94(8):2182–2186.
10. Mino M, Lauwers GY. Role of lymphocytic immunophenotyping in the diagnosis of gluten-sensitive enteropathy with preserved villous architecture. *Am J Surg Pathol*. 2003;27(9):1237–1242.
11. Robert ME, Ament ME, Weinstein WM. The histologic spectrum and clinical outcome of refractory and unclassified sprue. *Am J Surg Pathol*. 2000;24(5):676–687.
12. Cellier C, Delabesse E, Helmer C, et al. Refractory sprue, coeliac disease, and enteropathy-associated T-cell lymphoma. *Lancet*. 2000;356(9225):203–208.

Tropical Sprue

13. Brown IS, Bettington A, Bettington M, et al. Tropical sprue: revisiting an underrecognized disease. *Am J Surg Pathol.* 2014;38(5):666–672.
14. Ghoshal UC, Ghoshal U, Ayyagari A, et al. Tropical sprue is associated with contamination of small bowel with aerobic bacteria and reversible prolongation of orocecal transit time. *J Gastroenterol Hepatol.* 2003;18(5):540–547.

Small Intestinal Bacterial Overgrowth

15. Reddymasu SC, McCallum RW. Small intestinal bacterial overgrowth in gastroparesis: are there any predictors? *J Clin Gastroenterol.* 2010;44(1):e8–e13.
16. Vakiani E, Arguelles-Grande C, Mansukhani MM, et al. Collagenous sprue is not always associated with dismal outcomes: a clinicopathological study of 19 patients. *Mod Pathol.* 2009;23(1):12–26.
17. Maguire AA, Greenson JK, Lauwers GY, et al. Collagenous sprue: a clinicopathologic study of 12 cases. *Am J Surg Pathol.* 2009;33(10):1440–1449.

Olmesartan-Associated Sprue-Like Enteropathy

18. Rubio-Tapia A, Herman M, Ludvigsson J, et al. severe sprue-like enteropathy associated with olmesartan. *Mayo Clin Proc.* 2012;87(8):732–738.

Common Variable Immunodeficiency

19. Jørgensen SF, Reims HM, Frydenlund D, et al. A Cross-sectional study of the prevalence of gastrointestinal symptoms and pathology in patients with common variable immunodeficiency. *Am J Gastroenterol.* 2016;111(10):1467–1475.
20. Daniels JA, Lederman HM, Maitra A, et al. Gastrointestinal tract pathology in patients with common variable immunodeficiency (CVID): a clinicopathologic study and review. *Am J Surg Pathol.* 2007;31(12):1800–1812.

Autoimmune Enteropathy

21. Masia R, Peyton S, Lauwers GY, Brown I. Gastrointestinal biopsy findings of autoimmune enteropathy: a review of 25 cases. *Am J Surg Pathol.* 2014;38(10):1319–1329.
22. Akram S, Murray JA, Pardi DS, et al. Adult autoimmune enteropathy: Mayo Clinic Rochester experience. *Clin Gastroenterol Hepatol.* 2007;5(11):1282–1290.
23. Patey-Mariaud de Serre N, Canioni D, Ganousse S, et al. Digestive histopathological presentation of IPEX syndrome. *Mod Pathol.* 2009;22(1):95–102.
24. Bacchetta R, Passerini L, Gambineri E, et al. Defective regulatory and effector T cell functions in patients with FOXP3 mutations. *J Clin Invest.* 2006;116(6):1713–1722.
25. Singhi AD, Goyal A, Davison JM, et al. Pediatric autoimmune enteropathy: an entity frequently associated with immunodeficiency disorders. *Mod Pathol.* 2014;27(4):543–553.

Congenital Enteropathies

26. Shillingford NM, Calicchio ML, Teot LA, et al. Villin immunohistochemistry is a reliable method for diagnosing microvillus inclusion disease. *Am J Surg Pathol.* 2015;39(2):245–250.
27. Martin BA, Kerner JA, Hazard FK, et al. Evaluation of intestinal biopsies for pediatric enteropathy: a proposed immunohistochemical panel approach. *Am J Surg Pathol.* 2014;38(10):1387–1395.
28. Cortina G, Smart CN, Farmer DG, et al. Enteroendocrine cell dysgenesis and malabsorption, a histopathologic and immunohistochemical characterization. *Hum Pathol.* 2007;38(4):570–580.
29. Ranganathan S, Schmitt LA, Sindhi R. Tufting enteropathy revisited: the utility of MOC31 (EpCAM) immunohistochemistry in diagnosis. *Am J Surg Pathol.* 2014;38(2):265–272.
30. Goulet O, Salomon J, Ruemmele F, et al. Intestinal epithelial dysplasia (tufting enteropathy). *Orphanet J Rare Dis.* 2007;2(1):20.
31. Sivagnanam M, Mueller JL, Lee H, et al. Identification of EpCAM as the gene for congenital tufting enteropathy. *Gastroenterology.* 2008;135(2):429–437.
32. Wetterau JR, Aggerbeck LP, Bouma ME, et al. Absence of microsomal triglyceride transfer protein in individuals with abetalipoproteinemia. *Science.* 1992;258(5084):999–1001.

Crohn's Disease

33. Oberhuber G, Puspok A, Oesterreicher C, et al. Focally enhanced gastritis: a frequent type of gastritis in patients with Crohn's disease. *Gastroenterology.* 1997;112(3):698–706.
34. Crohn BB, Ginzburg L, Oppenheimer GD. Regional ileitis a pathologic and clinical entity. *J Am Med Assoc.* 1932;99(16):1323–1329.
35. Kugathasan S, Collins N, Maresso K, et al. CARD15 gene mutations and risk for early surgery in pediatric-onset Crohn's disease. *Clin Gastroenterol Hepatol.* 2004;2(11):1003–1009.
36. Pierik M, De Hertogh G, Vermeire S, et al. Epithelioid granulomas, pattern recognition receptors, and phenotypes of Crohn's disease. *Gut.* 2005;54(2):223–227.
37. Haskell H, Andrews CW, Reddy SI, et al. Pathologic features and clinical significance of "backwash" ileitis in ulcerative colitis. *Am J Surg Pathol.* 2005;29(11):1472–1481.
38. International Study Group for Behçet's Disease. Criteria for diagnosis of Behçet's disease. International Study Group for Behçet's Disease. *Lancet.* 1990;335(8697):1078–1080.
39. Ogura Y, Bonen DK, Inohara N, et al. A frameshift mutation in NOD2 associated with susceptibility to Crohn's disease. *Nature.* 2001;411(6837):603–606.

Graft-versus-Host Disease

40. Filipovich AH, Weisdorf D, Pavletic S, et al. National Institutes of Health Consensus Development Project on criteria for clinical trials in chronic graft-versus-host disease: I. Diagnosis and staging working group report. *Biol Blood Marrow Transplant.* 2005;11(12):945–956.
41. Selbst MK, Ahrens WA, Robert ME, et al. Spectrum of histologic changes in colonic biopsies in patients treated with mycophenolate mofetil. *Mod Pathol.* 2009;22(6):737–743.
42. Levine JE, Huber E, Hammer STG, et al. Low Paneth cell numbers at onset of gastrointestinal GVHD identify patients at high risk for non-relapse mortality. *Blood.* 2013;122(8):1505–1509.
43. Shulman HM, Cardona DM, Greenson JK, et al. NIH Consensus Development Project on Criteria for Clinical Trials in Chronic Graft-versus-Host Disease: II. The 2014 Pathology Working Group Report. *Biol Blood Marrow Transplant.* 2015;21(4):589–603.
44. Star KV, Ho VT, Wang HH, et al. Histologic features in colon biopsies can discriminate mycophenolate from GVHD-induced colitis. *Am J Surg Pathol.* 2013;37(9):1319–1328.
45. Nguyen T, Park JY, Scudiere JR, et al. Mycophenolic acid (cellcept and myofortic) induced injury of the upper GI tract. *Am J Surg Pathol.* 2009;33(9):1355–1363.
46. Parfitt JR, Jayakumar S, Driman DK. Mycophenolate mofetil-related gastrointestinal mucosal injury: variable injury patterns, including graft-versus-host disease-like changes. *Am J Surg Pathol.* 2008;32(9):1367–1372.

Eosinophilic Gastroenteritis

47. Klein NC, Hargrove RL, Sleisenger MH, Jeffries GH. Eosinophilic gastroenteritis. *Medicine (Baltimore).* 1970;49(4):299–319.
48. Talley NJ, Shorter RG, Phillips SF, et al. Eosinophilic gastroenteritis: a clinicopathological study of patients with disease of the mucosa, muscle layer, and subserosal tissues. *Gut.* 1990;31:54–58.

Ischemic Enteritis

49. Acosta S, Ögren M, Sternby NH, et al. Mesenteric venous thrombosis with transmural intestinal infarction: a population-based study. *J Vasc Surg.* 2005;41(1):59–63.

Lymphangiectasia

50. Uguralp S, Mutus M, Kutlu O, et al. Primary intestinal lymphangiectasia: a rare disease in the differential diagnosis of acute abdomen. *J Pediatr Gastroenterol Nutr.* 2001;33(October):508–510.

6

Neoplasms of the Small Intestine

■ **Reetesh K. Pai, MD**

The small intestine represents 75% of the length and 90% of the surface area of the gastrointestinal (GI) tract, yet neoplasms of the small intestine are rare, accounting for only 1% to 2% of all GI neoplasms and fewer than 1% of all cancers in the United States. Four major types of primary neoplasms arise in the small intestine. They are, in order of descending frequency, adenocarcinomas, neuroendocrine tumors (NETs; "carcinoid tumors"), lymphomas, and sarcomas. The small intestine is also the most common site in the GI tract for involvement by secondary tumors, which are more than twice as common as primary small intestinal tumors. This chapter discusses hyperplasias and heterotopias of the small intestine, polyps, primary adenocarcinomas, NETs, and common secondary tumors of the small intestine. Mesenchymal tumors and lymphomas and are discussed separately in Chapters 17 and 19, respectively.

■ BRUNNER'S GLAND HYPERPLASIA AND HAMARTOMA

Clinical Features

Brunner's glands can proliferate to create small polypoid excrescences, or the gland ducts can be blocked and present as small cystic nodules. These Brunner's gland lesions are commonly encountered in the duodenal bulb usually as an incidental finding at endoscopy. However, they may also be seen as one of a constellation of findings indicative of peptic duodenitis, including villous shortening and gastric foveolar mucous cell metaplasia of the villous epithelium. The nomenclature of Brunner's gland lesions is not well established, and a number of diagnostic terms, including *Brunner's gland hyperplasia, Brunner's gland adenoma*, and *Brunner's gland hamartoma*, have been used. The distinction between these diagnoses is arbitrary; however, the term *Brunner's gland adenoma* is potentially misleading because these lesions do not display epithelial dysplasia. The term *Brunner's gland hyperplasia* is preferred to highlight the non-neoplastic nature of the entity. The distinction between Brunner's gland hyperplasia and Brunner's gland hamartoma is of no clinical significance, and a diagnosis of Brunner's gland hyperplasia and hamartoma is usually sufficient in large polypoid lesions. *Brunner's gland cyst* may be used for the rare incidental cystic lesion that shows an ectatic Brunner's gland duct lined by a benign epithelium. Rare adenocarcinomas of the small intestine may show a gastric pyloric gland–like phenotype with small tubular glands and strong MUC6 positivity, which may be mistaken for Brunner's glands. However, these patients are symptomatic and typically show large, obstructing mass lesions on endoscopy unlike the incidental small nodules characteristic of Brunner's gland hyperplasia and hamartoma.

Pathologic Features

The diagnostic criteria for Brunner's gland hyperplasia are subjective because Brunner's glands may be normally seen in the lamina propria of the duodenum, particularly within the duodenal bulb. Brunner's gland hyperplasia may manifest as solitary or multiple nodules that are typically small (<1 cm) and characterized by lobules of glands that are increased in both size and number (Fig. 6.1). The lobules extend into the mucosa and are separated by delicate fibrous septa. Cystic dilation of Brunner's gland ducts may occur, and small case series of Brunner's gland cysts have also been reported. The cells are cytologically bland with abundant neutral mucin and small, basally located nuclei with minimal to absent mitotic activity.

Differential Diagnosis

If histologic features indicative of peptic-type duodenal injury are seen, the presence of Brunner's gland hyperplasia should be attributed to peptic duodenitis. Histologic features of peptic-type duodenal injury include active inflammation within the lamina propria or epithelium, Brunner's gland hyperplasia, and

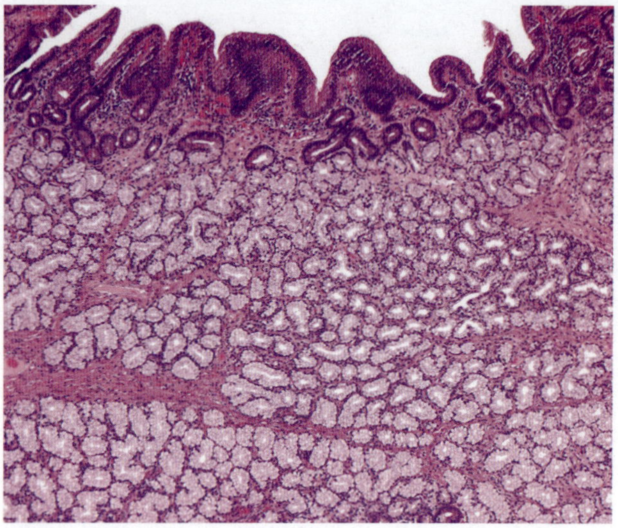

FIGURE 6.1

Brunner's gland hyperplasia: The lesion is characterized by prominent lobules of Brunner's glands within the submucosa and lamina propria.

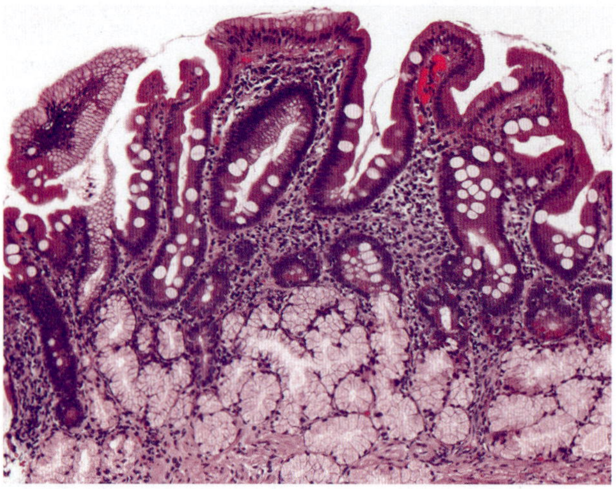

FIGURE 6.2

Peptic duodenitis: Prominent Brunner's glands within the submucosa and lamina propria associated with foveolar-type metaplasia on the villous surface of the duodenum and partial villous shortening are characteristic. In contrast to the absorptive cells of the small intestine, foveolar metaplastic cells have small apical mucin vacuoles (top left).

gastric foveolar metaplasia of the surface epithelium (Fig. 6.2).

GASTRIC HETEROTOPIA

Clinical and Endoscopic Features

Gastric heterotopias are most commonly identified in the duodenum and are usually incidental small (<1.0 cm) nodules. Gastric heterotopia may be associated with fundic gland polyps of the stomach, suggesting that the increased use of proton pump inhibitors (PPIs) in the general population may enhance its endoscopic detection. The presence of gastric foveolar metaplasia in duodenal biopsies should prompt a careful look for presence of heterotopic oxyntic glands because the increased acid secretion from these glands can also lead to metaplastic change of the surface epithelium.

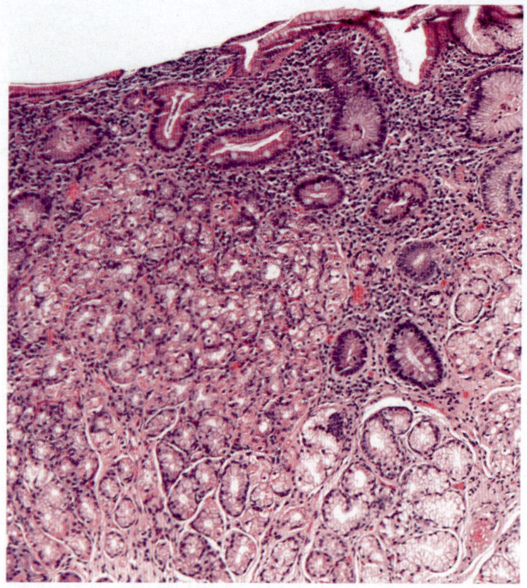

FIGURE 6.3

Gastric heterotopia: Tightly packed gastric oxyntic glands involving the duodenal mucosa. The surface epithelium also demonstrates gastric foveolar-type metaplasia.

Pathologic Features

Biopsies of gastric heterotopias display oxyntic glands composed of chief and parietal cells involving small intestinal mucosa (Fig. 6.3). Gastric foveolar-type mucin is often seen on the surface epithelium adjacent to normal intestinal villi.

Differential Diagnosis

Gastric heterotopia differs from gastric foveolar metaplasia, which is likely a metaplastic response to inflammation caused by peptic injury. Metaplastic gastric foveolar epithelium seen in the setting of peptic injury is not associated with the oxyntic glands characteristic of gastric heterotopia.

PANCREATIC HETEROTOPIA

Clinical and Endoscopic Features

Pancreatic heterotopia is synonymous with the terms *pancreatic rest* and *ectopic pancreas*. Pancreatic heterotopia of the small intestine is most commonly located in the proximal duodenum and is typically asymptomatic. Mural heterotopias may develop in the periampullary region and may be symptomatic resulting from duodenal obstruction, intussusception, and stricture or stenosis of the ampulla.

Pathologic Features

Pancreatic heterotopia is composed of pancreatic acini, ducts, or islets either alone or in combination and may be histologically indistinguishable from normal pancreas (Fig. 6.4). Most mucosa-based lesions are not associated with inflammation, and the duodenal mucosa is otherwise normal. Rare cases of ductal adenocarcinoma, mucinous neoplasms, and NETs have been reported to develop in pancreatic heterotopia.

Differential Diagnosis

Paraduodenal wall cyst ("groove pancreatitis") may be confused with mural pancreatic heterotopias because both may contain pancreatic ducts, acini, and islets. Paraduodenal wall cyst typically involves the area of the minor papilla where pancreatic tissue may be normally identified. Unlike pancreatic heterotopia, paraduodenal wall cyst shows significant inflammation and fibrosis and occurs in the so-called "groove" between the superior aspect of the pancreatic head, the common bile duct, and the duodenum. Most cases are characterized by multiple or solitary cysts varying in size from 1 to 10 cm within the duodenal wall and pancreas (Fig. 6.5). Cystically dilated ducts partially lined by ductal epithelium and containing inspissated eosinophilic material are characteristic of this entity. The adjacent stroma often shows pronounced myofibroblastic proliferation, which at times may be mistaken for a mesenchymal tumor.

PYLORIC GLAND ADENOMA

These polyps are more common in the stomach, but pyloric gland adenomas can also occur in the duodenum. They are composed of tightly packed glands lined by cuboidal epithelium with a monomorphic, monolayer of round nuclei located at the base of the glands with abundant eosinophilic to foamy cytoplasm reminiscent of pyloric-type glands (Fig. 6.6). Given their resemblance to Brunner's glands, the distinction between Brunner's gland hamartoma and hyperplasia can be difficult. However, pyloric gland adenomas often do not have overlying intestinalized epithelium when they occur in the duodenum. Furthermore, there is no lobular configuration in these lesions in contrast to Brunner's gland hamartoma and hyperplasia.

Pyloric gland adenomas exhibit dysplasia, classified as either low or high grade. Between 10% and 30% of pyloric gland adenomas are associated with invasive adenocarcinoma. Given their association with adenocarcinoma,

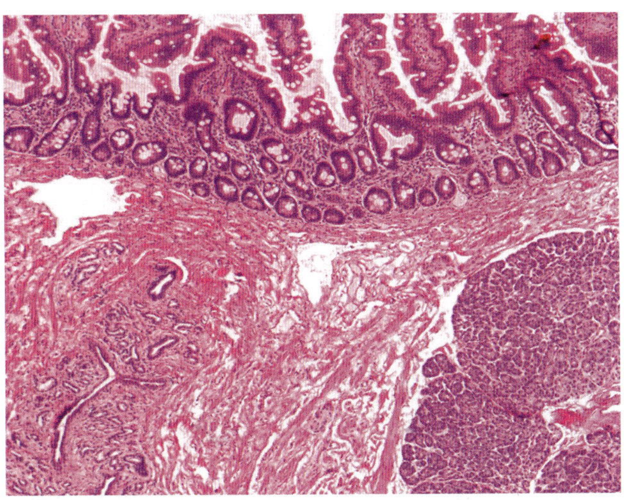

FIGURE 6.4

Pancreatic heterotopia: Lobules of ancreatic heterotopia consists of tightly packed pancreatic acini *(bottom right)* associated with pancreatic ducts *(bottom left)* located in the duodenum. In this image, the pancreatic heterotopia involves the duodenal submucosa, but it can involve any layer of the bowel wall.

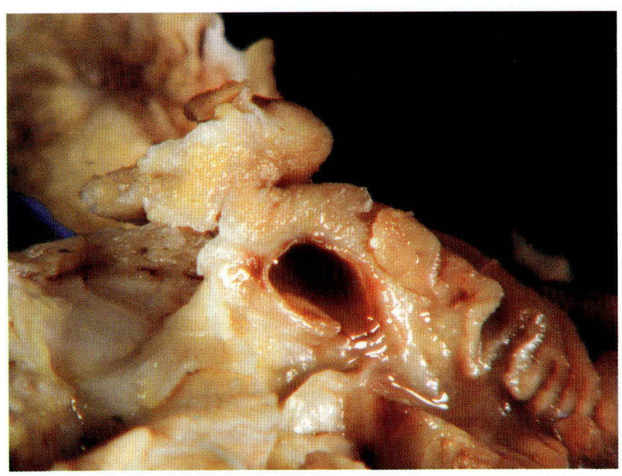

FIGURE 6.5

Solitary paraduodenal wall cyst ("groove pancreatitis") present at the minor papillae of the duodenum. This cyst was filled with proteinaceous debris and lined by fibrotic stroma with reactive myofibroblastic cells within the duodenal wall. Some cases of paraduodenal wall cyst may be characterized by multiple cysts that are partially lined by ductal-type epithelium.

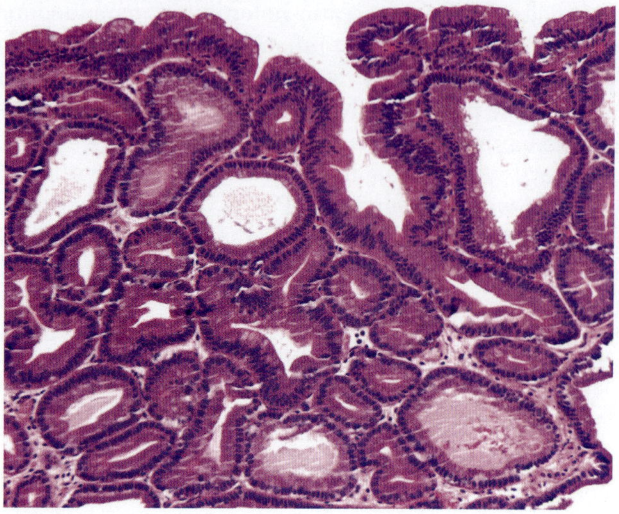

FIGURE 6.6

Pyloric gland adenoma: Tightly packed glands lined by cuboidal epithelium with basally located round nuclei. The epithelial cells have abundant eosinophilic cytoplasm with a "ground-glass" appearance and without an apical mucin cap.

complete endoscopic removal is advised for pyloric gland adenomas. Pyloric gland adenomas can also be seen as an upper GI tract manifestation of familial adenomatous polyposis (FAP), either classic or attenuated, and of Lynch syndrome.

CONVENTIONAL ADENOMA, SERRATED POLYPS, AND ADENOCARCINOMA OF THE SMALL INTESTINE

Clinical Features

Primary ("nonampullary") adenocarcinoma of the small intestine is rare, accounting for only 2 % of GI tract tumors and 1 % of all GI tract cancer deaths. They present in older adults (median age, 72 years) and with a nearly equal gender distribution. Compared with colorectal carcinoma, a higher proportion of small intestinal adenocarcinomas are seen in African Americans than in whites. Like colorectal adenocarcinomas, most small intestinal adenocarcinomas are sporadic and arise from adenomatous polyps. Serrated polyps, both hyperplastic polyps and traditional serrated adenoma-like lesions, may also occur in the duodenum, but are quite rare. Colonic sessile serrated polyp-like lesions have not been described in the duodenum.

Risk factors for sporadic small intestinal adenocarcinoma include smoking and consumption of alcohol, red meat, and fats. Increased body mass index may also be a risk factor. The remaining adenocarcinomas arise in the background of certain predisposing conditions, including polyposis syndromes, Crohn's disease, Lynch syndrome, gluten-sensitive enteropathy (GSE), and in ileostomies, and ileal conduits. FAP carries the greatest increase in risk for small intestinal adenocarcinoma (100- to 200-fold) followed by Crohn's disease and GSE, each of which increases the risk 80-fold. Other syndromes with increased risk include Lynch syndrome, Peutz-Jeghers syndrome, and juvenile polyposis syndrome.

The majority of small intestinal adenomas are located in the duodenum, and like their colonic counterparts, exhibit three major histologic types: tubular, tubulovillous, and villous (Fig. 6.7). True traditional serrated adenomas, similar to their colonic counterparts, are incredibly rare (Fig. 6.8). Most adenomas occur singly, and the presence of multiple adenomas in the small intestine is unusual in the absence of FAP, attenuated FAP, or *MUTYH*-associated polyposis. Because of their potential to undergo malignant transformation, adenomas should be removed completely. Endoscopic polypectomy is appropriate for pedunculated tumors, but large sessile lesions require endoscopic mucosal resection,

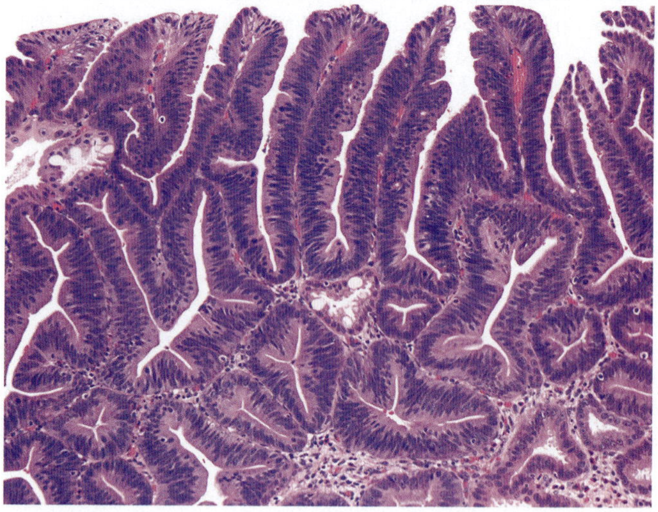

FIGURE 6.7

Duodenal adenoma with tubulovillous growth pattern and low-grade dysplasia characterized by pseudostratified, enlarged hyperchromatic nuclei. These cytologic changes extend from the crypts to involve the surface epithelium.

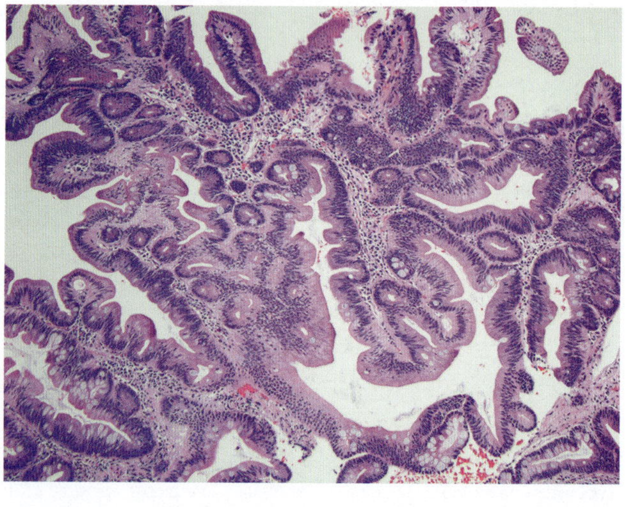

FIGURE 6.8

Traditional serrated adenoma of the small intestine is rare and poorly defined entity, unlike it's colorectal counterpart endoscopic submucosal dissection, or surgical resection. Adenocarcinomas arising sporadically and in the setting of most predisposing conditions also occur most frequently in the duodenum, where 65% are periampullary. The incidence decreases progressively through the rest of the small intestine. Adenocarcinoma arising in Crohn's disease is a notable exception to this rule. In Crohn's disease, 70% of adenocarcinomas are found in the ileum, the primary site of the inflammatory process (Fig. 6.9).

The most common presenting symptoms of small intestinal adenocarcinoma are abdominal pain, obstruction, and occult GI bleeding. Whereas patients with duodenal adenocarcinomas may present with gastric outlet obstruction, the combination of obstructive jaundice with occult GI bleeding is characteristic of ampullary tumors. More distal lesions tend to result in severe, cramping abdominal pain. Intestinal obstruction can be caused by progression of a constricting ("apple core") lesion or by a large intraluminal polypoid mass. Distal adenocarcinomas tend to present with advanced stage III or IV disease.

Duodenal lesions can typically be detected on routine endoscopy, whereas more distal lesions may require push or capsule enteroscopy, intraoperative endoscopy, or radiographic imaging modalities. Endoscopic ultrasound may be of use to assess depth of invasion and local lymph node metastasis.

Pathologic Features

Gross Findings

The macroscopic appearance depends largely on the site of the adenocarcinoma. The majority of the duodenal and ampullary tumors are small exophytic masses at the time of presentation. Distal tumors tend to be large, annular, constricting ("apple core") lesions with circumferential involvement of the bowel wall. Rarely, tumors can have a linitis plastica–like appearance. As in the colon, depth of invasion and serosal involvement must be documented.

Duodenal adenocarcinomas require additional sampling to evaluate the depth of retroperitoneal extension and involvement of the pancreas.

Microscopic Findings

Small intestinal adenocarcinomas are histologically similar to colorectal adenocarcinomas (Fig. 6.10). They are characterized by cellular pleomorphism, complex glandular architecture, luminal necrosis (so-called dirty necrosis), and invasion of the lamina propria or muscularis mucosae (intramucosal adenocarcinoma) or deeper into the bowel wall. Most adenocarcinomas are well- to moderately differentiated, and one-third are poorly differentiated. An extremely rare subset of these poorly differentiated tumors may be a manifestation of the recently described *SMARCA4* or *INI-1* deficient carcinomas, which must be excluded. Histologic grading and classification (e.g., mucinous, adenosquamous) have little bearing on prognosis, which is primarily dependent on anatomic extent, resectability, and lymph node involvement. The majority of small intestinal adenocarcinomas have invaded through the bowel wall at the time of diagnosis. Notably, intramucosal carcinomas of the small bowel are staged as T1a tumors rather than Tis. This is because of the presence of rich mucosal lymphatics that confer metastatic potential to these lesions. Residual adenomatous epithelium from a preexisting adenoma is present in the majority of proximal tumors but often cannot be demonstrated in large, distal small intestinal adenocarcinomas, presumably due to tumor

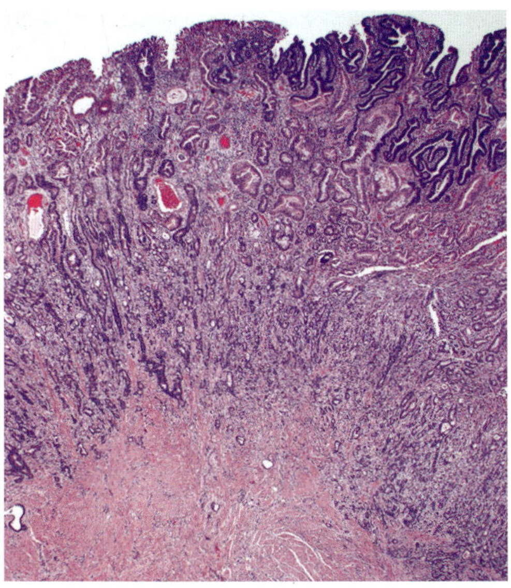

FIGURE 6.9

Adenocarcinoma of the terminal ileum in the setting of Crohn's disease. An invasive moderately differentiated adenocarcinoma invades the submucosa and muscularis propria and is present in association wtih dysplasia within the small intestinal mucosa.

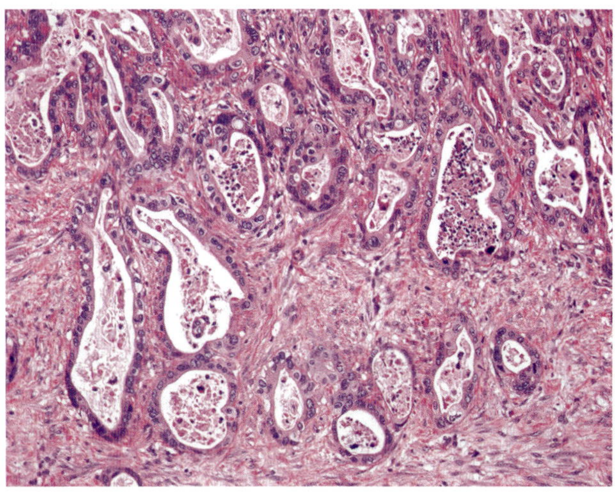

FIGURE 6.10

Adenocarcinoma of the terminal ileum in the setting of Crohn's disease. Invasive adenocarcinoma in submucosa characterized by irregular glands, luminal necrosis, and stromal desmoplasia.

overgrowth. Another subset of cases arise in a background of gastric type dysplasia, presumably likely secondary to peptic duodenitis and gastric heterotopia.

Adenocarcinoma subtypes in the small intestine are similar to those described in the colorectum (see Chapter 12) with a few exceptions: pancreatobiliary-type carcinoma and tubular adenocarcinoma have been more commonly recognized in the small intestine whereas serrated adenocarcinoma and micropapillary adenocarcinomas are more prevalent in the colorectum.

Differential Diagnosis

The main differential diagnostic consideration is metastatic carcinoma. Immunohistochemistry (IHC) can be helpful in excluding metastatic disease, specifically, metastatic adenocarcinomas (e.g., breast, lung) or other mimickers of poorly differentiated carcinoma (e.g., melanoma, lymphoma). Distinguishing small intestinal adenocarcinoma from metastatic colorectal adenocarcinoma can be challenging. It may be difficult to distinguish adenomatous precursors from colonization of the mucosa by the underlying invasive adenocarcinoma. Adenomatous epithelium can be mimicked by tumors metastatic to the GI mucosa, and a sharp transition from normal to overtly malignant epithelium should raise suspicion for secondary involvement of the mucosa (Fig. 6.11). Knowledge of clinical history in the patient, overall growth pattern (serosal predominant growth), and evidence of disseminated peritoneal disease may be helpful in establishing a diagnosis of metastatic adenocarcinoma to the small intestine. Secondary tumors of the small intestine are discussed in more detail later in this chapter.

The epithelioid variant of gastrointestinal stromal tumor (GIST) (discussed in Chapter 7) may also mimic an adenocarcinoma. In such cases, a more solid growth pattern with lack of gland formation and the relatively bland monotonous appearance of most GISTs, in combination with strong labeling for CD117 and DOG1 by IHC are helpful features. The epithelioid variant of peritoneal malignant mesothelioma may also resemble a primary adenocarcinoma. In contrast to primary small intestinal adenocarcinoma, peritoneal malignant mesothelioma diffusely involves visceral organs, forming either multiple small tumor nodules or completely encasing segments of the intestine. Notably, some epithelioid peritoneal malignant mesotheliomas may demonstrate cytoplasmic vacuolization reminiscent of gland formation and may be associated with extracellular mucoid material mimicking mucin. Most epithelioid malignant mesotheliomas demonstrate strong immunohistochemical labeling for one or more markers of mesothelial differentiation such as calretinin, D2–40, WT1, and cytokeratin 5/6 and do not express the epithelial markers BerEP4 and MOC31.

Endometriosis is a common disease that can involve the GI tract in between approximately 5% and 40% of cases. The small intestine is the second most frequently involved location after the colon. Endometriosis involving the small intestine is typically not a challenging diagnosis and is easy to recognize, given the combination of cellular endometrial stroma and endometrial glands. However, a subset of cases of endometriosis may demonstrate intestinal metaplasia and can mimic invasive adenocarcinoma. Typically, areas of conventional endometriosis will be present, and IHC for markers of endometriosis such as estrogen receptor, progesterone receptor, and CD10 can aid in the diagnosis.

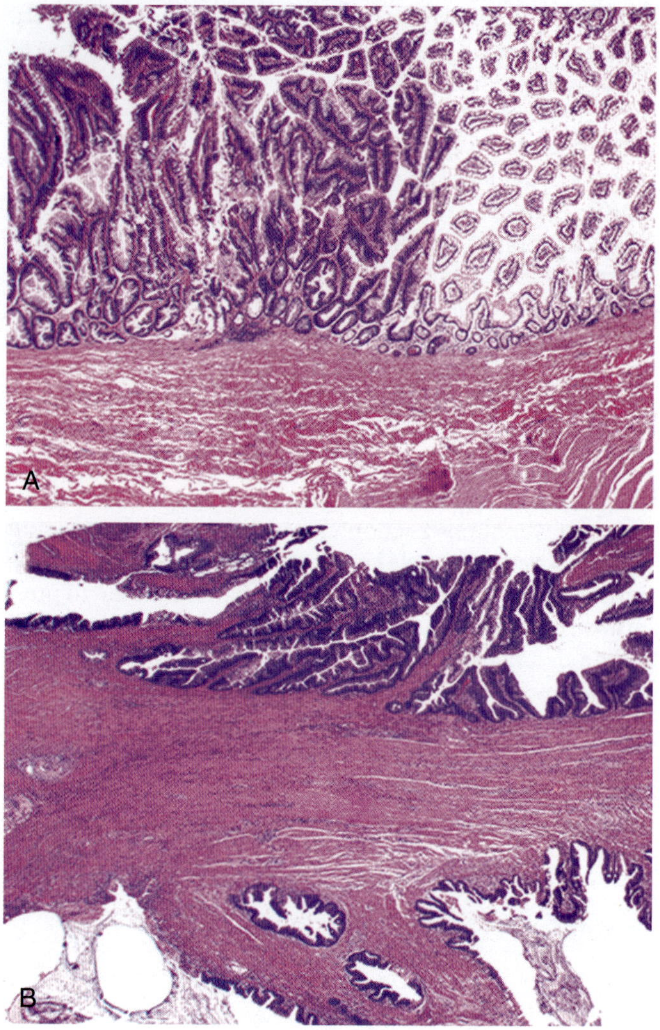

FIGURE 6.11

This patient had mucosal colonization of a segment of ileum that resembled a villous adenoma of the small intestine with a sharp transition from normal to overtly neoplastic epithelium (**A**). This patient had a known history of a primary appendiceal mucinous adenocarcinoma with evidence of disseminated peritoneal disease, numerous serosal tumor deposits, and one area of transmural invasion into the bowel wall (**B**), arguing against a primary small intestinal adenocarcinoma.

Prognosis and Therapy

Small intestinal adenomas can be resected endoscopically. Patients with FAP may have innumerable polyps in the duodenum, making endoscopic resection difficult. A

TABLE 6.1

Modified Spigelman Score[a] for Duodenal Adenomas in Patients with Familial Adenomatous Polyposis

Factor	1 Point	2 Points	3 Points
Polyp number	1–4	5–20	>20
Polyp size in millimeters	1–4	5–10	>10
Architecture	Tubular	Tubulovillous	Villous
Grade of dysplasia	Low grade (mild)	Low grade (moderate)	High grade

[a]Stage grouping: stage 0, no polyps; stage I, 1 to 4 points; stage II, 5 to 6 points; stage III, 7 to 8 points; stage IV, 9 to 12 points

Adapted from Saurin JC, Gutknecht C, Napoleon B, et al. Surveillance of duodenal adenomas in familial adenomatous polyposis reveals high cumulative risk of advanced disease. *J Clin Oncol*. 2002;22:493–498.

scoring scheme has been proposed (modified Spigelman scoring scheme) that takes into account polyp number, polyp size, polyp architecture (tubular, tubulovillous, and villous), and degree of dysplasia (low vs high) in an attempt to risk stratify patients with FAP for the development of invasive adenocarcinoma (Table 6.1). Some patients with modified Spigelman stage IV (e.g., with >20 polyps, polyps >10 mm in size, villous histology, and high-grade dysplasia) are at risk for developing adenocarcinoma and may benefit from pancreaticoduodenectomy.

Small intestinal adenocarcinomas are aggressive tumors, with a 5-year survival rate of approximately 35%. Survival is diminished in duodenal tumors and in patients older than 75 years of age. Surgery is the treatment of choice and the only modality with curative potential. Small polypoid or superficial tumors may be amenable to endoscopic polypectomy; endoscopic mucosal resection; or in the duodenum, submucosal dissection or a transduodenal resection. Larger proximal lesions may require pancreaticoduodenectomy, and distal tumors require segmental resection with accompanying mesentery. Of note, approximately 8% of small intestinal adenocarcinomas harbor deficient DNA mismatch repair, raising concern of Lynch syndrome. Thus, in the absence of known cancer-predisposing conditions such as Crohn's disease or FAP, screening of small intestinal adenocarcinomas for mismatch repair protein deficiency can be helpful in identifying patients with possible Lynch syndrome.

ADENOMA AND ADENOCARCINOMA OF THE AMPULLA OF VATER

The ampulla of Vater is the usual site for convergence of the common bile duct, main pancreatic duct (duct of Wirsung), and duodenum. The ampulla opens through the duodenal papilla and acts as a conduit for bile and pancreatic juices. This unique microenvironment may account for the disproportionate incidence of periampullary adenocarcinomas in the small intestine.

CLINICAL FEATURES

Adenocarcinoma of the ampulla of Vater is associated with adenomas in 80% to 90% of cases. The average age of presentation for ampullary adenomas is the mid-50s, whereas adenocarcinoma typically presents in the mid-60s. Adenocarcinoma is more common in whites than African Americans and more common in men than women. Ampullary adenomas and adenocarcinomas are far more likely to become symptomatic at an earlier stage than neoplasms at other locations in the small intestine. Obstruction of the ampulla frequently produces jaundice and bile duct dilation and occasionally results in pancreatitis, cholelithiasis, or choledocholithiasis. Other findings are nonspecific and include weight loss, abdominal pain, and occult bleeding. Ampullary adenomas and adenocarcinomas are visualized endoscopically or, if large enough, by radiographic imaging.

PATHOLOGIC FEATURES

GROSS FINDINGS

Sporadic ampullary adenomas (Fig. 6.12) usually present as polypoid masses, between 1 and 3 cm. Adenomas can also be located entirely intra-ampullary, in which case the gross appearance would be of a bulging ampulla

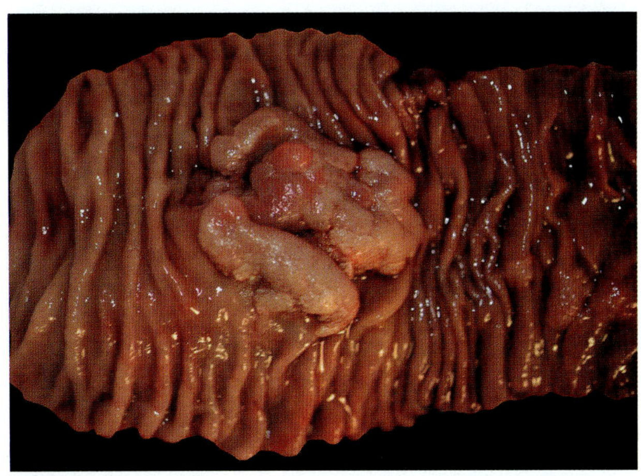

FIGURE 6.12

Ampullary adenoma: Gross evaluation of a pancreaticoduodenectomy specimen reveals an exophytic, broad-based lesion obstructing the common bile duct and resulting in dilation of the common bile duct. Adenomatous lesions are localized to the mucosa and are freely mobile on palpation. Any evidence of induration is an ominous finding and should raise suspicion for an underlying invasive adenocarcinoma.

rather than an exophytic mass. Adenocarcinomas appear as an infiltrating mass invading nearby structures.

At times, ampullary carcinomas can be difficult to distinguish from duodenal and pancreatic carcinoma. A tumor should be designated as primary to the ampulla in the following scenarios: (1) if the tumor epicenter is located in the lumen or walls of the distal ends (intra-ampullary component) of the bile duct or pancreatic duct or (2) if the epicenter is located at the junction of the duodenal and ampullary mucosa (the "papilla of Vater") and the ampullary orifice is located clearly within the tumor. Ampullary carcinoma has been further subdivided into four distinctive types primarily based on gross evaluation: (1) intra-ampullary type, defined as prominent intraluminal growth of preinvasive neoplasia in which nodules protrude into the lumen of the ampulla; (2) ampullary-ductal type, defined as infiltrative tumor centered on the walls of the distal ends of the bile duct or pancreatic duct, forming a firm, constrictive lesion; (3) periampullary duodenal type (Fig. 6.13), defined as exophytic growth on the duodenal surface of the ampulla surrounding the ampullary orifice and typically with minimal involvement of the intra-ampullary segment; and (4) ampullary, not otherwise specified (Fig. 6.14), defined as tumors of the papilla of Vater that do not show the characteristics of the other three subtypes.

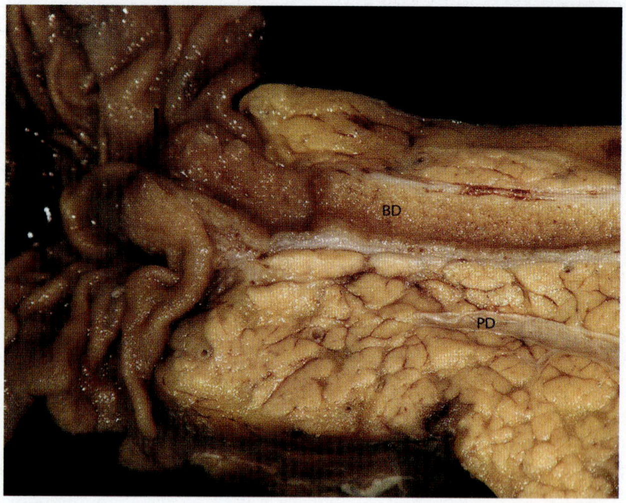

FIGURE 6.14

Gross appearance of an ampullary adenocarcinoma, not otherwise specified, with tumor centered on the papilla of Vater *(black arrow)* associated with a dilated common bile duct (BD) and pancreatic duct (PD).

Microscopic Findings

The duodenum-facing surface of the ampulla is lined by intestinal-type epithelium. The mucosa transitions to an admixture of gastric foveolar-type epithelium with intermixed goblet cells and then pancreaticobiliary-type epithelium contiguous with the common bile duct and main pancreatic duct. Most ampullary adenomas demonstrate intestinal-type epithelium similar to other intestinal adenomas. A smaller number of adenomas show a mixture of intestinal-type and pancreaticobiliary-type epithelium. Fewer than 10% of adenomas are composed entirely of pancreaticobiliary-type epithelium. These lesions resemble papillary tumors of the bile ducts and pancreas and have papillary projections with cuboidal epithelium and scant fibrous cores. They lack the abundant Paneth cells and mucin-depleted appearance of polypoid intestinal-type adenomas. The term *intra-ampullary papillary-tubular neoplasm* has also been proposed in the most recent World Health Organization classification (WHO; 2019) as a synonym for these pancreaticobiliary type ampullary lesions. By definition, the tumor should be confined almost exclusively within the ampulla with minimal extension into the main pancreatic duct, the distal common bile duct, or the duodenal papilla. In addition to typical adenomas, flat adenomas can also be seen in the ampulla.

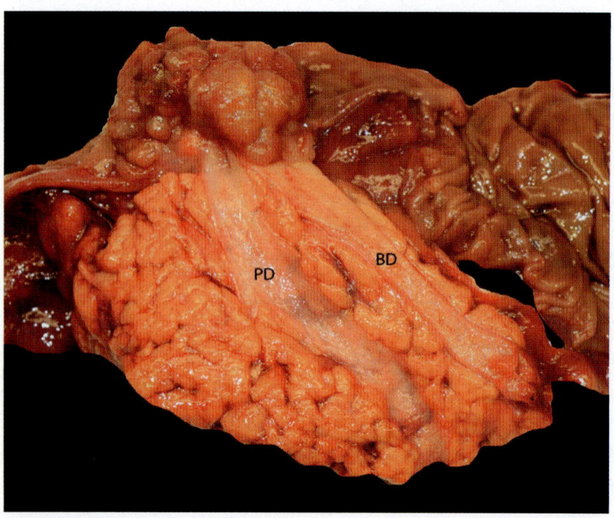

FIGURE 6.13

Gross appearance of an ampullary adenocarcinoma, periampullary duodenal type with tumor surrounding the papilla of Vater with prominent polypoid involvement of the duodenal surface of the papilla. Both the pancreatic duct (PD) and common bile duct (BD) are dilated.

Adenocarcinomas arising in the ampulla (Fig. 6.15) may be of intestinal type (Fig. 6.16) or pancreaticobiliary type (Fig. 6.17) or display hybrid histologic features. Intestinal-type adenocarcinomas of the ampulla of Vater are identical to those found elsewhere in the small and large intestines and are typically characterized by infiltrating glands lined by columnar cells with elongated, pseudostratified, hyperchromatic nuclei, often with luminal necrosis. The reported proportion of ampullary carcinomas with predominant intestinal-type morphology varies widely in the literature with a range between 30% and 70%. Pancreaticobiliary-type adenocarcinomas are very

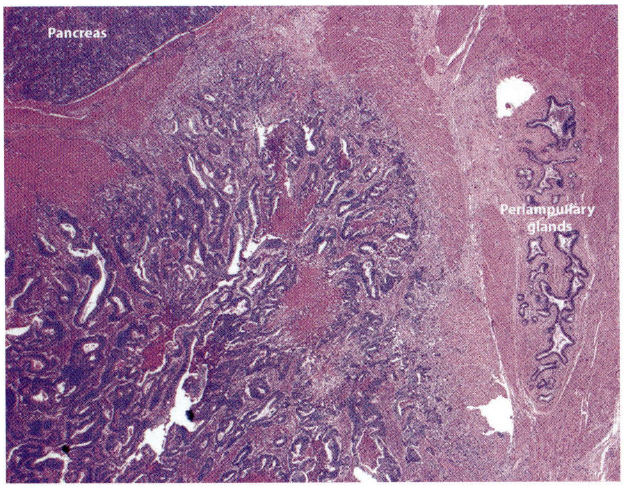

FIGURE 6.15

Ampullary adenocarcinoma invading through the muscle of the sphincter of Oddi, which contains periampullary glands. The invasive adenocarcinoma closely approaches adjacent pancreatic parenchyma.

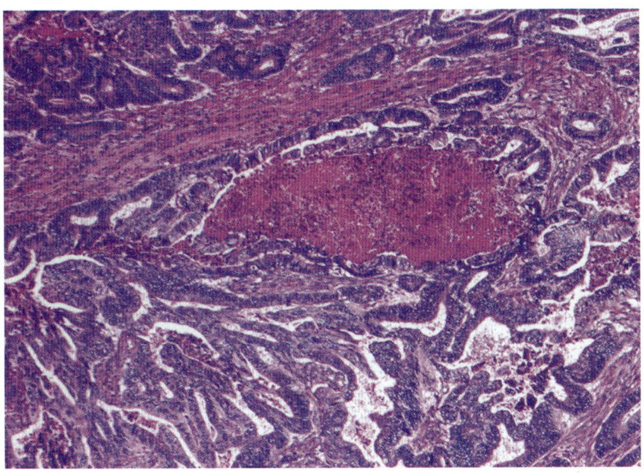

FIGURE 6.16

Ampullary adenocarcinoma, intestinal type, characterized by large glands lined by columnar cells with pseudostratified nuclei and associated with luminal necrosis.

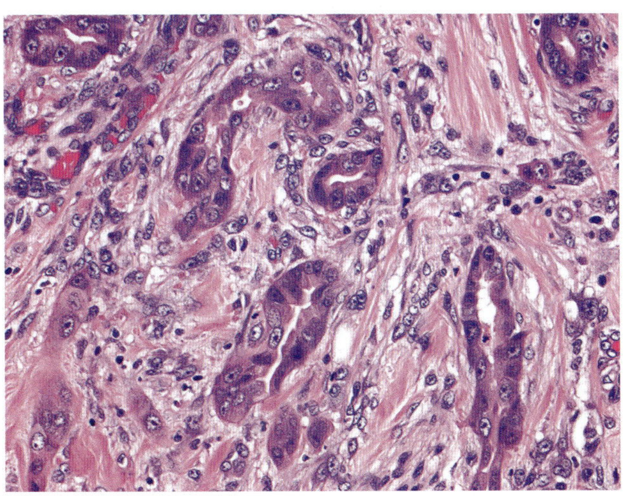

FIGURE 6.17

Ampullary adenocarcinoma, pancreaticobiliary type, characterized by small glands lined by cuboidal eosinophilic epithelium with irregular nuclear.

similar to adenocarcinomas of the pancreas and extrahepatic bile ducts and are composed of small glands lined by low cuboidal eosinophilic epithelium with high nuclear-to-cytoplasmic ratio, pleomorphic nuclei, vesicular chromatin, and irregular nuclear contours. The glands are surrounded by a prominent desmoplastic stroma, and features of intestinal adenocarcinomas, such as pseudostratification and luminal necrosis, are typically lacking. However, distinction between intestinal and pancreaticobiliary-type adenocarcinoma can be challenging with only moderate interobserver agreement noted in most studies. In addition, as many as 40 % of ampullary adenocarcinomas can display a hybrid intestinal and pancreaticobiliary morphology.

Immunohistochemistry using a panel of CDX2, MUC1, MUC2, and CK20 has been advocated to help subtype adenocarcinomas of the ampulla (Table 6.2). In general, intestinal-type adenocarcinoma is positive for CDX2, CK20, and MUC2 and negative for MUC1. Pancreaticobiliary-type adenocarcinomas are positive for MUC1 and negative for CDX2 and MUC2. However, IHC does not always allow for definitive subtyping, and a mixed or ambiguous immunophenotype is quite common. Other types of ampullary adenocarcinomas (e.g., mucinous, signet ring cell, medullary, adenosquamous, undifferentiated carcinoma) have also been described but are infrequent. Similarly, tumors with a rhabdoid phenotype with SMARCA4 or INI-1 loss are also rarely seen in the small intestine, either as primary or as metastasis from another site.

TABLE 6.2

Immunohistochemistry in the Subtyping of Adenocarcinoma of the Ampulla of Vater[a]

Immunohistochemical Subtype	Immunohistochemical Staining Pattern for CK20, CDX2, MUC2, and MUC1
Intestinal	1. Positive for CK20 or CDX2 or MUC2 and negative for MUC1 2. Positive for CK20, CDX2, and MUC2, irrespective of MUC1 staining pattern
Pancreaticobiliary	Positive for MUC1 AND negative for CDX2 and MUC2, irrespective of CK20 staining pattern
Ambiguous	Other combinations of phenotypes, including negative for all stains

[a]Positive staining is defined as more than 25% of tumor staining.
As advocated by Ang DC, Shia J, Tang LH, et al. The utility of immunohistochemistry in subtyping adenocarcinoma of the ampulla of Vater. *Am J Surg Pathol*. 2014;38:1371–1379.

Differential Diagnosis

Pancreaticobiliary neoplasms arising in the common bile duct or pancreas can colonize the ampullary epithelium or, if invasive, may directly involve the ampulla and be misdiagnosed as an ampullary adenoma or adenocarcinoma. Careful gross examination and review of clinical and imaging information are necessary when assigning the correct primary site to periampullary tumors. Metastasis from distant sites to the ampulla of Vater is rare but has been reported.

When adenomatous epithelium extends into periampullary glands in the smooth muscle of the sphincter of Oddi, care must be exercised to not misdiagnose the adenoma as an invasive carcinoma. Lack of a desmoplastic response and a clear continuity with low-grade dysplastic ductal epithelium supports a noninvasive diagnosis.

Prognosis and Therapy

Pedunculated ampullary adenomas without high-grade dysplasia can be resected endoscopically. Adenomas that are large or demonstrate high-grade dysplasia may be managed by transduodenal ampullectomy or pancreaticoduodenectomy.

Pancreaticoduodenectomy is the standard of care for resectable ampullary adenocarcinomas. Most studies have demonstrated that patients with intestinal-type ampullary adenocarcinomas have better overall survival than those with pancreaticobiliary-type ampullary adenocarcinoma, although not all studies have demonstrated that histologic subtype is an independent predictor of survival. At present, chemotherapeutic decision making is influenced by the histologic subtype of ampullary adenocarcinoma. Oncologists often use gemcitabine-based treatment regimens for pancreaticobiliary-type adenocarcinomas and fluorouracil-based treatment regimens for intestinal-type adenocarcinoma. Given the importance of histologic subtyping in selecting therapy, an attempt should be made to determine the predominant or favored histologic subtype for ampullary adenocarcinoma whether by using routine histology or by using one of the proposed immunohistochemical panels as detailed in Table 6.2. However, separation into histologic subtypes is not always possible, and an adenocarcinoma with hybrid histologic features should be classified as such.

NEUROENDOCRINE TUMORS OF THE SMALL INTESTINE

Neuroendocrine tumors of the small intestine represent approximately one-third of small intestinal neoplasms and 2% of all GI tumors. Small intestinal NETs are derived from two separate embryonic divisions of the alimentary tract: the foregut (duodenum) and the midgut (jejunum and ileum). Most NETs are encountered in the ileum (midgut). Duodenal NETs can be associated with clinical syndromes caused by hormone hypersecretion detected by serologic evaluation for elevated circulating hormones. Immunohistochemical staining for peptide hormones can be performed to confirm the clinical impression of a syndromic NET. However, specific functional terms such as *gastrinoma* should not be used to describe NETs in the absence of clinical and serologic findings indicative of a hormonal syndrome. Although the functional status of a NET is defined by the clinical and serologic findings, it is useful to divide NETs into categories based on location in the small intestine and corresponding cell subtype because it allows for discussion of site-related differences between NETs.

Clinical Features

Gastrin-producing NETs account for approximately two-thirds of NETs in the duodenum. Gastrin-producing NETs can be either nonfunctioning or associated with Zollinger-Ellison syndrome (ZES), a syndrome of hypergastrinemia, gastrin hypersecretion, and refractory peptic ulcer disease. The association with ZES is found in about 40% of duodenal gastrin-producing NET. Most ZES NETs are sporadic with approximately 25% associated with multiple endocrine neoplasia type 1 (MEN-1) (Fig. 6.18). Nonfunctional gastrin-producing NETs typically occur in the duodenal bulb and are normally confined to the lamina propria and submucosa. They are incidentally discovered during

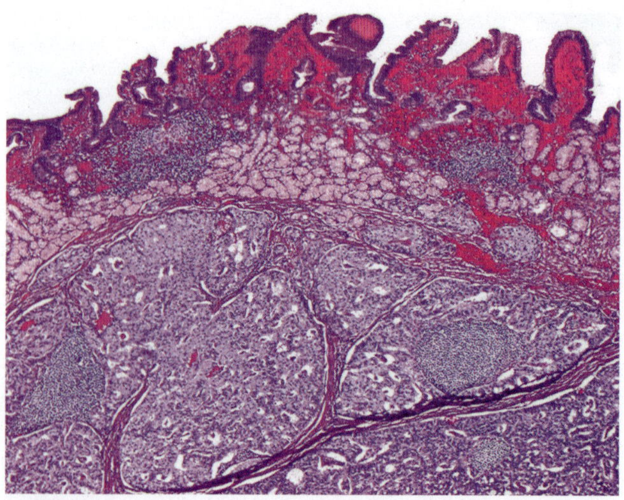

FIGURE 6.18
Well-differentiated neuroendocrine tumor of the duodenum located primarily in the duodenal submucosa. This neuroendocrine tumor was associated with elevated serum gastrin and Zollinger-Ellison syndrome.

endoscopy performed for other reasons or in surgical resections for unrelated causes. Nonfunctioning gastrin-positive NETs of the duodenum are frequently associated with *Helicobacter pylori* infection of the stomach or long-term PPI therapy.

Somatostatin-producing NETs account for approximately one-third of NETs in the duodenum and have a predilection for the ampulla and periampullary region, which can result in symptoms and signs of abdominal pain, obstructive jaundice, and biliary dilatation. The somatostatinoma syndrome consisting of diabetes mellitus (caused by inhibition of insulin secretion), steatorrhea (caused by inhibition of pancreatic enzyme secretion), hypochlorhydria or achlorhydria, and cholelithiasis (caused by suppression of cholecystokinin-pancreozymin release and gallbladder contraction) is rarely observed in duodenal somatostatin-producing NETs. One-third of somatostatin-producing ampullary or periampullary NETs have been associated with von Recklinghausen's disease (neurofibromatosis type 1 [NF1]).

The ileum is the single most common site for NETs in the GI tract. These tumors also elicit peritumoral or mesenteric fibrosis that may produce symptoms of recurrent small bowel obstruction, bowel ischemia and infarction, and protracted abdominal pain. NETs of the distal jejunum and ileum are serotonin-producing enterochromaffin cells and may produce the carcinoid syndrome that consists of watery diarrhea, flushing, and endocardial fibrosis. The carcinoid syndrome is usually, but not always, associated with metastasis to the liver and is seen in 5% to 7% of cases. Nearly one-third of patients diagnosed with a jejunoileal NET have a synchronous or metachronous carcinoma (e.g., colon, stomach, lung, or breast). Small (<1 cm) ileal NETs can give rise to large mesenteric tumor deposits and present as an occult primary.

PATHOLOGIC FEATURES

Neuroendocrine tumors are characterized by a monotonous proliferation of small bland polygonal cells with a moderate amount of cytoplasm and round regular nuclei with the typical "salt-and-pepper" chromatin (Fig. 6.19). NETs demonstrate variable architectural growth patterns, including insular or nested, trabecular, and acinar growth patterns. These patterns often overlap, and multiple patterns may be seen within any single tumor. Somatostatin-producing ampullary or periampullary NETs have characteristic morphologic features that help to distinguish these tumors from other NETs of the duodenum. Approximately 60% of somatostatin-producing NETs display a characteristic mixed pseudoglandular (Fig. 6.20) and trabecular architectural arrangement. The pseudoglandular structures have central lumens that frequently contain proteinaceous secretions and psammoma bodies (Fig. 6.21). Psammoma bodies are

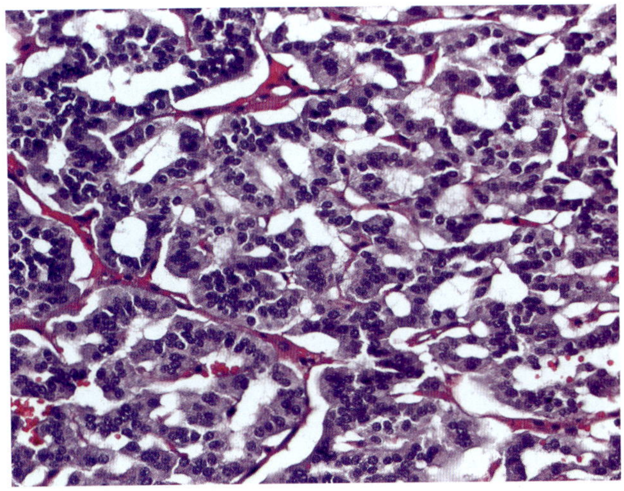

FIGURE 6.19

Well-differentiated neuroendocrine tumor of the duodenum characterized by cytologically bland tumor cells with bland, round nuclei, "salt-and-pepper" chromatin, and eosinophilic cytoplasm.

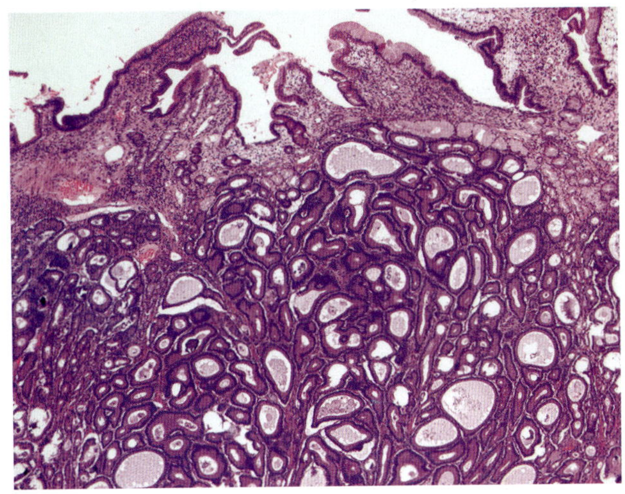

FIGURE 6.20

Periampullary somatostatin-producing well-differentiated neuroendocrine tumor with prominent pseudoglandular growth pattern involving the mucosa and submucosa of the periampullary duodenal mucosa.

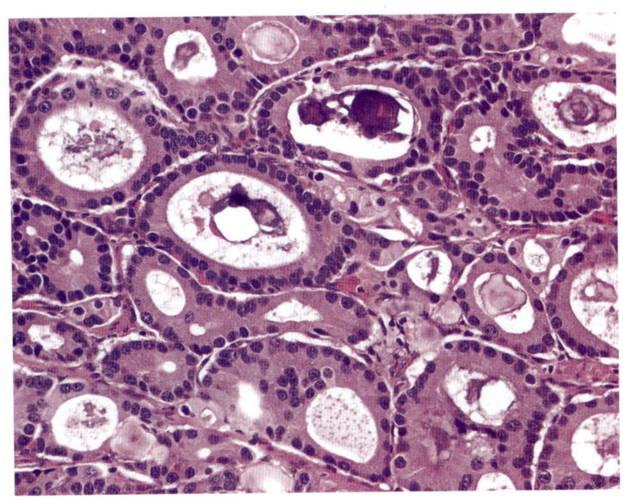

FIGURE 6.21

Periampullary somatostatin-producing well-differentiated neuroendocrine tumor with numerous intraluminal psammomatous calcifications.

seen in approximately 60% of sporadic somatostatin-producing ampullary and periampullary NETs and in almost all of NF1-associated somatostatin-producing NETs. However, psammoma bodies are not entirely specific for somatostatin-producing NETs and may also be seen in nonfunctioning NETs in the ileum or other sites within the GI tract.

Jejunoileal NETs may have a variable gross appearance, ranging from the presence of polypoid tan-yellow submucosal nodules to annular masses or strictures secondary to marked fibrosis characteristic of these lesions. One-quarter of tumors may present as multiple polypoid lesions (Fig. 6.22). Typically, the tumor cells are arranged in solid nests (Fig. 6.23) and are often associated with densely fibrotic stroma that may compress the tumor cells into a single-file and cordlike arrangement. Most tumors demonstrate perineural and lymphovascular invasion.

TABLE 6.3

World Health Organization (WHO) 2019 Grading of Neuroendocrine Tumors[a]

WHO Grade	Mitotic Count	Ki67 Index
G1	<2 per 2 mm^2	<3%
G2	2–20 per 2 mm^2	3%–20%
G3	>20 per 2 mm^2	>20%

[a]The grading requires mitotic count in at least 50 hpf (1 hpf = 2 mm^2) and Ki67 index using the MIB antibody as a percentage of 500 to 2000 cells counted in areas of strongest nuclear labeling ("hot spots"). If grade differs for mitotic count and Ki67 index, the higher grade should be assigned.
hpf, High-power field.

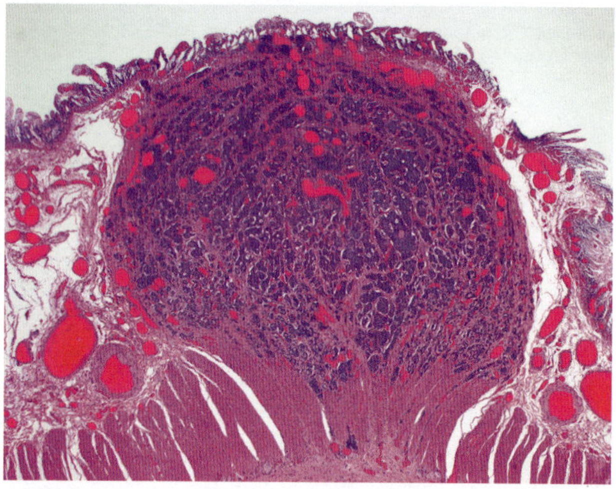

FIGURE 6.22

Well-differentiated neuroendocrine tumor involving the submucosa and muscularis propria of the ileum. Multiple polypoid lesions were identified in the small intestine of this patient, and the overlying ileal mucosa demonstrated necrosis resulting from mesenteric ischemia.

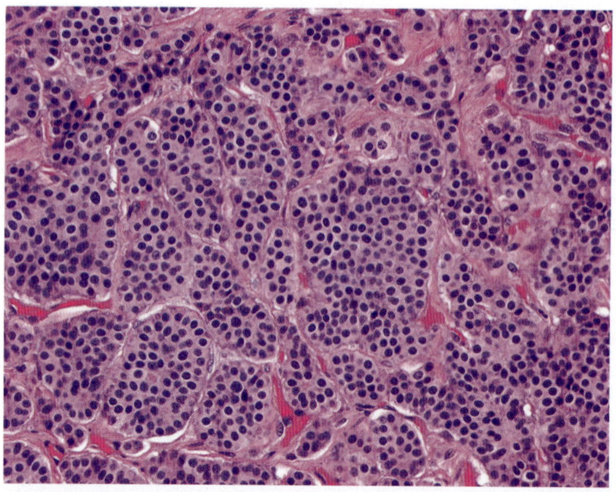

FIGURE 6.23

Well-differentiated neuroendocrine tumor of the ileum with a nested growth pattern. The tumor is composed of cells with bland, round nuclei, "salt-and-pepper" chromatin, and eosinophilic cytoplasm.

The WHO recommends grading NETs by the assessment of mitotic activity and Ki67 proliferation index (see Table 6.3). Well-differentiated NETs are defined by a nested, trabecular or tubular architecture and express markers of neuroendocrine differentiation such as chromogranin A and synaptophysin. The mitotic activity and proliferative index in well-differentiated tumors is typically low and encompasses WHO grade G1 (<2 mitoses per 2 mm^2 and <3% Ki67 index) and G2 (2–20 mitoses per 2 mm^2 and/or 3%–20% Ki67 index) (see Table 6.2). Rarely, tumors that are architecturally well differentiated may show high proliferative activity and qualify as WHO grade 3 (>20 mitosis per 2 mm^2 and/or >20% Ki67 index). In these cases, the Ki67 proliferation index is usually in the 30% to 50% range unlike typical high-grade neuroendocrine carcinomas, which more often show positive labeling in more than 75% of nuclei.

By IHC, small intestinal NETs express synaptophysin and chromogranin A. Jejunoileal NETs are typically strongly positive for CDX2. However, jejunoileal NETs are negative for PAX8, which may help to localize the primary site of a NET in the setting of metastatic disease to the liver with an unknown primary. Duodenal NETs infrequently label with CDX2 but may express PAX8 and PDX-1 by IHC. The adjacent duodenal mucosa can demonstrate gastrin-positive neuroendocrine hyperplasia in MEN1-associated gastrinomas and in sporadic nonfunctional gastrin-producing NETs associated with *H. pylori* gastritis and long-term PPI therapy. Although immunohistochemical stains are available for specific hormone products such as gastrin and somatostatin, functioning tumors are those associated with clinical manifestations of hormone production or secretion of measurable amounts of active hormone. Immunohistochemical expression of hormone does not correlate with clinical functionality and therefore is not recommended in daily practice.

Differential Diagnosis

Neuroendocrine tumors with a prominent acinar pattern may mimic adenocarcinoma. In such cases, the bland, monotonous appearance of the NET and the strong labeling for neuroendocrine markers are helpful features. The single-cell, linear growth pattern seen at the periphery of NETs may be confused with metastatic lesions such as lobular breast cancer. A nested pattern reminiscent of NETs can be mimicked by lamina propria and lymphatic invasion by melanoma, lymphoma, or other poorly differentiated carcinomas. The nuclear features are high grade in these latter instances, and when metastatic disease is a concern, IHC can easily provide a definitive answer.

Prognosis and Therapy

The overall behavior of NETs is difficult to predict but is dictated primarily by the stage of disease. Duodenal nonfunctioning gastrin-positive NETs of the duodenal bulb are generally indolent. In contrast, somatostatinoma-producing and ZES-associated NETs may behave in a clinically malignant fashion. Poor outcome in duodenal tumors is best predicted by invasion beyond the submucosa or by lymph node and distant metastases. Rarely, a gastrin-producing NET will be identified in lymph nodes in the pancreaticoduodenal region without a definite primary NET seen in the duodenum or pancreas. These so-called "primary lymph node gastrinomas" represent metastases, in most instances, from microscopic primary duodenal or pancreatic NETs that are easily overlooked on routine examination. However, rare patients who have done well clinically on follow up after resection of the nodal primary have also been described.

Because of their relatively small size and submucosal location, jejunoileal NETs are rarely diagnosed until the development of metastatic disease to lymph nodes or distant sites, particularly the liver. Jejunoileal NETs have a worse prognosis than those of the duodenum, with a 21% mortality rate. Survival is negatively correlated with tumor grade, distant metastases, multiple tumors, invasion beyond submucosa, and female gender. Patients with jejunoileal NETs should be treated with segmental resection of the bowel and associated mesentery. Even in those with metastatic disease, resection may be required for palliation to relieve obstruction.

GANGLIOCYTIC PARAGANGLIOMA

Clinical Features

Gangliocytic paragangliomas have a predilection for the ampulla or periampullary region and typically present as polypoid submucosal nodules. Some patients may present

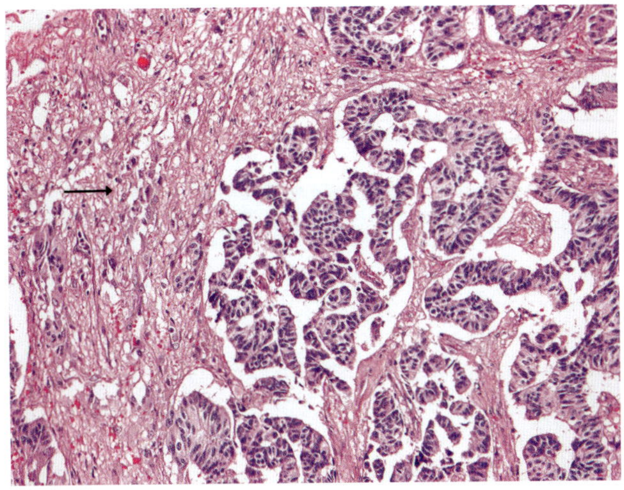

FIGURE 6.24

Gangliocytic paraganglioma of the periampullary duodenum. The neuroendocrine epithelioid cells are arranged in trabeculae and are set within spindled stromal cells with eosinophilic cytoplasm. Occasional ganglion-like cells *(black arrow)* are seen within the spindled stroma.

with GI bleeding caused by mucosal erosion or with obstructive jaundice. Gangliocytic paragangliomas may present as multiple lesions and may be associated with NF1.

Pathologic Features

Gangliocytic paragangliomas are composed of a variable mixture of (1) nests of uniform polygonal neuroendocrine cells, (2) ganglion-like cells, and (3) spindle cells with Schwannian differentiation arranged in fascicles (Fig. 6.24). The neuroendocrine cell population typically stains for both chromogranin A and synaptophysin. The spindle cells stain intensely for S100 and neurofilament protein. The ganglion cells may be seen dispersed singly or form small clusters and are positive for synaptophysin.

Prognosis and Therapy

Gangliocytic paragangliomas usually follow a benign course. However, there are reports of gangliocytic paragangliomas with metastasis to regional lymph nodes, particularly in large tumors (>2 cm). Most frequently, the metastatic tumor in lymph nodes consists of the neuroendocrine component of the tumor.

NEUROENDOCRINE CARCINOMA OF THE SMALL INTESTINE AND AMPULLA

Clinical Features

Within the small intestine, neuroendocrine carcinomas appear to more often occur in the ampulla or periampullary area. If the tumor contains a significant component (≥30%) of neuroendocrine carcinoma and adenocarcinoma, the term *mixed neuroendocrine–non-neuroendocrine neoplasm (MiNEN)* should be used.

Pathologic Features

Neuroendocrine carcinomas are poorly differentiated and composed of either small cells (small cell type) or intermediate to large cells (large cell type) with expression of markers of neuroendocrine differentiation, typically diffuse expression of synaptophysin and focal staining for chromogranin A. Neuroendocrine carcinomas also demonstrate a high mitotic rate (>20 per 2 mm^2) and greater than 20% Ki67 index, corresponding to WHO grade G3. These tumors should not be confused with the extremely rare examples of well-differentiated tumors that resemble typical carcinoids on morphology but show a high proliferative index that qualifies as grade 3. In well-differentiated grade 3 tumors, the proliferative index is usually in the 30% to 60% range and not extremely high as in typical small and large cell neuroendocrine carcinomas. The use of the diagnostic term *high-grade neuroendocrine carcinoma* is, therefore, discouraged because it can apply to both categories of grade 3 tumors with different genotypic abnormalities, treatment implications, and prognoses. Preliminary data suggest that well-differentiated grade 3 NETs have a better prognosis than poorly differentiated (small or large cell) grade 3 carcinomas but do not respond to platinum-based chemotherapy. The pathologic diagnosis in all NETs should clearly state the differentiation status (well or poor) and provide the WHO grade based on mitotic activity and/or Ki-67 immunostain to help guide therapy for these patients. Small cell neuroendocrine carcinoma tumor cells are typically less than three times the size of a small lymphocyte and are arranged in large sheets with areas of necrosis (Fig. 6.25). The nuclei display finely granular chromatin and inconspicuous nucleoli, and nuclear molding may be prominent. Large cell neuroendocrine carcinoma architecturally displays an organoid or trabecular architecture and may mimic a well-differentiated NET, but the tumor cells have large, vesicular nuclei; prominent nucleoli; and moderate amounts of cytoplasm. Both small cell and large cell neuroendocrine carcinoma can be associated with adenomas of the overlying surface epithelium.

Prognosis and Therapy

Neuroendocrine carcinomas are clinically aggressive, and patients typically present with advanced disease. The overall prognosis is dismal.

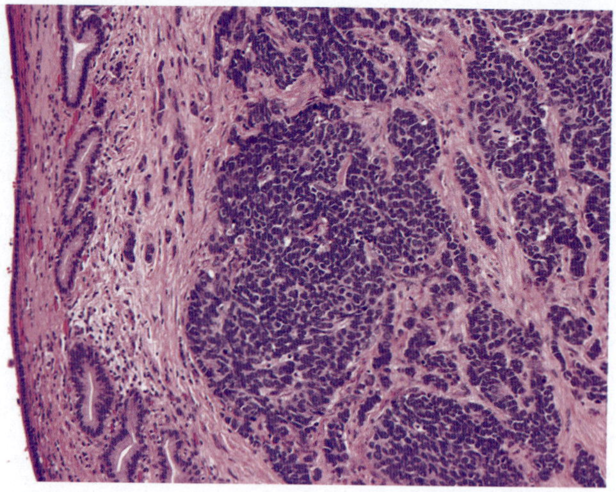

FIGURE 6.25

Poorly differentiated neuroendocrine carcinoma, small cell type, of the ampulla undermining ampullary mucosa. The tumor cells are arranged in large sheets with nuclear molding and scant cytoplasm. Numerous mitotic figures and a Ki67 index greater than 80% were identified. The tumor cells demonstrated strong, diffuse synaptophysin expression and focal chromogranin staining, confirming neuroendocrine differentiation.

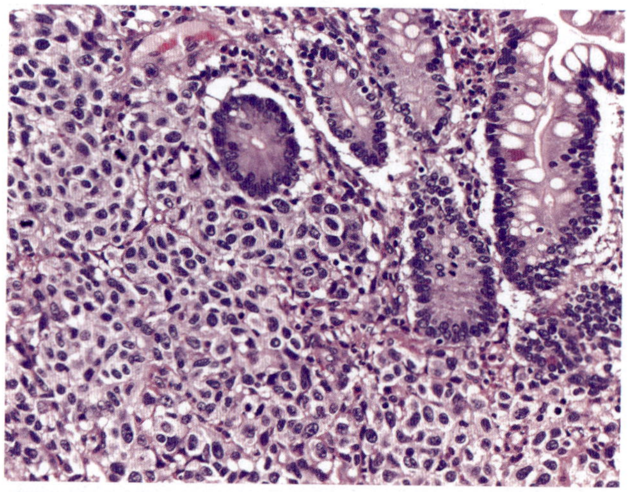

FIGURE 6.26

Metastatic melanoma to the small intestine can morphologically resemble a neuroendocrine tumor. This case demonstrates a nested growth pattern. Immunohistochemistry for markers of melanocytic differentiation (SOX10, S-100, Melan A, and/or HMB45) are helpful in confirming the diagnosis.

SECONDARY TUMORS

Secondary tumors are 2.5 times more common than primary small intestinal neoplasms. Involvement of the small intestine by secondary tumors can occur by direct extension, intraperitoneal spread, or lymphohematogenous metastasis. Virtually any type of malignancy may secondarily involve the small intestine. Melanoma (Fig. 6.26), breast, colon, and lung carcinoma are among the most common metastatic tumors involving the small intestine. Pancreatic and gastric carcinomas may also involve the small intestine by direct extension, whereas ovarian cancer is the mostly likely to involve the small intestine by serosal implantation. Secondary involvement of the small intestine may present as a thickened bowel wall or mass lesion with obstruction, intussusception, or perforation. Features favoring a metastatic tumor include the presence of multiple lesions, extensive mural and serosal disease with minimal mucosal involvement imparting a histologic appearance of tumor being "bottom heavy" or encroaching from serosal aspect to mucosal aspect of the bowel wall, and the absence of a dysplastic precursor. Small intestinal adenocarcinomas are of an intestinal type, and the presence of signet ring cell differentiation or a diffuse-type growth pattern is uncommon in primary carcinomas of the small intestine, especially in areas distal to the ampulla or in tumors unrelated to Crohn's disease. Frequently, metastatic adenocarcinoma to the small intestine can demonstrate maturation of the neoplastic epithelium as it grows from the serosa toward the bowel lumen. Metastatic carcinoma can also reach the mucosal surface of the small intestine and exhibit an in situ growth pattern along intact basement membranes, simulating a "precursor" dysplastic lesion (adenoma). Thus, the presence of an apparent "in situ" dysplastic lesion does not provide definitive evidence for a primary small intestinal carcinoma.

Immunohistochemistry should be used when the nature of the primary neoplasm is in doubt and is especially helpful in cases of poorly differentiated malignancies. Immunohistochemical stains are particularly helpful when considering metastasis from non-GI tract primary sites, such as the lung (often positive for thyroid transcription factor 1), breast (positive for GATA-3, gross cystic disease fluid protein [GCDFP] and variably positive for estrogen receptor [ER] and progesterone receptor [PR]), and ovary (often positive for ER, PR, and PAX8). However, IHC is not helpful in distinguishing primary small intestinal adenocarcinoma from metastatic GI tract adenocarcinomas. Primary small intestinal adenocarcinomas often demonstrate a CK7-positive/CK20-negative or CK7-positive/CK20-positive immunophenotype. However, colorectal adenocarcinomas, particularly those with high levels of microsatellite instability, can coexpress CK7 and CK20, limiting the utility of CK7 and CK20 IHC in this setting.

One of the most common malignancies to metastasize to the small intestine is malignant melanoma. Metastatic melanomas to the GI tract can be either pigmented or amelanotic and may mimic a variety of primary neoplasms, including carcinomas, sarcomas or GISTs, and large cell lymphoma. Immunohistochemical stains (S-100, HMB-45, A103 [MART-1], tyrosinase, microphthalmia transcription factor, and SOX10) have been shown to demonstrate high sensitivity and variable specificity for melanoma. Importantly, when evaluating high-grade spindle cell lesions for which GIST is in the differential diagnosis, one or more of melanoma stains should be included in the panel because up to 50% of malignant melanomas express CD117.

SMALL INTESTINAL ADENOCARCINOMA—FACT SHEET

Definition

- Primary malignant epithelial tumor of the small intestine

Incidence and Location

- Most common malignancy of the small intestine (30%–50% of small bowel malignancies)
- Overall rare lesions, 2% of gastrointestinal (GI) tumors, and 1% of GI cancer–related deaths

Gender, Race, and Age Distribution

- Presents in older adults (median, 72 years)
- Nearly equal gender distribution
- Compared with colorectal carcinoma, a higher proportion seen in African Americans than whites

Clinical Features

- Vast majority of cases are sporadic
- Similar to colorectal adenocarcinomas in risk factors and development from sporadic adenomatous polyps
- Minority arise in the background of predisposing hereditary or acquired risk factors: familial adenomatous polyposis, Crohn's disease, gluten-sensitive enteropathy, Lynch syndrome
- Combination of obstructive jaundice with occult GI bleeding characteristic of duodenal tumors
- 30% of patients present with stage IV disease

Prognosis and Therapy

- Poor outcome in all locations
- 5-year disease-free survival rate is approximately 35%

SMALL INTESTINAL ADENOCARCINOMA—PATHOLOGIC FEATURES

Gross Findings

- Duodenum (most in the periampullary region) > jejunum (first 30 cm) > ileum (Crohn's disease)
- Duodenal tumors: smaller exophytic masses
- Jejunoileal tumors: large, annular, constricting masses with circumferential bowel wall involvement
- Rarely, tumors can have a linitis plastica appearance
- Sampling background mucosa to assess for adenoma is important

Microscopic Findings

- Similar to colorectal adenocarcinomas and characterized by complex glandular architecture, luminal necrosis, and nuclear pleomorphism
- Most are moderately differentiated, and one-third are poorly differentiated
- Degree of differentiation and special histologic subsets (e.g., mucinous, adenosquamous) have little bearing on prognosis.
- The majority of small bowel adenocarcinomas have invaded through the bowel wall
- Preexisting adenoma is present in the majority of proximal tumors but often cannot be demonstrated in large distal tumors

Immunohistochemistry

- Immunohistochemistry is primarily used to exclude metastatic disease, specifically, metastatic adenocarcinoma (e.g., breast, lung) and other mimickers of poorly differentiated tumor (melanoma and lymphoma)

- Variable CK7 positivity (ranging from 30% to 60%), CK20 positivity (~60%) and CDX2 positivity (~70%)
- Distinguishing between primary small intestinal adenocarcinoma and metastatic colorectal adenocarcinoma can be very difficult

Differential Diagnosis

- Metastatic adenocarcinomas (e.g., colorectal, breast, ovary, lung)
- Poorly differentiated malignancies (e.g., lymphoma, melanoma)
- Epithelioid gastrointestinal stromal tumor
- Peritoneal malignant mesothelioma with epithelioid histology
- Endometriosis

AMPULLARY ADENOCARCINOMA—FACT SHEET

Definition

- Malignant epithelial tumor of the ampulla of Vater defined as
- Tumor epicenter in the lumen or walls of the very distal ends of the bile duct and/or pancreatic duct
- Tumor epicenter located at the junction of the duodenal and ampullary mucosa (the "papilla of Vater") with the ampullary orifice located within the tumor

Incidence and Location

- Rare lesions, 0.2% to 0.5% of gastrointestinal (GI) tumors and approximately 0.2% of GI cancer–related deaths

Gender, Race, and Age Distribution

- Presents in older adults (median, 65 years)
- Male predominance (male to female ratio, 1.5 to 1)

Clinical Features

- Vast majority of cases are sporadic
- Minority arise in the background of predisposing condition, such as familial adenomatous polyposis
- Common symptoms and signs: obstructive jaundice, occult GI bleeding, abdominal pain
- Many patients present with regional disease (stages I and II)

Prognosis and Therapy

- Pancreaticoduodenectomy for resectable tumors
- 5-year disease-free survival rate is approximately 40%
- Intestinal type has a better prognosis than pancreaticobiliary type
- Chemotherapy decision making is often affected by histologic subtype

AMPULLARY ADENOCARCINOMA—PATHOLOGIC FEATURES

Gross Findings

- Distinct types based primarily on gross appearance
- Intra-ampullary: prominent intraluminal growth of preinvasive neoplasia protruding into the lumen of the ampulla
- Ampullary ductal: firm, constrictive lesion within the walls of the very distal ends of the common bile duct or pancreatic duct
- Periampullary duodenal: exophytic growth on the duodenal surface of the ampulla surrounding the ampullary orifice
- Ampullary, not otherwise specified: tumors that do not show the characteristics of the other three subtypes
- Sampling background mucosa to assess for precursor neoplasia is important

Microscopic Findings

- Intestinal type characterized by large glands lined by columnar cells with elongated, pseudostratified hyperchromatic nuclei
- The pancreaticobiliary type arises either from intra-ampullary tubular and papillary neoplasms or from ampullary ductal neoplasia and are characterized by small glands lined by low cuboidal eosinophilic epithelium with high nuclear-to-cytoplasmic ratio; rounded, vesicular nuclei; and irregular nuclear contours
- Many adenocarcinomas have mixed intestinal and pancreaticobiliary histology
- The degree of differentiation and special histologic subsets (e.g., mucinous, adenosquamous) have little bearing on prognosis

Immunohistochemistry

- The intestinal type is usually positive for CK20, MUC2, and CDX2 and typically negative for MUC1 (see Table 6.2)
- The pancreaticobiliary type is usually positive for MUC1 and typically negative for CDX2 and MUC2
- Ambiguous or hybrid phenotypes are commonly seen, making definitive distinction between intestinal and pancreaticobiliary types difficult in some cases

Differential Diagnosis

- Ampullary adenoma involving periampullary glands in the smooth muscle of the sphincter of Oddi can mimic adenocarcinoma
- Distinction from duodenal, pancreatic ductal, and distal common bile duct adenocarcinoma requires careful gross evaluation to determine the tumor epicenter

NEUROENDOCRINE TUMORS OF THE SMALL INTESTINE—FACT SHEET

Definition

- Well-differentiated neuroendocrine neoplasm composed of cells with features similar to those of normal gut endocrine cells and expressing general markers of neuroendocrine differentiation (synaptophysin and chromogranin A)
- Encompasses neoplasms previously termed *carcinoid tumor*

Incidence and Location

- Represent 30% of small intestinal neoplasms and 40% of gastrointestinal neuroendocrine tumors (NETs)
- Seen primarily with roughly equal incidence in the duodenum and ileum

Gender, Race, and Age Distribution

- Median age of approximately 60 years
- Duodenal tumors more common in men (male-to-female ratio, 1.5 to 1), but no gender predilection is seen in jejunoileal tumors

Clinical Features

Duodenum

- Two-thirds of NETs of the duodenum are gastrin producing
- Approximately 40% of gastrin-producing NETs are functional and associated with Zollinger-Ellison syndrome (ZES; hypergastrinemia, gastric hypersecretion, refractory peptic ulcer disease). Twenty-five percent of ZES-associated gastrin-producing NETs are associated with multiple endocrine neoplasia type 1
- Approximately 60% of gastrin-producing NETs are nonfunctional, typically located in the duodenal bulb, smaller than 1 cm in size, and associated with *Helicobacter* infection or long-term proton pump inhibitor therapy

- One-third of NETs of the duodenum are somatostatin producing.
- Predilection for the ampullary and periampullary region
- Abdominal pain, obstructive jaundice, and biliary dilation are commonly seen
- One-third are associated with neurofibromatosis type 1
- Rarely functional

Jejunoileal

- Abdominal pain, bowel obstruction from fibrosis or intussusception, mesenteric ischemia
- Approximately 5% to 7% are associated with carcinoid syndrome (watery diarrhea, flushing, endocardial fibrosis)
- Often have metastasis to the liver and lymph nodes

Prognosis and Therapy

- Features associated with behavior, including World Health Organization grade (based on mitotic count and Ki67 index), size, extent of invasion, and lymph node involvement
- Duodenal nonfunctioning gastrin-producing NETs of the duodenal bulb are generally indolent
- Somatostatin-producing and ZES-associated NETs of the duodenum may behave in a malignant fashion
- Jejunoileal NETs have a worse prognosis than those of the duodenum and are treated by resection of the involved segment and small bowel mesentery

NEUROENDOCRINE TUMORS OF THE SMALL INTESTINE—PATHOLOGIC FEATURES

Gross Findings

Duodenum

- Nonfunctional gastrin-producing duodenal neuroendocrine tumors (NETs) located in the duodenal bulb
- Functional gastrin-producing NETs found in all parts of the duodenum
- Somatostatin-producing NETs have a predilection for the ampulla and periampullary region
- Submucosal-based lesions with an overlying mucosa that may be focally ulcerated
- Multicentricity of tumors is seen in 15% of cases

Jejunoileal

- Primarily located in the distal 60 cm of the ileum and less commonly the jejunum
- Multicentricity of tumors seen in 30% of cases
- Frequently locally advanced disease with mural, lymph node, and mesenteric involvement
- Submucosal-based lesions with an overlying mucosa that may be focally ulcerated

Microscopic Findings

- Monotonous proliferation of small bland polygonal cells with moderate amount of cytoplasm and round regular nuclei with "salt-and-pepper" chromatin
- Variable architectural growth patterns: nested, trabecular, acinar
- Multiple architectural growth patterns typically seen within a single tumor
- Typically poorly circumscribed and submucosal based with some mucosal extension
- Somatostatin-producing NETs often have a prominent pseudoglandular growth pattern with frequent intraluminal psammoma bodies
- Jejunoileal NETs and gastrin-producing NETs have variable histology and often a prominent nested growth pattern with more trabecular and acinar growth peripherally
- Jejunoileal NETs often invade deeply into the wall and can be associated with significant fibrosis

Immunohistochemistry

- Vast majority positive for synaptophysin and chromogranin
- CDX2 is positive in jejunoileal NETs but can be negative in duodenal NETs
- Immunohistochemical expression of peptide hormones (e.g., gastrin and somatostatin) can be performed but has limited utility because the functional status of tumors does not correlate with immunohistochemistry

Differential Diagnosis

- Somatostatin-producing NETs can superficially resemble adenocarcinoma because of a pseudoglandular growth pattern
- Other metastatic lesions (e.g., melanoma or lobular breast cancer) that can have a nested and trabecular growth pattern resembling NET

SUGGESTED READINGS

Hyperplasias and Heterotopias

Patel ND, Levy AD, Mehrotra AK, et al. Brunner's gland hyperplasia and hamartoma: imaging features with clinicopathologic correlation. *AJR Am J Roentgenol*. 2006;187:715–722.

Triadafilopoulos G. Clinical and pathologic features of the nodular duodenum. *Am J Gastroenterol*. 1993;88:1058–1064.

Genta RM, Kinsey RS, Singhal A, et al. Gastric foveolar metaplasia and gastric heterotopia in the duodenum: no evidence of an etiologic role for Helicobacter pylori. *Hum Pathol*. 2010;41:1593–1600.

Distler M, Rückert F, Aust D, et al. Pancreatic heterotopia of the duodenum: anatomic anomaly or clinical challenge? *J Gastrointest Surg*. 2011;15:631–636.

Pyloric Gland Adenoma

Chen Z-M, Scudiere JR, Abraham SC, Montgomery E. Pyloric gland adenoma: an entity distinct from gastric foveolar type adenoma. *Am J Surg Pathol*. 2009;33:186–193.

Wood LD, Salaria SN, Cruise MW, et al. Upper GI tract lesions in familial adenomatous polyposis (FAP): enrichment of pyloric gland adenomas and other gastric and duodenal neoplasms. *Am J Surg Pathol*. 2014;38:389–393.

Lee SE, Kang SY, Cho J, et al. Pyloric gland adenoma in Lynch syndrome. *Am J Surg Pathol*. 2014;38:784–792.

Conventional Adenoma and Adenocarcinoma of the Small Intestine

Arber N, Moshkowitz M. Small bowel polyposis syndromes. *Curr Gastroenterol Rep*. 2011;13:435–441.

Spigelman AD, Williams CB, Talbot IC, et al. Upper gastrointestinal cancer in patients with familial adenomatous polyposis. *Lancet*. 1989;2:783–785.

Chang H-K, Yu E, Kim J, et al. Adenocarcinoma of the small intestine: a multi-institutional study of 197 surgically resected cases. *Hum Pathol*. 2010;41:1087–1096.

Jun S, Kim M, Gu M, et al. Clinicopathologic and prognostic associations of KRAS and BRAF mutations in small intestinal adenocarcinoma. *Mod Pathol*. 2016;29:402–415.

Young JI, Mongoue-Tchokote S, Wieghard N, et al. Treatment and survival of small bowel adenocarcinoma in the United States: a comparison with colon cancer. *Dis Colon Rectum*. 2016;59:306–315.

Qubaiah O, Devesa SS, Platz CE, et al. Small intestinal cancer: a population based study of incidence and survival patterns in the

United States, 1992 to 2006. *Cancer Epidemiol Biomarkers Prev.* 2010;19:1908–1918.

Overman MJ, Pozadzides J, Kopetz S, et al. Immunophenotype and molecular characterization of adenocarcinoma of the small intestine. *Br J Cancer.* 2010;102:144–150.

Saurin JC, Gutknecht C, Napoleon B, et al. Surveillance of duodenal adenomas in familial adenomatous polyposis reveals high cumulative risk of advanced disease. *J Clin Oncol.* 2002;22:493–498.

Adenoma and Adenocarcinoma of the Ampulla

Klimstra DS, Albores-Saavedra J, Hruban RH, et al. Tumors of the *ampullary region: adenomas and other premalignant neoplastic conditions. In: WHO Classification of tumors of the digestive system.* 4th ed., *World Health Organization Classification of Tumors.* International Agency for Research on Cancer; 2010:83–86.

Adsay V, Ohike N, Tajiri T, et al. Ampullary region carcinomas: definition and site specific classification with delineation of four clinicopathologically and prognostically distinct subsets in an analysis of 249 cases. *Am J Surg Pathol.* 2012;36:1592–1608.

Reid MD, Balci S, Ohike N, et al. Ampullary carcinoma is often of mixed or hybrid histologic type: an analysis of reproducibility and clinical relevance of classification as pancreaticobiliary versus intestinal in 232 cases. *Mod Pathol.* 2016;29(12):1575–1585.

Ang DC, Shia J, Tang LH, et al. The utility of immunohistochemistry in subtyping adenocarcinoma of the ampulla of Vater. *Am J Surg Pathol.* 2014;38:1371–1379.

Chang DK, Jamieson NB, Johns AL, et al. Histomolecular phenotypes and outcome in adenocarcinoma of the ampulla of Vater. *J Clin Oncol.* 2013;31:1348–1356.

Albores-Saavedra J, Schwartz AM, Batich K, et al. Cancers of the ampulla of Vater: demographics, morphology, and survival based on 5,625 cases from the SEER program. *J Surg Oncol.* 2009;100:598–605.

Ohike N, Kim GE, Tajiri T, et al. Intra-ampullary papillary-tubular neoplasm (IAPN): characterization of tumoral intraepithelial neoplasia occurring within the ampulla: a clinicopathologic analysis of 82 cases. *Am J Surg Pathol.* 2010;34:1731–1748.

Neuroendocrine Tumor of the Small Intestine and Ampulla

WHO Classification of Tumours: Digestive Systems Tumours. International Agency for Research on Cancer; 2019:16-19. 5th ed.

Mocellin S, Nitti D. Gastrointestinal carcinoid: epidemiological and survival evidence from a large population based study (n = 25,531). *Ann Oncol.* 2013;24:3040–3044.

Randle RW, Ahmed S, Newman NA, et al. Clinical outcomes for neuroendocrine tumors of the duodenum and ampulla of Vater: a population-based study. *J Gastrointest Surg.* 2014;18:354–362.

Klöppel G, Rindi G, Anlauf M, et al. Site-specific biology and pathology of gastroenteropancreatic neuroendocrine tumors. *Virchows Arch.* 2007;451(suppl 1):S9–S27.

Merchant SH, VanderJagt T, Lathrop S, et al. Sporadic duodenal bulb gastrin-cell tumors: association with *Helicobacter pylori* gastritis and long-term use of proton pump inhibitors. *Am J Surg Pathol.* 2006;30:1581–1587.

Garbrecht N, Anlauf M, Schmitt A, et al. Somatostatin-producing neuroendocrine tumors of the duodenum and pancreas: incidence, types, biological behavior, association with inherited syndromes, and functional activity. *Endocr Relat Cancer.* 2008;15:229–241.

Scheithauer BW, Nora FE, LeChago J, et al. Duodenal gangliocytic paraganglioma. Clinicopathologic and immunocytochemical study of 11 cases. *Am J Clin Pathol.* 1986;86:559–565.

Sundararajan V, Robinson-Smith TM, Lowy AM. Duodenal gangliocytic paraganglioma with lymph node metastasis: a case report and review of the literature. *Arch Pathol Lab Med.* 2003;127:e139–e141.

Burke AP, Thomas RM, Elsayed AM, et al. Carcinoids of the jejunum and ileum: an immunohistochemical and clinicopathologic study of 167 cases. *Cancer.* 1997;79:1086–1093.

Yantiss RK, Odze RD, Farraye FA, et al. Solitary versus multiple carcinoid tumors of the ileum: a clinical and pathologic review of 68 cases. *Am J Surg Pathol.* 2003;27:811–817.

Saqi A, Alexis D, Remotti F, et al. Usefulness of CDX2 and TTF-1 in differentiating gastrointestinal from pulmonary carcinoids. *Am J Clin Pathol.* 2005;123:394–404.

Neuroendocrine Carcinoma of the Small Intestine and Ampulla

Albores-Saavedra J, Hart A, Chablé-Montero F, et al. Carcinoids and high-grade neuroendocrine carcinomas of the ampulla of Vater: a comparative analysis of 139 cases from the surveillance, epidemiology, and end results program—a population based study. *Arch Pathol Lab Med.* 2010;134:1692–1696.

Nassar H, Albores-Saavedra J, Klimstra DS. High-grade neuroendocrine carcinoma of the ampulla of Vater: a clinicopathologic and immunohistochemical analysis of 14 cases. *Am J Surg Pathol.* 2005;29:588–594.

Secondary Tumors of the Small Intestine

Washington K, McDonagh D. Secondary tumors of the gastrointestinal tract: surgical pathologic findings and comparison with autopsy survey. *Mod Pathol.* 1995;8:427–433.

Estrella JS, Wu T-T, Rashid A, et al. Mucosal colonization by metastatic carcinoma in the gastrointestinal tract: a potential mimic of primary neoplasia. *Am J Surg Pathol.* 2011;35:563–572.

7

Gastrointestinal Mesenchymal Tumors

David Papke, MD, PhD and Leona Doyle, MD

GASTROINTESTINAL STROMAL TUMOR

Gastrointestinal stromal tumors (GISTs) are the most common soft tissue tumors of the gastrointestinal (GI) tract, with a worldwide annual incidence of about 15 cases per million. Although there was historic controversy over the distinction between GIST, smooth muscle tumors, and nerve sheath tumors, by the late 1990s, it was established that GISTs exhibit differentiation of interstitial cells of Cajal and represent a distinct diagnostic entity. We now know that most GISTs harbor mutually exclusive mutations in *KIT* (80%) or platelet-derived growth factor receptor-α *(PDGFRA)* (~7%). The remaining 10% to 15% of so-called "wild-type GISTs" are a heterogeneous group of tumors that includes succinate dehydrogenase (SDH)–deficient GIST (accounting for 8% of GISTs), as well as neurofibromatosis-associated and *BRAF*-mutant GIST (Table 7.1). Correct subclassification is critical for determining the prognosis and appropriate treatment.

Clinical Features

In the United States, GIST has an estimated annual incidence of 3300 to 6000 cases per year and most commonly occurs in middle-aged to older adults (median age, 60 years). Clinically detected tumors in the GI tract most commonly occur in the stomach (60%) and small intestine (35%), with most remaining cases accounted for by colorectal tumors; GISTs of the esophagus and appendix are rare. GIST can also present as omental, peritoneal, and retroperitoneal tumors, although these are typically large tumors that very likely originally originated in the GI tract but may have detached from their point of origin. GIST exhibits a wide range of behavior, from benign "micro-GISTs," present in approximately 30% of the population based on autopsy series, to aggressive sarcomas. Prognosis depends in part on tumor location; for example, small intestinal GISTs are about twice as likely as gastric GISTs to behave in a clinically aggressive fashion.

Clinical presentation depends on tumor size and location. Large masses can cause abdominal pain, anemia, or GI bleeding. Micro-GISTs are found incidentally during surgery and may often be sent for frozen section analysis. GIST can also present as a component of multiple hereditary syndromes, including Carney-Stratakis syndrome, Carney triad, and neurofibromatosis. Carney-Stratakis syndrome (the dyad of gastric GIST and paraganglioma) is a familial syndrome caused by mutations in *SDHx* genes; these mutations account for about 65% of SDH-deficient GISTs. Patients with *SDHA* germline mutations mostly present with GISTs as young to middle-aged adults, whereas patients with other *SDH* germline mutations present in childhood and adolescence. Carney triad (gastric GIST, paraganglioma, and pulmonary chondroma) is a nonfamilial syndrome associated with *SDHC* promoter hypermethylation and not germline mutations. Neurofibromatosis type 1 (NF1) is the most common autosomal dominant genetic disorder and is associated with development of neurofibromas, ganglioneuromas, and malignant peripheral nerve sheath tumors (MPNSTs), among other tumor types. NF1 also predisposes patients to GISTs that are predominantly found in the small intestine and can be multiple in the same patient. These tumors are mostly low risk and are associated with interstitial cell hyperplasia. Last, there are rare instances of familial germline mutations in *KIT* and *PDGFRA*; patients with these mutations develop GISTs with nearly 100% penetrance, in a background of interstitial cell hyperplasia. Patients with *KIT* germline mutations also develop urticaria pigmentosa and cutaneous hyperpigmentation.

Radiologic Features

Radiologic features are not specific, but most large mural gastric masses are GISTs. An example of a gastric GIST is shown in Fig. 7.1.

TABLE 7.1

Prevalence of Genetic Subtypes in Clinically Identified Gastrointestinal Stromal Tumors[a]

Mutation	Prevalence (%)
KIT	80
Exon 9	8
Exon 11	70
Exon 13	1
Exon 17	1
PDGFRA	7
Exon 12	1.5
Exon 14	0.5
Exon 18	5
SDH Deficiency	8
SDHA inactivating mutation	~3
SDHB, *SDHC*, *SDHD* inactivating mutations	~2
SDHC promoter hypermethylation	~3
NF1 Biallelic Inactivation	2–3
BRAF V600E	<1

[a]*NF*, Neurofibromatosis; *PDGFRA*, platelet derived growth factor receptor alpha; *SDH*, succinate dehydrogenase (subunits A-C).

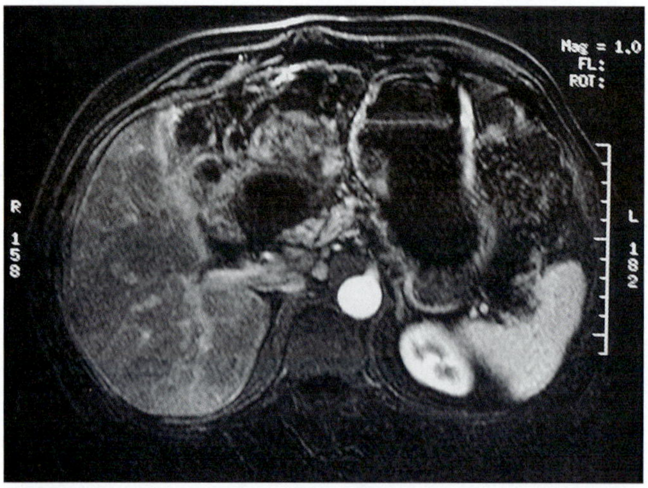

FIGURE 7.1

Imaging study from a patient with a large heterogenous gastric gastrointestinal stromal tumor, which was hard to distinguish from a primary liver lesion.

Pathologic Features

Gross Findings

Gastrointestinal stromal tumors vary in greatest dimension from smaller than 1 cm (micro-GISTs) to larger than 20 cm, and they can be submucosal, intramuscular, or subserosal, although most are centered in the muscularis propria. They can be solid or cystic with variable hemorrhage and necrosis, and there may be overlying mucosal ulceration. Generally, GISTs are well circumscribed. SDH-deficient GISTs have a characteristic multinodular or plexiform growth pattern. Fig. 7.2 shows a cross-section of a small intestinal GIST.

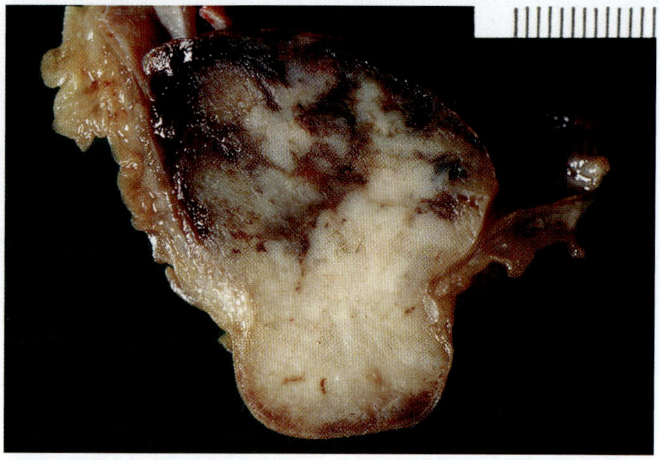

FIGURE 7.2

Small intestinal gastrointestinal stromal tumor involving the full thickness of the wall from mucosa to serosa, with hemorrhage at the serosal aspect.

Microscopic Findings

About 70 % of gastric GISTs and nearly all of those in the small and large intestine exhibit spindle cell morphology, with short fascicles of bland cells with indistinct cell borders, palely eosinophilic cytoplasm, and uniform, tapered nuclei with evenly dispersed chromatin (Figs. 7.3 and 7.4). Nuclear palisading is at least focally present in more than half of tumors. About 20 % of GISTs have purely epithelioid morphology; these tumors nearly all occur in the stomach and are associated with *PDGFRA* mutations (Fig. 7.5) or SDH deficiency (Fig. 7.6). Epithelioid GISTs are composed of sheets and nests of cells with palely eosinophilic cytoplasm and uniform nuclei, often in a myxohyaline stroma (Fig. 7.7; see also Figs. 7.5 and 7.6). The cell membranes are often better defined than spindle cell variants. SDH-deficient GIST has a characteristic multinodular or plexiform growth pattern and the cytomorphology is usually epithelioid (see Fig. 7.6). Gastric GISTs commonly have paranuclear vacuoles (see Figs. 7.3 and 7.7), and nearly half of small intestinal GISTs contain skeinoid fibers. Mitotic activity varies widely and is an important prognostic factor. Treatment effect can manifest as stromal hyalinization, decreased cellularity, or reduced mitotic activity. Rarely, tumors can develop heterologous rhabdomyosarcomatous differentiation after treatment, and both treated and treatment-naïve tumors can undergo dedifferentiation, in which there is a sharp transition from conventional morphology to high-grade pleomorphic regions that do not resemble GIST (Fig. 7.8). Both rhabdomyosarcomatous differentiation and dedifferentiation are associated with imatinib resistance and a poor prognosis.

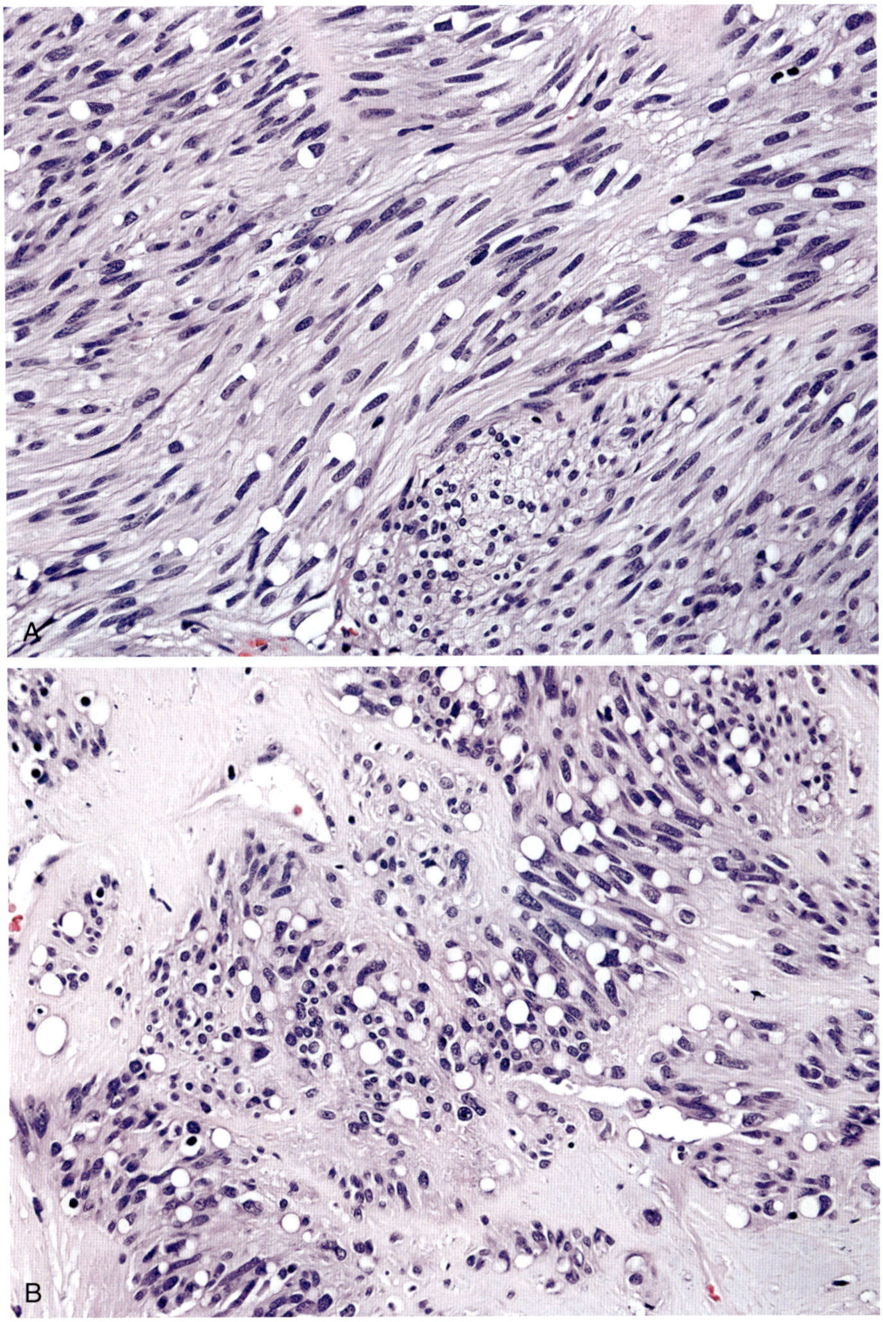

FIGURE 7.3

Gastric gastrointestinal stromal tumor (GIST) with spindle cell features exhibiting paranuclear vacuoles. **A**, Frequent vacuoles, as shown here, are a helpful feature within the differential diagnosis of spindle cell neoplasms of the stomach to support a diagnosis of GIST. Tapered nuclei are also a feature of GIST but not of leiomyoma or leiomyosarcoma. **B**, Myxoid stroma is seen in a subset of GISTs and is an uncommon finding in smooth muscle tumors.

Ancillary Studies

Immunohistochemistry

KIT (also known as CD117) is a receptor tyrosine kinase expressed in interstitial cells of Cajal, mast cells, melanocytes, a variety of epithelia, fetal endothelial cells, and a subset of CD34-positive hematopoietic stem cells. Oncogenic *KIT* mutations were discovered in the late 1990s to be present in the majority of GISTs, along with KIT overexpression. DOG1 (discovered on GIST1), a chloride channel normally expressed in the interstitial cells of Cajal, was also found to be expressed in GIST (hence the name "discovered on GIST 1"). Overall, KIT is positive in 95% of GISTs (Fig. 7.9), and DOG1 is also positive in 95% (Fig. 7.10). Fewer than 3% of tumors are negative for both markers; these tend to be epithelioid *PDGFRA*-mutant GISTs, and PDGFRA immunohistochemistry (IHC) is strongly and diffusely positive in essentially 100% of these tumors (see Fig. 7.5). PDGFRA is also weakly expressed in stromal cells, presenting a potential pitfall; only strong and diffuse staining should be used to support the diagnosis of GIST. CD34 is positive in about 70% of GISTs, although its diagnostic utility is now limited, given the superior sensitivity and specificity of KIT, DOG1, and PDGFRA IHC. Caldesmon is positive in 70% of GISTs, S-100 in 1% to 2% (especially duodenal GISTs), and desmin in 1% to 2% (but up to 10% in epithelioid *PDGFRA*-mutant GISTs; see Fig. 7.5D). Keratin positivity is rare.

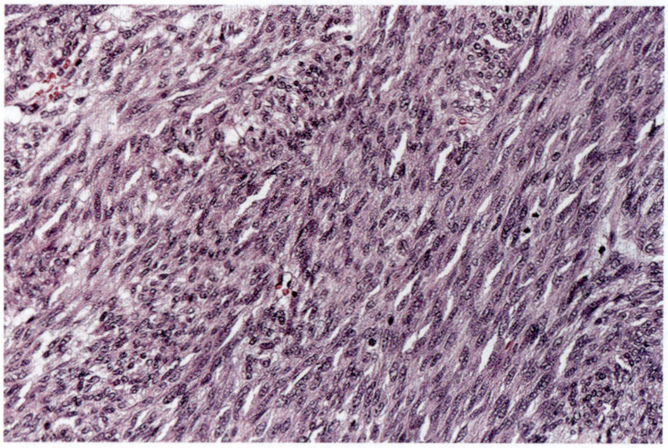

FIGURE 7.4

Small intestinal gastrointestinal stromal tumor (GIST). This spindle cell GIST is highly cellular and mitotically active.

Immunohistochemistry is also useful for diagnosing SDH-deficient GIST, which are generally positive for KIT and DOG1. The four SDH subunits (A–D) form a protein complex that is necessary to stabilize the SDHB protein. Therefore, loss of expression of any one of the subunits leads to loss of expression of SDHB. Thus, SDHB IHC can be used to screen for loss of expression of any subunit. SDHA expression is lost in about 35% of tumors, an event that is reliably detectable using SDHA IHC and that generally indicates underlying *SDHA* mutations. Of the 65% of SDH-deficient GISTs that express SDHA, about 30% have mutations in *SDHB*, *SDHC*, or *SDHD*, and the remaining 35% have *SDHC* promoter hypermethylation.

MOLECULAR GENETICS, PATHOLOGIC PHENOTYPES, AND PROGNOSIS

Gastrointestinal stromal tumors are not classified as benign or malignant tumors; instead, a risk

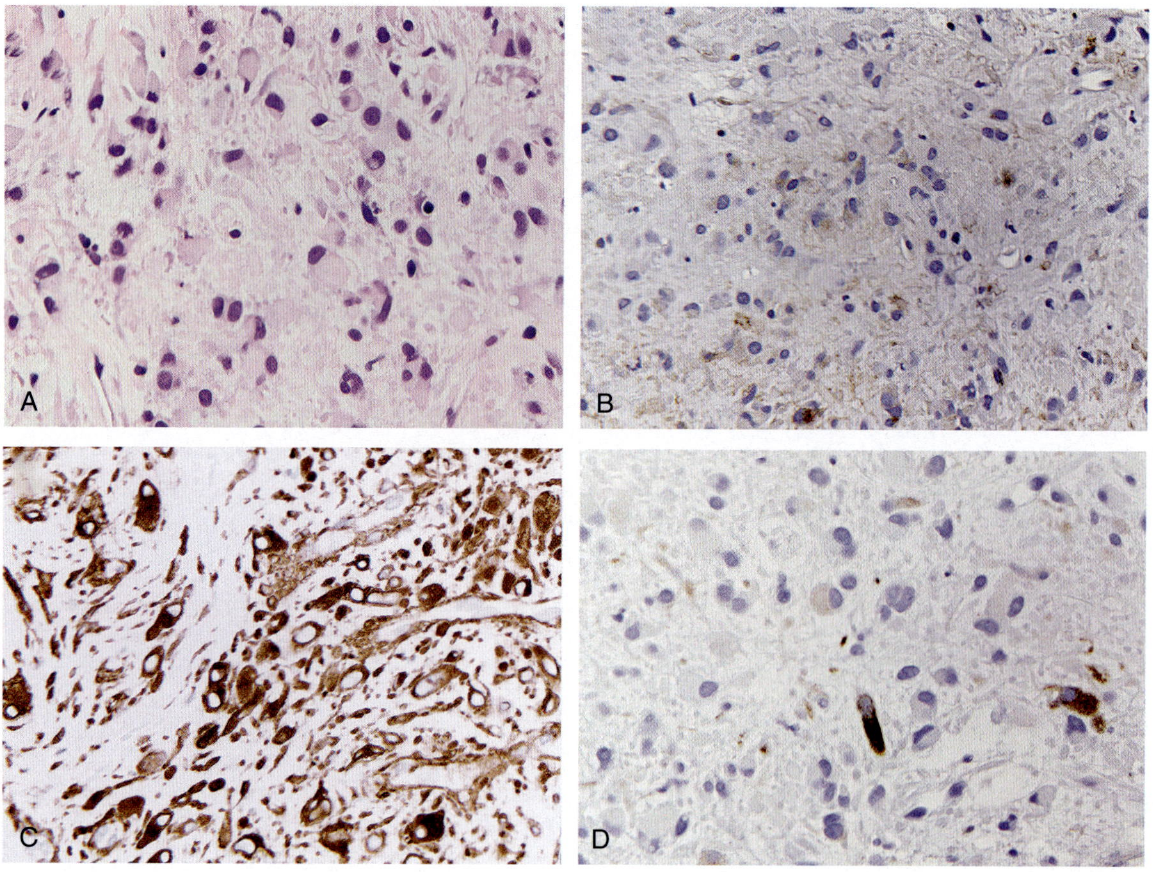

FIGURE 7.5

Platelet-derived growth factor receptor-α (*PDGFRA*)–mutant gastric gastrointestinal stromal tumor (GIST). **A**, The morphology shown here is typical of *PDGFRA*-mutant GIST, with epithelioid neoplastic cells dispersed singly and in small clusters within a myxohyaline stroma. Tumor cells have eosinophilic cytoplasm and relatively uniform nuclei with evenly dispersed chromatin. *PDGFRA*-mutant GIST has a striking predilection for the gastric wall, where this tumor occurred. **B**, In contrast to the *KIT*-mutant GIST in Fig. 7.9, KIT staining shows weak, scattered positivity in neoplastic cells. DOG1 (discovered on GIST1) was more diffusely positive (not shown). **C**, PDGFRA is strongly and diffusely positive in neoplastic cells. **D**, Desmin shows scattered positivity, a feature seen in about 10% of *PDGFRA*-mutant GISTs.

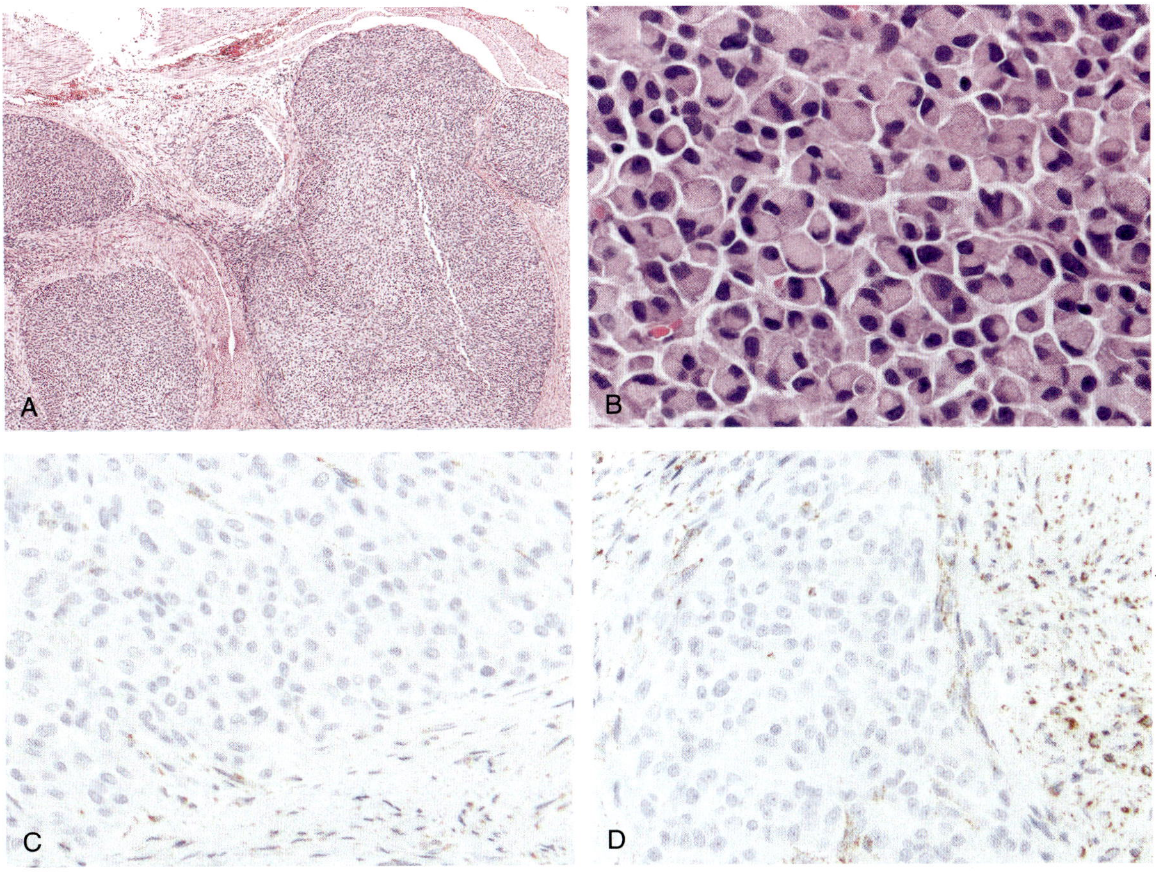

FIGURE 7.6

Succinate dehydrogenase (SDH)–deficient gastrointestinal stromal tumor (GIST). **A**, At low power, SDH-deficient GIST has a multinodular or plexiform growth pattern. **B**, The neoplastic cells are epithelioid, with abundant eosinophilic cytoplasm, relatively uniform nuclei, and a plasmacytoid appearance. **C**, SDH-B expression is lost in all SDH-deficient GISTs, regardless of the subunit mutation. **D**, SDH-A IHC is specifically negative in tumors with underlying *SDHA* mutations, which represent approximately 35% of SDH-deficient GISTs and are associated with Carney-Stratakis syndrome. Note that SDH-B and SDH-A are expressed in the mitochondria of adjacent non-neoplastic cells in *C* and *D*.

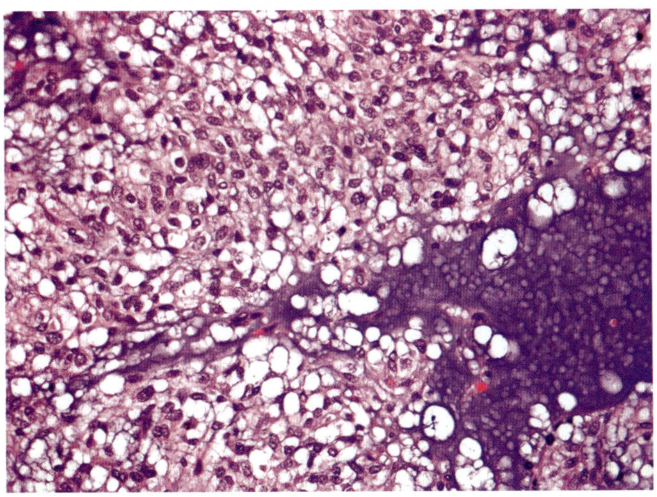

FIGURE 7.7

Epithelioid gastric gastrointestinal stromal tumor (GIST). Note the prominent paranuclear vacuoles and uniform nuclei; nuclear pleomorphism is unusual in GIST, and its presence should prompt consideration of other diagnoses.

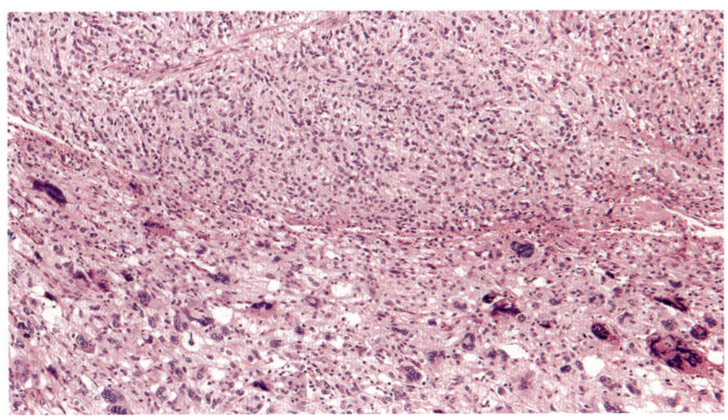

FIGURE 7.8

Dedifferentiated gastrointestinal stromal tumor (GIST). There is a sharp juxtaposition between conventional GIST (above) and dedifferentiated GIST (below), the latter of which appears to be a high-grade pleomorphic sarcoma that would not be easily recognized without the adjacent conventional component.

stratification scheme is used, with prognosis determined by using site, size, and mitotic index (Table 7.2). Mitoses should be counted in a 5-mm^2 area; on most modern microscopes, 5 mm^2 is close to 20 hpf. When GISTs behave in a clinically aggressive fashion, they most commonly metastasize to the abdominal cavity and liver. Metastasis can occur more than 10 years after surgical resection, underscoring the need for long-term follow-up.

Several studies have established relationships between specific GIST genotypes and their corresponding

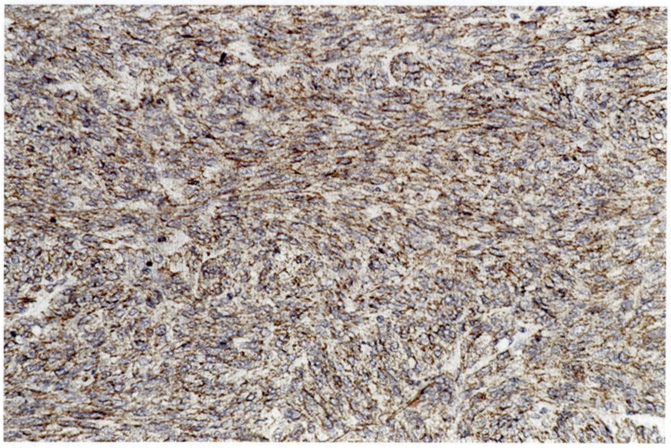

FIGURE 7.9

KIT staining in a *KIT*-mutant gastrointestinal stromal tumor (GIST). KIT shows diffuse membranous positivity in this tumor, and in general, it is positive in 95% of GISTs. KIT most commonly stains with a cytoplasmic pattern, although it can exhibit membranous (as shown here) and dot-like perinuclear staining.

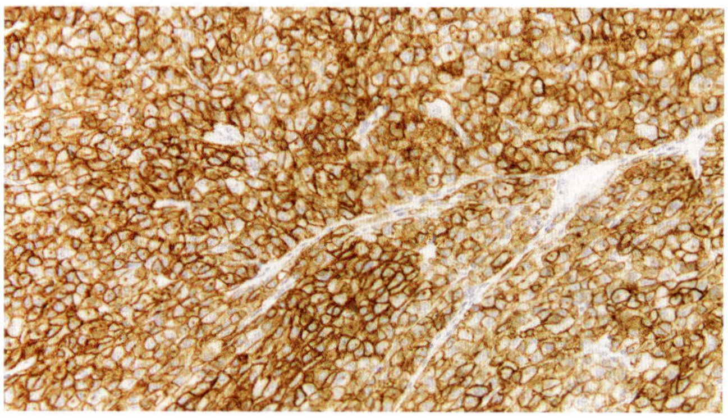

FIGURE 7.10

DOG1 (discovered on GIST1) staining in a succinate dehydrogenase–deficient gastrointestinal stromal tumor (GIST). DOG1 shows diffuse membranous positivity in this tumor along with scattered perinuclear dot-like positivity; cytoplasmic positivity is also seen in some tumors. In general, DOG1 is positive in about 95% of GISTs.

clinicopathologic phenotypes. The protein structures of KIT and PDGFRA receptors are similar, and activating a mutation in either one of these two genes leads to activation of similar signal transduction pathways and these mutations are thought to be initiating events in GIST tumorigenesis.

Eighty percent of GISTs have *KIT* mutations, and 7% have *PDGFRA* mutations. *KIT* mutations occur in exon 11 (overall accounting for 70% of GISTs), exon 9 (8%), exon 13 (1%), and exon 17 (1%) (see Table 7.1). Exon 11 (juxtamembrane domain) mutant GISTs occur in the stomach and small intestine, and they have spindle cell or mixed morphology. Exon 11 mutations include in-frame deletions (60%–70%), missense point mutations (20%–30%), and internal tandem duplications; whereas exon 11 point-mutant GISTs have a better prognosis than other GISTs, tumors with exon 11 deletions behave more aggressively. Recent clinical trials demonstrated that patients with exon 11 deletions benefit from an extended course of adjuvant imatinib therapy.

Exon 9 (dimerization motif domain) mutations occur in tumors typically located in the small and large intestines; these tumors have spindle cell or mixed morphology, and they require higher doses of imatinib to achieve treatment response. Exon 13 and exon 17 mutations together account for 2% of GISTs; these tumors mostly occur in the small intestine, have spindle cell morphology, and have inconsistent responses to imatinib.

About 8% of GISTs harbor mutations to *PDGFRA*; as in *KIT*-mutant GISTs, these occur in different exons corresponding to different protein domains. *PDGFRA* mutations occur in exon 18 (accounting for 7% of GISTs overall), exon 12 (1.5%), and exon 14 (0.5%). *PDGFRA*-mutant GISTs predominantly occur in the stomach, and essentially all have purely epithelioid morphology. A particular missense mutation (D842V) accounts for the majority of exon 18 mutations and confers imatinib resistance; recently, the Food and Drug Administration (FDA)-approved avapritinib to treat patients with these GISTs. Exon 12– and exon 14–mutant GISTs have variable responses to imatinib.

PDGFRA mutations, *KIT* mutations, and biallelic *NF1* inactivation are thought to be initiating events in GIST tumorigenesis; all three subtypes undergo the same additional chromosomal deletions as part of an apparent stepwise progression toward higher-risk tumor biology. Given that they share the same progression, it is perhaps not surprising that the prognosis of these three GIST subtypes can be determined using the same risk stratification system (see Table 7.2).

SDH deficiency is seen in about 8% of GISTs and is mutually exclusive with *PDGFRA* and *KIT* mutations and *NF1* inactivation. SDH-deficient GIST represents the majority of pediatric GIST but also occurs in a significant subset of adults. SDH-deficient GISTs are almost always gastric and show an epithelioid morphology with a unique plexiform architectural growth pattern (see Fig. 7.6). SDHA, SDHB, SDHC, and SDHD proteins form a multimeric complex in the inner mitochondrial membrane that is critical for cellular metabolism. Whereas *SDHA* mutations are present in about 35% of SDH-deficient GISTs, about 30% have mutations in *SDHB*, *SDHC*, or *SDHD*. The remaining 35% of SDH-deficient GISTs have *SDHC* promoter hypermethylation, which silences expression of SDHC, leading to SDH deficiency. *SDHB, SDHC*, or *SDHD* mutations are usually present in the germline, and these patients also develop paragangliomas in the familial Carney-Stratakis syndrome, as discussed earlier.

The prognosis of SDH-deficient GIST is different from the other described genetic subtypes, so

TABLE 7.2
Site-Specific Risk Stratification for Gastrointestinal Stromal Tumors[a]

Tumor Parameter		Risk of Progressive Disease[b] (%)			
Mitotic Index	**Size (cm)**	**Stomach**	**Duodenum**	**Jejunum/ileum**	**Rectum**
≤5 per 5 mm²	≤2	None (0%)	None (0%)	None (0%)	None (0%)
	>2–≤5	Very low (1.9%)	Low (8.3%)	Low (4.3%)	Low (8.5%)
	>5–≤10	Low (3.6%)	Insufficient data	Moderate (24%)	Insufficient data
	>10	Moderate (10%)	High (34%)	High (52%)	High (57%)
>5 per 5 mm²	≤2	None	Insufficient data	High	High (54%)
	>2–≤5	Moderate (16%)	High (50%)	High (73%)	High (52%)
	>5–≤10	High (55%)	Insufficient data	High (85%)	Insufficient data
	>10	High (86%)	High (86%)	High (90%)	High (71%)

[a]Does not apply to succinate dehydrogenase–deficient gastrointestinal stromal tumors.
[b]Defined as metastasis or tumor-related death.
Adapted from Demetri GD, von Mehren M, Antonescu CR, et al. NCCN Task Force report: update on the management of patients with gastrointestinal stromal tumors. *J Natl Compr Canc Netw*. 2010;8(suppl 2):S1–S41; quiz S42–S44 and Miettinen M, Lasota J. Gastrointestinal stromal tumors: pathology and prognosis at different sites. *Semin Diagn Pathol*. 2006;23(2):70–83.

the risk stratification system developed for *KIT*- and *PDGFRA*-mutant tumors does not apply. Instead, SDH-deficient GISTs frequently give rise to slowly growing lymph node metastases that progress over the course of several years to decades. SDH-deficient GISTs do not respond to imatinib therapy, and as of now, there is no targeted therapy to treat patients with these tumors.

BRAF-mutant GISTs are rare. Tumors harboring *BRAF* V600E occur in the small intestine and have spindle cell morphology. Although they do not respond to imatinib, they have been shown to respond to dabrafenib, a BRAF inhibitor.

Differential Diagnosis

The differential diagnosis for spindle cell GIST includes leiomyoma, leiomyosarcoma, schwannoma, and desmoid fibromatosis. Leiomyoma and leiomyosarcoma have more brightly eosinophilic cytoplasm, and they exhibit distinct cell borders in contrast to the indistinct cell borders of GIST. Leiomyoma and leiomyosarcoma also have blunt-ended nuclei, unlike the tapered nuclei of GIST. IHC is useful to resolve the differential diagnosis: leiomyoma and leiomyosarcoma commonly have diffuse desmin expression, which would be unusual in GIST, and they are negative for KIT and DOG1.

Gastric schwannoma typically has a peripheral cuff of lymphocytes and neural cytomorphology with buckled nuclei and mild atypia. The cells of schwannoma show diffuse S-100 expression and are negative for DOG1 and KIT.

Desmoid fibromatosis is more infiltrative than GIST and has longer fascicles. IHC demonstrates nuclear β-catenin positivity in 70% to 80% of desmoid fibromatoses, which is negative in GIST. Desmoid fibromatosis does not express KIT or DOG1.

The differential diagnosis for epithelioid GIST includes neuroendocrine tumors and gastric adenocarcinoma. Neuroendocrine tumors usually have smaller cells and darker nuclei with speckled chromatin. IHC for synaptophysin, chromogranin, KIT, and DOG1 readily distinguishes the two. Gastric adenocarcinoma exhibits significant nuclear pleomorphism and hyperchromasia, in contrast to the uniform nuclei and evenly dispersed chromatin of epithelioid GIST.

Treatment

Surgical excision is the treatment for patients with resectable GIST. Narrow margins suffice because tumors tend not to recur at the surgical site; the exception is SDH-deficient GISTs, likely because of their multinodular, infiltrative growth pattern. For most *KIT*-mutant GISTs and some *PDGFRA*-mutant GISTs, imatinib is the first-line therapy in the setting of metastases or locally advanced disease and as adjuvant therapy in GISTs that stratify into intermediate- or high-risk groups (see Table 7.2). Neoadjuvant imatinib is also used in some cases to reduce the size of locally advanced tumors prior to surgery. Imatinib resistance eventually develops in all treated GISTs, usually by means of secondary *KIT* mutations. Sunitinib and regorafenib are FDA-approved second- and third-line therapies, respectively, that are used in the setting of imatinib resistance. As mentioned earlier, avapritinib was recently FDA approved for first-line treatment of patients with *PDGFRA* exon 18–mutant GIST, which is resistant to imatinib, sunitinib, and regorafenib.

GASTROINTESTINAL STROMAL TUMORS—FACT SHEET

Definition

- Gastrointestinal stromal tumor (GIST) is the most common mesenchymal tumor in the gastrointestinal (GI) tract and exhibits differentiation of the interstitial cells of Cajal

Incidence and Location

- 3300 to 6000 cases per year in the United States
- Most commonly occurs in the stomach (60%) and small intestine (35%)

Morbidity and Mortality

- Tumor mortality depends in part on primary site: intestinal GISTs are about twice as likely to behave aggressively compared with gastric GISTs.
- Tumor size and mitotic count also influence clinical behavior

Gender, Race, and Age Distribution

- No sex predilection
- May be overrepresented in African Americans
- Most commonly occurs in adults, with a median age at presentation of 60 years
- Pediatric tumors are typically succinate dehydrogenase deficient

Clinical Features

- Clinical presentation depends on primary site but usually includes abdominal pain, symptoms of GI bleeding such as anemia or melena or obstruction
- Small tumors are often detected incidentally

Prognosis and Therapy

- Tumors are not classified as benign or malignant; instead, they are risk stratified based on anatomic site, tumor size, and mitotic activity (see Tables 7.2)
- Prognosis and treatment are determined based on the driving mutation and risk category
- Food and Drug Administration-approved treatment includes imatinib, sunitinib, and regorafenib (nonspecific tyrosine kinase inhibitors) and, more recently, avapritinib (used for *PDGFRA* exon 18-mutant GIST)

GASTROINTESTINAL STROMAL TUMORS—PATHOLOGIC FEATURES

Gross Findings

- Mural mass, sometimes with protrusion into the gastrointestinal lumen
- Fibrous to fleshy cut surface, with variable hemorrhage and/or cystic degeneration

Microscopic Findings

- Spindled or epithelioid cells with uniform nuclei and relatively limited atypia
- Nuclear palisading common
- Gastric gastrointestinal stromal tumors (GISTs) commonly have paranuclear vacuoles
- About half of small intestinal GISTs have skeinoid fibers

Immunohistochemistry

- Positive: DOG1 (discovered on GIST1; 95%), KIT (95%), CD34 (70
- Variable: smooth muscle actin (30%), S-100 (5%)
- Platelet-derived growth factor receptor-α (*PDGFRA*)–mutant GISTs: positive for PDGFRA (nearly 100%), DOG1 (95%), KIT (85%), desmin (≤10%)

Molecular Testing

- Determines optimal treatment
- *KIT* mutations (80%) in exon 11 (70%), exon 9 (8%), exon 13 (1%), exon 17 (1%), or exon 8 (rare)
- *PDGFRA* mutations (7%) in exon 18 (5%), exon 12 (1.5%), or exon 14 (0.5%)
- Succinate dehydrogenase (SDH) deficiency (8%): *SDHA* mutations (35%); *SDHB*, *SDHC*, or *SDHD* mutations (30%); *SDHC* promoter hypermethylation (35%); no *KIT* or *PDGFRA* mutations
- Biallelic *NF1* inactivation (2%–3%); no *KIT* or *PDGFRA* mutations
- *BRAF* V600E mutation (<1%)

Differential Diagnosis

- Spindle cell GIST: leiomyoma or leiomyosarcoma (desmin positive, KIT/DOG1 negative); schwannoma or malignant peripheral nerve sheath tumor (S-100 positive, KIT negative); desmoid fibromatosis (70%–80% nuclear β-catenin positivity; 95% negative for KIT)
- Epithelioid GIST: neuroendocrine tumor (synaptophysin and chromogranin positive, KIT and DOG1 negative), gastric adenocarcinoma (keratin positive, more atypical or pleomorphic)

SMOOTH MUSCLE TUMORS OF THE GASTROINTESTINAL TRACT

CLINICAL FEATURES

Smooth muscle tumors of the GI tract consist of leiomyoma and the much rarer leiomyosarcoma. Colonic leiomyomas classically arise in association with the muscularis mucosae and present as distal polyps on screening colonoscopy, usually in men in their seventh decade. Esophageal leiomyomas often present as intramural masses; patients have a median age of 35 years, there is a male predominance (~70%), and the clinical course is indolent. In the esophagus, the vast majority of spindle cell tumors are leiomyomas. Smooth muscle tumors of the stomach and small intestine are rare; GIST is much more common at these locations. Leiomyosarcoma of the GI tract is very rare and generally follows an aggressive course. Leiomyosarcoma of the colon shows a slight male predominance and presents in adults. Leiomyosarcoma is exceptional in the stomach. Leiomyomatosis has been described in the small intestine and colon.

RADIOLOGIC FEATURES

The radiologic features are not specific and are not distinguishable from those of GIST.

PATHOLOGIC FEATURES

GROSS FINDINGS

Esophageal leiomyomas form whorled white to pale yellow masses similar to uterine leiomyomas. Leiomyomas

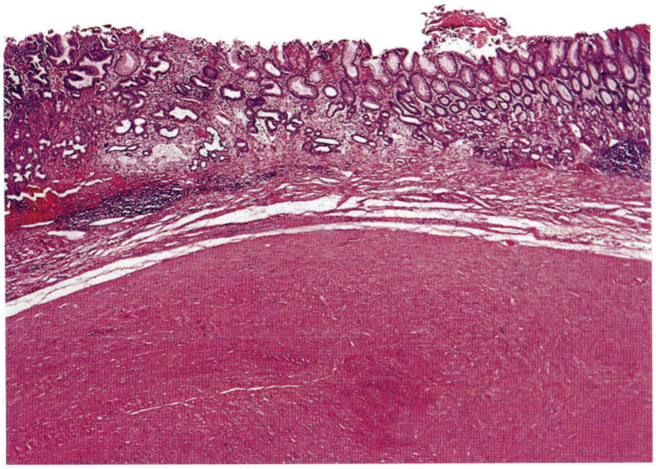

FIGURE 7.11

Gastric leiomyoma that has arisen in association with the muscularis mucosae. The bright eosinophilia of the cytoplasm is evident at low magnification.

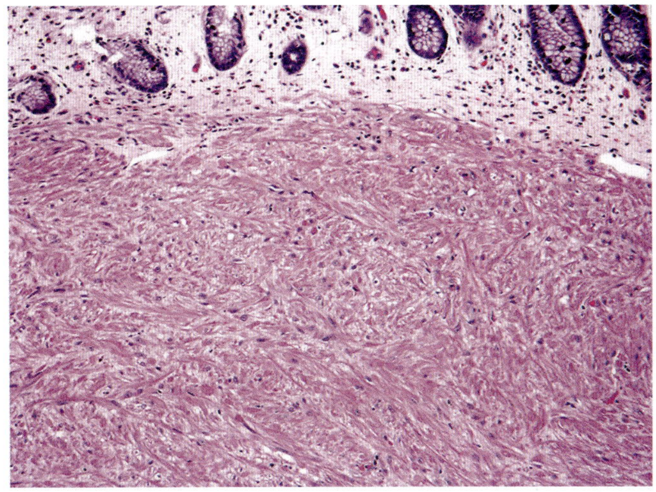

FIGURE 7.12

Submucosal leiomyoma of the colon. In contrast to leiomyomas in the esophagus, those in the colon tend have more ovoid nuclei and paler cytoplasm.

arising in the muscularis mucosae of the colorectum present as mucosal polyps, usually smaller than 1 cm. Leiomyosarcomas of the colorectum tend to be intraluminal bulging exophytic and polypoid masses, which may show necrosis and hemorrhage.

Microscopic Findings

Smooth muscle tumors of the GI tract have the same features of smooth muscle differentiation seen at other anatomic sites, namely perpendicularly oriented fascicles of spindle cells with distinct cell borders, brightly eosinophilic cytoplasm, longitudinal striations, and blunt-ended or cigar-shaped nuclei (Figs. 7.11 to 7.15). Leiomyomas are bland and resemble normal smooth muscle. They lack atypia and pleomorphism and generally show no or minimal mitotic activity. Leiomyosarcoma is characterized by conspicuous mitotic activity, cytologic atypia, and necrosis.

Ancillary Studies

Immunohistochemistry

Smooth muscle tumors show expression of smooth muscle actin (SMA), desmin, and caldesmon, but expression of the latter two markers may be variable in extent, especially in leiomyosarcoma. KIT, CD34, and S-100 protein are generally not expressed. Approximately 40% of leiomyosarcomas show variable keratin expression, which may be extensive occasionally and make distinction from sarcomatoid carcinoma difficult. Esophageal leiomyomas often contain numerous mast cells that are KIT positive, which may result in an erroneous diagnosis of GIST.

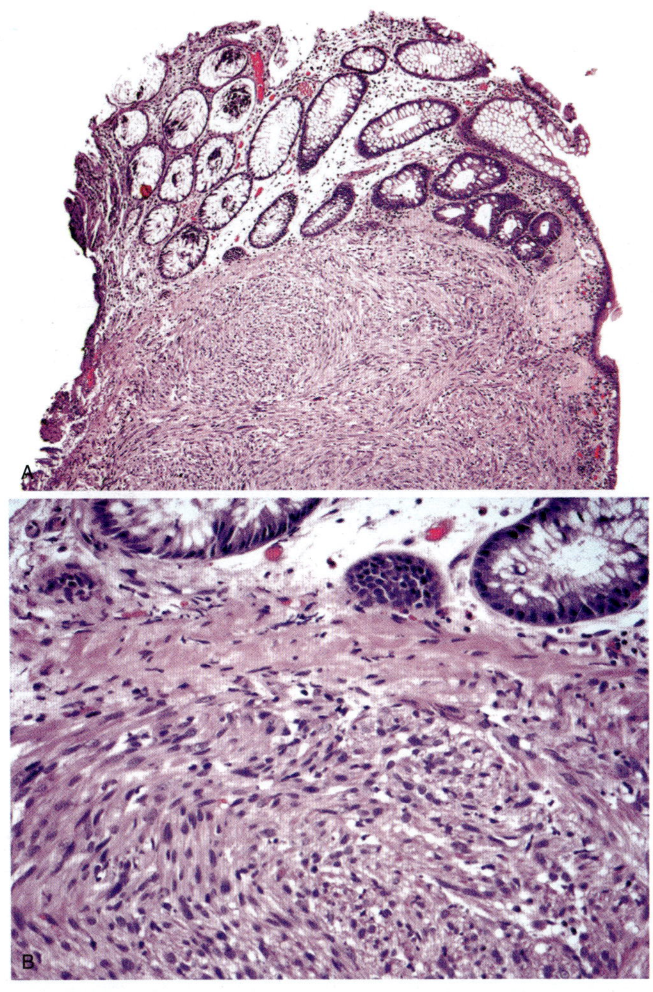

FIGURE 7.13

Leiomyosarcoma showing perpendicularly oriented fascicles of spindle cells with eosinophilic cytoplasm (A and B). Compare the cellularity of this lesion to that seen in Figs. 7.11 and 7.12.

Differential Diagnosis

The differential diagnosis is primarily with GIST and schwannoma, and the majority of lesions are readily separable by IHC. Sarcomatoid carcinoma may mimic leiomyosarcoma because both are composed of fascicles of atypical spindle cells, which may express keratins. Identification of a more epithelioid or conventional carcinomatous component allows for recognition of sarcomatoid carcinoma. In addition, the latter does not show desmin expression.

Prognosis and Therapy

The prognosis of leiomyomas is excellent in all sites because they are benign. In general, GI tract leiomyosarcomas have a poor prognosis, and about 75 % of patients die of disease.

SMOOTH MUSCLE TUMORS OF THE GASTROINTESTINAL TRACT—FACT SHEET

Definition

- Benign or malignant neoplasms with smooth muscle differentiation

Incidence and Location

- Leiomyoma is far more common than leiomyosarcoma, and leiomyoma is the most common spindle cell tumor of the esophagus.
- Small polypoid leiomyomas arise in association with the muscularis mucosae of the colorectum

Morbidity and Mortality

- Leiomyomas are benign; in contrast, 75% of patients with leiomyosarcomas of the gastrointestinal tract die of disease

Gender, Race, and Age Distribution

- Occur in adults (average, 60 years); slight male predominance

Clinical Features

- Whereas smooth muscle tumors of the esophagus present as an intramural mass, smooth muscle tumors of the colon present as polypoid lesions
- Smooth muscle tumors of the small intestine can present as either intramural masses or polypoid lesions

Prognosis and Therapy

- Poor prognosis for leiomyosarcomas; leiomyomas are benign.
- All lesions except small polypoid leiomyomas of the colorectum are treated surgically when possible; there is no targeted chemotherapy as there is for gastrointestinal stromal tumor

Smooth Muscle Tumors of The Gastrointestinal Tract—Pathologic Features

Gross Findings

- Esophageal leiomyomas are whorled, whitish masses
- Leiomyosarcomas are large, exophytic, mural-based masses, with variable amounts of necrosis and hemorrhage

Microscopic Findings

- Fascicular spindle cell neoplasm; tumor cells have brightly eosinophilic cytoplasm, distinct cell borders, and blunt-ended cigar-shaped nuclei
- Leiomyomas are bland, resemble normal smooth muscle, and lack atypia and necrosis
- Leiomyosarcomas show cytologic and nuclear pleomorphism and atypia, mitotic activity, and necrosis

Immunohistochemistry

- Positive for desmin, smooth muscle actin, caldesmon
- Negative for KIT, DOG1 and S-100 protein
- Focal keratin expression is common in leiomyosarcoma
- Usually negative for CD34

Differential Diagnosis

- Gastrointestinal stromal tumor: cytoplasm is paler; may show skeinoid fibers or paranuclear vacuoles; KIT and DOG1 positive and desmin negative
- Schwannoma: usually larger gastric lesions with a peripheral lymphoid cuff or smaller polypoid colonic lesions that entrap colonic crypts, different from the growth pattern of leiomyoma; tumor cells are positive for S-100
- Sarcomatoid carcinoma: may be difficult to distinguish from leiomyosarcoma, given that both can show keratin expression; identification of an epithelioid or overtly carcinomatous component is particularly helpful and may require extensive sampling

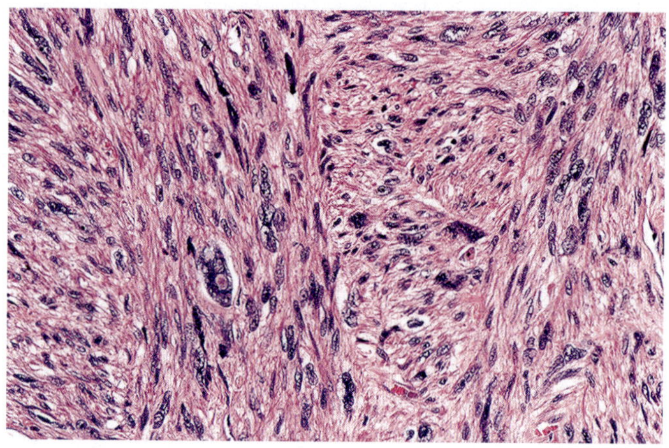

FIGURE 7.14

Leiomyosarcoma with marked pleomorphism and nuclear atypia.

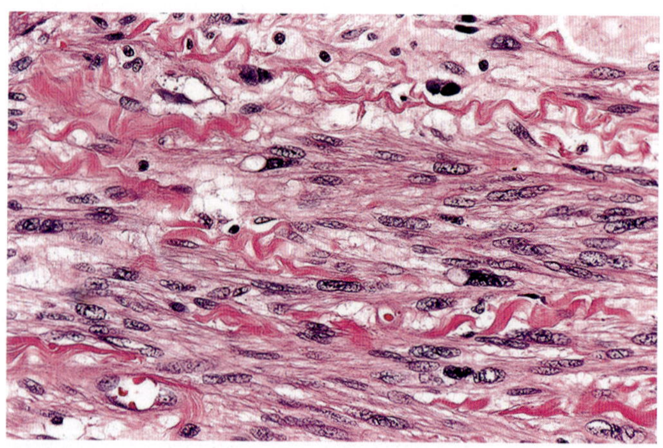

FIGURE 7.15

Leiomyosarcoma. The nuclei have blunt ends typical of smooth muscle differentiation, and there are scattered paranuclear vacuoles.

GRANULAR CELL TUMOR

CLINICAL FEATURES

Granular cell tumors are benign tumors that exhibit Schwannian differentiation. Although they can occur anywhere along the luminal GI tract, they have a striking predilection for the esophagus. Granular cell tumors usually occur in middle-aged adults and are more common in women and African Americans. Although they usually occur as unifocal tumors in the distal esophagus, they can also present as multiple sporadic esophageal tumors.

ENDOSCOPIC FEATURES

Granular cell tumors are often found incidentally on endoscopy, and they appear as small polyps or plaques.

PATHOLOGIC FEATURES

GROSS FINDINGS

Most granular cell tumors are small (<1 cm) with a yellow-white cut surface and infiltrative peripheral growth.

MICROSCOPIC FINDINGS

Granular cell tumors are composed of sheets and nests of large polygonal cells with brightly eosinophilic, granular cytoplasm, and centrally located, small, hyperchromatic nuclei (Figs. 7.16 and 7.17). There is frequently overlying squamous cell hyperplasia, a useful diagnostic clue. Occasionally, tumors can have spindle cell morphology, although the spindle cells still contain abundant granular cytoplasm. In conventional granular cell tumor, mitotic activity is low, and there is no necrosis.

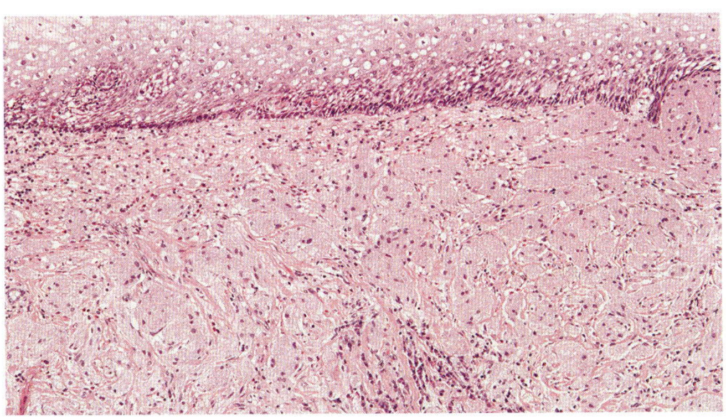

FIGURE 7.16
Granular cell tumor. Tumor cells are present in sheets and nests deep to the squamous epithelium.

ANCILLARY STUDIES

IMMUNOHISTOCHEMISTRY

Diffuse strong expression of S-100 protein and SOX10 is present in esophageal granular cell tumors (Fig. 7.18). Granular cell tumors also overexpress transcription factor enhancer 3 (TFE3), but they do not harbor underlying *TFE3* rearrangements.

MOLECULAR STUDIES

Granular cell tumors were recently found to have recurrent loss of function mutations in *ATP6AP1* and *ATP6AP2*, which are endosomal pH regulatory proteins; loss of expression of these proteins was shown to be oncogenic and to lead to accumulation of intracytoplasmic granules.

DIFFERENTIAL DIAGNOSIS

The differential diagnosis is limited because the cytomorphology of granular cell tumor is unique. Nested

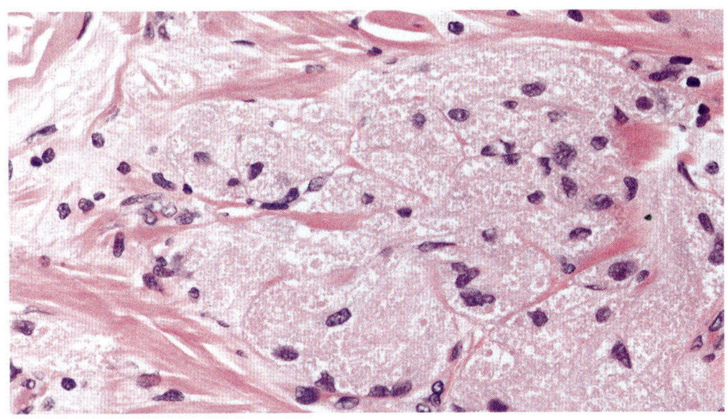

FIGURE 7.17
Granular cell tumor. Tumor cells have abundant granular cytoplasm and small hyperchromatic nuclei.

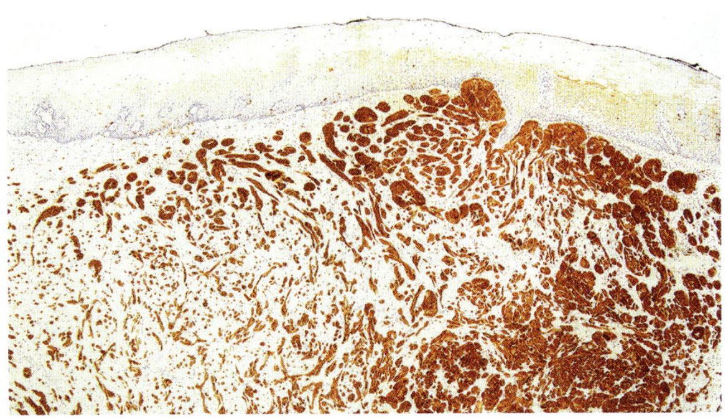

FIGURE 7.18
Granular cell tumor. S-100 is diffusely positive in tumor cells and highlights the predominantly nested tumor architecture.

examples can sometimes resemble alveolar soft part sarcoma, which also overexpresses TFE3; however, alveolar soft part sarcoma has significantly more cytologic atypia. Granular cell tumors with spindle cell morphology could be mistaken for schwannoma, but the latter does not contain abundant granular cytoplasm.

Prognosis and Therapy

The vast majority of granular cell tumors are benign and do not recur even if incompletely excised. The rare malignant granular cell tumors tend to have worrisome features such as increased mitotic activity and necrosis, neither of which are features of conventional granular cell tumor.

GRANULAR CELL TUMOR—FACT SHEET

Definition
- Benign neoplasm with Schwannian differentiation composed of large polygonal cells with bright eosinophilic granular cytoplasm

Incidence and Location
- Most commonly occur in the distal esophagus and rarely occur at other sites in the gastrointestinal tract

Gender, Race, and Age Distribution
- Wide age distribution, with a peak in middle age
- More common in women than men
- More common in African American patients

Clinical Features
- Small incidental polyps or plaques found during endoscopy

Prognosis and Therapy
- Mostly benign and do no recur even with positive margins
- Rare malignant granular cell tumors have worrisome features such as high mitotic activity and necrosis

Granular Cell Tumor—Pathologic Features

Gross Findings
- Subepithelial mass with a yellow cut surface and infiltrative borders

Microscopic Findings
- Sheets and nests of large polygonal cells with abundant eosinophilic granular cytoplasm; uncommonly, neoplastic cells can have spindled morphology
- Overlying squamous cell hyperplasia may be present

Immunohistochemistry
- Strong and diffuse expression of S-100 and SOX10

Differential Diagnosis
- Alveolar soft part sarcoma: both overexpress transcription factor enhancer 3 (TFE3), but granular cell tumor lacks the *TFE3* rearrangement of alveolar soft part sarcoma
- Schwannoma: can resemble spindle cell granular cell tumor, and both diffusely expression S-100 and SOX10; however, schwannoma lacks abundant granular cytoplasm

CLEAR CELL SARCOMA-LIKE TUMOR OF THE GASTROINTESTINAL TRACT/ MALIGNANT GASTROINTESTINAL NEUROECTODERMAL TUMOR

CLINICAL FEATURES

Clear cell sarcoma-like tumor of the GI tract, also known as malignant GI neuroectodermal tumor (malignant GNET), is a rare tumor with distinctive pathologic and genetic features, different from conventional clear cell sarcoma of tendons and aponeuroses. These tumors have also been called "osteoclast-rich tumors of the GI tract with features resembling clear cell sarcoma of soft parts." In contrast to conventional clear cell sarcoma of tendons and aponeuroses, these tumors usually show less nested growth pattern, contain osteoclast-like giant cells, and lack evidence of melanocytic differentiation ultrastructurally and immunohistochemically. They both, however, express S-100 and harbor the *EWSR1-ATF1* or *EWSR1-CREB1* fusion genes.

The most common site of involvement is the small intestine followed by the stomach and colon. Patients are usually young to middle-aged adults (mean age, 42 years; range, 17–77 years), and there is no apparent gender predilection. Presenting symptoms and signs include abdominal pain, intestinal obstruction, weight loss, anemia, and fever. Metastasis at the time of presentation is common.

Radiologic and Endoscopic Features

Tumors grow as exophytic masses that protrude into the lumen of the intestine. Overlying mucosal ulceration is often present. Tumors may also grow as circumferential masses, mimicking carcinoma or lymphoma.

Pathologic Features

Gross Findings

Tumors typically involve both submucosa and muscularis propria and range in size from 2 to 15 cm. Extension into mucosa may occur. Tumors are usually solid and firm, with a tan-white cut surface. Hemorrhage, necrosis, and cystic change may be present.

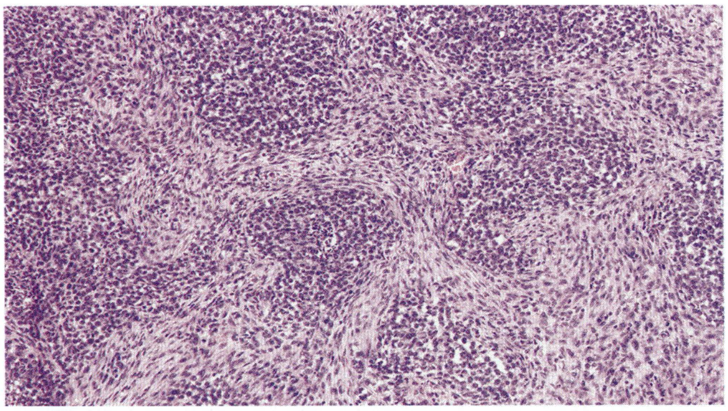

FIGURE 7.19

Malignant gastrointestinal neuroectodermal tumor (GNET). GNET is composed of sheets and large nests of epithelioid and spindle cells, in contrast to the smaller nests of clear cell sarcoma.

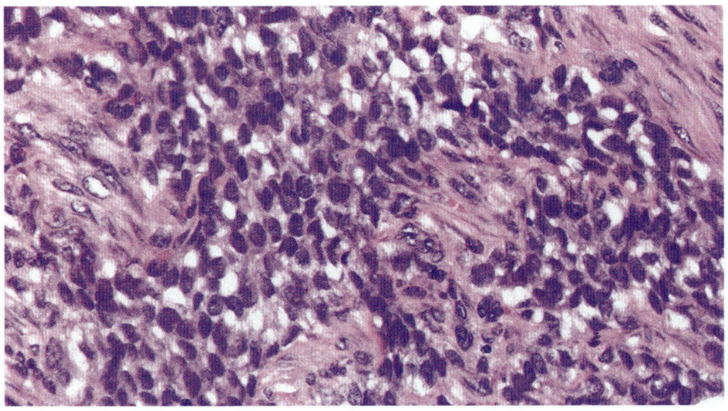

FIGURE 7.20

Malignant gastrointestinal neuroectodermal tumor (GNET). Whereas at low power, GNET resembles melanoma, at higher power, the tumor cells are usually less atypical. Rarely, GNET can exhibit pleomorphism, making the differential diagnosis with melanoma challenging to resolve.

Microscopic Findings

Malignant GNET is composed of sheets of round to epithelioid cells and in some cases ovoid to spindled cells (Fig. 7.19). Tumor cells have small amounts of pale eosinophilic cytoplasm and round to oval nuclei with vesicular chromatin and small nucleoli (Fig. 7.20). Mitotic activity is variable. The growth pattern is usually mixed, with focal areas of nested, pseudoglandular, pseudopapillary, microcystic, and fascicular architecture. Osteoclast-like giant cells are present in 50% of cases.

Ancillary Studies

Immunohistochemistry

Strong diffuse expression of S-100 is present in all cases (Fig. 7.21). SOX10 expression is also seen, reflecting the neuroectodermal differentiation of this tumor. In contrast, melanocytic markers HMB45 (human melanoma black), Melan-A, microphthalmia transcription factor (MiTF), and tyrosinase are negative. Tumor cells are also negative for KIT, DOG1, CD34, glial fibrillary acidic protein (GFAP), keratins, desmin, and SMA. Expression of synaptophysin and neuron-specific enolase (NSE) is seen in up to 50% of cases. Ultrastructural features of neural differentiation are seen by electron microscopy.

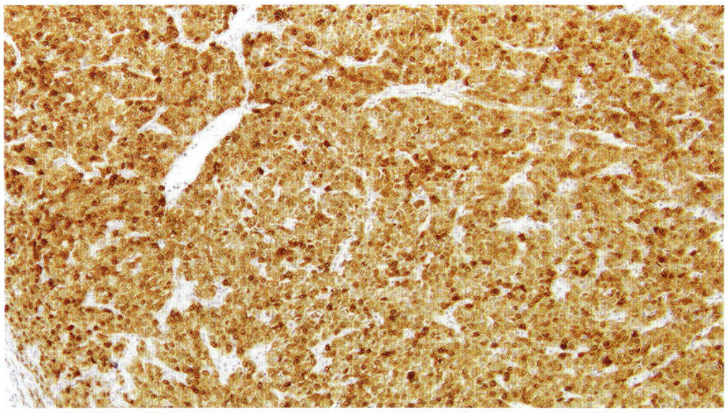

FIGURE 7.21

Malignant gastrointestinal neuroectodermal tumor (GNET) immunohistochemistry. GNET is diffusely positive for S-100 (pictured) and SOX10, but it is negative for secondary melanocytic markers such as HMB45 (human melanoma black) and Melan-A. Because melanoma can also lose expression of secondary melanocytic markers, fluorescence in situ hybridization for *EWSR1* rearrangement can be helpful when this differential diagnosis is otherwise difficult to resolve.

Molecular Genetics

Malignant GNET is a translocation-associated tumor, with *EWSR1-ATF1* and *EWSR1-CREB1* fusion genes in approximately 90% of cases caused by t(12;22)(q13;q12) or t(2;22)(q34;q12), respectively. FISH for *EWSR1* rearrangement is useful to exclude a diagnosis of malignant melanoma.

Differential Diagnosis

Conventional clear cell sarcoma typically arises in tendons or aponeuroses of the extremities of young adults and rarely involves the GI tract. Clear cell sarcoma is characterized by epithelioid or spindle-shaped tumor cells (or both) with clear or pale eosinophilic cytoplasm, in a nested or fascicular growth pattern with a delicate fibrovascular stroma. The nested growth pattern is more prominent than in malignant GNET. Melanin pigmentation is rarely seen, and osteoclast-like giant cells are not typical, in contrast to malignant GNET. In addition to S-100 protein expression, the tumor cells express secondary melanocytic markers such as HMB45, MART1, tyrosinase, and MiTF. Tumors usually harbor a t(12;22)(q13;q12), similar to malignant GNET.

Metastatic melanoma is common in the small intestine. Given the morphologic and immunohistochemical overlap, malignant GNET may easily be mistaken for metastatic melanoma and vice versa. As noted, malignant GNET lacks expression of secondary melanocytic markers, but this can also be the case in some metastatic melanomas. Clinical correlation to determine if there is a history of melanoma at other sites is essential, and demonstration of *EWSR1* rearrangement can confirm the diagnosis of malignant GNET.

Monophasic synovial sarcoma rarely involves the GI tract, but when it does, it has a predilection for the stomach. The spindled tumor cells of synovial sarcoma typically have overlapping nuclei and less cytoplasm than those of malignant GNET and show a more uniform fascicular growth pattern without the heterogeneity of the former. By IHC, the tumor cells are negative for S-100 and instead show expression of keratin, epithelial membrane antigen (EMA), and TLE1. Identification of *SS18 (SYT)* rearrangement can help confirm the diagnosis in difficult cases.

Gastrointestinal stromal tumors showing mixed epithelioid and spindled cell morphology may mimic malignant GNET. However, pseudoglandular areas and osteoclast-like giant cells are not typical of GIST. IHC readily distinguishes the two tumor types; expression of KIT, DOG1, and CD34 is seen in virtually all GIST but not in malignant GNET. Focal S-100 expression is seen in a small subset of duodenal GIST.

Prognosis and Therapy

Malignant GNET pursues an aggressive clinical course in most cases and has a poor prognosis. Metastasis to lymph nodes and liver is common. A study with clinical follow-up for 12 patients showed 50% died of disease with a mean survival period of 32 months.

MALIGNANT NEUROECTODERMAL TUMOR—FACT SHEET

Definition

- Malignant neuroectodermal tumor

Incidence and Location

- Extremely rare; usually arises in the small intestine

Morbidity and Mortality

- Malignant tumors with frequent metastases and death from disease

Gender, Race, and Age Distribution

- No gender predilection
- Young to middle-aged adults

Clinical Features

- Pain, gastric outlet obstruction, bleeding, anemia, fever

Prognosis and Therapy

- Aggressive tumors with frequent metastasis

Malignant Neuroectodermal Tumor—Pathologic Features

Gross Findings

- Intramural, 2- to 15-cm, solid masses, often with hemorrhage or necrosis

Microscopic Findings

- Sheets of epithelioid, round or spindled cells
- Osteoclast-like giant cells in 50%
- Mixed growth patterns: sheets-like, pseudoglandular, pseudopapillary, or nested

Immunohistochemistry

- Positive for S-100
- Negative for secondary melanocytic markers, KIT, DOG1 (discovered on GIST1), and CD34

Molecular Genetics

- *EWSR1-ATF1* and *EWSR1-CREB1* fusion genes in 90%

Differential Diagnosis

- Gastrointestinal stromal tumor: especially myxoid or succinate dehydrogenase–deficient types: positive for KIT and DOG1
- Metastatic melanoma: may be positive for secondary melanocytic markers; lacks EWSR1 rearrangement
- Conventional clear cell sarcoma: rarely involves the gastrointestinal tract; more prominent nested growth pattern; also expresses HMB45 (human melanoma black), MART1, tyrosinase
- Synovial sarcoma: more uniform fascicular growth pattern; lacks osteoclast-like giant cells; positive for EMA and TLE1; *SS18* gene rearrangement

INFLAMMATORY FIBROID POLYP

CLINICAL FEATURES

Inflammatory fibroid polyp is a benign tumor that most commonly arises in the gastric antrum or ileum and rarely in other intestinal locations. Patients usually present in their sixth decade, and there is a slight female predominance. Large gastric tumors can cause abdominal pain, gastric outlet obstruction, and GI bleeding, and large intestinal tumors commonly cause intussusception, often requiring emergent surgery. Smaller tumors can be found incidentally during endoscopy.

Radiologic and Endoscopic Features

Endoscopically, there may be a small polypoid mass or a larger mass bulging into the lumen, with or without mucosal ulceration.

Pathologic Features

Gross Findings

Gastric tumors are typically small (<3 cm) polypoid masses; small intestinal tumors tend to be larger (3 to >10 cm). They involve the lamina propria or submucosa and can extend into muscularis propria or serosa. The cut surface appears glistening and fleshy, consistent with the edematous stroma microscopically.

Microscopic Findings

Tumors exhibit a diffuse growth pattern of stellate, ovoid or short spindled fibroblastic cells, most commonly in an edematous or myxoid stroma (Fig. 7.22). Sometimes the stroma can appear more collagenous, and some tumors exhibit perivascular onion-skinning fibrosis. Inflammatory fibroid polyp is usually hypocellular, and neoplastic cells have at most minimal atypia. The lesion can resemble a non-neoplastic inflammatory lesion. Mitotic activity is low or absent. There are frequently admixed eosinophils, a useful diagnostic clue, as well as lymphocytes and histiocytes (Fig. 7.23A).

Ancillary Studies

Immunohistochemistry

Neoplastic cells are positive for CD34 and, in 20 % of cases, SMA. They are virtually always negative for KIT, DOG1, desmin, and S-100, which can be useful to exclude histologic mimics. IHC for PDGFRA, when available, is helpful as it is diffusely positive in essentially all inflammatory fibroid polyps; because background stromal cells express PDGFRA at lower levels, it is important to only interpret strong diffuse positivity as a positive result (Fig. 7.23B).

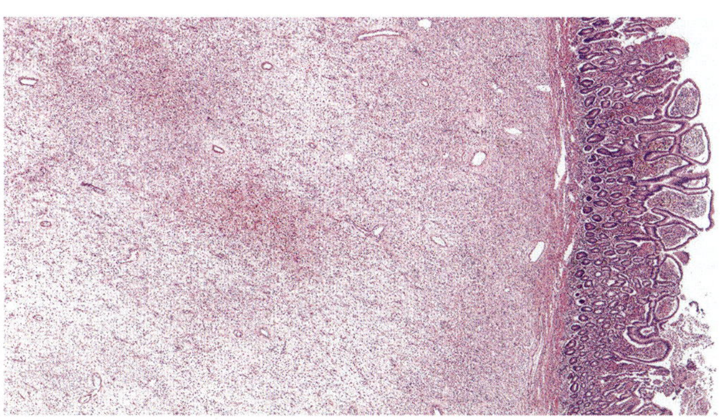

FIGURE 7.22

Inflammatory fibroid polyp. Inflammatory fibroid polyp commonly occurs in the stomach and small intestine. When tumors arise in the small intestine, patients frequently present with intussusception, as happened with this ileal tumor. At low power, this tumor contains scattered vessels in an edematous stroma.

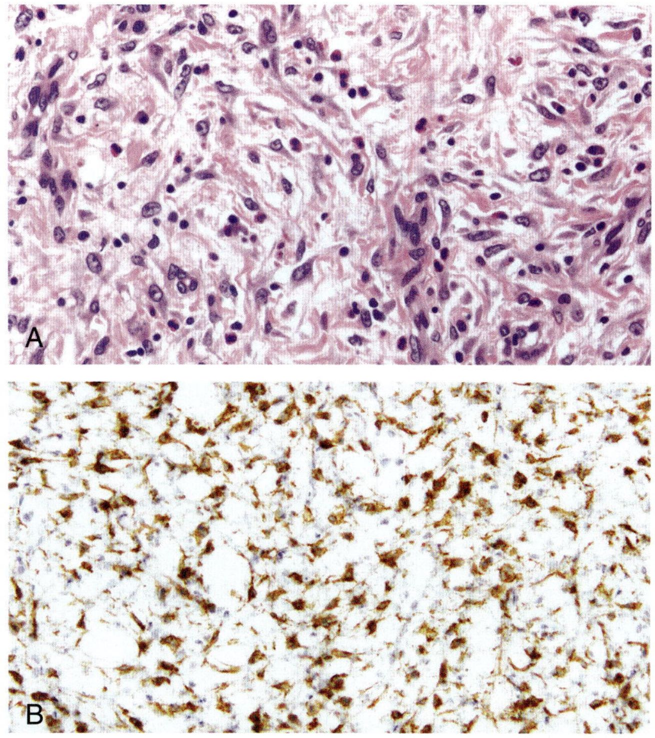

FIGURE 7.23

Inflammatory fibroid polyp. **A**, At higher power, neoplastic cells are stellate, with vesicular nuclei and small nucleoli. There are admixed eosinophils, a useful diagnostic clue when present. **B**, The tumor cells typically show strong diffuse expression of platelet-derived growth factor receptor-α (PDGFRA), reflecting the presence of *PDGFRA* mutations.

Molecular Studies

Inflammatory fibroid polyp harbors mutations in *PDGFRA*, including some of the same mutations present in *PDGFRA*-mutant GIST. The exonic mutations correlate with tumor location, with mutations in exon 12 more commonly occurring in small intestinal tumors and exon 18 more commonly occurring in gastric tumors.

Differential Diagnosis

Myxoid GIST can appear similar to inflammatory fibroid polyp but is typically more densely cellular and lacks an eosinophil-rich inflammatory infiltrate. Many myxoid GISTs are PDGFRA mutant, such that PDGFRA IHC is not useful to resolve this differential diagnosis. However, in contrast to inflammatory fibroid polyp, the tumor cells of GIST are positive for KIT and DOG1.

Plexiform fibromyxoma arises in the gastric antrum, but in contrast to inflammatory fibroid polyp, it exhibits a multinodular or plexiform growth pattern and is predominantly located in the muscularis propria. Although plexiform fibromyxoma is also composed of bland spindle cells, it does not have the eosinophil-rich inflammatory infiltrate characteristic of inflammatory fibroid polyp. IHC for PDGFRA can be used to distinguish these entities.

Inflammatory myofibroblastic tumor (IMT) also contains an inflammatory infiltrate, but its neoplastic cells exhibit a fascicular growth pattern. IHC for PDGFRA and anaplastic lymphoma kinase (ALK) can discriminate between these tumor types.

Prognosis and Therapy

Complete excision is curative. Very rarely, inflammatory fibroid polyp occurs in the inherited Devon polyposis syndrome.

INFLAMMATORY FIBROID POLYP—FACT SHEET

Definition

- Benign fibroblastic proliferation that commonly manifests as a gastric antral polyp or an intestinal mass causing intussusception

Incidence and Location

- Rare tumor that typically arises in the lamina propria/submucosa of the gastric antrum, ileum, or, less commonly, other intestinal sites

Morbidity and Mortality

- Inflammatory fibroid polyps are benign and only rarely occur in a familial syndromic setting (Devon polyposis syndrome)

Gender, Race, and Age Distribution

- Slight female predominance
- Wide age range, with peak in the sixth decade of life

Clinical Features

- Gastric tumors sometimes present with pain, gastric outlet obstruction, or bleeding
- Small intestinal tumors can present with intussusception
- Small tumors can be incidentally found during endoscopy

Prognosis and Therapy

- Benign and cured by simple excision

Inflammatory Fibroid Polyp—Pathologic Features

Gross Findings

- Wide size range (1–>10 cm); gastric tumors tend to be smaller than intestinal tumors
- Uniform fleshy or glistening cut surface

Microscopic Findings

- Submucosal location, sometimes with infiltration into the muscularis propria
- Hypocellular neoplasm with edematous or myxoid stroma rich in eosinophils
- Bland stellate, ovoid, or short spindled neoplastic cells
- Perivascular onion-skinning fibrosis is common

Immunohistochemistry

- Positive for CD34, platelet-derived growth factor receptor-α (PDGFRA), and smooth muscle actin (20%)
- Negative for S-100, KIT, DOG1 (discovered on GIST1), and desmin

Molecular Genetics

- Mutations in *PDGFRA* gene, with a different but somewhat overlapping exonic distribution compared with *PDGFRA*-mutant gastrointestinal stromal tumor (GIST)

Differential Diagnosis

- GIST: especially myxoid or *PDGFRA*-mutant GIST, which is usually more cellular; positive for KIT and DOG1; both inflammatory fibroid polyp and *PDGFRA*-mutant GIST are positive for PDGFRA
- Plexiform fibromyxoma: usually intramural rather than submucosal, has plexiform growth, lacks prominent inflammatory infiltrate
- Inflammatory myofibroblastic tumor: more cellular, with fascicles of neoplastic myofibroblasts; negative for PDGFRA, 50% positive for anaplastic lymphoma kinase

PLEXIFORM FIBROMYXOMA

CLINICAL FEATURES

Plexiform fibromyxoma is a benign tumor that virtually always arises in stomach, most often at the gastric antrum. Very rare cases arise in the small intestine. Patients are usually in their fifth decade, and there is no gender predilection. Presenting symptoms include abdominal pain, gastric outlet obstruction, and GI bleeding.

Radiologic and Endoscopic Features

Endoscopically, there may be a bulging mass into the gastric lumen, with or without mucosal ulceration.

Pathologic Features

Gross Findings

Tumors usually measure between 2 and 15 cm. They are typically intramural but may extend into mucosa or serosa. Tumors are lobulated and the cut surface variably red, tan, or white, with a gelatinous and glistening appearance because of the myxoid stroma.

Microscopic Findings

Tumors arise within the muscularis propria and show a multinodular or plexiform growth pattern on low power examination, resulting in separation of smooth muscle bundles (Fig. 7.24). The nodules are relatively hypocellular and contain bland oval-spindled tumor cells with at most minimal atypia, within a variably myxoid and collagenous stroma (Fig. 7.25). There is typically a prominent capillary proliferation. The tumor cells have indistinct cytoplasm and small nuclei. Mitotic activity is low or absent. Extension into mucosa may result in mucosal ulceration. Subserosal or serosal tumor nodules may be present.

Ancillary Studies

Immunohistochemistry

The immunoprofile is nonspecific: the spindled cells express SMA, either diffusely or focally, and are virtually always negative for KIT, DOG1, CD34, and S-100 protein. Focal expression of desmin or caldesmon has been reported in a small subset of tumors. IHC may be helpful to exclude histologic mimics.

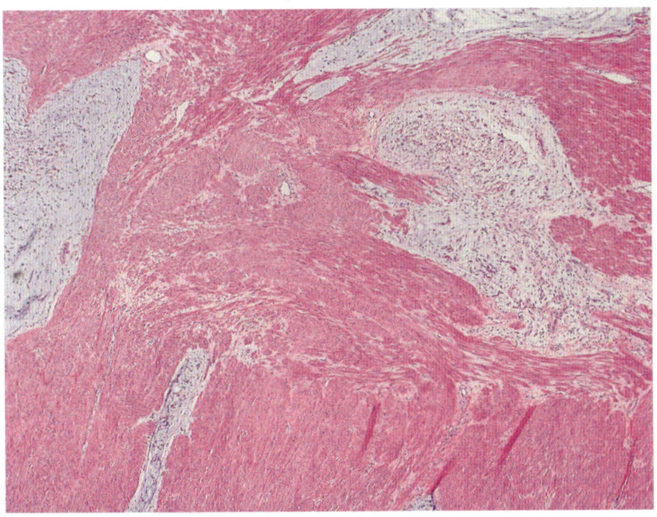

FIGURE 7.24

Plexiform fibromyxoma. Plexiform fibromyxoma has a characteristic plexiform growth pattern and is composed of bland fibroblastic cells in a variably myxoid or collagenous stroma.

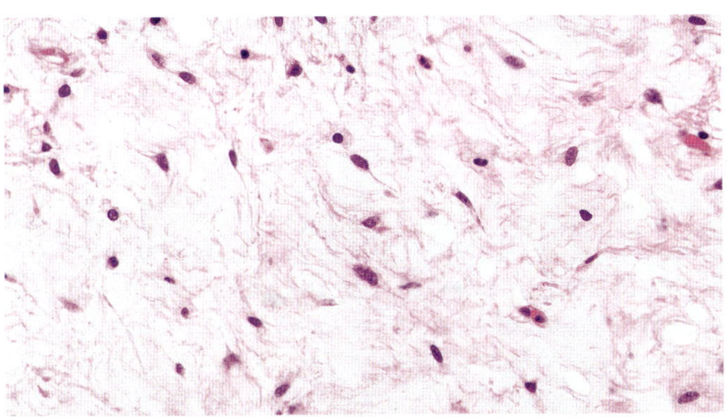

FIGURE 7.25

Plexiform fibromyxoma cytomorphology. Neoplastic cells in this tumor appear myofibroblastic, with eosinophilic cytoplasm and cytoplasmic tails.

Molecular Studies

A subset of tumors harbor *MALAT1-GLI1* fusion, *GLI1* polysomy, or *PTCH1* loss, all of which are expected to activate the hedgehog pathway.

Differential Diagnosis

Purely myxoid GIST is uncommon but can mimic plexiform fibromyxoma. Myxoid GIST lacks the multinodular or plexiform growth pattern of plexiform fibromyxoma and is composed of a uniform proliferation of spindled or epithelioid tumor cells. Many myxoid GIST are PDGFRA mutant. SDH-deficient GIST also shows a plexiform growth pattern but is less often myxoid and is usually more cellular, and the tumor cells are usually epithelioid. Unlike plexiform fibromyxoma, tumor cells of GIST are positive for KIT, DOG1, and CD34. Additional IHC for SDHB can confirm a diagnosis of SDH-deficient GIST.

Inflammatory fibroid polyp also arises in the gastric antrum but in contrast to plexiform fibromyxoma is predominantly submucosal in location. Inflammatory fibroid polyp is also composed of bland spindle cells, but the cells form a characteristic "onion-skin" pattern of condensation around blood vessels, and the tumor lacks a plexiform growth pattern. In addition, the characteristic inflammatory infiltrate associated with inflammatory fibroid polyp is not present in plexiform fibromyxoma.

Desmoid fibromatosis lacks a multinodular or plexiform growth pattern and is composed of more uniformly cellular long fascicles of bland spindled cells with small nucleoli and variable amounts of palely eosinophilic cytoplasm. IHC for β-catenin, which shows nuclear expression in 70% to 80% of desmoid fibromatoses can be helpful in making this distinction.

Prognosis and Therapy

Complete excision is curative. Vascular invasion is often present and has no apparent significance; metastasis has not been described.

PLEXIFORM FIBROMYXOMA–FACT SHEET

Definition

- Benign fibroblastic proliferation with a multinodular growth pattern and myxoid stroma

Incidence and Location

- Rare tumor that typically arises in the gastric antrum

Morbidity and Mortality

- Plexiform fibromyxomas are benign and not syndromic

Gender, Race, and Age Distribution

- No gender predilection
- Most common in adults in fifth decade of life

Clinical Features

- Pain, gastric outlet obstruction, bleeding

Prognosis and Therapy

- Benign and cured by simple excision

PLEXIFORM FIBROMYXOMA–PATHOLOGIC FEATURES

Gross Findings

- Intramural, nodular, 2 to 15 cm

Microscopic Findings

- Multinodular or plexiform lesion
- Bland spindle cells with no or minimal atypia
- Prominent capillary proliferation
- Variably myxoid and collagenous stroma

Immunohistochemistry

- Positive for smooth muscle actin
- Negative for S-100, KIT, DOG1 (discovered on GIST1), and CD34

Molecular Genetics

- Hedgehog pathway activation through *MALAT1-GLI1* fusion, *GLI1* polysomy, or *PTCH1* inactivation in subset of cases

Differential Diagnosis

- Gastrointestinal stromal tumor: especially myxoid or succinate dehydrogenase–deficient types, usually more cellular; positive for KIT and DOG1
- Inflammatory fibroid polyp: lacks plexiform growth; shows perivascular condensation of spindled cells and a prominent inflammatory infiltrate
- Desmoid fibromatosis: long sweeping fascicles, nuclear β-catenin expression in 70% to 80%

CALCIFYING FIBROUS TUMOR

CLINICAL FEATURES

Calcifying fibrous tumor is a rare benign mesenchymal lesion that typically involves serosal surfaces (pleura, peritoneum), but it can also arise in viscera and soft tissue. Within the GI tract, the most common site of involvement is the small intestine followed by colon and stomach. Most tumors are either submucosal or mesenteric, with a smaller number being serosal. Peritoneal tumors may be multifocal.

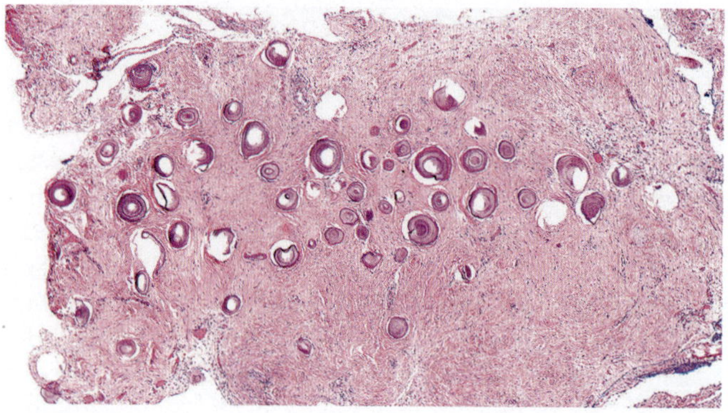

FIGURE 7.26

Calcifying fibrous tumor. This example contains numerous psammomatous calcifications in a hypocellular collagenous stroma.

There is a wide age range, there is no gender predilection, and tumors are rarely familial (usually multiple lesions in young adults). Presenting symptoms depend on the site and depth of involvement but include pain, obstruction, and intussusception. Small tumors are often detected incidentally. These are benign lesions, and recurrence is rare.

MICROSCOPIC FINDINGS

Histologically these tumors are usually paucicellular and have abundant hyalinized collagen. The lesional cells are bland spindled CD34 positive fibroblasts. A plasma cell infiltrate is common. Dystrophic or psammomatous calcifications are present in most cases (Fig. 7.26), but 20 % lack calcifications, making recognition difficult. IHC is helpful to exclude other tumors that may fall into the differential diagnosis, particularly GIST, schwannoma, and IMT.

SCHWANNOMA OF THE GASTROINTESTINAL TRACT

CLINICAL FEATURES

Schwannomas are benign nerve sheath tumors, and when located in the GI tract, they harbor features distinctive from schwannomas occurring at other sites. Almost all schwannomas of the GI tract arise in the stomach and involve the submucosa and muscularis propria. Rare cases involve the colon. Tumors usually occur in middle-aged or older adults (50–70 years). Gastric schwannomas are more common in women than men and present with symptoms of upper GI tract bleeding, abdominal pain, or obstructive symptoms. Colonic cases may be detected incidentally or may present with lower GI tract bleeding. There is no known association between isolated schwannoma of the GI tract and neurofibromatosis.

Radiologic and Endoscopic Features

Gastric schwannomas are usually not distinguishable from GISTs by imaging. Endoscopically, there is a submucosal mass with or without overlying mucosal ulceration.

Pathologic Features

Gross Findings

Tumors are well circumscribed and have a yellow fleshy cut surface. Cystic change may be present. The average size is 3 cm, with a range of 0.5 to 11 cm.

Microscopic Findings

Gastrointestinal tract schwannomas are not encapsulated and there is a peripheral cuff of lymphocytes, which may show germinal center formation. There may also be intratumoral lymphocytes, scattered plasma cells, and aggregates of foamy histiocytes. Tumors have a fascicular or whorled growth pattern of spindled cells with tapering nuclei, uniform fine chromatin with a small nucleolus and indistinct pale cytoplasm. (Figs. 7.27 to 7.30). Nuclear typia may be present but is usually mild and degenerative in nature. Mitotic activity is low, and necrosis is not

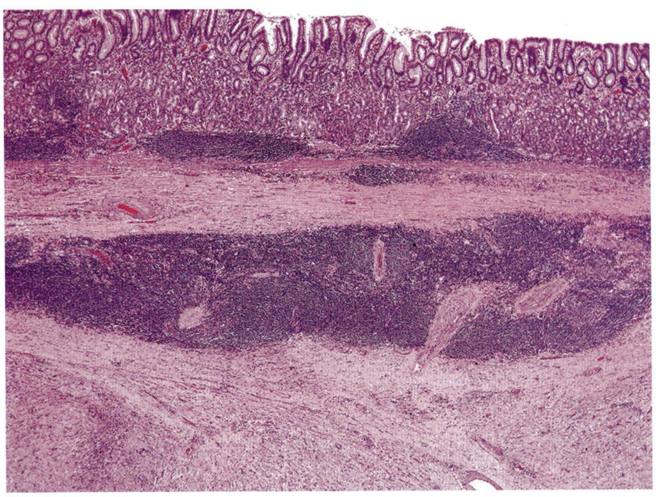

FIGURE 7.27
Gastric schwannoma. Note the striking lymphoid cuff at low magnification, a helpful diagnostic feature.

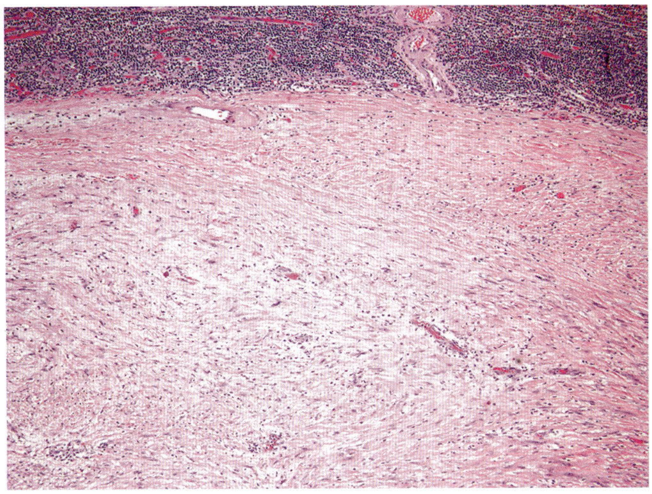

FIGURE 7.28
Gastric schwannoma. The cellularity is usually moderate, with mild atypia on low power.

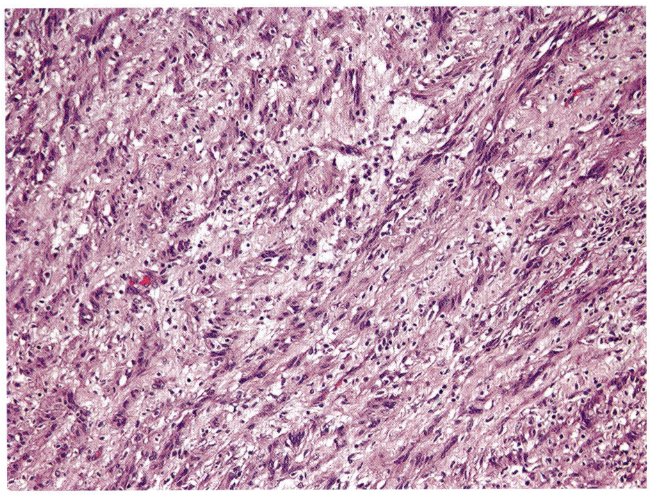

FIGURE 7.29
Gastric schwannoma. At intermediate magnification, a lymphocytic infiltrate is apparent.

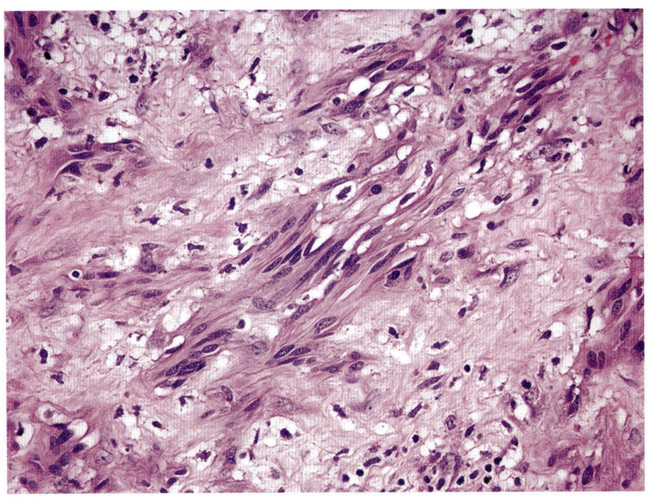

FIGURE 7.30
Gastric schwannoma cytomorphology. Neoplastic cells have palely eosinophilic, fibrillary cytoplasm, and nuclei with tapered ends.

present. Additional distinguishing features from conventional schwannoma are less conspicuous thick-walled or hyaline vessels and an absence of nuclear palisading and Verocay bodies. Finally, schwannomas of the GI tract lack alternating Antoni A and B patterns and instead tend to be uniformly cellular. The tumor stroma is usually collagenous and may show myxoid change.

Ancillary Studies

Immunohistochemistry

Diffuse strong expression of S-100 protein and SOX10 is characteristic (Fig. 7.31). Focal expression of CD34 and GFAP may be present. Schwannomas of the GI tract lack an EMA-positive capsule. Schwannoma is negative for KIT, DOG1, secondary melanocytic markers, keratins, and desmin.

Molecular Studies

Gastric schwannomas lack alterations in the *NF2* gene, in contrast to somatic soft tissue schwannomas; instead, about half of the cases exhibit *NF1* inactivation.

Differential Diagnosis

Particularly in small biopsies, the morphologic differential diagnosis of schwannoma includes GIST, metastatic melanoma, and clear cell sarcoma-like tumor of the GI tract/malignant GNET. IMT and smooth muscle neoplasms may also show some histologic similarities to schwannoma.

Gastrointestinal stromal tumors also arise in the muscularis propria but lack a peripheral lymphoid cuff. The tumor cells may be spindled or epithelioid and are usually more monotonous than the tumor cells of schwannoma. IHC is helpful in this differential diagnosis; the tumor cells of GIST are positive for KIT and DOG1 in 95% of cases.

Metastatic melanoma frequently involves the GI tract and usually presents as a well-circumscribed intramucosal nodule. Melanoma typically shows marked cytologic pleomorphism, nuclear atypia, and high mitotic activity and lacks a peripheral lymphoid cuff. Although the tumor cells of both lesions have diffuse expression of S-100, in contrast to schwannoma, melanoma shows expression of second-line melanocytic markers, such as HMB45 and Melan-A/MART1.

Malignant GNET/CCS-like tumor of the GI tract may potentially mimic gastric schwannoma, particularly because both show diffuse S-100 positivity. However, malignant GNET shows infiltrative growth; a mixed nested, sheet-like, and pseudoglandular growth patterns; and greater cytologic atypia. Identification of *EWSR1* gene rearrangement helps confirm this diagnosis.

Inflammatory myofibroblastic tumor may mimic schwannoma in that it is also a fascicular spindle cell neoplasm with a prominent inflammatory infiltrate. IMT is usually less circumscribed and lacks a peripheral lymphoid cuff, but because these features cannot be evaluated in small biopsies, IHC is particularly helpful. The tumor cells express SMA, desmin, and ALK (50% of tumors) and are negative for S-100 and SOX10.

Pure smooth muscle tumors are very rare in the stomach. The tumor cells have brightly eosinophilic cytoplasm, and the nuclei are blunt ended, unlike the buckled wavy and tapering nuclei of schwannoma cells. The tumor cells express SMA, desmin, and caldesmon and are negative for S-100 and SOX10. Neurofibroma is exceptionally rare in the stomach. It is composed of a mixed population of Schwann cells, perineural cells, and fibroblasts, which is reflected in the more heterogeneous staining pattern for S-100, EMA, and CD34. There is a syndromic association with NF1.

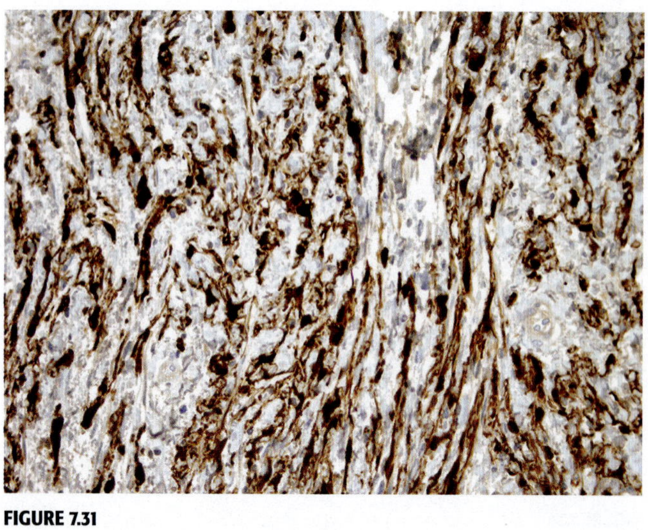

FIGURE 7.31
Gastric schwannoma. There is diffuse nuclear and cytoplasmic S-100 protein expression.

Prognosis and Therapy

Gastrointestinal schwannomas are benign, and excision is curative.

SCHWANNOMA OF THE GASTROINTESTINAL TRACT—FACT SHEET

Definition

- Benign nerve sheath tumors that differ from schwannoma of other sites by the absence of a capsule, absence of Antoni A and B zonation, and presence of a prominent peripheral lymphocytic infiltrate

Incidence and Location

- Rare and usually arise in the gastric wall

Gender, Race, and Age Distribution

- Occur in adults
- Gastric schwannomas are more common in women

Clinical Features

- Site specific, often incidental
- May present with symptoms of gastrointestinal tract bleeding or obstruction

Prognosis and Therapy

- Benign and treated by simple excision
- No syndromic associations

SCHWANNOMA OF THE GASTROINTESTINAL TRACT—PATHOLOGIC FEATURES

Gross Findings

- Well circumscribed but not encapsulated, in contrast to most schwannomas at other sites
- Generally intramural in the stomach and polypoid in the colon

Microscopic Findings

- Unencapsulated uniformly cellular spindle cell neoplasm
- Tumor cells have indistinct pale cytoplasm and tapering nuclei with uniform fine chromatin and small nucleoli
- Striking lymphoid cuff at periphery of tumor
- Lack palisading, hyalinized vessels, and alternating Antoni A and B zonation

Immunohistochemistry

- Strong diffuse S-100 protein and SOX10
- May be positive for CD34
- Negative for KIT, desmin, and caldesmon

Differential Diagnosis

- Gastrointestinal stromal tumor: lacks a lymphoid cuff and is more likely to show palisading; positive for KIT and DOG1 (discovered on GIST1), usually negative for S-100
- Metastatic melanoma: greater cytologic atypia, may have epithelioid as well as spindled morphology, and lacks a lymphoid cuff; secondary melanocytic markers (HMB45 [human melanoma black], MART1) are positive
- Malignant gastrointestinal neuroectodermal tumor: infiltrative; heterogenous growth pattern; *EWSR1* gene rearrangement
- IMT: less circumscribed; variable expression of smooth muscle actin (SMA), desmin, and anaplastic lymphoma kinase; negative for S-100 and SOX10
- Smooth muscle tumors: very rare in the stomach; tumor cells have brightly eosinophilic cytoplasm, and the nuclei are blunt ended; express SMA and desmin and are negative for S-100 and SOX10

MUCOSAL PERINEURIOMA ("BENIGN FIBROBLASTIC POLYP")

CLINICAL FEATURES

Mucosal perineurioma is a benign nerve sheath tumor showing perineurial cell differentiation. Although most present as small intramucosal polyps, occasional cases involve the submucosa and are similar to perineurioma of soft tissue. Tumors can arise in the colon or small intestine, but most are colonic and occur in the rectosigmoid region and are typically identified during screening colonoscopy. The tumor shows a female predominance, and patients are usually in their sixth decade. Most lesions previously described as "benign fibroblastic polyp of the colon" represent perineuriomas.

ENDOSCOPIC FEATURES

Colonic mucosal perineuriomas are small and sessile polyps, usually around 0.4 cm in greatest dimension. Submucosal lesions may be significantly larger, in the range of 3 to 5 cm.

PATHOLOGIC FEATURES

GROSS FINDINGS

The tumors often present as colonic polyps with size ranging from 0.2 to 0.6 cm (median, 0.4 cm). Rarely, tumors arise as submucosal masses and may be significantly larger, between 3 and 5 cm. The cut surface of larger tumors is well circumscribed and has a white, solid, myxoid appearance without necrosis.

MICROSCOPIC FINDINGS

The lesion is composed of a monotonous population of bland spindle cells with oval to elongated nuclei and pale eosinophilic cytoplasm (Figs. 7.32 and 7.33). Elongated cytoplasmic processes may be seen by hematoxylin and

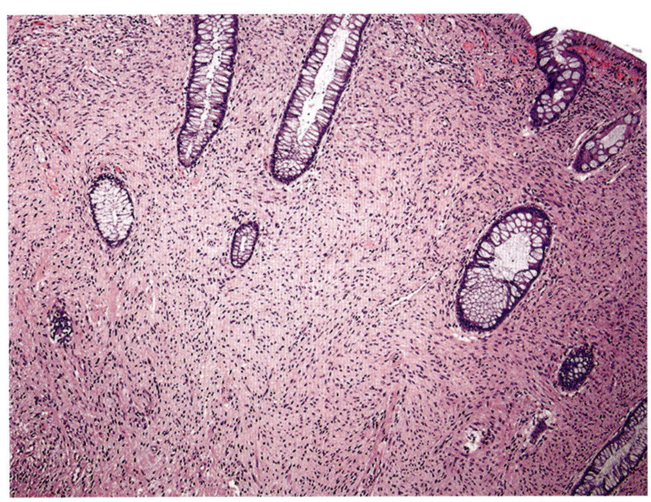

FIGURE 7.32

Mucosal perineurioma of the colon. The proliferating cells expand the lamina propria.

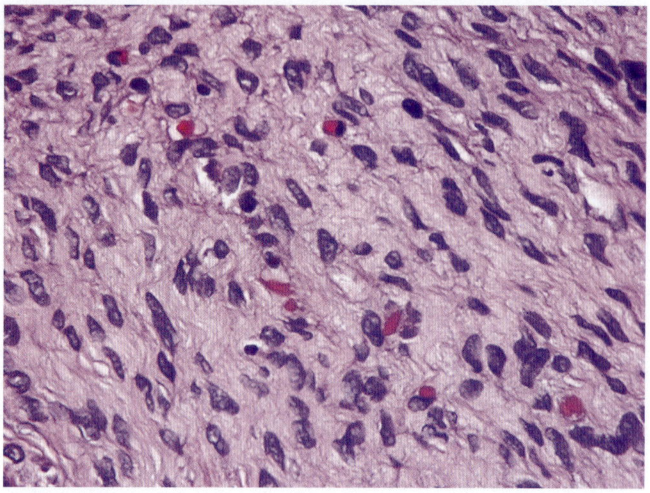

FIGURE 7.33

Higher magnification of a mucosal perineurioma of the colon. The cells have pale eosinophilic cytoplasm and bland nuclei.

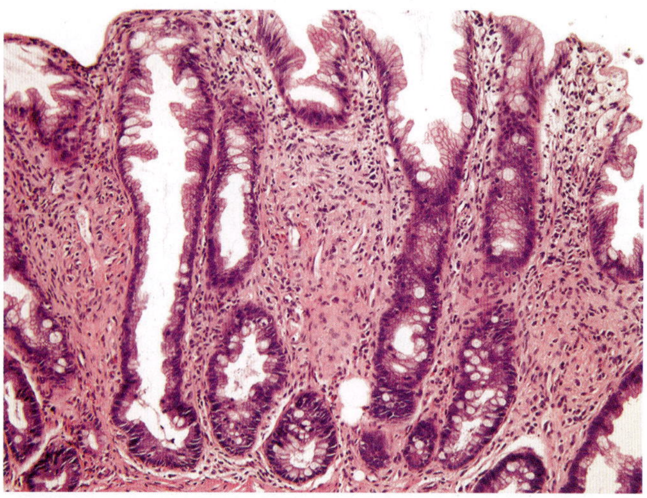

FIGURE 7.34

Mucosal perineuriomas are frequently associated with serrated polyps.

eosin but are highlighted by immunohistochemical stains EMA and CD34. The cells grow in a whorled pattern, entrapping colonic crypts. The stroma is collagenous. There is generally no cytologic atypia, necrosis, or mitotic activity. The adjacent crypt epithelium may show hyperplastic change (Fig. 7.34), or the perineural proliferation may be present in association with a serrated polyp, either hyperplastic polyp or sessile serrated polyp, in which case it seems to be a secondary process induced by the epithelial proliferation.

Ancillary Studies

Immunohistochemistry

Perineurioma shows expression of markers of perineural differentiation: EMA, claudin-1, and CD34. Expression of the latter two may be variable in extent. The cells do not express S-100, GFAP, SMA, CD117/KIT, or pan-keratin.

Differential Diagnosis

The differential diagnosis includes Schwann cell hamartoma, ganglioneuroma, neurofibroma, and leiomyoma.

Schwann cell hamartoma may be very difficult to distinguish morphologically from perineurioma, but Schwann cells are plumper and lack the long cytoplasmic processes of perineurial cells. IHC readily distinguishes the two: whereas Schwann cell hamartoma shows diffuse expression of S-100, perineurioma is negative.

Ganglioneuroma is distinguished by the presence of ganglion cells and admixed Schwann cells, both of which are S-100 positive, as well as neurofilament protein (NFP) positive axons.

Neurofibroma of the GI tract is extremely rare and is highly associated with NF1. Most mucosal lesions previously classified as neurofibroma likely represent Schwann cell hamartomas. Neurofibroma is composed of a mixed population of Schwann cells, perineurial cells, fibroblasts, and axons; this mixed population of cell types is reflected in the immunohistochemical profile, with expression of S-100, NFP, and EMA.

Leiomyoma also presents a small polypoid lesion in the colon but is usually readily distinguished by obvious smooth muscle differentiation—bright eosinophilic cytoplasm and cigar-shaped nuclei, as well as positivity for SMA, desmin, and caldesmon.

Prognosis and Therapy

Mucosal perineurioma is a benign tumor; local recurrences after excision or polypectomy have not been reported.

MUCOSAL PERINEURIOMA—FACT SHEET

Definition

- Benign nerve sheath tumor composed of perineurial cells

Incidence and Location

- Tumor arises in the colon and less often the small intestine
- Most common location is the rectosigmoid region

Gender, Race, and Age Distribution

- Female predominance
- Median age is 51 years

Clinical Features

- Usually incidentally detected during colonoscopy

Prognosis and Therapy

- Benign tumor; excision is curative

MUCOSAL PERINEURIOMA—PATHOLOGIC FEATURES

Gross Findings

- Present as small colonic polyps or as intramural mass arising in submucosa of the colorectum or, rarely, the small bowel

Microscopic Findings

- Proliferation of bland spindle cells centered in the lamina propria, muscularis mucosae, and superficial submucosa, sometimes with adjacent serrated polyp

Immunohistochemistry

- Tumor cells express epithelial membrane antigen, claudin-1, and CD34, the latter two sometimes variably in extent

Differential Diagnosis

- Mucosal Schwann cell hamartoma: plumper cells; S-100 positive
- Ganglioneuroma: mixed population of cells including S-100–positive ganglion and Schwann cells
- Neurofibroma: mixed population of Schwann cell, perineurial cells, fibroblasts, and axons
- Leiomyoma: bright eosinophilic cytoplasm; smooth muscle actin and desmin positive

MUCOSAL SCHWANN CELL HAMARTOMA

CLINICAL FEATURES

This benign intramucosal Schwann cell proliferation differs from schwannoma, perineurioma, and neurofibroma. It is a sporadic rather than syndromic lesion. These lesions arise in the colon and are usually detected during screening endoscopy; the lesion appears as a small (<1 cm) polyp. The mean age at presentation is about 60 years, and there is a slight female predominance.

PATHOLOGIC FEATURES

MICROSCOPIC FINDINGS

These mucosal lesions are variably circumscribed, and the spindle cells usually show entrapment of colonic crypts (Fig. 7.35). The cells are spindled to ovoid and tend to be plumper than perineurial cells, which they may otherwise resemble. The cells show Schwannian morphology in that they have wavy nuclei, eosinophilic cytoplasm, and indistinct cell borders. There is no cytologic atypia or pleomorphism, and mitoses are generally not seen.

The relationship between Schwann cell hamartoma and GI schwannoma is unclear, but the differing histologic features favor classification as distinct entities. Although both lesions are composed of a pure population of Schwann cells, Schwann cell hamartoma lacks the circumscription, peritumoral lymphoid aggregates, dense collagenous stroma, and nuclear heterogeneity of GI schwannoma and usually presents as a small polypoid lesion in the colon, unlike GI schwannoma, which involves stomach and is submucosal or mural.

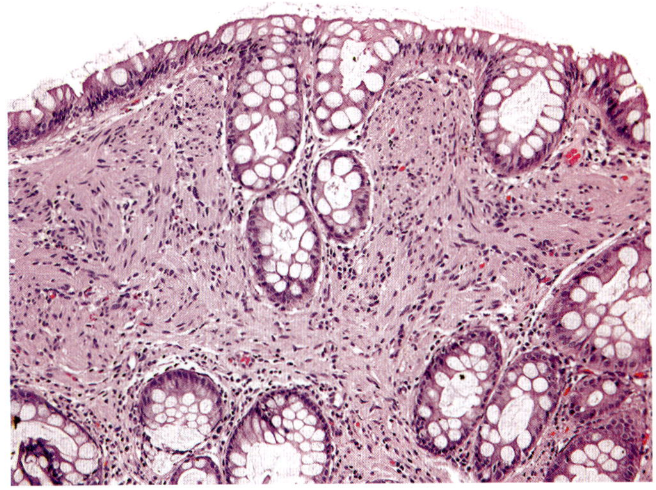

FIGURE 7.35

Mucosal Schwann cell hamartoma. Short fascicles of Schwann cells entrap colonic crypts. The lesional cells are spindled to ovoid with pale, fibrillary cytoplasm and no significant nuclear atypia.

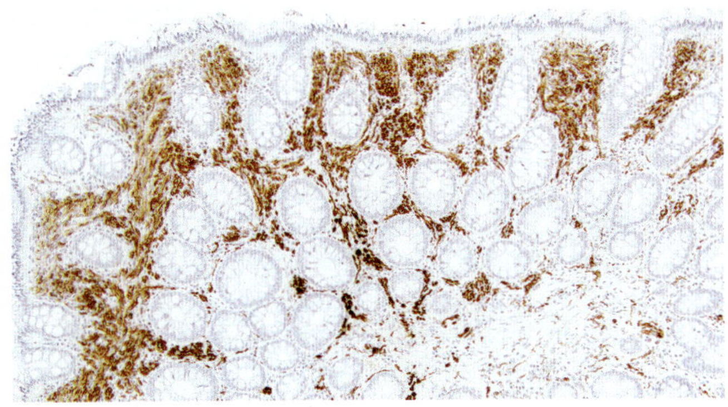

FIGURE 7.36

S-100 is diffusely positive in mucosal Schwann cell hamartoma and is negative in mucosal perineurioma, its closest differential diagnostic consideration.

ANCILLARY STUDIES

IMMUNOHISTOCHEMISTRY

Lesional cells show diffuse expression of S-100 protein, consistent with their Schwannian origin (Fig. 7.36). The cells are negative for KIT, CD34, EMA, claudin-1, and SMA.

DIFFERENTIAL DIAGNOSIS

Other mucosal benign nerve sheath tumors may mimic mucosal Schwann cell hamartoma. Mucosal perineurioma also shows entrapment of colonic crypts by bland spindle cells. Perineurial cells are less plump than those of Schwann cell hamartoma and have elongated cytoplasmic processes that are highlighted by CD34 and EMA. Expression of S-100 is not seen in perineurioma.

Mucosal neuroma occurs in the oral cavity in patients with multiple endocrine neoplasia IIb (MEN2B) on the lips or tongue and is extremely rare in the GI tract. Many Schwann cell hamartomas were previously classified as "neuroma," but true mucosal neuroma is composed of bundles of hyperplastic nerves with admixed axons, which are highlighted by NFP IHC.

Schwann cell hamartoma is distinguished from neurofibroma by the following features: (1) most neurofibromas of the GI tract are mural lesions involving submucosa or muscularis propria, which may extend into the overlying mucosa; (2) neurofibroma is composed of a mixed population of Schwann cell, perineurial-like cells, fibroblasts, and axons, in contrast to the single Schwann cell population of Schwann cell hamartoma; (3) expression of S-100 is present in only a subset of cells in neurofibroma, in contrast to the diffuse staining pattern seen in Schwann cell hamartoma; and (4) neurofibromas of the GI tract are strongly associated with NF1.

Polypoid ganglioneuroma may resemble mucosal Schwann cell hamartoma because there is usually a predominance of Schwann cells; however, ganglioneuroma also contains ganglion cells and axons.

Mucosal benign epithelioid nerve sheath tumor is a similar and possibly related lesion composed of Schwann cells with epithelioid features entrapping colonic crypts.

PROGNOSIS AND THERAPY

Schwann cell hamartoma is benign and managed by polypectomy.

MUCOSAL SCHWANN CELL HAMARTOMA—FACT SHEET

Definition
- Benign Schwann cell proliferation

Incidence and Location
- Rare; arises in colonic mucosa

Gender, Race, and Age Distribution
- Slight female predominance

Clinical Features
- Incidental finding, small (<1 cm) mucosal polyp

Prognosis and Therapy
- Benign tumor

MUCOSAL SCHWANN CELL HAMARTOMA—PATHOLOGIC FEATURES

Microscopic Findings
- Small proliferations of Schwann cells in the lamina propria that entrap colonic crypts

Immunohistochemistry
- Diffuse expression of S-100 protein
- Negative for C34, CD117, epithelial membrane antigen, smooth muscle actin, and claudin-1

Differential Diagnosis
- Perineurioma
- Neurofibroma
- Ganglioneuroma

GANGLIONEUROMA

CLINICAL FEATURES

Ganglioneuromas occur in two general settings: (1) sporadically as solitary lesions and (2) syndromically as multiple lesions either producing multiple exophytic polyps (ganglioneuromatous polyposis, Cowden syndrome) or poorly demarcated transmural proliferations (diffuse ganglioneuromatosis; MEN2B and NF1). For solitary cases, there is no gender predominance, and lesions occur in adults over a broad age range, with a peak incidence between 40 and 60 years. The majority are found in the colon, usually on the left side; are asymptomatic; and are detected during screening colonoscopy. Solitary lesions are not associated with genetic syndromes.

In contrast, ganglioneuromatous polyposis is associated with Cowden syndrome (PTEN hamartoma syndrome) and familial adenomatous polyposis (FAP), and diffuse ganglioneuromatosis is associated with MEN2B and with NF1 (von Recklinghausen's disease). Diffuse ganglioneuromatosis is found in virtually all patients with MEN2B and often antedates the development of the endocrine neoplasms. Patients with MEN2B and ganglioneuromatosis present with diverse GI symptoms, likely reflecting disruption of the myenteric plexus, including constipation, diarrhea, vomiting, and crampy abdominal pain. Most syndromic GI tract ganglioneuromas are found in the colorectum and in younger patients (mean age, ~35 years). Other conditions that have been reported to associate with ganglioneuromatosis include tuberous sclerosis and juvenile polyposis.

PATHOLOGIC FEATURES

GROSS FINDINGS

Polypoid isolated ganglioneuroma presents as a small sessile or pedunculated polyp (usually <2 cm) that grossly

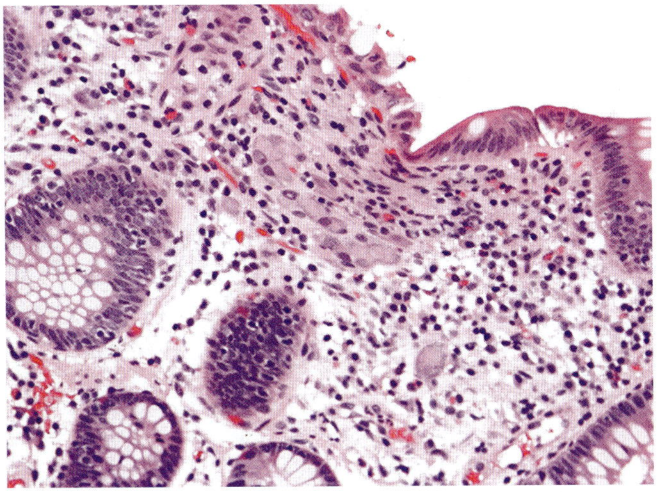

FIGURE 7.37
Ganglioneuroma. Ganglioneuroma is composed of spindled Schwann cells expanding the lamina propria, with admixed ganglion cells.

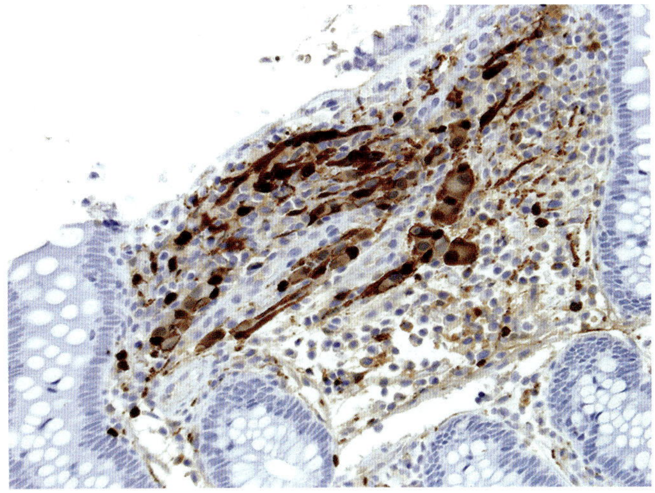

FIGURE 7.38
Ganglioneuroma immunohistochemistry. S-100 protein is diffusely positive in spindled Schwann cells and ganglion cells.

resembles juvenile polyp or adenoma. The polyps in ganglioneuromatous polyposis are multiple (20–40) and may be larger than sporadic cases. Diffuse ganglioneuromatosis results in a poorly demarcated mural thickening.

Microscopic Findings

Polypoid ganglioneuromas (sporadic or syndromic) are mucosal. They are poorly circumscribed and show an expanded lamina propria and entrapment of colonic crypts by a mixed population of spindled Schwann cells, axons, and ganglion cells, which may be clustered or present as scattered isolated cells (Fig. 7.37). Occasionally, polypoid lesions may extend into submucosa. In diffuse ganglioneuromatosis, the same mixed cell population is centered around the myenteric plexus.

Ancillary Studies

Immunohistochemistry

These lesions are easily diagnosed without IHC, but the spindle cells react with S-100 protein and GFAP (Fig. 7.38); the ganglion cells with S-100 protein, NSE, and synaptophysin; and axons with NFP.

Differential Diagnosis

The main mimics are mucosal Schwann cell hamartoma and neurofibroma. Schwann cell hamartoma lacks ganglion cells and is composed of a pure population of Schwann cells, which are also S-100 positive. Neurofibroma of the GI tract is very rare and is associated with NF1. Neurofibromas are composed of Schwann cells, perineurial cells, fibroblasts, and axons and show a correspondingly mixed immunoprofile with expression of S-100, NFP, and EMA.

Prognosis and Therapy

Sporadic isolated ganglioneuromas are treated by polypectomy and seldom recur. These polyps are not associated with MEN2B and NF1. Patients with syndromic ganglioneuromas must be carefully followed based on their specific syndromes. Multiple polypoid ganglioneuromas are associated with Cowden syndrome, whereas the diffuse type is most likely associated with NF1 and MEN2B. The latter may cause strictures requiring resection, but the ganglioneuromas themselves are benign. Patients with NF1 may develop other neural lesions, including malignant peripheral sheath tumors, and those with MEN2B may develop endocrine neoplasms.

GANGLIONEUROMA—FACT SHEET

Definition

- Ganglioneuromas are composed of a mixed population of S-100-positive Schwann cells, neurofilament protein–positive axons, and ganglion cells. Multiple lesions are usually syndromic

Incidence and Location

- Rare
- Majority arise in the left colon

Gender, Race, and Age Distribution

- No gender or racial predominance
- Syndromic lesions present at an earlier age (mean, 35 years) than sporadic examples (mean, 48 years)

Clinical Features

- Most polypoid lesions detected during routine colonoscopy
- Solitary lesions not associated with genetic syndromes
- Ganglioneuromatous polyposis associated with Cowden syndrome
- Diffuse ganglioneuromatosis associated with multiple endocrine neoplasia IIb and neurofibromatosis type 1
- Patients with ganglioneuromatosis present with diverse gastrointestinal symptoms

Prognosis and Therapy

- Benign
- Sporadic cases are treated by polypectomy
- Because diffuse ganglioneuromas may be transmural, there can be associated strictures requiring surgery

GANGLIONEUROMA—PATHOLOGIC FEATURES

Gross Findings

- Solitary or multiple mucosal polyps
- Diffuse lesions are transmural

Microscopic Findings

- Spindled Schwann cells with admixed ganglion cells
- In diffuse ganglioneuromatosis, the lesion is centered around the myenteric plexus

Immunohistochemistry

- Schwann cell population expresses S-100 and glial fibrillary acidic protein
- Ganglion cells express S-100, neuron-specific enolase, synaptophysin and axons stain with neurofilament protein

Differential Diagnosis

- Usually easy to recognize; lesions that have few ganglion cells may mimic neurofibromas

GANGLIOCYTIC PARAGANGLIOMA

CLINICAL FEATURES

These are rare tumors, the vast majority of which are found in the duodenum in adult patients (average age, 54 years). They typically arise in the ampullary region as polypoid submucosal masses. Extremely rare cases have been reported to occur in the jejunum, pylorus, colon, and appendix. The typical presentation is bleeding caused by overlying mucosal ulceration, but because of their ampullary location, some patients may present with painless jaundice. The majority of cases are sporadic, with a small subset being associated with neurofibromatosis.

PATHOLOGIC FEATURES

GROSS FINDINGS

These lesions are typically centered in the submucosa, with extension into the mucosa, and measure 3 to 4 cm in diameter. The cut surface is pale yellow, and they are usually soft in consistency. They have infiltrative borders.

MICROSCOPIC FINDINGS

Tumors are composed of three cell types: (1) spindled Schwann cells with eosinophilic cytoplasm arranged in fascicles or whorls; (2) ganglion cells with round nuclei and prominent nucleoli, scattered throughout the lesion or arranged in clusters; and (3) epithelioid neuroendocrine cells arranged in nests, trabeculae, or papillae. The proportion of the cell types is variable (Figs. 7.39 to 7.42). Psammomatous calcifications may be present.

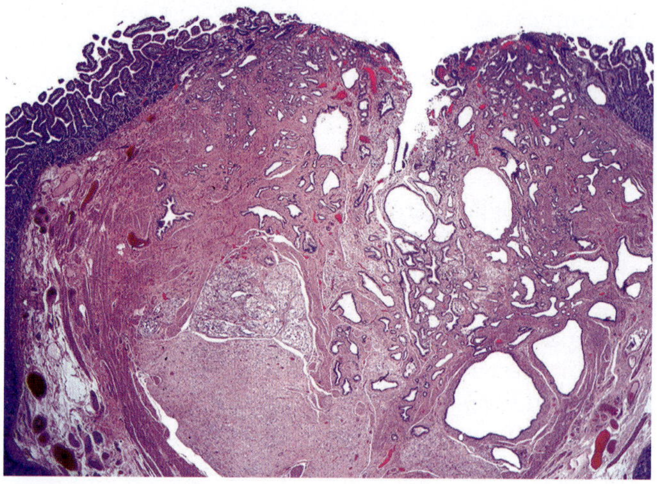

FIGURE 7.39

This gangliocytic paraganglioma arose in the ampulla. Disorganized ampullary (biliary type) glands are at the right side of the field; the lesion is at the lower left.

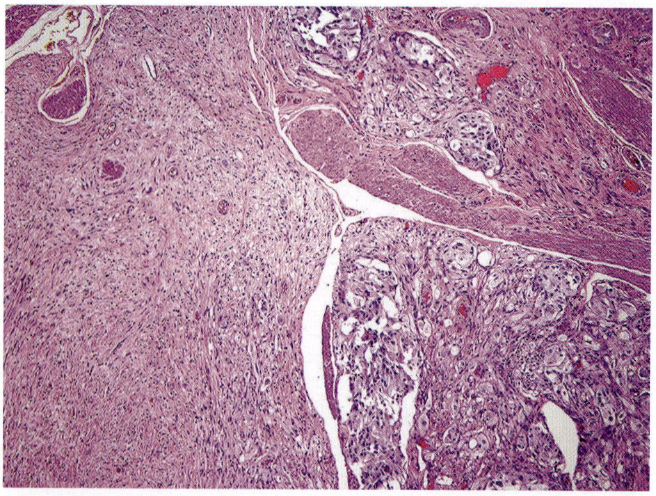

FIGURE 7.40

This gangliocytic paraganglioma shows spindle cells similar to those of a schwannoma, nests of epithelioid cells, and dysmorphic ganglion cells.

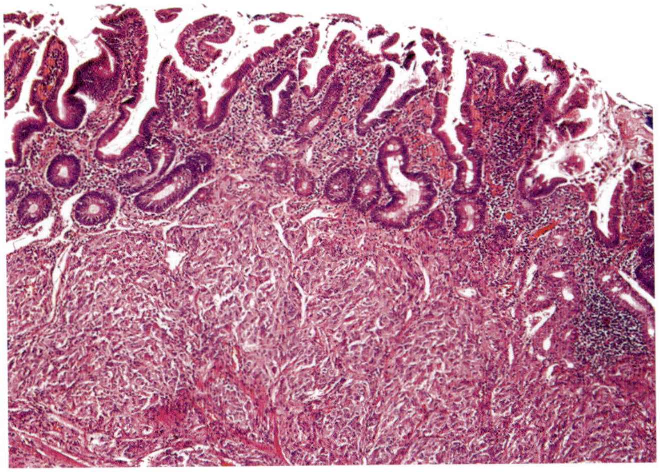

FIGURE 7.41

Epithelioid cells predominate in this gangliocytic paraganglioma; this lesion could be mistaken for a carcinoid tumor on a small mucosal biopsy.

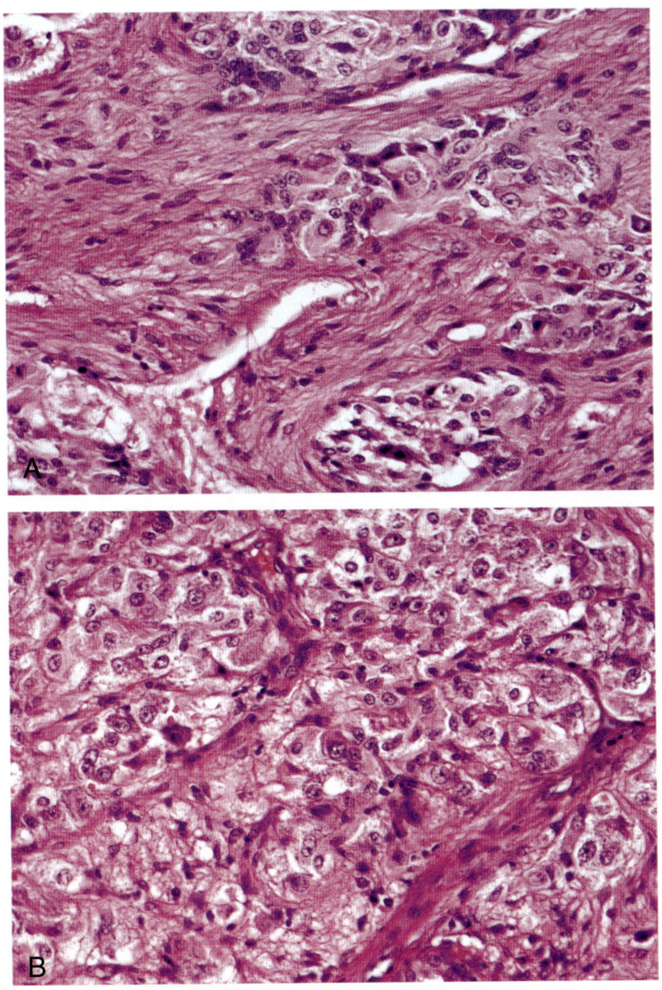

FIGURE 7.42

Gangliocytic paraganglioma. This field is from a more diagnostic area of the neoplasm depicted in Fig. 7.41. **A**, Numerous spindle cells. **B**, Epithelioid nests are predominant.

Ancillary Studies

Immunohistochemistry

Immunohistochemically, the tumors show S-100 protein expression in spindled Schwann cells, synaptophysin in ganglion cells, and synaptophysin and chromogranin in the epithelioid neuroendocrine cells. About half of cases show keratin expression in the epithelioid cells. The neuroendocrine cells can express a variety of hormones, including somatostatin, human pancreatic polypeptide, serotonin, gastrin, glucagon, insulin, and vasoactive intestinal peptide.

Differential Diagnosis

In spindle cell–predominant lesions, the differential diagnosis includes GIST and nerve sheath tumors: S-100 protein expression virtually excludes GIST, and finding the admixture of other cell types excludes other nerve sheath tumors. Epithelioid-predominant lesions are distinguished from carcinoid tumors and carcinomas by the admixture of other cell types and prominent S-100 expression.

Prognosis and Therapy

Gangliocytic paragangliomas are benign and surgical excision is curative. There are rare reports of regional lymph node metastases but not of tumor-associated deaths.

GANGLIOCYTIC PARAGANGLIOMA–FACT SHEET

Definition
- Unusual neoplasm displaying "triphasic" differentiation

Incidence and Location
- Rare tumors that almost always occur in the duodenum

Morbidity and Mortality
- Vast majority are benign
- Morbidity is generally related to surgical removal

Gender, Race, and Age Distribution
- No reported gender or race predilection
- Occurs in adults (average age, 54 years)

Clinical Features
- Abdominal pain, gastric outlet obstruction, or bleeding
- Rare association with neurofibromatosis

Prognosis and Therapy
- Treatment is excision
- Rare reports of regional spread to lymph nodes but no disease-associated reported deaths

Gangliocytic Paraganglioma—Pathologic Features

Gross Findings

- Centered in submucosa with infiltrative borders and yellowish surface

Microscopic Findings

- Three cell types: (1) S-100–positive spindle cells, (2) ganglion cells, and (3) epithelioid neuroendocrine cells in variable proportions
- Psammoma bodies may be present

Immunohistochemistry

- Spindle cells are positive for S-100
- Ganglion cells are positive for synaptophysin
- Epithelioid component expressed neuroendocrine markers and variably keratin

Differential Diagnosis

- Spindle cell–predominant lesions are distinguished from schwannomas by identifying the other cellular components
- Epithelioid-predominant lesions are distinguished from neuroendocrine tumors by identifying the admixed spindle cell population

GLOMUS TUMOR

CLINICAL FEATURES

Glomus tumor is composed of modified perivascular smooth muscle cells, and although far more common in somatic soft tissue sites, they also occur in the GI tract. The stomach is the most common site, antrum more than corpus, but there are reports of glomus tumor arising in the small intestine and colon. There is a slight female predominance, and the median age at presentation is 53 years. Presenting symptoms include ulcer-like pain; severe bleeding producing melena, anemia; or hematemesis; and obstructive symptoms. Some cases are incidentally detected at the time of surgery or endoscopy for other reasons.

Pathologic Features

Gross Findings

Tumors are circumscribed intramural masses with a median diameter of 2.5 cm. They can bulge either into the mucosa or externally toward the serosa. They are yellowish and occasionally calcified or cystic on cut surface.

Microscopic Findings

Glomus tumors are composed of multiple nodules separated by strands of residual muscularis propria. There may be ulceration of the overlying mucosa. The tumor cells within the nodules are organized in solid sheets or nests surrounding dilated capillaries that show branching or hemangiopericytoma-like features (Fig. 7.43). Tumor cells also tend to be present in the muscular walls of larger vessels. The tumor cells are round with sharply defined cell membranes, pale cytoplasm, and uniform round nuclei with fine chromatin (Figs. 7.44 and 7.45). In some cases, the tumor cells have oncocytic cytoplasm. Myxoid change, calcification, and metaplastic bone may be present. Within somatic soft tissue, features associated with malignant clinical course include large tumor size (>5 cm), nuclear atypia, spindled morphology, and high mitotic activity. However, these criteria for malignancy do not appear to apply to GI glomus tumors, and the vast majority of glomus tumors greater than 2 cm in size pursue a benign clinical course.

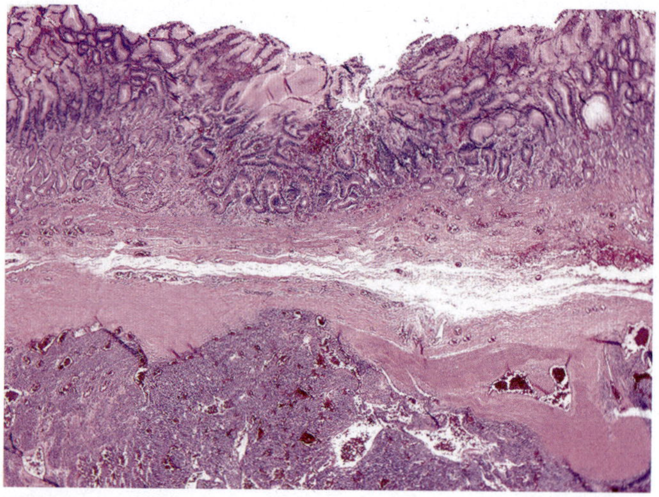

FIGURE 7.43

Glomus tumor. Glomus tumors are composed of uniform small neoplastic cells with round nuclei; neoplastic cells are prominent around hemangiopericytoma-like vessels.

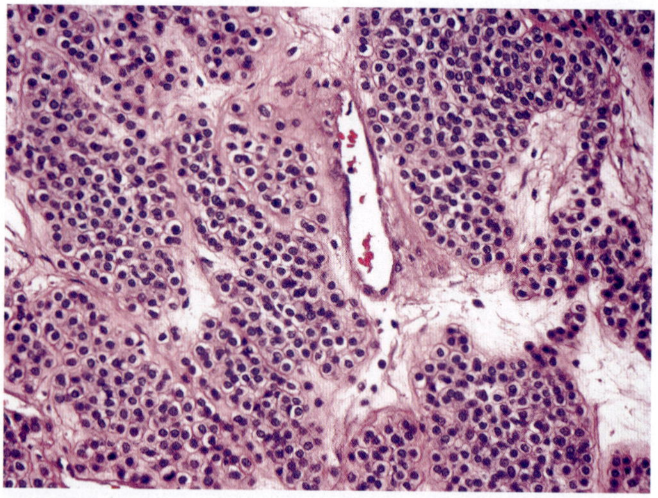

FIGURE 7.44

Glomus tumor. Note the prominent cell borders.

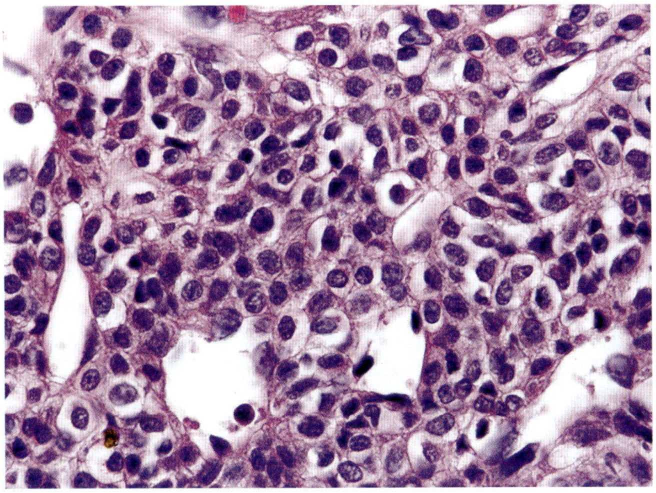

FIGURE 7.45

Glomus tumor. This lesion has somewhat clear cells and characteristic prominent cell borders.

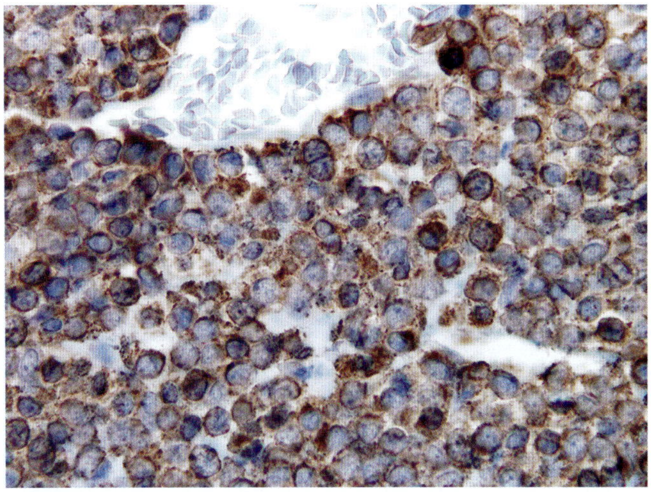

FIGURE 7.46

Glomus tumor immunohistochemistry. Gastric glomus tumors consistently express smooth muscle actin but not desmin.

Ancillary Studies

Immunohistochemistry

The tumor cells express SMA (Fig. 7.46) in virtually all cases, and h-caldesmon in 60% but usually lack desmin expression. SMA and caldesmon expression usually highlights the well-defined cell borders of the tumor cells. Some cases show focal CD34 expression. Glomus tumors are negative for KIT. Approximately 20% of cases show synaptophysin expression (usually weak or focal), which can lead to an erroneous diagnosis of neuroendocrine tumor, especially in small biopsies, but glomus tumors are negative for chromogranin and keratin.

Molecular Genetics

A small subset has *MIR143-NOTCH* gene fusion.

Differential Diagnosis

The differential diagnosis includes neuroendocrine tumor and GIST with epithelioid features. Neuroendocrine tumors are usually mucosal based, lack the distinctive membranous pattern of SMA expression seen in glomus tumors, and typically show chromogranin expression. Epithelioid GIST is also easily distinguished by IHC, but because many epithelioid GIST (those with *PDGFRA* mutations) are KIT negative, DOG1 should be evaluated if KIT is negative and the suspicion for GIST remains.

Prognosis and Therapy

Most glomus tumors behave in a benign fashion. However, rare cases pursue an aggressive clinical course. It is difficult to predict which tumors will have an unfavorable outcome, but some histologic features have been associated with malignant behavior.

Glomus Tumors—Fact Sheet

Definition

- Mesenchymal neoplasms composed of perivascular smooth muscle cells; gastrointestinal tract glomus tumors resemble their peripheral soft tissue counterparts

Incidence and Location

- Rare, usually arise in the stomach

Gender, Race, and Age Distribution

- Tumors of adults (median age, 53 years)
- Slight female predominance

Clinical Features

- Gastrointestinal bleeding is common, and some are associated with ulcer-like pain
- About 20% are found incidentally

Prognosis and Therapy

- The vast majority are benign
- Treatment is surgical
- Histologic features do not reliably predict the rare occurrence of metastasis

Glomus Tumors—Pathologic Features

Gross Findings

- Tumors are usually circumscribed with a yellowish often lobulated cut surface
- Some have calcifications

Microscopic Findings

- Uniform round cells with sharply defined cell membranes and uniform nuclei
- Cells condense around vessels that show a hemangiopericytoma-like pattern

Immunohistochemistry

- Positive for smooth muscle actin and caldesmon
- Negative for desmin, endocrine markers, keratin, and KIT

Differential Diagnosis

- Gastrointestinal stromal tumor with epithelioid features: positive for KIT and DOG1 (discovered on GIST1), with variable smooth muscle actin expression
- Neuroendocrine tumors (carcinoids): keratin positive, usually express both synaptophysin and chromogranin, and are negative for smooth muscle actin

INTRAABDOMINAL DESMOID FIBROMATOSIS

CLINICAL FEATURES

Intraabdominal (desmoid) fibromatosis may involve mesentery of the small intestine, abdominal wall, or retroperitoneum. It usually presents as a slowly growing mass, and in some cases, there is a history of prior surgery such as cesarean section. A subset of patients, especially young patients, have Gardner's syndrome, an autosomal dominant familial disease with a female predilection consisting of colorectal adenomatous polyposis, osteomas, cutaneous cysts, and desmoid fibromatosis. Gardner's syndrome is related to FAP, a disorder caused by germline adenomatous polyposis coli (*APC*) gene mutations. It is associated with a 7% to 12% incidence of developing fibromatosis. Desmoid fibromatosis in patients with Gardner's syndrome appears to have a higher recurrence rate than in patients without this syndrome.

RADIOLOGIC FEATURES

Although not specific, imaging studies show a mass lesion with a mesenteric epicenter, an infiltrative pattern, and a low signal on all magnetic resonance imaging sequences.

PATHOLOGIC FEATURES

GROSS FINDINGS

Grossly, the tumor is firm with coarse white trabeculation resembling a scar, and a gritty texture is detected when the tumor is cut.

MICROSCOPIC FINDINGS

Microscopically, the lesion is usually poorly defined with infiltrative margins; even tumors that are grossly circumscribed usually show infiltrative edges. Tumors are composed of long fascicles of uniform bland spindled fibroblasts separated by a dense collagenous stroma (Fig. 7.47). Scattered thin-walled (Fig. 7.48), elongated, and compressed vessels are seen. The tumor cells have tapering nuclei with delicate nucleoli and smooth nuclear membranes (Fig. 7.49). Mitotic figures are infrequent. Fasciitis-like features, with storiform growth and looser myxoid matrix, are common in mesenteric fibromatosis. Keloid-like hyalinization is often present and may be so extensive as to obscure the original pattern of the tumor. Rarely, calcification or chondro-osseous metaplasia is present.

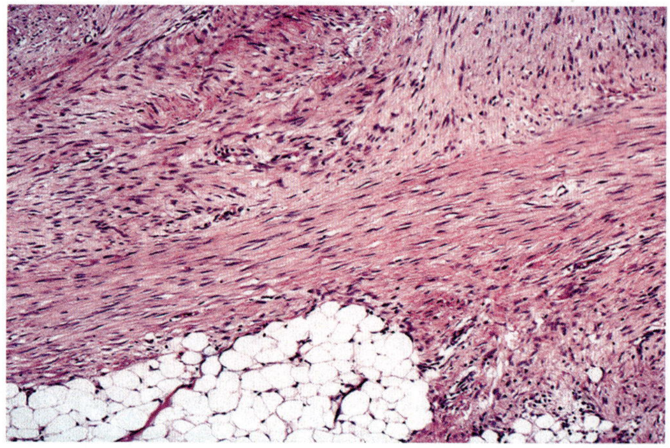

FIGURE 7.47

Desmoid fibromatosis. Desmoid fibromatosis is composed of long, sweeping fascicles of myofibroblasts with abundant stromal collagen deposition.

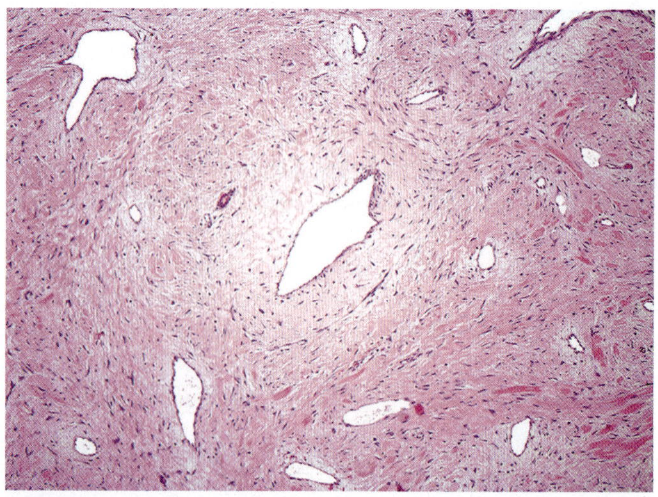

FIGURE 7.48

Desmoid fibromatosis. When it involves the mesentery, desmoid fibromatosis tends to exhibit thin-walled vessels that appear to be "pulled open" by the proliferating myofibroblasts.

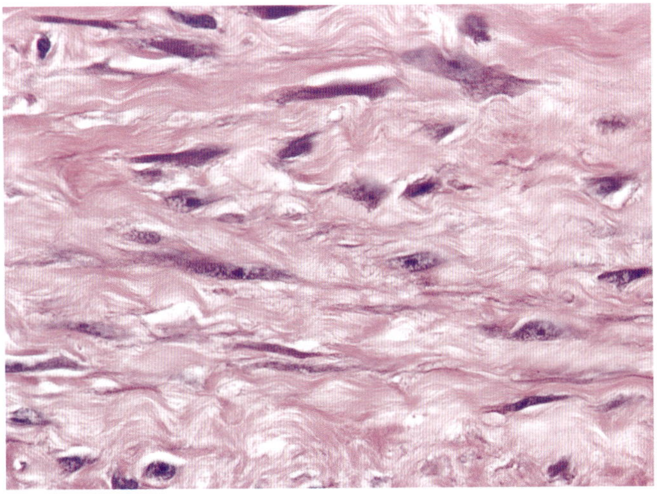

FIGURE 7.49

Desmoid fibromatosis. Desmoid fibromatoses typically have small pinpoint nucleoli and bland cytologic features at high magnification.

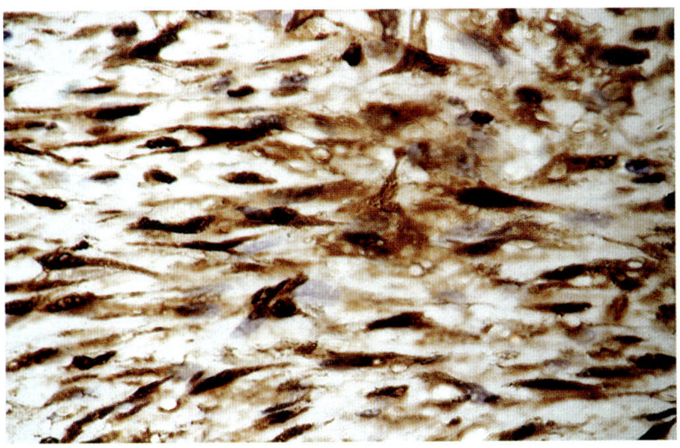

FIGURE 7.50

Nuclear β-catenin staining in fibromatoses. Cytoplasmic staining is not specific; only nuclear staining should be used to support a diagnosis of fibromatosis.

Ancillary Studies

Immunohistochemistry

Because fibromatoses are myofibroblastic lesions, they express SMA and less frequently desmin. They typically lack CD34. Nuclear β-catenin is detected in 70% to 80% of fibromatosis cases (Fig. 7.50) and is not present in most histologic mimics.

Other Studies

Molecular Genetics

Among patients with FAP, intestinal and extraintestinal neoplasms typically arise through biallelic (germline then somatic) inactivation of the *APC* gene, whereas tumors in non-FAP patients occur either through somatic biallelic *APC* inactivation or somatic mutation of a single β-catenin allele.

Differential Diagnosis

The differential diagnosis includes low-grade dedifferentiated liposarcoma and benign fibroblastic proliferative lesions. Dedifferentiated liposarcoma is distinguished from fibromatoses by having at least scattered hyperchromatic nuclei in contrast to the bland nuclei of fibromatosis. Identification of areas of well-differentiated liposarcoma is obviously helpful, but if not present, then identification of *MDM2* gene amplification or MDM2 and CDK4 nuclear expression by IHC helps confirm the diagnosis. Reactive myofibroblastic proliferations after surgery or trauma may be histologically very similar, especially on small biopsies. The presence of associated fat necrosis and lack of β-catenin expression favors a reactive process. Correlation with clinical history is essential. Sclerosing mesenteritis or idiopathic retroperitoneal fibrosis is also in the differential diagnosis and is discussed in the following section.

Prognosis and Therapy

Desmoid fibromatoses show locally aggressive growth and frequent recurrence but do not metastasize. Although surgical excision used to be the mainstay of therapy, now a more conservative approach is followed, with observation or chemotherapy with doxorubicin for cases that show aggressive growth. Surgery is still performed in certain patients, but there is no longer a need to obtain wide margins, given the recent recognition that margin status is less predictive of recurrence than mutation type.

INTRAABDOMINAL DESMOID FIBROMATOSIS—FACT SHEET

Definition

- Myofibroblastic proliferation that shows locally aggressive behavior but does not metastasize

Incidence and Location

- Usually arise in somatic soft tissue, but a subset is found intraabdominally or in the mesentery

Gender, Race, and Age Distribution

- No gender predominance in childhood; female predominance during young adulthood; no gender predominance in older adults
- No report of racial predilection
- Arises in patients of all ages

Clinical Features

- Mass lesions; may be a component of familial adenomatous polyposis or Gardner's syndrome

Prognosis and Therapy

- Local recurrence is common, and aggressive growth may be associated with significant morbidity and even mortality
- Treatment was traditionally surgical, but contemporary approaches are conservative
- Chemotherapy with doxorubicin is used for some locally aggressive cases
- Risk of recurrence is better predicted by specific mutation type rather than margin status
- Mesenteric fibromatoses in Gardner's syndrome more likely to recur

Intraabdominal Desmoid Fibromatosis—Pathologic Features

Gross Findings

- Large infiltrative masses with firm, white cut surfaces

Microscopic Findings

- Long fascicles of bland spindled myofibroblasts

Immunohistochemistry

- May be positive for actin
- Most lack desmin
- 80% show nuclear β-catenin positivity

Differential Diagnosis

- Low-grade dedifferentiated liposarcoma: atypical hyperchromatic cells; may be identifiable well-differentiated component; positive for *MDM2* gene amplification
- Gastrointestinal stromal tumor: lacks long sweeping fascicles; cytoplasm is slightly more eosinophilic; KIT and DOG1 (discovered on GIST1) expression, and absence of nuclear β-catenin
- Reactive myofibroblastic proliferations: associated fat necrosis; shorter fascicles, lacks β-catenin expression or *CTNNB1* mutations

SCLEROSING MESENTERITIS

CLINICAL FEATURES

Sclerosing mesenteritis is a non-neoplastic fibroinflammatory lesion that most commonly affects mesentery of the small intestine, presenting as an isolated large mass, although 20% of patients have multiple lesions. The cause of these lesions remains unknown, and although they are assumed to reflect a reparative response, usually to trauma or surgery, in many cases, no such history is found. A subset of patients with sclerosing mesenteritis are found to have immunoglobulin (Ig) G4-related sclerosing disease, have elevated serum IgG4 levels, and often have additional histologic features characteristic of this entity. However, whereas most patients with classic IgG4-related sclerosing disorders respond to systemic steroid therapy, patients with sclerosing mesenteritis usually do not.

In one large study, the patient age ranged from 23 to 87 years (mean, 60 years) without a gender predilection. Most patients presented with nonspecific symptoms such as abdominal pain, palpable mass, and symptoms related to bowel obstruction.

RADIOLOGIC FEATURES

The computed tomography appearance of sclerosing mesenteritis can vary from subtle increased attenuation in the mesentery to a solid soft tissue mass. Sclerosing mesenteritis most commonly appears as a soft tissue mass in the small bowel mesentery, although infiltration of the region of the pancreas or porta hepatis is also possible. The mass may envelop the mesenteric vessels, and over time, collateral vessels may develop. There may be preservation of fat around the mesenteric vessels, a phenomenon that is referred to as the *fat ring sign*. This finding may help distinguish sclerosing mesenteritis from other mesenteric processes such as lymphoma, carcinoid tumor, or carcinomatosis. A tumoral pseudocapsule may be present.

PATHOLOGIC FEATURES

GROSS FINDINGS

Lesions typically consist of a whitish, firm mass with extensions of firm, fibrous tissue into surrounding normal-appearing fat or adherent to adjacent tissues.

MICROSCOPIC FINDINGS

Lesions consist of fascicles of bland spindled fibroblasts and myofibroblasts infiltrating fat (Figs. 7.51 to 7.53) with associated fat necrosis. There may be admixed inflammatory cells, typically lymphocytes, plasma cells, and eosinophils. Obstructive phlebitis and prominent plasma cell infiltrate with storiform fibrosis suggests the possibility of IgG4-related sclerosing disorder (see Fig. 7.53).

ANCILLARY STUDIES

IMMUNOHISTOCHEMISTRY

The spindle cells are fibroblastic or myofibroblastic, and this is reflected by expression of SMA and rarely desmin. S-100, caldesmon, KIT, ALK, and β-catenin are negative. If there is suspicion for IgG4-related sclerosing disease, then evaluation of the IgG/IgG4 ratio in admixed plasma cells can be helpful, with a ratio greater than 40% suggestive of the latter (Fig. 7.54).

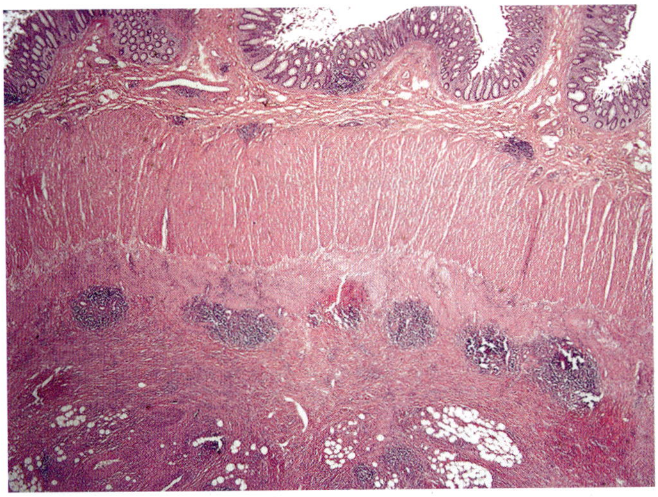

FIGURE 7.51

Sclerosing mesenteritis. A disorganized sclerotic process involves mesenteric fat, usually accompanied by a lymphoplasmacytic inflammatory response but not by neutrophils.

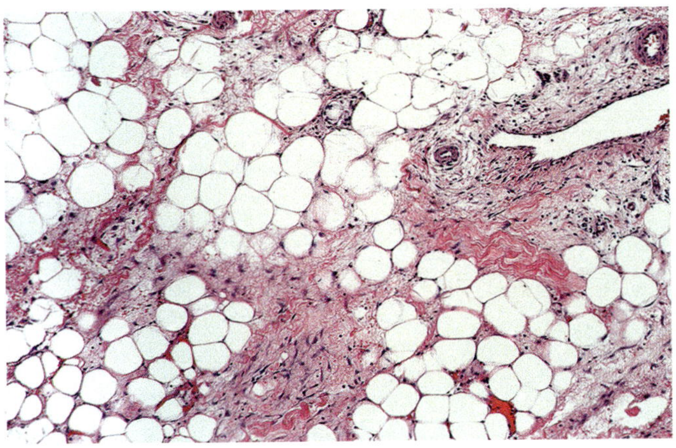

FIGURE 7.52

Sclerosing mesenteritis. Note the bland cytologic features in a sclerotic area.

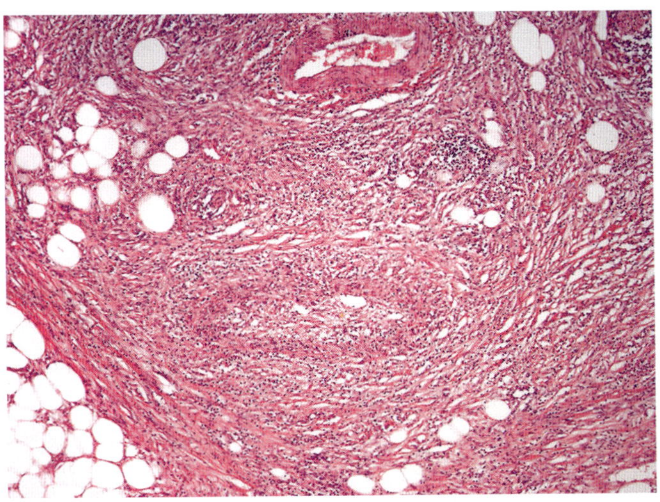

FIGURE 7.53

Many examples of sclerosing mesenteritis display a lymphocytic phlebitis pattern. Note the damaged inflamed vein beneath the uninvolved artery in this field.

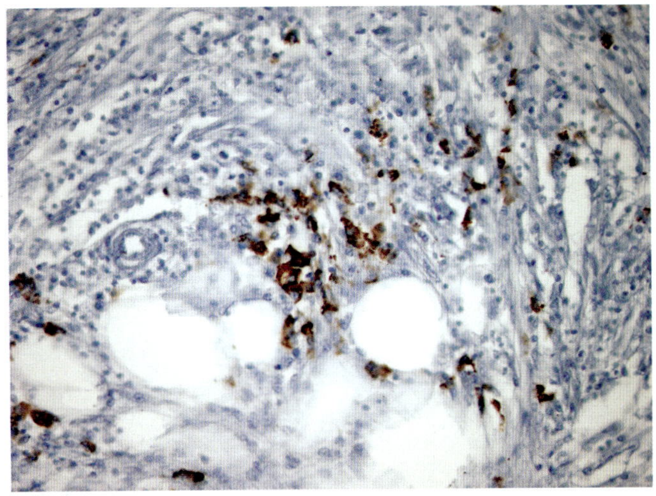

FIGURE 7.54

Sclerosing mesenteritis. Prominent immunoglobulin G4 expression can be encountered in these lesions, although its significance remains unclear.

Differential Diagnosis

Sclerosing mesenteritis is distinguished from desmoid fibromatosis by its abundance of inflammation and fat entrapment with fat necrosis. Fibromatosis, although infiltrative at its periphery, grows as a solid mass composed of sweeping fascicles of fibroblasts with minimal inflammation. Inflammatory well- or dedifferentiated liposarcoma can appear similar but differs by the presence of enlarged hyperchromatic cells. Expression of MDM2 and CDK4 or identification of *MDM2* gene amplification can help confirm a diagnosis of well- or dedifferentiated liposarcoma. Care should be taken when interpreting MDM2 because expression is common in histiocytes, which may be abundant in sclerosing mesenteritis; therefore, CDK4 should also be evaluated and fluorescence in situ hybridization performed if there is any ambiguity.

Prognosis and Therapy

Treatment has included medical therapy alone, surgery alone, and surgery followed by medical therapy, but about half of patients seem to require no treatment. Tamoxifen in combination with prednisone has resulted in improvement in 60% of patients. Sclerosing mesenteritis can have a prolonged debilitating course in a subset of patients, but the overall prognosis is favorable.

SCLEROSING MESENTERITIS–FACT SHEET

Definition

- A fibroinflammatory condition of uncertain etiology affecting the mesentery
- A subset of cases may represent immunoglobulin G4–related sclerosing disease

Incidence and Location

- Rare and usually involves small bowel mesentery

Gender, Race, and Age Distribution

- No gender or racial predominance
- Adults affected (average age, 60 years)

Clinical Features

- Patients present with abdominal pain, abdominal mass, or obstruction
- May be a history of trauma or prior surgery

Radiologic Features

- Soft tissue mass in mesentery, sometimes with preservation of fat around mesenteric vessels ("fat ring sign")

Prognosis and Therapy

- Treatment can be surgical or medical using steroids and tamoxifen
- Recurrence is uncommon, and only rare cases are associated with significant morbidity, usually because of obstructive symptoms

SCLEROSING MESENTERITIS—PATHOLOGIC FEATURES

Gross Findings

- Infiltrative solitary (80%) whitish mass lesion with extension into surrounding fat

Microscopic Findings

- Fascicles of bland spindle cells with associated fat necrosis
- Variable degree of admixed inflammatory cells

Immunohistochemistry

- Spindle cells show variable expression of smooth muscle actin
- Negative for keratin, S-100 protein, KIT, and β-catenin

Differential Diagnosis

- Desmoid fibromatosis: lacks associated fat necrosis and prominent inflammation; 70% to 80% show nuclear β-catenin expression
- Inflammatory myofibroblastic tumor: lacks associated fat necrosis, anaplastic lymphoma kinase positive in 50%
- Dedifferentiated liposarcoma: at least focal atypical hyperchromatic nuclei, presence of a well-differentiated liposarcoma component; MDM2 and CDK4 expression or *MDM2* gene amplification

INFLAMMATORY MYOFIBROBLASTIC TUMOR

CLINICAL FEATURES

Inflammatory myofibroblastic tumor (historically also referred to as inflammatory pseudotumor or inflammatory fibrosarcoma) is a mesenchymal neoplasm of intermediate biologic potential with a tendency for local recurrence but rare metastasis. Half of the cases harbor *ALK* gene rearrangement, and a smaller subset harbor rearrangements in other receptor tyrosine kinases such as *ROS* and *RET*. IMT most often arises in lung or abdominal soft tissues (omentum, retroperitoneum, viscera) of children and young adults, but there is a wide age range and anatomic distribution. Patients with IMT of the GI tract are usually older, with an average age of 43 years. Within the GI tract, the colon and small intestine are most often involved, followed by the stomach and esophagus. The clinical presentation may be with abdominal pain or mass, and some patients have systemic symptoms such as fever and weight loss. Abnormalities in serologic inflammatory markers, including elevated erythrocyte sedimentation rate and hypergammaglobulinemia, may be found and typically resolve after tumor resection. Epithelioid inflammatory myofibroblastic sarcoma is a distinct variant of IMT that usually arises in the abdominal cavity of young men and pursues a very aggressive clinical course. A *RANBP2-ALK* fusion gene is commonly identified in this variant.

RADIOLOGIC FEATURES

Imaging studies show poorly marginated mass, and a small number of cases have calcifications.

PATHOLOGIC FEATURES

GROSS FINDINGS

These tumors form firm white infiltrative masses (average, 6–7 cm) that appear fibrous, myxoid, or occasionally fleshy on cut surface. Within the tubal gut, the tumors may involve any layer from serosa to mucosa (Fig. 7.55).

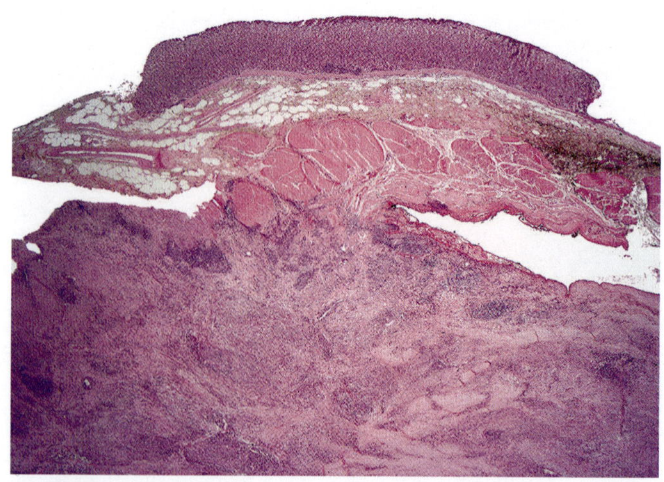

FIGURE 7.55

Inflammatory myofibroblastic tumor centered in the adipose tissue outside the gastric muscularis propria (although it has focally extended into the smooth muscle). In contrast to gastric schwannoma, the inflammation is more uniformly distributed throughout the tumor rather than forming a peritumoral cuff.

Microscopic Findings

Histologically, IMT is composed of fascicles of spindle cells with eosinophilic cytoplasm and ovoid to tapered nuclei (Fig. 7.56). Typically, there is admixed prominent chronic inflammation. IMT can range from highly cellular to paucicellular, and some tumors have prominent myxoid stroma.

Epithelioid inflammatory myofibroblastic sarcoma exhibits epithelioid to round cell cytomorphology in an abundant myxoid stroma, and in contrast to IMT, it most commonly features a neutrophilic inflammatory infiltrate (Fig. 7.57). Neoplastic cells have pink cytoplasm, vesicular nuclei, and prominent nucleoli.

Ancillary Studies

Immunohistochemistry

Smooth muscle actin expression is seen in 80% to 90% of cases and desmin and HHF35 in 60%. Approximately one-third show expression of keratins. ALK protein expression is present in approximately 50% of cases (more common in younger patients) and reflects the presence of *ALK* gene rearrangement (Fig. 7.58). Similarly, approximately 5 % to 10% show expression of ROS1. Epithelioid inflammatory myofibroblastic sarcoma has a characteristic nuclear membranous staining pattern in most cases and a cytoplasmic pattern with Golgi dot-like accentuation in the remaining minority of cases (Fig. 7.59).

Other Studies

Gene fusions involving the *ALK* gene, a receptor tyrosine kinase at chromosome 2p23, occur in approximately 50% of cases. A smaller number of tumors have rearrangements of other receptor tyrosine kinases such as *ROS*, *RET*, and *NTRK*, and treatment with crizotinib can be effective in advanced disease. The fusion partners with ALK include *ATIC, CARS, CLTC, TPM3, TPM4, CLTC, RANB2*, and *SEC31L*.

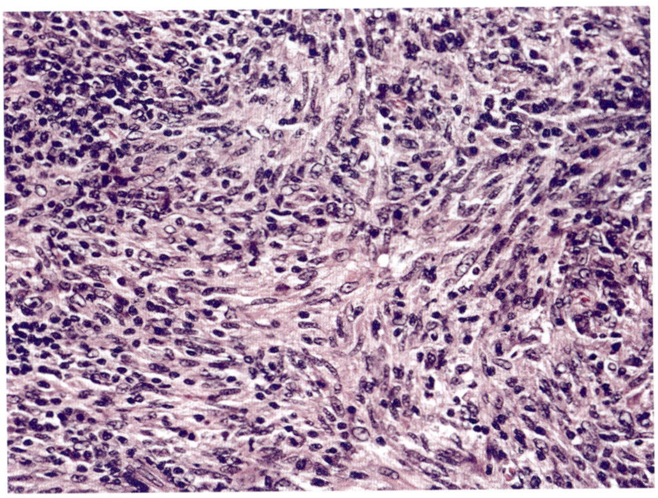

FIGURE 7.56

Inflammatory myofibroblastic tumor consisting of a storiform proliferation of spindle cells with abundant plasma cells.

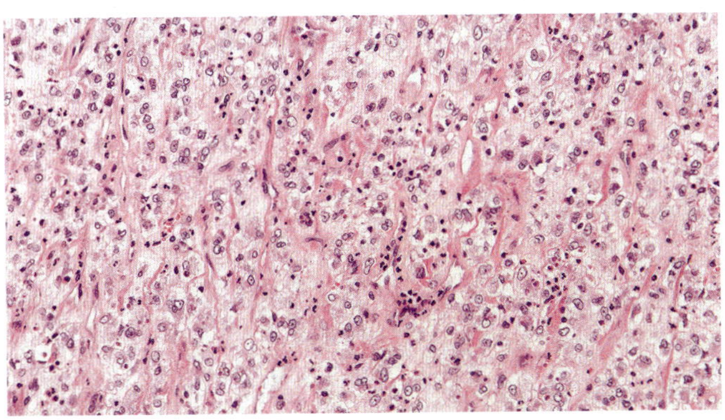

FIGURE 7.57

Epithelioid inflammatory myofibroblastic sarcoma. Neoplastic cells are epithelioid, with palely eosinophilic cytoplasm, vesicular nuclei, and prominent nucleoli. There is a background myxohyaline stroma, and there are scattered admixed inflammatory cells, including a prominent neutrophilic component, typical of this entity.

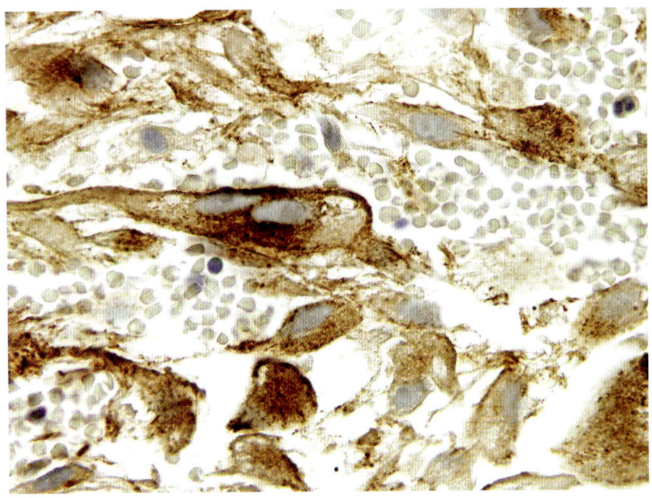

FIGURE 7.58

Inflammatory myofibroblastic tumor immunohistochemistry. Anaplastic lymphoma kinase is positive in approximately 50% of inflammatory myofibroblastic tumors.

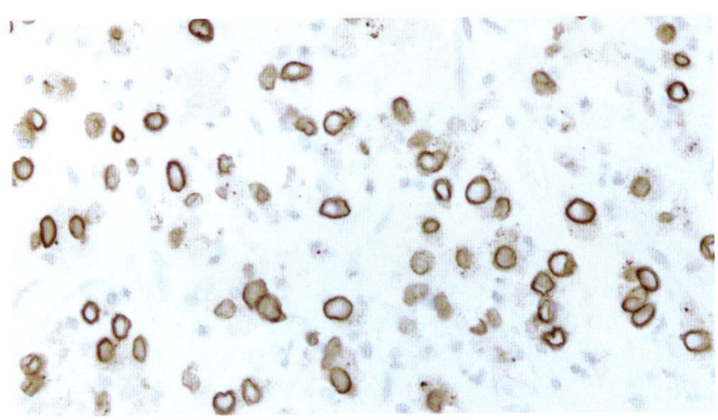

FIGURE 7.59

Epithelioid inflammatory myofibroblastic sarcoma immunohistochemistry. Perinuclear anaplastic lymphoma kinase staining is characteristic in epithelioid inflammatory myofibroblastic sarcoma.

Differential Diagnosis

The differential diagnosis of IMT can sometimes be difficult to resolve, particularly in cases negative for ALK or ROS1 by IHC. The differential diagnosis includes inflammatory well-differentiated liposarcoma (WDLPS), dedifferentiated liposarcoma, desmoid fibromatosis and inflammatory leiomyosarcoma, as well as inflammatory conditions including retroperitoneal fibrosis and sclerosing mesenteritis.

Inflammatory WDLPS is a distinctive variant of WDLPS with prominent mixed inflammation containing scattered neoplastic cells. The neoplastic cells are much more atypical than those of IMT, exhibiting prominent nuclear pleomorphism and hyperchromasia. DDLPS can also closely mimic IMT because it can exhibit fascicles of mildly atypical spindle cells with admixed inflammation. The inflammatory component in WDLPS is usually lymphoplasmacytic, whereas in DDLPS, it is usually neutrophilic. IHC for MDM2 and CDK4 is useful to resolve this differential diagnosis because it is positive in most cases of WDLPS and DDLPS.

Desmoid fibromatosis is also composed of myofibroblastic neoplastic cells, but it does not have a prominent inflammatory infiltrate, and it has longer fascicles and usually no significant cytologic atypia. There is nuclear β-catenin expression in 70% to 80% of cases but not in IMT. Inflammatory leiomyosarcoma contains prominent mixed inflammatory infiltrates that can sometimes make it difficult to recognize the admixed neoplastic cells. However, the neoplastic cells are more myoid, with brightly eosinophilic cytoplasm and blunt-ended nuclei.

Retroperitoneal fibrosis and sclerosing mesenteritis both contain spindle cells with admixed chronic inflammation. However, retroperitoneal fibrosis is clinically distinctive, presenting with bilateral retroperitoneal involvement, often including bilateral ureteral obstruction. In contrast to IMT, sclerosing mesenteritis has associated fat necrosis.

Prognosis and Therapy

Inflammatory myofibroblastic tumor of the abdomen and pelvis has one of the highest recurrence rates among all IMT at 25%. Metastasis occurs in fewer than 5% of patients. The much rarer epithelioid inflammatory myofibroblastic sarcoma pursues a much more aggressive course, with early recurrences and death from disease in almost all patients. Surgical excision is often performed. Targeted tyrosine kinase inhibitor therapy (e.g., crizotinib) has shown efficacy in patients with advanced disease.

INFLAMMATORY MYOFIBROBLASTIC TUMOR—FACT SHEET

Definition

- Neoplasm composed of cells with myofibroblastic differentiation, usually with a prominent inflammatory infiltrate

Incidence and Location

- Rare; occurs in mesentery, omentum, and retroperitoneum (>80% of cases), with occasional cases in the mediastinum, abdominal wall, liver, and gastrointestinal (GI) tract proper
- Most tubal gut lesions arise in the colon or small intestine

Morbidity and Mortality

- Multicentricity may be a feature
- Patients may die of local disease rather than systemic spread

Gender, Race, and Age Distribution

- Average age of patients with GI tract tumors is 43 years, but the range is wide
- No gender or race predominance

Clinical Features

- Patients present with mass lesions, abdominal pain, or constitutional symptoms (anemia, weight loss, malaise)

Prognosis and Therapy

- Local recurrence or local growth is the main cause of morbidity
- Metastases are rare but do occur
- Most examples are indolent; treatment is surgical and relatively conservative

Inflammatory Myofibroblastic Tumor—Pathologic Features

Gross Findings

- Firm, white infiltrative mass

Microscopic Findings

- Inflammatory myofibroblastic tumor (IMT): fascicular spindle cell neoplasm with admixed chronic inflammatory infiltrate
- Epithelioid inflammatory myofibroblastic sarcoma: epithelioid neoplastic cells in abundant myxoid stroma with admixed neutrophils

Immunohistochemistry

- Positive: smooth muscle actin (80%–90%), desmin (60%), HHF35 (60%), keratin (~30%), anaplastic lymphoma kinase (ALK) (50% of IMT, approaching 100% of epithelioid inflammatory myofibroblastic sarcoma), ROS1 (5%–10%)

Differential Diagnosis

- Fibromatosis; less inflamed, express β-catenin in 70% to 80% of cases and lack expression of ALK or ROS
- Sclerosing mesenteritis: older patients; associated fat necrosis is common

LYMPHANGIOMA

CLINICAL FEATURES

Lymphangioma is a benign proliferation of lymphatic spaces lined by a single layer of endothelium and is relatively rare in the GI tract. Lymphangiomatosis is a multicentric lymphatic proliferation. However, the incidence of small lesions has increased, probably because of increased detection. Lymphangiomas can occur at any site in the GI tract but are most common in small intestine followed by the large intestine and esophagus. In the abdominal cavity, most occur within the mesentery and retroperitoneum. Diffuse lymphangiomatosis involves either a single organ or multiple organs, such as the liver, spleen, lungs, or bones.

Lymphangiomas primarily occur in children and young adults, although the age range is wide, and there is an overall slight male predominance. Presentation may be with bleeding, intussusception, or an acute abdomen. Small lesions are usually incidentally detected.

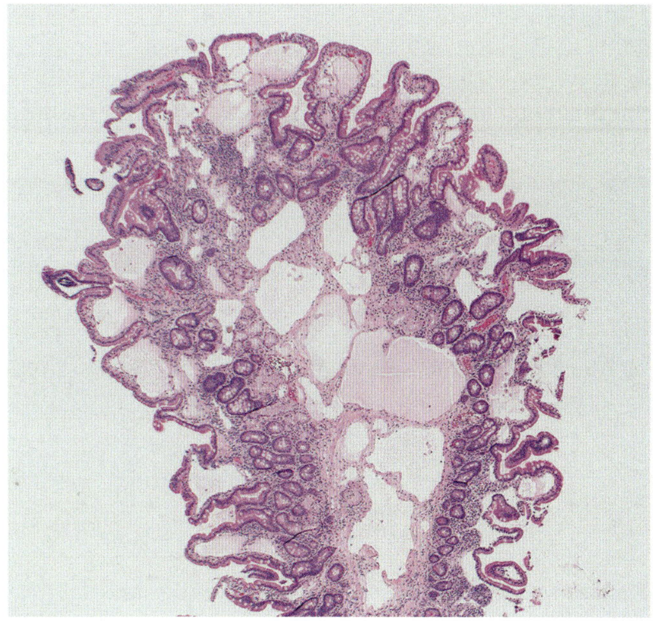

FIGURE 7.60

Lymphangioma of the duodenum. Dilated lymphatics are present in the lamina propria and submucosa of this polypoid duodenal lesion. Lymphatic fluid can be seen in some vessels.

RADIOLOGIC AND ENDOSCOPIC FEATURES

Lymphangiomas of the GI tract occur in two main forms: (1) small (<2 cm) polypoid white or yellow mucosal lesions that are usually incidentally detected at endoscopy and (2) larger masses that may be transmural or may involve mesenteric fat.

PATHOLOGIC FEATURES

GROSS FEATURES

Lymphangiomas are usually polypoid with a soft, spongy texture. Thick gelatinous or milky fluid is seen in the cystic spaces.

HISTOLOGIC FEATURES

Lesions can involve one or all layers of the GI tract, usually mucosa, submucosa, or muscularis propria (Fig. 7.60), and consist of dilated cystic lymphatic channels lined by a simple layer of bland lymphatic endothelial cells (Fig. 7.61). Some lymphatic channels are partially surrounded by a layer of smooth muscle. The spaces contain clear lymphatic fluid, prominent foamy histiocytes, or both (see Figs. 7.60 and 7.61). Deep lesions may be associated with overlying mucosal clusters of small lymphatics. Scattered lymphoid aggregates, granulation tissue, or foci of xanthogranulomatous inflammation may be present, especially in mesenteric or retroperitoneal lesions, and can obscure the underlying lymphatic abnormality. Other associated vascular abnormalities may be present, such as vascular malformations with thick-walled arteries, aneurysm-like cavities, and vessel abnormalities such as shunt vessels and wall excrescences. Esophageal lesions can sometimes display cavernous morphology. Lymphangioma of the liver is usually multiloculated and composed of cystically dilatated lymphatic vessels within hepatic parenchyma.

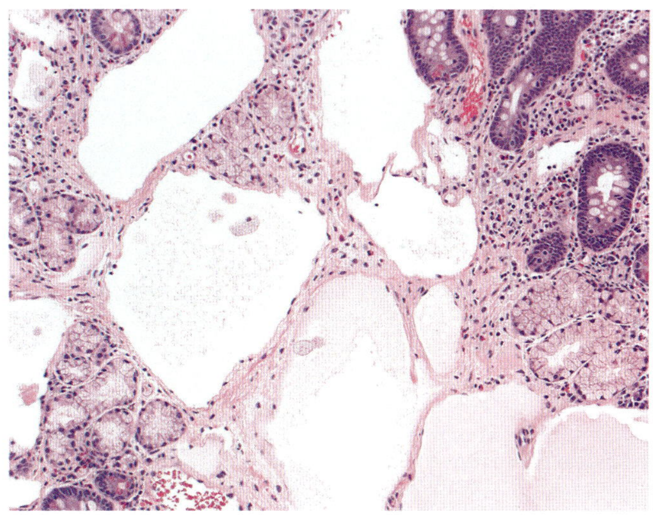

FIGURE 7.61

Lymphangioma. The dilated lymphatics are lined by simple inconspicuous endothelial cells, and some contain intraluminal foamy histiocytes.

ANCILLARY STUDIES

IMMUNOHISTOCHEMISTRY

The endothelial cells express CD31, D2-40, and podoplanin and show variable CD34 expression. SMA is positive in smooth muscle cells around larger lymphatics. The smooth muscle component where present is negative for melanocytic markers, distinguishing it from lymphangioleiomyomatosis (perivascular epithelioid cell tumor [PEComa]).

Differential Diagnosis

Distinction from hemangiomas is aided by detection of blood in the dilated spaces in hemangioma and expression of D2-40 in lymphangioma.

Prognosis and Therapy

Endoscopic removal of small polypoid lesions and surgical excision of larger lesions is curative, and lesions usually do not recur. Lymphangiomatosis with visceral involvement often pursue a more aggressive clinical course.

LYMPHANGIOMA—FACT SHEET

Definition

- Benign proliferation of lymphatic spaces
- Lymphangiomatosis is multicentric or extensively infiltrating lymphangioma

Incidence and Location

- Rare
- Most common in small intestine; also arise in mesenteric fat

Gender, Race, and Age Distribution

- Slight male predominance
- Wide age range but usually children and young adults

Clinical Features

- Incidental or bleeding, intussusception

Prognosis and Therapy

- Benign; majority cured by simple excision
- Lymphangiomatosis may pursue a more aggressive clinical course

Lymphangioma—Pathologic Features

Gross Findings

- Wide size range; mucosal polypoid lesions are usually smaller than2 cm, but mural or mesenteric masses may be significantly larger

Microscopic Findings

- Dilated lymphatic channels lined by a single of bland lymphatic endothelial cells
- May involve any layer of the intestine
- Spaces contain clear lymphatic fluid and/or prominent foamy histiocytes
- Other associated vascular abnormalities may be present

Immunohistochemistry

- Positive for CD31, D2-40, and podoplanin, with variable CD34 expression

Differential Diagnosis

- Hemangioma: vascular spaces contain blood; lining endothelial cells are negative for D2-40
- Lymphangioleiomyomatosis: usually occurs in lung; perivascular condensation of spindle myoid cells; expression of HMB45 (human melanoma black), Melan-A, and smooth muscle actin, and desmin in lesional cells

PECOMA

CLINICAL FEATURES

PEComas are mesenchymal neoplasms that show an unusual line of differentiation toward modified perivascular smooth muscle cells that also show melanocytic differentiation; there is no known normal counterpart to the tumor cells. PEComas can arise at virtually any anatomic site, but within the GI tract, the most common site is the colon followed by the small intestine and stomach. The PEComa family of tumors includes angiomyolipoma of the kidney and liver. Tumors usually arise in adults, and occurrence in children is rare. Whereas PEComas generally show a female predilection, this difference is not so clear in tumors of the GI tract. There is a wide spectrum of biologic behavior, from benign to highly aggressive tumors. Most PEComas of the GI tract are sporadic, with only a small subset being associated with the tuberous sclerosis complex, in contrast to the more significant association with PEComas at other sites. Presenting symptoms depend on the site of involvement and can include pain, obstruction, and bleeding.

Radiologic and Endoscopic Features

Tumors may present as polypoid or intramural masses. Imaging studies may identify features of increased vascularity within the mass but are often nonspecific.

Pathologic Features

Gross Findings

Tumors are usually well circumscribed but unencapsulated and may involve any layer of the GI wall but most often involve muscularis propria and subserosa. They may also involve the mesentery without definite attachment to the bowel wall. The cut surface is white and solid, and necrosis or hemorrhage may be present. There is a wide size range (1–22 cm), but tumors usually measure between 3 and 8 cm.

Microscopic Findings

The growth pattern of PEComa is usually nests or sheets of epithelioid cells (Fig. 7.62). Less often, a fascicular spindle cell growth pattern may be present. The tumor cells, epithelioid or spindled, classically have eosinophilic or granular cytoplasm (Fig. 7.63), prominent nucleoli, and variable degrees of pleomorphism. A prominent delicate capillary network surrounds tumor cells, often resulting in the nested pattern. A perivascular growth pattern is characteristic, with tumor cells arranged radially around vessel walls and replacing the muscular wall of larger vessels (Fig. 7.64). Necrosis may be present. The sclerosing variant virtually always occurs in retroperitoneal soft tissue and shows a spindled cytomorphology. Angiomyolipoma of the liver consists of thick-walled vessels, admixed epithelioid or spindled tumor cells, and variable amounts of mature fat. Malignant PEComa of the GI tract shows diffuse pleomorphism, marked cytologic atypia, and mitotic activity of 2/10 hpf or greater.

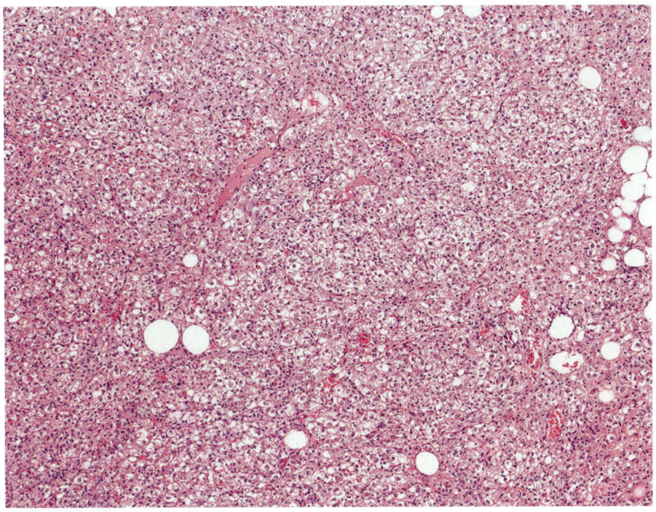

FIGURE 7.62

Perivascular epithelioid cell tumor (PEComa). Sheet-like and vaguely nested growth pattern of PEComa of the liver with epithelioid cytomorphology.

Ancillary Studies

Immunohistochemistry

Immunohistochemistry is usually needed to confirm the diagnosis given the wide differential considerations. A panel that encompasses myoid and melanocytic markers is recommended, including HMB45, Melan-A/MART1, MiTF, SMA, desmin, and caldesmon. Expression of these markers is usually variable in terms of intensity and extent; expression of just one muscle or one melanocytic marker may be seen (Figs. 7.65 and 7.66). S-100 may show focal positivity in 10% to 20% of cases. TFE3 expression is present in 5% to 10%, is associated with *TFE3* gene rearrangements, and is usually mutually exclusive with MiTF expression. KIT, keratin, and CD34 expression is typically absent.

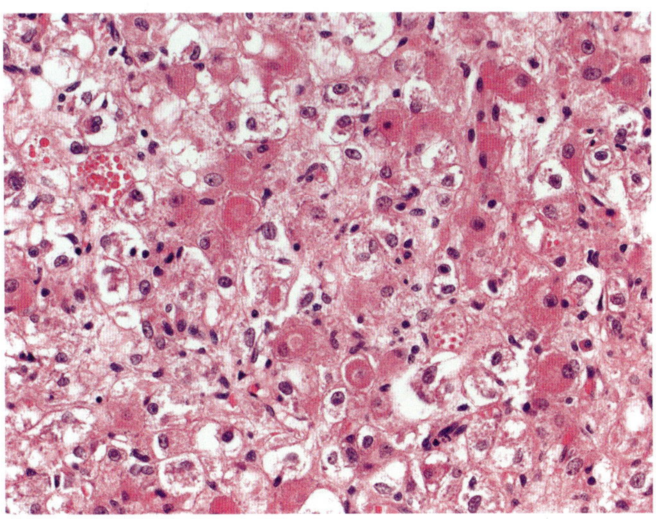

FIGURE 7.63

Perivascular epithelioid cell tumor (PEComa). Characteristic granular and eosinophilic cytoplasm of the tumor cells of PEComa; the nuclei have small nucleoli, and there is cytologic pleomorphism.

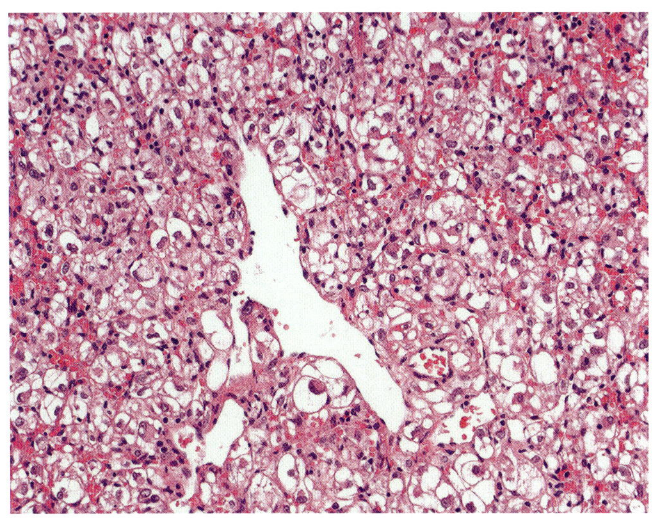

FIGURE 7.64

Perivascular epithelioid cell tumor (PEComa). The tumor cells of PEComa often show an intimate association with vessels, being radially arranged and appearing to replace the vessel wall.

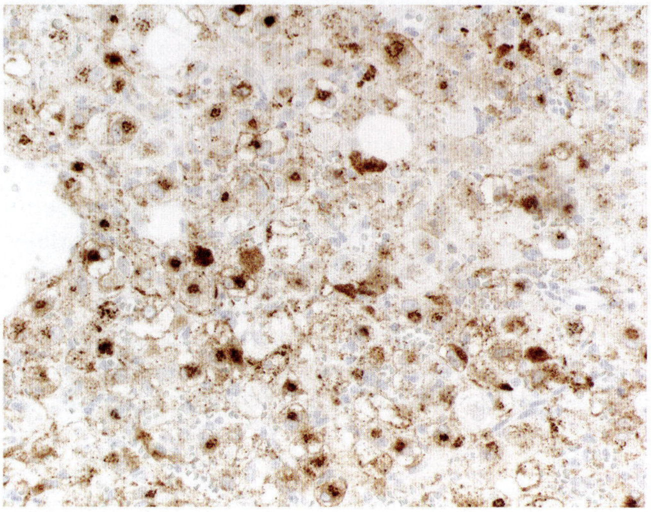

FIGURE 7.65

Perivascular epithelioid cell tumor (PEComa). Diffuse cytoplasmic expression of HMB45 (human melanoma black) in PEComa with epithelioid features.

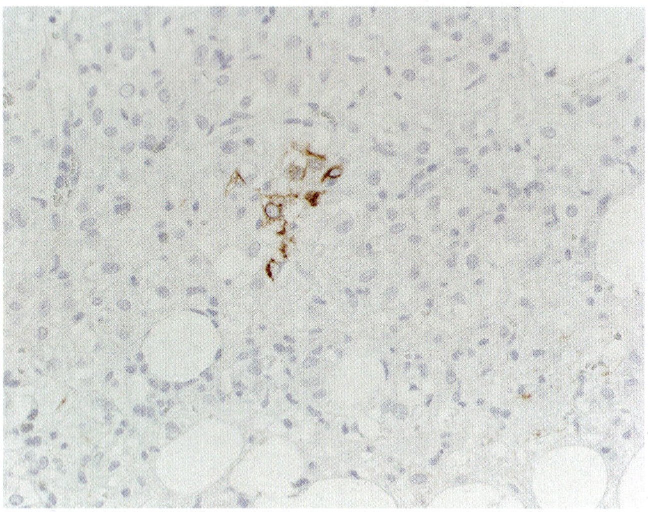

FIGURE 7.66

Perivascular epithelioid cell tumor (PEComa). Focal cytoplasmic expression of desmin in PEComa with epithelioid features.

Molecular Genetics

Both sporadic and syndromic cases are associated with abnormalities in the tuberous sclerosis gene complex. Mutations in *TSC2* (less often *TSC1*) are present in approximately 80% of cases and result in activation of the mTOR (mammalian target of rapamycin) pathway. A smaller subset of PEComas has *TFE3* gene rearrangements; the most common fusion partner with *TFE3* is *PSF/SFPQ*.

Differential Diagnosis

Pure smooth muscle tumors of the GI tract include the more common leiomyoma and far less common leiomyosarcoma. When PEComa is composed entirely of spindled cells, distinction from pure smooth muscle tumor may be impossible without IHC that demonstrates expression of melanocytic markers.

Metastatic renal cell carcinoma and metastatic melanoma may mimic PEComa with their typical nested growth pattern, epithelioid cells with variable amounts of clear or palely eosinophilic cytoplasm, and a prominent vascular network among tumor cells. Correlation with clinical history is crucial. Renal cell carcinoma is positive for PAX8 and EMA, unlike PEComa. Melanoma is more likely to show diffuse S-100 and SOX10 protein expression and is usually negative for SMA and desmin.

Epithelioid GIST may mimic PEComa; however, the tumor cells of GIST are usually less pleomorphic and lack the granular cytoplasm and the perivascular arrangement of tumor cells present in PEComa. Although there may be expression of SMA and desmin in GIST, the cells are negative for melanocytic markers. PEComa may rarely show focal expression of DOG1.

PEComa may show similar morphologic features to malignant GNET or clear cell sarcoma-like tumor of the GI tract in that both tumors are typically composed of an admixture of spindled and epithelioid cells, with varying degrees of atypia. Furthermore, PEComa may show focal expression of S-100. Distinction is made by careful morphologic evaluation and further aided by IHC and molecular tests when necessary. GNET frequently contains osteoclast-like giant cells and pseudoglandular areas, and the tumor cells do not show the close association with vessel walls typical of PEComa. The tumor cells show strong diffuse S-100 positivity and are negative for SMA, desmin, and melanocytic markers (unlike conventional clear cell sarcoma). Molecular studies to evaluate for *EWSR1* rearrangement (caused by the presence of *EWSR1-ATF1* or *EWSR1-CREB1* fusion genes) can help confirm a diagnosis of malignant GNET.

Immunohistochemistry can also distinguish PEComa from paraganglioma because the cells of paraganglioma are positive for synaptophysin and chromogranin and negative for smooth muscle and melanocytic markers.

Prognosis and Therapy

PEComas may be benign or may pursue a clinically aggressive course. The most common metastatic sites are the liver, lymph nodes, lungs, and bone. mTOR pathway inhibitors such as sirolimus and everolimus have shown efficacy in advanced disease. In a series of 35 patients with PEComa of the GI tract, 13 (37%) developed metastases, and 5 died of disease, with a median interval from time of diagnosis to death of 22 months.

PECOMA—FACT SHEET

Definition

- Mesenchymal neoplasm showing dual myoid and melanocytic differentiation

Incidence and Location

- Rare; in the gastrointestinal (GI) tract, colon is the most common site
- Angiomyolipoma is a subtype of perivascular epithelioid cell tumor (PEComa) that occurs in the liver and kidney

Morbidity and Mortality

- Symptoms depend on specific site and tumor size
- Behavior ranges from benign to malignant

Gender, Race, and Age Distribution

- Overall female predilection but less so in the GI tract
- Young to middle-aged adults

Clinical Features

- Pain, obstructive symptoms, bleeding, anemia, fever

Prognosis and Therapy

- Behavior ranges from benign to malignant
- Surgical excision is standard of care
- mTOR (mammalian target of rapamycin) inhibitors may show efficacy in the management of advanced disease

PECOMA—PATHOLOGIC FEATURES

Gross Findings

- 3 to 6 cm but wide size range
- Solid white mass; may involve any later of the intestinal wall

Microscopic Findings

- Nests or sheets of epithelioid cells; sometimes with admixed or predominance of spindled cells
- Granular, pale cytoplasm
- Radial arrangement of tumor cells around blood vessels
- Variable mitotic activity
- Malignant forms may show marked cytologic atypia and pleomorphism and increased mitotic activity
- Prominent vascular network composed of capillaries and small-medium sized thin-walled vessels

Immunohistochemistry

- Variable expression of smooth muscle actin, desmin and caldesmon, and HMB45 (human melanoma black), Melan-A/MART-1, microphthalmia transcription factor (MiTF)
- Transcription factor enhancer 3 (TFE3)expression in a subset of cases, often with *TFE3* gene rearrangement
- S-100 expression is uncommon and if present is usually focal
- Negative for secondary melanocytic markers, KIT, keratin, and CD34

Molecular Genetics

- *TSC2* (and less often *TSC1*) mutations in 80%
- *TFE3* gene rearrangements in around 10%; the most common fusion partner is *PSF/SFPQ*

Differential Diagnosis

- Gastrointestinal stromal tumor: especially myxoid or succinate dehydrogenase–deficient types: positive for KIT and DOG1
- Metastatic melanoma: may be positive for secondary melanocytic markers; lacks EWSR1 rearrangement
- Conventional clear cell sarcoma: rarely involves the gastrointestinal tract; more prominent nested growth pattern; also expresses HMB45, MART1, and tyrosinase

SUGGESTED READINGS

1. Fletcher CD, Berman JJ, Corless C, et al. Diagnosis of gastrointestinal stromal tumors: a consensus approach. *Human Pathol.* 2002;33(5):459–465.
2. Andersson J, Bumming P, Meis-Kindblom JM, et al. Gastrointestinal stromal tumors with KIT exon 11 deletions are associated with poor prognosis. *Gastroenterology.* 2006;130(6):1573–1581.
3. Wagner AJ, Remillard SP, Zhang YX, et al. Loss of expression of SDHA predicts SDHA mutations in gastrointestinal stromal tumors. *Mod Pathol.* 2013;26(2):289–294.
4. Antonescu CR, Romeo S, Zhang L, et al. Dedifferentiation in gastrointestinal stromal tumor to an anaplastic KIT-negative phenotype: a diagnostic pitfall: morphologic and molecular characterization of 8 cases occurring either de novo or after imatinib therapy. *Am J Surg Pathol.* 2013;37(3):385–392.
5. Duensing A, Medeiros F, McConarty B, et al. Mechanisms of oncogenic KIT signal transduction in primary gastrointestinal stromal tumors (GISTs). *Oncogene.* 2004;23(22):3999–4006.
6. Lasota J, Corless CL, Heinrich MC, et al. Clinicopathologic profile of gastrointestinal stromal tumors (GISTs) with primary KIT exon 13 or exon 17 mutations: a multicenter study on 54 cases. *Mod Pathol.* 2008;21(4):476–484.
7. Lasota J, Miettinen M. Clinical significance of oncogenic KIT and PDGFRA mutations in gastrointestinal stromal tumours. *Histopathology.* 2008;53(3):245–266.
8. Liegl B, Kepten I, Le C, et al. Heterogeneity of kinase inhibitor resistance mechanisms in GIST. *J Pathol.* 2008;216(1):64–74.
9. Miettinen M, Makhlouf H, Sobin LH, et al. Gastrointestinal stromal tumors of the jejunum and ileum: a clinicopathologic, immunohistochemical, and molecular genetic study of 906 cases before imatinib with long-term follow-up. *Am J Surg Pathol.* 2006;30(4):477–489.
10. West RB, Corless CL, Chen X, et al. The novel marker, DOG1, is expressed ubiquitously in gastrointestinal stromal tumors irrespective of KIT or PDGFRA mutation status. *Am J Pathol.* 2004;165(1):107–113.
11. Doyle LA, Nelson D, Heinrich MC, et al. Loss of succinate dehydrogenase subunit B (SDHB) expression is limited to a distinctive subset of gastric wild-type gastrointestinal stromal tumours: a comprehensive genotype-phenotype correlation study. *Histopathology.* 2012;61(5):801–809.
12. Miettinen M, Sarlomo-Rikala M, Sobin LH, et al. Gastrointestinal stromal tumors and leiomyosarcomas in the colon: a clinicopathologic, immunohistochemical, and molecular genetic study of 44 cases. *Am J Surg Pathol.* 2000;24(10):1339–1352.
13. Miettinen M, Sarlomo-Rikala M, Sobin LH, et al. Esophageal stromal tumors: a clinicopathologic, immunohistochemical, and molecular genetic study of 17 cases and comparison with esophageal leiomyomas and leiomyosarcomas. *Am J Surg Pathol.* 2000;24(2):211–222.
14. Miettinen M, Furlong M, Sarlomo-Rikala M, et al. Gastrointestinal stromal tumors, intramural leiomyomas, and leiomyosarcomas in the rectum and anus: a clinicopathologic, immunohistochemical, and molecular genetic study of 144 cases. *Am J Surg Pathol.* 2001;25(9):1121–1133.
15. Miettinen M, Sarlomo-Rikala M, Sobin LH. Mesenchymal tumors of muscularis mucosae of colon and rectum are benign leiomyomas that should be separated from gastrointestinal stromal tumors—a clinicopathologic and immunohistochemical study of eighty-eight cases. *Mod Pathol.* 2001;14(10):950–956.

16. Alpert L, Al-Sabti R, Graham RP, et al. Smooth muscle tumors of the gastrointestinal tract: an analysis of prognostic features in 407 cases. *Mod Pathol*. 2020;33(7):1410–1419.
17. Antonescu CR, Nafa K, Segal NH, et al. EWS-CREB1: a recurrent variant fusion in clear cell sarcoma—association with gastrointestinal location and absence of melanocytic differentiation. *Clin Cancer Res*. 2006;12(18):5356–5362.
18. Kosemehmetoglu K, Folpe AL. Clear cell sarcoma of tendons and aponeuroses, and osteoclast-rich tumour of the gastrointestinal tract with features resembling clear cell sarcoma of soft parts: a review and update. *J Clin Pathol*. 2010;63(5):416–423.
19. Stockman DL, Miettinen M, Suster S, et al. Malignant gastrointestinal neuroectodermal tumor: clinicopathologic, immunohistochemical, ultrastructural, and molecular analysis of 16 cases with a reappraisal of clear cell sarcoma-like tumors of the gastrointestinal tract. *Am J Surg Pathol*. 2012;36(6):857–868.
20. Daum O, Hes O, Vanecek T, et al. Vanek's tumor (inflammatory fibroid polyp). Report of 18 cases and comparison with three cases of original Vanek's series. *Ann Diagn Pathol*. 2003;7(6):337–347.
21. Pantanowitz L, Antonioli DA, Pinkus GS, et al. Inflammatory fibroid polyps of the gastrointestinal tract: evidence for a dendritic cell origin. *Am J Surg Pathol*. 2004;28(1):107–114.
22. Huss S, Wardelmann E, Goltz D, et al. Activating PDGFRA mutations in inflammatory fibroid polyps occur in exons 12, 14 and 18 and are associated with tumour localization. *Histopathology*. 2012;61(1):59–68.
23. Lasota J, Wang ZF, Sobin LH, et al. Gain-of-function PDGFRA mutations, earlier reported in gastrointestinal stromal tumors, are common in small intestinal inflammatory fibroid polyps. A study of 60 cases. *Mod Pathol*. 2009;22(8):1049–1056.
24. Takahashi Y, Suzuki M, Fukusato T. Plexiform angiomyxoid myofibroblastic tumor of the stomach. *World J Gastroenterol*. 2010;16(23):2835–2840.
25. Pailoor J, Mun KS, Chen CT, et al. Plexiform angiomyxoid myofibroblastic tumour of the stomach. *Pathology*. 2009;41(7):698–699.
26. Miettinen M, Makhlouf HR, Sobin LH, et al. Plexiform fibromyxoma: a distinctive benign gastric antral neoplasm not to be confused with a myxoid GIST. *Am J Surg Pathol*. 2009;33(11):1624–1632.
27. Voltaggio L, Murray R, Lasota J, et al. Gastric schwannoma: a clinicopathologic study of 51 cases and critical review of the literature. *Human Pathol*. 2012;43(5):650–659.
28. Miettinen M, Shekitka KM, Sobin LH. Schwannomas in the colon and rectum: a clinicopathologic and immunohistochemical study of 20 cases. *Am J Surg Pathol*. 2001;25(7):846–855.
29. Agaimy A, Stoehr R, Vieth M, et al. Benign serrated colorectal fibroblastic polyps/intramucosal perineuriomas are true mixed epithelial-stromal polyps (hybrid hyperplastic polyp/mucosal perineurioma) with frequent BRAF mutations. *Am J Surg Pathol*. 2010;34(11):1663–1671.
30. Eslami-Varzaneh F, Washington K, Robert ME, et al. Benign fibroblastic polyps of the colon: a histologic, immunohistochemical, and ultrastructural study. *Am J Surg Pathol*. 2004;28(3):374–378.
31. Hornick JL, Fletcher CD. Intestinal perineuriomas: clinicopathologic definition of a new anatomic subset in a series of 10 cases. *Am J Surg Pathol*. 2005;29(7):859–865.
32. Lewin MR, Dilworth HP, Abu Alfa AK, et al. Mucosal benign epithelioid nerve sheath tumors. *Am J Surg Pathol*. 2005;29(10):1310–1315.
33. Gibson JA, Hornick JL. Mucosal Schwann cell "hamartoma": clinicopathologic study of 26 neural colorectal polyps distinct from neurofibromas and mucosal neuromas. *Am J Surg Pathol*. 2009;33(5):781–787.
34. Shekitka KM, Sobin LH. Ganglioneuromas of the gastrointestinal tract. Relation to Von Recklinghausen disease and other multiple tumor syndromes. *Am J Surg Pathol*. 1994;18(3):250–257.
35. Burke 1 AP, Helwig EB. Gangliocytic paraganglioma. *Am J Clin Pathol*. 1989;92(1):1–9.
36. Appelman HD, Helwig EB. Glomus tumors of the stomach. *Cancer*. 1969;23(1):203–213.
37. Miettinen M, Paal E, Lasota J, et al. Gastrointestinal glomus tumors: a clinicopathologic, immunohistochemical, and molecular genetic study of 32 cases. *Am J Surg Pathol*. 2002;26(3):301–311.
38. Folpe AL, Fanburg-Smith JC, Miettinen M, et al. Atypical and malignant glomus tumors: analysis of 52 cases, with a proposal for the reclassification of glomus tumors. *Am J Surg Pathol*. 2001;25(1):1–12.
39. Makhlouf HR, Sobin LH. Inflammatory myofibroblastic tumors (inflammatory pseudotumors) of the gastrointestinal tract: how closely are they related to inflammatory fibroid polyps? *Human Pathol*. 2002;33(3):307–315.
40. Folpe AL, Mentzel T, Lehr HA, et al. Perivascular epithelioid cell neoplasms of soft tissue and gynecologic origin: a clinicopathologic study of 26 cases and review of the literature. *Am J Surg Pathol*. 2005;29(12):1558–1575.
41. Doyle LA, Hornick JL, Fletcher CD. PEComa of the gastrointestinal tract: clinicopathologic study of 35 cases with evaluation of prognostic parameters. *Am J Surg Pathol*. 2013;37(12):1769–1782.

8

Non-Neoplastic and Neoplastic Disorders of the Appendix

■ **Deepa T. Patil, MD**

■ CONGENITAL AND ACQUIRED ANATOMIC ANOMALIES OF THE APPENDIX

Abnormal Location, Size, and Absence of the Appendix

The appendix can have a host of anatomic abnormalities, including atypical location, duplication, and congenital absence. The position of appendix is determined by the rotation of the gut and position of the cecum during embryonic development. Retrocecal appendix is the most common abnormal location of the appendix. An abnormally long appendix (normal is 7–10 cm) has been linked to primary acute torsion, although torsion has also been reported in appendices of normal length. There can be complete or incomplete septa, which are seen principally in children and young adults and associated with acute appendicitis. Complete absence of appendix or atresia is extremely rare. This diagnosis in only made after a thorough search of the ileocecal region has failed to reveal an abnormally located appendix.

Diverticular Disease

Diverticula of the appendix can be congenital, in which case the muscularis propria is part of the diverticular wall, or acquired, in which case the diverticulum results from increased intraluminal pressure and mucosal herniation through a defect in the muscularis propria. This defect usually corresponds to the site of a penetrating artery. Acquired diverticula are more common than congenital diverticula and are seen in 1% to 2% of the population. However, acquired diverticula are greatly increased in patients with cystic fibrosis (CF), in whom they are found in up to 22% of appendectomy specimens. Patients may be completely asymptomatic or may present with signs and symptoms of acute appendicitis.

Grossly, the appendix may appear edematous and dilated. However, in most cases, diverticula cannot be easily identified. In case of perforation, the serosa shows purulent exudate. In the presence of dilated appendix, the lumen may be filled with mucin, and there may be evidence of extraappendiceal mucin. Histologically, there is outpouching of appendiceal mucosa through the muscularis propria, with or without periappendiceal fibrosis (Fig. 8.1). The muscularis propria is usually attenuated. The epithelium may show reactive or hyperplastic epithelial changes that may be difficult to distinguish from low-grade appendiceal mucinous neoplasm. Diverticular disease can be associated with acellular mucin within the appendiceal wall, resulting in diagnostic mimicry with an appendiceal mucinous neoplasm. Preservation of the mucosal architecture with intact lamina propria and muscularis mucosae and lack of unequivocal cytologic dysplasia support a diagnosis of diverticular disease.

■ FIBROUS OBLITERATION OF THE APPENDICEAL LUMEN (NEURAL HYPERPLASIA)

CLINICAL FEATURES

There are no specific features because this is typically an incidental finding in about one-third of appendices excised for a variety of reasons.

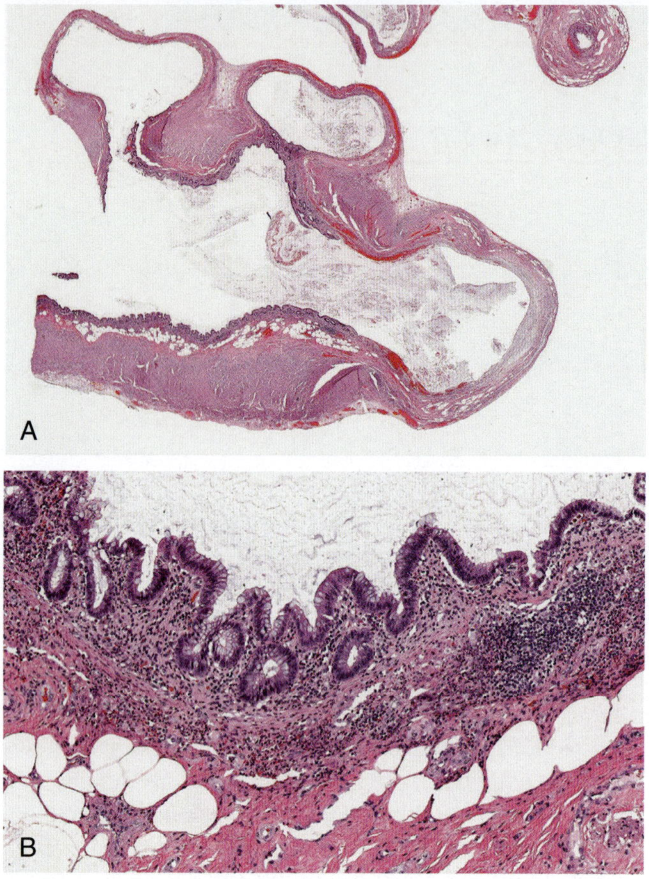

FIGURE 8.1

A, Appendiceal diverticular disease. The appendiceal tip shows numerous outpouchings composed of mucosa and submucosal tissue with attenuation of the corresponding muscularis propria. **B**, Higher magnification of the mucosa shows normal epithelial lining with intact lamina propria and muscularis mucosae.

FIBROUS OBLITERATION OF THE APPENDICEAL LUMEN (NEURAL HYPERPLASIA)—FACT SHEET

Definition

- A spindle cell proliferation that fills and "obliterates" the appendix lumen, usually at the tip

Incidence and Location

- Found in about one-third of excised appendices

Morbidity and Mortality

- None

Gender, Race, and Age Distribution

- All ages, without race or gender predisposition

Clinical Features

- Incidental finding in appendices excised for all reasons

Pathologic Features

Gross Findings

The tip of the appendix is usually affected. No definite lumen is identified. Instead, the cut surface appears tan to white.

Microscopic Findings

The appendiceal lumen is obliterated by a proliferation of bland spindle cells in a collagenous and myxoid background. The individual cells may have "wavy" or "buckled" nuclei (Fig. 8.2). These cells consist of an admixture of fibroblasts, Schwann cells, and axons. The process may be confined to the mucosa ("intramucosal variant") or may replace the entire lumen. These phenomena are believed to be overall proliferative, with attendant phases of growth, involution, and finally fibrosis. Immunohistochemical staining shows S-100 protein and neuron-specific enolase–reactive spindle cells (intermingled Schwann cells and axons, respectively), and scattered endocrine cells. The fibroblasts may be positive for CD34.

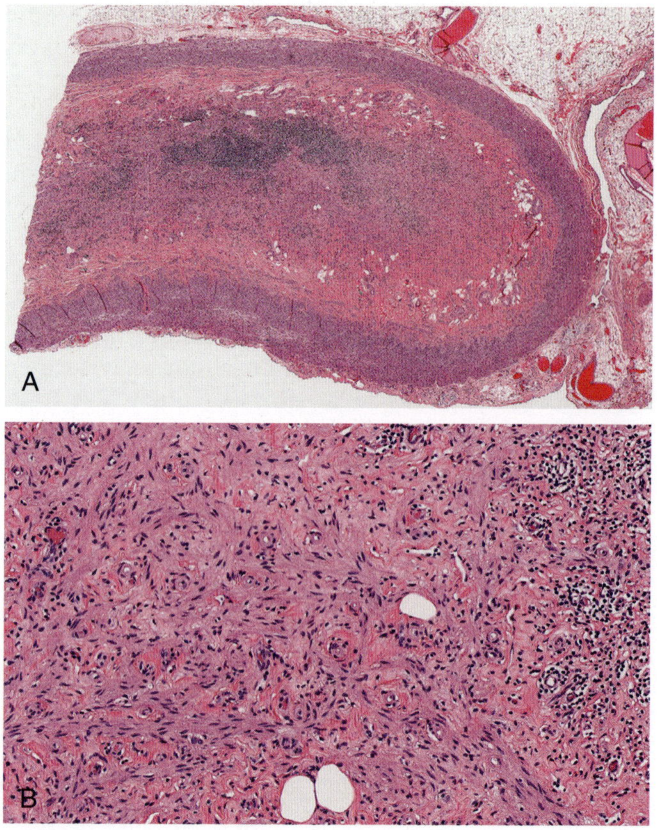

FIGURE 8.2

Fibrous obliteration of appendix. **A**, The bisected appendiceal tip shows completer obliteration of the appendiceal lumen by spindle cells and inflammatory cells. **B**, Higher magnification shows that the spindle cell population is composed of bland cells with wavy nuclei. These cells express S-100 protein and are often admixed with fibroblasts.

Fibrous Obliteration of the Appendiceal Lumen (Neural Hyperplasia)—Pathologic Features

Gross Findings

- Normal appendix diameter with lumen being replaced by tan-white fibrous tissue

Microscopic Findings

- Bland spindle cell proliferation amid fibromyxoid stroma

Immunohistochemistry

- S-100– and neuron-specific enolase–positive cells with scattered endocrine cells

Differential Diagnosis

- With benign mesenchymal tumors, the luminal location is the key

Differential Diagnosis

The differential diagnosis is with the host of spindle cell tumors of the gastrointestinal (GI) tract that are discussed in Chapter 7. However, the location (with its epicenter in the lumen of the appendix) and nature of the spindle cell proliferation are helpful in distinguishing it from other mesenchymal neoplasms, especially those of neural origin.

Prognosis and Therapy

Fibrous obliteration is a benign and incidental lesion.

ACUTE APPENDICITIS

CLINICAL FEATURES

Acute appendicitis most commonly affects children and adolescents (5–15 years) but occasionally may present in older individuals as well. The approximate incidence of acute appendicitis is 7% to 10%. It results from mucosal injury secondary to luminal obstruction by a fecalith, parasite, fragment of undigested food, or lymphoid hyperplasia followed by bacterial infection that progressively spreads from the mucosa to involve the appendiceal wall. Perforation is more common in the very young and in the older age groups. In older patients, the inflammatory process is often associated with neoplasms. Some observers believe that all appendices should be removed during surgery for suspected acute appendicitis, even when grossly normal, because nearly 20% of normal-appearing appendices may have acute inflammation on microscopic examination. A possible exception is patients who might require urologic surgery in the future because their appendices may later serve as urinary conduits.

Both ultrasound and computed tomography (CT) are useful in diagnosing acute appendicitis. The only sonographic sign that is specific for appendicitis is an enlarged, noncompressible appendix measuring greater than 6 mm in maximal diameter. CT signs of acute appendicitis include a distended appendix greater than 7 mm in maximal diameter, appendiceal wall thickening and enhancement, an appendicolith, circumferential or focal cecal apical thickening, pericecal fat stranding, adjacent bowel wall thickening, focal or free peritoneal fluid, mesenteric lymphadenopathy, and intraperitoneal phlegmon or abscess.

ACUTE APPENDICITIS—FACT SHEET

Definition

- An acute inflammatory process attributed to local obstruction and infection involving the appendix

Incidence and Location

- Involves the appendix
- Incidences reported up to 7%

Morbidity and Mortality

- Complications include wound infection, urinary retention, bowel obstruction, intraabdominal abscesses, urinary tract infections, and pneumonia, all more likely if the appendix has perforated
- Overall mortality rate for appendectomy is about 0.3%; in individuals older than 65 years, this percentage is closer to 5%

Gender, Race, and Age Distribution

- Peak presentation is from 5 to 15 years, but it occurs at any age
- Male predominance in all races, but acute appendicitis is more common in whites than in African Americans and Asian Americans

Clinical Features

- Classically, right lower quadrant pain accompanied by fever and elevated white blood cell count, but many variants occur

Prognosis and Therapy

- Treatment is appendectomy
- Preoperative antibiotics followed by appendectomy ("interval appendectomy") have been advocated in patients with perforated appendices
- Overall prognosis is good

Pathologic Features

Gross Findings

The appendix may appear grossly normal when inflammation is limited to the mucosa and submucosa. However, when inflammation extends into the muscularis propria, the appendix frequently becomes swollen and erythematous. When the serosa is affected, the serosal aspect is initially dull and gray followed by a fibrinous or purulent exudate. Gangrenous appendicitis may show a purple, green, or blackish discoloration. Perforation secondary to mural necrosis can follow, which may lead to abscess formation. Cut surface shows edema and hyperemia of the wall, with or without intraluminal purulent contents. At times, an appendix resected in the clinical setting of acute appendicitis is grossly and histologically normal, even after submission of the complete specimen for histologic examination. In these cases, a cause is rarely found.

MICROSCOPIC FINDINGS

Early acute suppurative appendicitis (phlegmonous appendicitis) usually shows mucosal erosions and scattered cryptitis and crypt abscesses (Figs. 8.3 and 8.4). Later, the inflammation extends to involve the appendiceal wall. Collection of neutrophils within the appendiceal lumen is considered insufficient for a diagnosis of acute appendicitis. Gangrenous appendicitis is associated with transmural necrosis extensive serosal fibroinflammatory reaction and can lead to perforation if left untreated.

As the appendix heals, two basic patterns may be seen. In the first, more typical pattern, there is a mixed inflammatory infiltrate ranging from patchy and mild to diffuse and transmural inflammation. Intramural or serosal foreign body–type giant cells surrounded by granulation tissue indicate prior rupture. Submucosal fibrosis, serositis, and fibrous adhesions can be present as well. In some cases, mucin extravasation may be a prominent feature and may lead to confusion with an appendiceal mucinous neoplasm. However, typical appendiceal mucinous neoplasms, even those that perforate, seldom show a prominent acute inflammatory component within the wall of the appendix and often display a dense fibrocollagenous stroma that is distinct from the acute edematous appearance of the stroma in acute appendicitis. A second pattern, which has been termed *xanthogranulomatous appendicitis*, consists of an inflammatory infiltrate rich in foamy histiocytes, multinucleate giant cells, abundant hemosiderin, and luminal obliteration with sparing of lymphoid follicles. These latter cases share features with Crohn's disease but differ by lacking epithelioid granulomas, having fewer lymphoid aggregates, and having less profound subserosal fibrosis.

Commonly, patients who present with ruptured acute appendicitis are treated with antibiotic therapy and drainage followed by a delayed or "interval appendectomy" (Figs. 8.5 and 8.6). In this setting, about two-thirds

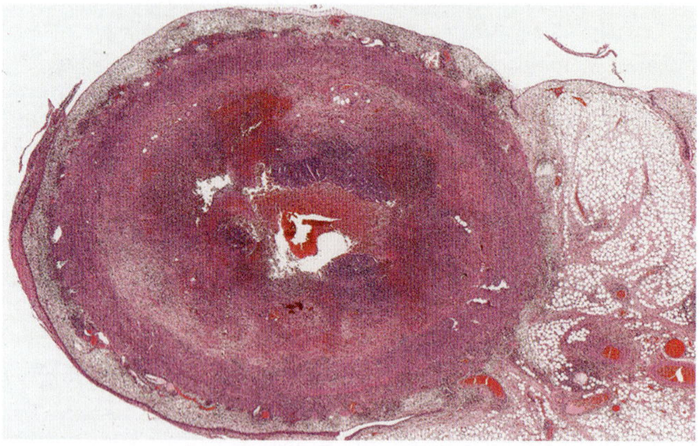

FIGURE 8.3

Acute appendicitis. The appendix shows an edematous and thickened wall with extensive mucosal ulceration and transmural suppurative inflammation. There is marked serosal fibroinflammatory reaction.

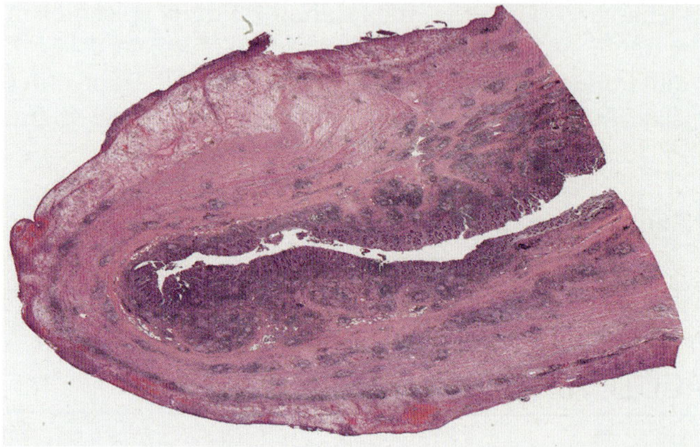

FIGURE 8.5

Gross specimen prepared from an "interval appendix." Antibiotic treatment was carried out for 4 weeks prior to appendectomy. Note the fibrous thickened wall, which suggests the possibility of Crohn's disease.

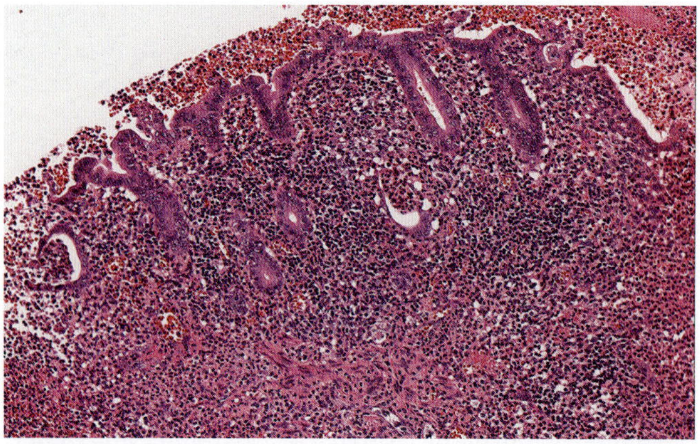

FIGURE 8.4

Acute appendicitis. Higher magnification of the mucosa shows reactive epithelial changes characterized by loss of mucin, cytoplasmic eosinophilia, slight nuclear hyperchromasia, and nuclear enlargement. There are neutrophilic cryptitis and crypt abscess formation.

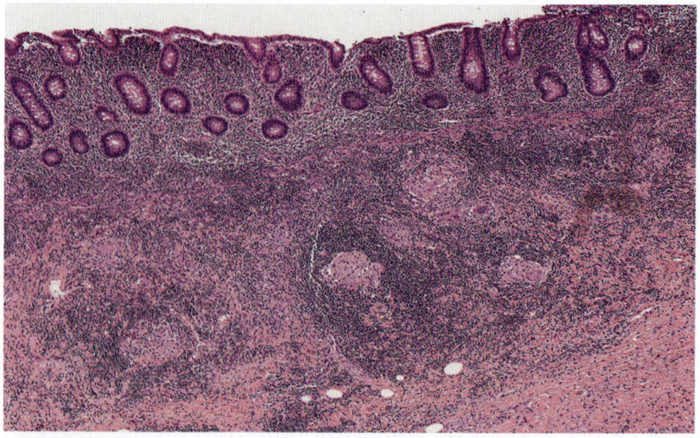

FIGURE 8.6

"Interval appendix." **A**, Low magnification shows thickened appendiceal wall with mural lymphoid aggregates arranged in a concentric pattern. This pattern has been linked to a "string of pearls." **B**, Higher magnification shows giant cells and epithelioid granulomas within the appendiceal submucosa.

of patients have granulomas compared with fewer than 10% of acute appendicitis control participants. About one-third of interval appendectomy patients have xanthogranulomatous inflammation, and about half show a Crohn's-like infiltrate. This is analogous to changes seen in sigmoid colon resections after antibiotic therapy for acute diverticulitis and should not be misinterpreted as manifestations of Crohn's disease.

It is common for patients with neoplastic processes to present with clinical signs and symptoms of acute appendicitis only to reveal a neuroendocrine tumor (NET) or goblet cell neoplasm within the wall of the appendix. These cases require careful histologic evaluation to prevent misdiagnosis.

ACUTE APPENDICITIS—PATHOLOGIC FEATURES

Gross Findings

- Thickened diameter, depending on severity of process, with or without perforation. Serosa may be dull from periappendicitis

Microscopic Findings

- Early lesions display mucosal erosions and scattered crypt abscesses; later, the inflammation extends into the wall of the appendix
- When the inflammation extensively damages the muscularis propria, mural necrosis can lead to perforation
- In appendectomies performed in patients with prior appendicitis, there are mixed inflammatory infiltrates ranging from patchy and mild to diffuse and transmural
- In some appendices, there may be intramural or serosal foreign body–type giant cells surrounded by granulation tissue suggestive of prior rupture
- Serositis and fibrous adhesions, as well as prominent submucosal fibrosis, may be present
- Mucin extravasation is often seen but is admixed with a prominent inflammatory component, which is helpful in distinguishing this from a ruptured low-grade appendiceal mucinous neoplasm
- Xanthogranulomatous appendicitis: features an infiltrate of foam cells, scattered multinucleated histiocytes, abundant hemosiderin, and luminal obliteration with spared lymphoid follicles

Differential Diagnosis

- Interval appendectomy specimens share features with Crohn's disease but differ by lacking epithelioid granulomas and having fewer lymphoid aggregates and less mural fibrosis, and these patients lack prior and concurrent clinical symptoms and endoscopic or radiologic signs of Crohn's disease
- Appendiceal involvement as part of an infectious enterocolitis and mechanical trauma associated with fecaliths. Both these conditions can cause superficial cryptitis and crypt abscesses. However, mural inflammation is typically present only in acute appendicitis. Inflammatory bowel disease involving the appendix is also in the differential (discussed later)

PROGNOSIS AND THERAPY

The definite form of treatment is appendectomy. Complications include wound infection, urinary retention, bowel obstruction, intraabdominal abscesses, urinary tract infections, and pneumonia, all more likely if the appendix has perforated. Rarer complications include fistula formation, pylephlebitis, and liver abscesses. The overall mortality rate for appendectomy is about 0.3%. In individuals older than 65 years, the mortality rate approaches 5%.

PERIAPPENDICITIS

Periappendicitis is characterized by serosal fibroinflammatory reaction with or without adhesions in the absence of mucosal or mural inflammation. Although intraoperative mechanical manipulation of the appendix alone may result in mild granulocytic infiltration of the serosa, the presence of fibrinous exudate is a potentially clinically significant finding. Periappendicitis is found in 1% to 5% of appendices resected for clinically acute appendicitis. The vast majority of cases are secondary to salpingitis. In two large series, the causes of periappendicitis included gonococcal and chlamydial salpingitis, yersiniosis, Meckel's diverticulitis, and associated intraperitoneal abscess, urologic disorders, colon neoplasms, infectious colitis, abdominal aortic aneurysm, bacterial peritonitis, and GI perforation.

Grossly, the appendix is normal in size, and depending on the severity of periappendicitis, the serosal surface appears dull or tan to gray. The lumen and mucosa appear normal. Histologically, there is a serosa-confined (or possibly with extension into muscularis propria) inflammatory cell infiltrate consisting of neutrophils and fibrin if the process is acute (Fig. 8.7) or with adhesions and chronic inflammation if the process is chronic. The lumen is unaffected. The pathologist's finding of periappendicitis on an appendectomy specimen in the absence of luminal disease should alert the surgeon to take measures to identify the source of the serosal injury. If the patient is a woman, the genital tract is a likely source, but as noted previously,

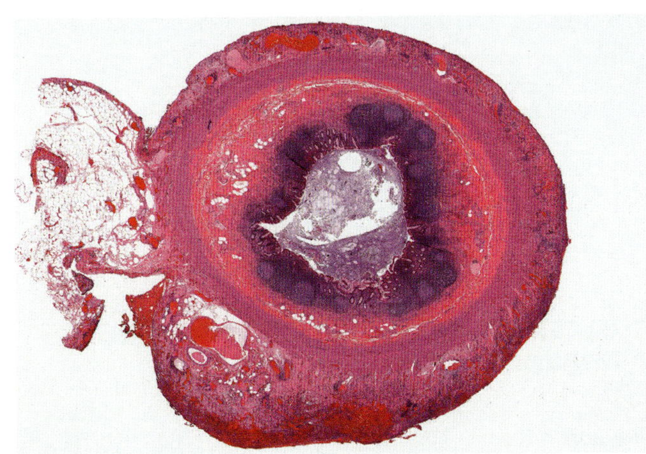

FIGURE 8.7

Periappendicitis with acute and chronic serositis with fibrosis and adhesions. In these cases, the mucosa is usually completely normal.

any abdominal process may result in periappendicitis. The treatment and prognosis depend on the inciting extraappendiceal lesion.

PERIAPPENDICITIS—FACT SHEET

Definition

- Inflammatory process confined to the appendix serosa without luminal involvement (and thus with an extraappendiceal source)

Incidence and Location

- Periappendicitis alone is found in 1% to 5% of appendices resected for clinically acute appendicitis, the majority of which are attributable to salpingitis

Morbidity and Mortality

- Depends on the source of the periappendicitis

Clinical Features

- Attributable to a variety of processes: gonococcal and chlamydial salpingitis; yersiniosis, Meckel's diverticulitis, and associated intraperitoneal abscess; urologic disorders; colon neoplasms; infectious colitis; abdominal aortic aneurysm; bacterial peritonitis; and gastrointestinal perforation

Prognosis and Therapy

- Depends on the source of the periappendicitis

PERIAPPENDICITIS—PATHOLOGIC FEATURES

Gross Findings

- Serosal thickening or exudates with normal muscularis propria and mucosa

Microscopic Findings

- Serosal fibroinflammatory process with normal rest of the appendiceal wall

Differential Diagnosis

- Acute appendicitis
- Chronic appendicitis: The term *chronic appendicitis* has been variably used in the past to describe pathologic changes following recurrent episodes of acute appendicitis, for interval appendectomy when resection for perforated appendix is delayed as a result of initial conservative therapy with antibiotics and drainage, and other chronic inflammatory conditions of the appendix, such as ulcerative colitis, Crohn's disease, granulomatous appendicitis, infections, diverticular disease, and cystic fibrosis

ULCERATIVE COLITIS INVOLVING THE APPENDIX

The appendix has been shown to play a protective role in ulcerative colitis. The prevalence of prior appendectomy is lower in patients with ulcerative colitis than in the general population. Ulcerative appendicitis, the appendiceal counterpart of ulcerative colitis, is typically present in patients with pancolitis but is also common as a "skip lesion" in patients who have left-sided or rectal disease. It has an overall prevalence of 50% in patients with ulcerative colitis.

Grossly, the appendiceal mucosa appears erythematous and ulcerated. Ulcerative appendicitis shows the same histologic features as ulcerative colitis. Active mucosal inflammation is characterized by cryptitis and crypt abscesses. Chronic changes include crypt architectural distortion, basal lymphoplasmacytosis, and basal lymphoid aggregates. Ulcerative appendicitis is distinguished from early acute appendicitis partly on the basis of clinical history, although early acute appendicitis shows minimal crypt architectural distortion and basal plasmacytosis.

ULCERATIVE COLITIS INVOLVING THE APPENDIX—FACT SHEET

Definition

- Appendiceal inflammatory disease (usually chronic active) in patient with ulcerative colitis

Incidence and Location

- Common in patients with ulcerative colitis and predominantly involving the orifice rather than the appendiceal tip

Morbidity and Mortality

- Same as for ulcerative colitis

Gender, Race, and Age Distribution

- Same as for ulcerative colitis

ULCERATIVE COLITIS INVOLVING THE APPENDIX—PATHOLOGIC FEATURES

Gross Findings

- Found either in continuity with pancolitis in ulcerative colitis or as a "skip" lesion in left-sided disease

Microscopic Findings

- Similar to those of ulcerative colitis elsewhere, featuring cryptitis, crypt distortion, and basal plasmacytosis

Differential Diagnosis

- Acute appendicitis

CROHN'S DISEASE INVOLVING THE APPENDIX

Most appendices resected in patients with Crohn's disease are unremarkable. Appendiceal involvement by Crohn's disease has been reported in up to 20% of patients and is typically associated with extensive ileocolonic involvement. Most patients who present with *granulomatous appendicitis* do not later manifest typical Crohn's disease elsewhere in the GI tract.

CROHN'S DISEASE INVOLVING THE APPENDIX—FACT SHEET

Definition

- Appendiceal inflammatory disease in a patient known to have Crohn's disease

Incidence and Location

- Uncommon; may be found in any part of the appendix

Morbidity and Mortality

- Same as for Crohn's disease

Gender, Race, and Age Distribution

- Same as Crohn's disease: Grossly, the appendiceal wall is thick and fibrotic in patients with Crohn's disease, and involvement may be patchy. In patients with clinical Crohn's disease, the appendices have the typical histologic features of Crohn's seen elsewhere in the gastrointestinal tract, with fissures, ulcers, active or chronic active inflammation, lymphoid aggregates, and occasional granulomas (see Figs. 8.8 and 8.9 and Table 8.1). Diagnosis of Crohn's disease of the appendix requires clinicopathologic correlation. Determination of the type of inflammatory bowel disease should not be performed based on the findings in an appendectomy specimen because several causes may result in granulomatous appendicitis (see later). The prognosis for patients with Crohn's disease of the appendix is that of Crohn's disease in general (see Chapter 10) because those with appendiceal involvement usually have extensive ileocolic involvement

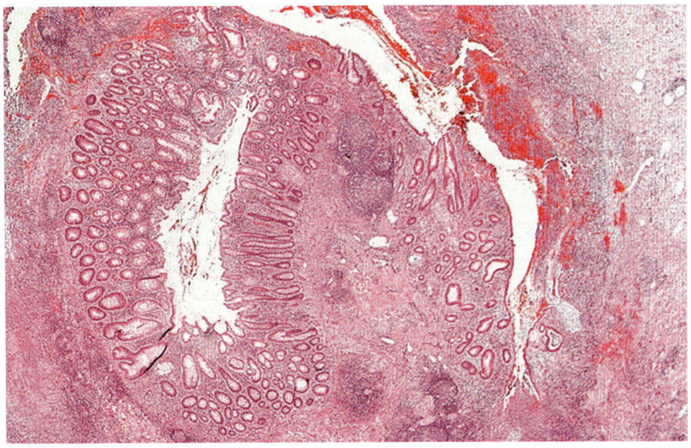

FIGURE 8.8

Appendiceal Crohn's disease. The specimen shows presence of active inflammation along with a deep fissuring ulcer.

CROHN'S DISEASE INVOLVING THE APPENDIX—PATHOLOGIC FEATURES

Gross Findings

- Thickened appendix, usually without grossly visible mucosal lesions

Microscopic Findings

- Segmental involvement with fissuring ulcers, chronic active inflammation, transmural lymphoid aggregates, epithelioid granulomas, and mural fibrosis

Differential Diagnosis

- If disease is limited to the appendix, one should not label a de novo patient as having Crohn's disease, and "interval" appendicitis should be considered
- Sarcoidosis

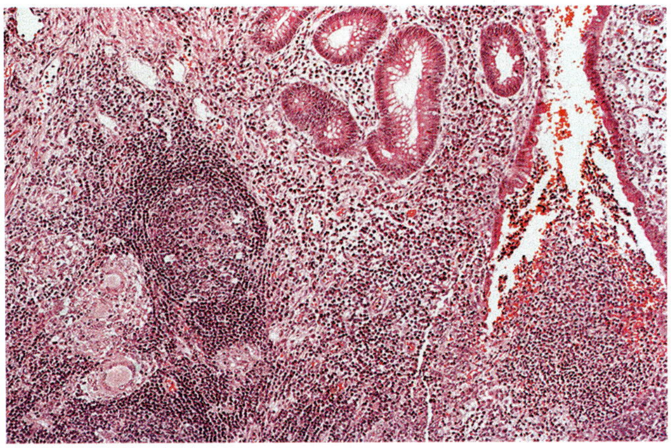

FIGURE 8.9

Appendiceal Crohn's disease. The specimen shows chronic active colitis with granulomatous inflammation.

TABLE 8.1

Chronic Inflammatory Disorders of the Appendix

Finding	Idiopathic Granulomatous Appendicitis	Crohn's Disease	Healing Acute Appendicitis
Neutrophilic cryptitis or crypt abscesses	+	+	+
Fissures or fistulae	Occasional fissures	+	-
Transmural lymphoid aggregates	Often	Often	Occasionally
Fibrosis	Often	Often	Often
Granulomas	Numerous	Occasional	No, but may have numerous foam cells

Other Studies

Newer microbiologic techniques may provide some clues to the causes of granulomatous appendicitis. For example, in a 2001 study by Lamps and her colleagues, 10 of 40 (25%) cases of granulomatous appendicitis were found to have evidence of pathogenic *Yersinia* species by polymerase chain reaction. However, now that some of the features of Crohn's disease are believed to reflect an immunologic defect in processing organisms that do not affect normal individuals, the interest in search for a unifying infectious cause of Crohn's disease has diminished greatly.

Granulomatous Appendicitis

Granulomatous appendicitis was first described in 1953 by Meyerding and Bertram and was initially believed to be a manifestation of Crohn's disease. However, studies that have appendiceal pathology in patients with documented idiopathic inflammatory bowel disease have shown that only a minority of patients with granulomatous appendicitis are a true manifestation of Crohn's disease. Based on our current understanding, granulomatous appendicitis results from several conditions such as interval appendicitis, infections (bacterial—*Yersinia* spp., tuberculosis; parasitic—schistosomiasis, strongyloidosis; fungal—*Candida* spp., *Histoplasma* spp.), sarcoidosis, Crohn's disease, and foreign body reaction. When a cause cannot be found, the condition is termed *idiopathic granulomatous appendicitis*. This histologic hallmark is the presence of granulomas that may involve any layer of the appendiceal wall. The presence of numerous granulomas, large-sized granulomas (>200 microns), and those with caseous necrosis or suppurative inflammation should prompt a search for infectious pathogens. The management of granulomatous appendicitis depends on the underlying cause, so appropriate ancillary infectious work-up and clinical information is essential.

CYSTIC FIBROSIS

Clinical Features

Cystic fibrosis occurs in approximately 1 of every 3200 live white births (in 1 of every 3900 live births of all Americans). Approximately 1000 new cases of CF are diagnosed each year. More than 80% of patients are diagnosed by age 3 years; however, nearly 10% of newly diagnosed patients are age 18 years or older. People with CF have a variety of symptoms, including very salty-tasting skin; persistent coughing, at times with phlegm; wheezing, or shortness of breath; an excessive appetite but poor weight gain; and greasy, bulky stools. Symptoms vary from person to person owing in part to the more than 1000 mutations of the *CFTR gene*. The sweat chloride test is the standard diagnostic test for CF.

Although recurrent pulmonary infections and pulmonary insufficiency are the hallmarks, GI symptoms commonly antedate the pulmonary findings and may suggest the diagnosis in infants and young children. The protean GI manifestations of CF result primarily from abnormally viscous luminal secretions within hollow viscera and the ducts of solid organs. Bowel obstruction may be present at birth because of meconium ileus or meconium plug syndrome. Overall, patients with CF have a lower frequency of acute appendicitis (1.5%) than the general population (~7%). In some cases, the engorged appendix itself can cause clinical symptoms of appendicitis even though histologic examination reveals no inflammation. The incidence of acquired appendiceal diverticula is also markedly increased in patients with CF.

CYSTIC FIBROSIS INVOLVING THE APPENDIX—FACT SHEET

Definition

- Involvement of the appendix in a patient known or subsequently found to have cystic fibrosis (CF)
- Gastrointestinal tract involvement may be the first presentation

Incidence and Location

- CF occurs in approximately 1 in every 3200 live white births (1 in every 3900 live births of all Americans)

Morbidity and Mortality

- Same as for CF in general
- Patients usually have numerous respiratory infections and gastrointestinal (GI) tract complications
- Adults are prone to diabetes, osteoporosis, and GI tract malignancies

Gender, Race, and Age Distribution

- Most cases of CF are diagnosed in early childhood
- No gender prevalence
- Most common in white populations

Clinical Features

- Patients with CF have a variety of symptoms, including very salty-tasting skin; persistent coughing, at times with phlegm; wheezing or shortness of breath; excessive appetite but poor weight gain; and greasy, bulky stools
- Symptoms vary owing in part to the more than 1000 mutations of the *CFTR* gene. Many patients present with GI tract symptoms, but the incidence of appendicitis is lower in these people than in control subjects (1%–2% vs 7%–10%)

Prognosis and Treatment

- Same as for CF
- Treatment of the underlying disease is directed at reducing pulmonary infections
- Most patients with CF live into their 30s

Pathologic Features

Gross Findings

On gross examination, the appendiceal lumen contains thick viscous tenacious mucus. In some cases, there may be evidence of a mucus plug. This abnormal mucin can cause marked engorgement of the appendix and can lead to a "sausage-like" appendix.

Microscopic Findings

In CF, the most common histologic finding is enlarged and distended goblet cells containing normal-appearing mucin, although this can be a subtle finding in many cases. The most readily identifiable abnormality is the presence of the thick inspissated eosinophilic mucin in the appendiceal lumen as well as within the crypts (Fig. 8.10).

Cystic Fibrosis Involving the Appendix—Pathologic Features

Gross Findings

- The appendix is enlarged and distended with mucus

Microscopic Findings

- Enlarged and distended goblet cells containing normal-appearing mucin along with thick inspissated eosinophilic mucin in the lumen as well as within the crypts

Differential Diagnosis

- Evaluation of the epithelium excludes neoplasms (sometimes multiple sections are required), and correlation with the clinical history is best in establishing a diagnosis of cystic fibrosis

Differential Diagnosis

Patients without CF sometimes have prominent inspissated mucus in their appendices. The clinical history is helpful in this regard. CF involving the appendix should also be differentiated from mucinous neoplasms of the appendix, which are typically associated with abundant luminal mucin. Evaluation of the epithelium helps exclude mucinous neoplasms.

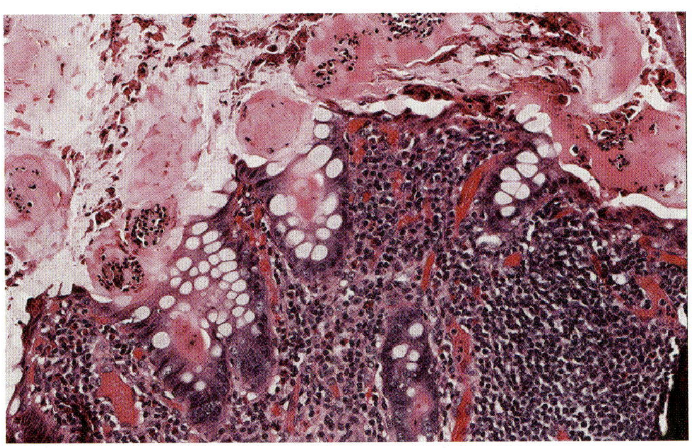

FIGURE 8.10

Cystic fibrosis (CF). The goblet cells are more prominent, and the luminal surface as well as the crypts contain thick inspissated mucin characteristic of CF.

Prognosis and Therapy

The treatment of patients with CF depends on the stage of the disease and the organs involved. Chest physical therapy, TOBI (tobramycin solution for inhalation), dornase alfa (Pulmozyme), and azithromycin are administered with the goal of clearing and thinning mucus secretions and controlling bacterial (especially *Pseudomonas aeruginosa*) infections.

INFECTIOUS CAUSES OF ACUTE APPENDICITIS

CLINICAL FEATURES

Infections of the appendix can be caused by bacteria, viruses, fungi, or parasites. In most cases of acute appendicitis, no organisms are identified by histology. Although specific infectious causes of acute appendicitis are only rarely identified, certain agents can occasionally be implicated. A few specific infections are noted in the following sections (see Chapter 9 for more details).

Actinomyces spp.

Actinomyces israelii is a rare cause of appendicitis. *A. israelii* can rarely lead to infections of the small intestine, appendix, or colon. Histologically, the long filamentous organisms stain dark blue on routine hematoxylin and eosin preparations and are particularly easy to recognize when associated with characteristic sulfur granules. Active inflammation in the mucosal wall is typically present, and fistula formation, rupture of the appendix, and abscess formation may complicate the clinical course. *Actinomyces turicensis* has also been implicated in appendicitis and is frequently accompanied by aerobic bacterial isolates of the *Streptococcus anginosus* group.

Malakoplakia

Malakoplakia is most commonly seen in the urinary tract but can occasionally be found in the appendix (Figs. 8.11 and 8.12). In general, malakoplakia results from an abnormal immune response in which bacteria are incompletely digested and accumulate in histiocytes.

The histologic findings typically consist of a diffuse or nodular thickening of the mucosal wall resulting from the accumulation of numerous macrophages, including many that are eosinophilic, with scattered lymphocytes and plasma cells. Most characteristics are the admixed Michaelis-Gutmann bodies, which are round, laminated, bluish-black structures with a targetoid appearance that can be highlighted with iron or calcium stains.

Parasite Infections

Enterobius vermicularis is one of the most common parasites seen in the appendix. Individuals in late childhood and early adolescence have the highest frequency of infection (ages 5–15 years). The organism is most commonly found in the lumen with no mucosal inflammatory response (Figs. 8.13 and 8.14). In one study, in which close to 22,000 appendices were evaluated, granulomatous inflammation and increased eosinophils in the lamina propria were quite rare and were both noted in fewer than 2 % of infections. There is an inverse relationship between active mucosal inflammation and pinworm infection. Mucosal inflammation, when present, has been more strongly linked to the presence of parasite ova.

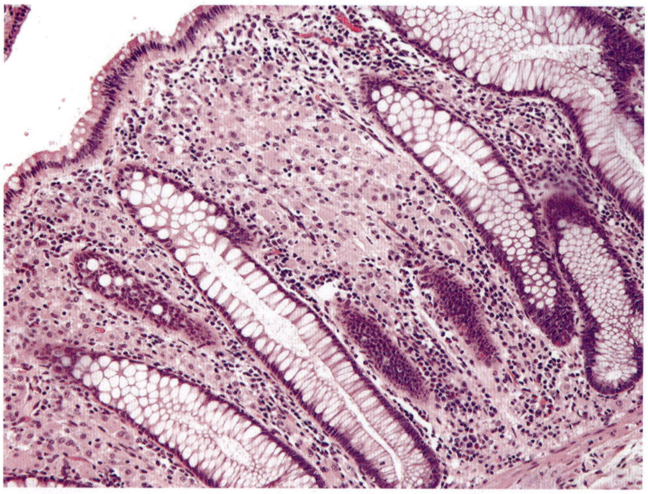

FIGURE 8.11

Malakoplakia showing sheets of histiocytes expanding the lamina propria.

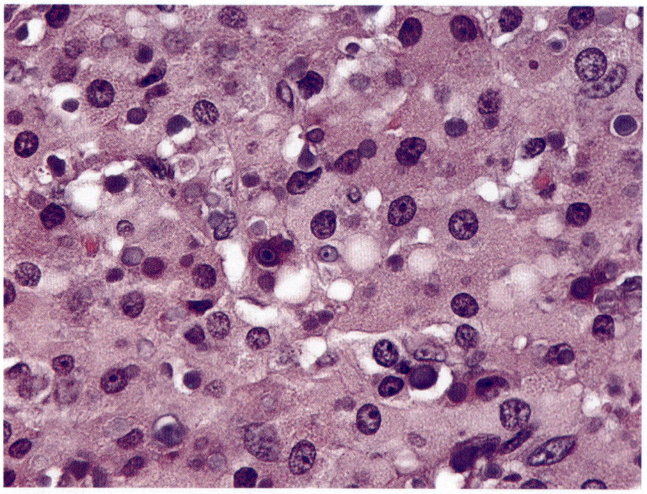

FIGURE 8.12

Malakoplakia. Note the admixed Michaelis-Gutmann bodies in this example of malakoplakia (round, laminated bluish-black structures with a targetoid appearance).

Viral Infections

Viral gastroenteritis does not typically result in appendectomy. Viral enteritis classically results in surgical excision of the appendix when it leads to ileocecal

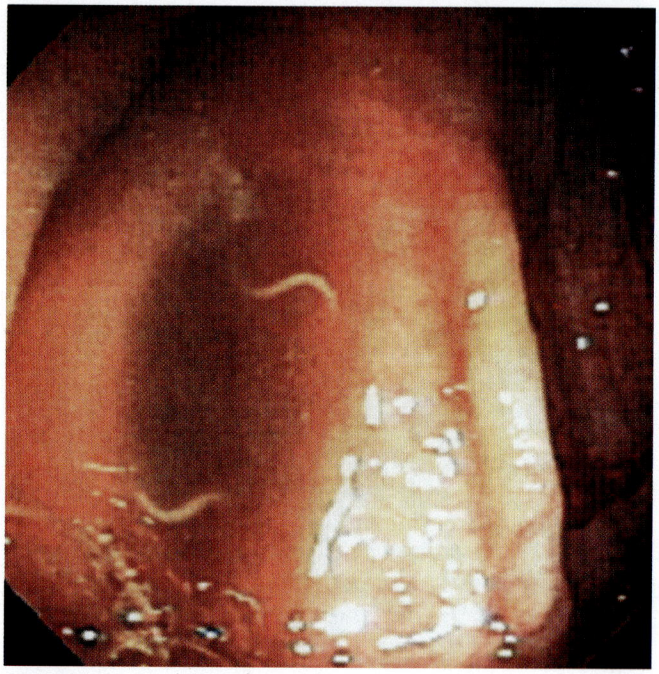

FIGURE 8.13

Enterobius vermicularis. Endoscopic appearance of the cecum in a patient with appendiceal disease. The image shows tiny, white parasites adherent to the mucosal surface.

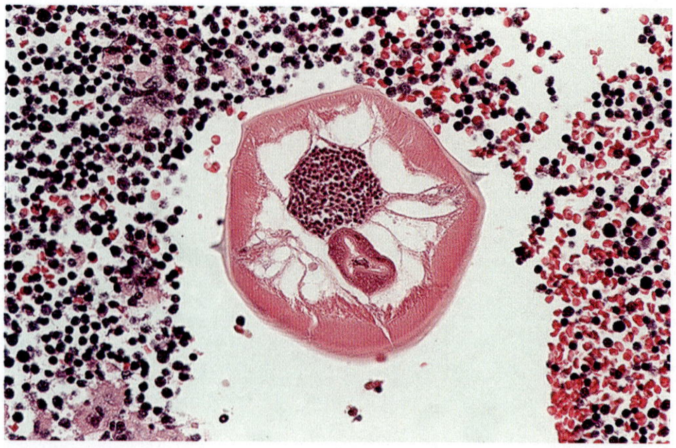

FIGURE 8.14

Enterobius vermicularis in the appendiceal lumen. Note the characteristic cuticular crests.

intussusception. Intussusception is common in infants and young children and is most often attributable to lymphoid hyperplasia in the terminal ileum, which can form a "leading edge." The viral agents implicated in this setting are rotavirus, echovirus, and adenovirus, of which adenovirus is the most common infectious agent. In appendices infected with adenovirus, in addition to prominent lymphoid hyperplasia, erosions may be identified. However, viral inclusions are usually found only in intact epithelial cells. Zones in which inclusions are more likely to be found are selected by scanning for areas with frayed-appearing epithelium showing loss of nuclear polarity and an eosinophilic appearance imparted by reactive mucin loss. Such zones are frequently seen in close association with lymphoid follicles. Intranuclear adenovirus inclusions are typically of the Cowdry B type, consisting of basophilic inclusions with nuclear smudging, although Cowdry A inclusions, featuring sharply demarcated globules surrounded by a clear zone, may be found in a minority of cases (Figs. 8.15 and 8.16).

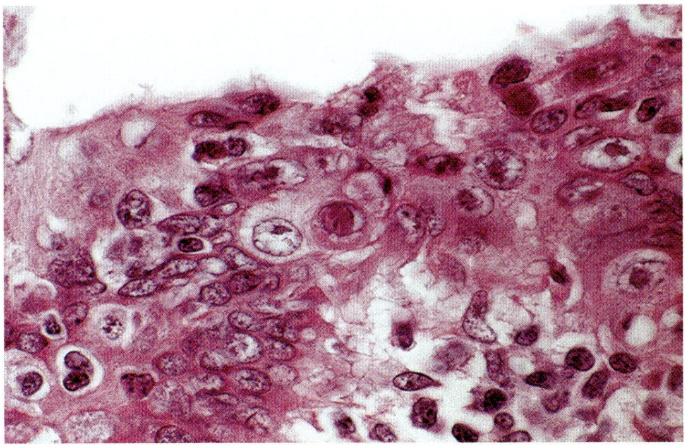

FIGURE 8.15

Adenovirus infection with epithelial cells containing both Cowdry A and B inclusions.

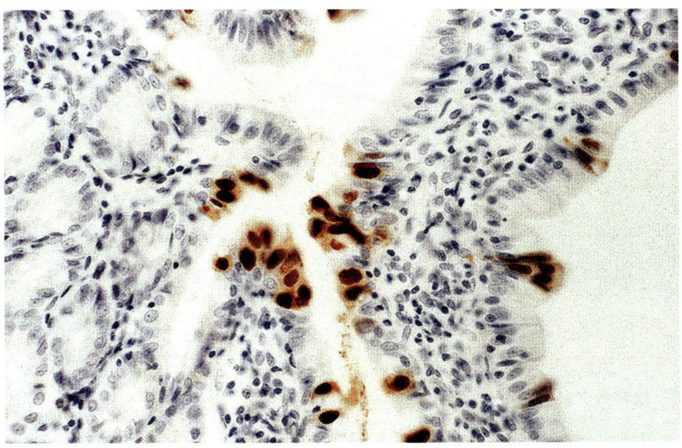

FIGURE 8.16

Strong nuclear expression of adenovirus on immunohistochemical staining.

ENDOMETRIOSIS, DECIDUOSIS, GLIOMATOSIS

CLINICAL FEATURES

Endometriosis affects the GI tract in up to 40% of patients with pelvic endometriosis. The sigmoid colon is the most common site, but the appendix may be involved in up to 15% of cases. Although appendiceal endometriosis can masquerade clinically as acute appendicitis, it usually has a nonspecific presentation. In some instances, there may be history of pain that waxes and wanes with the menstrual cycle.

A similar phenomenon, termed *deciduosis* (ectopic decidua), has been found in the appendices of pregnant women. In contrast to endometriosis, deciduosis typically presents with signs and symptoms of acute appendicitis.

When present, pelvic gliomatosis can also affect the serosal aspect of the appendix. Gliomatosis peritonei is found in patients with ovarian teratomas and manifests as foci of mature glial tissue deposited ubiquitously over the serosal surfaces. It has been reported to be a rare complication of ventricular shunts, and cases of malignant transformation have also been recorded.

ENDOMETRIOSIS, DECIDUOSIS, GLIOMATOSIS—FACT SHEET

Definition

- Deposition of endometrial-type glands and stroma, decidualized endometrial-type tissue, or glial tissue in the appendix

Incidence and Location

- Affects the gastrointestinal tract in about 40% of patients with endometriosis; appendix in 15%
- Deciduosis and gliomatosis are rare

Morbidity and Mortality

- Benign processes that can result in adhesions and obstruction

Gender, Race, and Age Distribution

- Affects women in their reproductive years

Clinical Features

- Patients have nonspecific symptoms that may wax and wane with the menstrual cycle
- Deciduosis presents with symptoms and signs of acute appendicitis
- Gliomatosis presentation is nonspecific

Prognosis and Treatment

- Benign clinical course
- Rarely, carcinomas can arise in association with endometriosis and malignant degeneration may be seen in patients with gliomatosis
- Treatment is same as that for endometriosis (hormonal manipulation, lysis of adhesions)

Pathologic Features

Gross Findings

On gross examination, endometriosis appears as hemorrhagic areas that may contain cysts filled with brown fluid. The appearances of deciduosis and gliomatosis are less specific; both appear as whitish plaques.

Microscopic Findings

Most examples of endometriosis affect the serosa or muscularis propria and are accompanied by abundant fibrosis and adhesions. The characteristic histologic features include endometrial-type glands and stroma associated with hemosiderin deposition. (Figs. 8.17 and 8.18). The endometrial-type epithelium changes with the menstrual cycle. A stromal decidual reaction may be found in endometriotic foci in pregnant patients. In some instances, there may be prominent smooth muscle hyperplasia of the appendiceal wall (Fig. 8.19). Repeated foci of hemorrhage, fibrosis, and smooth muscle hyperplasia may result in focal, complete obstruction of the appendiceal lumen and marked dilation of the proximal appendix. The latter findings mimic an appendiceal mucinous neoplasm, especially when endometriosis is associated with significant subepithelial fibrosis, flattening of the appendiceal luminal epithelium, and foci of intestinal metaplasia within endometrial glands. Lack of cytologic atypia within the lining epithelium is helpful in excluding an appendiceal mucinous neoplasm.

Deciduosis is characterized by the presence of nests and sheets of large polyhedral cells with abundant glassy eosinophilic cytoplasm and bland round to oval nuclei (Fig. 8.20). These foci are usually located within in the serosa or outer muscularis propria. Such cells can sometimes be mistaken for malignant (often epithelial) lesions. If deciduosis raises a concern for carcinoma, immunohistochemical stains may be performed to aid this distinction. Decidualize cells usually express vimentin but are negative for keratin. They may show desmin or smooth muscle actin positivity.

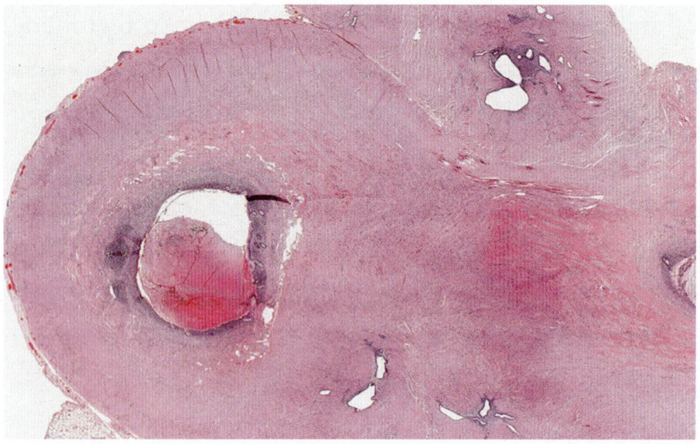

FIGURE 8.17

Endometriosis. The appendix shows marked thickening of the appendiceal wall with cystically dilated glands surrounded by cellular stroma within the muscularis propria.

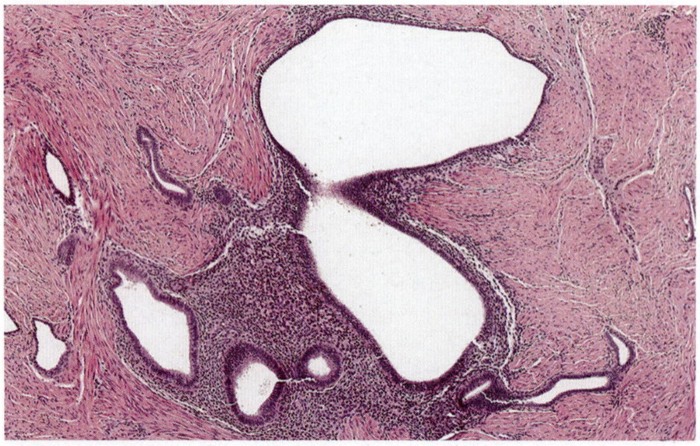

FIGURE 8.18

Endometriosis. Higher magnification shows benign endometrial-type glands surrounded by endometrial stroma.

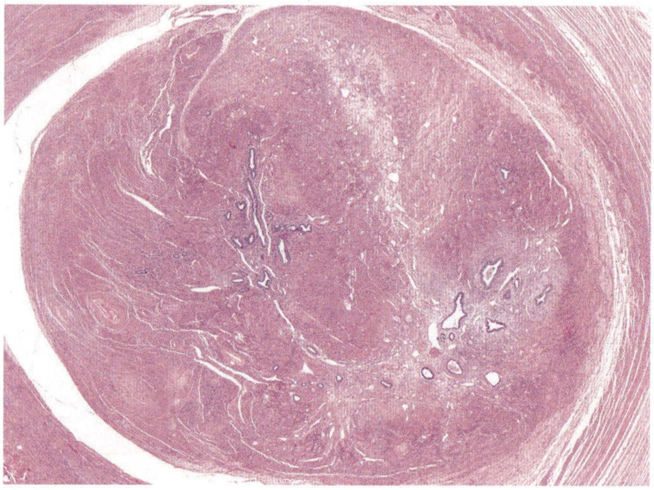

FIGURE 8.19

Appendiceal endometriosis with smooth muscular hyperplasia causing complete obliteration of the appendiceal lumen.

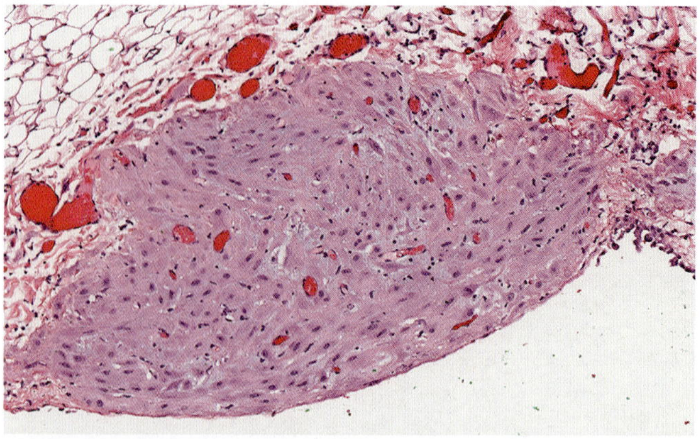

FIGURE 8.20

Deciduosis. The image shows appendiceal serosa with a nodule composed of bland epithelioid or polygonal cells with abundant eosinophilic glassy cytoplasm. Multiple such nodules were identified on the serosal aspect of this appendectomy specimen from a 30-year-old pregnant woman.

Endometriosis, Deciduosis, Gliomatosis—Pathologic Features

Gross Findings

- Endometriosis: hemorrhagic lesions, often with cysts containing brown fluid
- Deciduosis and gliomatosis: white plaques

Microscopic Findings

- Endometriosis: endometrial glands and stroma with associated fibrosis and adhesions (usually serosal)
- Deciduosis: large polyhedral cells with glassy eosinophilic cytoplasm arranged in sheets
- Gliomatosis: nodules of glial tissue localized to the serosa

Differential Diagnosis

- Endometriosis: adenocarcinoma (lacks stroma), appendiceal mucinous neoplasm (when intestinal metaplasia is present and the appendix is significantly dilated)
- Deciduosis: epithelioid malignant neoplasms (lacks mitoses)
- Gliomatosis: spindle cell neoplasms

Differential Diagnosis

The appearances of endometriosis, deciduosis, and gliomatosis are quite characteristic.

Prognosis and Therapy

These processes are benign, but endometriosis of the appendix is associated with adhesions (just as endometriosis in general).

EPITHELIAL NEOPLASMS OF THE APPENDIX (NONENDOCRINE)

The nomenclature and classification of appendiceal mucinous neoplasms have been subjects of considerable controversy. This is primarily because of variability in histologic criteria, sampling, and clinical follow-up across clinical studies. In an effort to develop a standardized system, the Peritoneal Surface Oncology Group International (PSOGI) proposed guidelines to report appendiceal neoplasms and pseudomyxoma peritonei (PMP) (Table 8.2). Based on this system, epithelial neoplasms of the appendix are classified into adenoma, serrated polyp, low-grade appendiceal mucinous neoplasm (LAMN), high-grade appendiceal mucinous neoplasm (HAMN), and invasive adenocarcinoma (mucinous or non-mucinous type). The term *adenoma* has been removed from the fifth edition of the Digestive System World Health Organization (WHO) Classification of Tumours but still remains in use in clinical practice. An algorithmic approach to these lesions is presented in Fig. 8.21.

TABLE 8.2

The Peritoneal Surface Oncology Group International Consensus Classification of Noncarcinoid Epithelial Neoplasia of the Appendix

Lesion	Terminology
Adenoma, resembling traditional colorectal type, confined to the mucosa; muscularis mucosae intact	Tubular, tubulovillous or villous adenoma, low-grade or high-grade dysplasia
Tumor with serrated features, confined to the mucosa; muscularis mucosae intact	Serrated polyp with or without dysplasia (low or high grade)
Mucinous neoplasm with low-grade cytologic atypia and any of Loss of muscularis mucosae Fibrosis of submucosa "Pushing invasion" (expansile or diverticulum-like growth) Dissection of acellular mucin in wall Undulating or flattened epithelial growth Rupture of appendix Mucin and/or cells outside appendix	Low-grade appendiceal mucinous neoplasm (LAMN)
Mucinous neoplasm with the architectural features of LAMN and no infiltrative invasion but with high-grade cytologic atypia	High-grade appendiceal mucinous neoplasm (HAMN)
Mucinous neoplasm with infiltrative invasion (tumor budding and/or small, irregular glands within a desmoplastic stroma)	Mucinous adenocarcinoma: well, moderately, or poorly differentiated
Neoplasm with signet ring cells (≤50% of cells)	Poorly differentiated (mucinous) adenocarcinoma with signet ring cells
Neoplasm with signet ring cells (>50% of cells)	(Mucinous) signet ring cell carcinoma
Nonmucinous adenocarcinoma resembling traditional colorectal type	Adenocarcinoma: well, moderately, or poorly differentiated

Adapted from Carr NJ, Cecil TD, Mohamed F, et al. A consensus for classification and pathologic reporting of pseudomyxoma peritonei and associated appendiceal neoplasia: the results of the Peritoneal Surface Oncology Group International (PSOGI) Modified Delphi Process. *Am J Surg Pathol*. 2016;40:14–26.

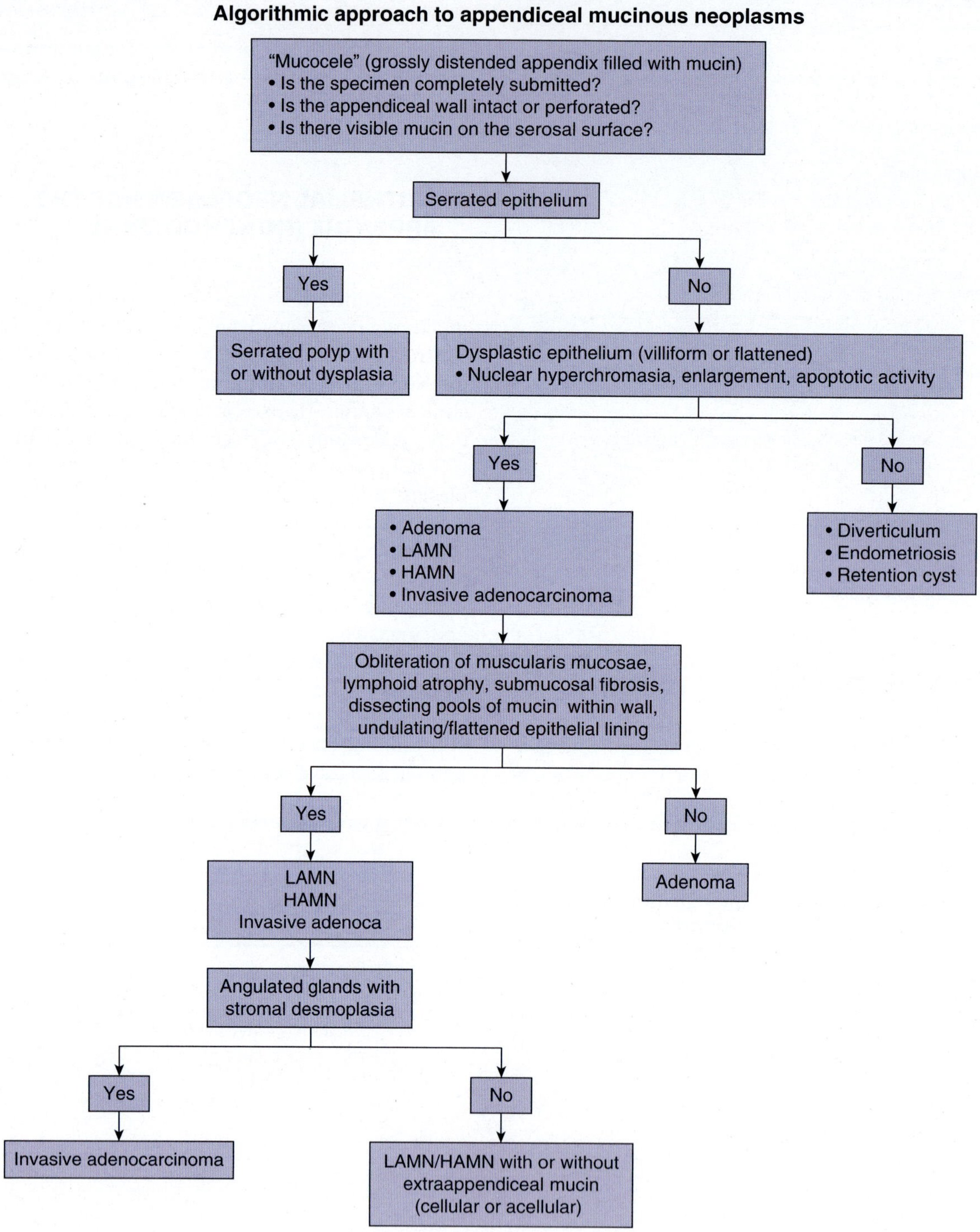

FIGURE 8.21

Algorithmic approach to appendiceal mucinous neoplasms.

ADENOMA

CLINICAL FEATURES

Adenomas that resemble conventional colorectal adenoma are rare in the appendix. These lesions were formerly known as mucinous cystadenoma. They are frequently encountered as incidental findings. Most manifest clinically with appendicitis related to neoplastic luminal obstruction.

ADENOMA—FACT SHEET

Definition
- Epithelial neoplasm resembling traditional colorectal adenoma

Incidence and Location
- Less common than low-grade appendiceal mucinous neoplasm

Morbidity and Mortality
- Causes acute appendicitis

Gender, Race, and Age Distribution
- Males more than females
- No clear racial difference

Clinical Features
- Most are incidental findings
- Patients may present with acute appendicitis

Prognosis and Treatment
- Complete excision is curative for adenomas

PATHOLOGIC FEATURES

GROSS FINDINGS

Gross examination may show features similar to those found in the colon, including a visible lesion within the mucosa. However, in most instances, these are incidental lesions found in a dilated appendix. Compared with LAMNs and NETs, which are frequently found in the tip of the appendix, colonic-type adenomas reside at the appendiceal orifice. The term *mucocele* does not describe a histologic entity but rather a gross finding describing a cystically dilated appendix containing mucin and should be reserved for clinicians, radiologists, and gross descriptions. Superimposed appendicitis may be associated with a purulent exudate.

MICROSCOPIC FINDINGS

The lesions consist of conventional tubular, tubulovillous, or villous adenomas with or without high-grade dysplasia, similar to those encountered in the rest of the colon (Fig. 8.22). All of these lesions are restricted to the mucosa; the lamina propria is preserved, and the muscularis mucosae is intact. This finding is helpful in distinguishing conventional adenomatous lesions from LAMNs. The finding of adenomatous change should prompt submission of the entire appendix to exclude a higher grade lesion.

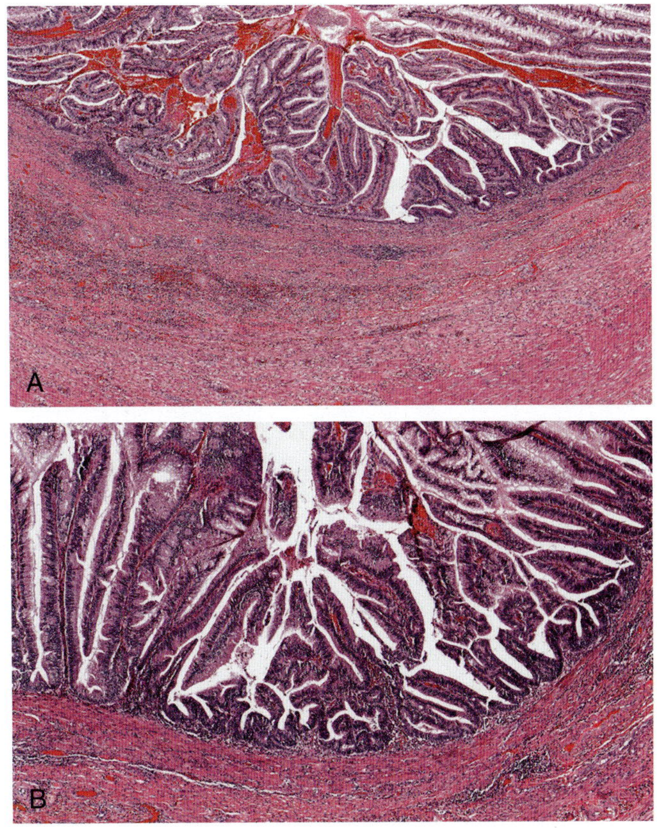

FIGURE 8.22
Adenoma of the appendix.

The descriptive term *cystadenoma* was to describe an adenomatous lesion that grows and causes cystic dilation of the appendix but shows intact lamina propria. However, the use of the term mucinous *cystadenoma* is no longer recommended by the PSOGI consensus guidelines published in 2016. Using the diagnosis of LAMN in this scenario can result in an unnecessary concern for subsequent pseudomyxoma in these patients who are essentially cured and do not need any future surveillance.

ADENOMA—PATHOLOGIC FEATURES

Gross Findings
- Mucosal thickening or ulceration
- Rarely has mucocele formation
- Rarely has a polypoid lesion

Microscopic Findings
- Identical to adenomas found in colon

Differential Diagnosis
- Adenomas should be differentiated from retention cysts and low-grade appendiceal mucinous neoplasms

Differential Diagnosis

Retention cysts also form a dilation of the appendix. However, although the epithelial lining of a retention cyst is attenuated and not dysplastic, a cause of luminal obstruction, such as an incidental well-differentiated NET or serosal adhesion, is often found. Simple retention cysts rarely exceed 2 cm in diameter.

Prognosis and Therapy

Adenomatous lesions are treated with appendectomy alone and require no additional follow-up. Colonoscopy should be considered to exclude synchronous colorectal neoplasia.

SERRATED POLYPS

Serrated epithelial polyps of the appendix show a spectrum of morphologic features that resemble serrated polyps of the colorectum. The most recent WHO Digestive System Tumours Classification further divides these into hyperplastic polyps (HPs) and sessile serrated lesions (SSLs) with and without dysplasia. For the purpose of the discussion in this chapter, these two categories are discussed together as a group. Recent molecular studies have shown that serrated lesions of the appendix harbor different mutations compared with their colonic counterparts. In particular, a large proportion of appendiceal serrated lesions do not harbor either *KRAS* or *BRAF* mutations. When present, harbor *KRAS* mutations are common, but *BRAF* are relatively infrequent. Therefore, the PSOGI consensus panel recommends using a descriptive term *serrated polyp with or without dysplasia* for serrated lesions of the appendix. A pathologist may choose to specify the type of dysplasia as resembling a colorectal adenoma (conventional adenomatous dysplasia) or traditional serrated adenoma.

CLINICAL FEATURES

Serrated appendiceal polyps usually affect older adults (mean age, 60 years) and do not show any gender predilection. Nearly half of the patients may present with signs and symptoms of acute appendicitis. However, most are incidentally discovered in resection specimens. They are usually not associated with concurrent colorectal neoplasia.

Serrated Polyps of the Appendix—Fact Sheet

Definition

- Epithelial neoplasm characterized by serrated crypt architecture either focally or diffusely involving the circumference of the appendiceal lumen
- Harbor molecular alterations that are differ from their colonic counterparts (*KRAS* more common than *BRAF*)

Incidence and Location

- Rare neoplasm; incidental finding

Morbidity and Mortality

- Appendectomy is usually curative

Gender, Race, and Age Distribution

- No clear gender predilection
- Mean age is the sixth decade

Clinical Features

- Patients may present with acute appendicitis

Prognosis and Treatment

- Complete excision is curative

Pathologic Features

Gross Findings

Depending on the indication for surgery, the appendix may show a completely normal appearance or show congested and edematous appearance. On cut section, there is only slight luminal dilation. The mucosa may show foci of hemorrhage, and there may be luminal purulent material. Mucin or mass formation is generally not present.

Microscopic Findings

Serrated nondysplastic polyps resemble conventional HPs or SSLs seen in the colorectum (Fig. 8.23). HPs are usually smaller in size (<1 cm); SSLs tend to be larger. Both these lesions may either present as solitary polyps (approximately one-third of cases) or as diffuse circumferential proliferations (approximately two-thirds of cases). Cytologic atypia is only present within the proliferative compartment of the crypts. The surface epithelium shows an admixture of goblet cells, tall columnar cells with or without eosinophilic cytoplasm.

Serrated dysplastic polyps often show circumferential involvement of the appendiceal lumen with serrated luminal architecture. Histologically, they show low- or high-grade cytologic dysplasia that resembles a conventional adenomatous polyp or traditional serrated adenoma seen in the colorectum (see Chapter 13).

Serrated Polyps of the Appendix—Pathologic Features

Gross Findings

- Normal or dilated, cystic appendix, typically without significant mucin

Microscopic Findings

- Serrated nondysplastic polyps resemble hyperplastic polyps and sessile serrated lesions (SSLs) of the colorectum
- Serrated nondysplastic polyps may either present as solitary, discrete polyps (one-third of cases) or occupy the entire circumference of the appendiceal lumen (two-thirds of cases)
- Serrated dysplasia polyps show dysplasia resembling conventional adenomatous dysplasia or traditional serrated adenoma of the colorectum

Differential Diagnosis

- Reactive hyperplastic epithelial changes in acute appendicitis
- Adenoma
- Low- or high-grade appendiceal mucinous neoplasm
- Serrated polyps should be distinguished from reactive hyperplastic epithelial changes that are often encountered within mucosa adjacent to an ulcer. Within these areas, the surface epithelium shows luminal serrations, and the individual cells harbor mild cytologic atypia with or without loss of mucin. Because these cytoarchitectural changes are only present adjacent to inflamed and ulcerated mucosa, they can be readily distinguished from hyperplastic or serrated polyps that present as discrete lesions in noninflamed mucosa
- Similar to colonic counterparts, tubular, tubulovillous and villous adenomas need to be differentiated from serrated dysplastic polyps with low- or high-grade dysplasia. Dysplasia in this setting is usually of the conventional adenomatous type, and a diagnosis of SSL with low or high-grade dysplasia is typically rendered only when cytologic atypia is present in continuity with a nondysplastic serrated polyp
- It is important to distinguish serrated polyps from low- or high-grade appendiceal mucinous neoplasms because the latter are now considered "low-grade carcinoma" per the American Joint Committee on Cancer staging system and have their own staging system. The key distinguishing feature of serrated polyps is that these proliferations are confined to the mucosa and show intact muscularis mucosae. Appendiceal mucinous neoplasms are characterized by loss of muscularis mucosae, submucosal fibrosis with or without expansile growth pattern, and dissection of acellular mucin within the appendiceal wall. Furthermore, true villi and copious amounts of cytoplasmic mucin is generally a feature of appendiceal mucinous neoplasms rather than serrated polyps

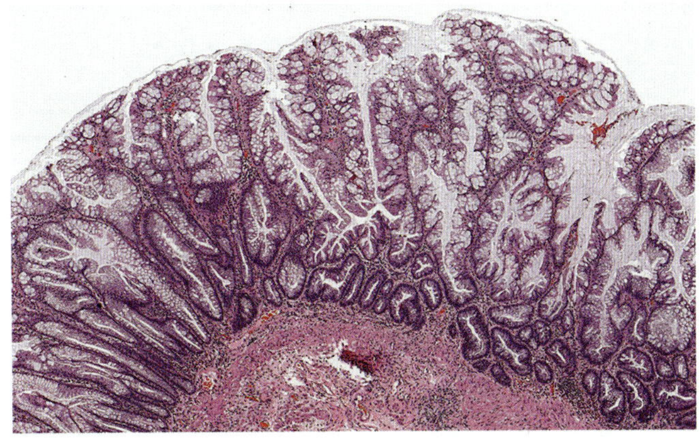

FIGURE 8.23

Serrated polyp of the appendix. The specimen shows a lesion composed of serrated crypts lined by cells with mucinous cytoplasm. In some areas, the serrations reach the basal aspects of the crypts. This lesion resembles a sessile serrated polyp of the colon. Per the Peritoneal Surface Oncology Group International Consensus recommendations, these lesions are classified as serrated polyps with or without dysplasia.

LOW-AND HIGH-GRADE APPENDICEAL MUCINOUS NEOPLASMS

Appendiceal mucinous neoplasms are a group of epithelial neoplasms that demonstrate banal cytoarchitectural features but are associated with extraappendiceal spread in a minor subset of cases. In perforated lesions with cellular extraappendiceal spread, these lesions often pursue an indolent but progressive clinical course with significant morbidity and mortality. A multitude of potentially confusing terms and competing classification schemes have been used to characterize these lesions, including terms such as *pseudomyxoma peritonei*, *disseminated peritoneal adenomucinosis*, *cystadenoma*, *low-grade appendiceal mucinous neoplasm*, *mucinous borderline tumor of the appendix*, *mucinous tumor of uncertain malignant potential*, and *low-grade mucinous carcinoma*. The PSOGI consensus guidelines now classify these neoplasms into LAMN and HAMN. By definition, these neoplasms are considered mostly low-grade carcinomas but lack the infiltrative invasion characteristic of conventional adenocarcinoma.

CLINICAL FEATURES

Mucinous neoplasms are detected in only 0.3% of surgically removed appendices but account for nearly one-third of all appendiceal epithelial tumors. Patients may present with symptoms of acute appendicitis, obstruction, or a palpable mass. Intussusception into the colon is a rare but well-recognized complication of appendiceal *mucocele*. Patients late in the disease process may present with *pseudomyxoma peritonei* (meaning false mucinous tumor of the peritoneum), a term that should be reserved for the clinical syndrome in which patients experience slowly increasing abdominal girth caused by mucinous ascites resulting from prior "mucocele" rupture or transmural extension. The abdominal cavity relentlessly fills with mucin produced by the neoplastic cells.

LOW-AND HIGH-GRADE APPENDICEAL MUCINOUS NEOPLASMS—FACT SHEET

Definition

- Epithelial neoplasm usually demonstrating low- or high-grade mucinous morphology but associated with extraappendiceal spread

Incidence and Location

- Rare neoplasm (0.3% of appendectomies)
- Outnumbers colonic-type epithelial neoplasms in appendix by 9 to 1

Morbidity and Mortality

- Peritoneal spread leads to clinical syndrome of pseudomyxoma peritonei
- Spread to ovaries can cause confusion regarding primary site of peritoneal disease
- Spread is usually via direct extension and infrequently by lymphatic or hematogenous routes

Gender, Race, and Age Distribution

- Females more than males
- No clear racial difference
- Mean age sixth decade

Clinical Features

- Patients present with acute appendicitis, obstruction, palpable mass, and intussusception
- Mucinous ascites (*pseudomyxoma peritonei*) is a late, uncommon finding

Prognosis and Treatment

- Patients with periappendiceal spread of acellular mucin have an excellent prognosis
- Patients with periappendiceal spread of mucin with neoplastic cells (even if paucicellular) are more likely to develop mucinous ascites
- Complete excision of a confined appendiceal neoplasm is curative; hemicolectomy is not recommended
- Follow-up includes regular computed tomography and tumor marker evaluation
- After peritoneal spread, aggressive surgical debulking (cytoreduction) and hyperthermic chemotherapy are treatments of choice

Pathologic Features

Gross Findings

On gross examination, the appendix is often dilated or cystic with tenacious mucin in the lumen. The wall is thick and fibrotic, sometimes with mural calcification ("porcelain appendix"). The term *mucocele* is used to describe the gross and clinical appearance of a dilated, mucin-filled appendix but does not indicate whether the histologic appearance is benign or malignant.

When a *mucocele*-like gross appearance is encountered, it is extremely important to determine whether the wall of the appendix is intact or disrupted (Fig. 8.24). A gross assessment of the appendix at the time of surgery and at the grossing bench is essential. Proper surgical management of the *mucocele* is essential because iatrogenic rupture of the LAMN may lead to pelvic or peritoneal dissemination.

Microscopic Findings

Peritoneal Surface Oncology Group International consensus guidelines classify appendiceal mucinous neoplasms as LAMN or HAMN. Both LAMN and HAMN frequently show effacement of the lamina propria with obliteration of the muscularis mucosae and submucosal fibrosis. There is decreased lymphoid tissue, and the appendiceal wall is fibrotic and can even be hyalinized.

Low-grade appendiceal mucinous neoplasms are composed of a villous, undulating, or flat proliferation of mucinous epithelium that shows circumferential involvement of the dilated appendiceal lumen. The epithelial cells show uniform, hyperchromatic, stratified nuclei with only mild nuclear enlargement. Nucleoli are usually inconspicuous, and nuclear polarity is preserved (Figs. 8.25 and 8.26). The cells show abundant intracytoplasmic mucin. Regardless of the overall growth pattern (villous, undulating, or flat), the cells are generally arranged in a monolayer.

High-grade appendiceal mucinous neoplasms have cytoarchitectural atypia in the form of markedly hyperchromatic and enlarged nuclei, prominent nucleoli, loss of nuclear polarity, numerous or atypical mitotic figures, and cribriform or micropapillary growth patterns.

The dilation of the appendix causes weakness of the muscular wall, leading to extension of neoplastic epithelium into the appendiceal wall. This may occur in two forms: (1) pushing invasion characterized by tongue-like protrusions, diverticulum-like structures or broad-based extensions of epithelium and (2) dissecting

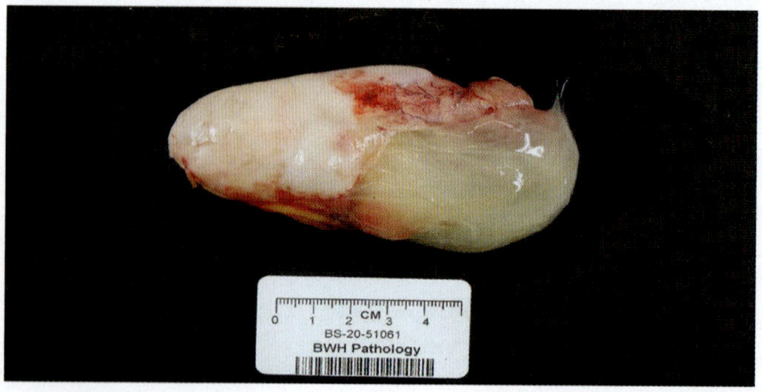

FIGURE 8.24

Low-grade appendiceal mucinous neoplasm. The appendectomy specimen shows glistening mucin confined to the lumen (the appendix has been opened longitudinally). The serosal surface appears to be uninvolved by this process. Clinically, a dilated appendix containing mucin is referred to as a *mucocele*.

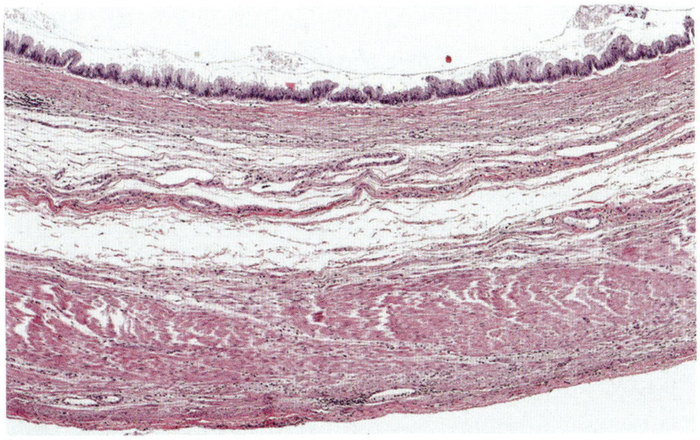

FIGURE 8.25

Low-grade appendiceal mucinous neoplasm. A representative section of the dilated lumen shows an undulated epithelial lining composed of cells with stratified and hyperchromatic nuclei. There are fibrosis of the lamina propria and obliteration of the muscularis mucosae. The rest of the wall appears unremarkable.

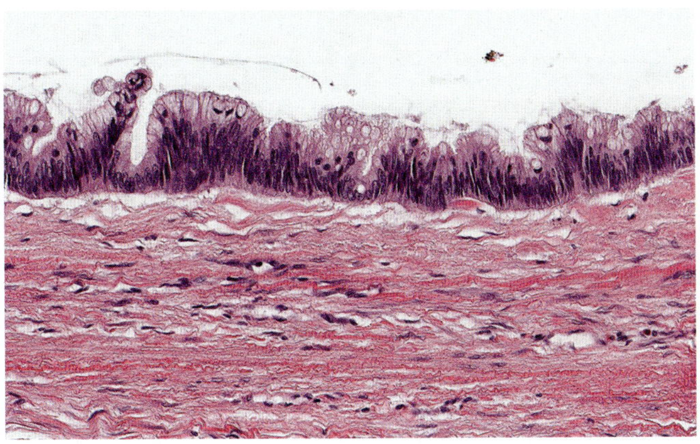

FIGURE 8.26

Low-grade appendiceal mucinous neoplasm. Higher magnification shows cells with enlarged, hyperchromatic, and stratified nuclei with maintained nuclear polarity consistent with low-grade dysplasia. Most of the cells still retain their mucinous cytoplasm.

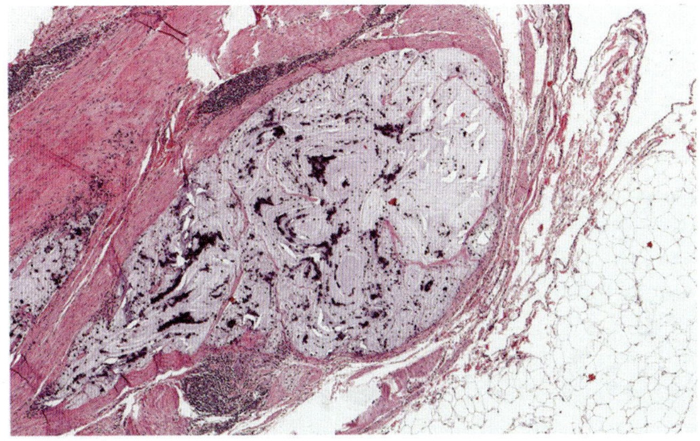

FIGURE 8.27

Low-grade appendiceal mucinous neoplasm with acellular mucin dissecting through the muscularis propria.

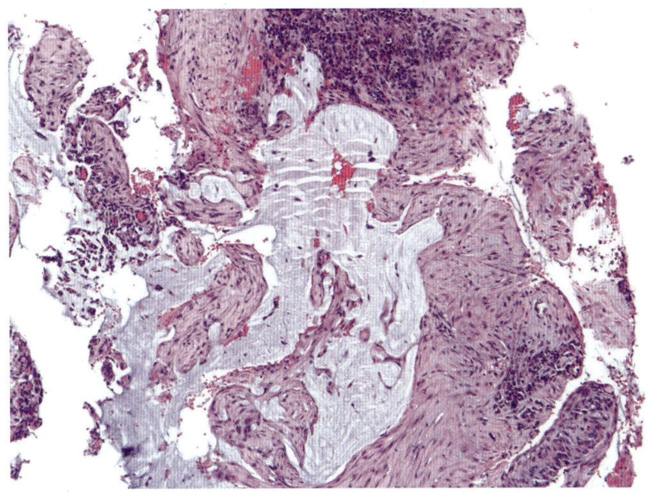

FIGURE 8.28

Extraappendiceal mucin in a case of low-grade appendiceal mucinous neoplasm. This finding should be distinguished from artifactual "carry-over" contamination from tissue sectioning or processing. To qualify as extraappendiceal mucin, the mucinous deposits should be located beyond the muscular wall of the appendix and should be associated with a granulation tissue–like response or neovascularization.

pools of acellular mucin through the appendiceal wall (Fig. 8.27). Both these processes of epithelial extension can lead to intraperitoneal spread either through direct rupture with or without concurrent appendicitis.

Rupture or extraappendiceal spread of mucin may be localized to the periappendiceal area. This periappendiceal spread may contain mucin that is acellular (Fig. 8.28) or cellular, harboring strips or clusters of neoplastic epithelia. Because patients with acellular mucin have an excellent prognosis, it is critical to accurately assess the presence or absence of epithelial elements. Microscopic examination of the entire appendix as well as all of the periappendiceal mucin is necessary because lesions with cellular extraappendiceal mucin are more likely to progress to disseminated disease and result in the death of the patient, even if the mucin is paucicellular and confined to the periappendiceal region.

Appendiceal mucinous neoplasms are now staged according to the American Joint Committee on Cancer (AJCC) staging system for LAMNs. LAMN or HAMNs that extend only up to the muscularis propria are staged as pTis (LAMN), regardless of whether the extension is merely acellular mucin or contains mucinous epithelium. T1 and T2 stages are not applicable to LAMN or HAMN. Acellular mucin or mucinous epithelium that extends into the subserosa or serosa should be classified as T3 or T4a, respectively.

Differential Diagnosis

The differential diagnosis for appendiceal mucinous neoplasms, especially LAMN, include adenoma and invasive mucinous adenocarcinoma as well as a variety of non-neoplastic entities such as retention cyst, appendicitis and diverticulitis with mucin extravasation, and endometriosis with intestinal metaplasia.

It is important to distinguish LAMN from an adenoma because LAMNs now need to be staged in the AJCC eighth edition. Whereas adenomas (tubular, tubulovillous, or villous) are usually confined to the mucosa and do not show gross luminal dilation, LAMNs are characteristically associated with dilated lumen that is filled with copious amounts of mucin. Histologically, adenomas retain muscularis mucosae as well as lymphoid tissue, but LAMNs by definition show obliteration of the lamina propria, muscularis mucosae, and submucosal fibrosis or hyalinization.

Pushing type or broad-based invasion can mimic invasive mucinous adenocarcinoma. However, the pattern of invasion is key in differentiating these entities. Invasive adenocarcinoma is diagnosed only on the basis of an infiltrative pattern of invasion in which the glands show angulated profiles or tumor budding and are surrounded by stromal desmoplasia. The pushing invasion of LAMNs or HAMNs is usually associated with fibrosis or hyalinization that is dense and paucicellular compared to stromal desmoplasia.

Retention cyst of the appendix can show marked dilation of the lumen and can present as a mucocele. Retention cysts are rare and are generally smaller than 2 cm in diameter. Lack of atypia within this epithelial lining as well as presence of intact muscularis mucosae supports a diagnosis of retention cyst rather than LAMN (Figs. 8.29–8.31). Distinguishing these from LAMN can be particularly challenging in cases that show extensive denudation and ulceration of the epithelial lining. If the entire appendix has been sampled and there is no evidence of a neoplasm, the possibility of a retention cyst should be considered.

Appendiceal diverticular disease can be associated with mild cytologic atypia, hyperplastic epithelial changes, and extravasation of mucin within the appendiceal wall or into the periappendiceal tissue. In well-oriented sections, one may see two distinct lumens or even multiple luminal profiles with intact mucosal architecture that suggest diverticular disease. Similar to the colon, an attenuated muscularis propria may be present as well. Diverticular disease usually lacks villous architecture, effacement of lamina propria, crowded crypts, and cytologic dysplasia that are typically associated with LAMN.

Rarely, endometriosis with intestinal metaplasia may be associated with dissecting acellular mucin and mimic LAMN. In most instances, endometriosis is readily recognized by the presence of endometrial stroma surrounding these glands.

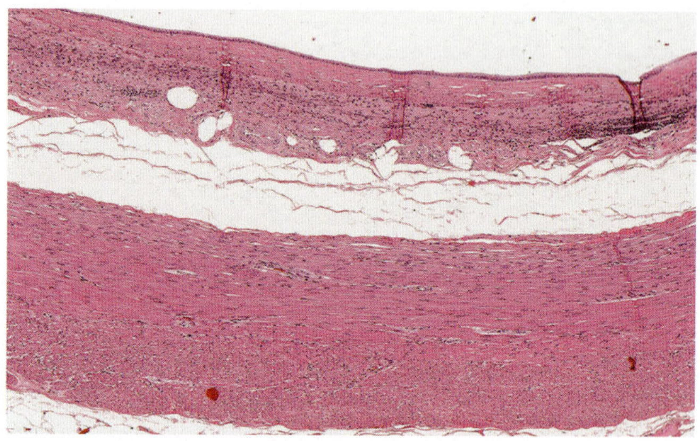

FIGURE 8.30

Retention cyst of the appendix. A representative section of the appendiceal wall shows flattened epithelial lining without cytologic atypia. The underlying lamina propria is somewhat fibrotic. However, the muscularis mucosae is intact.

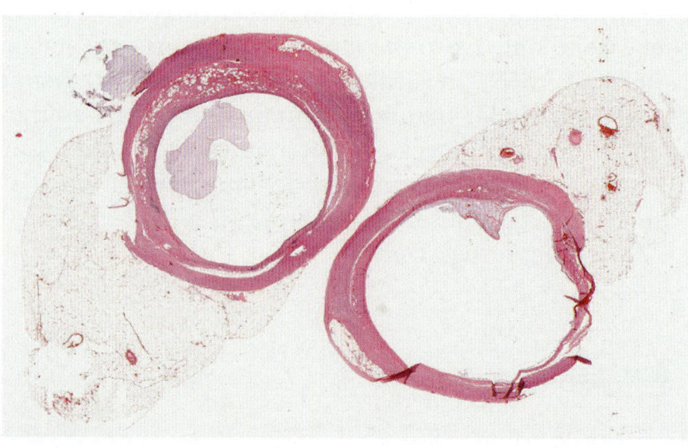

FIGURE 8.29

Retention cyst of the appendix. The specimen shows cystically dilated appendiceal lumen. Grossly, the lumen shows abundant mucin.

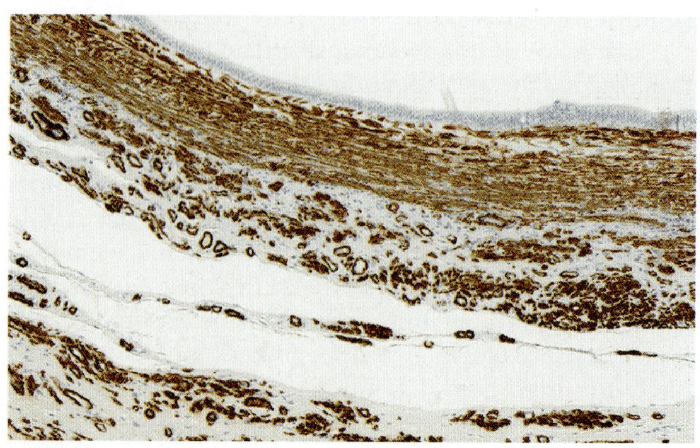

FIGURE 8.31

Retention cyst of the appendix. Desmin immunohistochemical stain highlights the intact muscularis mucosae.

Appendiceal Mucinous Neoplasm—Pathologic Features

Gross Findings

- Dilated, cystic appendix filled with mucin
- Thickened wall, sometimes with mural calcification (porcelain appendix)
- Status of intact vs ruptured appendix is critical to patient outcome

Microscopic Findings

- Mucinous neoplasm with no invasion but with any of the following features:
  - Loss of muscularis mucosae
  - Fibrosis of submucosa
  - Expansile or diverticulum-like growth
  - Dissection of acellular mucin in wall
  - Undulating or flattened epithelial growth
  - Rupture of appendix
  - Mucin and/or cells outside appendix
- Low-grade appendiceal mucinous neoplasm: epithelial lining composed of low-grade cytologic atypia: hyperchromasia, stratification of nuclei, no architectural complexity
- High-grade appendiceal mucinous neoplasm shows severe cytologic abnormalities: loss of nuclear polarity, prominent nucleoli, complex cribriform and papillary architecture
- Extension of mucin outside of appendix may be acellular or have strips, clusters, or single epithelial cells
- Involvement of peritoneum may be acellular or show cells with low- or high-grade morphology

Differential Diagnosis

- Adenoma of colonic type (tubular, tubulovillous or villous)
- Invasive adenocarcinoma
- Retention cyst
- Diverticular disease
- Endometriosis

Prognosis and Therapy

Gross examination of the appendix at the time of appendectomy and an assessment of the size of the *mucocele* cannot determine whether the *mucocele* is benign or malignant. The prudent surgical approach is to regard every *mucocele* of the appendix as potentially malignant. This means that special care in the resection of an appendiceal *mucocele* must occur to avoid trauma and possible rupture of the appendix as it is removed. Often, this means conversion of a laparoscopic appendectomy to an open laparotomy.

Unfortunately, there is a paucity of evidence-based literature regarding appropriate clinical management and surveillance of appendiceal mucinous neoplasms that are confined to the appendix. It is important to sample all of the appendiceal tissue and periappendiceal mucin to provide accurate information for predicting clinical behavior of these lesions. Involvement of the proximal margin by appendiceal mucinous neoplasm does not seem to result in recurrent disease based on limited data. Residual tumor has been documented in follow-up resection specimens and reported to be associated with poor disease-free survival.

The PSOGI consensus guidelines do not recommend routine right hemicolectomy for LAMN because these neoplasms usually do not show lymph node involvement. Furthermore, there is always a potential that subsequent treatment consisting of peritonectomy and heated intraperitoneal chemotherapy (HIPEC) may not reach the extraappendiceal neoplastic cells that are embedded in scar tissue from previous surgery. Thus, patients diagnosed with LAMN or HAMN must be followed to exclude development of PMP. The risk of PMP is low when the lesion is confined to the appendix and there is no extraappendiceal mucin. However, there is a small risk in patients with acellular mucin and a significant risk in those with cellular extraappendiceal mucin. Per PSOGI guidelines, the follow-up schedule for LAMN includes abdominopelvic CT scans and tumor markers at 1 year, annually at first, and then with decreasing frequency over time. If there is no evidence of cells or mucin beyond the appendix, a 5- to 10-year follow-up is considered appropriate.

Aggressive surgical debulking for mucinous-type tumors improves survival rate and reduces recurrence rates in patients with generalized PMP compared with simple appendectomy. Intraperitoneal hyperthermic

APPENDICEAL ADENOCARCINOMA—FACT SHEET

Definition

- Neoplastic proliferation of epithelium characterized by angulated, atypical glands showing an infiltrative growth pattern and surrounded by stromal desmoplastic response

Incidence and Location

- 0.97 per 100,000 population

Morbidity and Mortality

- Related to depth of invasion and nodal stage
- May be associated with peritoneal implants or pseudomyxoma peritonei

Gender, Race, and Age Distribution

- Females more than males
- No clear racial difference
- Peak age of incidence in the sixth decade of life

Clinical Features

- Abdominal mass, acute appendicitis, or diffuse enlargement of abdominal girth caused by pseudomyxoma peritonei

Prognosis and Treatment

- Right hemicolectomy with lymph node dissection
- Treated similar to colonic adenocarcinoma
- If evidence of peritoneal implants or pseudomyxoma peritonei, cytoreductive therapy with heated intraperitoneal chemotherapy

chemotherapy after cytoreduction of tumor bulk is the current standard of treatment for patients with peritoneal spread.

Appendiceal Adenocarcinoma

Adenocarcinomas of the appendix are defined by the presence of infiltrative invasion and desmoplastic stromal response. They are categorized into mucinous or nonmucinous type. Similar to their colonic counterparts, mucinous adenocarcinomas are defined as malignant tumors in which more than 50% of the cross-sectional area of the lesion is composed of extracellular mucin.

CLINICAL FEATURES

The incidence of appendiceal adenocarcinoma has gradually increased since the year 2000, such that the reported incidence in year 2009 was 0.97 per 100,000 population. Women are more commonly affected than men, and the peak age of incidence is during the sixth decade of life. Patients may present with signs and symptoms of acute appendicitis, obstruction, or palpable mass or with a diffuse increase in abdominal girth.

Pathologic Features

Gross Findings

Grossly, the appendix is enlarged and may show presence of extraappendiceal mucin. Cut section often reveals extensive luminal mucin, a thickened appendiceal wall with or without a distinct mass.

Microscopic Findings

Similar to colorectal adenocarcinomas, adenocarcinomas of the appendix show an infiltrative pattern of invasion characterized by angulated atypical glands surrounded by desmoplastic stromal response (Fig. 8.32). These changes may be accompanied by foci of tumor budding or single cell infiltration.

If more than 50% of the neoplastic cells show signet ring cell morphology, the tumor should be classified as signet ring cell carcinoma. The nonmucinous adenocarcinomas are classified similar to colorectal

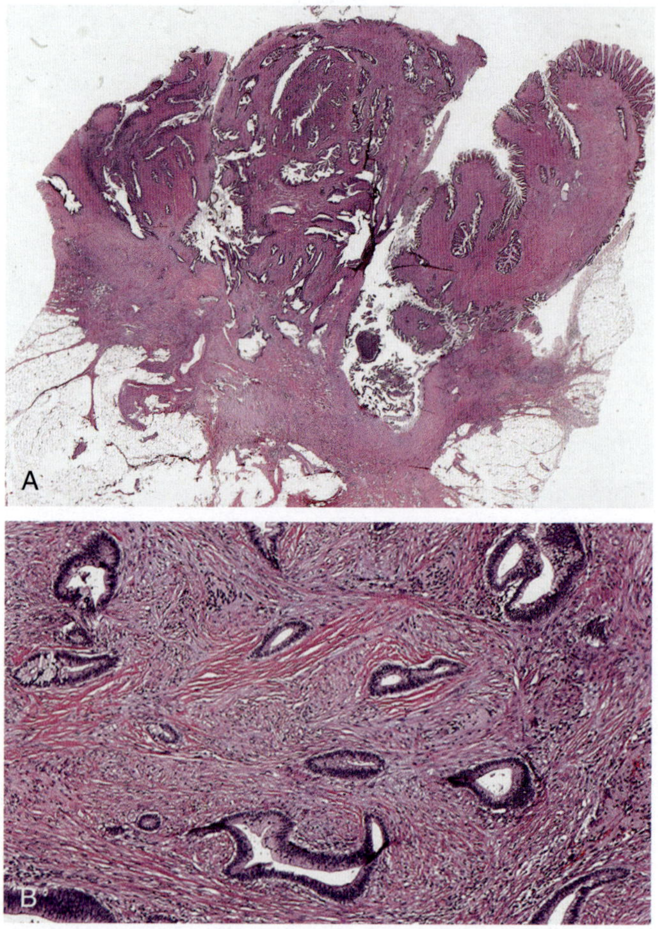

FIGURE 8.32

Invasive adenocarcinoma of the appendix. **A**, An invasive adenocarcinoma infiltrating transmurally into the periappendiceal adipose tissue. **B**, Higher magnification of the neoplastic glands. Similar to conventional colonic adenocarcinoma, the neoplastic glands show angulated, infiltrative profiles and are surrounded by desmoplastic stroma.

Appendiceal Adenocarcinoma—Pathologic Features

Gross Findings

- Dilated appendix with mucin
- Circumferential thickening with or without a distinct mass

Microscopic Findings

- Infiltrative invasion characterized by angulated, atypical glands surrounded by stromal desmoplasia
- Tumor budding or single-cell infiltration may be present
- Two subtypes: mucinous and nonmucinous adenocarcinoma
  - Mucinous adenocarcinoma
    - >50% of cross-sectional area contains extracellular mucin
    - Signet ring cell carcinoma: if more than 50% of tumor is composed of signet ring cells
    - Often associated with serrated polyps, low-grade appendiceal mucinous neoplasms (LAMNs) or high-grade appendiceal mucinous neoplasms (HAMNs)
  - Nonmucinous adenocarcinoma
    - Shows morphologic features that are similar to colonic counterparts
    - Often associated with an adenomatous precursor

Differential Diagnosis

- LAMN or HAMN
- Diverticular disease

adenocarcinomas. They are more likely to be associated with an adenomatous precursor, but mucinous adenocarcinomas usually arise in a background of serrated polyps, and rarely LAMNs or HAMNs.

Differential Diagnosis

The differential diagnosis includes appendiceal mucinous neoplasms and diverticular disease. Mucinous adenocarcinomas can be difficult to distinguish from LAMNs. In contrast to invasive adenocarcinoma, which at least focally shows infiltrative and angulated glandular contours with stromal desmoplasia, the advancing edge of LAMNs is associated with paucicellular hyaline stroma.

Diverticular disease can be associated with dissecting pools of mucin and thus mimic invasive adenocarcinoma. However, lack of cytologic atypia, preservation of the mucosal architecture, lack of an infiltrative glandular pattern, or stromal desmoplasia supports diverticular disease-related changes rather than invasive mucinous adenocarcinoma.

Last, poorly differentiated adenocarcinoma may raise the possibility of undifferentiated carcinoma. As in other sites of the GI tract, undifferentiated carcinomas lack any glandular, squamous, or neuroendocrine differentiation and can also rarely occur in the appendix.

Prognosis and Therapy

Right hemicolectomy with lymph node dissection is the treatment of choice. In general, the treatment is similar to that of colonic adenocarcinoma. If there is evidence of peritoneal implants or PMP, cytoreductive therapy with HIPEC is indicated.

Pseudomyxoma Peritonei

Pseudomyxoma peritonei is not a histologic term and is used to describe a clinical syndrome characterized by development of mucinous ascites and peritoneal implants. Underlying this phenomenon is invariably a ruptured appendiceal mucinous neoplasm with peritoneal spread or mucinous adenocarcinoma arising from the appendix. Mucin usually accumulates within the pelvis, paracolic gutters, liver capsule, and omentum. The ovaries may show involvement by low- or high-grade lesions and often appear as multiloculated masses.

The reported incidence is 0.2 per 100,000 per year. Patients present with abdominal distension or symptoms related to intestinal obstruction. Most cases of PMP are appendiceal in origin. Rarely, mucinous neoplasms originating from the colon, ovary, pancreas, and urachus may result in PMP. Based on multiple studies, we now know that primary mucinous neoplasms of the ovary are not the most common source of PMP. In fact, patients with borderline mucinous tumors or mucinous adenocarcinoma of the ovary either do not progress or tend to follow a course that is similar to conventional adenocarcinoma rather than PMP. Therefore, it is extremely important to sample the appendix completely even if the appendix appears grossly unremarkable.

The diagnostic criteria and classification of intraabdominal mucin and PMP proposed by PSOGI are outlined in Table 8.3. Histologically, the neoplastic cells may be extremely scant within abundant mucinous material (Figs. 8.33 and 8.34). Extensive sampling may be required to demonstrate them.

Low-grade mucinous carcinoma typically has a scant epithelial component, arranged in strips or rare gland-like structures. Cytologic atypia is mild, and cells may appear really bland. High-grade lesions show increased cellularity and cytologic atypia characterized by enlarged, vesicular nuclei with prominent nucleoli, loss of nuclear polarity, and cribriform growth pattern. Destructive invasion of underlying or adjacent organs is also a feature of high-grade disease. Tumors that contain signet ring cells should be classified separately from other high-grade lesions because they have a worse prognosis.

TABLE 8.3

The Peritoneal Surface Oncology Group International Consensus Classification of Pseudomyxoma Peritonei (PMP; Peritoneal Disease Component)

Lesion	Terminology
Mucin without epithelial cells	Acellular mucin
PMP with low-grade histologic features	Low-grade mucinous carcinoma peritonei *or* Disseminated peritoneal adenomucinosis (DPAM)
PMP with high-grade histologic features	High-grade mucinous carcinoma peritonei *or* Peritoneal mucinous carcinomatosis (PMCA)
PMP with signet ring cells	High-grade mucinous carcinoma peritonei with signet ring cells *or* Peritoneal mucinous carcinomatosis with signet ring cells (PMCA-S)

Adapted from Carr NJ, Cecil TD, Mohamed F, et al. A consensus for classification and pathologic reporting of pseudomyxoma peritonei and associated appendiceal neoplasia: the results of the Peritoneal Surface Oncology Group International (PSOGI) Modified Delphi Process. *Am J Surg Pathol.* 2016;40:14–26.

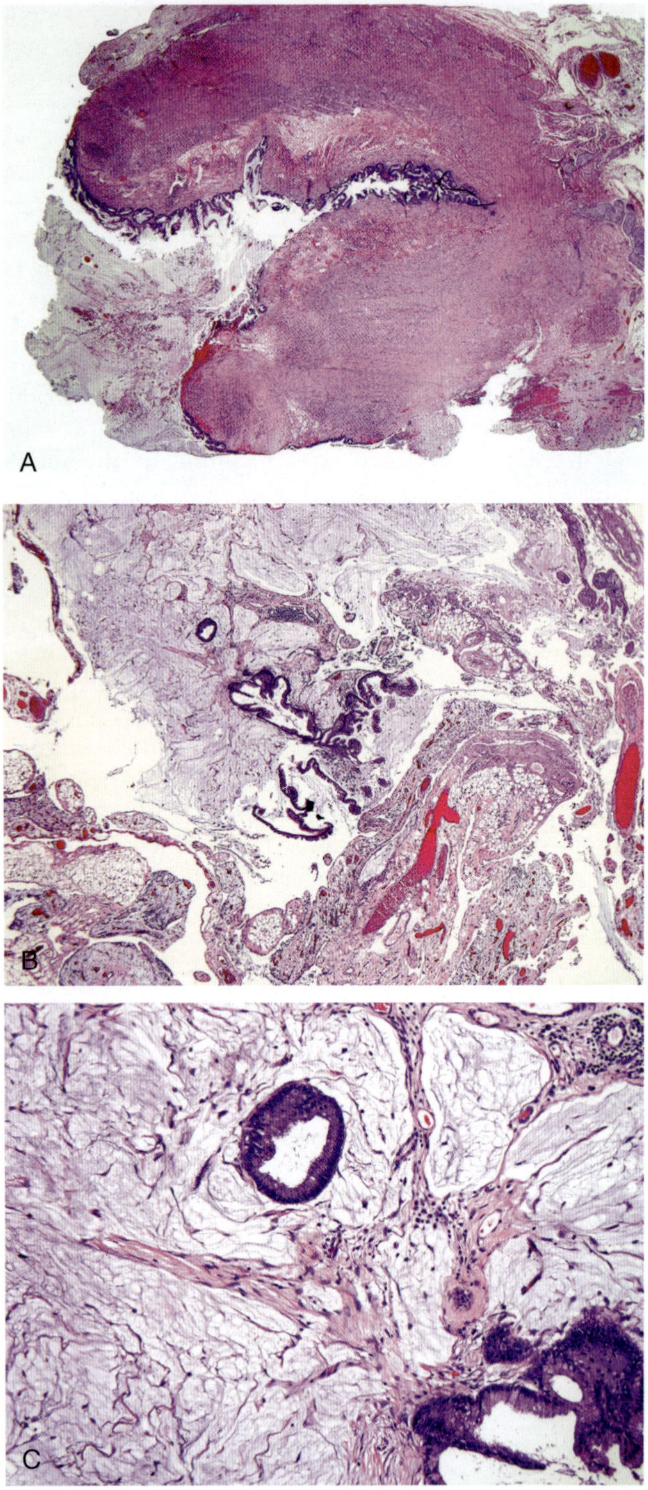

FIGURE 8.33

A patient with clinical pseudomyxoma peritonei syndrome. **A**, Examination of the appendix shows a low-grade appendiceal mucinous neoplasm with rupture and extraappendiceal spread of tumor cells. **B**, A sample from the peritoneum shows abundant mucin with free-floating clusters of epithelial cells, which can be called *diffuse peritoneal adenomucinosis* or *low-grade mucinous carcinoma peritonei*. **C**, On high power, the epithelial cells have low-grade cytology and are identical to the mucinous neoplasm found in the appendix.

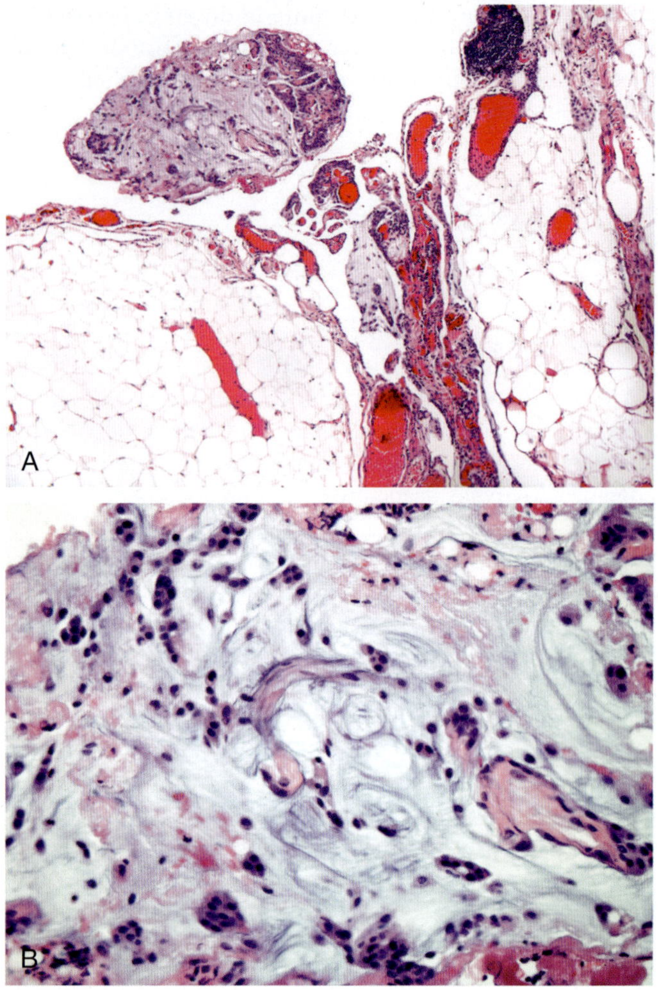

FIGURE 8.34

Another patient with pseudomyxoma peritonei. **A**, Sampling of the peritoneal cavity shows clusters of epithelial cells in abundant mucin. **B**, A high-power view of sample in **A** shows high-grade cytology with loss of polarity, high nuclear-to-cytoplasmic ratio, and pleomorphism. Patients with this unfavorable histology have a significantly worse prognosis. These lesions are referred to as *peritoneal mucinous carcinomatosis* or *high-grade mucinous carcinoma peritonei*.

Based on the eighth edition classification for appendiceal adenocarcinomas and LAMNs, in cases in which an appendectomy shows a mucinous neoplasm that has ruptured with extraappendiceal cells and mucin, the term *PMP* should only be used if there is evidence of spread beyond the right lower quadrant of the abdomen. Histological grade is a component of the TNM classification of stage IV appendiceal neoplasms without nodal metastasis.

Because of prognostic implications, it is prudent for the pathologist to indicate whether the lesional cells have histology that correlates with an aggressive or an indolent clinical course and whether the mucin is acellular or cellular. The initial treatment of choice is surgical debulking for symptomatic disease. This treatment is not curative but aims to resect gross disease to limit the accumulation of abdominal mucin and prevent the ensuing complications. A more aggressive approach includes radical resection of all intraabdominal and pelvic disease and the administration of HIPEC. However, despite this radical therapy, the penetration of HIPEC into tumor tissue is limited to a maximum depth of 1 to 2 mm. The outcome of this therapy depends on completeness of cytoreduction, the histopathology of the appendiceal malignancy, and the extent of previous surgical interventions. Studies have shown that whereas patients who underwent complete cytoreduction for PMP with low-grade histologic features had a 5-year survival rate of 86%, those with higher grade features had a 5-year survival rate of 50%.

NEUROENDOCRINE TUMORS OF THE APPENDIX

The pathogenesis of appendiceal NETs is unknown. The majority show either enterochromaffin (EC) or L-cell differentiation. Similar to the rest of the GI tract, NETs of the appendix are graded based on mitotic activity and Ki-67 index.

CLINICAL FEATURES

Neuroendocrine tumors can be found throughout the GI tract and are detected in 1.8% of all appendectomies. The appendix follows small intestine (41.8%) and rectum (27.4%) in frequency. Well-differentiated NETs comprise 75% of all neoplasms found in the appendix. Patients tend to be much younger compared with those diagnosed with other appendiceal neoplasms or NETs at other sites—approximately 20 years younger than for NETs from other sites. These tumors occur more often in women, with a male-to-female ratio of 1 to 2. Appendiceal NETs are also the most common GI neoplasm in childhood. It is unclear whether these demographic data represent the actual distribution of tumor or the age range of the population that typically undergoes appendectomy for inflammatory appendicitis or incidental appendectomy during pelvic surgery for other reasons.

The most common clinical presentation is that of an incidental nodule detected at the time of appendectomy for presumed appendicitis. Others may be found incidentally during laparotomy or at autopsy. Rarely, patients present with an abdominal mass, pain, or the carcinoid syndrome.

NEUROENDOCRINE TUMORS OF THE APPENDIX—FACT SHEET

Definition

- A neuroendocrine tumor showing enterochromaffin cell or L-cell differentiation

Incidence and Location

- Most frequent tumor of the appendix, occurring in 0.2% to 1.8% of all appendectomy specimens

Morbidity and Mortality

- Metastasis is rare, usually to regional nodes
- Hematogenous spread is exceptional

Gender, Race, and Age Distribution

- Females more than males (2:1 ratio)
- No clear racial difference
- Can occur at any age; peak incidence in young adults; mean age is 42 years

Clinical Features

- Most are incidental findings
- Often occurs in children and have excellent long-term outcomes
- Carcinoid syndrome is very rare and is associated with metastatic liver disease

Prognosis and Treatment

- Complete excision is curative
- Incomplete resection or tumors larger than 2 cm should be staged with computed tomography or magnetic resonance imaging. If no distant disease is identified, reexploration with right hemicolectomy is performed

PATHOLOGIC FEATURES

GROSS FINDINGS

The majority of appendiceal NETs are localized to the tip of appendix at the time of diagnosis. Therefore, it is a common protocol to bisect and sample the tip of the appendix in its entirety. The majority of the lesions are smaller than 1 cm in diameter. They are round or oval and sometimes palpable. The cut surface is tan to yellow.

MICROSCOPIC FINDINGS

Neuroendocrine tumors of the appendix are morphologically similar to their small intestinal and rectal counterparts (Fig. 8.35). They are characterized by a monotonous proliferation of uniform cells with a moderate amount of eosinophilic to amphophilic cytoplasm. Nuclei are round with inconspicuous nucleoli and finely stippled chromatin ("salt and pepper" chromatin).

Pleomorphism and mitoses are rare. Morphologic features of the cells do not differ by cell of origin. NETs demonstrate variable architectural growth patterns including nested (insular), trabecular, acinar, and tubular (Fig. 8.36). Trabecular and glandular growth patterns are more common in L-cell NETs. These tumors usually secrete proglucagon-related peptides such as glucagon-like peptide 1. EC cell NETs may show S-100 positive sustentacular-like cells. These patterns do not have prognostic significance. The stroma can range from delicate and vascular to dense and fibrous. The vast majority of NETs are diffusely positive for chromogranin and synaptophysin, as well as CD56 (Fig. 8.37). However, per recent National Comprehensive Cancer Network guidelines, these ancillary stains are not required to diagnose NETs when sufficient histologic material is available for review.

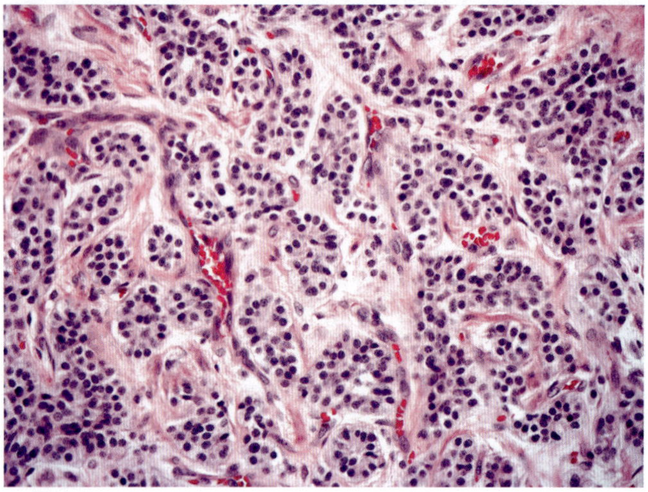

FIGURE 8.35

Well-differentiated neuroendocrine tumor. The neoplasm is composed of nested of uniform cells with round to oval nuclei and a distinct stippled or "salt and pepper" chromatin pattern.

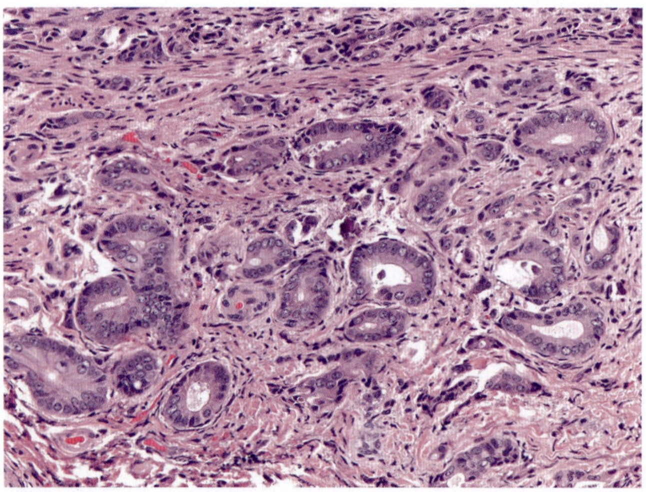

FIGURE 8.36

Tubular pattern of neuroendocrine tumor (NET). As the name indicates, this variant of NET is composed of small acini or tubules of neuroendocrine cells within a loose stroma.

Similar to rest of the NET in the GI tract, the College of American Pathologists recommends the following grading system for well-differentiated NETs:

- Well-differentiated NET (grade 1): mitotic rate, less than 2 per 2 mm^2 and/or Ki-67 index less than 3 %

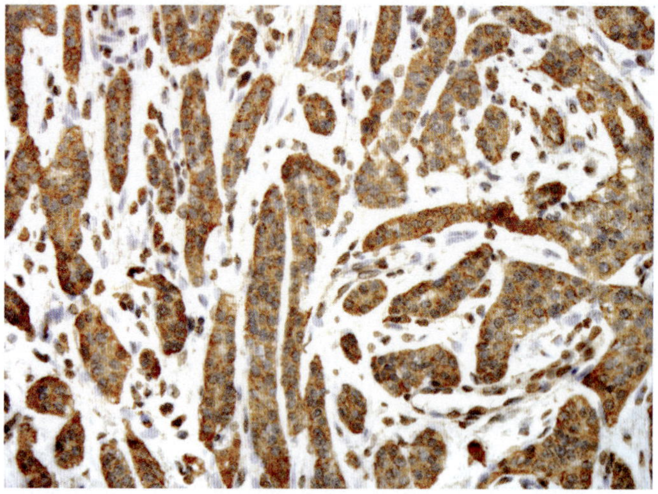

FIGURE 8.37

Well-differentiated neuroendocrine tumor with strong, diffuse chromogranin immunoreactivity.

NEUROENDOCRINE TUMORS OF THE APPENDIX—PATHOLOGIC FEATURES

Gross Findings

- Round or oval lesion usually found at the tip of the appendix
- Most are smaller than 1 cm in diameter
- Cut surface is gray or yellow

Microscopic Findings

- Nested and insular pattern, sometimes with acinar or tubular structures
- Cells are uniform, round to polygonal
- Nuclei are round with inconspicuous nucleoli and speckled chromatin
- Eosinophilic or amphophilic cytoplasm may contain small granules
- Variants include tubular or clear cell neuroendocrine tumor
- Grading is performed based on mitotic activity (per 10 hpf) and Ki-67 index (per College of American Pathologists guidelines)
  - Grade 1 (well-differentiated NET): <2 mitoses/10 hpf and/or <3% Ki-67 index
  - Grade 2 (well-differentiated NET): 2–20 mitoses/10 hpf and/or 3%–20% Ki-67 index
  - Grade 3 (well-differentiated NET): >20 mitoses/10 hpf and/or >20% Ki-67 index

Differential Diagnosis

- Goblet cell adenocarcinoma
- Adenocarcinoma

- Well-differentiated NET (grade 2): mitotic rate, 2 to 20 per mm^2 and/or Ki-67 index, 3% to 20%
- Well-differentiated NET (grade 3): mitotic rate, greater than 20 per 2 mm^2 and/or Ki-67 index greater than 20%

Poorly differentiated neuroendocrine carcinomas (large cell and small cell type) are now staged as colorectal carcinomas. Mixed adenocarcinoma-large (or small) cell neuroendocrine carcinomas are rare and reminiscent of their colonic counterparts.

Differential Diagnosis

Most cases of NETs do not pose any diagnostic problem. Goblet cell adenocarcinoma (GCA) remains in the differential diagnosis because of its appendiceal origin and reactivity to synaptophysin and chromogranin. However, GCAs have well-defined goblet cells with eccentric nuclei that are displaced and compressed by cytoplasmic mucin, which is not present in appendiceal neuroendocrine neoplasms. The cytoplasmic mucin can be demonstrated with a mucicarmine or Alcian blue stain. Neuroendocrine neoplasms with a predominantly tubular architecture may mimic an adenocarcinoma. However, the presence of more conventional foci of invasive adenocarcinoma is helpful in distinguishing it form NET.

Prognosis and Therapy

The prognosis for patients with well-differentiated appendiceal NETs is better than that for those in all other anatomic sites and demonstrates a 5-year survival rate greater than 95%. Clinical behavior and prognosis are best predicted by tumor size. Tumors smaller than 2 cm (found in ~95% of patients) are unlikely to have metastasized, but up to one-third of larger lesions are metastatic at diagnosis, usually to regional nodes rather than to the liver.

Treatment by appendectomy is curative in most cases, particularly for tumors smaller than 2 cm in greatest dimension that are confined to the appendix because metastasis is very uncommon in these patients. However, some controversy exists regarding the management of appendiceal NETs measuring less than 2 cm with more aggressive histologic features. Patients with an incomplete resection or tumors larger than 2 cm are at risk for locoregional or distant metastases. These patients should be staged with abdominal or pelvic CT or magnetic resonance imaging with contrast. If no distant disease is identified, they should undergo reexploration with right hemicolectomy.

GOBLET CELL ADENOCARCINOMA

Appendiceal GCA (formerly known as goblet cell carcinoid and adenocarcinoma ex goblet cell carcinoid) was first recognized as a distinct entity in 1969 and remains a rare appendiceal neoplasm with uncertain histogenesis. These infiltrative tumors have a mixed phenotype, with partial neuroendocrine differentiation and intestinal-type goblet cell morphology. As such, they have been classified in the past with other neoplasms that show both neuroendocrine and glandular differentiation as *adenocarcinoid tumors*, a term that encompasses biologically diverse neoplasms such as tubular pattern NET and a collision tumor of typical NET with a de novo adenocarcinoma. The term *adenocarcinoid* is no longer used by the WHO and is termed *goblet cell adenocarcinoma* and graded as low or high, recognizing that both goblet cell carcinoid and adenocarcinoma ex goblet cell carcinoid are part of the same spectrum of tumors and not two separate histologic types. Distinguishing GCA from these other entities is important because the clinical characteristics and prognoses are distinct. In the past, GCA has also been proposed as crypt cell carcinoma, mucinous carcinoid, microglandular carcinoid, or amphicrine carcinoma to distinguish the entity from classical NET tumor of the appendix.

CLINICAL FEATURES

Goblet cell adenocarcinomas occur in adults, with a mean age of 50 years. There is a female predominance with a male-to-female ratio of about 1 to 2. The most common clinical presentation is abdominal pain and a palpable mass (50%). Other patients present with symptoms related to acute appendicitis, and only 3% of patients are diagnosed incidentally. Patients with advanced disease most frequently present with abdominal masses. In female patients with stage IV disease, 83% present with ovarian masses and a presumptive diagnosis of a primary ovarian neoplasm. Overall, fewer than 1% of patients have a preoperative diagnosis of a primary appendiceal tumor.

Pathologic Features

Gross Findings

The appendix in patients with GCA can appear grossly unremarkable. A discrete nodule or mass is only rarely identified. Because of the circumferential pattern of involvement, there may be some thickening of the wall. Most tumors are larger than 2 cm in size (representing length of tumor extension rather than diameter).

GOBLET CELL ADENOCARCINOMA—FACT SHEET

Definition

- Appendiceal tumor with mixed phenotype: partial neuroendocrine differentiation and intestinal-type goblet cell morphology of uncertain histogenesis

Incidence and Location

- Rare; essentially exclusive to the appendix

Morbidity and Mortality

- Metastatic spread is present in more than half of patients at time of presentation (peritoneum, omentum, ovaries)
- Commonly has direct extension into the right colon
- Lymph node metastasis is present in more than one-third of cases

Gender, Race, and Age Distribution

- Females more than males (2:1 ratio)
- Occurs in adults; mean age is 50 years

Clinical Features

- Nearly 50% patients present with abdominal pain and a palpable mass
- Forty percent present with acute appendicitis symptoms
- Fewer than 5% are incidental

Prognosis and Treatment

- Prognosis is related to tumor stage at presentation and histologic grade
- Nearly 95% of patients have transmural invasion at the time of diagnosis
- Surgical resection is the most effective treatment for early-stage disease
- Advanced disease and peritoneal spread may require additional debulking, oophorectomy, and intraperitoneal chemotherapy

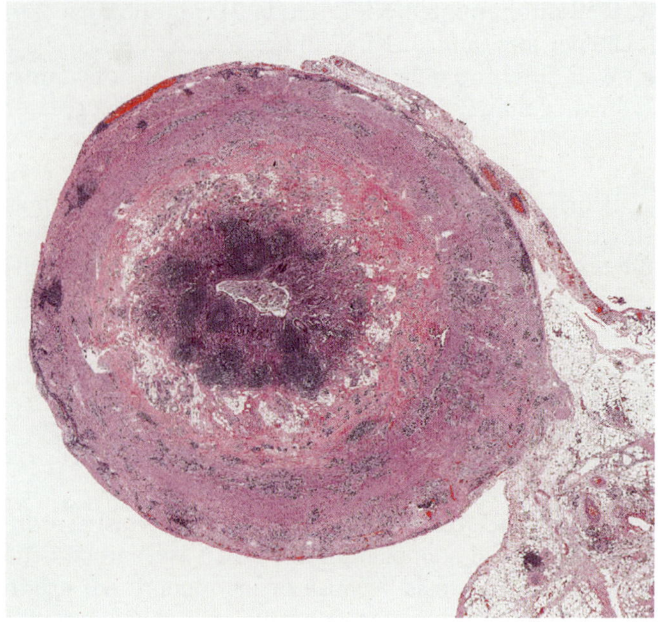

FIGURE 8.38

Goblet cell adenocarcinoma. Low-power view of the appendix emphasizes the subtle, concentric infiltrating pattern of this tumor.

Microscopic Findings

Goblet cell adenocarcinomas arise without a recognizable precursor lesion. These tumors infiltrate in a concentric manner with small clusters, linear rows, or single cells that can be difficult to appreciate on low-power examination (Fig. 8.38). They usually appear to be most prominent along the deep aspect of lamina propria and submucosa and display a wide range of histologic patterns. For a lesion to be classified as a GCA, the tumor must demonstrate a component of classic low-grade GCA characterized by tubules composed of goblet-like mucinous cells, variable numbers of endocrine cells, and Paneth cells. There is minimal cytologic atypia, and mitoses are infrequent (Fig. 8.39). Some lesions may show extensive extracellular mucin.

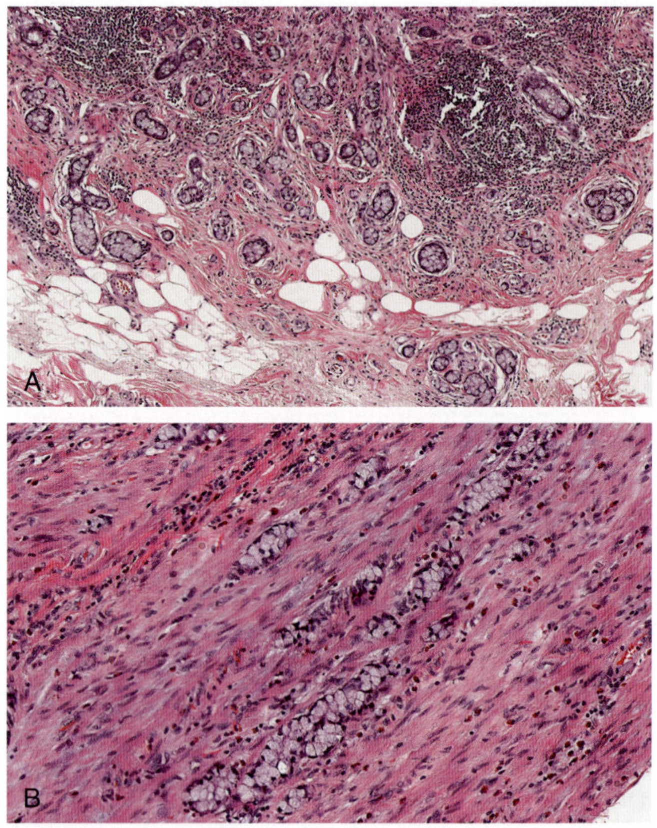

FIGURE 8.39

Goblet cell adenocarcinoma with low-grade features **A**, Well-defined goblet cells are arranged in tight clusters. **B**, The cells may also show a cohesive linear pattern with minimal atypia and no desmoplasia.

High-grade histologic features include complex anastomosing tubules, tumor infiltrating as single mucinous

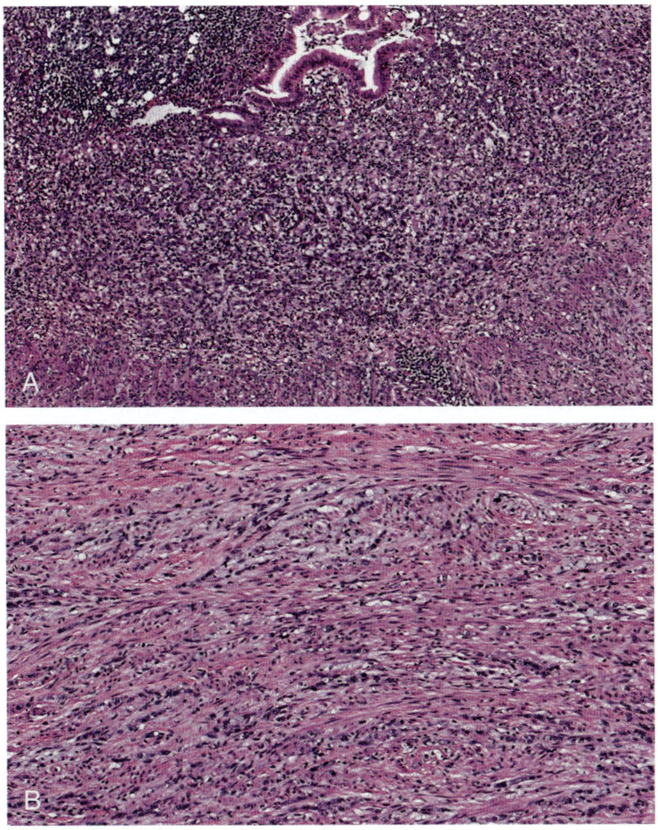

FIGURE 8.40

Goblet cell adenocarcinoma with high-grade features **A**, The neoplastic goblet cells or signet ring cells are arranged in irregular, large, disorganized clusters that have lost cohesion. **B**, The individual cells show a discohesive growth pattern and infiltrate as single atypical cells.

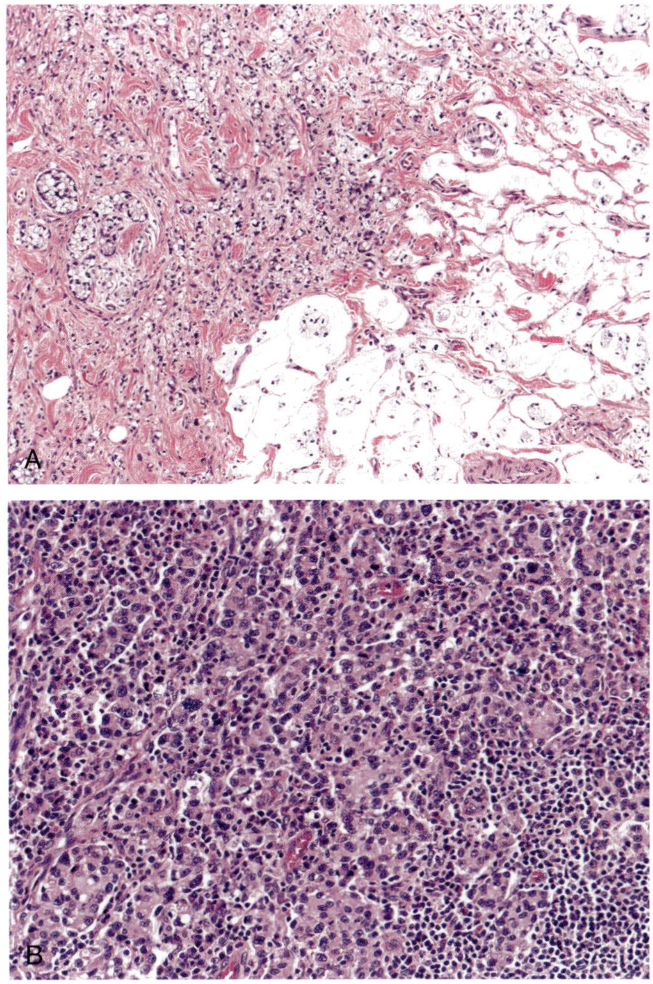

FIGURE 8.41

Goblet cell adenocarcinoma with high-grade features. **A**, The poorly differentiated tumor cells are present in the form of a mucinous adenocarcinoma. The left half of the image shows well-formed clusters of goblet cells **B**, An example of an undifferentiated carcinoma arising from a goblet cell carcinoid. Although this area does not demonstrate signet ring or goblet cell features, other areas of the same tumor had focal goblet cell morphology.

or nonmucinous cells, cribriform architecture, sheets of tumor cells, and large aggregates of goblet-like or signet ring–like cells. (Figs. 8.40 and 8.41) In some cases, there may be foci of conventional adenocarcinoma. Desmoplasia, cytologic atypia, numerous mitoses, and atypical mitotic figures may be seen.

Unlike classic NET, mitotic count or Ki-67 index is not used to classify or predict clinical behavior of GCAs. They are graded using a three-tiered system (Table 8.4) They are staged using the TNM (tumor, node, metastasis) system for appendiceal carcinoma.

Nearly all GCAs stain for cytokeratin (CK) 20, and up to 70% coexpress CK7. The neoplastic cells at least focally show immunoreactivity with endocrine markers chromogranin and synaptophysin (Fig. 8.42). Intracytoplasmic mucin can be demonstrated with mucicarmine.

TABLE 8.4

Three-Tiered Grading system for Goblet Cell Adenocarcinoma

Grade	Tubular or Clustered Growth (Low-Grade Pattern) (%)	Loss of Tubular or Clustered Growth (Any Combination of High-Grade Patterns) (%)
1	>75	<25
2	50–75	25–50
3	<50	>50

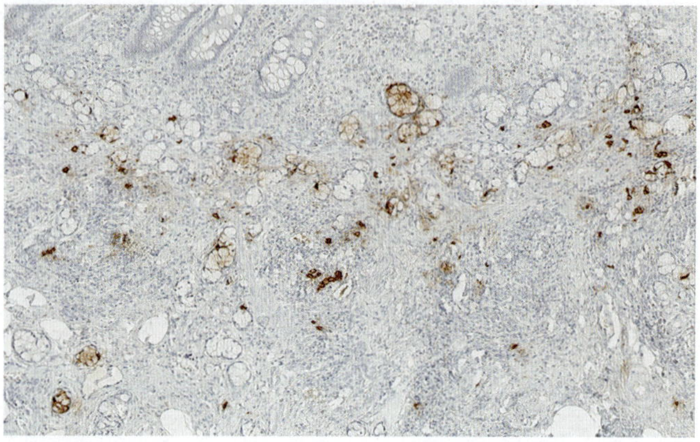

FIGURE 8.42

Goblet cell adenocarcinoma with patchy chromogranin immunoreactivity. In comparison, typical neuroendocrine tumors express strong, diffuse staining of these endocrine markers.

Goblet Cell Adenocarcinoma—Pathologic Features

Gross Findings

- Does not produce a discrete mass lesion; appendix may look normal
- Circumferential thickening with longitudinal infiltration
- Most are larger than 2 cm (tumor involvement along length of appendix)

Microscopic Findings

- Arises within the deep lamina propria or submucosa without a precursor lesion
- Concentric, infiltrative growth pattern of goblet-shaped or signet-ring cells and neuroendocrine cells

Morphologic Subtypes

- Low-grade features
  - Minimal cytologic atypia
  - Tubules of goblet-like mucinous cells with variable endocrine and Paneth cells
  - Mitoses infrequent
  - High-grade features
  - Discohesive single file or single infiltrating cells of mucinous or nonmucinous cells
  - Significant cytologic atypia
  - Desmoplasia and destruction of the appendiceal wall
  - Sheets of atypical cells
  - Cribriform pattern
  - Large clusters of goblet-like cells

Immunohistochemistry

- Cytokeratin (CK) 20 positive (with coexpression of CK7 in 70%)
- Patchy, focal reactivity with endocrine markers (chromogranin, synaptophysin)

Differential Diagnosis

- Tubular pattern classical neuroendocrine tumor (NET)
- Collision tumor of adenocarcinoma and NET
- Classical NET with entrapped benign epithelium
- Metastatic adenocarcinoma with signet ring features

Differential Diagnosis

Neuroendocrine tumor with a tubular pattern (tubular carcinoid) was previously regarded as "adenocarcinoid" tumor. These can be distinguished from GCAs by their formation of glandular structures, lack of prominent goblet or signet ring cells, and strong diffuse staining with endocrine markers. GCAs, by comparison, have a patchy or focal staining pattern with endocrine markers. Tubular NETs behave indolently like classical NETs and should not be confused with the more aggressive GCA.

Prognosis and Therapy

Compared with classic NETs of the appendix, GCAs behave more aggressively. Most patients (97%) have transmural extension of the tumor at the time of diagnosis, and more than half present with metastatic disease. Metastatic disease to other solid organs (e.g., lung, liver, bone) is exceptionally rare. The most commonly involved extraappendiceal sites include direct extension into the right colon and ileum followed by spread to the peritoneum and omentum. The ovary is the most common site of metastasis in women (88%), usually presenting as Krukenberg tumor. Lymph node metastases are detected in more than one-third of patients, depending on the histologic subtype.

Surgical management with right hemicolectomy is recommended after appendectomy. Additional debulking procedures may be needed, followed by chemotherapy. Chemotherapy regimens are similar to those used for colonic adenocarcinomas. Intraperitoneal spread may warrant oophorectomy and intraperitoneal chemotherapy.

SUGGESTED READINGS

1. Lamps LW, Gray Jr GF, Dilday BR, et al. The coexistence of low-grade mucinous neoplasms of the appendix and appendiceal diverticula: a possible role in the pathogenesis of pseudomyxoma peritonei. *Mod Pathol*. 2000;13(5):495–501.
2. Sahami S, Kooij IA, Meijer SL, et al. The link between the appendix and ulcerative colitis: clinical relevance and potential immunological mechanisms. *Am J Gastroenterol*. 2016;111(2):163–169.
3. Bronner MP. Granulomatous appendicitis and the appendix in idiopathic inflammatory bowel disease. *Semin Diagn Pathol*. 2004;21(2):98–107.
4. Guo G, Greenson JK. Histopathology of interval (delayed) appendectomy specimens: strong association with granulomatous and xanthogranulomatous appendicitis. *Am J Surg Pathol*. 2003;27(8):1147–1151.
5. Misdraji J, Yantiss RK, Graeme-Cook FM, et al. Appendiceal mucinous neoplasms: a clinicopathologic analysis of 107 cases. *Am J Surg Pathol*. 2003;27(8):1089–1103.
6. Misdraji J, Young RH. Primary epithelial neoplasms and other epithelial lesions of the appendix (excluding carcinoid tumors). *Semin Diagn Pathol*. 2004;21(2):120–133.

7. Misdraji J, Graeme-Cook FM. Miscellaneous conditions of the appendix. *Semin Diagn Pathol*. 2004;21(2):151–163.
8. Yantiss RK, Panczykowski A, Misdraji J, et al. A comprehensive study of nondysplastic and dysplastic serrated polyps of the vermiform appendix. *Am J Surg Pathol*. 2007;31(11):1742–1753.
9. Yantiss RK, Shia J, Klimstra DS, Hahn HP, Odze RD, Misdraji J. Prognostic significance of localized extra-appendiceal mucin deposition in appendiceal mucinous neoplasms. *Am J Surg Pathol*. 2009;33(2):248-255.
10. Arnason T, Kamionek M, Yang M, et al. Significance of proximal margin involvement in low-grade appendiceal mucinous neoplasms. *Arch Pathol Lab Med*. 2015;139(4):518–521.
11. Pai RK, Beck AH, Norton JA, et al. Appendiceal mucinous neoplasms: clinicopathologic study of 116 cases with analysis of factors predicting recurrence. *Am J Surg Pathol*. 2009;33(10):1425–1439.
12. Pai RK, Hartman DJ, Gonzalo DH, et al. Serrated lesions of the appendix frequently harbor KRAS mutations and not BRAF mutations indicating a distinctly different serrated neoplastic pathway in the appendix. *Hum Pathol*. 2014;45(2):227–235.
13. Carr NJ, Bibeau F, Bradley RF, et al. The histopathological classification, diagnosis and differential diagnosis of mucinous appendiceal neoplasms, appendiceal adenocarcinomas and pseudomyxoma peritonei. *Histopathology*. 2017;71(6):847–858.
14. Carr NJ, Cecil TD, Mohamed F, et al. Peritoneal Surface Oncology Group International. A consensus for classification and pathologic reporting of pseudomyxoma peritonei and associated appendiceal neoplasia: the results of the Peritoneal Surface Oncology Group International (PSOGI) Modified Delphi Process. *Am J Surg Pathol*. 2016;40(1):14–26.
15. Barrios P, Losa F, Gonzalez-Moreno S, et al. Recommendations in the management of epithelial appendiceal neoplasms and peritoneal dissemination from mucinous tumours (pseudomyxoma peritonei). *Clin Transl Oncol*. 2016;18(5):437–448.
16. Moris D, Tsilimigras DI, Vagios S, et al. Neuroendocrine neoplasms of the appendix: a review of the literature. *Anticancer Res*. 2018;38(2):601–611.
17. Tang LH, Shia J, Soslow RA, et al. Pathologic classification and clinical behavior of the spectrum of goblet cell carcinoid tumors of the appendix. *Am J Surg Pathol*. 2008;32(10):1429–1443.

9

Infectious Diseases of the Gastrointestinal Tract

■ Nicole C. Panarelli, MD

Surgical pathologists who evaluate specimens from the gastrointestinal (GI) tract for possible infections must first attempt to differentiate histologic changes suggesting infection from other inflammatory processes. After this determination, dedicated attempts must be made to diagnose the specific infectious organisms. The surgical pathologist's ability to detect infectious processes in tissue sections has grown exponentially with the advent of new histochemical and immunohistochemical stains, in situ hybridization, and polymerase chain reaction (PCR) analysis. Of note, multiplexed PCR assays performed on stool samples have become widely available and are slowly replacing traditional stool culture for identification of causative bacterial and viral pathogens in many centers. Use of these techniques has resulted in an increase in our knowledge of the pathologic features of specific infections.

Most GI infections are self-limited. Patients who undergo endoscopic evaluation and biopsy generally have unusual clinical features such as debilitating diarrhea, evidence of systemic disease, or a history of immunocompromise. One of the most valuable (and least expensive) diagnostic aids for a surgical pathologist is a discussion with the gastroenterologist regarding specific symptoms, colonoscopic findings, travel history, food intake history (e.g., sushi, poorly cooked beef), sexual practices, and immune status.

VIRAL INFECTIONS

A wide variety of viruses affect the GI tract. Manifestations of disease vary with the type of virus, specific site of infection, and immune status of the patient.

■ CYTOMEGALOVIRUS

Cytomegalovirus (CMV) infection occurs in both immunocompromised and immunocompetent persons and may be found throughout the GI tract. The pathogenesis in truly healthy patients is poorly understood. An underlying immunocompromised state should be considered when CMV infection is diagnosed because it is an opportunistic pathogen in patients with many conditions that compromise immunity, including those with acquired immunodeficiency syndrome (AIDS) or solid organ or bone marrow transplant recipients, as well those who receive prolonged immunomodulator or steroid therapy for immune-mediated or autoimmune disorders.

■ CLINICAL FEATURES

Symptoms vary with the immune status of the patient and the specific site of infection. In immunocompromised individuals, CMV esophagitis causes odynophagia, whereas gastroenteritis is marked by abdominal pain, diarrhea (either bloody or watery), fever, and weight loss. Hypertrophic gastropathy with protein-losing enteropathy resembling Menetrier's disease has rarely been reported in association with CMV gastritis. Primary infections in healthy, immunocompetent persons are often self-limited. CMV superinfection is known to exacerbate other chronic GI diseases, such as ulcerative colitis and Crohn's disease; in such cases, it is associated with toxic megacolon, refractoriness to medical therapy, and high mortality.

CYTOMEGALOVIRUS—FACT SHEET

Definition

- Viral infection

Incidence and Location

- Anywhere in the gastrointestinal tract

Clinical Features

- Most common in, but not limited to, immunocompromised patients
  - Odynophagia, diarrhea (with or without blood), abdominal pain, fever, weight loss
    - May cause an ischemic picture, both clinically and pathologically
- May be reactivated in Crohn's disease or ulcerative colitis after immunosuppressive therapy

Prognosis and Therapy

- Infections in healthy persons are usually self-limiting
- Ganciclovir often in combination with newer drugs

PATHOLOGIC FEATURES

GROSS FINDINGS

Cytomegalovirus causes a wide variety of gross lesions with ulcers being the most common finding (Fig. 9.1); they may be single or multiple and either superficial or deep. The ulcers often have a well-demarcated, "punched-out" appearance. Other gross findings include hemorrhagic colitis, pseudomembranous colitis, and obstructive mass lesions.

Segmental colonic involvement with linear ulcers mimicking Crohn's disease have been well documented in colonic CMV infection. Rarely, severe ulcerative CMV infection may lead to bowel perforation.

MICROSCOPIC FINDINGS

The histologic spectrum of CMV infection also varies widely, often depending on the patient's immune status. Typical histologic features include mixed inflammation with numerous neutrophils and mucosal ulceration with prominent granulation tissue. Epithelial cell apoptosis may be prominent (Fig. 9.2A). Virtually no associated inflammatory reaction may be seen in severely immunocompromised patients. Inclusions are preferentially found in endothelial cells and stromal cells and only rarely in epithelial cells; thus, they are usually seen deep in ulcer bases.

The characteristic "owl's eye" intranuclear inclusions are visible on routine (hematoxylin and eosin) preparations, as are brightly eosinophilic, granular intracytoplasmic inclusions (Fig. 9.2B). Occasionally, CMV infection of endothelial cells of mucosal and submucosal vessels of the bowel initiates inflammatory mediators, leading to vascular thrombosis and subsequent bowel ischemia. Segmental bowel ischemia caused by infection with CMV shows histologic features that are similar to other causes of ischemia (hemorrhagic necrosis and crypt withering). In addition to CMV inclusions, the vessels may show marked inflammation and necrosis.

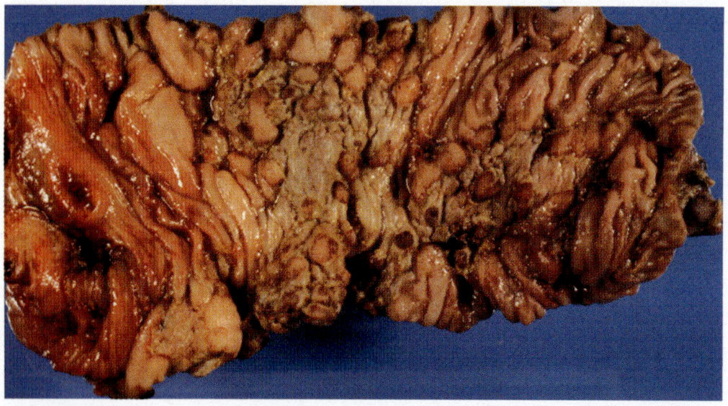

FIGURE 9.1

Colon resected from a renal transplant patient with cytomegalovirus colitis. Note the sharply demarcated area of coalescing ulcers.

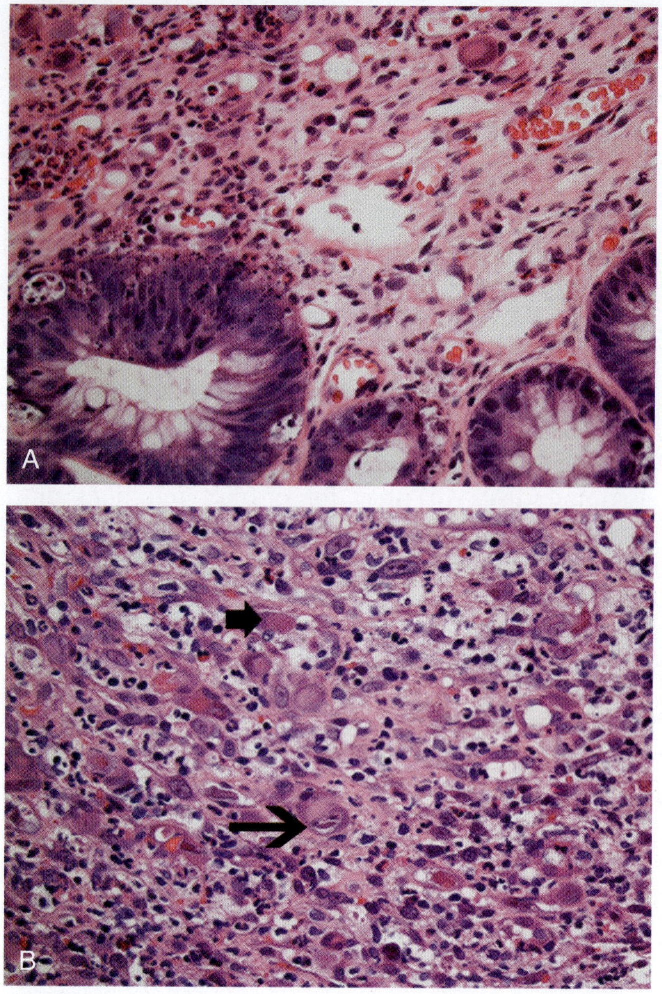

FIGURE 9.2

A, Abundant apoptotic crypt epithelial cells simulate graft-versus-host disease in cytomegalovirus infection (hematoxylin and eosin [H&E]). **B**, Characteristic "owl's eye" inclusions *(thin arrow)* are seen within the nuclei of endothelial and mesenchymal cells in the lamina propria. The cytoplasm contains granular eosinophilic inclusions *(thick arrow)* (H&E).

CYTOMEGALOVIRUS—PATHOLOGIC FEATURES

Gross Findings

- Most commonly ulcers, single or multiple, shallow or deep
- May also manifest as colitis (hemorrhagic or pseudomembranous) or obstructive mass
- Segmental or linear ulceration may mimic Crohn's disease grossly

Microscopic Findings

- Characteristic inclusions: "owl's eye" inclusions in the nuclei of endothelial and stromal cells
- Granular eosinophilic inclusions in the cytoplasm of endothelial and stromal cells
- Mixed inflammation with prominent neutrophils and apoptosis
- No associated inflammatory reaction may be seen, particularly in severely immunocompromised patients
- Endothelial infection may cause ischemia

Differential Diagnosis

- Other viral infections, particularly adenovirus
- Crohn's disease
- Graft-versus-host disease
- Ischemic colitis

Ancillary Studies

Examination of multiple levels and immunohistochemical stains facilitates detection of rare CMV inclusions in cases when clinical suspicion is high but characteristic findings are lacking or when exuberant inflammation obscures diagnostic features, such as in samples from patients with corticosteroid-dependent IBD. Detection of isolated CMV-positive cells may be of clinical import for patients with GI complaints because some experience symptomatic improvement with antiviral therapy. Findings on immunohistochemical stains should always be correlated with routine sections because granulocytes and plasma cells may show nonspecific staining. Other useful diagnostic aids include viral culture, PCR assays, and in situ hybridization. Isolation of CMV in culture, however, does not imply active infection because virus may be excreted for months to years after a primary infection. Similarly, positive serologic studies may indicate prior or primary infection.

Differential Diagnosis

The differential diagnoses are primarily other viral infections, particularly adenovirus. CMV inclusions and are present within both the nucleus and cytoplasm. Adenovirus inclusions, by comparison, are crescent shaped or have irregular outlines, are generally within surface epithelium, and are only intranuclear. The distinction between CMV infection and graft-versus-host disease (GVHD) in bone marrow transplant patients may be particularly difficult because both clinical and histologic features are similar. Immunohistochemistry (IHC) may be used to rule out CMV infection in this setting. As mentioned previously, CMV infection may produce architectural distortion, deep "fissuring" ulcers, and skip lesions that simulate Crohn disease but does not produce neural hyperplasia, transmural lymphoid aggregates, muscularis mucosae hypertrophy, or pyloric metaplasia. Of course, a careful search for inclusions should confirm the diagnosis of CMV infection in cases with features of both disorders (although the two may coincide; Fig. 9.3).

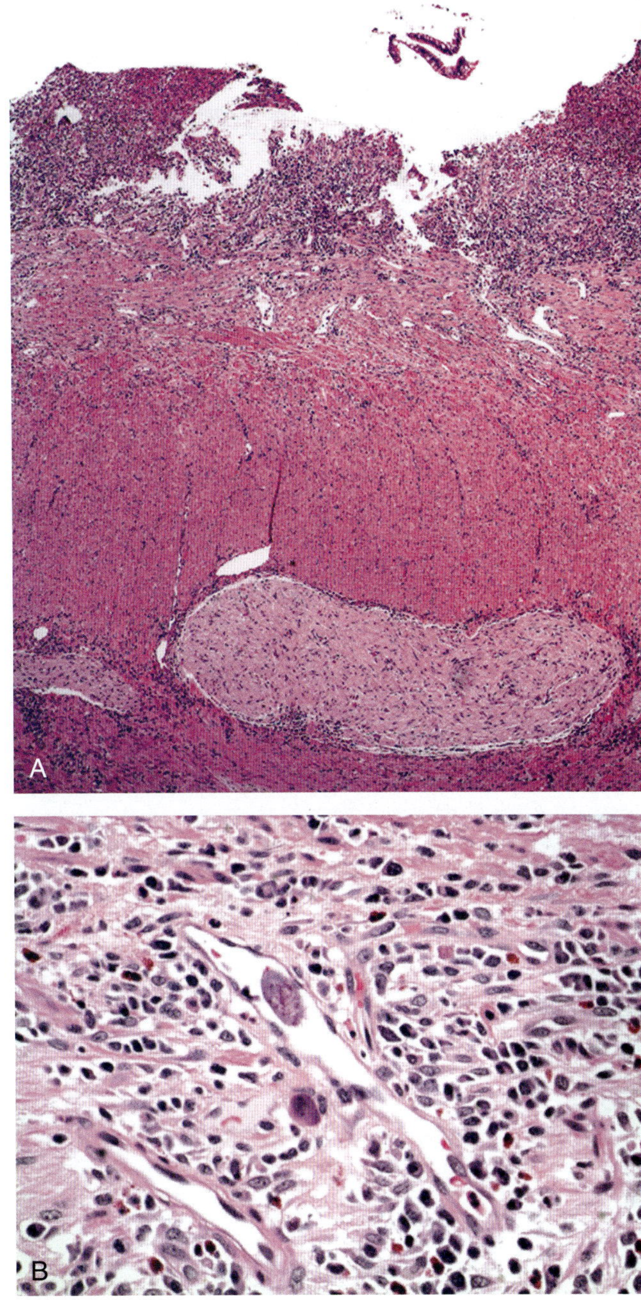

FIGURE 9.3

Cytomegalovirus (CMV) infection superimposed on chronic Crohn's disease. **A**, Note active ulcer overlying thickened colon wall with marked neural hyperplasia (hematoxylin and eosin [H&E]). **B**, CMV inclusions are seen within endothelial cells at the base of the ulcer (H&E). Case courtesy of Dr. Brian Quinn.

Prognosis and Therapy

The vast majority of infections in healthy persons are self-limiting. Ganciclovir has historically been the mainstay of medical therapy, but this drug has problems with toxicity and poor oral bioavailability, and resistant strains are evolving. Newer drugs such as foscarnet are now often used in combination with ganciclovir.

HERPESVIRUS

Herpetic infection is most commonly seen in the esophagus and anorectum. The symptoms and pathologic features of herpes simplex virus type 1 (HSV-1) versus HSV-2 are indistinguishable. Herpetic proctitis is the most common cause of nongonococcal proctitis in homosexual men. In immunocompetent patients, herpes outbreaks are often self-limiting; immunocompromised persons may be at risk for dissemination and life-threatening illness.

Clinical Features

Herpetic esophagitis causes dysphagia, vomiting, and hematemesis. Proctitis presents with severe anorectal pain, bloody discharge or frank bleeding, tenesmus, constipation, and fever. Concomitant neurologic symptoms (difficulty in urination and paresthesias of the buttocks and upper thighs) are well described, as is inguinal lymphadenopathy. Herpes colitis is most often seen in immunocompromised patients and may be a fulminant, life-threatening condition.

HERPES SIMPLEX VIRUS—FACT SHEET

Definition

- Viral infection, often in immunocompromised patients

Incidence and Location

- Predominantly esophageal and anorectal; rarely colonic
- Most common cause of nongonococcal proctitis in homosexual men

Clinical Features

- Most common in, but not limited to, immunocompromised patients
  - Esophagitis: dysphagia, vomiting, hematemesis
  - Proctitis: anorectal pain, discharge, often with neurologic symptoms, and inguinal lymphadenopathy; perianal vesicles
  - Colitis: diarrhea, lower gastrointestinal bleeding; fulminant colitis with perforation may develop

Prognosis and Therapy

- Acyclovir is first line of medical therapy; surgery may be required if fulminant colitis or perforation develops

Pathologic Features

Gross Findings

Ulcers are the most common findings in the esophagus, but one may also see intact vesicles. Severe cases may be characterized by diffuse erosive esophagitis. In herpetic proctitis, perianal vesicles are common, and they may extend into the anal canal and rectum. In herpetic colitis, the most typical finding is multiple and confluent ulcers. The surrounding mucosa is often hemorrhagic and friable, and "cobblestoning" of the mucosa may be seen.

Microscopic Findings

Ulcers are associated with increased neutrophils in the lamina propria, and perivascular lymphocytic cuffing. The inflammatory exudate often contains sloughed epithelial cells. Two types of characteristic nuclear inclusions may be found: (1) the more common smudged, ground-glass nuclear inclusion with peripheral darker, marginated chromatin (Fig. 9.4), and (2) the acidophilic inclusions with a surrounding clear halo and peripheral chromatin margination (Cowdry type A inclusion). They are usually present in squamous epithelial cells at the edges of ulcers and are often multiple.

Ancillary Studies

Fewer than half of biopsy specimens contain inclusions. Viral culture is the most valuable aid to diagnosis; IHC, in situ hybridization, and PCR assays may also be of use.

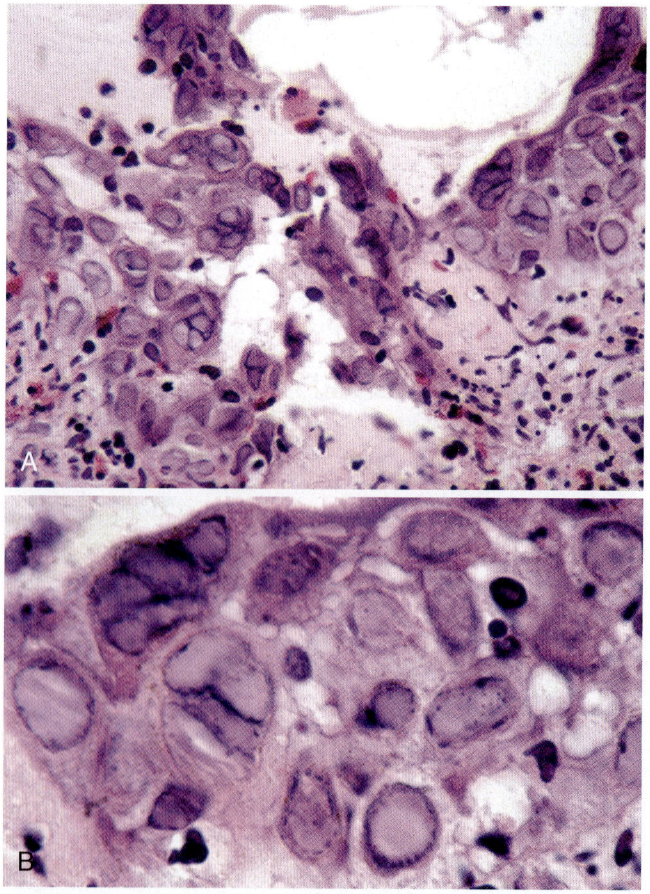

FIGURE 9.4

Typical herpes simplex virus inclusions. Note the smudged, ground-glass nuclei with peripheral darker, marginated chromatin (hematoxylin and eosin).

Herpes Simplex Virus—Pathologic Features

Gross Findings
- Ulcers, vesicles
- Mucosal friability and hemorrhage, "cobblestoned" mucosa in the colon

Microscopic Findings
- Ulceration, inflammatory exudate with sloughed epithelial cells
- Viral inclusions in epithelial cells, consisting of a smudged, ground-glass nucleus with peripheral darker, marginated chromatin

Differential Diagnosis
- Other viral infections, particularly varicella
- Crohn's disease

Differential Diagnosis

The differential diagnosis predominantly includes other viral infections, such as CMV and varicella zoster (VZV). Morphology and location of the inclusions distinguishes HSV from CMV. Herpetic inclusions are most often in the epithelial cells of the mucosa, whereas CMV preferentially involves the endothelial and stromal cells. Co-infection may also occur, particularly in the immunocompromised. Rarely, segmental ulceration and cobblestoning of mucosa may mimic Crohn's disease, as in the case of CMV infection. Unlike CMV infection, HSV complicating idiopathic IBD is rare, and data are limited to case reports. Serologic studies play a limited role in the diagnosis of HSV colitis owing to the high prevalence of HSV seropositivity overall; IHC may be used when suspicion is raised on morphologic grounds. HSV may be detected in colonic tissue samples via PCR but is not routinely used. Varicella zoster inclusions are indistinguishable from HSV on H&E sections, but tend to be occur at all levels in infected mucosa, rather than in a superficial distribution. Patients often have a skin rash. VZV inclusions are negative on HSV immunostains; immunostains targeting VZV are available.

Prognosis and Therapy

Acyclovir is the mainstay of medical therapy. Segmental resection to control bleeding and prevent perforation may be required in severe cases of herpetic colitis.

ADENOVIRUS

Adenovirus infection is second only to rotavirus as a cause of self-limiting childhood diarrhea. However, it has recently gained much attention as a cause of diarrhea in immunocompromised patients, especially those with AIDS and patients who have undergone transplantation (particularly bone marrow transplantation). Adenovirus infection of the GI tract is strongly associated with concomitant acute GVHD.

CLINICAL FEATURES

Virtually all patients present with diarrhea, sometimes accompanied by fever, weight loss, lower GI bleeding, and abdominal pain.

ADENOVIRUS—FACT SHEET

Definition
- Viral infection, often in immunocompromised or transplant patients

Incidence and Location
- Small intestine, colon

Clinical Features
- Diarrhea sometimes accompanied by fever, weight loss, abdominal pain, or gastrointestinal bleeding

Prognosis and Therapy
- Ribavirin

Pathologic Features

Gross Findings

Endoscopic findings typically include erythematous, friable, and granular mucosa.

Microscopic Findings

Histologic features of adenovirus infection include epithelial changes such as superficial cellular degeneration, apoptosis of epithelial cells, and focal acute inflammation. Severe cases may show ulceration and exudate. Characteristic homogeneous, smudgy, eosinophilic inclusions may be seen lining the nucleus. Adenovirus inclusions are, except in rare circumstances, limited to epithelial cells; inclusions are most common within surface epithelium but may also be seen in the crypt epithelium. Inclusions are particularly common in surface goblet cells, in which they are often crescent shaped (Fig. 9.5).

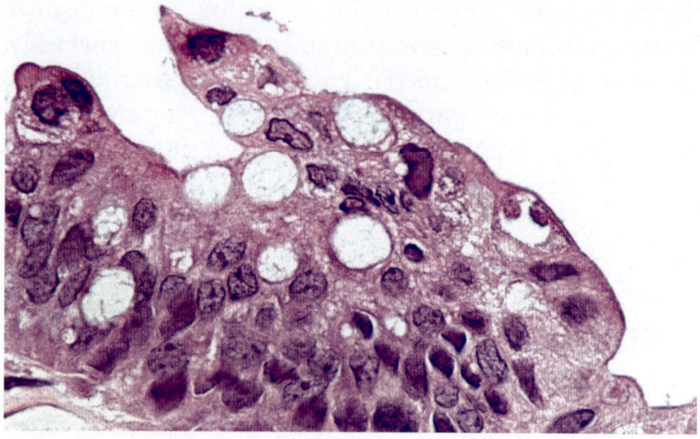

FIGURE 9.5

Homogeneous, smudgy, eosinophilic inclusions fill the nuclei of the surface enterocytes in adenovirus infection (hematoxylin and eosin). Courtesy of Dr. Joel Greenson.

Adenovirus—Pathologic Features

Gross Findings

- Erythematous, friable, and granular mucosa

Microscopic Findings

- Superficial cellular degeneration, apoptosis of epithelial cells, and focal acute inflammation; severe cases may show ulceration and exudate
    - Inclusions
    - Homogeneous, smudgy, eosinophilic inclusions fill the nucleus.
    - Inclusions can be crescent shaped or targetoid
    - Most common within surface epithelium, particularly goblet cells, but can be seen in crypt epithelial cells; almost never in endothelial and mesenchymal cells

Differential Diagnosis

- Other viral infections, particularly cytomegalovirus

Ancillary Studies

Immunohistochemistry is useful aid for adenovirus detection.

Differential Diagnosis

The differential diagnosis primarily includes other viral infections, especially CMV. Morphologic differences between the two viruses, as well as differences in location within the gut (epithelium vs endothelium or stromal cells) usually help resolve the differential diagnosis. Because adenovirus often coexists with GVHD, it may be overlooked if a careful search for inclusions is not undertaken. Adenovirus inclusions also show morphologic overlap with reactive and degenerative nuclear changes in intestinal epithelia and may be easily overlooked; a high index of suspicion should be maintained in immunosuppressed populations.

Prognosis and Therapy

The antiviral drug ribavirin is the mainstay of therapy.

Human Immunodeficiency Virus–Associated Ulcerative Esophagitis

Human immunodeficiency virus (HIV) has been implicated in the pathogenesis of chronic esophageal ulcers in infected patients, due, in part, to detection of viral proteins in ulcerated mucosa. The diagnosis is one of exclusion; thus, one should thoroughly evaluate other possibilities, including other viral infections and medication-induced injuries. Ulcers may contain atypical-appearing fibroblasts, and the associated squamous mucosa may be atrophic.

AIDS Enterocolopathy

AIDS enterocolopathy is a term that describes morphologic changes seen in the gut of patients with HIV/AIDS and chronic diarrhea, for which no other infectious cause has been identified. Some argue that these changes represent either primary infection of gut epithelial cells with HIV or a secondary autoimmune reaction to viral infection. Others believe that this is a poorly understood term that does not clearly represent a specific disease entity and thus should not be used at all. The controversy arises because asymptomatic patients may have similar morphologic findings on biopsy, and conversely, severely symptomatic patients may have normal biopsy findings. In addition, there is always the added concern that a causative pathogen simply has been missed.

Patients with AIDS enterocolopathy often have chronic diarrhea, but some are asymptomatic. Colonoscopy is usually normal. The small bowel is more commonly affected than the colon. Histologic features include increased apoptotic activity (Fig. 9.6) and decreased numbers of mitotic figures relative to extent of mucosal injury; the changes resemble those seen in mild GVHD and chemotherapy-related mucosal injuries. The differential diagnosis includes conditions that are associated with prominent apoptosis, such as GVHD, chemotherapy- and drug-related injury, and other viral infections Other infectious agents should be rigorously excluded.

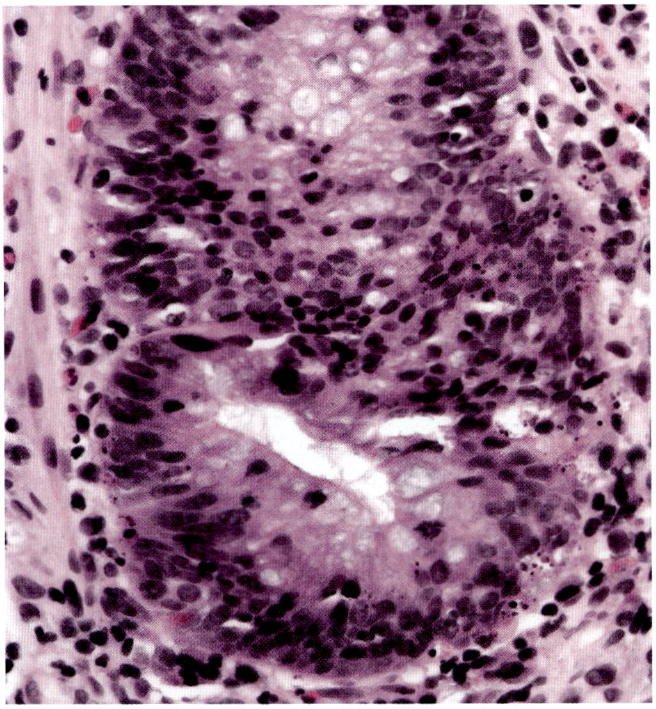

FIGURE 9.6
Numerous apoptotic enterocytes are present in this case of AIDS-related enterocolopathy (hematoxylin and eosin).

BACTERIAL INFECTIONS

A seemingly endless array of bacterial species are pathogenic in the GI tract. Many produce nonspecific changes, but others may be identified in tissue sections or produce inflammatory patterns that are suggestive of specific infections. This section covers major bacterial pathogens, emphasizing features that guide pathologists and clinicians in reaching a correct diagnosis.

SARCINA VENTRICULI AND RELATED ORGANISMS

Sarcina spp. are gram-positive cocci that may be found associated with ulcerated gastric mucosa. Severe complications for *S. ventriculi* infection are rare, and the organism is found in stool of healthy individuals; thus, its pathogenicity remains controversial.

CLINICAL FEATURES

Sarcina organisms are identified in patients with delayed gastric emptying and gastric outlet obstruction, often in the setting of an obstructing mass, stricture, or prior surgery. Clinical and imaging findings usually reveal an alternate explanation for gastric obstruction, raising the possibility that *Sarcina* organisms do not cause disease but are a marker of luminal stasis. Patients report epigastric pain, dyspepsia, bloating, and vomiting. *Sarcina* organisms have been implicated in rare cases of acute emphysematous gastritis.

SARCINA VENTRICULI—FACT SHEET

Definition
- Gram-positive anaerobic coccus that can grow in acidic environments

Incidence and Location
- Stomach
- Infection is rare

Clinical Features
- Nausea, vomiting
- Abdominal pain
- Melena, hematemesis
- Emphysematous gastritis
- Perforation
- May be asymptomatic
- History of prior gastric surgery
- Presence of an obstructing mass

Prognosis and Therapy
- Metronidazole with or without other antibiotics
- Relief of gastric outlet obstruction
- Antiacid therapy

PATHOLOGIC FEATURES

GROSS FINDINGS

Endoscopic findings include retained food and bile, masses, gastritis, and ulcers.

MICROSCOPIC FINDINGS

Sarcina organisms do not invade the gastric mucosa and do not typically evoke an inflammatory response. This supports the notion that the organisms are not pathogenic; however, they may colonize preexisting ulcers, which increases the risk of perforation or emphysematous gastritis (Fig. 9.7A). They are spherical to cuboidal organisms that span 1.8 to 3 μm and have refractile cell walls, resembling vegetable matter (Fig. 9.7B). They occur in a "tetrad packet" arrangement of four organisms or multiples of four, reflecting cell division in multiple planes.

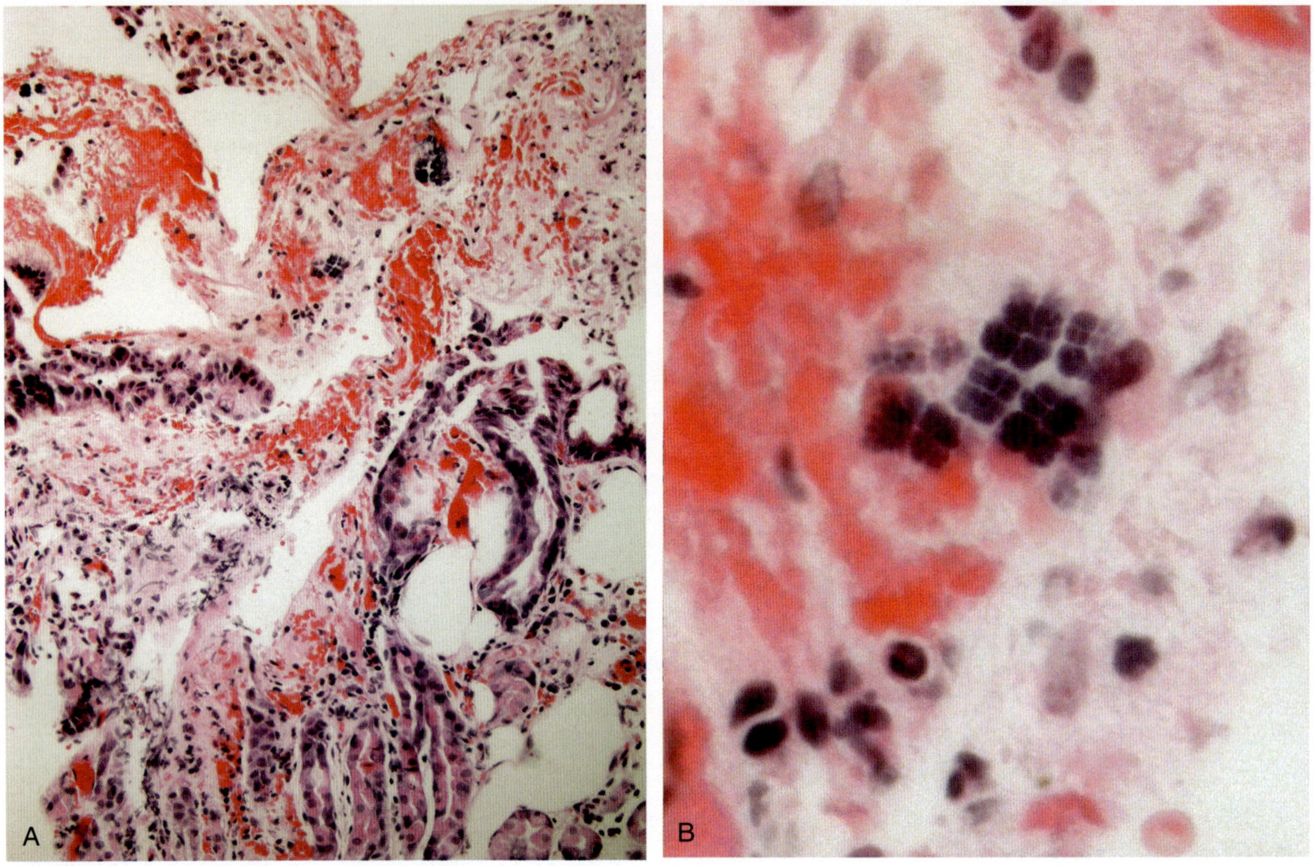

FIGURE 9.7

A, *Sarcina* organisms are present in surface debris of a gastric ulcer. **B**, High magnification shows tetrads of the bacteria clustered into larger groups (hematoxylin and eosin). Courtesy of Dr. Kathryn E. Tanaka.

SARCINA VENTRICULI—PATHOLOGIC FEATURES

Gross Findings

- Ulcers
- Gastritis
- Retained food

Microscopic Findings

- Tetrads of non-invasive spherical to cuboidal organisms
- Associated mucosal ulceration
- Differential Diagnosis
- *Micrococcus*
- *Staphylococcus*

ANCILLARY STUDIES

S. ventriculi can usually be diagnosed in routine sections, but tissue Gram stain may highlight the organisms. If necessary, PCR amplification of the 16S rRNA gene can confirm the diagnosis.

DIFFERENTIAL DIAGNOSIS

Micrococcus spp. are also gram-positive cocci that occur in tetrads, but they are considerably smaller (0.5 µm) than *S. ventriculi* and are aerobes. *Staphylococci* are also gram positive but measure only 1 µm and occur in grape-like clusters rather than tetrads.

PROGNOSIS AND THERAPY

Therapy is aimed at eliminating the underlying cause of gastric outlet obstruction. Eradication of the organisms with metronidazole therapy in combination with other antibiotics has been reported. Some patients report symptomatic relief with proton pump inhibitors, H2 receptor blockers, and antiemetic therapy.

TROPHERYMA WHIPPLEI (WHIPPLE DISEASE)

Whipple disease is a rare, multisystemic infectious disorder caused by the bacillus, *Tropheryma whipplei* (formerly *T. whippelii*). The disease predominantly occurs in middle-aged white men; however, recent studies show increased incidence in women. It has historically shown a predilection for farmers and carpenters. Some point to detection of *T. whipplei* in asymptomatic individuals and familial cases as evidence of a possible genetic susceptibility to a commensal organism.

CLINICAL FEATURES

Whipple disease may affect virtually any organ system, but the classic presentation includes diarrhea, weight loss, fever, abdominal lymphadenopathy, and arthralgia. A substantial proportion of patients experience cardiovascular and pulmonary symptoms. The most severe form of disease includes neuropsychiatric manifestations, such as ophthalmoplegia, myoclonus, and dementia.

TROPHERYMA WHIPPLEI–FACT SHEET

Definition

- Gram-positive bacillus responsible for rare multisystem disorder characterized by diarrhea and malabsorption

Incidence and Location

- Small intestine; rarely the esophagus stomach, colon, and mesenteric lymph nodes

Clinical Features

- Diarrhea, weight loss, abdominal lymphadenopathy
- Fever
- Arthralgias
- Cardiac failure, pericarditis
- Cough and pleuritic chest pain
- Dementia and neuromuscular symptoms

Prognosis and Therapy

- Months to years of antibiotic therapy may be necessary
- Supportive care for malabsorption
- Relapse may occur

PATHOLOGIC FEATURES

GROSS FINDINGS

The duodenal mucosa may show thickened small intestinal folds that are coated with yellow-white plaques. The adjacent mucosa may appear erythematous or friable.

MICROSCOPIC FINDINGS

Whipple disease is most commonly diagnosed in duodenal biopsy specimens. Involvement of the liver, esophagus, stomach, colon, and mesenteric lymph nodes has also been documented. In small bowel biopsies, the villi are blunted by expansion of the lamina propria with foamy macrophages (Fig. 9.8A). In addition, there may be neutrophilic activity, fat vacuoles (small collections of extracellular lipid droplets), and lymphangiectasia. Foamy macrophages contain periodic acid–Schiff (PAS)–positive bacillary organisms (Fig. 9.8B).

TROPHERYMA WHIPPLEI–PATHOLOGIC FEATURES

Gross Findings

- Enlarged mucosal folds
- Yellow-white plaques

Microscopic Findings

- Villous blunting
- Foamy macrophages expand the lamina propria and submucosa
- Periodic acid–Schiff–positive bacillary organisms within foamy macrophages
- Neutrophilic infiltrates
- Fat droplets and lymphangiectasia in the mucosa

Differential Diagnosis

- *Histoplasma capsulatum*
- *Mycobacterium avium-intracellulare* complex

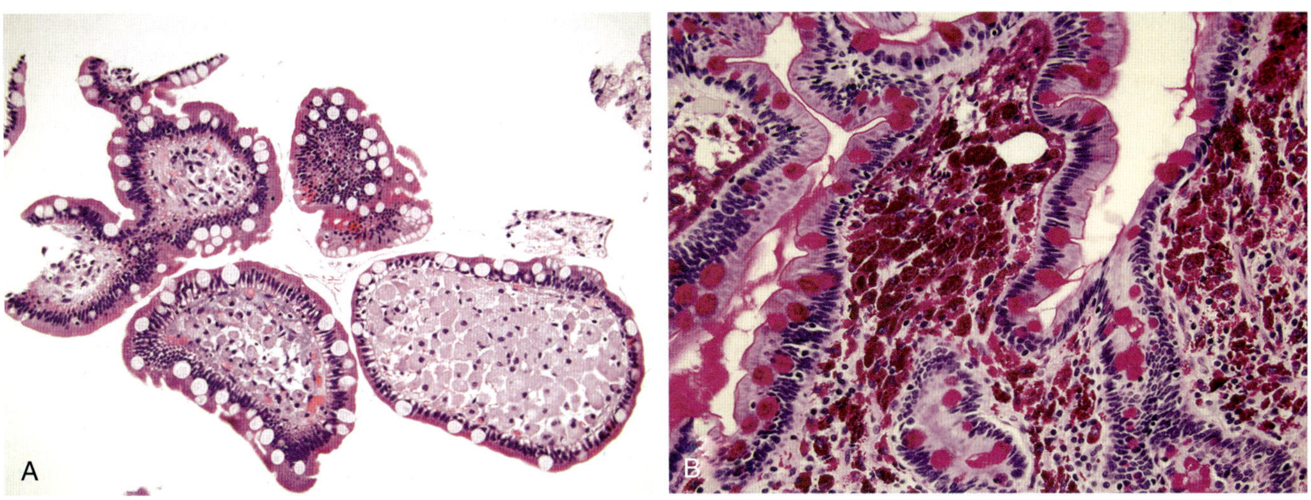

FIGURE 9.8

A, The duodenal lamina propria is filled with abundant macrophages in a case of Whipple disease (hematoxylin and eosin). **B**, The macrophages contain periodic acid–Schiff–positive bacteria, consistent with Tropheryma whipplei. Courtesy of Dr. Maria Westerhoff.

Differential Diagnosis

The differential diagnosis includes other organisms that infect the mononuclear phagocytic system. *Histoplasma capsulatum* organisms are ovoid with a surrounding halo and stain with Gomori methenamine silver (GMS). *Mycobacterium avium-intracellulare* (MAI) are filamentous, pale blue intracellular organisms on H&E stain. They can be PAS positive but are distinguished from *T. whipplei* by positive staining with Ziehl-Neelsen or other acid-fast stains. Both of these infections may elicit granulomatous inflammation in immunocompetent hosts.

Ancillary Studies

Culture of *T. whipplei* has met with limited success because of the organism's slow growth and need for an acidic environment that simulates intracellular conditions. IHC is available to confirm this diagnosis. PCR assay is a highly sensitive and specific method to confirm this diagnosis in suspicious cases. Given the availability of IHC and PCR assays, electron microscopy is less commonly used for confirmation.

BACTERIAL ENTEROCOLITIS

Diarrhea resulting from bacterial infection is a significant worldwide health problem. *Escherichia coli* and *Salmonella, Shigella*, and *Campylobacter* spp. are the most commonly identified pathogens. Many bacterial infections of the gut are related to ingestion of contaminated water or food or travel to countries where these organisms are endemic. Although bacteria are often recovered by culture or identified by molecular means, surgical pathologists may play a valuable role in diagnosis. A general classification of colonic bacterial infections by histologic pattern is given in Table 9.1.

Despite the large number of infectious agents that may affect the colon, the histologic features that they produce may be generally categorized as follows:

1. Organisms producing very mild or no histologic changes (e.g., enteroadherent *E. coli* [EAEC])
2. Organisms producing the histologic features of acute infectious/self-limited colitis or focal active colitis, such as *Campylobacter* spp.
3. Organisms producing suggestive or diagnostic histologic features, such as pseudomembranes, granulomas, or ischemic changes

The pattern of acute self-limited colitis or focal active colitis is one of the most common seen in infectious colitis. Typical histologic features include cryptitis, with or without increased neutrophils in the lamina propria and crypt abscesses; preservation of crypt architecture; and lack of basal plasmacytosis. The acute inflammatory component may be most prominent in the mid to upper crypts. The lack of crypt distortion and basal lymphoplasmacytosis helps distinguish acute self-limited colitis from early IBD.

ESCHERICHIA COLI

Diarrheagenic *E. coli* organisms are classified into five groups: enterotoxigenic, enteropathogenic, enteroadherent, enteroinvasive, and enterohemorrhagic. If pathogenic *E. coli* is suspected, the clinical laboratory should be notified to search for it specifically because cultures may be a valuable diagnostic aid.

Enterotoxigenic *E. coli* is a major cause of traveler's diarrhea, but patients are seldom examined via biopsy, and the pathology has not been well characterized in humans. Enteropathogenic *E. coli* (EPEC) predominantly affects infants and neonates. Biopsy is not generally performed and is not diagnostically useful, although occasionally gram-negative rods may be seen at the surface of the mucosa (Fig. 9.9). EAEC is similar to the enteropathogenic group and is also an important cause of traveler's diarrhea and pediatric diarrhea worldwide. Both EPEC and EAEC have been increasingly recognized as causes of chronic diarrhea and wasting in AIDS patients. Endoscopic findings are usually unremarkable, but histologic examination shows a coating of adherent bacteria at the surface epithelium, which may stain gram negative. Degenerated surface epithelial cells with associated intraepithelial inflammatory cells may also be present. Enteroinvasive *E. coli* (EIEC) is similar to *Shigella* both genetically and in its clinical presentation and pathogenesis. Given its capacity for invasion, EIEC produces a severe dysentery-like diarrheal illness that can be a particular problem in patients with AIDS. The gross and microscopic pathology of EIEC has not been well described.

ENTEROHEMORRHAGIC *ESCHERICHIA COLI*

The most common strain of EHEC is 0157:H7. This infectious disease is probably markedly underdiagnosed. This organism adheres to intestinal epithelial cells and produces a cytotoxin similar to that produced by *Shigella dysenteriae*; however, there is no invasion. Although contaminated meat is the most frequent mode of transmission, infection may also occur through contaminated water, milk, produce, and person-to-person contact.

TABLE 9.1

Classification of Bacterial Infections of the Colon According to Histologic Pattern

Minimal or No Inflammatory Change	Acute Self-Limited Colitis Pattern	Pseudomembranous Pattern	Predominantly Granulomatous	Diffuse Histiocytic	Predominantly Lymphohistiocytic	Marked Architectural Distortion	Ischemic Pattern
Enteropathic *Escherichia coli* Enteroadherent *E. coli* Spirochetosis *Neisseria* spp. *Vibrio cholerae*	*Shigella* spp. *Campylobacter* spp. *Aeromonas* spp. *Salmonella* spp. (nontyphoid) Occasionally *Clostridioides difficile* Syphilis (± increased plasma cells)	Enterohemorrhagic *E. coli* C. difficile Occasionally *Shigella* spp.	*Yersinia* spp. *Mycobacterium tuberculosis* Actinomycosis (mixed suppurative and granulomatous) MAI (immunocompetent patients) Rarely syphilis	*Rhodococcus equi* MAI (immuno-compromised patients)	LGV *Salmonella typhimurium*	*S. typhimurium* *Shigella* spp.	Enterohemorrhagic *E. coli* *Klebsiella oxytoca*

LGV, Lymphogranuloma venereum; MAI, Mycobacterium avium-intracellulare complex.

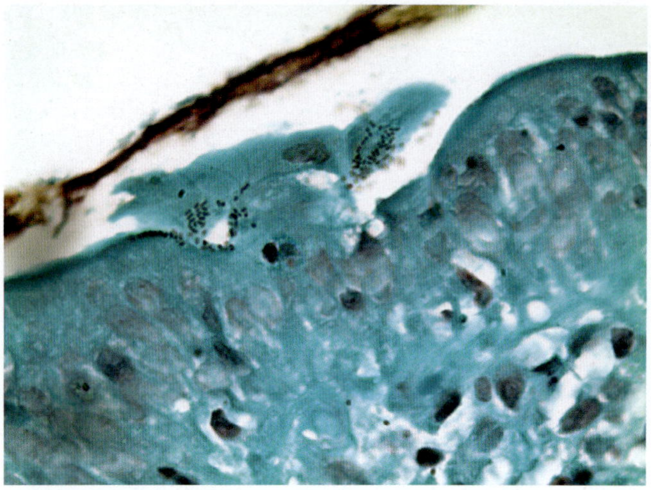

FIGURE 9.9

Enteroadherent Escherichia coli in a patient with AIDS. A coating of gram-negative rods with little inflammatory reaction is noted at the surface of the colonic mucosa (Twort Gram stain with oil immersion).

CLINICAL FEATURES

Symptoms usually consist of bloody diarrhea with severe abdominal cramps and mild or no fever. Nonbloody, watery diarrhea may occur, however. Only one-third of patients have fecal leukocytes. Rarely, this infection leads to frank lower GI bleeding. Affected persons may develop hemolytic-uremic syndrome or thrombotic thrombocytopenic purpura, and children and older adults are at particular risk for serious, systemic illness.

ENTEROHEMORRHAGIC *ESCHERICHIA COLI*–FACT SHEET

Definition

- Diarrheagenic *Escherichia coli* strain producing hemorrhagic colitis

Incidence and Location

- Preferentially involves the right colon

Clinical Features

- Bloody diarrhea with severe abdominal cramps
- Mild or no fever
- Sometimes leads to obstructive edema or massive bleeding
- Patients at risk for hemolytic-uremic syndrome and thrombotic thrombocytopenic purpura

Prognosis and Therapy

- Mainly supportive care
- Role of antibiotics controversial
- Surgery may be required to relieve obstruction or control bleeding

PATHOLOGIC FEATURES

GROSS FINDINGS

Endoscopically, patients have colonic edema, erosions, ulcers, and hemorrhage, and the right colon is usually more severely affected. The edema may be so marked as to cause obstruction.

MICROSCOPIC FINDINGS

The histopathologic features are those of ischemic colitis because the toxin is believed to induce an ischemic insult. These features include lamina propria and submucosal hemorrhage (Fig. 9.10), with associated mucosal acute inflammation, crypt withering, and necrosis. Intimal thickening and luminal thrombi may be seen in small vessels, and pseudomembranes are occasionally present (Fig. 9.11). Necrosis and hemorrhage

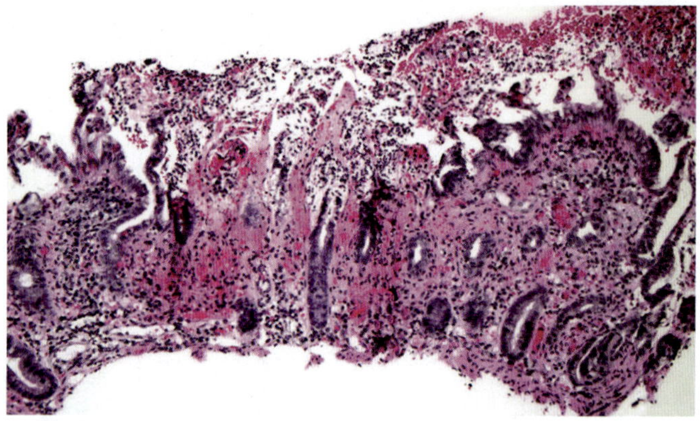

FIGURE 9.10

Enterohemorrhagic *Escherichia coli* infection. Hemorrhagic mucosal necrosis of the upper epithelium, crypt withering, lamina propria hyalinization, and microthrombi (hematoxylin and eosin).

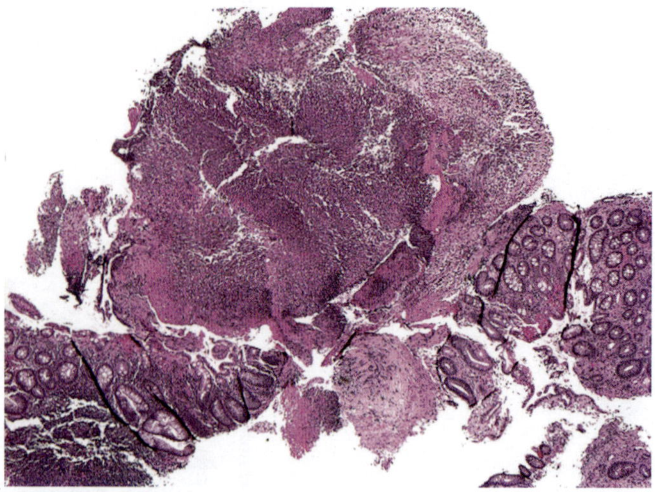

FIGURE 9.11

Enterohemorrhagic *Escherichia coli* can have prominent necroinflammatory exudates that resemble pseudomembranes (hematoxylin and eosin).

of the superficial colonic crypts with sparing of the deeper compartment is characteristic of enterohemorrhagic *E. coli* but may also be seen in other types of ischemia. A combination of ischemic changes and features of acute colitis should raise suspicion for infection.

ENTEROHEMORRHAGIC *ESCHERICHIA COLI*—PATHOLOGIC FEATURES

Gross Findings

- Colonic edema, erosions, ulcers, and hemorrhage

Microscopic Findings

- Mimics ischemic colitis of other causes
- Microthrombi may be seen within small vessels
- Pseudomembranes may be present

Differential Diagnosis

- Ischemic colitis of other causes
- *Clostridioides difficile*–related pseudomembranous colitis
- Rarely, idiopathic inflammatory bowel disease

ANCILLARY STUDIES

Examination of stool samples by PCR has recently become a crucial diagnostic aid. Routine stool cultures do not distinguish 0157:H7 from normal intestinal flora, and successful culture may be impossible more than 4 days after onset of symptoms. Microbiologic diagnosis requires screening on sorbitol–MacConkey agar and testing of colonies with antisera. An immunohistochemical stain for this organism is described, but is not used in clinical practice.

DIFFERENTIAL DIAGNOSIS

The differential diagnosis includes ischemic colitis, *Clostridioides difficile*–related colitis, and idiopathic IBD. Histologic features of ischemia in the right colon, particularly in patients who are not at risk for atherosclerotic disease, should prompt consideration of EHEC and the appropriate cultures. The histologic features of ischemia generally serve to distinguish EHEC from idiopathic IBD. If pseudomembranes are present, differentiation from *C. difficile*–related colitis may be difficult, and cultures or the *C. difficile* toxin assay may be required.

PROGNOSIS AND THERAPY

There is no proven therapy for EHEC, and the role of antibiotic treatment is controversial, although most strains are susceptible. Surgical resection of the affected colon may be required to relieve obstruction from edema or to control bleeding.

SALMONELLOSIS

Salmonella, which are gram-negative bacilli, are transmitted through food and water and are particularly prevalent where sanitation is poor. They are an important cause of both food poisoning and traveler's diarrhea. The discussion of *Salmonella* spp. may be generally divided into typhoid and nontyphoid species. Enteric (typhoid) fever is usually caused by *S. typhi*; the most common nontyphoid species include *Salmonella enteritidis, Salmonella typhimurium, Salmonella muenchen, Salmonella anatum, Salmonella paratyphi*, and *Salmonella give*. Although historically enteric fever was considered much more severe than nontyphoid salmonellosis, more recent literature suggests a greater degree of overlap (both clinically and pathologically). The infective dose is relatively low ($\sim 10^3$ organisms may cause human disease). Patients with low gastric acidity and patients with AIDS have a greater risk for *Salmonella* infection and associated complications.

CLINICAL FEATURES

There are numerous manifestations of *Salmonella* infection, including an asymptomatic carrier state (often the organism is harbored in the gallbladder), a self-limited gastroenteritis, typhoid fever, and septicemia. Patients with typhoid (enteric) fever typically present with fever (which generally rises over several days), abdominal pain, headache, and occasionally initial constipation. Abdominal rash ("rose spots"), delirium, hepatosplenomegaly, and leukopenia are fairly common. The diarrhea, which begins in the second or third week of infection, is first watery but may progress to severe GI bleeding and perforation. Nontyphoid *Salmonella* spp. generally cause a milder, self-limited gastroenteritis with vomiting, nausea, fever, and watery diarrhea. Occasionally, these species cause bloody diarrhea or toxic megacolon.

SALMONELLOSIS—FACT SHEET

Definition

- Gram-negative enteric bacterium causing typhoid (enteric) fever or milder gastroenteritis

Incidence and Location

- Any segment of colon; typhoidal form typically involves ileum, right colon, and appendix

Clinical Features

- Typhoidal form
- Fever (rising over several days), abdominal pain, headache, and occasionally constipation
- Abdominal rash (rose spots) and leukopenia
- Diarrhea begins in the second or third week
- Diarrhea is initially watery but may progress to severe gastrointestinal bleeding
- Nontyphoidal form
- Milder, self-limited gastroenteritis with vomiting, nausea, fever, and watery diarrhea
- More clinical and pathologic overlap between the typhoidal and nontyphoidal forms than previously thought

Prognosis and Therapy

- Antibiotics, supportive care

Pathologic Features

Gross Findings

In enteric fever, any anatomic segment of the alimentary tract may be involved, but the characteristic pathology is most prominent in the ileum, appendix, and right colon and is associated with Peyer's patches. Grossly, the bowel wall is thickened, and raised nodules may be seen corresponding to hyperplastic Peyer's patches. Aphthoid ulcers overlying Peyer's patches, linear ulcers, discoid ulcers, or full-thickness ulceration and necrosis are common as disease progresses. Perforation and toxic megacolon may also be seen, as may suppurative mesenteric lymphadenitis. Occasionally, the mucosa is grossly normal or only mildly inflamed and edematous. Endoscopic findings in nontyphoid salmonellosis include mucosal redness, ulceration, and exudates, but the characteristic nodularity and marked edema are not generally seen.

Microscopic Findings

Macrophages predominate in enteric fever (Fig. 9.12A). Peyer's patches become hyperplastic, and then acute inflammation of the overlying epithelium is seen (Fig. 9.12B). Eventually, the lymphoid follicles are infiltrated and obliterated by macrophages. Necrosis begins in the Peyer's patch and spreads to surrounding mucosa, which eventually ulcerates. The ulcers are typically deep, with the base at the muscularis propria. Typhoid fever may also show features more consistent with acute self-limited colitis, including prominent neutrophils, cryptitis, crypt abscesses, and overlying fibrinous exudate. Granulomas are occasionally seen. In nontyphoid salmonellosis, the pathologic features are those of acute self-limited colitis of any infectious cause. Occasionally, significant crypt distortion may be seen.

***Salmonellosis*—Pathologic Features**

Gross Findings

- Typhoid
- Characteristic pathology most prominent in ileum, appendix, and right colon
- Markedly thickened bowel, raised nodules correspond to hyperplastic Peyer's patches
- Aphthoid ulcers overlying Peyer's patches, linear ulcers, discoid ulcers, or full-thickness ulceration and necrosis are common
- Perforation and toxic megacolon rarely seen
- Suppurative mesenteric lymphadenitis may be present
- Nontyphoid
- Generally milder findings, including mucosal redness, ulceration, and exudates

Microscopic Findings

- Typhoid
- Macrophage is the predominant inflammatory cell
- Hyperplastic Peyer's patches with overlying acute inflammation; eventually, frank ulceration begins in Peyer's patch and spreads to surrounding mucosa
- Lymphoid follicles are infiltrated and obliterated by macrophages
- Neutrophils are usually limited to erosions overlying hyperplastic Peyer's patches
- Ulcers are typically very deep, with the base at the muscularis propria.
- Rare granulomas
- Nontyphoid
- Features of acute self-limited colitis

Differential Diagnosis

- Other bacterial infections (*Yersinia* spp., *Shigella* spp.)
- Crohn's disease
- Ulcerative colitis

Ancillary Studies

Stool cultures followed by serologic typing are the gold standard for detection, and blood cultures may also be of use if the patient is septic.

Differential Diagnosis

The differential diagnosis of typhoid fever includes yersiniosis and other infectious processes, as well as Crohn's disease, and there may be significant histologic

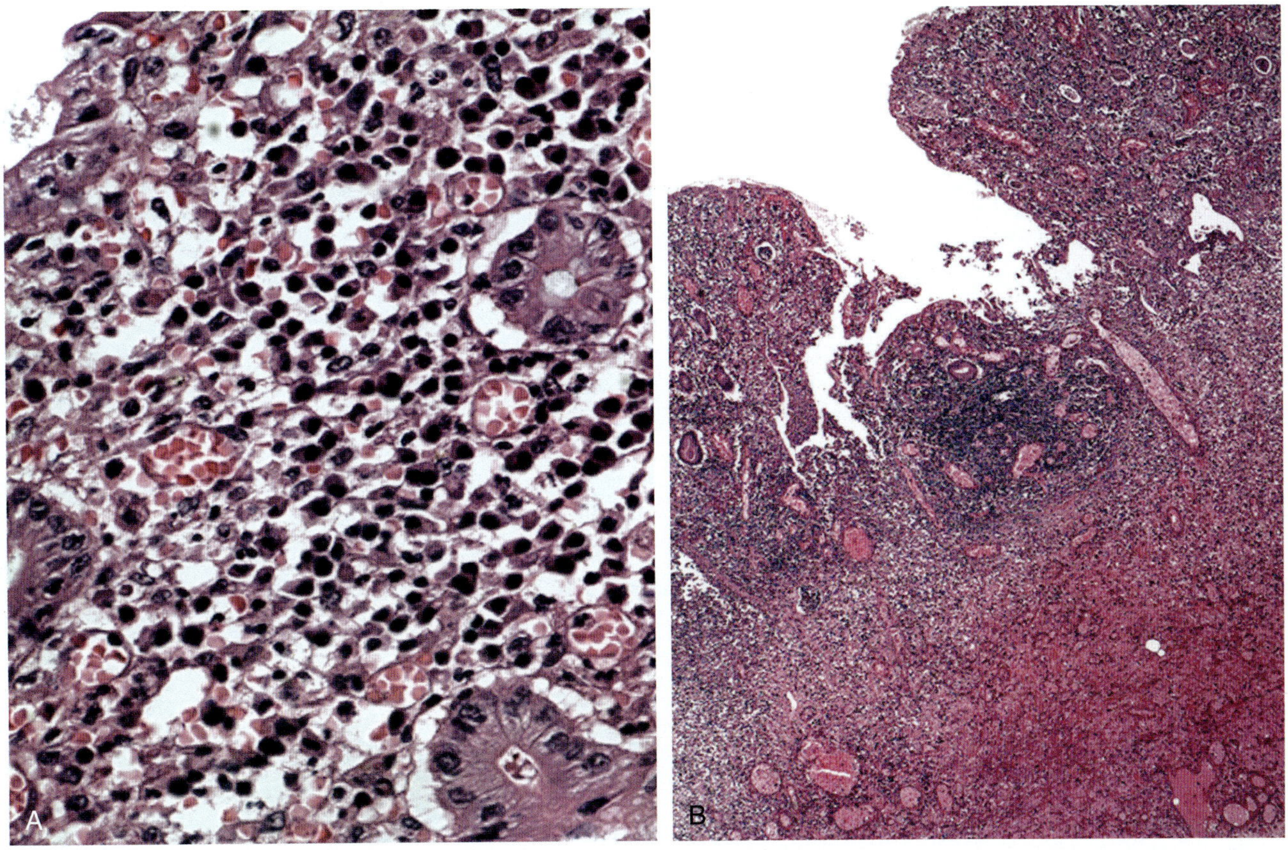

FIGURE 9.12
Mononuclear cells comprise the inflammatory infiltrate in enteric fever, with a dearth of neutrophils (hematoxylin and eosin [H&E]) (**A**). Ulcer overlying a Peyer's patch in typhoid fever (H&E) (**B**). Case courtesy of Dr. A. Brian West.

overlap. Neutrophils and granulomas are often more prominent in the latter two diseases. The differential diagnosis of nontyphoid *Salmonella* infection also includes other causes of acute self-limited infectious colitis, as well as ulcerative colitis. In addition, *Salmonella* infection may complicate preexisting idiopathic IBD. Although significant crypt distortion has been reported in some cases of salmonellosis, it is likely to be more pronounced in ulcerative colitis. Clinical presentation and stool culture may be helpful in resolving the differential diagnosis.

Prognosis and Therapy

Although the vast majority of *Salmonella* infections in developed countries resolve with antibiotics and supportive care, illness may progress to septicemia and death, particularly in older adults and very young people and in patients who are ill for other reasons. Delayed treatment is associated with higher mortality rates, and antibiotics are particularly important for neonates, older patients, immunocompromised persons, and patients with cardiac valve abnormalities or indwelling prostheses. *Salmonella* spp. are sensitive to several antibiotics, including ciprofloxacin, penicillins, and quinolones.

SHIGELLOSIS

Shigella spp. are virulent, invasive, gram-negative bacilli that cause severe bloody diarrhea. They are a major cause of infectious diarrhea worldwide. *Shigella dysenteriae* is the most common species isolated, although *Shigella sonnei* and *Shigella flexneri* are increasingly reported in the United States. The infective dose is low (as few as 10–100 in S. dysenteriae type 1). *Shigella* spp. are generally ingested from water contaminated with feces, but person-to-person transmission is also possible through the fecal–oral route. Infants; young children; and malnourished, immunocompromised, and debilitated patients are most commonly affected in developed countries. Like salmonellosis, rare cases of chronic shigellosis may simulate IBD grossly and microscopically.

CLINICAL FEATURES

Symptoms include abdominal pain, fever, and watery diarrhea followed by bloody diarrhea. Chronic disease is rare. Perforation and hemolytic-uremic syndrome associated with *Shigella* infection have been rarely described. Most studies of mortality in shigellosis were performed in underdeveloped nations, and figures range from 2% to 10%. The mortality rate is significantly higher (>20%) if patients become septic.

SHIGELLOSIS—FACT SHEET

Definition

- Gram-negative bacterium causing severe bloody diarrhea

Incidence and Location

- Colon, with the left colon most severely affected

Clinical Features

- Abdominal pain, fever
- Watery diarrhea followed by bloody diarrhea
- Chronic disease is rare (and may mimic ulcerative colitis and Crohn's disease)
- Perforation and hemolytic-uremic syndrome occasionally develop
- Severity worse in debilitated or immunocompromised patients

Prognosis and Therapy

- Supportive care
- Selected antibiotics because *Shigella* organisms have multidrug resistance

PATHOLOGIC FEATURES

GROSS FINDINGS

The large bowel is typically affected, with the left colon more severely involved. The mucosa is hemorrhagic, with exudates that may form pseudomembranes. Ulcerations may be present as well.

MICROSCOPIC FINDINGS

Early infection manifests as acute self-limited colitis with cryptitis, crypt abscesses (often superficial), and ulceration. Pseudomembranes similar to *C. difficile* infection may be seen, as may aphthoid ulcers similar to those of Crohn's disease. As disease progresses, there is increased mucosal destruction with a mixed inflammatory infiltrate containing many neutrophils in the lamina propria. Marked architectural distortion to an extent that mimics idiopathic IBD is the best-described histologic pattern in mucosal biopsies, most likely because patients do not typically undergo colonoscopy early in the disease course.

SHIGELLOSIS—PATHOLOGIC FEATURES

Gross Findings

- Hemorrhagic mucosa, with exudates that may form pseudomembranes
- Ulcerations may be present

Microscopic Findings

- Early infection
- Acute self-limited colitis with cryptitis, crypt abscesses, ulceration
- Pseudomembranes or aphthoid ulcers may be seen
- Later infection
- Increased mucosal destruction with a predominantly neutrophilic inflammatory infiltrate
- Marked architectural distortion to an extent that mimics idiopathic inflammatory bowel disease

Differential Diagnosis

- Other infections, especially *Clostridioides difficile* and enteroinvasive *Escherichia coli*
- Inflammatory bowel disease

ANCILLARY STUDIES

Stool culture *requires* rapid inoculation onto appropriate culture plates because *Shigella* organisms are fastidious and die quickly. Multiple cultures may be necessary. Stool cultures are more sensitive than rectal swabs. PCR, DNA probes, and serologic studies are also available.

DIFFERENTIAL DIAGNOSIS

The differential diagnosis of early shigellosis is primarily that of other infections, particularly EIEC and *C. difficile*. As disease progresses, it may be extremely difficult to distinguish shigellosis from Crohn's disease or ulcerative colitis both endoscopically and histologically. Stool cultures and clinical presentation may be helpful in this instance.

PROGNOSIS AND THERAPY

Treatment includes supportive care with fluid and electrolyte replacement and antibiotics, particularly in children, people who are severely ill, and HIV-positive patients. Antibiotics lessen the mortality rate and shorten the duration of the illness. Most *Shigella* spp. have at least some degree of antibiotic resistance; trimethoprim–sulfamethoxazole, third-generation cephalosporins, and some fluoroquinolones are drugs of choice.

CAMPYLOBACTER SPP.

Campylobacter spp., particularly *Campylobacter jejuni*, are major causes of diarrhea worldwide. *Campylobacter* is the most common stool isolate identified in the United States. It is transmitted by the fecal–oral route; is found in contaminated meat, water, and milk; and is a common animal pathogen. *C. jejuni* is most commonly associated with gastroenteritis; *Campylobacter fetus* and the other less common species are more often seen in immunosuppressed patients and homosexual men. The importance of *C. fetus* may be underrecognized as a result of the difficulty of culturing it under conditions used for other *Campylobacter* strains. The infective dose is low (ingestion of as few as 500 organisms may cause disease), and invasion may occur.

CLINICAL FEATURES

Patients typically have fever, malaise, abdominal pain (often severe), and watery diarrhea, often bloody and with fecal leukocytes. Symptoms generally present within 1 to 5 days of exposure and last for 4 to 10 days. Relapse is common, although it is usually less severe than the original attack. Immunosuppressed patients have a higher incidence of symptomatic infection, and symptoms are more severe. Most infections are self-limited, especially in healthy patients. Of note, Guillain-Barré syndrome and reactive arthropathy are associated with *Campylobacter* infection.

CAMPYLOBACTER SPP.—FACT SHEET

Definition
- Gram-negative bacterium
- Most common stool isolate in United States

Incidence and Location
- Colon

Clinical Features
- Fever, malaise, abdominal pain, watery diarrhea, often bloody and with fecal leukocytes
- Symptoms generally present within 1 to 5 days of exposure and last for 4 to 10 days
- Infection is generally self-limited, although relapse is frequent

Prognosis and Therapy
- Supportive care in most cases
- Erythromycin in severe cases and in immunocompromised patients

PATHOLOGIC FEATURES

GROSS FINDINGS

Endoscopic findings include friable colonic mucosa with associated erythema and hemorrhage.

MICROSCOPIC FINDINGS

Histologic examination most frequently shows features of acute infectious or self-limited colitis, including cryptitis, crypt abscesses, surface epithelial damage, and a lymphoplasmacytic infiltrate in the lamina propria (Fig. 9.13). Marked edema and superficial mucosal erosion with associated hemorrhage may be seen. Findings may be patchy. Although the mucosal architecture is usually well-preserved in *Campylobacter* infection, mild crypt distortion may occasionally be seen.

CAMPYLOBACTER SPP.—PATHOLOGIC FEATURES

Gross Findings
- Friable colonic mucosa
- Erythema and hemorrhage

Microscopic Findings
- Acute self-limited colitis pattern

Differential Diagnosis
- Other infections that cause the acute self-limited colitis pattern

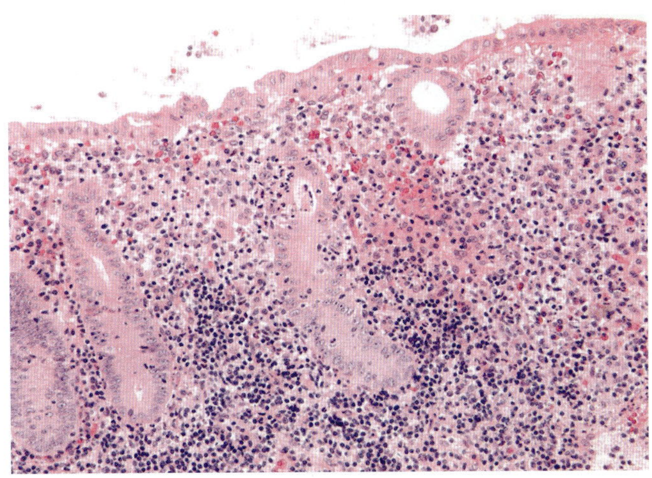

FIGURE 9.13
Campylobacter jejuni infection showing cryptitis, surface epithelial injury, and preservation of crypt architecture (hematoxylin and eosin).

Ancillary Studies

Culture and PCR on stool specimens are mainstays culture of *Campylobacter* detection. Preliminary diagnosis may be made by detection of organisms in fresh stool smears by dark-field microscopy. Rapid enzyme immunoassay tests have also been developed, but should be correlated with culture results.

Differential Diagnosis

The differential diagnosis primarily includes other forms of infectious enterocolitis that produce the acute self-limited colitis pattern; stool culture may be essential to resolving the differential diagnosis.

Prognosis and Therapy

In most uncomplicated cases of *Campylobacter* infection, fluid and electrolyte replacement is the principal therapy. Antibiotics are not generally indicated unless there is high fever, severe or bloody diarrhea, or symptoms longer than 1 week or the patient is immunocompromised or septic. Erythromycin is the antibiotic of choice.

YERSINIOSIS

Yersinia enterocolitica and *Yersinia pseudotuberculosis* are the two *Yersinia* species pertinent to human GI disease. *Yersinia* is one of the most common causes of bacterial enteritis in Western and Northern Europe, and numerous cases have been documented in North America and Australia. *Yersinia* spp. may be found in many food products, including meats (particularly undercooked pork), dairy products, and water.

CLINICAL FEATURES

These gram-negative coccobacilli are causative agents in appendicitis, ileitis, colitis, and mesenteric lymphadenitis. In addition, they are responsible for many cases of isolated granulomatous appendicitis. Infection with either species may cause symptoms and signs of an acute abdomen, chronic abdominal pain, and diarrhea. Although yersiniosis is usually a self-limited process, chronic infections (including chronic colitis) and persistent abdominal pain have been well documented. Immunocompromised and debilitated patients, as well as patients on deferoxamine or with iron overload resulting from other causes, are at significant risk for serious disease.

YERSINIA SPP.—FACT SHEET

Definition

- Common cause of granulomatous appendicitis, enterocolitis in the United States and Europe

Incidence and Location

- Ileum, appendix, and colon

Clinical Features

- Signs and symptoms of enterocolitis, acute appendicitis
- Usually self-limiting; occasionally causes chronic disease
- May have mesenteric adenopathy

Prognosis and Therapy

- Usually self-limiting
- Severe cases and debilitated patients require antibiotics

Pathologic Features

Gross Findings

Grossly, involved bowel has a thickened, edematous wall with nodular inflammatory masses centered around Peyer's patches. Aphthoid and linear ulcers may be seen. Involved appendices are enlarged and mimic suppurative granulomatous appendicitis; perforation is often seen. Involved lymph nodes may show gross foci of necrosis.

Microscopic Findings

Both suppurative and granulomatous patterns of inflammation may be seen, and a mixture of the two is common. GI infection with *Y. pseudotuberculosis* has characteristically been described as a granulomatous process with central microabscesses, almost always accompanied by mesenteric adenopathy. Infection with *Y. enterocolitica* has not typically been associated with discrete granulomas but has been characterized by hyperplastic Peyer's patches with overlying ulceration and accompanying acute inflammation, hemorrhagic necrosis, and palisading histiocytes. Recent studies have shown that there is significant overlap between the histologic features of *Y. enterocolitica* and *Y. pseudotuberculosis* infection and that either species may show epithelioid granulomas (Fig. 9.14A), lymphoid hyperplasia (see Fig. 9.13B), epithelioid granulomas with prominent lymphoid cuffing (see Fig. 9.13C), transmural lymphoid aggregates, giant cells, mucosal ulceration, cryptitis, and concomitant lymph node involvement. Some cases show only nonspecific features of acute self-limited colitis.

YERSINIA SPP.—PATHOLOGIC FEATURES

Gross Findings

- Thickened, edematous wall with nodular inflammatory masses centered around Peyer's patches
- Aphthoid and linear ulcers may be seen
- Involved appendices are enlarged and mimic typical suppurative appendicitis; perforation is frequent
- Mesenteric lymph node involvement is common

Microscopic Findings

- Often mix of both suppurative and granulomatous patterns of inflammation
- Lymphoid hyperplasia, epithelioid granulomas with prominent lymphoid cuffing and sometimes central abscesses, transmural lymphoid aggregates, giant cells, mucosal ulceration, and cryptitis
- There is significant overlap between the histologic features of *Yersinia enterocolitica* and *Yersinia pseudotuberculosis* infection
- Rare cases show only acute self-limited colitis

Differential Diagnosis

- Primarily Crohn's disease
- Other infections such as *Mycobacterium tuberculosis*, *Salmonella* spp.

ANCILLARY STUDIES

Cultures, serologic studies, and particularly PCR assays are the most useful diagnostic aids.

DIFFERENTIAL DIAGNOSIS

The major differential diagnoses of *Yersinia* infection include other similar infectious processes, particularly mycobacterial infection and salmonellosis. Acid-fast stains and culture results should help to distinguish mycobacterial infection; clinical features and the presence of granulomas may help to distinguish yersiniosis from salmonellosis.

Crohn's disease and yersiniosis have a long and complicated relationship. Both may show similar histologic features, and, in fact, isolated granulomatous appendicitis has in the past frequently been interpreted as primary Crohn's disease of the appendix. However, patients with granulomatous inflammation confined to the appendix rarely develop idiopathic IBD. Features that may favor Crohn's disease include cobblestoning of mucosa and creeping fat grossly and changes of chronicity microscopically, including crypt distortion, thickening of the muscularis mucosa, and prominent neural hyperplasia. However, some cases are indistinguishable on histologic grounds alone.

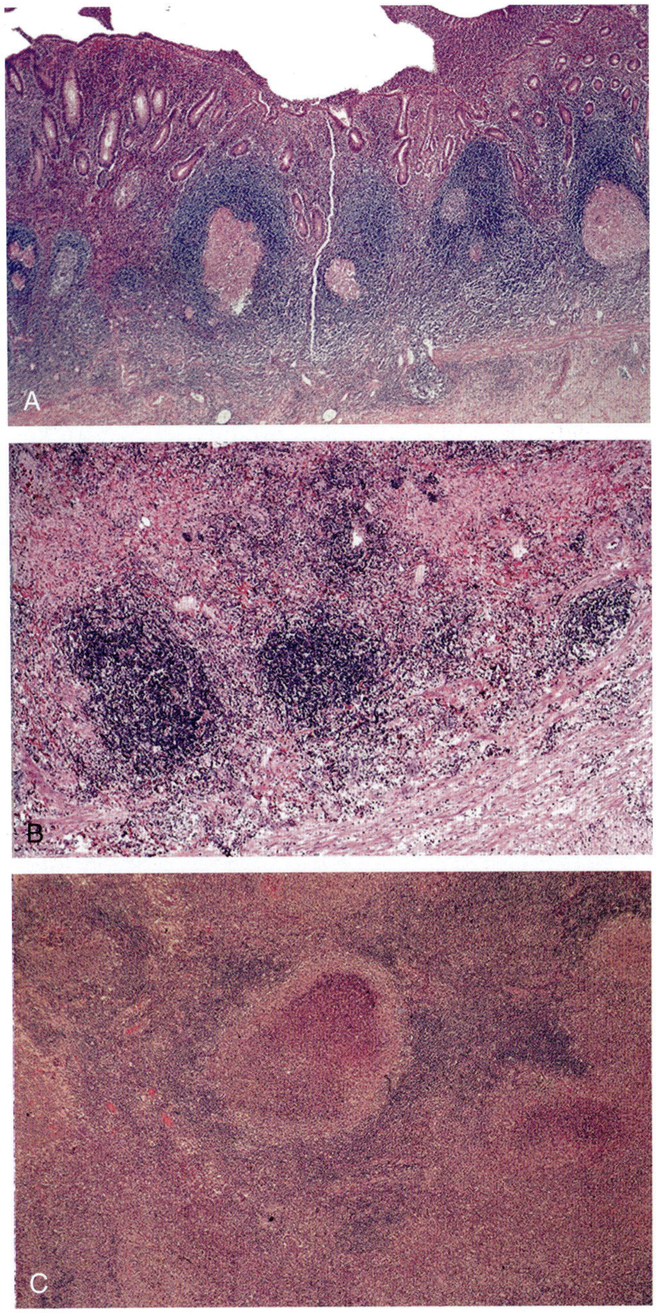

FIGURE 9.14

Yersinia enterocolitica infection. **A**, Mucosal ulceration, lymphoid hyperplasia, and epithelioid granulomas are seen (hematoxylin and eosin [H&E]). **B**, Linear arrangement of mural and serosal lymphoid aggregates in *Yersinia* infection can mimic Crohn's disease (H&E). **C**, *Yersinia pseudotuberculosis* infection. Granulomatous inflammation with central microabscess formation (H&E).

PROGNOSIS AND THERAPY

Most cases of yersiniosis resolve spontaneously. *Yersinia* spp. are susceptible to many antibiotics, and therapy is recommended in patients with severe infections or bacteremia and in the context of immunocompromise or debilitation.

VIBRIO CHOLERAE AND RELATED ORGANISMS

Vibrio cholerae and other members of the genus, *Vibrio* (*Vibrio parahaemolyticus*, *Vibrio vulnificus*, *Vibrio alginolyticus*), are gram-negative bacilli found in saltwater environments. Consequently, infection is usually acquired from consumption of contaminated raw or undercooked seafood. The illness known as cholera is caused by toxigenic serogroups of *V. cholerae* O1 and O139. Toxigenic *V. cholerae* has been responsible for several global pandemics of life-threatening gastroenteritis. The O75 and O141 serogroups produce less severe disease. In the United States, the Florida Gulf coast and Atlantic coast are the most common sources of infection.

CLINICAL FEATURES

Cholera is characterized by voluminous watery diarrhea, sometimes exceeding 1 L/hr, in the absence of pain or fever. The intestinal mucosal lining may also be shed, appearing as white flecks of tissue in so-called "rice water stool". Vomiting is also common. The copious release of fluids can lead to severe dehydration and electrolyte imbalance.

VIBRIO CHOLERAE—FACT SHEET

Definition
- Gram-negative bacillus found in saltwater environments

Incidence and Location
- Small intestine

Clinical Features
- Voluminous watery diarrhea
- Vomiting
- Dehydration
- Electrolyte imbalances
- Absence of pain and fever

Prognosis and Therapy
- May lead to hypovolemic shock or cardiac arrest
- Antibiotics (tetracyclines, fluoroquinolones, macrolides)

PATHOLOGIC FEATURES

GROSS FINDINGS

Despite the severity of disease, *Vibrio* spp. are noninvasive; thus, colonoscopic findings are usually normal.

MICROSCOPIC FINDINGS

The small intestinal mucosa usually appears unremarkable. Mucin depletion of the small intestinal epithelium, increased chronic inflammation in the lamina propria, and epithelial cell disarray have been reported.

VIBRIO CHOLERAE—PATHOLOGIC FEATURES

Gross Findings
- Colonoscopy is usually unremarkable

Microscopic Findings
- Usually normal
- Mucin depletion
- Increased lamina propria inflammation
- Degenerative epithelial cell changes

Differential Diagnosis
- Other cause of bacterial enterocolitis

ANCILLARY STUDIES

Culture, PCR, and serologic studies may aid the diagnosis.

DIFFERENTIAL DIAGNOSIS

V. cholerae is indistinguishable from other causes of bacterial enterocolitis that produce minimal changes in the intestinal mucosa. Enterocolitis caused by some non-O1 strains of *V. cholerae* and other *Vibrio* spp. assumes an acute self-limited colitis pattern.

PROGNOSIS AND THERAPY

Antibiotic therapy (tetracyclines, fluoroquinolones, macrolides) can shorten the course and reduce the volume of diarrhea. Untreated cases of cholera may result in death from hypovolemic shock or cardiac arrest.

AEROMONAS SPP.

Aeromonas spp., initially thought to be nonpathogenic gram-negative bacteria, are increasingly recognized as causes of gastroenteritis in both children and adults. The motile *Aeromonas hydrophila* and *Aeromonas sobria* most often cause GI disease in humans.

CLINICAL FEATURES

The typical presentation is bloody diarrhea, sometimes chronic, accompanied by nausea, vomiting, and cramping pain. The diarrhea may contain mucus as well as blood. The duration of illness varies widely, ranging from a few days to several years, indicating that *Aeromonas* infection can cause a chronic colitis.

AEROMONAS SPP.—FACT SHEET

Definition

- Gram-negative bacterium initially believed nonpathogenic; now increasingly recognized as cause of infectious enterocolitis

Incidence and Location

- Colon; often segmental distribution

Clinical Features

- Bloody diarrhea, which can be chronic; nausea, vomiting, cramping pain

Prognosis and Therapy

- Most cases resolve spontaneously; susceptible to multiple antibiotics if needed

PATHOLOGIC FEATURES

GROSS FINDINGS

Endoscopically, signs of colitis may be seen, including edema, friability, erosions, exudates, and loss of vascular pattern; the features are often segmental and may mimic ischemic colitis or Crohn's disease. A pancolitis mimicking ulcerative colitis has also been described.

MICROSCOPIC FINDINGS

The histologic features are usually those of acute self-limited colitis. However, basal lymphoplasmacytosis may be seen (Fig. 9.15).

AEROMONAS SPP.—PATHOLOGIC FEATURES

Gross Findings

- Edema, friability, erosions, exudates, and loss of vascular pattern
- Often segmental
- Pancolitis mimicking ulcerative colitis has been seen

Microscopic Findings

- Usually those of acute self-limited colitis
- Ulceration and basal lymphoplasmacytosis may be seen

Differential Diagnosis

- Crohn's disease
- Ischemic colitis (particularly grossly)
- Ulcerative colitis (grossly, if pancolitis present)

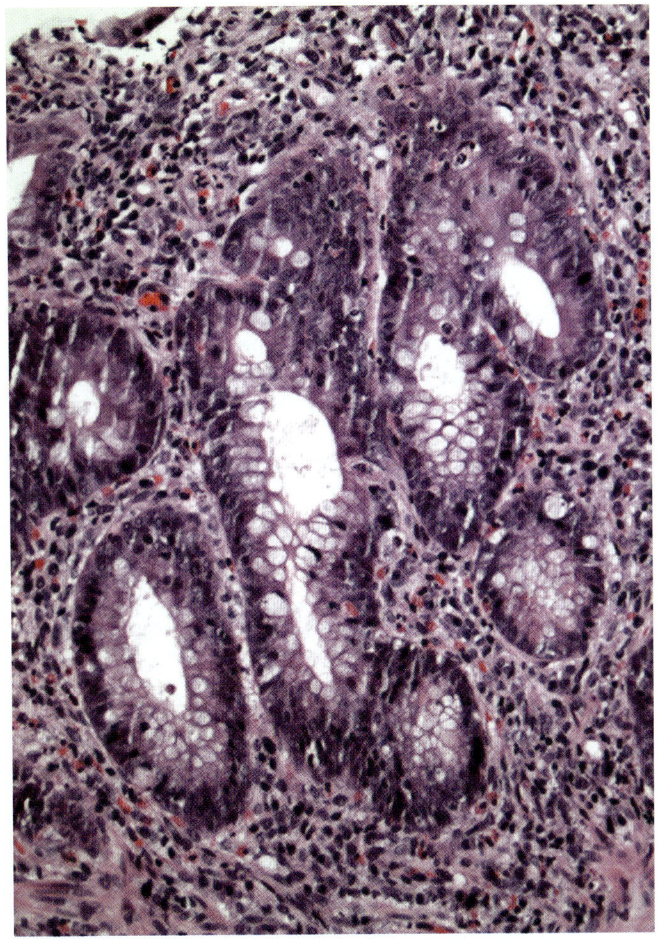

FIGURE 9.15
Cryptitis and mucosal ulceration with slight basal lymphoplasmacytosis in culture-proven *Aeromonas* infection (hematoxylin and eosin).

ANCILLARY STUDIES

PCR or stool cultures are used to make the diagnosis.

DIFFERENTIAL DIAGNOSIS

The differential diagnosis includes other infectious processes, ischemic colitis, and chronic idiopathic IBD. Culture should help exclude other infections, and typical features of ischemia (crypt withering, mucosal necrosis) are not present with *Aeromonas* spp. When architectural distortion is present in a patient with chronic symptoms, it may be very difficult to resolve the issue of Aeromonas infection versus Crohn's disease or ulcerative colitis. Some authorities recommend culturing for *Aeromonas* spp. in all patients with refractory chronic IBD.

PROGNOSIS AND THERAPY

Most cases resolve spontaneously. *Aeromonas* spp. are susceptible to many antibiotics, which can be used in severe or chronic infections.

CLOSTRIDIAL INFECTIONS OF THE GUT

Clostridial organisms are some of the most potent collections of toxigenic bacteria in existence. The most important GI pathogens are *Clostridioides difficile* and *Clostridium septicum*, as discussed subsequently. *Clostridium perfringens* (*welchii*) causes a rare form of life-threatening necrotizing enteritis. The largest outbreaks have been reported in Papua New Guinea among patients who consumed large amounts of sweet potatoes and inadequately cooked pork contaminated with pig intestine; the infection has been referred to as "pigbel" in this region. Cases in developed countries have been reported in patients who consume large amounts of food after starvation or who have diabetes. Resected small intestinal segments are dusky red with serosal exudate. The mucosa may contain pseudomembranes. Microscopic examination reveals transmural necrosis with hemorrhage and mucosal and submucosal pneumatosis. Gram stains reveal club-shaped gram-positive organisms adherent to necrotic mucosa.

CLINICAL FEATURES

C. difficile is the most common nosocomial GI pathogen. Infection is usually related to prior antibiotic exposure (especially orally administered antibiotics) because the organisms cannot infect in the presence of normal colonic flora.

The majority of patients are old, although infection is certainly not limited to this group. In addition, the incidence of *C. difficile* infection has increased in patients with chronic idiopathic IBD and negatively affects clinical outcome in terms of both increased hospitalization and need for colectomy.

Recurrent disease is common despite successful treatment and is seen in up to 50% of cases; the incidence of recurrent disease appears to be increasing. Furthermore, the incidence of severe or life-threatening *C. difficile* colitis in North America has increased recently. This increase has been linked to an epidemic strain of *C. difficile* known as strain BI/NAP1; this strain is hypervirulent, with increased production of both toxins A and B, and is resistant to fluoroquinolones.

Presentation ranges from mild diarrhea to pseudomembranous to fulminant colitis with perforation or toxic megacolon. Watery diarrhea is most common initially and may be accompanied by abdominal pain, cramping, fever, and leukocytosis (sometimes marked). Bloody diarrhea is variably seen. Symptoms can occur up to several weeks after discontinuation of antibiotic therapy. Patients with more severe disease may not have diarrhea, and the only clues to diagnosis may be fever, marked leukocytosis, and a markedly tender, distended abdomen. An associated reactive polyarthritis also has been described.

Necrotizing enterocolitis (typhlitis) is a serious complication of neutropenia as a result of chemotherapy in patients with hematopoietic and solid tumors, as well as in patients with primary neutropenia. Most patients have received chemotherapy within the previous month before the onset of colitis. *C. septicum* has been frequently reported as a causative organism, especially in adults. *C. septicum* infection is also associated with malignancies (particularly adenocarcinoma) in the colon and distal ileum. Patients usually present with the abrupt onset of GI hemorrhage, fever, abdominal pain and distention, and diarrhea. Perforation is a complication that may result in peritonitis, sepsis, and death.

CLOSTRIDIOIDES DIFFICILE–RELATED PSEUDOMEMBRANOUS COLITIS—FACT SHEET

Definition

- Colitis caused by overgrowth of *Clostridioides difficile*, usually after antibiotic administration
- Most common nosocomial gut pathogen

Incidence and Location

- Anywhere in colon, often patchy distribution; the rectum may be spared

Clinical Features

- Usually prior, orally administered antibiotic exposure; diarrhea can happen weeks after antibiotic therapy
- Ranges from mild diarrhea to fulminant colitis with toxic megacolon
- Watery diarrhea initially; may be accompanied by abdominal pain, cramping, fever, and leukocytosis
- Bloody diarrhea sometimes seen

Prognosis and Therapy

- Remove offending drug
- Supportive measures
- Oral vancomycin or Flagyl

CLOSTRIDIUM SEPTICUM–RELATED NECROTIZING ENTEROCOLITIS—FACT SHEET

Definition

- Neutropenic enterocolitis
- Usually in the context of previous chemotherapy

Incidence and Location

- Right colon preferentially involved

Clinical Features

- Gastrointestinal hemorrhage, with fever, abdominal pain and distention, diarrhea
- Perforation a frequent complication

Prognosis and Therapy

- Antibiotics and supportive measures
- Surgery may be required to prevent or treat perforation

Pathologic Features

Gross Findings

Endoscopically, classic pseudomembranous colitis shows yellow-white pseudomembranes, most commonly in the left colon. The plaques bleed when scraped. The distribution may be patchy, and the rectum may be spared. Less striking findings may also be seen, including erythema and friability of the mucosa without pseudomembranes. Typical histologic findings may be seen, however, even in the absence of grossly visible pseudomembranes.

The right colon is preferentially involved in necrotizing enterocolitis, although the ileum and other sites in the colon may be affected. Gross findings include diffuse dilation and edema of the bowel, with varying severity of ulceration and hemorrhage. Exudates and pseudomembranes resembling *C. difficile* colitis may be seen.

Microscopic Findings

Classic pseudomembranous colitis features "volcano" lesions with intercrypt necrosis and ballooned crypts giving rise to the typical laminated pseudomembrane composed of fibrin, mucin, and neutrophils (Fig. 9.16). Dilated crypts lined by attenuated epithelium are filled with neutrophils and mucin. They may also contain sloughed epithelial cells in their lumina or near the mucosal surface that simulate signet ring cells. More severe and prolonged pseudomembranous colitis may lead to full-thickness mucosal necrosis. Less characteristic lesions, usually focal active colitis with occasional crypt abscesses but lacking pseudomembranous features, have been well described in association with other evidence of *C. difficile* infection. *C. difficile* infection can complicate idiopathic IBD. Unfortunately, pseudomembranes are inconsistently present in biopsy samples from these patients and, in fact, may be present in active IBD in the absence of *C. difficile* infection. Biopsy samples from patients with persistent or recurrent *C. difficile* colitis may display overlapping features with IBD. Stool-based diagnostic assays are thus invaluable for confirming the diagnosis of *C. difficile* infection.

In necrotizing enterocolitis, microscopic changes range from mild hemorrhage to prominent submucosal edema, ulceration, marked hemorrhage, and focal necrosis, often with a striking absence of neutrophils and other inflammatory cells (Figs. 9.17 and 9.18). However, neutrophils are sometimes present despite peripheral neutropenia, although the severity of mucosal and mural damage appears out of proportion to inflammation. A pseudomembranous exudate resembling *C. difficile*–related colitis may be seen. Sometimes organisms can be detected in the wall of the bowel on Gram stain.

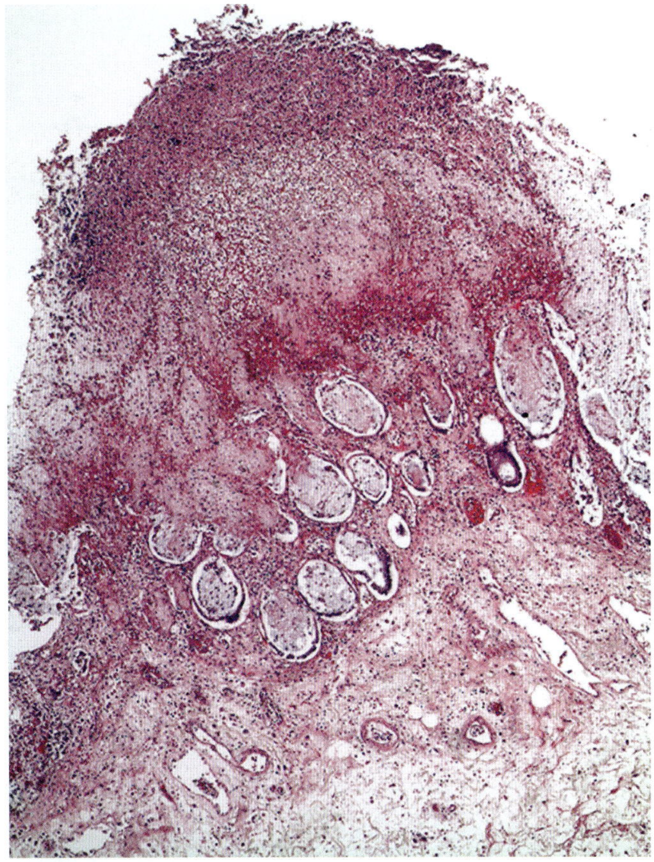

FIGURE 9.16

"Volcano" lesion of *Clostridioides difficile*–related pseudomembranous colitis. Note the ballooned crypts containing neutrophils, intercrypt necrosis, and laminated pseudomembrane composed of fibrin, mucus, and neutrophils (hematoxylin and eosin).

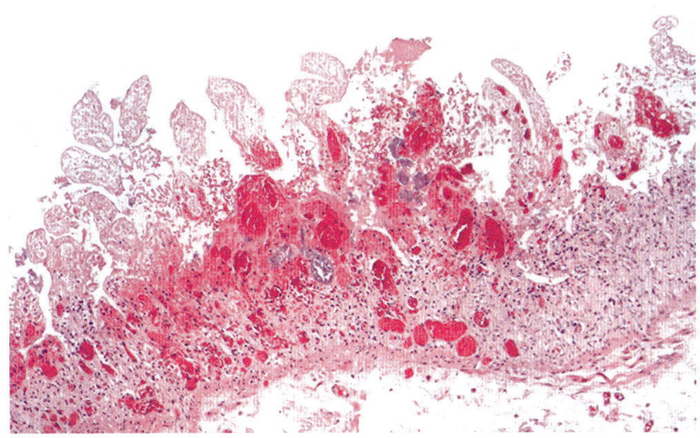

FIGURE 9.17

Necrotizing enterocolitis in a chemotherapy patient. Note the sections of ileum and cecum with ulceration, hemorrhagic necrosis, and a coating of surface bacteria (hematoxylin and eosin).

Clostridioides difficil–Related Pseudomembranous Colitis—Pathologic Features

Gross Findings

- Yellow-white pseudomembranes, most commonly in the left colon; distribution may be patchy
- Plaques bleed when scraped
- Erythema and friability of the mucosa may be present, without pseudomembranes

Microscopic Findings

- Classic features
  - "Volcano" lesions with intercrypt necrosis and ballooned crypts giving rise to laminated pseudomembrane composed of fibrin, mucin, and neutrophils
  - Dilated crypts filled with neutrophils and mucin
- Exceptions
  - Severe and prolonged pseudomembranous colitis may lead to full-thickness mucosal necrosis
  - Some cases show only focal active colitis and lack pseudomembranes
  - Stool-based assays are the key to diagnosis

Differential Diagnosis

- Ischemia
- Other infections, including Shigella spp. and enterohemorrhagic *Escherichia coli*

Clostridium septicum–Related Necrotizing Enterocolitis—Pathologic Features

Gross Findings

- Right colon is preferentially involved
- Diffuse dilation and edema of bowel; varying severity of ulceration and hemorrhage
- Exudates and pseudomembranes common

Microscopic Findings

- Range from mild hemorrhage to prominent submucosal edema, ulceration, marked hemorrhage, and focal necrosis
- Often with a striking absence of inflammatory cells
- Neutrophils sometimes found despite peripheral neutropenia
- Overall, severity of injury out of proportion to inflammation
- Pseudomembranous exudate resembling *Clostridioides difficil*–related colitis may be seen
- Sometimes organisms are seen in the bowel wall with Gram stain

Differential Diagnosis

- Ischemic colitis
- Pseudomembranous colitis

Ancillary Studies

The *C. difficile* toxin enzyme immunoassays and nucleic acid amplification tests are the most helpful diagnostic aids in pseudomembranous colitis. Culture is the most helpful technique for confirming the diagnosis of *C. septicum* infection.

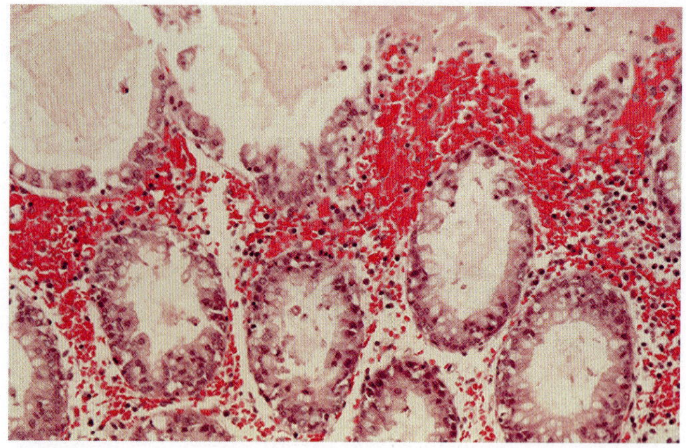

FIGURE 9.18

Necrotizing enterocolitis. Note the lack of neutrophils (hematoxylin and eosin).

Differential Diagnosis

The term pseudomembranous colitis is a description of an inflammatory pattern, not a specific diagnosis. Although most cases of pseudomembranous colitis are related to *C. difficile* infection, other infectious entities as well as ischemic colitis may have similar appearances. A hyalinized lamina propria favors the diagnosis of ischemia; other features, such as crypt withering, pseudomembranes, and mucosal necrosis, may be seen in either entity. Endoscopically, pseudomembrane formation is also seen more often in pseudomembranous colitis, although this finding may be present in ischemia as well.

History of antibiotic use and stool assay for *C. difficile* toxin may be invaluable in sorting out this differential diagnosis. Early laboratory tests for *C. difficile* involved enzyme immunoassays for toxins A and B produced by the bacteria but displayed suboptimal sensitivity. Adding detection of glutamate dehydrogenase, an enzyme produced by *C. difficile*, improved sensitivity but did not distinguish toxigenic from nontoxigenic strains. Highly sensitive and specific PCR-based assays that detect genes for toxins A, B, and C are now the preferred definitive tests, and enzyme immunoassays may be used for rapid screening.

The differential diagnosis for necrotizing enterocolitis includes ischemic colitis and pseudomembranous colitis. The appropriate clinical setting is most helpful is supporting a diagnosis of necrotizing enterocolitis.

Prognosis and Therapy

Treatment of pseudomembranous colitis includes a combination of removal of the offending drug, supportive measures, and antibiotics (oral vancomycin or metronidazole). Treatment of necrotizing enterocolitis is controversial; whereas some recommend antibiotics and supportive measures, others recommend segmental resection of the involved bowel. Surgery may be required to prevent or treat perforation in severe cases.

KLEBSIELLA OXYTOCA

Klebsiella oxytoca is a cytotoxin-producing gram negative bacillus. It causes antibiotic-associated diarrhea, usually in young, otherwise healthy individuals who take penicillin and its derivatives. *K. oxytoca* has also been isolated from the stools of healthy patients and thus may not be pathogenic in the absence of antibiotic treatment.

Patients experience bloody diarrhea and abdominal cramps within 3 to 7 days of starting antibiotic treatment. Laboratory findings include leukocytosis and elevated C-reactive protein. Most patients recover completely within 4 days of stopping antibiotic treatment.

Colonoscopy reveals segmental hemorrhagic colitis with rectal sparing. The right colon is preferentially affected, but disease may extend to the transverse and descending segments. Mucosal edema, erosion, and longitudinal ulcers are also typical, but pseudomembranes are not usually observed. The histologic picture is that of ischemic colitis, including "withered" crypts with increased mitotic figures, crypt loss and apoptosis, and mucosal hemorrhage

The differential diagnosis includes ischemia and other infections. The distinction between EHEC colitis or Shigellosis and *K. oxytoca* is best made using culture results; furthermore, the former two infections are not associated with antibiotic use. Finally, *C. difficile* colitis is antibiotic associated but usually occurs in ill and hospitalized patients and shows pseudomembranes endoscopically and histologically.

MYCOBACTERIAL INFECTIONS OF THE GUT

Although more common in developing countries and immigrant populations, there has been a remarkable resurgence of tuberculosis in Western countries largely because of AIDS but also because of institutional overcrowding and immigrant populations. Although many patients present with pulmonary symptoms, GI symptoms may be the initial presenting findings in these patients, and primary GI tuberculosis has been well documented. The ileocecal and jejunoileal areas are the most commonly involved areas of the gut in *M. tuberculosis* infection followed by the appendix and ascending colon; duodenal, gastroesophageal, and anorectal involvement are much less common. This distribution is probably caused by the organism's affinity for lymphoid tissue.

Mycobacterium avium-intracellulare complex is the most common atypical *Mycobacterium* organism isolated from the GI tract. The small bowel is preferentially involved, but colonic involvement may also be present, as may mesenteric adenopathy.

Clinical Features

Symptoms of colonic tuberculosis are nonspecific and include weight loss, fever, abdominal pain, diarrhea, or a palpable abdominal mass. Complications include hemorrhage, perforation, obstruction, or malabsorption. Mesenteric adenopathy is common. Symptoms in MAI infection are similar and often reflect systemic disease.

MYCOBACTERIAL INFECTIONS OF THE GUT—FACT SHEET

Location

- *Mycobacterium tuberculosis*: anywhere in colon, but ileocecum preferentially involved
- *Mycobacterium avium-intracellulare complex*: small bowel more often involved than the colon

Clinical Features

- *Mycobacterium tuberculosis*: weight loss, fever, abdominal pain, diarrhea, or a palpable abdominal mass
- Complications include hemorrhage, perforation, obstruction, and malabsorption
- Mesenteric adenopathy is common
- *Mycobacterium avium-intracellulare complex*: similar to *M. tuberculosis*; often reflects systemic disease

Prognosis and Therapy

- Multidrug antimycobacterial regimens
- Surgery required for obstruction, perforation, and bleeding

Pathologic Features

Gross Findings

The ileocecal valve is often deformed and gaping in cases of ileocecal *M. tuberculosis* infection. Multiple and segmental lesions with skip areas are common. Strictures and ulcers are the most common endoscopic findings, along with thickened mucosal folds and inflammatory nodules. The ulcers are often circumferential and transverse. Large inflammatory masses, usually involving the ileocecum, may be seen. Endoscopic findings with MAI infection are usually unremarkable, except for occasional white nodules, small ulcers, or hemorrhages.

Microscopic Findings

In *M. tuberculosis* infection, the characteristic histologic lesion is caseating granulomas, which may be present at any level of the wall of the gut (Fig. 9.19). Granulomas are often confluent, with a peripheral rim of lymphocytes. Granulomas may be hyalinized and calcified. Aphthoid ulcers or frank ulceration, as well as inflammation of submucosal vessels, may be seen as well. Acid-fast stains may demonstrate organisms, but culture may be required; in addition, excellent PCR assays are available. Purified protein derivative tests are unreliable in immunocompromised and debilitated patients.

In MAI infection, histology varies with immune status. Immunocompetent patients show a granulomatous response (Fig. 9.20), either necrotizing or non-necrotizing. Immunocompromised patients generally have a diffuse infiltration of histiocytes containing the bacilli, with little inflammatory response (Fig. 9.21). Rarely, poorly formed granulomas occur in immunocompromised patients.

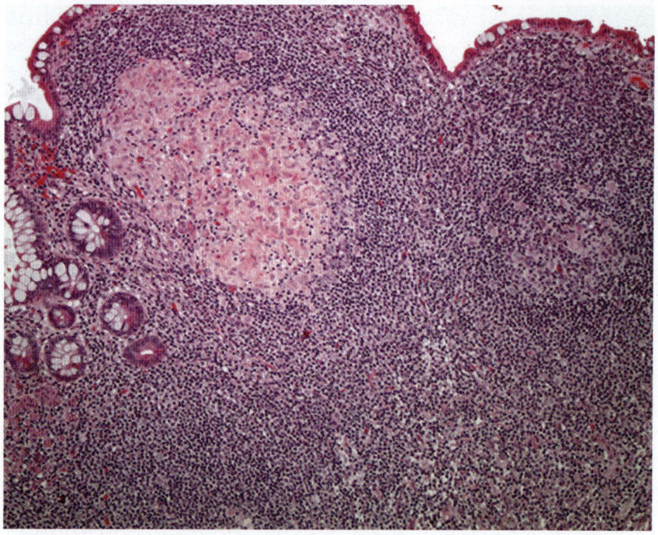

FIGURE 9.20

Mycobacterium avium-intracellulare complex infection. Note the epithelioid, noncaseating granulomas in the ileocecum of an immunocompetent person (hematoxylin and eosin).

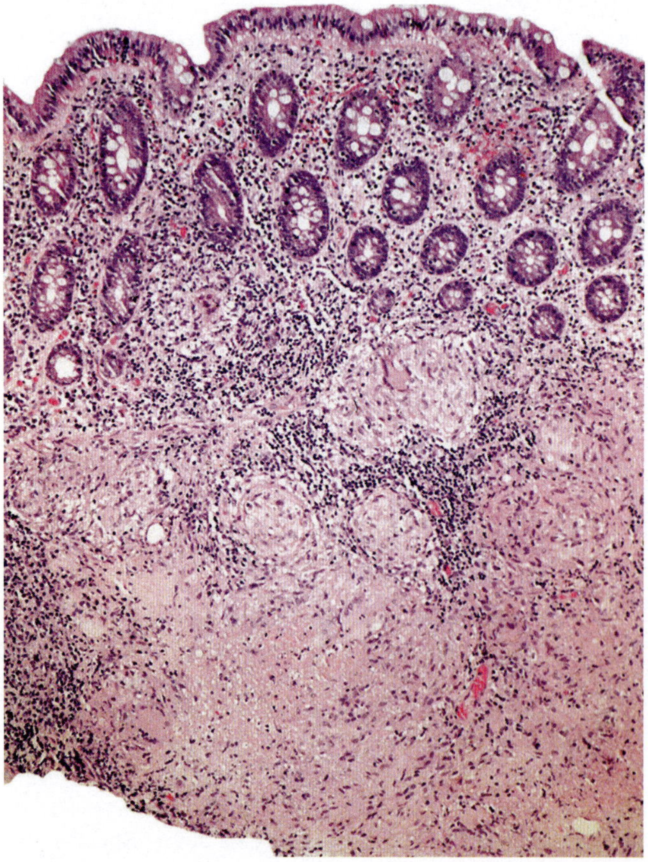

FIGURE 9.19

Colonic Mycobacterium tuberculosis with confluent caseating granulomas in the mucosa (hematoxylin and eosin).

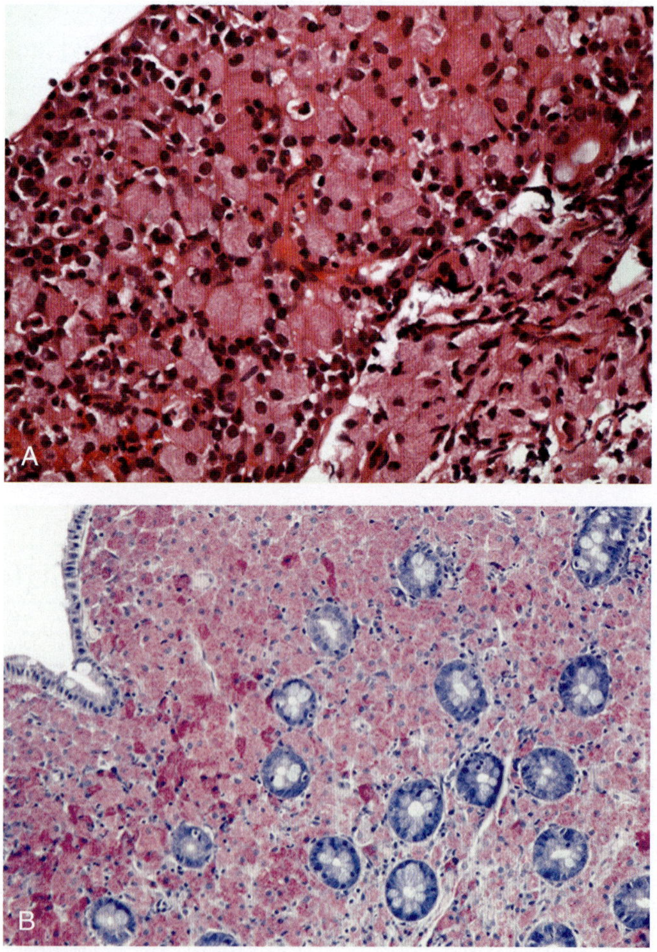

FIGURE 9.21

Gastrointestinal *Mycobacterium avium-intracellulare* complex infection. **A**, Infiltrate of foamy macrophages in a patient with AIDS (hematoxylin and eosin). **B**, Numerous acid-fast bacilli within foamy macrophages (Ziehl-Neelsen).

MYCOBACTERIAL INFECTIONS OF THE GUT—PATHOLOGIC FEATURES

Gross Findings

- *Mycobacterium tuberculosis*
  - Deformed and gaping ileocecal valve
  - Segmental lesions with skip areas, thickened mucosal folds, and raised nodules
  - Strictures and ulcers are the most common endoscopic findings; ulcers are often circumferential and transverse
  - Large, obstructing inflammatory masses
- *Mycobacterium avium-intracellulare* complex
  - Usually normal colonoscopy; rare findings include white nodules, small ulcers, or hemorrhages

Microscopic Findings

- *Mycobacterium tuberculosis*
  - Characteristic histologic lesion is caseating granulomas in any part of gut wall
  - Often confluent, with a rim of lymphocytes at the periphery
  - May be rare or hyalinized and calcified
  - Inflammation of submucosal vessels
  - Acid-fast stains may demonstrate organisms
- *Mycobacterium avium-intracellulare* complex
  - Immunocompetent patients show a granulomatous response, either necrotizing or non-necrotizing
  - Immunocompromised patients have a diffuse infiltration of histiocytes containing the bacilli, with little inflammatory response

Differential Diagnosis

- Other infectious processes causing granulomas, histiocytic infiltrate
- Crohn's disease

ANCILLARY STUDIES

The bacilli stain with acid-fast stains, as well as PAS stains. Organisms are generally abundant in immunocompromised patients but may be hard to detect in healthy patients. Culture and PCR assays may also be helpful.

DIFFERENTIAL DIAGNOSIS

The differential diagnosis of *M. tuberculosis* infection includes other granulomatous infections, especially yersiniosis and fungal diseases. The granulomas of yersiniosis are typically noncaseating, but there may be considerable histologic overlap. Crohn's disease may be difficult to distinguish from tuberculosis; features favoring Crohn's disease are linear rather than circumferential ulcers, transmural lymphoid aggregates, and deep fistulas and fissures. Tuberculosis also commonly lacks mucosal cobblestoning. Atypical mycobacteria, such as *Mycobacterium kansasii* and *Mycobacterium bovis*, may yield a similar histologic picture. The differential diagnosis of MAI includes other infectious processes causing a histiocytic infiltrate, such as infection with *Rhodococcus equi*.

PROGNOSIS AND THERAPY

Gastrointestinal tuberculosis responds to the same medication regimen as pulmonary tuberculosis. Surgical therapy may be required for obstructive disease, perforation, or hemorrhage. MAI of the GI tract is also treated a with multidrug antimycobacterial regimens.

SYPHILIS (*TREPONEMA PALLIDUM*)

Gastrointestinal syphilis commonly involves the anorectum. Homosexual men are at particularly high risk of infection, and many authorities believe that syphilis, particularly anorectal syphilis, is markedly underdiagnosed as a result of the variability of the clinical findings and a low index of suspicion.

CLINICAL FEATURES

Patients are often asymptomatic, but common presenting symptoms in patients with syphilitic proctitis include pain, often with defecation; tenesmus; constipation; bleeding; and anal discharge, which may be mucoid or bloody.

SYPHILIS—FACT SHEET

Definition

- Sexually transmitted infection with *Treponema pallidum*

Incidence and Location

- Usually anorectal

Clinical Features

- Often asymptomatic
- Bleeding, discharge, ulceration may be present

Prognosis and Therapy

- Penicillin is the treatment of choice

PATHOLOGIC FEATURES

GROSS FINDINGS

Gross findings in primary anorectal syphilis include anal chancres (indurated, circular lesions, single or multiple, with variable tenderness) or a mild proctitis. Signs of secondary syphilis typically present 6 to 8 weeks later and include masses, mucocutaneous rash, or condyloma lata (raised, moist, smooth warts that secrete mucus and are associated with itching and a foul odor). Inguinal adenopathy is typical. The gross features of primary and secondary infection sometimes coexist. The mass lesions of secondary syphilis may mimic malignancy, and surgical removal without a prior biopsy should be avoided.

Microscopic Findings

Histologically, syphilitic proctitis features lymphohistiocytic infiltrate with prominent plasma cells and lymphoid aggregates, mild acute inflammation, crypt distortion, and rare, poorly formed granulomas., Prominent capillary endothelial cells with perivascular plasma cells (proliferative endarteriolitis) are a clue to the diagnosis. Syphilitic proctitis may be nonspecific, showing only features of acute infectious-type colitis without a significant increase in plasma cells (Fig. 9.22). Gastritis is a rare complication of syphilis and incites a similar inflammatory reaction, including intense lymphoplasmacytic inflammation and occasional granulomas.

Syphilis—Pathologic Features

Gross Findings
- Primary syphilis: anal chancres and/or an associated mild proctitis
- Secondary syphilis: masses, a mucocutaneous rash, or condyloma lata
- Inguinal adenopathy is typical

Microscopic Findings
- Syphilitic chancres: dense mononuclear cell infiltrate with prominent plasma cells
- Syphilitic proctitis: nonspecific, with features of acute self-limited or focal active colitis with or without increase in plasma cells
- Granulomas have been reported

Differential Diagnosis
- Other infectious processes
- Anal fissures, fistulas, and traumatic lesions
- Condyloma acuminata

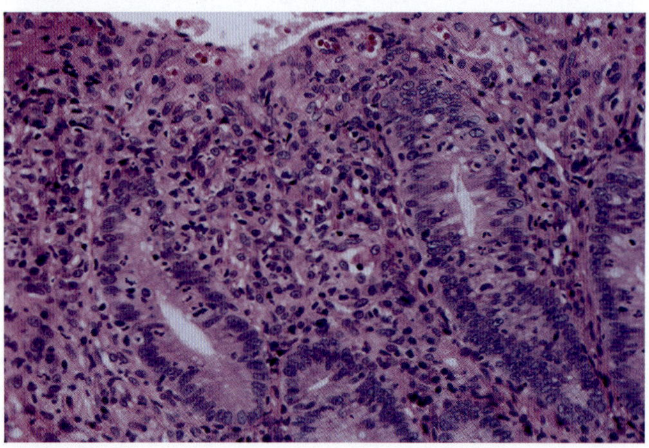

FIGURE 9.22
Syphilitic proctitis with increased plasma cells in the lamina propria (hematoxylin and eosin). Courtesy of Drs. Rodger C. Haggitt and Mary P. Bronner.

Ancillary Studies

Immunohistochemical stains for *T. pallidum* are available but results are negative in the majority of cases. When present, spirochetes cluster at the junction of the lamina propria and anal squamous epithelium.

Differential Diagnosis

The gross differential diagnosis of chancre includes anal fissures, fistulas, and traumatic lesions. Condyloma acuminata are drier and more keratinized than condyloma lata.

Several other types of infectious proctocolitis are common among homosexual men and should be considered in the differential diagnosis of sexually acquired infectious proctocolitis. Patients generally present with similar symptoms regardless of infectious agent, including anal discharge, pain, diarrhea, constipation, bloody stools, and tenesmus. Proctoscopic findings range from normal to mucosal friability, erosions, and erythema.

Substantial overlap between the features of syphilitic proctitis and IBD underscores the need for pathologists to maintain a high index of suspicion for infectious causes of proctitis and obtain clinical history that includes HIV infection status and sexual practices if infection is suspected. Idiopathic IBD is observed to display more active cryptitis, crypt architectural distortion, and basally oriented inflammation than syphilis. Unfortunately, reliable distinguishing features are yet to be identified.

Prognosis and Therapy

Penicillin is the treatment of choice in most cases of syphilis. HIV-positive patients should be monitored particularly closely because the infection may have a more aggressive course in this population.

CHLAMYDIA TRACHOMATIS

Chlamydia trachomatis (serotypes L1, L2, and L3) is the causative agent of lymphogranuloma venereum (LGV). Although the anorectum is the most common site, LGV has been described in the ileum and colon as well. It also causes periappendicitis in women with pelvic inflammatory disease. Most patients have a lymphoplasmacytic infiltrate in the mucosa and submucosa, but neutrophils may also be prominent. Granulomatous inflammation is sometimes present. Crypt distortion, crypt abscesses, ulceration, fissuring ulcers, neural hyperplasia, and fibrosis have also been described. In addition, LGV may produce a striking follicular proctitis. Because of these latter features, LGV may be difficult to distinguish from Crohn's disease or ulcerative colitis, and culture, direct immunofluorescence studies, and IHC may provide valuable diagnostic aids. *Granuloma inguinale (Calymmobacterium granulomatis)* may cause anal and perianal disease that can be clinically and histologically similar to LGV, although rectal involvement favors LGV. *Chlamydia* infection should also be considered in the setting of periappendicitis, in which it may be seen as a complication of pelvic inflammatory disease. Warthin-Starry or Giemsa stains may aid in visualizing the Donovan bodies typical of granuloma inguinale.

NEISSERIA GONORRHEAE

Gonorrhea has been reported in up to 20% of homosexual men and is frequently asymptomatic. The anorectum (alone or in combination with pharyngitis and urethritis) is a common site of gonorrheal infection. Proctoscopic examination is usually unremarkable. Most histologic biopsy results in rectal gonorrhea are normal; some contain a mild increase in neutrophils and mononuclear cells or focal cryptitis. Gram-negative cocci can occasionally be seen on Gram stain of anal discharge, and culture can also be a valuable diagnostic aid.

INTESTINAL SPIROCHETOSIS

Intestinal spirochetosis is primarily seen in homosexual men, although it has been described in a wide variety of other conditions, including diverticular disease, ulcerative colitis, and adenomas. Spirochetosis represents infection by a heterogeneous group of related organisms, most importantly *Brachyspira aalborgi* and *Brachyspira pilosicoli*, which are genetically unrelated to *T. pallidum*. Patients with spirochetosis may harbor one or both of these species.

CLINICAL FEATURES

Although patients with this histologic finding often have symptoms such as diarrhea or anal pain and discharge, it is not clear that spirochetosis causes these symptoms. Many patients have concomitant infections (especially gonorrhea), thus complicating the clinical picture.

INTESTINAL SPIROCHETOSIS—FACT SHEET

Definition

- Coating of the colonic luminal surface with spirillar bacteria, primarily in homosexual men

Incidence and Location

- Colon and appendix

Clinical Features

- Usually asymptomatic; some patients have diarrhea

Prognosis and Therapy

- Metronidazole or other antimicrobials; treatment of asymptomatic persons is controversial

PATHOLOGIC FEATURES

GROSS FINDINGS

Endoscopic abnormalities are mild or absent.

MICROSCOPIC FINDINGS

On H&E, spirochetosis resembles a fuzzy, "fringed" blue line at the luminal border of the colonic mucosa (Fig. 9.23A). Invasion is not seen. The changes can be very focal. Most show no associated inflammatory infiltrate, although occasionally an associated cryptitis may be seen. Warthin-Starry or similar silver stains stain the organisms intensely (Fig. 9.23B). The organisms will also stain with Alcian blue (pH, 2.5) and PAS.

INTESTINAL SPIROCHETOSIS—PATHOLOGIC FEATURES

Gross Findings

- Usually normal colonoscopy

Microscopic Findings

- Fuzzy, "fringed" blue line at the luminal border of the colonic mucosa
- Invasion is not seen
- May be focal
- Most have little or no associated inflammatory infiltrate
- Warthin-Starry or similar silver stains highlight organisms

Differential Diagnosis

- Enteroadherent *Escherichia coli*
- Prominent glycocalyx of colonic mucosa

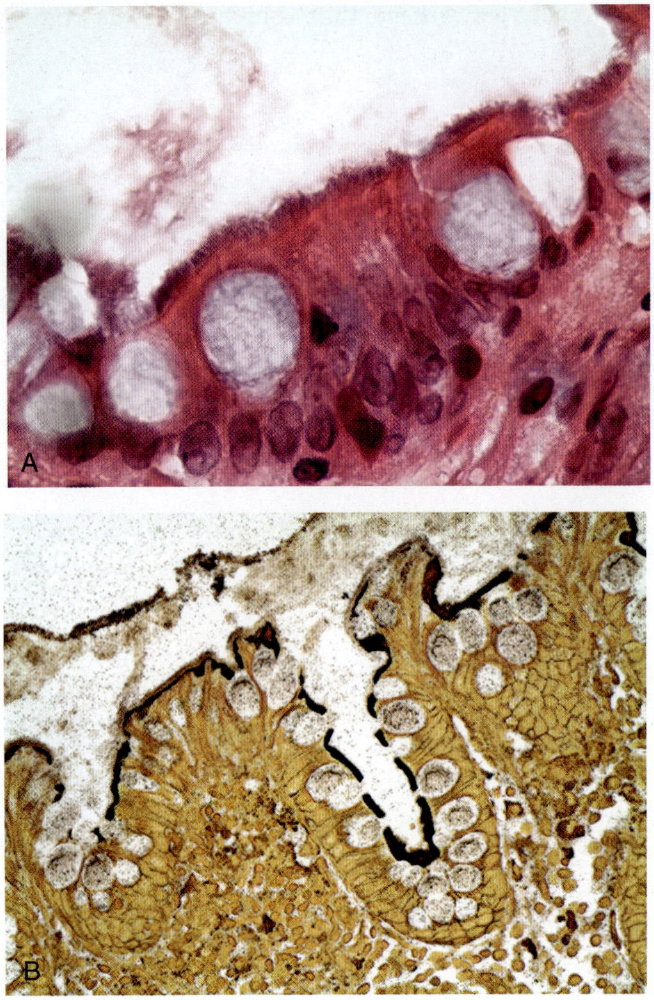

FIGURE 9.23

A, "Fringe" of bacteria along luminal surface in spirochetosis. No attendant inflammation (hematoxylin and eosin with oil immersion). **B**, Spirochetes are intensely positive with silver impregnation staining (Warthin-Starry).

Differential Diagnosis

The differential diagnosis primarily consists of a prominent glycocalyx, which should not stain with Warthin-Starry stains. Occasionally EAEC can give a similar appearance, but *E. coli* should stain gram negative and not have spirillar morphology.

Prognosis and Therapy

Treatment is somewhat controversial. Some authorities do not advocate treating asymptomatic patients. Others advocate treatment with metronidazole or other antimicrobials. There are few long-term follow-up data on treatment effects.

ACTINOMYCOSIS

Actinomycosis is caused by *Actinomyces* spp., filamentous anaerobic gram-positive bacteria that are normal inhabitants of the oral cavity and upper GI tract. They rarely cause disease of the alimentary tract, usually as a chronic, nonopportunistic infection, particularly *Actinomyces israelii*. Infection may be at any level of the GI tract but is usually in a solitary site. Sometimes this infection is associated with diverticular disease. Symptoms include fever, weight loss, abdominal pain, and sometimes a palpable mass. Perianal fistulas and chronic (often granulomatous) appendicitis resulting from actinomycosis have also been described.

Grossly, *Actinomyces* spp. Often produce a large, solitary mass, with or without ulceration, usually with significant mural infiltration that may extend into surrounding structures and grossly mimic carcinoma. The organisms typically produce actinomycotic ("sulfur") granules consisting of irregularly rounded clusters of bacteria bordered by eosinophilic, clublike projections (Splendore-Hoeppli material). The inflammatory reaction is predominantly neutrophilic, with abscess formation (Fig. 9.24). Palisading histiocytes and giant cells, as well as frank granulomas, often surround the neutrophilic inflammation. There may be a marked associated fibrotic response.

Gram stains will reveal the filamentous, gram-positive organisms (Fig. 9.25). GMS and Warthin-Starry stains also stain actinomycosis. Immunofluorescence studies are also available.

The gross differential diagnosis includes abscess of other infectious causes, lymphoma, and carcinoma. The histologic differential primarily includes other infectious processes, particularly *Nocardia* spp. Unlike *Nocardia* spp., this organism is not at all acid fast. Care should also be taken not to confuse actinomycosis with fungi or other bacteria that may form clusters and chains but

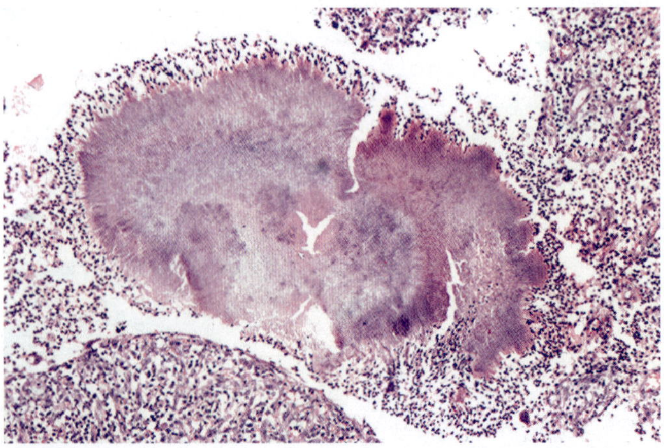

FIGURE 9.24

Clusters of *Actinomyces* with associated Splendore-Hoeppli material and acute inflammation (hematoxylin and eosin). Courtesy of Dr. George F. Gray, Jr.

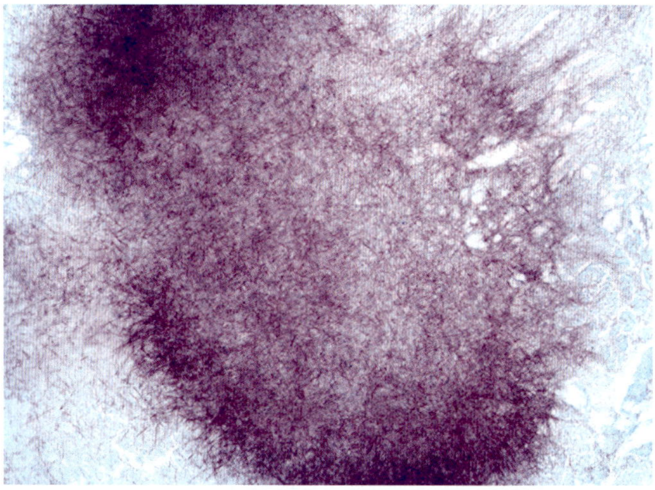

FIGURE 9.25

Filamentous gram-positive bacteria characteristic of actinomycosis are seen on Gram stain (Twort Gram stain).

are not truly filamentous, such as *Pseudomonas* spp. and *E. coli*. Most cases require surgical removal of the affected area or at least drainage of any abscess. Prolonged antibiotic therapy, often intravenous (IV) in route and for several months to 1 year, is recommended after surgical therapy. *Actinomyces* spp. Are susceptible to many antimicrobial agents. Follow-up computed tomography is recommended to assess therapy.

FUNGAL INFECTIONS

The importance of fungal infections of the GI tract has increased in parallel with the numbers of patients with organ transplants, AIDS, and other immunodeficiency states. Signs and symptoms of GI fungal infections are generally similar regardless of type of fungus and include diarrhea, vomiting, melena, frank GI bleeding, abdominal pain, and fever. Although fungal infections of the GI tract are often a part of a disseminated disease process, GI symptoms and signs may well be the presenting manifestations of disease.

Fungi can often be appreciated in routine H&E sections in fulminant infections, but GMS and PAS stains remain invaluable diagnostic aids. Fungi can also be correctly classified in tissue sections based on morphologic criteria. It should be stressed, however, that if there is any doubt as to classification, fungal culture should be relied on as the gold standard for speciation; antifungal therapy may vary according to the type of fungus identified. The differential diagnosis of the various types of fungal infection (Table 9.2) as well as helpful ancillary studies are discussed at the end of this section.

FUNGAL INFECTIONS—FACT SHEET

Location

- Anywhere in the gastrointestinal (GI) tract

Clinical Features

- Usually occurs in immunocompromised patients
- Signs and symptoms of GI fungal infections are similar regardless of type of fungus: diarrhea, vomiting, melena, frank GI bleeding, abdominal pain, and fever
- Occasionally mass lesions may form, obstructing the bowel
- Often a part of a disseminated disease process
- GI symptoms and signs may be the presenting manifestations of disease

PROGNOSIS AND THERAPY

Most commonly, IV amphotericin B is used.

CANDIDA SPP.

Candida spp. may be seen at any level of the GI tract, and the GI tract is a major entryway for disseminated candidiasis. Although immunocompromised patients are most frequently affected, immunocompetent patients can also contract GI candidiasis. Infection with *Candida albicans* is most common, but *Candida tropicalis* and *Candida* (*torulopsis*) *glabrata* may produce similar infections. It is unclear whether *Candida* organisms produce a true primary infection or rather secondarily superinfect preexisting ulcerative lesions of any cause.

PATHOLOGIC FEATURES

GROSS FINDINGS

Candida is the most common infection of the esophagus. The squamous mucosa is coated with white plaques that may be peeled off to reveal ulcerated mucosa. Gross features of colonic candidiasis include ulceration, enterocolitis that may feature pseudomembranes, and inflammatory masses. If vascular invasion is prominent, the gross appearance of infarcted bowel may be seen. Involvement may be diffuse or segmental; by some reports, *C. tropicalis* is more likely to be diffuse, more extensively invasive, and involve the entire alimentary tract.

TABLE 9.2
Morphologic Features of Fungi Involving the Colon

Organism	Morphologic Features	Histologic Response	Major Differential Diagnoses
Aspergillus spp.	Hypha-septate uniform width Branching-regular acute angles Conidial head formation in cavitary lesions	Ischemic necrosis with angioinvasion Acute inflammation Occasionally granulomatous	Mucormycosis *Fusarium* spp. *Pseudallescheria boydii*
Mucormycosis	Hypha-pauciseptate ribbon-like thin walls Branching-haphazard Optically clear on cut section	Similar to *Aspergillus* spp.	Similar to *Aspergillus* spp.
Basidiobolus ranarum	Thin walled, broad, pauciseptate hyphae	Hyphae surrounded by a radiating, intensely eosinophilic cuff (Splendore-Hoeppli phenomenon) Necrotizing granulomas	Mucormycosis
Candida albicans *Candida tropicalis*	Mixture of budding yeast and pseudohyphae; occasional septate hypha	Usually suppurative May be necrotic and ulcerative Occasionally granulomatous	*Trichosporon* spp.
Candida glabrata	Budding yeast; no true hyphae; no "halo" effect	Similar to other *Candida* spp.	Histoplasmosis *Cryptococcus* spp.
Cryptococcus neoformans	Pleomorphic Narrow-based buds Usually mucicarmine positive Variable in size	Usually suppurative May have extensive necrosis Sometimes granulomatous	Histoplasmosis Blastomycosis *C. glabrata*
Histoplasma capsulatum	Ovoid, narrow-based buds Intracellular "Halo" effect around organism on H&E	Lymphohistiocytic infiltrate with parasitized histiocytes Occasional granulomas	*Cryptococcus* spp. *P. marneffei* *C. glabrata* Intracellular parasites *P. carinii*
Penicillium marneffei	Round and elongated ("pill capsule") yeast forms within macrophages	Diffuse macrophage infiltrates Granulomas Neutrophilic inflammation	*Leishmania donovani* *Histoplasma* spp. *capsulatum* *Cryptococcus neoformans*

H&E, Hematoxylin and eosin staining.

Microscopic Findings

The associated inflammatory response ranges from minimal if any tissue reaction to organisms (especially in immunocompromised patients) to prominent neutrophilic infiltrates, erosion or ulceration, abscess formation, and necrosis. Granulomas are not usually seen. A characteristic feature of esophageal candidiasis is pseudohyphae and yeast forms within exfoliated squamous cells and keratin debris. Pseudohyphae are often arranged perpendicular to keratin fibers (Fig. 9.26). Fungi may invade to any level of the wall, from submucosa to transmural invasion and perforation. Invasion of mucosal and submucosal blood vessels is also a prominent feature of invasive candidal infection. *C. albicans* and *C. tropicalis* produce a mixture of budding yeast forms, hyphae, and pseudohyphae. *C.* (*torulopsis*) *glabrata* features tiny budding yeast forms similar to *Histoplasma* spp. and does not produce hyphae or pseudohyphae.

CANDIDIASIS SPP.—PATHOLOGIC FEATURES

Gross Findings

- White plaques in the esophagus
- Enterocolitis that may feature pseudomembranes or inflammatory masses
- Involvement may be diffuse or segmental
- Appearance of infarction if vascular invasion is prominent

Microscopic Findings

- Yeasts and pseudohyphae: often found in sloughed keratin in the esophagus
- Prominent neutrophilic infiltrates, erosion or ulceration, abscess formation, and necrosis
- Granulomas rare
- Minimal tissue reaction in many immunocompromised patients
- Fungi may invade to any level of the gut wall, from submucosa to transmural invasion and perforation; may also invade vessels

Differential Diagnosis

- Other fungi (see Table 9.2)

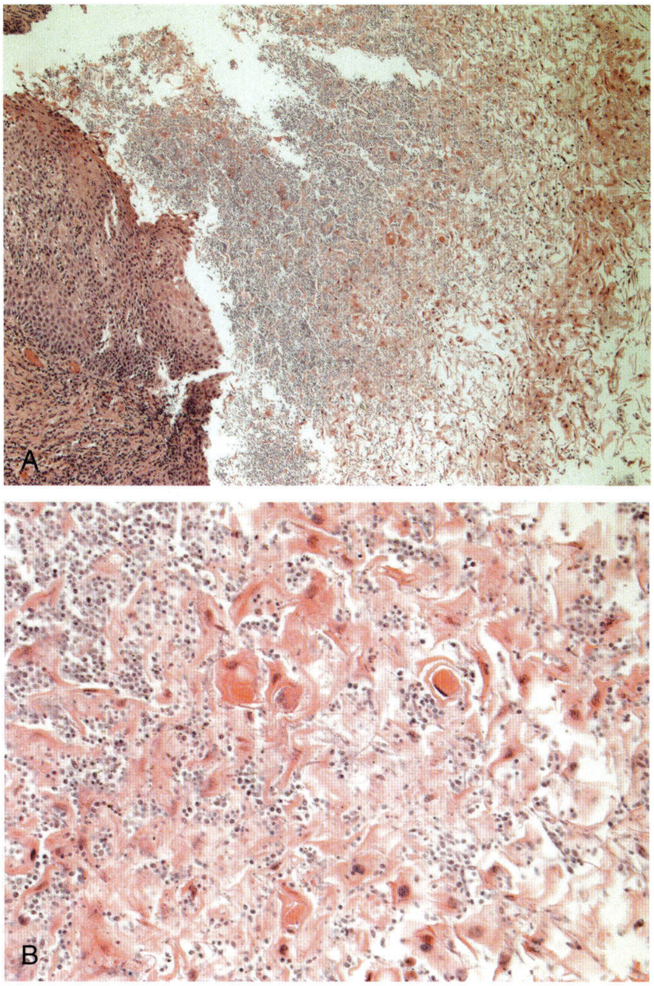

FIGURE 9.26

A, *Candida* infection with active esophagitis and abundant luminal keratin debris. Abundant yeast forms are present in the debris. **B**, Pseudohyphae are arranged perpendicularly to the keratin and desquamated epithelial cells (hematoxylin and eosin).

Prognosis and Therapy

Intravenous amphotericin B is the treatment of choice for invasive candidiasis.

ASPERGILLUS SPP.

Aspergillus species infection of the GI tract occurs almost exclusively in immunocompromised patients. The majority of patients with GI *Aspergillus* infection have coexistent lung lesions. GI signs and symptoms and gross pathologic findings are similar to infection with *Candida* spp.

Pathologic Features

Gross Findings

Invasion of vessels often produces the classic "target lesion" consisting of a necrotic central area surrounded by hemorrhage (Fig. 9.27). The bowel may appear grossly infarcted, and transmural infarction is common.

Microscopic Findings

The characteristic histologic lesion of aspergillosis is a nodular infarction consisting of a zone of ischemic necrosis centered on a blood vessel containing fungal organisms (Figs. 9.28 and 9.29). The fungal hyphae

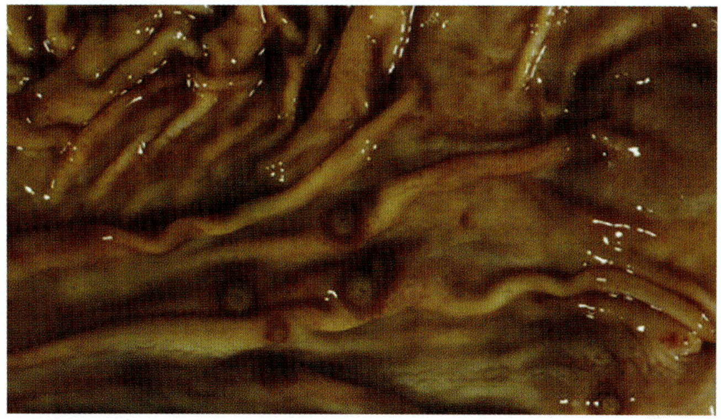

FIGURE 9.27

Targetoid lesions in the stomach represent vascular thrombosis and surrounding infarcted tissue produced by invasive *Aspergillus* spp. (Courtesy Dr. Laura W. Lamps.)

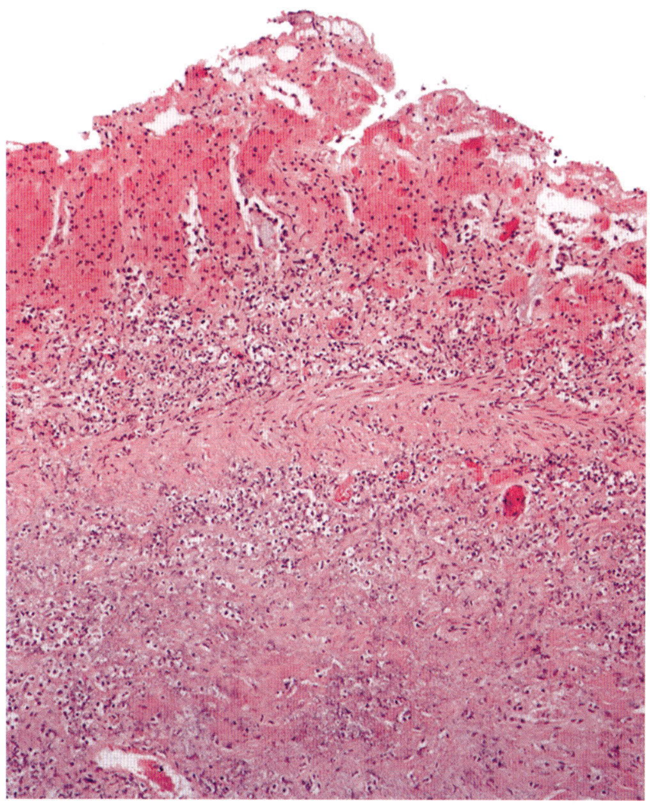

FIGURE 9.28

Bowel infarction due to aspergillosis. Note nodular focus of ischemic necrosis (hematoxylin and eosin).

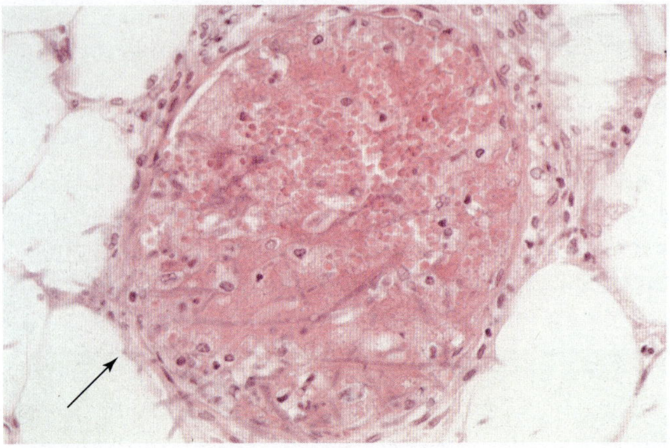

FIGURE 9.29
Aspergillus organisms penetrate a submucosal vessel (hematoxylin and eosin).

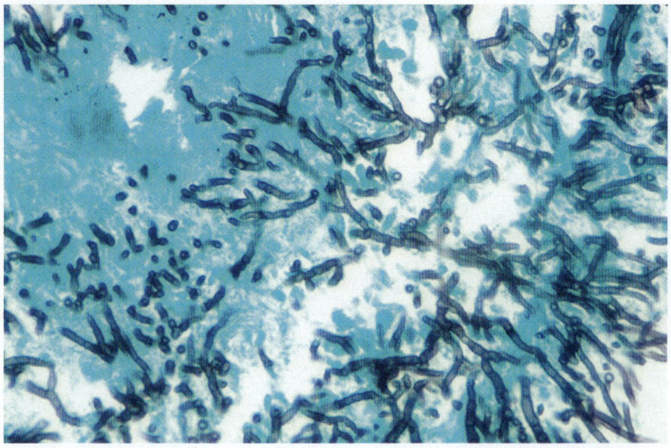

FIGURE 9.30
Aspergillus organisms have septate hyphae that branch at acute angles (Gomori methenamine silver).

often extend outward from the infarct in parallel or radial arrays. Inflammatory response ranges from minimal to marked neutrophilic infiltrate; granulomatous inflammation is occasionally seen. The typical hyphae of *Aspergillus* spp. are septate and branch at acute angles (Fig. 9.30).

Aspergillus spp.—Pathologic Features

Gross Findings
- Prominent neutrophilic infiltrates, erosion or ulceration, abscess formation, and necrosis
- Granulomas rare
- Target lesions resulting from vascular invasion
- Bowel appears grossly infarcted

Microscopic Findings
- Characteristic nodular infarction consisting of a zone of ischemic necrosis centered on a blood vessel containing fungal organisms
- Fungal hyphae extend outward from the infarct in parallel or radial arrays
- Inflammatory response ranges from minimal to a marked neutrophilic infiltrate
- Granulomatous inflammation is occasionally seen
- Typical hyphae of *Aspergillus* spp. are septate and branch at acute angles

Differential Diagnosis
- Other fungal infections (see Table 9.2)

Differential Diagnosis

The differential diagnosis consists primarily of other fungal infections (see Table 9.2).

Prognosis and Therapy

Amphotericin B is the most commonly used antifungal agent for *Aspergillus* infection, particularly in neutropenic patients. Other useful antifungal agents include ketoconazole, fluconazole, and itraconazole.

MUCORMYCOSIS AND RELATED INFECTIONS

Mucormycosis (previously called zygomycosis) are ubiquitous soil fungi. They are uncommon pathogens in the GI tract and are seen predominantly in immunocompromised patients. Infections are usually caused by species in the *Rhizopus* and *Mucor* genera. These fungi usually superinfect tissues that have been previously ulcerated; invasive disease is often fatal. Although many cases of GI mucormycosis are part of a disseminated fungal infection, infection limited to the GI tract has been described.

CLINICAL FEATURES

Immunocompromised patients, particularly those with diabetes or other causes of systemic acidosis, appear to be at increased risk for developing mucormycosis.

Pathologic Features

Gross Findings

Any segment of the GI tract may be involved, and the cecum is a common location. The gross features are similar to those produced by *Aspergillus* spp. Ulcerative lesions are the most common gross manifestation, and ulcers containing these organisms tend to be large with rolled, irregular edges that may mimic malignancy. The often invades through the wall to involve and destroy other structures and may produce large, obstructive masses. Similar to aspergillosis and candidiasis, if large vessels are penetrated and occluded by fungi, infarction may develop, and the gross picture is that of ischemia.

MICROSCOPIC FINDINGS

The inflammatory reaction and presence of intravascular thrombotic lesions are markedly similar to that seen in aspergillosis. Typical organisms have broad, ribbonlike, pauciseptate hyphae that branch randomly at various angles. Transected hyphae have optically clear centers in tissue sections (Fig. 9.31).

MUCORMYCOSIS—PATHOLOGIC FEATURES

Gross Findings
- Similar to *Aspergillus* spp., often mimicking infarction
- Ulcerative lesions are the most common gross manifestation, often large with rolled, irregular edges
- Process often invades through wall to involve and destroy other structures
- May produce large, obstructive masses
- If vessels are penetrated, produces ischemic picture

Microscopic Findings
- Inflammatory reaction and presence of intravascular thrombotic lesions are markedly similar to aspergillosis
- Typical organisms have broad, ribbon-like, pauciseptate hyphae that branch randomly at various angles
- Transected hyphae have optically clear centers in tissue sections

Differential Diagnosis
- Other fungi (see Table 9.2)

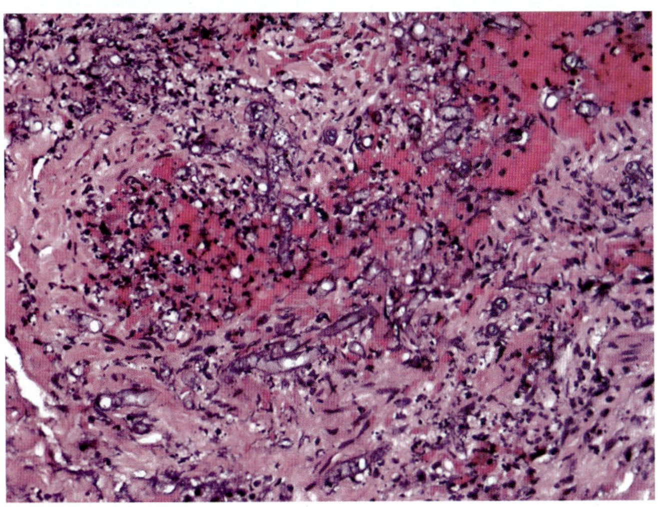

FIGURE 9.31
Mucor organisms, present within a vessel, have broad, ribbon-like pauciseptate hyphae with optically clear centers on cut section (hematoxylin and eosin). (Courtesy of Dr. Neriman Gokden.)

DIFFERENTIAL DIAGNOSIS

The differential diagnosis is that of other fungal infections (see Table 9.2).

PROGNOSIS AND THERAPY

Amphotericin B and posaconazole are the most commonly used antifungal agents in invasive mucormycosis.

BASIDIOBOLUS RANARUM

Basidiobolus ranarum is an environmental fungus found in soil and decaying organic matter. Although it has historically been limited to tropical and subtropical climates, including Africa, the Middle East, and Southeast Asia, *B. ranarum* is now recognized as an emerging fungal pathogen in the American southwest.

CLINICAL FEATURES

B. ranarum usually causes chronic subcutaneous mycosis, and extracutaneous involvement is rare. GI disease is marked by abdominal pain and tenderness, sometimes associated with a palpable mass that creates the clinical impression of malignancy or IBD. Risk factors include pediatric age group, peptic ulcer disease, and diabetes. Infection is usually seen in immunocompetent hosts.

***BASIDIOBOLUS RANARUM*—FACT SHEET**

Definition
- Environmental fungus in the order *Entomophthorales*

Incidence and Location
- Colon and rectum

Clinical Features
- Abdominal pain
- Nausea, vomiting
- Palpable mass

Prognosis and Therapy
- Posaconazole is the drug of choice
- Surgical resection of involved bowel segment is sometimes necessary

Pathologic Features

Gross Findings

Endoscopically, infection produces a mass, strictures, or adhesions. Resection specimens reveal mural thickening and yellowish transmural nodules.

Microscopic Findings

The inflammatory reaction is characterized by transmural necrotizing granulomas (see Table 9.2). Thin walled, broad, pauci-septate fungal hyphae, often surrounded by a cuff of radiating, intensely eosinophilic material (Splendore-Hoeppli phenomenon), are key to the diagnosis (Fig. 9.32). Tissue eosinophilia and Charcot-Leyden crystals may also be seen.

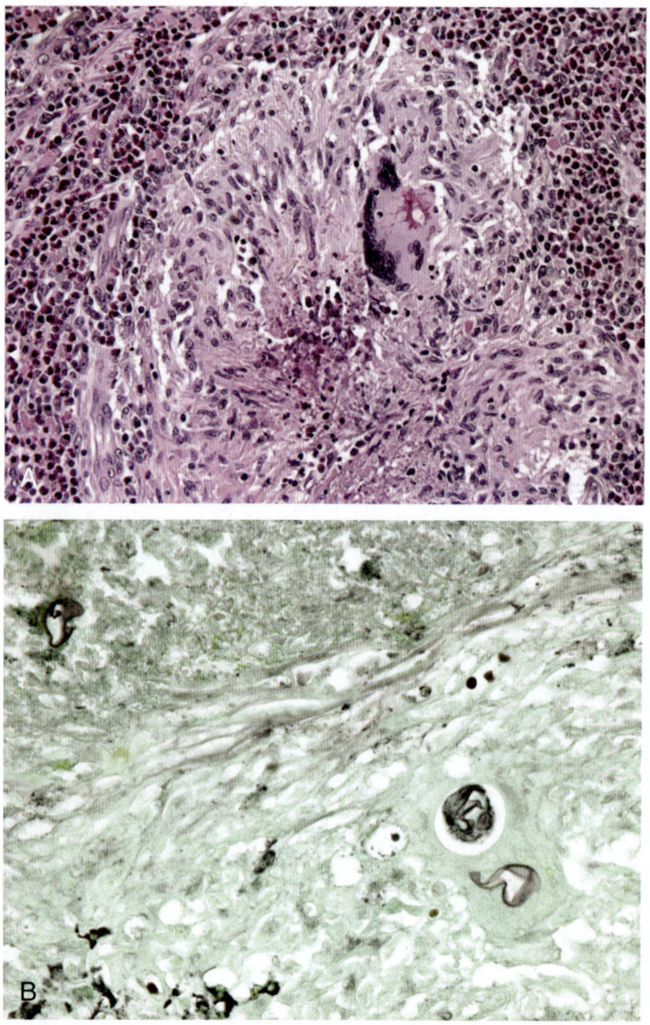

FIGURE 9.32

A, Granulomatous inflammation and striking tissue eosinophilia are characteristic of basidiobolomycosis (hematoxylin and eosin). **B**, Gomori methenamine silver stain demonstrates the "cellophane ball" appearance of *B. ranarum* hyphae. Courtesy of Dr. Laura W. Lamps.

***Basidiobolus ranarum*—Pathologic Features**

Gross Findings

- Masses
- Strictures, adhesions
- Yellow-white nodules in all levels of the colon wall

Microscopic Findings

- Thin walled, broad, pauci-septate hyphae
- Splendore-Hoeppli phenomenon
- Necrotizing granulomas
- Tissue eosinophilia
- Charcot-Leyden crystals
- Differential Diagnosis
- Other fungal infections, especially mucormycosis

Ancillary Studies

Fungal culture is the best means of making an unequivocal diagnosis of basidiobolomycosis.

Differential Diagnosis

The main differential diagnosis is mucormycosis, which also form broad, pauci-septate hyphae; however, *B. ranarum* is not angioinvasive and therefore is not associated with intestinal infarction. Mucormycosis, on the other hand, does not elicit intense eosinophilic infiltrates and necrotizing granulomatous inflammation and may show little inflammatory response, particularly in immunocompromised patients.

Prognosis and Therapy

Surgical resection of the affected bowel segment with debridement of involved tissue in combination with long-term antifungal therapy appears to be effective treatment of patients with GI disease. Rare cases have proven fatal because of delayed diagnosis and subsequent disseminated disease.

HISTOPLASMOSIS

Histoplasma capsulatum is endemic to the central United States but has been described in many nonendemic areas as well. It is most abundant in soil enriched with bat or avian droppings. Although disseminated histoplasmosis occurs mostly in immunocompromised patients, immunocompetent patients may be affected as well, especially young children and older adults. GI involvement occurs in approximately 80% or more of patients with disseminated infection. Patients may initially present with signs and symptoms of GI illness and do not always have concomitant pulmonary involvement.

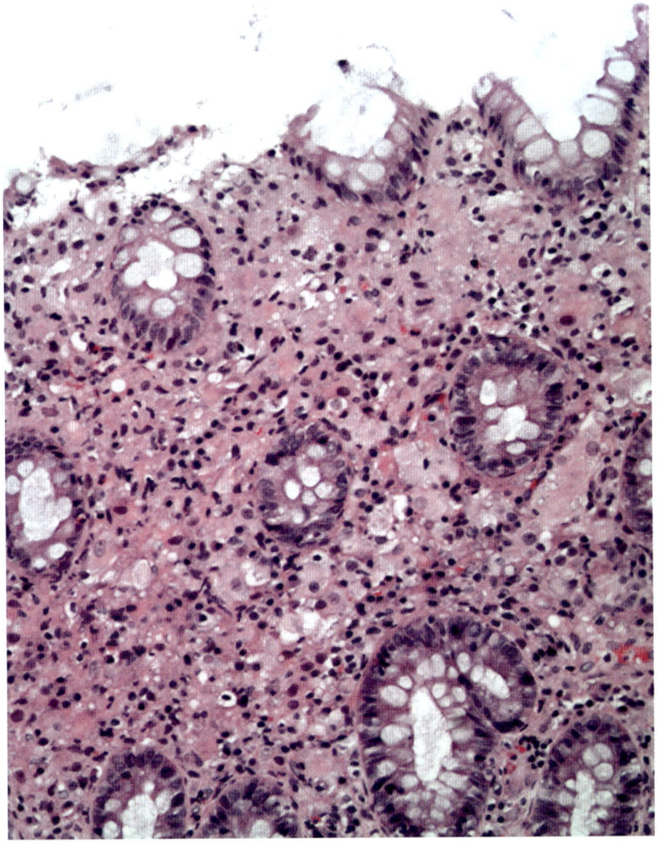

FIGURE 9.33
Histiocytic infiltrate in a colon biopsy from a patient with AIDS with disseminated histoplasmosis. Note the "halo" around the organisms (hematoxylin and eosin).

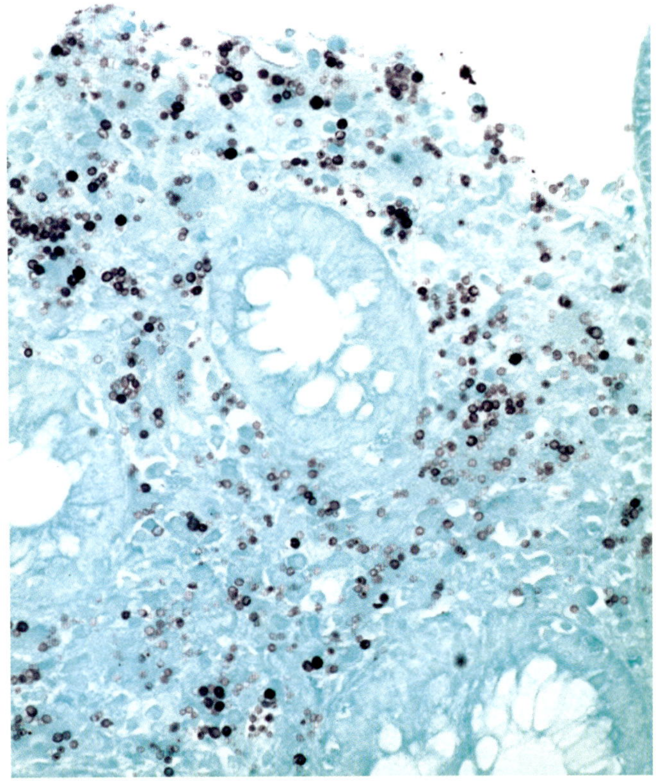

FIGURE 9.34
Fungal stain shows uniformly small yeast forms with buds at the more pointed pole, consistent with histoplasmosis (Gomori methenamine silver).

Pathologic Features

Gross Findings

Any part of the GI tract may be involved, but the terminal ileum is the most common site. Gross lesions include ulcers, nodules, obstructive mass lesions, and normal mucosa (often in immunocompromised patients). A combination of these lesions is commonly seen in a single patient.

Microscopic Findings

Histologic findings include diffuse lymphohistiocytic infiltrates (Fig. 9.33) and nodules, usually involving the mucosa and submucosa, with associated ulceration. Often these lesions are present overlying Peyer's patches. Discrete granulomas and giant cells are seen in only a minority of cases. In immunocompromised patients, large numbers of organisms may be seen with virtually no tissue reaction. Histoplasma organisms typically are small, ovoid, usually intracellular yeast forms with small buds at the more pointed pole (Fig. 9.34).

Histoplasmosis—Pathologic Features

Gross Findings
- Terminal ileum most commonly involved
- Ulcers, nodules, obstructive mass lesions most common gross lesions; often a combination
- Normal mucosa in immunocompromised patients

Microscopic Findings
- Diffuse lymphohistiocytic infiltrates and nodules, usually involving the mucosa and submucosa, with associated ulceration
- Discrete granulomas and giant cells seen in only a minority of cases
- In immunocompromised patients, large numbers of organisms may be seen with virtually no tissue reaction
- *Histoplasma* organisms are small, ovoid, usually intracellular yeast forms with small buds at the more pointed pole

Differential Diagnosis
- Other fungal infections (see Table 9.2)

Differential Diagnosis

The differential diagnosis is primarily that of other fungal infections (see Table 9.2).

Prognosis and Therapy

Amphotericin is the most commonly used antifungal agent in histoplasmosis.

PENICILLIUM MARNEFFEI

Penicillium marneffei is a dimorphic fungus and intracellular pathogen. It causes disseminated infection in endemic areas, including southeast Asia, southern China, and Hong Kong, and travelers to these areas. *P. marneffei* is an increasingly important cause of invasive mycosis in immunocompromised hosts, particularly those with AIDS. The infection usually affects the lungs and liver followed by the GI tract. Patients experience respiratory distress and may require intubation. Those with GI disease experience abdominal cramping and watery or bloody diarrhea. Dissemination occurs rapidly in immunocompromised hosts and may be fatal if untreated.

Gross abnormalities may be seen at any level of the GI tract. Endoscopic abnormalities include ulcers, erosions, and petechiae. Mass lesions that simulate malignancy have been reported in several cases. Most cases show diffuse macrophage infiltrates. Macrophages are distended by intracellular, 2- to 5-µm yeast forms. The macrophages may lyse and release free organisms. Occasional elongated ("pill capsule") forms with central septation may be seen and can span up to 20 µm. *P. marneffei* reproduce by fission; budding is not seen. The inflammatory response may include granulomas and neutrophils, particularly in immunocompetent patients. Similar to other fungi, the organisms can be highlighted by GMS and PAS stains. Fungal culture confirms the diagnosis but may take weeks to produce results.

The differential diagnosis includes other yeasts (see Table 9.2). *H. capsulatum* are also intracellular and of similar size (2–4 µm) but are endemic to the central United States. Unlike *P. marneffei*, *H. capsulatum* have easily identifiable buds at their pointed poles. Intracellular *H. capsulatum* yeast have a surrounding "halo," reflecting their cell walls. *Cryptococcus neoformans* frequently infects immunocompromised patients but is a rare pathogen in the GI tract. It also appears as small yeast forms (4–7 µm) and shows narrow-based budding. *C. neoformans* is extracellular and has a mucopolysaccharide capsule that creates a halo effect on H&E and stains magenta with mucicarmine.

CRYPTOCOCCUS SPP.

C. neoformans is an unusual but important cause of GI infection, particularly in immunocompromised patients. Cryptococci have a global distribution and are abundant in avian (especially pigeon) habitats. Virtually all patients with GI cryptococcosis have hematogenously disseminated disease with multisystem organ involvement, and most have pulmonary and meningeal disease.

Pathologic Features

Gross Findings

The colon is the most common site of cryptococcal infection followed by the esophagus. Endoscopic lesions include nodules and ulcers, sometimes associated with a thick white exudate; however, no mucosal abnormalities are present in many cases of GI cryptococcosis.

Microscopic Findings

Histologic features include typical round to oval yeast forms with narrow-based budding; cryptococci may show considerable variation in size. Occasionally, cryptococci produce hyphae and pseudohyphae. Often a "halo" effect can be seen on H&E staining, representing the capsule of the organism. Both superficial and deep involvement may occur, and lymphatic involvement is frequent. The inflammatory reaction is variable and depends on the immune status of the host, ranging from a suppurative, necrotizing inflammatory reaction often with granulomatous features to virtually no reaction at all in anergic hosts. The mucopolysaccharide capsular material stains with Alcian blue, Fontana-Masson, mucicarmine (Fig. 9.35), and colloidal iron; GMS stains are, of course, positive as well. Capsule-deficient cryptococcal infection may present a diagnostic challenge, but most have sufficient capsular material left to be seen on mucin stains.

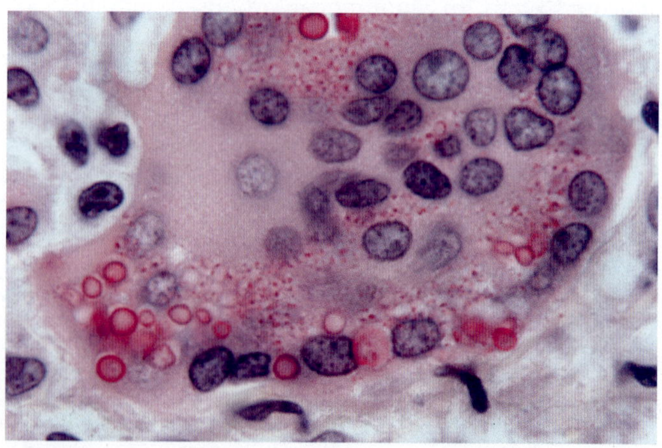

FIGURE 9.35
Cryptococcus within a giant cell (mucicarmine). Courtesy of Dr. George F. Gray, Jr.

CRYPTOCOCCUS SPP.—PATHOLOGIC FEATURES

Gross Findings

- Present in the colon and/or esophagus
- Endoscopic lesions include nodules and ulcers, sometimes associated with a thick white exudate
- No mucosal abnormalities are present in many cases

Microscopic Findings

- Round-to-oval yeast forms with narrow-based budding and considerable variation in size
- Often a "halo" effect can be seen on hematoxylin and eosin staining, representing the capsule
- Both superficial and deep involvement may occur, and lymphatic involvement is frequent
- The inflammatory reaction ranges from a suppurative, necrotizing inflammatory reaction, often with a granulomatous feature, to virtually no reaction at all in anergic hosts
- Organisms are Gomori methenamine silver positive; mucopolysaccharide capsular material stains with Alcian blue, mucicarmine, and colloidal iron

Differential Diagnosis

- Other fungal infections (see Table 9.2)

DIFFERENTIAL DIAGNOSIS

The differential diagnosis consists of other fungal infections (see Table 9.2).

PROGNOSIS AND THERAPY

Amphotericin B is the most commonly used antifungal agent.

The differential diagnosis of fungal infections most often includes other infectious processes; occasionally Crohn's disease, ulcerative colitis, sarcoidosis, and ischemic colitis enter the differential diagnosis as well. The bigger challenge, after a fungus has been identified, is to properly classify it. Although definite speciation must rely on culture techniques, some attempt can and should be made to classify the organisms on morphologic grounds (see Table 9.2; Fig. 9.36). It is important to remember that fungi exposed to antifungal therapy or ambient air may produce bizarre

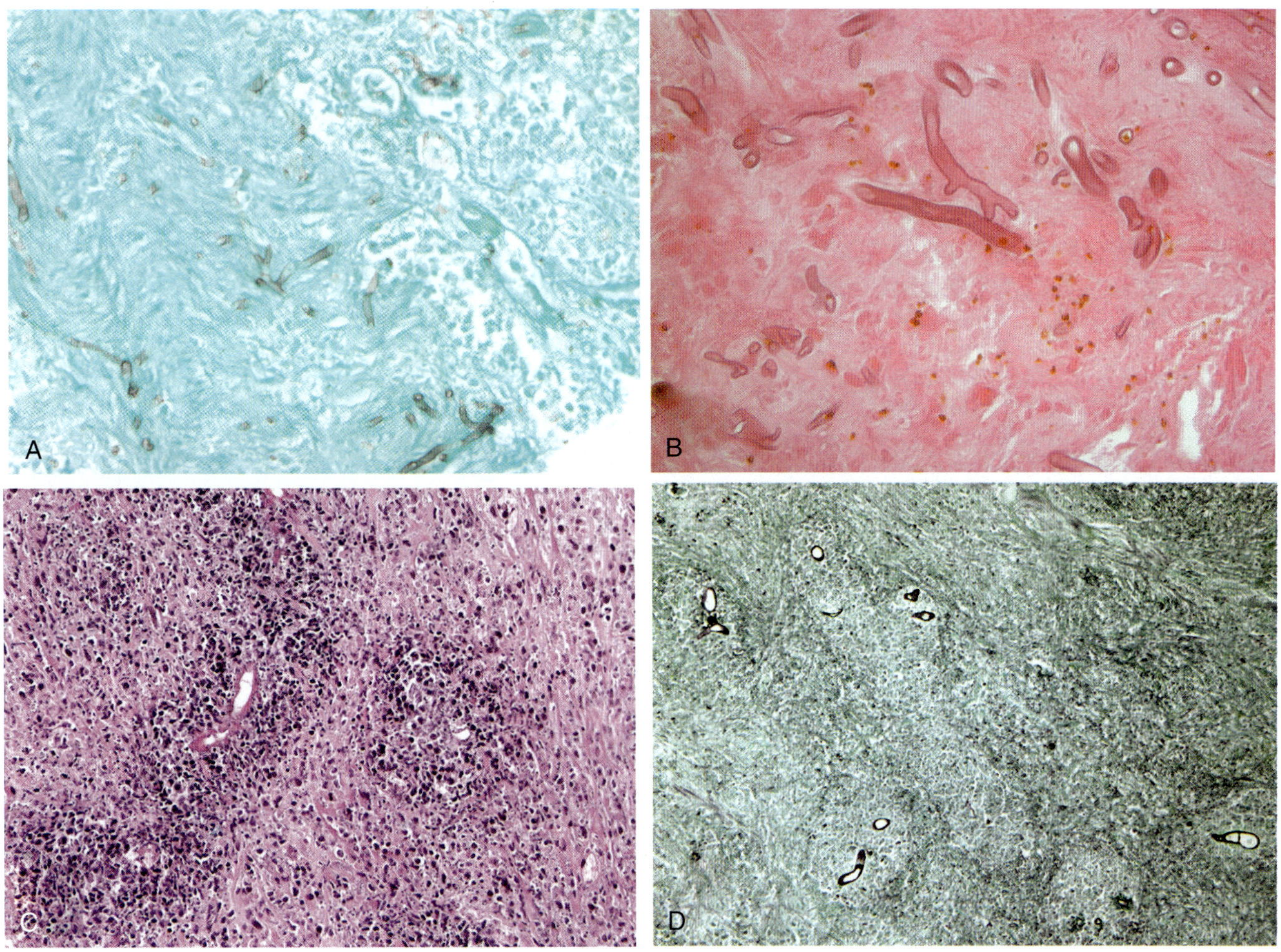

FIGURE 9.36
(Continued)

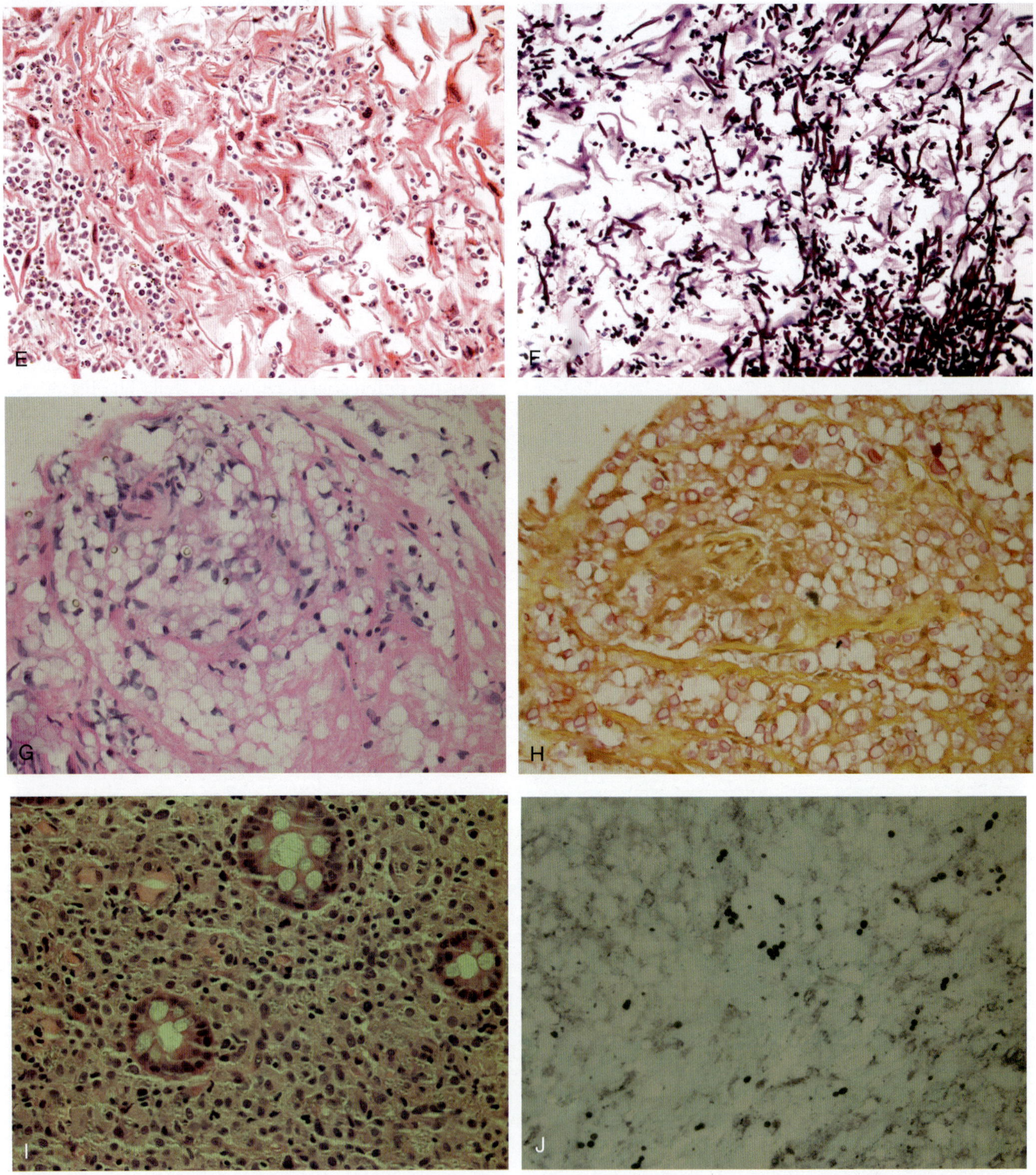

FIGURE 9.36

A, *Aspergillus* spp. have septate hyphae that branch at acute angles (Gomori methenamine silver [GMS]). **B**, The hyphae of *Mucor* are broader and pauci-septate. They branch at irregular angles and appear clear when sectioned transversely (hematoxylin and eosin [H&E]). **C**, *Basidiobolus ranarum* are often associated with granulomatous and eosinophil-rich inflammation (H&E). **D**, Their hyphae are broader than those of *Mucor* and have thinner walls (Gomori methenamine silver [GMS]). (Courtesy of Dr. Laura W. Lamps.) **E**, The yeast and pseudohyphae of *Candida* spp. are admixed with keratin debris in the esophagus (H&E). **F**, Periodic acid–Schiff D stain highlights elongated pseudohyphae and round yeast forms. **G**, *Cryptococcus neoformans* are variably sized and round (H&E). **H**, A mucicarmine stain highlights their mucopolysaccharide capsule (mucicarmine). **I**, Foamy macrophages fill the lamina propria in a case of histoplasmosis (H&E). **J**, A GMS stain reveals yeasts with narrow-based budding (GMS).

and unusual forms. Helpful diagnostic aids, in addition to culture, include serologic assays and antigen tests.

PARASITIC INFECTIONS OF THE GASTROINTESTINAL TRACT

PROTOZOA

ENTAMOEBA HISTOLYTICA

Approximately 10% of the world's population is infected with this parasite, and the prevalence is much higher in tropical and subtropical locations. Homosexual men are also at increased risk for harboring this pathogen.

CLINICAL FEATURES

Many infected patients are asymptomatic or have only vague, nonspecific GI complaints that may mimic irritable bowel syndrome. Symptomatic patients most commonly have diarrhea, abdominal cramps, and variable right lower quadrant tenderness; this may be referred to as "nondysenteric" amebiasis. Invasive disease, most often manifested as amoebic dysentery or liver abscess, reportedly occurs in fewer than 10% of infected persons. Amebic dysentery presents suddenly, approximately 1 to 3 weeks after exposure, with severe abdominal cramps, tenesmus, fever, and diarrhea (which may be mucoid or bloody).

AMEBIASIS—FACT SHEET

Definition

- Common protozoal infection, affecting approximately 10% of the population worldwide

Incidence and Location

- Any level of the colon or appendix; cecum most frequent

Clinical Features

- Many patients asymptomatic or with vague, nonspecific gastrointestinal symptoms
- Some patients have fulminant colitis
- May form large inflammatory masses
- Homosexual men at increased risk for infection

Prognosis and Therapy

- Antiparasitic drugs such as metronidazole

Complications of intestinal amebiasis include bleeding; perforation; dissemination to other sites, particularly the liver; fistula formation between the intestine and the skin, peritoneum, and urogenital tract; and toxic megacolon. The latter complication is often associated with corticosteroid use. Rarely, large inflammatory masses (amebomas) may be formed.

PATHOLOGIC FEATURES

GROSS FINDINGS

Small ulcers are the early lesion, which may coalesce to form large, irregular ulcers that are often "geographic" or serpiginous. Intervening mucosa is often normal. The ulcers have associated inflammatory exudate or adjacent inflammatory polyps. Ulcers may undermine adjacent mucosa to produce the classic "flask-shaped" lesion. The cecum is the most common site of involvement. Indeed, the presence of multiple ulcers in the ileocecal region may simulate Crohn's disease endoscopically, particularly when aphthae are present. Any part of the colon or appendix may be involved. Fulminant colitis resembling ulcerative colitis, pseudomembranous colitis resembling that caused by *C. difficile*, and toxic megacolon have been described. Colonoscopy may be normal in asymptomatic patients and those with mild disease.

MICROSCOPIC FINDINGS

The earliest lesion is a mild neutrophilic infiltrate. In more advanced disease, ulcers are often deep, extending at least into the submucosa (Fig. 9.37), with undermining of adjacent normal mucosa. There is associated necroinflammatory debris; the organisms are generally found within this purulent material (Fig. 9.38). Invasive amebae are occasionally seen within the bowel wall. The adjacent mucosa is usually normal but may show gland distortion and inflammation. The organisms, which may be very few in number, resemble macrophages with foamy cytoplasm and a round, eccentric nucleus; the presence of ingested red blood cells is pathognomonic of *Entamoeba histolytica*. In patients who are asymptomatic or have mild symptoms, histologic changes may range from normal to a heavy mixed inflammatory infiltrate. Organisms may be particularly difficult (if not impossible) to find in these patients.

AMEBIASIS—PATHOLOGIC FEATURES

Gross Findings

- Early lesion: small ulcers, may coalesce to form larger ones
- Ulcers may undermine adjacent mucosa to form classic "flask-shaped" ulcer
- Normal intervening mucosa
- May grossly resemble ulcerative colitis, pseudomembranous colitis, Crohn's disease
- Colonoscopy may be normal in asymptomatic patients or those with mild disease

Microscopic Findings

- Early lesion: mild neutrophilic infiltrate
- Advanced disease: deep ulcers, undermining adjacent normal mucosa

- Associated necroinflammatory debris, which may harbor organisms
- Intervening mucosa may have architectural distortion, inflammation
- Organisms resemble macrophages with foamy cytoplasm and round, eccentric nucleus
- Ingested red blood cells pathognomonic of *Entamoeba histolytica*
- Amebas are trichrome positive

Differential Diagnosis

- Ulcerative colitis
- Crohn's disease
- *Balantidium coli*

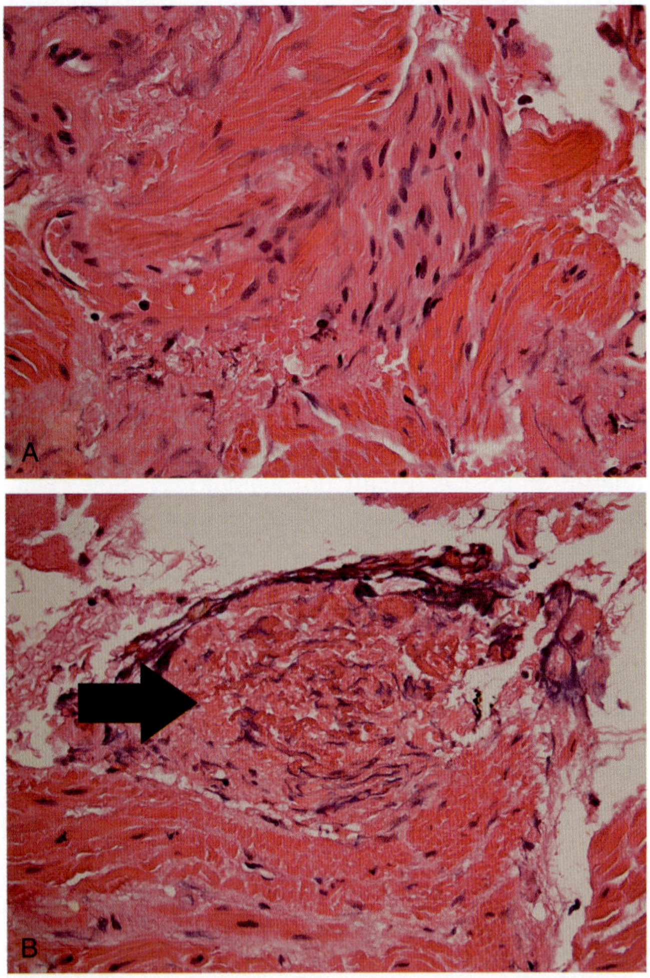

FIGURE 9.37

A, Chagas disease results in absence of ganglion cells in the myenteric plexus (hematoxylin and eosin [H&E]). **B**, Over time, nerves may exhibit fibrosis with collagen deposits (H&E).

Ancillary Studies

Examination of stool for parasites is a helpful diagnostic test, and serologies are also available.

Differential Diagnosis

The differential diagnosis most often is that of amebae versus macrophages within an inflammatory exudate. *Amebae* are trichrome positive. Amebiasis can also be confused with Crohn's disease or ulcerative colitis, as well as other types of infectious colitis. The ciliate *Balantidium coli* produces a spectrum of clinical and pathologic changes similar to that of *E. histolytica*. However, *B. coli* organisms are distinguished from amebae by their larger size, kidney bean–shaped nuclei, and cilia (Fig. 9.39).

Two other species of amoeba, *Entamoeba dispar* and *Entamoeba moshkovskii*, which are histologically indistinguishable from *E. histolytica*, have recently received attention because they have been recovered from the stool of patients with GI symptoms. To date, there is no convincing evidence that *E. dispar* causes symptomatic GI disease, and many studies on both species are confounded by coinfection with *E. histolytica* and other GI pathogens. Some authorities refer to the organism as

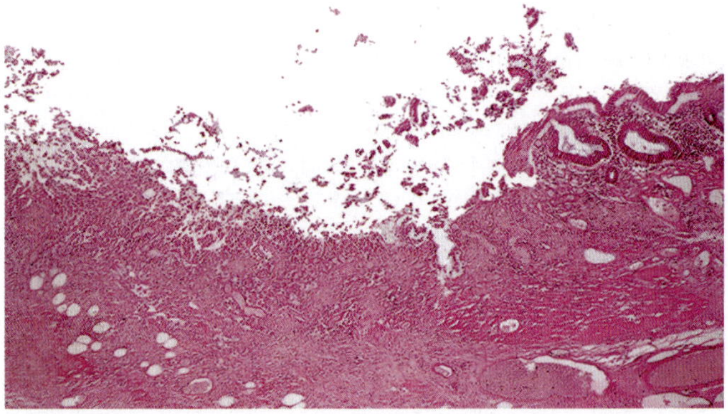

FIGURE 9.38

Colonic amebiasis. Deep ulcer with overlying exudate (hematoxylin and eosin).

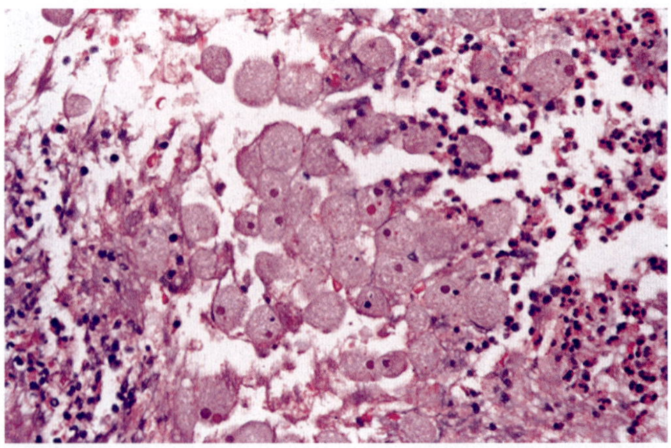

FIGURE 9.39

Entamoeba histolytica organisms have foamy cytoplasms and a round, eccentric nucleus. The presence of ingested red blood cells is pathognomonic of E. histolytica (hematoxylin and eosin). Case courtesy of Dr. Rickey Ryals.

"*E. histolytica–E. dispar*" complex, resulting from the high rate of coinfection.

Prognosis and Therapy

Antiparasitic drugs such as metronidazole are effective, even against invasive amebiasis.

TRYPANOSOMA CRUZI (CHAGAS DISEASE)

Chagas disease is caused by infection with the protozoan parasite *Trypanosoma cruzi*, which is transmitted by insect vectors and affects several million people in Latin America. The disease may also be transmitted through blood transfusion, organ transplantation, and congenitally. Intestinal dysfunction is caused by damage to the enteric nervous system induced by T cell–mediated inflammatory response to *T. cruzi* proteins. Acute infection with Chagas disease is usually subclinical, and most patients develop lifelong asymptomatic infection. Those who develop chronic disease most commonly experience cardiac and intestinal complications. Upper digestive tract involvement takes the form of secondary achalasia or megaesophagus, causing dysphagia, odynophagia, and severe reflux and regurgitation. Colonic involvement results in megacolon, constipation, obstipation, and abdominal pain. The disease may be successfully eradicated with adequate antiparasitic therapy with benznidazole and nifurtimox. Most deaths from Chagas disease are caused by cardiac complications.

The esophagus and colon are markedly dilated. The esophageal squamous mucosa may appear thickened and irregular because of stasis of luminal contents. Histologic findings include smooth muscle fibrosis and lymphocytic inflammation and fibrosis around the myenteric and submucosal plexuses, which contain reduced numbers of neurons and ganglion cells (Fig. 9.40). The esophageal squamous mucosa also often shows striking lymphocyte-rich inflammation. The organisms are rarely identified histologically but when present are seen in ganglion cells. Helpful laboratory assays include PCR, serologic studies, and culture. Infection may be difficult to detect serologically, however, because circulating organisms are usually relatively scarce.

The main differential diagnosis is primary achalasia and causes of pseudoachalasia, such as diffuse esophageal spasm, hypertensive lower esophageal sphincter, and malignant infiltration of the distal esophagus. Other causes of neuronal dysfunction in the colon, such as Hirschsprung disease, are usually easily excluded on clinical grounds because manifestation of Chagas disease is rarely isolated to the GI tract.

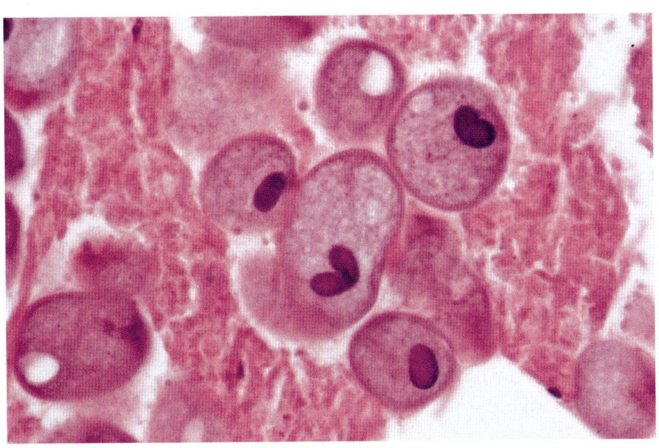

FIGURE 9.40

The ciliate *Balantidium coli* is distinguished from *Entamoeba histolytica* by its larger size, kidney bean–shaped nucleus, and cilia (hematoxylin and eosin). Case courtesy of Dr. David Owen.

FLAGELLATES

Giardia Lamblia

Giardia lamblia is a flagellated protozoan parasite that is a common cause of diarrheal disease worldwide. It is spread via fecal–oral transmission through contaminated water and food. *G. lamblia* are ingested as cysts and complete their life cycle in the intestine. Cysts are also found in the stool of farm animals and household pets. Illness is more common among children. Patients with primary immunodeficiencies may experience repeated or prolonged *G. lamblia* infections.

Clinical Features

Up to 40% of *Giardia* infections are asymptomatic. Symptomatic patients present with explosive, foul-smelling, watery diarrhea. Symptoms also include cramps, bloating, nausea, and vomiting. Infections are usually self-limiting, but chronic diarrhea may develop, especially in children and immunocompromised patients.

GIARDIA LAMBLIA—FACT SHEET

Definition

- Flagellated protozoan with worldwide distribution

Incidence and Location

- Duodenum, terminal ileum

Clinical Features

- Explosive watery diarrhea
- Abdominal cramping
- Bloating
- Nausea, vomiting

Prognosis and Therapy

- Usually self-limited
- Metronidazole

PATHOLOGIC FEATURES

GROSS FINDINGS

Endoscopy is usually unremarkable or reveals non-specific findings, such as edema and patchy erythema.

MICROSCOPIC FINDINGS

Giardiasis is most commonly diagnosed in duodenal biopsy specimens; however, terminal ileal biopsies may reveal *G. lamblia* trophozoites, especially in the chronic phase of infection. The duodenal mucosa often appears unremarkable; however, biopsy samples may show villous blunting and increased lamina propria inflammation, including lymphocytes, plasma cells, and eosinophils, and lymphoid aggregates (Fig. 9.41A). In some cases, intraepithelial lymphocytes may also be increased. The diagnostic finding is trophozoites clustered at the tips of villi or in the intervillous spaces (Fig. 9.41B). The organisms are pear shaped when viewed en face or may appear crescentic or "kite shaped" when tangentially sectioned. They contain two ovoid nuclei and a central karyosome. Flagella are usually not appreciable in routine sections.

GIARDIA LAMBLIA—PATHOLOGIC FEATURES

Gross Findings
- Endoscopy is usually unremarkable

Microscopic Findings
- Preserved villous architecture
- Increased lamina propria inflammation, lymphoid aggregates
- Increased intraepithelial lymphocytes
- Pear- or kite-shaped trophozoites in intervillous spaces

Differential Diagnosis
- Sloughed epithelial cells
- Extruded mucin

ANCILLARY STUDIES

Trichrome stains may help to highlight *G. lamblia* in cases with rare organisms. Stool antigen tests and PCR assays are also available.

DIFFERENTIAL DIAGNOSIS

Giardia organisms may be easily overlooked in biopsy samples, particularly when the duodenal mucosa appears normal. Organisms may be few and inconspicuous. Poorly preserved organisms may resemble sloughed epithelial cells or extruded mucin. Pathologists should consider a diagnosis of giardiasis when the clinical history is suggestive of infection and be mindful of organisms in intervillous spaces because tissue invasion is not a feature of giardiasis.

PROGNOSIS AND THERAPY

Treatment is recommended only if patients develop prolonged disease and typically includes a course of metronidazole and supportive care. Disease eradication is particularly important for children, as chronic giardiasis has been associated with cognitive impairment.

VISCERAL LEISHMANIASIS (KALA-AZAR) CAUSED BY *LEISHMANIA DONOVANI* AND RELATED SPECIES

The prevalence of leishmaniasis is increasing worldwide as a result of immigration, urbanization, and increased numbers of immunocompromised patients. It is endemic in more than 80 countries in Africa, Asia, South and Central America, and Europe. The causative parasite, *Leishmania* spp., is transmitted via sandfly bites.

CLINICAL FEATURES

Gastrointestinal involvement is generally part of widely disseminated disease. GI signs and symptoms include fever, abdominal pain, diarrhea, dysphagia, malabsorption, and weight loss.

LEISHMANIASIS—FACT SHEET

Definition
- Parasitic infection transmitted by sandfly bites, endemic in more than 80 countries in Africa, Asia, South and Central America, and Europe

Incidence and Location
- Anywhere in the bowel; rarely the esophagus

Clinical Features
- Part of widely disseminated disease
- Fever, abdominal pain, diarrhea, dysphagia, malabsorption, and weight loss

Prognosis and Therapy
- Pentavalent antimony, amphotericin, pentamidine

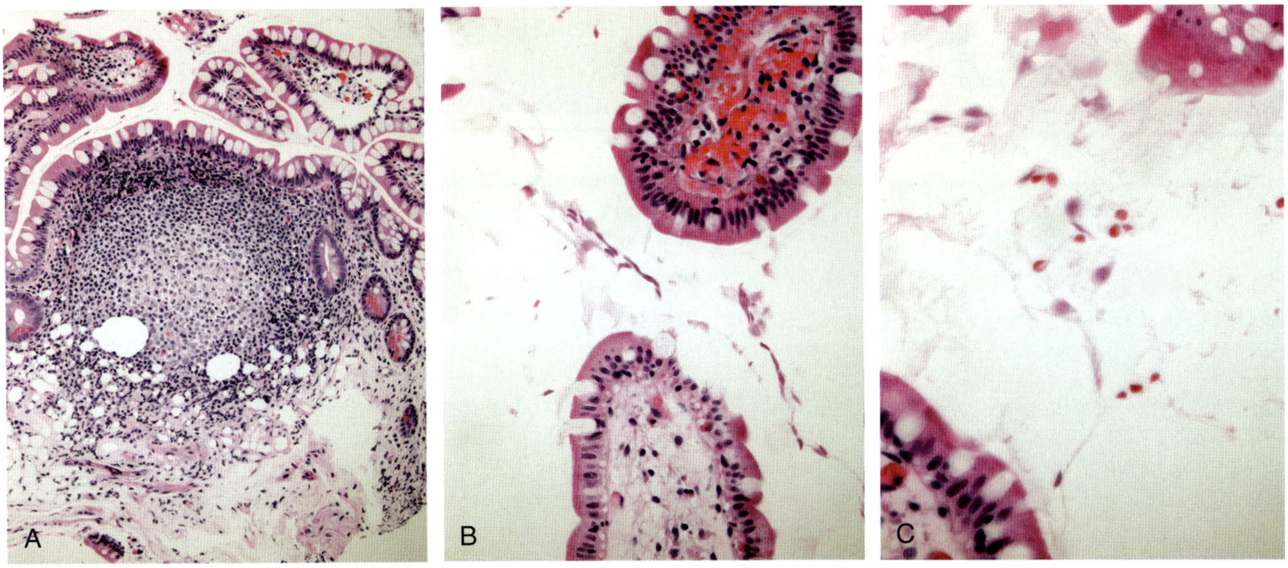

FIGURE 9.41

A, A reactive lymphoid aggregate is present in the duodenal mucosa of a patient with giardiasis. **B**, *Giardia lamblia* organisms in the intervillous space have a crescentic contour in some sections. **C**, The organisms are pear shaped when sectioned lengthwise (hematoxylin and eosin).

Pathologic Features

Gross Findings

Leishmania organisms may be found anywhere in the small intestine and colon, and rarely in the esophagus. Endoscopic findings include normal examination, focal ulceration, and changes grossly consistent with enteritis.

Microscopic Findings

Histologic changes in immunocompetent and immunocompromised persons are similar. Histologic features typically consist of macrophages within the lamina propria containing amastigotes. Often, an associated inflammatory infiltrate is absent. The amastigotes are round to oval, tiny organisms with a nucleus and kinetoplast in a "double-knot" configuration.

Leishmaniasis—Pathologic Features

Gross Findings

- Range from normal to focal ulceration, changes of enteritis

Microscopic Findings

- Macrophages within the lamina propria containing amastigotes
- Amastigotes are round to oval, tiny organisms with a nucleus and kinetoplast in a "double-knot" configuration
- Histologic changes in immunocompetent and immunocompromised persons are similar
- Inflammatory infiltrate is often absent

Differential Diagnosis

- *Histoplasma capsulatum*
- *Trypanosoma cruzi* (Chagas disease)

Ancillary Studies

Serologic studies and IHC may aid in diagnosis.

Differential Diagnosis

The differential diagnosis is primarily that of other parasitic and fungal infections, and *Leishmania* spp. may be confused with similar organisms such as *Histoplasma* spp. and *T. cruzi*. All but *T. cruzi* lack a kinetoplast, and Leishmania spp. are GMS, mucicarmine, and PAS negative. *T. cruzi* is seldom visualized in the GI tract, and the resultant inflammatory lesion affects the myenteric plexus rather than the lamina propria.

Prognosis and Therapy

Pentavalent antimonial compounds are the first line of therapy in most cases. Other drugs such as amphotericin B and pentamidine are also used.

COCCIDIANS AND RELATED ORGANISMS

Unicellular protozoa formerly considered coccidians have recently undergone substantial reclassification. These organisms, including *Cryptosporidium parvum*, *Cryptosporidium hominis*, *Cryptosporidium meleagridis*, *Cyclospora cayetanensis*, *Cystoisospora belli*, and *Microsporidia* spp. are important causes of malabsorptive diarrhea worldwide. *Cryptosporidia* spp. are now classified as gregarines, a subclass of conoidasida related to coccidians. *C. cayetanensis* and *C. belli* remain in the coccidians class, whereas *Microsporidia* spp. are now considered fungi. These organisms are discussed as a group herein because of their overlapping clinical and morphologic features.

CLINICAL FEATURES

Coccidians, conoidasida, and *Microsporidia* spp. often produce asymptomatic infections in both immunocompromised and healthy patients. All except *Microsporidia* spp. (which is thought to be limited to immunocompromised individuals) can cause diarrhea (often prolonged) in healthy patients, especially infants and children, travelers, and institutionalized people. Diarrhea may be accompanied by fever, weight loss, abdominal pain, and malaise. The stool does not usually contain red blood cells or leukocytes. In immunocompetent persons, infection is usually self-limited. Immunocompromised patients are at risk for chronic, severe diarrhea with malabsorption, dehydration, and death.. They are worldwide pathogens that are more common in, but not limited to, developing countries. Transmission is via the fecal–oral route, either directly or via contaminated food and water.

COCCIDIANS AND RELATED ORGANISMS–FACT SHEET

Definition

- Unicellular organisms causing chronic diarrhea, most often in immunocompromised patients; transmitted through fecal–oral route and contaminated food and water

Incidence and Location

- Most commonly the small bowel; rarely the colon and gallbladder

Clinical Features

- Chronic diarrhea, with or without fever, weight loss, abdominal pain, and malaise
- Stool lacks red blood cells and leukocytes
- Infection is self-limited in immunocompetent persons
- Immunocompromised patients are at risk for chronic, severe diarrhea with malabsorption, dehydration, and death

Prognosis and Therapy

- *Cryptosporidium*: no effective treatment
- *Microsporidium*: some efficacy with drugs such as albendazole
- *Toxoplasmosis*: numerous effective antibiotics, especially sulfa drugs
- *Cyclospora*: sulfa drugs
- *Cystoisospora*: sulfa drugs

PATHOLOGIC FEATURES

GROSS FINDINGS

Endoscopic findings are usually absent or mild. When present, they may include mild erythema, mucosal granularity, mucosal atrophy, and mild erosions.

MICROSCOPIC FINDINGS

1. *C. parvum*. Although most commonly seen in the small bowel, *Cryptosporidium* spp. may be seen in the colon as well. The characteristic appearance of the organism is a 2- to 5-µm basophilic spherical body protruding from the apex of the enterocyte (Fig. 9.42). It can be found in the crypts or at the surface. Associated mucosal changes include a mixed inflammatory infiltrate, and crypt abscesses. Organisms stain with the Giemsa stain. *Cryptosporidium* spp. may be distinguished by their unique apical location; although *Cyclospora* organisms are similar in appearance, they are much larger, and some forms are banana shaped.
2. *Toxoplasma gondii*. GI toxoplasmosis is primarily a disease of immunocompromised persons. Intestinal involvement is a rare feature. Ulcers have been described in the bowel, with Toxoplasma organisms in the ulcer base. Both crescent-shaped tachyzoites and cysts containing bradyzoites may be seen within tissue sections.
3. *Microsporidia* spp. *Enterocytozoon bieneusi* and *Encephalitozoon intestinalis* are the most commonly seen in human infection. They are usually seen in the small bowel, but the colon and biliary tree may be affected. These stain with modified trichrome (Fig. 9.43), tissue Gram stain, and silver impregnation stains. *Microsporidia* organisms can be very

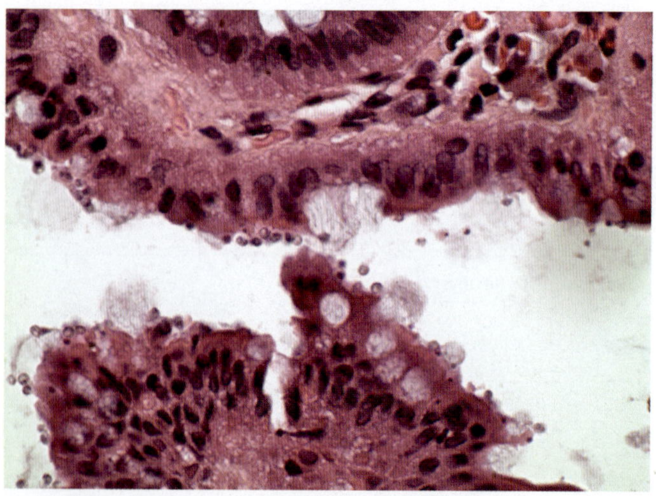

FIGURE 9.42

Colon biopsy from a patient with AIDS. Numerous *Cryptosporidia* organisms are seen bulging beneath the surface of enterocytes (hematoxylin and eosin).

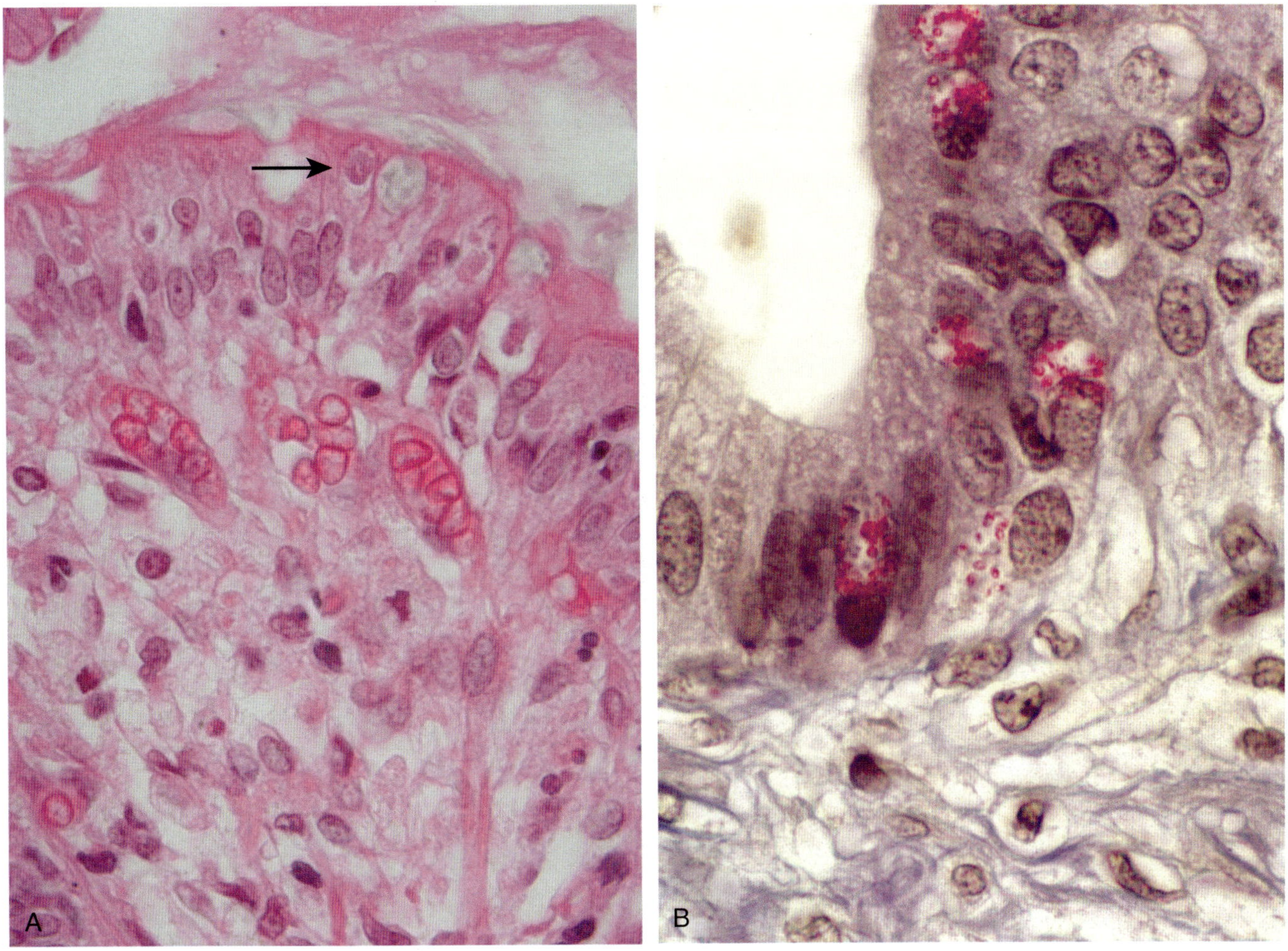

FIGURE 9.43

A, *Microsporidia* infection produces epithelial disarray; the organisms may be appreciable as tiny clusters of intracytoplasmic "dots" on hematoxylin and eosin *(arrow)*. **B**, Tiny *Microsporidia* organisms are present within enterocytes, with minimal inflammatory response (modified trichrome).

difficult to detect in H&E sections. The histologic features include a subtle vacuolization of the surface epithelium and a patchy lymphoplasmacytic infiltrate in the lamina propria. Sometimes *Microsporidia* spp. polarize within tissue biopsies because the chitin-rich internal polar filament of the organism is birefringent under polarized light. However, this method is unreliable because of the unpredictability of spore birefringence, as well as variability depending on the microscope and light source used.

4. *Cyclospora cayetanensis* can infect immunocompetent or immunocompromised patients. The organisms appear as 2- to 3-μm schizonts or 5- to 6-μm banana-shaped merozoites within a parasitophorous vacuole in enterocytes (Fig. 9.44).
5. *Cystoisospora belli* is usually found in the small bowel but may also involve the colon or gallbladder. It is the largest coccidian, appearing as 15- to 20-μm forms at all stages of the organism's life cycle. Whereas schizonts and merozoites are crescent shaped, the sexual forms are round with prominent nuclei. They may be found in epithelial cells or macrophages, often within a parasitophorous vacuole (Fig. 9.45).

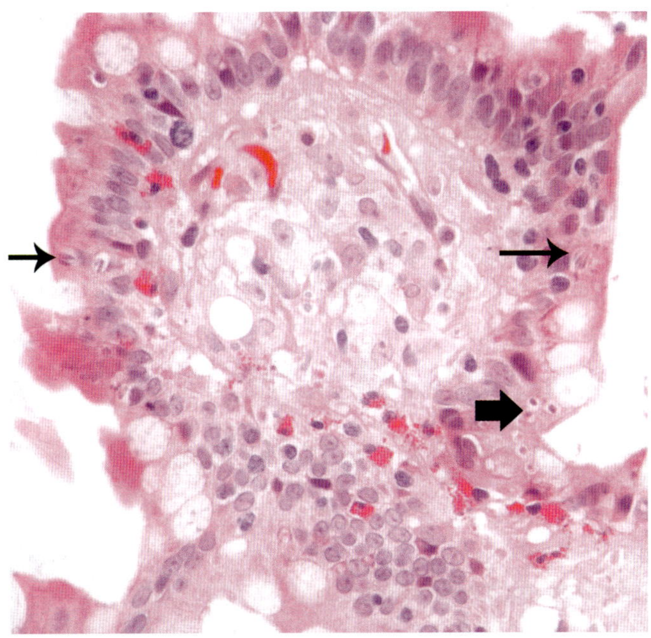

FIGURE 9.44

Cyclospora cayetanensis organisms are present within intracytoplasmic vacuoles. Both round schizonts *(thick arrow)* and elongated merozoites *(thin arrow)* can be seen.

Coccidians And Related Organisms—Pathologic Features

Gross Findings

- Usually absent or mild
- Can have mild erythema, mucosal granularity, mucosal atrophy, and mild erosions

Microscopic Findings

- *Cryptosporidium parvum*
  - 2- to 5-mm basophilic spherical body protruding from the apex of the enterocyte
  - In the crypts or at the surface
  - Tissue reaction includes mixed inflammatory infiltrate, crypt abscesses
- *Toxoplasma gondii*
  - Almost always immunocompromised
  - Intestinal involvement is a rare feature
  - Both crescent-shaped tachyzoites and cysts containing bradyzoites can be seen
- *Microsporidia* spp.
  - Tiny organisms in apex of enterocytes
  - Stain with modified trichrome, tissue Gram stain, and silver impregnation stains
- *Cyclospora cayetanensis*
  - 2- to 3-μm schizonts or 5- to 6-μm banana-shaped merozoites within a parasitophorous vacuole in enterocytes
  - Gomori methenamine silver (GMS), periodic acid–Schiff, Gram, and trichrome negative
- *Cystoisospora belli*
- Intracellular crescent-shaped schizonts and merozoites, often within a parasitophorous vacuole
- Crescent-shaped schizonts and merozoites
- Round sexual forms with prominent nuclei
- Highlighted with GMS and Giemsa stains

Differential Diagnosis

- Primarily other unicellular protozoa

Ancillary Studies

Although electron microscopy was once considered the gold standard for diagnosis of these organisms, it is expensive, subject to sampling bias, and not widely used. Examination of stool specimens may be helpful in many cases. Enzyme-linked immunosorbent assay techniques, IHC, and PCR studies have been developed, although these tests are not widely available to practicing pathologists.

Differential Diagnosis

The differential diagnosis is primarily other unicellular protozoa.

Prognosis and Therapy

Most antimicrobial agents are ineffective against cryptosporidial infection, although antimotility agents may provide symptomatic relief. Agents such as albendazole are at least anecdotally effective against microsporidial infection in some studies. Antibiotics may be effective against *Cyclospora* spp., *Cystoisospora* spp., and toxoplasmosis.

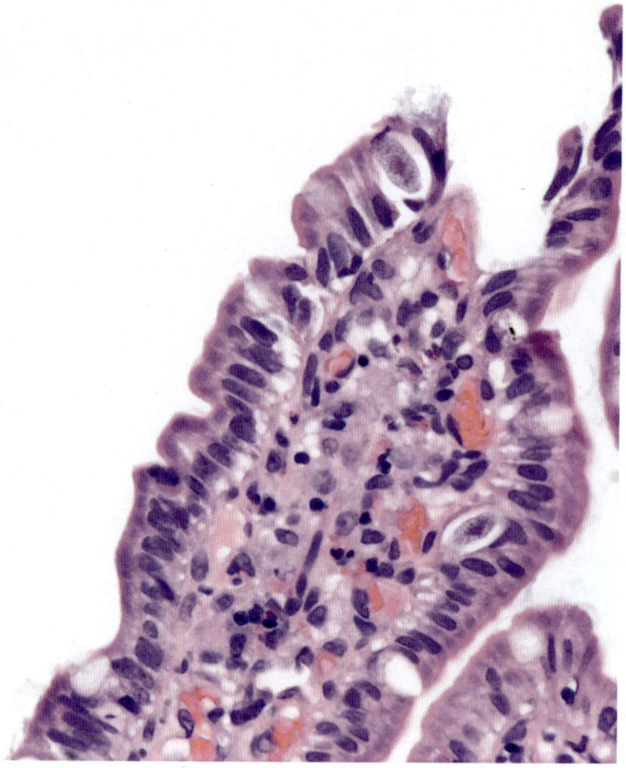

FIGURE 9.45

Cystoisospora belli are round to banana-shaped eosinophilic organisms with prominent nucleoli found within parasitophorous vacuoles (hematoxylin and eosin). (Courtesy of Dr. Laura W. Lamps.)

HELMINTHS (NEMATODES, TREMATODES, AND CESTODES)

Although the most common method of diagnosing GI helminth infections is examination of stool for ova and parasites, these organisms are occasionally seen in biopsy or resection specimens. GI helminths have a worldwide distribution, but their clinical importance varies with geographic region. They are more often a cause of serious disease in underdeveloped nations because deficient sanitation systems; poor socioeconomic status; and hot, humid climates are predisposing factors. Helminthic infections are becoming an increasingly important problem in immunocompromised patients. The nutritional problems caused by helminths can be severe and even life threatening, particularly in children. The anatomic site of infection is most often the small bowel, although the large bowel may certainly be involved.

The differential diagnosis of helminthic infections often involves differentiating between types of worm. Other entities to be considered include other causes of ulcerative inflammation, eosinophilic infiltration, and granulomatous inflammation, such as tuberculosis, amebiasis, allergic enteritides, and Crohn's disease.

NEMATODES

ENTEROBIUS VERMICULARIS (PINWORMS)

Pinworms are one of the most common parasites affecting humans. They have a worldwide distribution but are more common in cold or temperate climates and developed countries. They are extremely common in the United States and Northwestern Europe. The infective larva-containing egg resides in dust and soil, and transmission is believed to be fecal–oral. School children and adolescents, especially those who live in institutions, have the highest prevalence of infection. The worms live and reproduce in the ileum, cecum, proximal colon, and appendix, and the female migrates to the anus to lay her eggs and die. The ability of *Enterobius* spp. to cause colitis and actual mucosal damage is controversial. However, they have been noted to rarely invade the GI mucosa.

CLINICAL FEATURES

The eggs and worms produce the classic symptom of nocturnal pruritus ani. Many infections are asymptomatic, but heavy infections may cause abdominal pain, nausea, and vomiting. Appendicitis, vulvovaginitis, colitis, and peritoneal involvement have been described secondary to pinworm infection.

ENTEROBIASIS—FACT SHEET

Definition
- Common helminthic infection; rarely causes colitis

Incidence and Location
- Anus, appendix, large bowel

Clinical Features
- Perianal itching, primarily nocturnal
- Rarely, colitis and appendicitis

Prognosis and Therapy
- Antiparasitic drugs such as mebendazole

PATHOLOGIC FEATURES

GROSS FINDINGS

Grossly, the worms are 2 to 5 mm in length and may be seen with the naked eye. Although the mucosa of the GI tract often appears normal upon examination, hemorrhage and ulceration are occasionally seen in invasive infection.

MICROSCOPIC FINDINGS

Although even invasive pinworms usually incite little or no inflammatory reaction, as discussed previously, an inflammatory infiltrate composed predominantly of eosinophils may occasionally be seen. Granulomas, sometimes with necrosis, may be seen as well, often associated with degenerating worms or eggs. These lesions have been described within the omentum and peritoneum, as well as in the appendix, anus, and colon in rare cases.

ENTEROBIASIS—PATHOLOGIC FEATURES

Gross Findings
- Worms are 2 to 5 mm in length
- Mucosa often appears normal on examination
- Hemorrhage and ulceration are occasionally seen in invasive infection

Microscopic Findings
- Usually little or no inflammatory reaction
- Rarely, an inflammatory infiltrate composed of neutrophils is present
- Granulomas, sometimes with necrosis, can be associated with degenerating worms or eggs
- Worm morphology: lateral ala with easily visible intestine and uterus (in the female); eggs are ovoid with one flat side and have a bilayered refractile shell

Differential Diagnosis
- Other helminths

ANCILLARY STUDIES

Stool examination for ova and parasites has a relatively low yield. Inspection of the perianal area for worms, and the anal "scotch tape test" are the most helpful diagnostic aids.

DIFFERENTIAL DIAGNOSIS

The differential diagnosis is primarily other types of worms. Pinworms have lateral ala (Fig. 9.46) with an

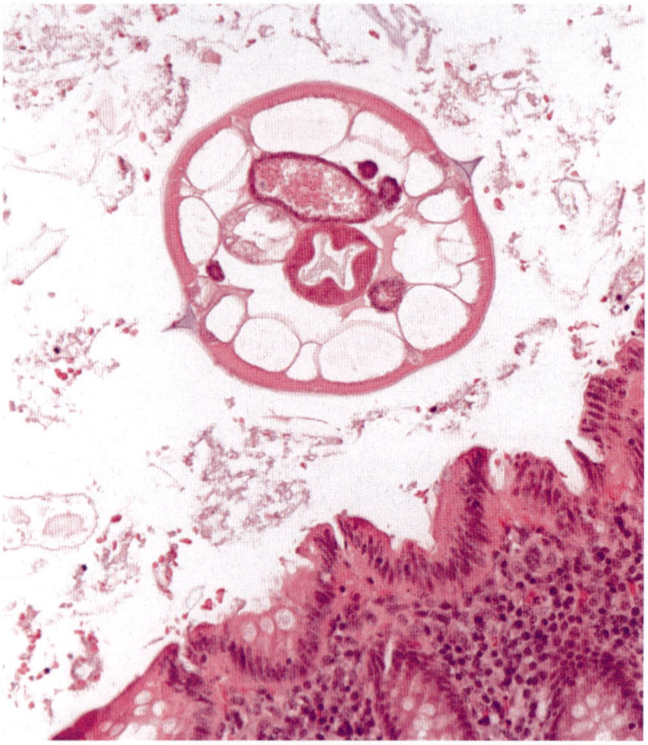

FIGURE 9.46

Pinworms have prominent lateral ala and an easily visible intestine (hematoxylin and eosin).

easily visible intestine and uterus (in the female). The eggs are ovoid with one flat side and have a bilayered refractile shell. It may be difficult to distinguish between primary *Enterobius* infection and infection complicating a preexisting inflammatory lesion such as an inflamed anal fissure.

Prognosis and Therapy

Most infections clear spontaneously, although this may require several weeks. However, treatment with antiparasitic drugs such as mebendazole is recommended to prevent transmission to others, and for symptomatic cases.

ASCARIS LUMBRICOIDES (ROUNDWORM), *ANCYLOSTOMA DUODENALE* (HOOKWORM), AND *TRICHURIS TRICHIURA* (WHIPWORM)

These worms are rarely a problem in diagnostic biopsies but may cause significant GI complications, including bleeding, malabsorption, anemia, obstruction, and diarrhea. *Ascaris* spp. are some of the most frequent parasites in humans. It has a worldwide distribution but is most common in the tropics. These worms are ingested from soil contaminated with feces. Hookworms (*Necator americanus* and *Ancylostoma duodenale*) are a common parasite in virtually all tropical and subtropical countries. Whipworms (*T. trichiura*) are also soil-borne helminths with a worldwide distribution.

CLINICAL FEATURES

Clinical findings in *Ascaris* infection are variable and include appendicitis, massive infection with obstruction and perforation, childhood growth retardation, and pancreaticobiliary obstruction. Hookworms attach to the intestinal wall and suck blood from villous capillaries, resulting in anemia. Other clinical symptoms include abdominal pain, diarrhea, hypoproteinemia, and an associated cough with eosinophilia as the worms migrate. Mesenteric adenitis secondary to hookworm infection has also been described. The anemia may lead to significant growth retardation in children. Whipworm infection is often asymptomatic, but infection may cause diarrhea, GI bleeding, malabsorption, anemia, and appendicitis.

ROUNDWORM, HOOKWORM, WHIPWORM—FACT SHEET

Definition

- Common helminthic infections with a worldwide distribution

Incidence and Location

- Small and large bowel

Clinical Features

- In general, bleeding, malabsorption, anemia, obstruction, and diarrhea
- *Ascaris* spp. may cause bowel obstruction
- Hookworm known to cause anemia
- All may cause significant growth problems in children

Prognosis and Therapy

- Antihelminthic drugs; surgery if obstructed; iron supplementation if anemic

Pathologic Features

Ascaris organisms are very large worms (≤20 cm) that may be identified endoscopically or at resection if obstruction occurs (Fig. 9.47). Tissue damage occurs primarily at attachment sites. Hookworms affect all levels of the GI tract. Endoscopically, the worms (~1 cm in length) are visible to the naked eye. Pieces of worm may be visible on biopsy; although other histologic changes are usually

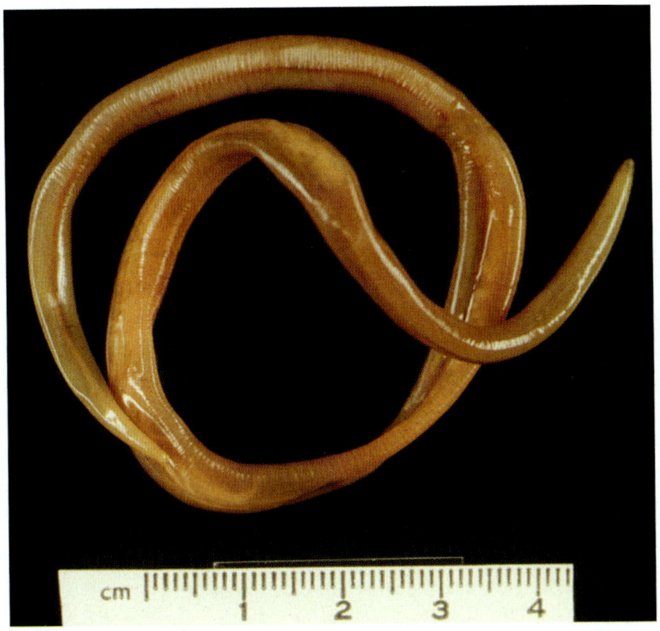

FIGURE 9.47

Ascaris organisms measure up to 20 cm in length and are easily seen with the naked eye.

minimal, an eosinophilic infiltrate is sometimes seen. Whipworms are found predominantly in the right colon and ileum. They may cause gross mucosal hemorrhage and ulceration; the worms are 3 to 5 mm long with a characteristic whiplike tail and can be seen endoscopically. Histologically, the worms thread their anterior ends under mucosal epithelium, which may produce enterocyte atrophy and an associated mixed inflammatory infiltrate; crypt abscesses may be present as well. Whipworm infection also may rarely mimic Crohn's disease.

ROUNDWORM, HOOKWORM, WHIPWORM—PATHOLOGIC FEATURES

Gross Findings

- *Ascaris* spp. are very large worms (≤20 cm)
- Hookworms measure about 1 cm in length
- Whipworms are 3 to 5 mm long, with whiplike tails (Fig. 9.48)
- Hookworm- and whipworm-associated tissue damage may mimic Crohn's disease grossly

Microscopic Findings

- *Ascaris*-related tissue damage occurs primarily at attachment sites
- Hookworm causes minimal histologic change; rarely an eosinophilic infiltrate
- Whipworm may cause mixed inflammatory infiltrate and crypt abscesses, usually associated with attachment site

Differential Diagnosis

- Other helminths
- Crohn's disease

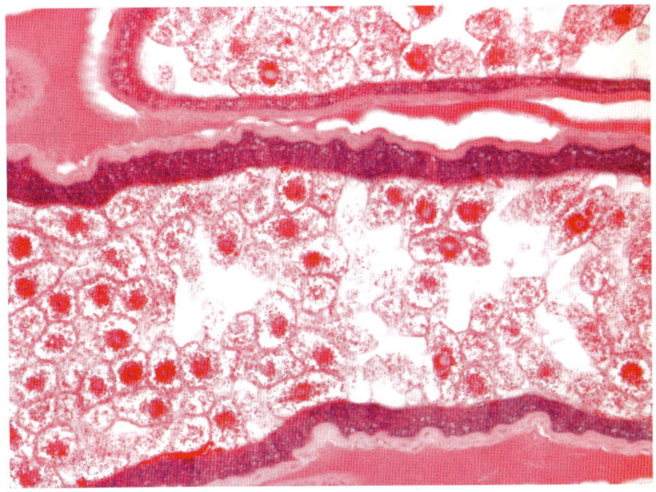

FIGURE 9.48

Numerous eggs are seen in a cross section of *Trichuris trichiura* (whipworm) (hematoxylin and eosin).

ANCILLARY STUDIES

Stool examination for ova and parasites is a helpful diagnostic test.

DIFFERENTIAL DIAGNOSIS

The differential diagnosis is primarily that of other helminthic infections. An ulcerative inflammatory process similar to Crohn's disease has been described associated with both whipworm and hookworm infection.

PROGNOSIS AND THERAPY

Antihelminthic treatment is recommended, and similar drugs may be used against all three worms. Intestinal obstruction (particularly in *Ascaris* infection) may require surgery. Iron supplementation may be required for infections causing anemia.

STRONGYLOIDES STERCORALIS

This nematode has a worldwide distribution. In the United States, it is endemic in the Southeast, urban areas with large immigrant populations, and mental institutions. This infection occurs primarily in adults, many of whom are hospitalized, have chronic illnesses, or are immunocompromised. Strongyloides stercoralis penetrates the skin, enters the venous system, travels to the lungs, and then migrates up the respiratory tree and down the esophagus to eventually reach the small intestine. The female lives in the small intestine and lays eggs there, thus perpetuating the cycle. This capability of autoinfection allows it to reside in the host and produce illness for upwards of 30 years.

CLINICAL FEATURES

Symptoms and signs include diarrhea, abdominal pain and tenderness, nausea, vomiting, weight loss, malabsorption, and GI bleeding. GI symptoms may be accompanied by rash, eosinophilia, urticaria, pruritus, and pulmonary symptoms. However, many patients are asymptomatic. S. stercoralis can disseminate in immunocompromised patients, causing severe and even fatal illness.

STRONGYLOIDIASIS—FACT SHEET

Definition

- Helminthic infection infecting the bowel; may cause fatal disseminated disease in immunocompromised patients

Incidence and Location

- Large bowel, small bowel, stomach

Clinical Features

- Diarrhea, abdominal pain and tenderness, nausea, vomiting, weight loss, malabsorption, and gastrointestinal bleeding
- Often accompanied by rash, eosinophilia, urticaria, pruritus, and pulmonary symptoms
- Many patients are asymptomatic
- May disseminate in immunocompromised patients, causing fatal illness

PATHOLOGIC FEATURES

GROSS FINDINGS

Lesions may be seen in the stomach, as well as the small and large intestines. Endoscopically, colonic findings include ulcers, which may be aphthoid, and pancolitis; features of pseudomembranous colitis have also been reported.

MICROSCOPIC FINDINGS

Histologically, both adult worms and larvae may be found in the crypts (Fig. 9.49), but they may be difficult to detect. Adult worms typically have sharply pointed tails that may be curved. Other histologic features include ulcers (which may be fissuring), edema, and a dense eosinophilic and neutrophilic infiltrate. Granulomas may also be seen, often mixed with eosinophilic and neutrophilic infiltrates. In biopsies with an eosinophil-rich inflammatory infiltrate, step sectioning may reveal degenerating parasitic forms or eggs.

STRONGYLOIDIASIS—PATHOLOGIC FEATURES

Gross Findings

- Ulcers, which may be aphthoid
- Pancolitis
- Pseudomembranous colitis rarely reported

Microscopic Findings

- Both adult worms and larvae may be found in the crypts
- Adult worms typically have sharply pointed tails that may be curved
- Histologic features include ulcers (which may be fissuring), edema, and a dense eosinophilic and neutrophilic infiltrate
- Granulomas may also be seen

Differential Diagnosis

- Other infectious processes, especially other helminthic infections
- Crohn's disease
- Ulcerative colitis
- Pseudomembranous colitis from other causes

ANCILLARY STUDIES

Stool examination is the primary ancillary technique for diagnosis.

DIFFERENTIAL DIAGNOSIS

The differential diagnosis is primarily that of other helminthic infections and infectious processes, although the histologic inflammatory pattern may mimic pseudomembranous colitis, Crohn's disease, and ulcerative colitis.

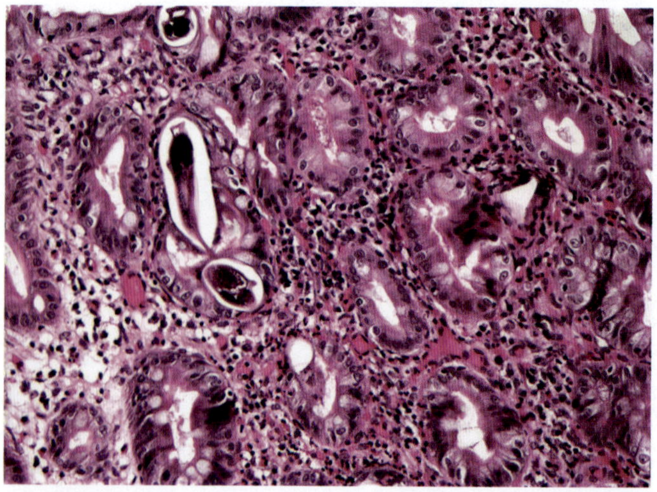

FIGURE 9.49
Strongyloides organisms within colonic crypts have pointed tails (hematoxylin and eosin).

Prognosis and Therapy

Antihelminthic treatment with agents such as thiabendazole is required.

ANISAKIS SIMPLEX (ANISAKIASIS) AND RELATED SPECIES

These nematodes parasitize fish and sea mammals, and humans generally ingest them when eating raw and pickled fish.

CLINICAL FEATURES

The most common clinical manifestations are those of acute gastric anisakiasis, including epigastric pain, nausea, and vomiting, often within 12 hours of consuming contaminated food. Colonic manifestations have also been well described, presenting with abdominal pain and distention, often accompanied by peripheral eosinophilia. *Anisakis* spp. also have allergenic potential, and some patients with gastroallergic anisakiasis manifest both GI and hypersensitivity symptoms such as urticaria, angioedema, eosinophilia, and anaphylaxis.

ANISAKIASIS—FACT SHEET

Definition
- Parasitic infection most often associated with consumption of raw fish

Incidence and Location
- Common in stomach; rare in colon and small bowel

Clinical Features
- Abdominal pain and distention
- Peripheral eosinophilia
- May cause gastroallergic anisakiasis, featuring both gastrointestinal and hypersensitivity symptoms

Prognosis and Therapy
- Endoscopic or surgical removal of worm

Pathologic Features

Gross Findings

The stomach is the most frequent site of involvement, although the small bowel, colon, and appendix may also be involved. Endoscopic findings include mucosal edema, friability, hemorrhage, erosions, and ulcers. Sometimes larvae may be seen endoscopically.

Microscopic Findings

Histologic findings include an inflammatory infiltrate rich in eosinophils, which often extends transmurally into serosal and mesenteric tissues. Eosinophilic microabscesses, granulomas, and giant cells may also be seen. The inflammatory changes may be centered around a worm. Larvae (ranging from 0.5–3.0 cm in length) are occasionally seen in tissue sections.

ANISAKIASIS—PATHOLOGIC FEATURES

Gross Findings
- Mucosal edema, friability, hemorrhage, erosions, and ulcers
- Larvae may be seen endoscopically

Microscopic Findings
- Inflammatory infiltrate rich in eosinophils, often extends transmurally into serosal and mesenteric tissues
- Eosinophilic microabscesses, granulomas, and giant cells may also be seen
- Inflammatory changes may be centered around a worm
- Larvae are occasionally seen in tissue sections

Differential Diagnosis
- Primarily other helminths

Ancillary Studies

No ancillary studies are helpful in anisakiasis because worms and larvae are rarely seen in stool samples.

Differential Diagnosis

The differential diagnosis primarily includes other worms. The size and morphology of the worm usually confirm the diagnosis.

Prognosis and Therapy

Endoscopic removal of the worm is the therapy of choice.

TREMATODES

SCHISTOSOMIASIS

All species of *Schistosoma* are capable of causing significant GI disease. In addition, patients with Schistosoma-related liver disease may also have associated portal colopathy and GI bleeding.

CLINICAL FEATURES

Patients generally present with diarrhea (often bloody) accompanied by anemia, weight loss, and protein-losing enteropathy. More dramatic GI presentations have also been described, including profound dysentery-like illness, obstruction, perforation, intussusception, rectal prolapse, fistulas, and perianal abscesses. Intestinal schistosomiasis is most often caused by *Schistosoma mansoni*, *Schistosoma japonicum*, *Schistosoma mekongi*, and *Schistosoma intercalatum*. *Schistosoma haematobium* may cause appendicitis.

PATHOLOGIC FEATURES

GROSS FINDINGS

Any level of the alimentary tract may be affected. Endoscopically, schistosomiasis can cause a striking inflammatory polyposis (particularly in the distal colon) with associated mucosal granularity, friability, and punctate ulcers and hemorrhages.

MICROSCOPIC FINDINGS

Histologically, inflammatory polyps and mucosal ulcers with associated granulomatous inflammation and eosinophilic infiltrates are typical. Eggs are occasionally seen in histologic specimens, and sometimes they are calcified. Remote disease may show only calcified eggs with no inflammatory infiltrate (Fig. 9.50). Eggs of different *Schistosoma* spp. may be distinguished from one another by the presence and location of spines. For example, *Schistosoma mansoni* eggs have a lateral spine, whereas *S. haematobium* eggs have a terminal spine, and spine are minute or absent on *S. japonicum* eggs. Schistosome eggs are variably acid fast.

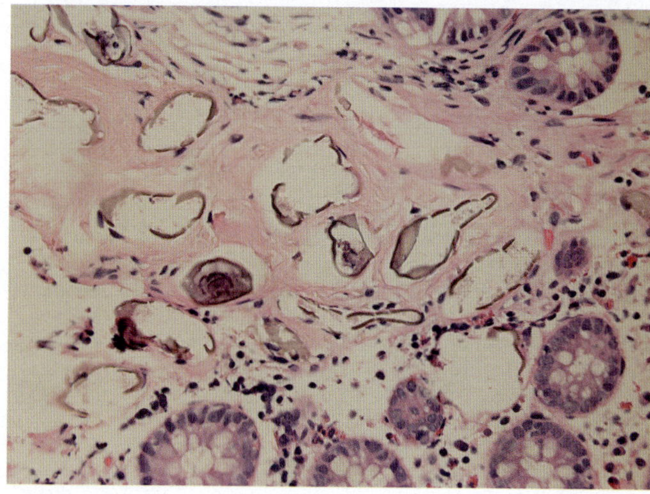

FIGURE 9.50

Remote colonic infection with schistosomes may show calcified eggs with no inflammatory reaction (hematoxylin and eosin).

SCHISTOSOMIASIS—FACT SHEET

Definition
- Parasitic disease causing numerous gastrointestinal and hepatic manifestations

Incidence and Location
- Any level of the alimentary tract

Clinical Features
- Diarrhea (often bloody), accompanied by anemia, weight loss, and protein-losing enteropathy
- Profound dysentery-like illness, obstruction, perforation, intussusception, rectal prolapse, fistulas, and perianal abscesses have also been described
- Patients with schistosome-related cirrhosis may have varices and portal colopathy

Prognosis and Therapy
- Antiparasitic agents such as praziquantel

SCHISTOSOMIASIS—PATHOLOGIC FEATURES

Gross Findings
- Any level of the alimentary tract may be affected
- Striking inflammatory polyposis (particularly in the distal colon) with associated mucosal granularity, friability, and punctate ulcers and hemorrhages

Microscopic Findings
- Inflammatory polyps and mucosal ulcers with associated granulomatous inflammation and an eosinophilic infiltrate
- Eggs are occasionally seen in histologic specimens
- Remote disease may show only calcified eggs with no inflammatory infiltrate

Differential Diagnosis
- Other helminthic infections

ANCILLARY STUDIES

Stool for ova and parasites is a helpful ancillary test. Serologic testing may also be helpful, especially outside of endemic areas. History of travel to an endemic area may be invaluable.

DIFFERENTIAL DIAGNOSIS

The differential diagnosis is primarily that of other helminthic infections or other granulomatous infections if eggs or worms are not visible.

PROGNOSIS AND THERAPY

Antiparasitic agents, such as praziquantel, are the treatment for schistosomiasis.

ACKNOWLEDGEMENT

The author thanks Dr. Laura W. Lamps for her work on this chapter in previous editions and for her guidance in creating this revision.

SUGGESTED READINGS

General

1. Lai KK, Lamps LW. Enterocolitis in immunocompromised patients. *Semin Diagn Pathol.* 2014;31:176–191.
2. Lamps LW. Infectious diseases of the lower gastrointestinal tract. *Surg Pathol Clin.* 2010;3:297–326.
3. Lamps LW. Update on infectious enterocolitides and the diseases that they mimic. *Histopathology.* 2015;66:3–14.
4. Nostrant TT, Kumar NB, Appelman HD. Histopathology differentiates acute self-limited colitis from ulcerative colitis. *Gastroenterology.* 1987;92:318–328.

Cytomegalovirus

5. Chetty R, Roskell DE. Cytomegalovirus infection in the gastrointestinal tract. *J Clin Pathol.* 1994;47:968–972.
6. Kambham N, Vig R, Cartwright CA, et al. Cytomegalovirus infection in steroid-refractory ulcerative colitis; a case-control study. *Am J Surg Pathol.* 2004;28:365–373.
7. Keates J, Lagahee S, Crilley P, et al. CMV enteritis causing segmental ischemia and massive intestinal hemorrhage. *Gastrointest Endosc.* 2001;53:355–359.
8. Mills AM, Guo FP, Copland AP, et al. A comparison of CMV detection in gastrointestinal mucosal biopsies using immunohistochemistry and PCR performed on formalin-fixed, paraffin-embedded tissue. *Am J Surg Pathol.* 2013;37:995–1000.

Herpes Simplex Virus

9. Colemont LJ, Pen JH, Pelckmans PA, et al. Herpes simplex virus type 1 colitis: an unusual cause of diarrhea. *Am J Gastroenterol.* 1990;85:1182–1185.
10. Goodell SE, Quinn TC, Mkrtichian E, et al. Herpes simplex virus proctitis in homosexual men. clinical, sigmoidoscopic, and histopathological features. *N Eng J Med.* 1983;308:868–871.
11. Greenson JK, Beschorner WE, Boitnott JK, Yardley JH. Prominent mononuclear cell infiltrate is characteristic of herpes esophagitis. *Hum Pathol.* 1991;22:541–549.

Adenovirus

12. Shayan K, Saunders F, Roberts E, et al. Adenovirus colitis in pediatric patients following bone marrow transplantation: report of 2 cases and review of the literature. *Arch Pathol Lab Med.* 2003;127:1615–1618.
13. Yan Z, Nguyen S, Poles M, et al. Adenovirus colitis in human immunodeficiency virus infection. an underdiagnosed entity. *Am J Surg Pathol.* 1998;22:1101–1106.

AIDS Enterocolopathy

14. Rabeneck L. AIDS enteropathy. what's in a name? *J Clin Gastroenterol.* 1994;19:154–157.

Sarcina spp

15. Al Rasheed MR, Senseng CG. Sarcina ventriculi: review of the literature. *Arch Pathol Lab Med.* 2016;140(12):1441–1445.
16. Lam-Himlin D, Tsiatis AC, Montgomery E, et al. Sarcina organisms in the gastrointestinal tract: a clinicopathologic and molecular study. *Am J Surg Pathol.* 2011;bi35(11):1700–1705.

Escherichia coli

17. Johnson KE, Thorpe CM, Sears CL. The emerging clinical importance of non-O157 Shiga toxin-producing Escherichia coli. *Clin Infect Dis.* 2006;43:1587–1595.
18. Kelly J, Oryshak A, Wenetsek M, et al. The colonic pathology of E. coli 0157:H7 infection. *Am J Surg Pathol.* 1990;14:87–92.

Salmonellosis

19. Dougan G, Baker S. Salmonella enterica serovar typhi and the pathogenesis of typhoid fever. *Annu Rev Microbiol.* 2014;68:317–336.
20. Kraus MD, Amatya B, Kimula Y. Histopathology of typhoid enteritis. morphologic and immunophenotypic findings. *Mod Pathol.* 1999;12:949–955.

Shigellosis

21. Mathan MM, Mathan VI. Morphology of rectal mucosa of patients with shigellosis. *Rev Infect Dis.* 1991;13(suppl 4):314–318.
22. Speelman P, Kabir I, Islam M. Distribution and spread of colonic lesions in shigellosis: a colonoscopic study. *J Infect Dis.* 1984;150:899–903.

Campylobacter spp

23. Price AB, Jewkes J, Sanderson PJ. Acute diarrhoea. Campylobacter colitis and the role of rectal biopsy. *J Clin Pathol.* 1979;32:990–997.
24. Schneider EN, Havens JM, Goldblum JR, et al. Molecular detection of Campylobacter infection in cases of focal active colitis. *Mod Pathol.* 2007;31(1):160.

Yersinia spp

25. Gleason TH, Patterson SD. The pathology of Yersinia enterocolitica ileocolitis. *Am J Surg Pathol.* 1982;6:347–355.
26. Lamps LW, Madhusudhan KT, Greenson JK, et al. The role of Y. enterocolitica and Y. pseudotuberculosis in granulomatous appendicitis. a histologic and molecular study. *Am J Surg Pathol.* 2001;25: 508–515.
27. Lamps LW, Madhusudhan KT, Havens JM, et al. Pathogenic Yersinia enterocolitica and Yersinia pseudotuberculosis DNA is detected in bowel and mesenteric nodes from Crohn's disease patients. *Am J Surg Pathol.* 2003;27:220–227.

Clostridial Diseases of the Gut

28. Aslam S, Musher DM. An update on the diagnosis, treatment, and prevention of Clostridium-difficile associated disease. *Gastroenterol Clin North Am.* 2006;35:315–335.
29. Dignan CR, Greenson JK. Can ischemic colitis be differentiated from C. difficile colitis in biopsy specimens. *Am J Surg Pathol.* 1997;21:706–710.
30. Rodemann JF, Dubberke ER, Reske KA, et al. Incidence of Clostridium difficile infection in inflammatory bowel disease. *Clin Gastroenterol Hepatol.* 2007;5:339–344.
31. Sachak T, Arnold MA, Naini BV, et al. Neutropenic enterocolitis: new insights into a deadly entity. *Am J Surg Pathol.* 2015;39 1635-1342.

Klebsiella oxytoca

32. Hogenauer C, Langner C, Beubler E, et al. Klebsiella oxytoca as a causative organism of antibiotic-associated hemorrhagic colitis. *N Engl J Med.* 2006;355:2418–2426.

Mycobacterial Infections of the Intestine

33. Donoghue HD, Holton J. Intestinal tuberculosis. *Curr Opin Infect Dis.* 2009;22:490–496.
34. Farhi DC, Mason UG, Horsburgh CR. Pathologic findings in disseminated Mycobacterium avium-intracellulare infection. a report of 11 cases. *Am J Clin Pathol.* 1986;85:67–72.
35. Makharia GK, Srivastava S, Das P, et al. Clinical, endoscopic, and histological differentiations between Crohn's disease and intestinal tuberculosis. *Am J Gastroenterol.* 2010;105:642–651.
36. Roth RI, Owen RL, Keren DF, et al. Intestinal infection with MAI in acquired immune deficiency syndrome (AIDS): histological and clinical comparison with Whipple's disease. *Dig Dis Sci.* 1985;5:497–504.

Syphilis and Sexually Acquired Proctocolitis

37. Arnold CA, Roth R, Arsenescu R, et al. Sexually transmitted infectious colitis vs inflammatory bowel disease: distinguishing features from a case-controlled study. *Am J Clin Pathol.* 2015;144(5):771–781.

38. Arnold CA, Limketkai BN, Illei PB, et al. Syphilitic and lymphogranuloma venereum (LGV) proctocolitis: clues to a frequently missed diagnosis. *Am J Surg Pathol*. 2013;37(1):38–46.
39. Voltaggio L, Montgomery EA, Ali MA, et al. Sex, lies, and gastrointestinal tract biopsies: a review of selected sexually transmitted proctocolitides. *Adv Anat Pathol*. 2014;21:83–93.
40. Korner M, Gebbers JO. Clinical significance of human intestinal spirochetosis—a morphologic approach. *Infection.*. 2003;31: 341–349.

Fungal Infection of the Gastrointestinal Tract

41. Deng ZL, Connor DH. Progressive disseminated penicilliosis caused by Penicillium marneffei. Report of eight cases and differentiation of the causative organism from Histoplasma capsulatum. *Am J Clin Pathol*. 1985;84:323–327.
42. Dioverti MV, Cawcutt KA, Abidi M, et al. Gastrointestinal mucormycosis in immunocompromised hosts. *Mycoses.*. 2015;58:714–718.
43. Geramizadeh B, Foroughi R, Keshtkar-Jahromi M, et al. Gastrointestinal basidiobolomycosis, an emerging infection in the immunocompetent host: a report of 14 patients. *J Med Microbiol*. 2012;61(Pt 12):1770–1774.
44. Lamps LW, Molina CP, West AB, et al. The pathologic spectrum of gastrointestinal and hepatic histoplasmosis. *Am J Clin Pathol*. 2000;113:64–72.
45. Lamps LW, Lai KK, Milner Jr. DA. Fungal infections of the gastrointestinal tract in the immunocompromised host: an update. *Adv Anat Pathol*. 2014;21:217–227.

Parasitic Infections of the Gastrointestinal Tract

46. Cama VA, Mathison BA. Infections by Intestinal Coccidia and Giardia duodenalis. *Clin Lab Med*. 2015;35:423–444.
47. Cao J, Liu WJ, Xu XY, Zou XP. Endoscopic findings and clinicopathologic characteristics of colonic schistosomiasis: a report of 46 cases. *World J Gastroenterol*. 2010;16:723–727.
48. Cook GC. The clinical significance of gastrointestinal helminths—a review. *Trans R Soc Trop Med Hyg*. 1986;80:675–685.
49. Daschner A, Alonso-Gomez A, Cabanas R, et al. Gastroallergic anisakiasis. borderline between food allergy and parasitic disease—clinical and allergologic evaluation of 20 patients with confirmed acute parasitism. *J Allergy Clin Immunol*. 2000;105:176–181.
50. de Oliveira RB, Troncon LEA, Dantas RO, et al. Gastrointestinal manifestations of Chagas' disease. *Am J Gastroenterol*. 1998;93: 884–889.
51. da Silveira AB, Lemos EM, Adad SJ, et al. Megacolon in Chagas disease: a study of inflammatory cells, enteric nerves, and glial cells. *Hum Pathol*. 2007;38(8):1256–1264.
52. Keiser PB, Nutman TB. Strongyloides stercoralis in the Immunocompromised Population. *Clin Microbiol Rev*. 2004;17: 208–217.
53. Oberhuber G, Mesteri I, Kopf W, Muller H. Demonstration of trophozoites of G. lamblia in ileal mucosal biopsy specimens may reveal giardiasis in patients with significantly inflamed parasite-free duodenal mucosa. *Am J Surg Pathol*. 2016;90:1280–1285.
54. Variyam EP, Gogate P, Hassan M, et al. Nondysenteric intestinal amebiasis. colonic morphology and search for Entamoeba histolytica adherence and invasion. *Dig Dis Sci*. 1989;34:732–740.

10

Non-neoplastic Disorders of the Colon

Rish K. Pai, MD, PhD

Mucosal biopsies from the colon are obtained most commonly (1) in acutely symptomatic patients with the possibility of an ischemic, infectious, or drug-induced colitis; (2) when graft-versus-host disease (GVHD) needs to be ruled out; or (3) in those with chronic symptoms in whom the main consideration is inflammatory bowel disease (IBD). In other instances, patients with diarrhea and normal colonoscopy results are biopsied to rule out lymphocytic or collagenous ("microscopic") colitis. An understanding of normal variations and artifacts is essential while interpreting mucosal biopsies from the colon. The bowel preparation itself induces some artifacts, and minor foci of lamina propria hemorrhage, surface erosion without lamina propria inflammation, and scattered crypt epithelial apoptosis are common and should not be misinterpreted as abnormal findings. Similarly, knowledge of normal variations in histology is also helpful to avoid misdiagnosis. The cecal and right colon mucosa normally has a higher density of lamina propria mononuclear cell infiltrate, which should not be confused with a colitis, and the rectal mucosa often shows slight architectural disarray that must not be misinterpreted as manifestation of a chronic colitis.

Despite the wide array of underlying causes, the histologic alterations in inflammatory disorders of the colon are limited and can be classified only into one of few categories. The pattern of colitis may be categorized as focal or diffuse (Fig. 10.1A and B) based on the extent of inflammatory lymphoplasmacytic infiltrate in the lamina propria. Diffuse colitis is graded into mild, moderate, or severe depending on the degree of activity, which in the vast majority of cases implies neutrophilic infiltration into the surface or crypt epithelium (or both). Rarely, eosinophils may be the predominant acute inflammatory cell type in the lamina propria with significant intraepithelial infiltration, a pattern that can be classified as eosinophilic colitis. Abnormal neoplastic infiltrate in the lamina propria in systemic mastocytosis or Langerhans cell histiocytosis may also induce a prominent eosinophilic infiltrate and mimic a colitis and should be considered in the differential diagnosis of an eosinophilic colitis. A diffuse colitis may also be associated with increased intraepithelial lymphocytes or an abnormal subepithelial collagen layer and defines lymphocytic and collagenous colitis (CC), respectively. A diagnosis of chronic colitis is based on inflammatory, architectural, or metaplastic features (Fig. 10.1C) and is discussed in greater detail later. Epithelial injury from vascular causes typically results in an ischemic or hemorrhagic pattern of colitis (Fig. 10.1D). Finally, a spectrum of disorders may be associated with minimal or no inflammation and should be considered before diagnosing a biopsy as within normal limits. Common disorders in this category include infections in immunocompromised hosts, GVHD (Fig. 10.1E) and its mimics, and amyloidosis. A mucosal biopsy diagnosis based on the specific morphologic pattern of injury rather than a descriptive one greatly aids gastroenterologists in formulating a differential diagnosis and working up patients with any ancillary testing that may be needed. Whereas focal or diffuse active colitis is usually associated with infections, drugs, or early IBD, chronic colitis is a hallmark of IBD or one of its mimics. Infectious colitis is discussed in detail in Chapter x, and the distinction of acute self-limited colitis from IBD is discussed in detail later under the differential diagnosis of IBD.

IDIOPATHIC INFLAMMATORY BOWEL DISEASE

Chronic injury in mucosal biopsies is typically diagnosed based on inflammatory, architectural, or metaplastic features. Basal lymphoplasmacytosis is by far the most useful inflammatory feature that helps in establishing the diagnosis of a chronic colitis and manifests as a deep band of lymphocytes and plasma cells that separates the base of the crypts from the muscularis mucosae. Architectural crypt disarray; crypt branching, shortening, or loss; and pyloric gland or Paneth cell metaplasia are also features typically used to favor a chronic colitis. A diagnosis of chronic colitis usually implies a high probability of IBD, but a number of well-defined IBD mimics are known that should always be ruled out before giving patients a serious diagnosis that carries important lifelong surveillance implications.

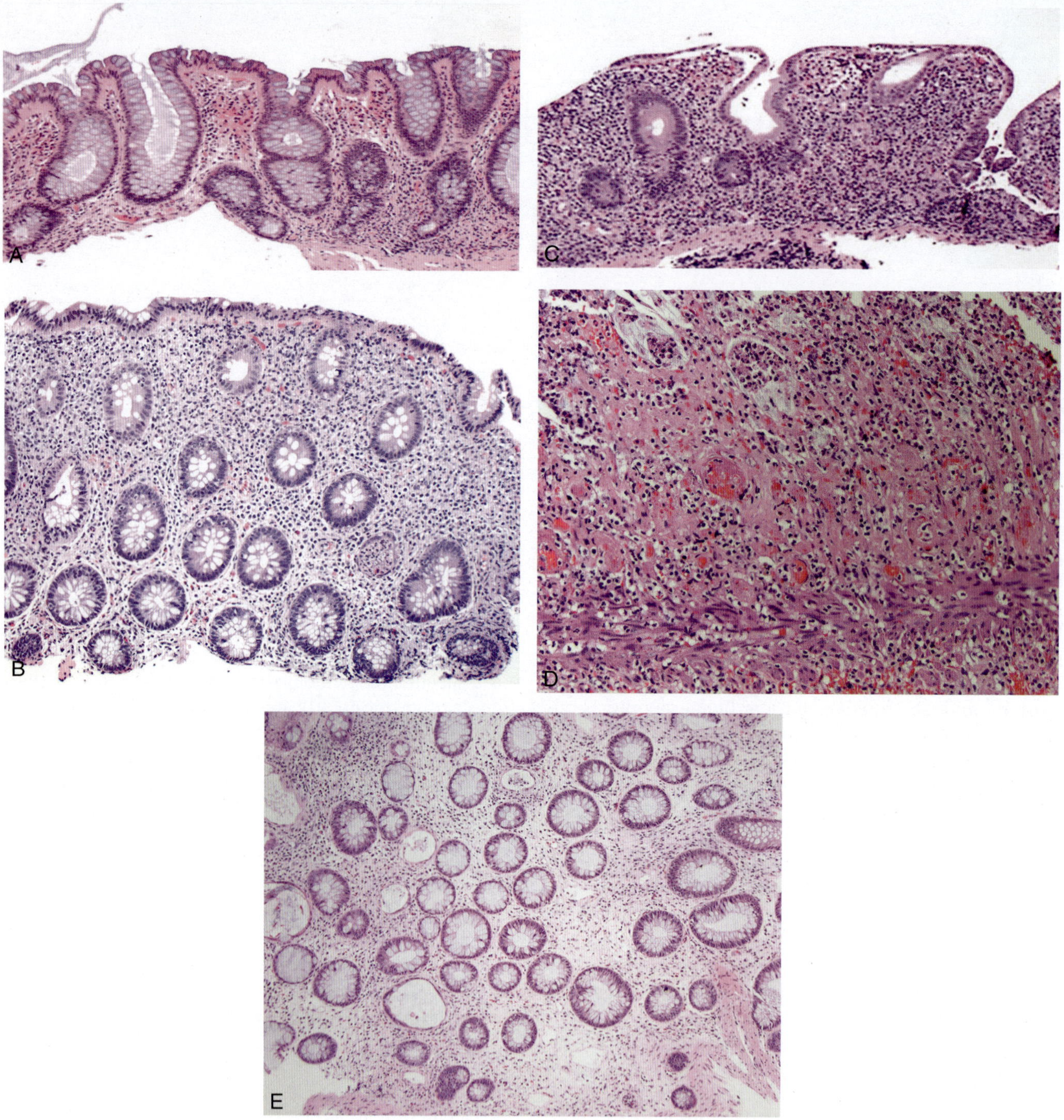

FIGURE 10.1

Common morphologic patterns of injury in mucosal biopsies from the colon. Focal active colitis shows a localized, sharply demarcated increase in lamina propria inflammation that may be associated with cryptitis, crypt abscess or erosion (**A**). Diffuse active colitis shows a uniformly increased lamina propria infiltrate with variable degrees of activity (**B**). Chronic colitis is characterized by a basal lymphoplasmacytic infiltrate that separates the base of the crypts from the muscularis mucosae (**C**). Architectural disarray is not necessary for a diagnosis of chronic colitis. Lamina propria hemorrhage or hyalinization is typical for acute ischemic colitis pattern of injury (**D**), but some disorders such as graft-versus-host disease are quite pauciinflammatory and may be mistaken for a normal biopsy (**E**).

Ulcerative colitis and Crohn's disease are the two most common manifestations of IBD and differ significantly in their clinical presentation, morphologic patterns of injury, natural history, therapy, and response to treatment. These differences, particularly with regard to recommended treatment options and surveillance strategies, underscore the importance of distinguishing between the two entities. Although classic cases can be easily separated, there may be gross, clinical, and histologic overlap not only between ulcerative colitis and Crohn's disease but also with other inflammatory disorders of the colon.

ULCERATIVE COLITIS

Ulcerative colitis is a chronic colitis of unknown cause characterized by bloody diarrhea, mucosa-limited disease, and a fluctuating clinical course.

CLINICAL FEATURES

Ulcerative colitis has a slightly higher incidence in males and occurs at all ages, with the major peak incidence in the age range of 15 to 25 years and a minor peak in the seventh decade of life. There is a familial association, with up to 25% of patients having a family member affected with IBD.

Clinically, ulcerative colitis is characterized by recurrent episodes of bloody diarrhea that can undergo spontaneous or therapy-induced remission. The initial presentation may be indolent in onset or severe and acute, presenting with a fulminant colitis. Ulcerative proctitis occurs in 30% to 50% of patients at presentation. Approximately one-third present with left-sided colitis and the remaining with a pancolitis. The terminal ileum may also be involved in a subset of those with a severe pancolitis and rarely upper gastrointestinal (GI) involvement may be present in an otherwise typical ulcerative colitis. However, the distribution of disease is not static and may change over time. Between 20% and 30% of patients with ulcerative colitis require a colectomy during the course of their disease.

RADIOLOGIC FEATURES

Endoscopy with biopsy has replaced radiology in the initial diagnosis of IBD. Features that may be seen radiographically in patients with ulcerative colitis include continuous involvement of the colon with ulcers or polyps and the occasional finding of megacolon. Strictures, fistulas, "thumbprinting," and skip areas are not seen.

ENDOSCOPIC FEATURES

The gross endoscopic appearance of ulcerative colitis varies with the degree of activity, duration of disease, and response to therapy. It is characterized by diffuse disease, with rectal involvement extending proximally. In the more active phases, the mucosa is typically erythematous and friable, with a granular appearance (Fig. 10.2). Erosions and ulcers are common. Quiescent disease may appear normal or granular with areas of punctuate erythema (Fig. 10.3). Pseudopolyps that represent mucosal remnants and inflammatory polyps may be seen in active or quiescent disease (Fig. 10.4). In most cases, the normal submucosal vascular pattern is lost and is an important clue to the endoscopist in favor of a chronic colitis. In patients who have had repeated bouts of colitis, the normal haustral folds may be lost, giving the lumen a tubelike appearance. The transition between normal and abnormal mucosa is generally gradual but may be abrupt. Variations to this classic appearance may occur in some patients and are discussed next.

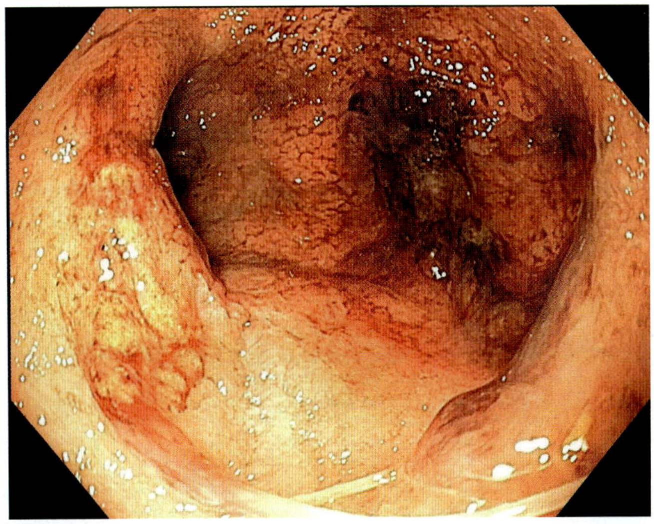

FIGURE 10.2
Chronic ulcerative colitis. Colonoscopy image with diffuse erythema and granular appearance

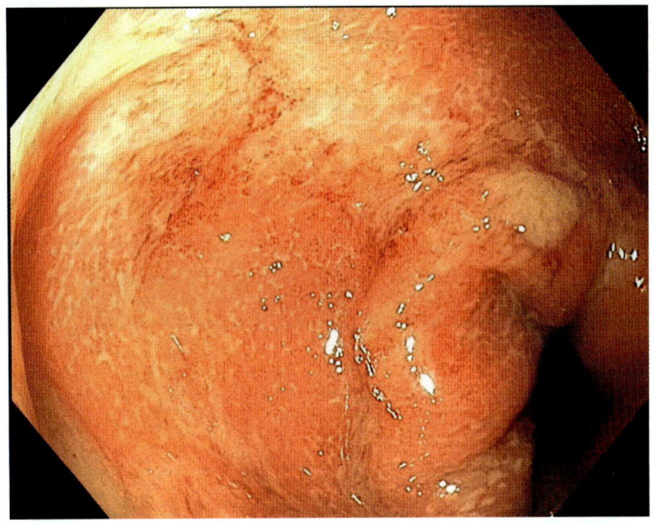

FIGURE 10.3
Quiescent chronic ulcerative colitis. Mucosa is granular with minimal erythema and friability. Mucosal folds are flattened, and the submucosal vascular pattern is lost.

PATHOLOGIC FEATURES

GROSS FINDINGS

The colonic wall is usually of normal thickness with an unremarkable serosa, and strictures are rare in patients

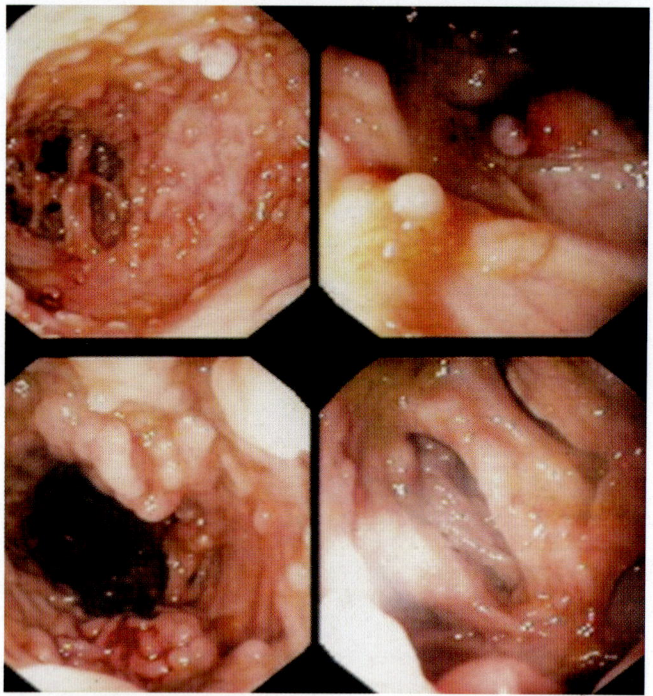

FIGURE 10.4

Chronic ulcerative colitis. Mucosa is diffusely involved by polyps and areas of bridging.

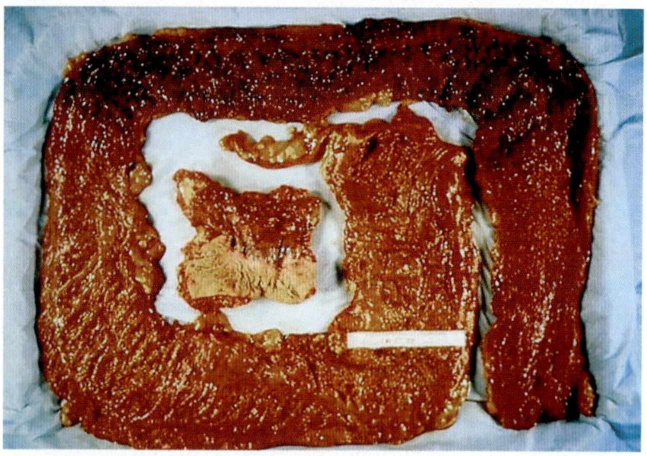

FIGURE 10.5

Ulcerative colitis. Diffusely hemorrhagic mucosa extends from the anorectal junction to the cecum. The bowel wall thickness is grossly normal.

with ulcerative colitis. The mucosa may be flattened, hemorrhagic, and friable (Fig. 10.5) with numerous inflammatory polyps. Disease involvement grossly extends in a continuous manner from the rectum proximally and may involve the entire colon and appendix and even the terminal ileum ("backwash ileitis"). Skip areas are not a feature of ulcerative colitis outside of well recognized exceptions to the rule, discussed in greater detail later.

Microscopic Findings

Biopsy Findings. Morphologically, diagnostic features of a chronic colitis can be broadly divided into architectural, inflammatory, and metaplastic. Architectural features include crypt disarray and branching and result from cycles of recurrent mucosal injury and inadequate repair. Most patients with suspected IBD undergo colonoscopy much earlier in their disease course than in the past. As a result, architectural features of chronicity are seldom pronounced in mucosal biopsies at initial presentation, and pathologists often rely merely on inflammatory and metaplastic features to make a diagnosis of a chronic colitis. Inflammatory features of a chronic colitis include basal lymphoplasmacytosis, which results from a marked increase in lamina propria inflammatory cells involving the entire thickness of the mucosa and creates a distinct band of lymphoplasmacytic inflammation between the base of the crypts and the muscularis mucosa (Fig. 10.6). The lamina propria infiltrate is heterogeneous with a variable number of lymphocytes, plasma cells, and eosinophils. Eosinophils and lymphoid aggregates at the mucosal–submucosal interface can be quite prominent in some cases. Neutrophils are the hallmark of disease activity and may be present within the lamina propria, crypt epithelium (cryptitis), or crypt lumens (crypt abscesses) (Fig. 10.7). Disease activity in chronic colitis is subjectively graded in mucosal biopsies as mild (cryptitis only), moderate (crypt abscesses), and severe (ulcerated mucosa). A loose collection of histiocytes may be present around ruptured crypts and is variously referred to as *mucin granulomas* or *crypt rupture reaction* (Fig. 10.8) and should not be confused with compact sarcoid-like granulomas of Crohn's disease. The injured colonic epithelium is mucin depleted and attenuated, but these findings are not helpful in distinguishing

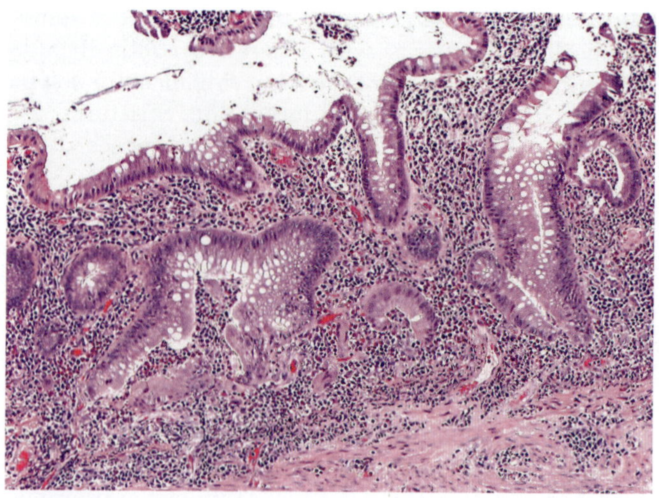

FIGURE 10.6

Ulcerative colitis. Biopsy shows crypt architectural distortion and branching. Crypt abscess extends into lamina propria; basal plasmacytosis diagnostic of a chronic colitis is present.

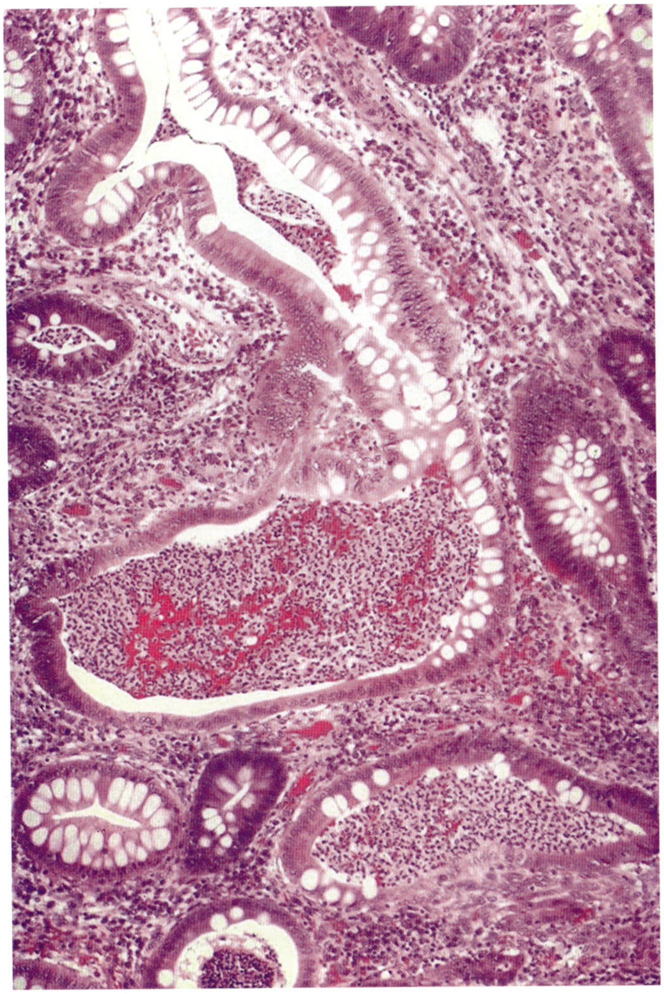

FIGURE 10.7

Ulcerative colitis. Biopsy shows marked inflammation, crypt distortion, and crypt abscesses.

an acute from a chronic colitis. Metaplastic features of chronicity include pyloric gland metaplasia, which is more common in terminal ileum biopsies, and Paneth cell metaplasia, which is helpful in left colon and rectal biopsies. Paneth cells are normal in the proximal colon but are an indicator of chronic mucosal injury and repair in the distal colon. It is important to emphasize that low-grade ischemic injury, radiation, GVHD, and medications can also result in architectural and metaplastic features similar to IBD, and an initial diagnosis of untreated ulcerative colitis or Crohn's disease should not be rendered in the absence of diagnostic inflammatory features of a chronic colitis.

Posttreatment biopsies in patients with IBD may show complete normalization of the mucosa, continued disease activity similar to the initial biopsies, or partial resolution with some evidence of residual injury. The latter group may show a chronic inactive colitis with increased lymphoplasmacytic infiltrate but without neutrophilic infiltration in the epithelium or a chronic quiescent colitis with only mild architectural disarray and/or Paneth cell metaplasia but without any increase in lamina propria inflammation (Fig. 10.9).

Flares of ulcerative colitis occur quite commonly. Endoscopic evaluation with biopsy is done to confirm active ulcerative colitis and to exclude other causes such as *Clostridium difficile* colitis and cytomegalovirus (CMV) infection. CMV infection is quite common in patients with ulcerative colitis, and the presence of numerous CMV inclusions in a patient with active colitis warrants treatment with antiviral medications (Fig. 10.10). The significance of only rare CMV inclusions in an otherwise typical active ulcerative colitis biopsy is less clear, although these patients are often treated with both immunosuppression and antiviral

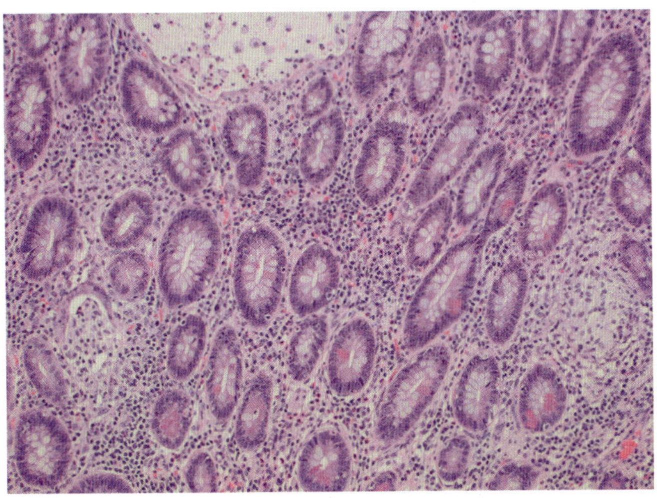

FIGURE 10.8

Rupture of inflamed crypts may lead to mucin extravasation and a loose histiocytic reaction ("crypt rupture reaction") that should not be mistaken for compact sarcoid-like granulomas of Crohn's disease.

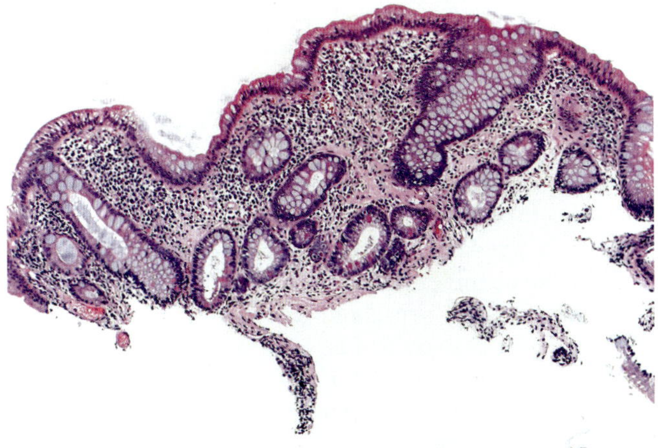

FIGURE 10.9

Quiescent ulcerative colitis. Mild crypt distortion, minimal inflammation, and Paneth cell metaplasia.

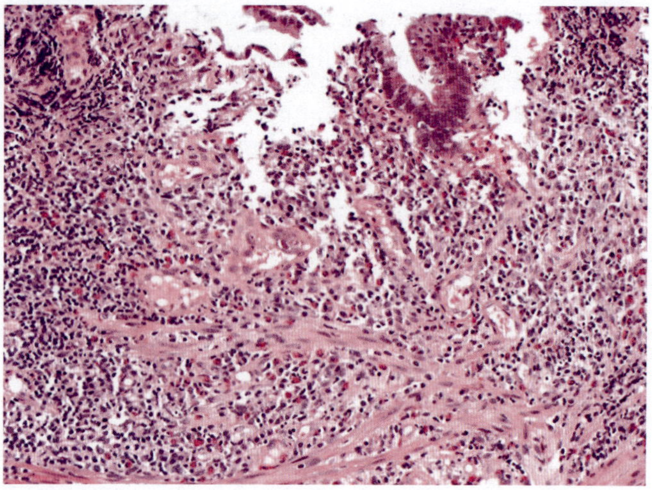

FIGURE 10.10

Cytomegalovirus (CMV) infection in ulcerative colitis. A singe CMV inclusion is seen in the background of severe chronic active colitis.

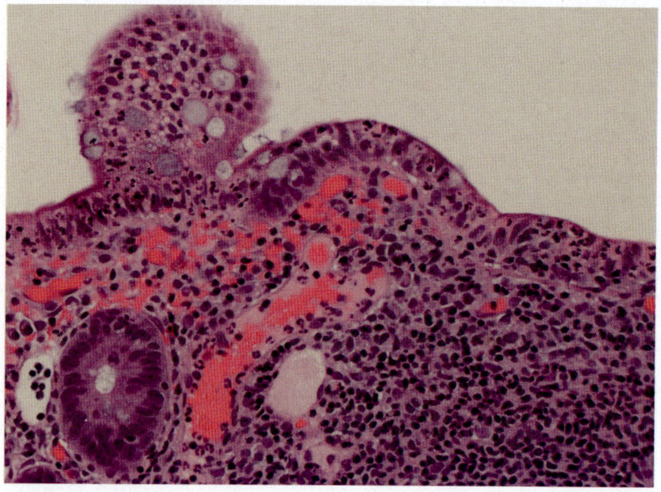

FIGURE 10.11

Backwash ileitis in ulcerative colitis. Mild active inflammation is present in the surface epithelium. Rarely, features of a chronic ileitis may also be present.

medications. Corticosteroids are often used to induce remission of the underlying IBD.

Variants of Ulcerative Colitis

There are defined variants of ulcerative colitis that deviate from the typical appearance already described and deserve mention. Up to 30% of patients with left-sided colitis may have patches of active disease in the right colon, particularly in the cecum near the appendiceal orifice. This finding, often referred to as the *cecal patch*, should not be confused with Crohn's disease. Similarly, patchy disease involvement may be seen in patients with severe fulminant ulcerative colitis who present acutely and undergo a total colectomy to prevent perforation or in patients who have undergone treatment. Ulcerative colitis in the pediatric population may show relative or complete rectal sparing. In adults, rare cases may show relative rectal sparing with decreased disease activity compared with the more proximal colon, but complete rectal sparing is not seen. Ileal involvement by ulcerative colitis ("backwash ileitis") may occur in patients who have severe pancolitis, and this should not be confused with Crohn's disease (Fig. 10.11). Inflammation in the ileum in this setting is often mild, limited to the distal few centimeters, and characterized by mild inflammation in the lamina propria and active neutrophilic infiltration in the crypt or villous epithelium. Chronic changes such as pyloric gland metaplasia, reminiscent of Crohn's disease, may also be seen but are rare. Finally, biopsies from the upper GI tract may show histologic abnormalities in a subset of patients with ulcerative colitis, the most common being a focal active gastritis. A diffuse duodenitis and even a pan-enteritis have been described in rare patients with ulcerative colitis after total colectomy and ileal pouch anal anastomosis. The cause of this diffuse enteritis is unclear.

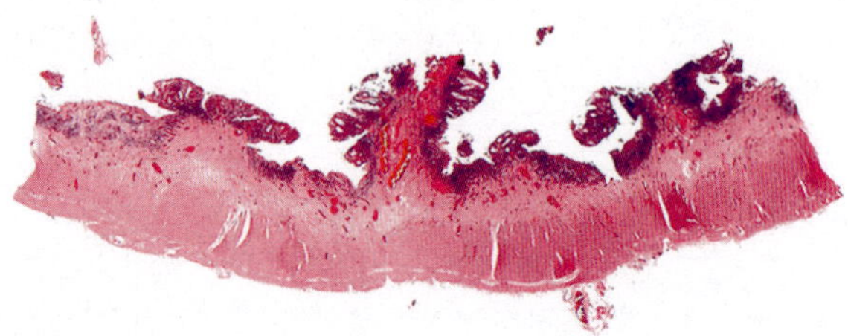

FIGURE 10.12

Ulcerative colitis, resection specimen. Low-power shows diffuse mucosal inflammation that abruptly stops at the mucosa–submucosa interface.

Resection Findings. The inflammatory process is confined to the mucosa in most cases (Fig. 10.12) and shows a cellular inflamed lamina propria on low power, often with crypt architectural disarray and crypt loss. Lymphoid aggregates at the mucosal–submucosal interface may be present and can be numerous in some cases. Disease activity can be variable, ranging from mild cryptitis to mucosal ulcers with associated granulation tissue. Mounds of residual mucosal remnants surrounded by ulcer may stand out as pseudopolyps. (Fig. 10.13). Most patients receive some form of medical therapy before a colectomy, so it is not unusual to see patchy disease involvement in resection specimens. The submucosa may be edematous and congested but is typically without significant inflammation or fibrosis. Lymphoid aggregates may be prominent underneath areas of mucosal ulceration and should not be mistaken for Crohn's disease.

Occasionally, resection specimens for presumed ulcerative colitis show atypical histologic features that preclude a definitive diagnosis of ulcerative colitis and raise the possibility of Crohn's disease. The presence of strictures, fistulas, perianal disease, transmural lymphoid aggregates, granulomas away from injured crypts or deeper in the intestinal wall, and segmental disease in

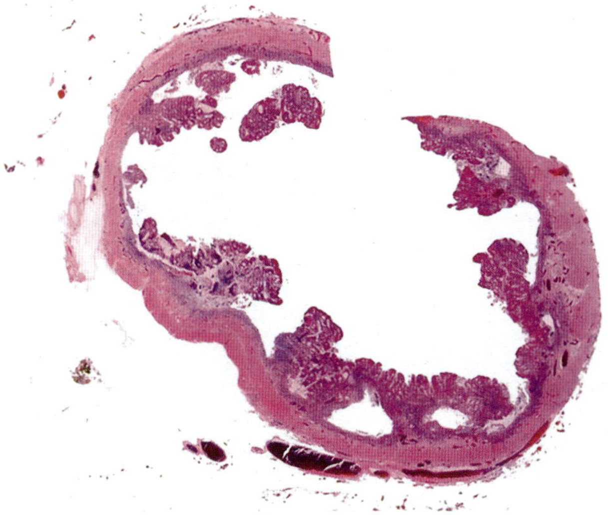

FIGURE 10.13

Ulcerative colitis, resection specimen. Low power shows diffuse involvement by inflammatory polyps and pseudopolyps with mucosal bridging. Inflammation is confined to the mucosa.

an untreated setting are diagnostic features in favor of Crohn's disease. A diagnosis of Crohn's disease in a total colectomy for presumed ulcerative colitis has significant clinical consequences because these patients are not considered candidates for ileal pouch anal anastomosis at most centers. Conversely, defined histologic variants of ulcerative colitis described in the previous section should not be mistaken for Crohn's disease. Despite meticulous work-up and systematic review, rare cases are difficult to classify, and such resection specimens may be diagnosed as IBD, unclassified type. The use of the term *indeterminate colitis* is discouraged. At most centers, these patients are followed closely for definitive signs of Crohn's disease, and an ileal pouch anal anastomosis is eventually performed if no signs of Crohn's disease are seen on follow-up.

Differential Diagnosis. In the early phase of the disease, features of chronicity may not be well established in mucosal biopsies obtained from patients with ulcerative colitis. In this scenario, the main differential diagnosis is with acute self-limited colitis and drug-induced colitis. *Acute self-limited colitis* is a clinical term often used for diarrheal disorders of short duration related to an infectious cause. The biopsy findings in acute self-limited colitis are those of a focal or diffuse active colitis of varying severity. The increased lymphoplasmacytic infiltrate in the lamina propria is typically described as being confined to the upper half of the mucosa but may be full thickness in severe cases. However, the characteristic basal lymphoplasmacytosis of a chronic colitis is absent, and normal colonic crypt architecture is preserved. Similarly, a variety of medications may cause a similar pattern of injury. The most recent addition to this group are immune checkpoint receptor inhibitors that are being used with increasing frequency in the management of a variety of solid tumors.

In the chronic phase of the disease, the differential diagnosis is limited to a chronic infectious colitis or a handful of well-recognized IBD mimics. Infections that can have a chronic relapsing course, such as *C. difficile*, may induce mucosal changes that mimic IBD. Similarly, architectural changes of IBD may be seen in radiation or low-grade ischemic injury, but these can be easily distinguished based on the lack of a prominent inflammatory component. The distinction from diverticular disease associated colitis and diversion colitis can be challenging and is discussed in detail under these entities later.

Ancillary Studies

No specific tests for ulcerative colitis are available. Initially, patients should be tested for infectious causes that are known to be associated with long-standing colitis, particularly to exclude *Shigella* spp., *Salmonella* spp., *Escherichia coli* O157:H7, *Campylobacter jejuni*, and *C. difficile*. Stool studies for ova and parasites as well as exclusion of *Giardia* spp. may be warranted in patients with specific risk factors or relevant travel history. Patients who have a flare of ulcerative colitis while being treated with immunosuppressive therapy may also benefit from testing for CMV and *C. difficile* infection, which can present with deep ulcers in the background of ulcerative colitis. *C. difficile* infections in the setting of ulcerative colitis seldom show the typical pseudomembranous colitis pattern, and microbiologic work-up is necessary for diagnosis. Results of serologic tests for perinuclear antineutrophil cytoplasmic antibody are often positive in patients with ulcerative colitis but have limited utility in differentiating ulcerative colitis from Crohn's disease in difficult cases.

DYSPLASIA IN ULCERATIVE COLITIS

Long-standing ulcerative colitis is associated with an increased risk for dysplasia and adenocarcinoma. This risk is even higher in patients with concurrent ulcerative colitis and primary sclerosing cholangitis. Periodic surveillance biopsies are the mainstay of management for early detection of dysplasia and adenocarcinoma. Four quadrant biopsies every 10 cm of colon that has been involved by disease are usually recommended, in addition to sampling or removal of any visible lesions. Pathologists should record any evidence of chronic colitis, degree of activity, and the presence or absence of dysplasia in their reports from surveillance biopsies. Dysplasia is categorized into negative, indefinite, low grade, and high grade. Intramucosal or invasive adenocarcinoma may also be seen in surveillance biopsies, the latter usually in tissue obtained from visible lesions.

Pathologic Features

Gross Findings

Dysplasia can be found in two distinct forms: endoscopically invisible (also described as "flat") dysplasia that are picked up in random biopsies and endoscopically visible dysplasia that may present as a discrete polypoid lesion or a sessile ill-defined mass. The endoscopic findings are critical, even more so than the grade of dysplasia, when deciding management of patients. This is discussed in greater detail later.

Microscopic Findings

Dysplasia in ulcerative colitis may show cytologic and architectural changes that vary with grade of dysplasia. Architecturally, the crypts may be normal or show crypt budding, crowding, or prominent serration, the latter in the case of serrated dysplasia. Nuclear hyperchromasia, enlargement, and irregularity are often present, and the cytoplasmic features are variable and range from complete mucin depletion to abundant eosinophilic, hypermucinous, or clear cytoplasm reminiscent of foveolar type dysplasia seen in the upper GI tract. Low-grade dysplasia is similar to sporadic tubular adenomas and is characterized by elongated penicillate, hyperchromatic nuclei perpendicular to the basement membrane with variable degree of pseudostratification. An abrupt change from adjacent normal mucosa is helpful in diagnosis of dysplasia (Fig. 10.14). High-grade dysplasia is characterized by more pronounced nuclear changes, including round nuclei no longer perpendicular to the basement membrane (loss of polarity), nuclear pleomorphism, marked hyperchromasia, and nucleolar prominence (Fig. 10.15). In many instances, high-grade dysplasia in the setting of IBD, particularly flat invisible dysplasia, may not show architectural features of crypt crowding and budding. Diagnostic cytologic features described earlier are sufficient to classify such biopsies as high-grade dysplasia. Surveillance biopsies in ulcerative colitis, particularly those obtained during chromoendoscopy, may show serrated lesions with morphological appearance similar to sporadic hyperplastic polyps, sessile serrated adenoma or polyp (SSP), or a traditional serrated adenoma (TSA). The presence of hyperplastic polyp-like change in flat mucosal biopsies in IBD has been referred to as *serrated epithelial change* and does not lead to increased surveillance. SSP and TSA morphology in IBD is almost always seen in biopsies obtained from endoscopically visible lesions. The significance of hyperplastic polyp or SSP in patients with IBD with respect to recommended surveillance intervals is unclear, but the overall risk of cancer appears to be low as long as complete excision of visible lesions is performed.

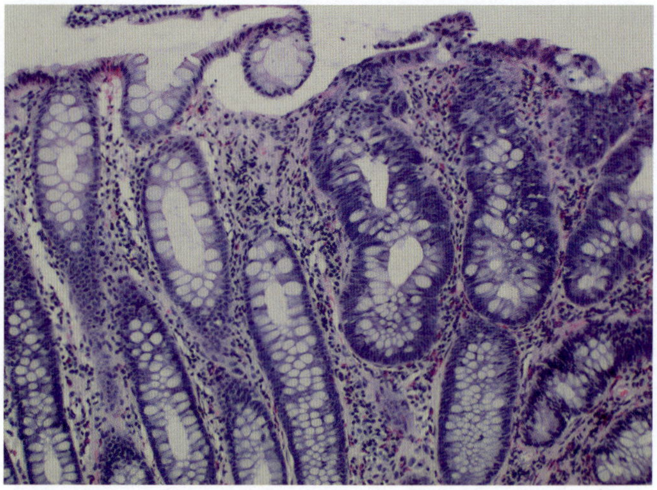

FIGURE 10.14

Invisible low-grade dysplasia in ulcerative colitis. A random colonic biopsy demonstrating nuclear enlargement, nuclear stratification, and loss of surface maturation. Note the abrupt change from adjacent normal colonic mucosa, which is helpful in the diagnosis of dysplasia.

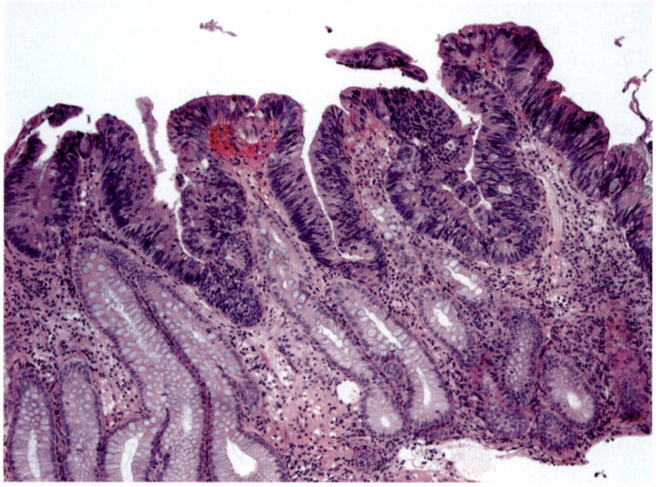

FIGURE 10.15

Dysplasia in ulcerative colitis, high grade. Hyperchromatic and enlarged nuclei, with loss of polarity and marked pleomorphism.

The presence of a visible dysplastic lesion in the background of ulcerative colitis may either represent a sporadic adenoma or colitis-associated dysplasia. Although some molecular differences exist between these two forms of visible dysplasia, it is impossible to separate these lesions based on morphology alone. Fortunately, making this distinction is of little practical importance because management of visible lesions in the setting of ulcerative colitis depends mostly on the endoscopic appearance. Patients with well-circumscribed lesions (Fig. 10.16) that can be removed endoscopically can be safely followed with surveillance after complete polypectomy. Irregular lesions with indistinct borders often require surgical intervention, although advanced endoscopic techniques such as endoscopic mucosal resection and endoscopic submucosal dissection

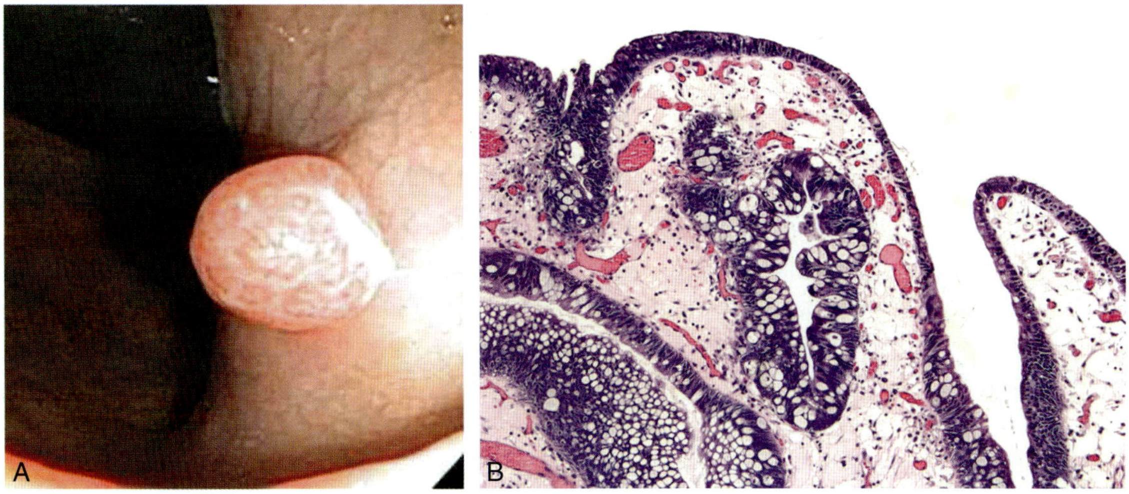

FIGURE 10.16

Visible dysplasia in ulcerative colitis. **A**, Low-grade dysplasia arising in a well-circumscribed polyp. **B**, Nuclear hyperchromasia and stratification and dystrophic goblet cells in low-grade dysplasia.

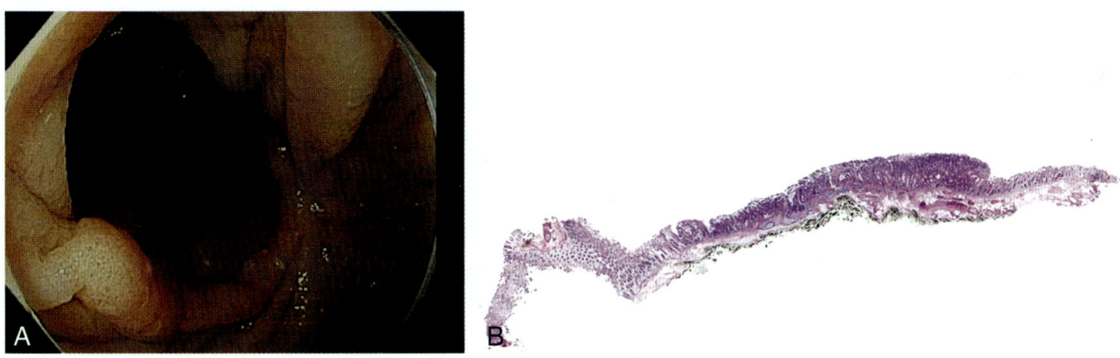

FIGURE 10.17

Visible dysplasia in ulcerative colitis. **A**, A large, flat, irregular plaque-like lesion in ulcerative colitis. **B**, These lesions can now be treated by endoscopic submucosal dissection, which allows complete removal with negative margins.

(Fig. 10.17) are increasingly used at tertiary academic centers.

Invisible dysplasia is becoming increasingly less common with the advent of chromoendoscopy. A single focus of invisible low-grade dysplasia may be followed by increased surveillance. Persistent or multifocal flat low-grade dysplasia and invisible high-grade dysplasia usually warrant a colectomy because of the high risk of concurrent adenocarcinoma.

Differential Diagnosis

Ulcerative colitis must be distinguished from a large number of mimics, including infectious colitis, medication-induced colitis, ischemic colitis, Crohn's disease, diversion colitis, and diverticular disease associated colitis, among others. Long-standing infectious colitis may have many of the features of ulcerative colitis, including increased chronic inflammation, neutrophils, and diffuse colonic involvement. The clinical setting, lack of significant basal lymphoplasmacytosis, and microbiologic work-up are all key to avoiding a misdiagnosis of IBD at initial presentation. Medications, particularly nonsteroidal antiinflammatory drugs (NSAIDs), may present with focal active colitis, chronic active colitis, or one or many ulcers throughout the colon. Histologically, NSAID ulcers are small and discrete and lack the confluent mucosal involvement typically seen in ulcerative colitis on endoscopy. Recently, chronic colitis has also been described in patients on immune checkpoint receptor inhibitor–associated chemotherapy. The presence of a concomitant increase in intraepithelial lymphocytes and prominent apoptosis along with features of a chronic colitis are helpful features in favor of an immunotherapy-associated colitis. Like with other drug-induced colitides, correlation with timeline of disease course and resolution of symptoms after cessation of drug or immunosuppression is needed to establish the diagnosis. Chronic ischemic or radiation colitis can also be mistaken for ulcerative colitis, particularly because ischemia resulting from low vascular flow often affects the left colon, and repeated injury and repair may lead to architectural changes of a chronic colitis. However, these cases lack the typically inflammatory component of ulcerative colitis, and an initial diagnosis of IBD should never be made only on architectural features in an untreated patient. The patchy distribution of the disease is only helpful in distinguishing Crohn's disease from ulcerative colitis at initial presentation. After institution of medical therapy, the mucosa of patients with ulcerative colitis often heals in a patchy distribution. Diverticular disease–associated colitis can have features identical to ulcerative colitis. The distribution of the colitis involving the interdiverticular mucosa in a colonic segment involved with diverticular disease and sparing of the rectum and remaining colon are helpful in making this distinction. Segments of colon that are excluded from the fecal stream develop a diversion colitis characterized by marked lymphoid hyperplasia, cryptitis, and crypt architectural distortion, which mimics ulcerative colitis. Knowledge of the clinical setting is important to avoid misdiagnosis.

Prognosis and Therapy

The goals of medical treatment in ulcerative colitis include inducing and maintaining remission, minimizing side effects, and improving the quality of life. Standard therapy includes antiinflammatory drugs, specifically, the 5-aminosalicylic acid (5-ASA) compounds (sulfasalazine and other salicylates), which are effective in preventing exacerbations in patients in remission. Steroids, either topical (enemas) or systemic, are effective in treating acute flares of disease. Biologic therapy is becoming increasingly common, particularly antibodies against tumor necrosis factor-α (TNF-α) and antibodies against adhesion molecules that affect lymphocyte trafficking. Patients with acute fulminant colitis, refractory disease, or persistent invisible dysplasia or endoscopically unresectable visible dysplasia are all treated with total colectomy. Resection with subsequent ileal pouch anal pouch anastomosis allows the patient to have relatively normal bowel function by maintaining the anal sphincter after colectomy.

Patients who are detected to have adenocarcinoma on surveillance have a significantly better prognosis than those in whom carcinoma is detected after the development of clinical symptoms. Additional long-term complications and associated conditions of ulcerative colitis include chronic anemia, hypoalbuminemia, sclerosing cholangitis, ankylosing spondylitis, arthritis, uveal disease, arthritis, vasculitis, and drug-associated complications.

ULCERATIVE COLITIS—FACT SHEET

Definition

- Idiopathic chronic colitis that presents with bloody diarrhea and is histologically characterized by a chronic colitis limited to the mucosa with continuous involvement from the rectum extending proximally

Incidence and Location

- Uncommon (4–20 per 100,000 population annually)
- Higher incidence in North America, Western Europe, South Africa

Age, Gender, and Race, Distribution

- Rare in first decade of life
- Major peak at 15 to 25 years of age
- Minor peak at 60 to 70 years of age
- Incidence slightly higher in men than women
- Whites show higher incidence than other ethnic groups
- Jews have a higher incidence than other religious groups
- 25% have an affected relative with inflammatory bowel disease

Clinical Features

- Recurrent episodes of bloody diarrhea

Endoscopic Features

- Active phase: erythema, abnormal vascular pattern, spontaneous bleeding, friability, granularity, erosions, and ulcers
- Quiescent phase: may appear normal; often there are granularity and erythema; loss of haustral folds (tubelike appearance)
- Polyps: pseudopolyps (mucosal remnants) and inflammatory polyps in active disease and postinflammatory polyps in active or quiescent disease
- All phases: submucosal vascular network is usually abnormal

Prognosis and Therapy

- Low mortality, high morbidity
- Treatment: antiinflammatory and immunosuppressive drugs; surgery if not responsive to medications and may be potentially curative
- Increased risk for dysplasia and adenocarcinoma
- Surveillance for dysplasia annually, starting 8 years after initiation presentation
- Total colectomy for fulminant ulcerative colitis, adenocarcinoma, and endoscopically invisible ("flat") dysplasia or endoscopically unresectable visible dysplasia
- Ileal pouch (J-pouch) anal anastomosis performed in most instances

Ulcerative Colitis—Pathologic Features

Gross Findings

- Mucosa flattened, bloody, friable, and granular with variable numbers of polyps
- Continuous involvement from rectum proximally but may have patchy appearance due to medical therapy or in acute fulminant cases
- May involve terminal ileum in cases with severe pancolitis
- Cecal or appendiceal involvement may be present in patients with left sided ulcerative colitis

- Relative or absolute rectal sparing may be present; more commonly in children
- Upper gastrointestinal tract involved in rare cases

Microscopic Findings

Biopsy

- Architectural features include crypt distortion, branching, loss, or shortening
- Inflammatory features include basal lymphoplasmacytosis, with variable activity
- Neutrophils, the hallmark of active disease, are located within crypt epithelium (cryptitis) and crypt lumens (crypt abscesses)
- Eosinophils and intraepithelial lymphocytes may be prominent in posttreatment biopsies
- Lymphoid aggregates may be seen at the mucosal–submucosal interface
- Inflammation is usually more severe distally
- Metaplastic features include pyloric gland metaplasia in the ileum or colon or Paneth cell metaplasia in left colon biopsies

Resection

- Inflammatory process is confined to mucosa; deeper layers may be involved in fulminant cases with broad ulcers but do not show transmural lymphoid aggregates
- Superficial fissuring ulcers may be present in fulminant colitis cases in areas of confluent mucosal denudation
- Architectural, inflammatory, and metaplastic features of chronic injury are present
- Pseudopolyps and inflammatory polyps present in variable numbers
- Transmural lymphoid aggregates, deep fissuring ulcers, strictures, fistulas, and granulomas away from ruptured crypts or deep to the mucosa not present

Differential Diagnosis

- Infectious colitis
- Medication-induced colitis
- Chronic low-grade ischemic colitis
- Crohn's disease
- Diverticular disease–associated colitis
- Diversion colitis

CROHN'S DISEASE

Crohn's disease, also referred to as *regional enteritis*, *granulomatous enterocolitis*, and *terminal ileitis*, is a chronic relapsing and remitting inflammatory disease of unknown cause that is often multifocal and can affect any portion of the GI tract. It is typically characterized by aphthous erosions, serpiginous ulcers, chronic mucosal injury, and transmural lymphoid aggregates with or without granulomas, strictures, fistulas, and perianal disease.

CLINICAL FEATURES

Crohn's disease has a slightly higher incidence in females and occurs at all ages, with the major peak incidence between 20 and 30 years of age. The initial presentation may be indolent in onset or may be acute and severe. The symptoms are variable but often include cramping abdominal pain, typically localized to the right lower quadrant; nonbloody diarrhea; and fever, malaise, and anorexia. These findings may mimic acute appendicitis. Although the appendix may be involved with Crohn's disease, appendicitis as a presenting feature is rare. Hemorrhage and hematochezia are uncommon, but chronic blood loss can occur as a result of bleeding erosions and ulcers. Patients with upper intestinal disease may present with dyspepsia, weight loss, hypoalbuminemia, and iron-deficiency anemia mimicking celiac disease. Patients with strictures present with symptoms and signs of bowel obstruction. Enterovaginal, enterovesical, and enterocutaneous fistulas may result in the passage of blood, feces, pus, and air from the vagina, urethra, or perineal skin. Inflammatory changes can occur in joints, eyes, liver, and skin. The genetic association is stronger in Crohn's disease compared with ulcerative colitis with 10% of the patients having another affected family member.

RADIOLOGIC FEATURES

As with ulcerative colitis, endoscopy has replaced radiology in the diagnosis of Crohn's disease; however, visualization of small bowel lesions often requires radiologic imaging, particularly with magnetic resonance imaging or computed tomography (CT) enterography. Radiographic features typical of Crohn's disease include asymmetric ileal involvement, longitudinal ulcers, cobblestone appearance, mural thickening and fat stranding, segmental stenosis and fistulas.

ENDOSCOPIC FEATURES

The gross endoscopic appearance of Crohn's disease is most consistently characterized as a multifocal process. Aphthous erosions (Fig. 10.18), longitudinal ulcers (train track or rake ulcers) (Fig. 10.19), and adjacent areas of erythematous or unremarkable mucosa are characteristic of Crohn's disease. Additional endoscopic findings include cobblestoning resulting from alternating ulcers and edematous mucosa, strictures, fissures, and fistula. The rectum is often spared, unlike in ulcerative colitis. A variable number of inflammatory polyps may be present and are at times large and numerous, a phenomenon described as *giant filiform polyposis* in the literature. In both Crohn's disease and ulcerative colitis, the normal submucosal vascular network is lost in the involved areas, assisting the endoscopist in the diagnosis of chronic colitis.

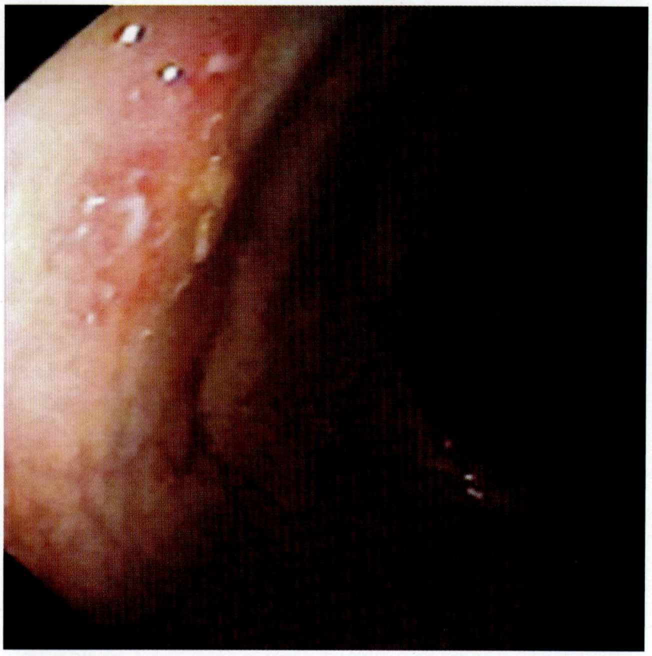

FIGURE 10.18

Crohn's enterocolitis. Aphthous erosions: small, irregular white mucosal erosions with erythematous borders.

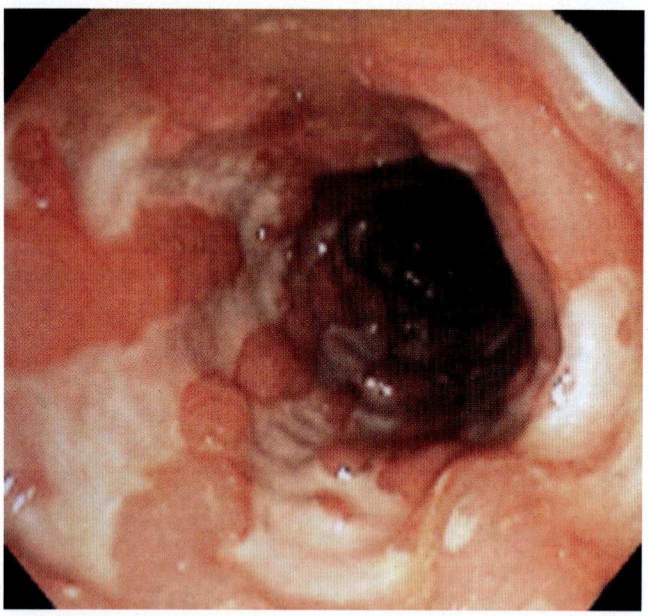

FIGURE 10.19

Crohn's enterocolitis. Longitudinal "rake" ulcers with intervening normal-appearing mucosa.

Pathologic Features

Gross Findings

Resection is typically performed only in patients who have severe complications such as obstruction resulting from strictures, abscess, fistulas, or perforation. Because the milder forms of the disease are not resected, the gross pathologic findings in resection specimens

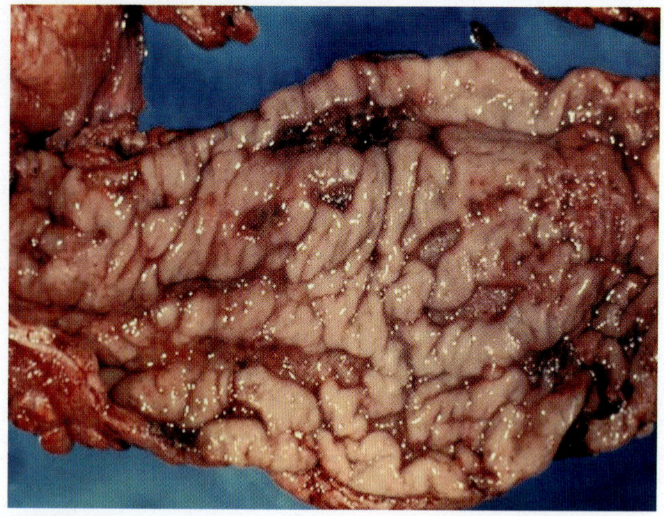

FIGURE 10.20

Crohn's enterocolitis. Narrow, constricted lumen with greatly thickened wall, "pipe stem" bowel.

are usually prominent. The subserosal fat is often firm and contracted over stenotic areas of involvement, so-called *creeping fat*. Longitudinal opening of the bowel may reveal areas with normal bowel wall thickness and other areas of the bowel that are firm, thick, and pipelike (Fig. 10.20). Interloop adhesions may occur. The mucosa may show a variety of changes, including aphthous erosions, longitudinal ulcers, cobblestoning, polyps, fissures, and fistulas. The process is usually multifocal, often with rectal sparing, but may become confluent. When confluent, the firm, pipelike nature of the bowel may help to distinguish Crohn's disease from ulcerative colitis, in which fibrosis is unusual.

Microscopic Findings

Biopsy Findings. It is hard to distinguish Crohn's disease from ulcerative colitis based on microscopic findings in mucosal biopsies since the characteristic features are present deeper in the bowel wall. The presence of granulomas away from inflamed crypts or in superficial submucosa is helpful but is seen only in a minority of patients. In most instances, knowledge of clinical and endoscopic findings is critical for diagnosing Crohn's disease. Aphthous erosions or ulcers, characterized by focal surface epithelial injury associated with a mixed inflammatory infiltrate and sometimes associated with underlying lymphoid aggregates, are typical early lesions. Variability of inflammation within a single biopsy sample and among several biopsy fragments from the same anatomic location is often seen but not diagnostic because acute fulminant or early ulcerative colitis and posttreatment biopsies in ulcerative colitis may show the same pattern of injury. The areas of inflammation show architectural changes of chronic crypt destructive colitis, but adjacent crypts may appear totally normal (Fig. 10.21). Granulomas tend to occur

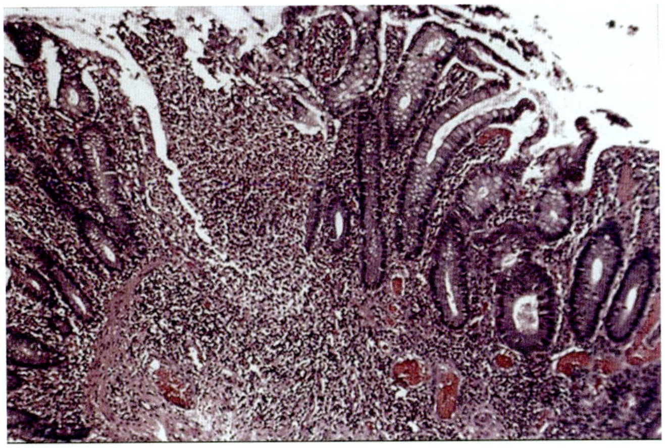

FIGURE 10.21

Crohn's enterocolitis. Biopsy of an aphthous erosion with focal mucosal disruption and polymorphs over a lymphoid nodule. Adjacent crypts appear relatively normal.

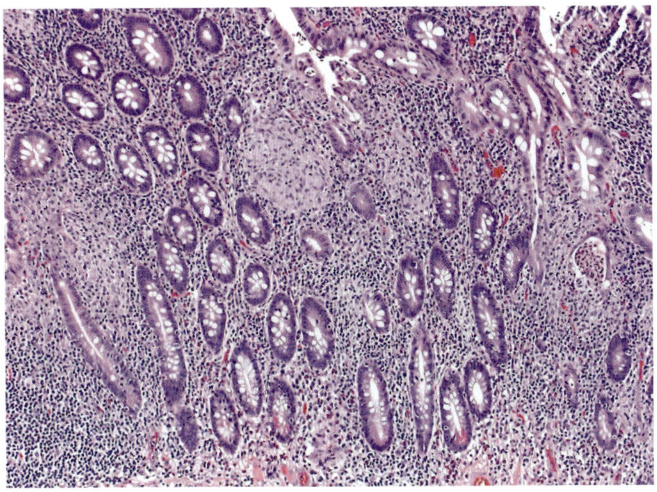

FIGURE 10.22

Crohn's enterocolitis. Poorly formed, non-necrotizing granuloma associated with marked chronic inflammation.

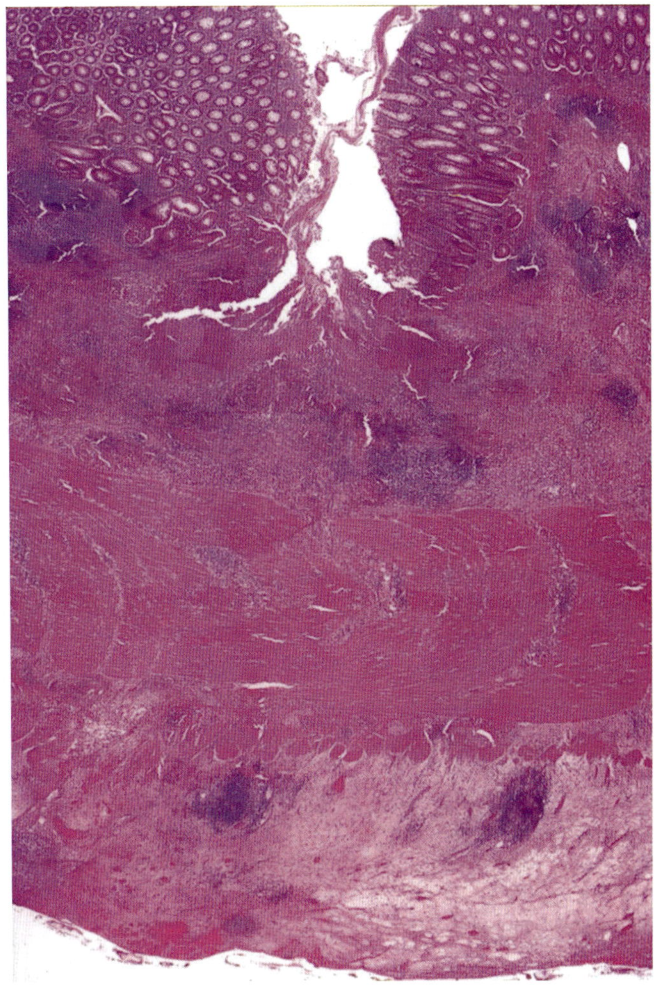

FIGURE 10.23

Crohn's enterocolitis resection. Aphthous erosion associated with transmural inflammation and submucosal fibrosis.

more frequently in pediatric patients, usually present away from inflamed crypts and in the submucosa, and are non-necrotizing (Fig. 10.22).

Crohn's disease involving the terminal ileum may show a focal active ileitis or a chronic active ileitis pattern of injury. Aphthous erosions, increased lamina propria infiltrate leading to villous blunting, and cryptitis are often seen at initial presentation. Crypt disarray is often difficult to assess in the small intestine in the presence of marked inflammation, but metaplastic features are very helpful in this setting. Pyloric gland metaplasia consisting of simple mucus glands reminiscent of the antral or pyloric mucosa are the most reproducible features of chronicity in ileal biopsies. Peyer's patches are a normal component of the terminal ileum, particularly in young individuals, and should not be mistaken for increased lymphoplasmacytic inflammation of Crohn's disease. The mucosa over Peyer's patches may be distorted with flattened villi resulting from underlying expansion of lymphoid nodules in nonspecific reactive hyperplasia or from infections such as *Yersinia* spp.

Resection Findings. The inflammatory process is typically multifocal with a chronic enteritis or colitis, superficial and deep fissures, fistulas, and prominent transmural lymphoid aggregates (Figs. 10.23 to 10.25). Ulcers are typically longitudinally oriented, separated by histologically normal edematous mucosa. Granulomas, when present, may be located at any level of the bowel wall. Lymphoid aggregates are often around dilated lymphatics or nerves. Neural hyperplasia is common in the submucosa and muscularis propria.

Ancillary Studies

No specific tests for Crohn's colitis are available. However, as with ulcerative colitis, exclusion of infectious causes is important, particularly *Yersinia* infection. Antibodies to *Saccharomyces cerevisiae* are present

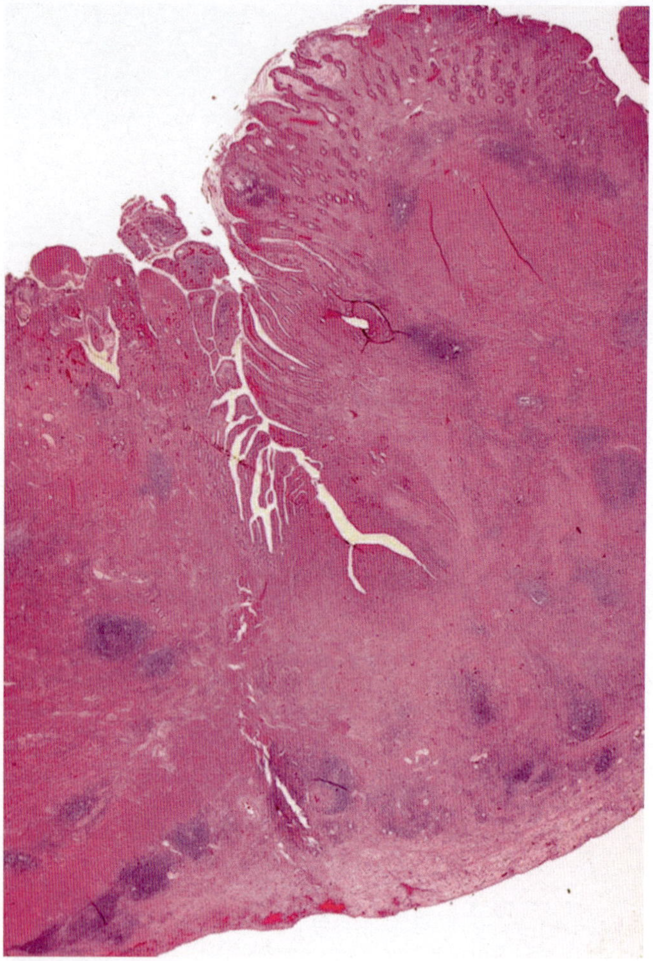

FIGURE 10.24

Crohn's enterocolitis resection. Marked submucosal fibrosis associated with transmural and subserosal lymphoid aggregates. Fissuring ulceration.

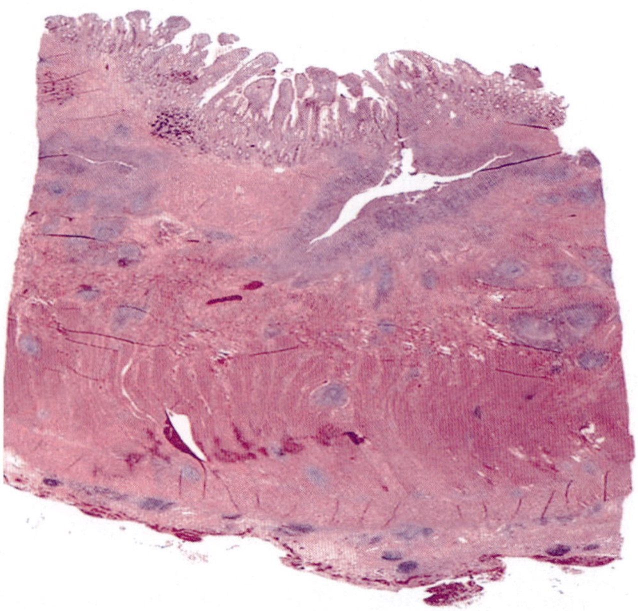

FIGURE 10.25

Crohn's enterocolitis resection. Greatly thickened bowel wall with distorted mucosa, fissure, submucosal fibrosis, and transmural lymphoid aggregates.

in approximately 70% of patients with Crohn's disease and are usually absent in patients with ulcerative colitis. In contrast, p-ANCA test results are positive in approximately 70% of patients with ulcerative colitis and in 10% to 30% of patients with Crohn's disease. There is overlap of results between Crohn's disease and ulcerative colitis, and although these tests may be helpful in rare instances, they are seldom performed to distinguish ulcerative colitis from Crohn's disease.

Differential Diagnosis

Crohn's disease must be distinguished from infections, ulcerative colitis, ischemic colitis, medication-associated injury, diverticular disease–associated colitis, and isolated asymptomatic ileitis. The endoscopic finding of focal aphthous erosions of early Crohn's disease may be similar to erosions caused by medications and infections. Histologically, the erosions of Crohn's colitis and ileitis are associated with a dense lymphoplasmacytic infiltrate. Focal active ileitis is most commonly caused by medications, particularly NSAIDs, but a small subset may be associated with Crohn's disease, which is why correlation with clinical and endoscopic findings is essential. Isolated chronic active ileitis in an asymptomatic patient may be seen in patients undergoing routine screening colonoscopy and is associated with chronic NSAID use or low-grade ischemia and is not a manifestation of Crohn's disease (Fig. 10.26). Biopsies from other sites of the GI tract, including upper tract biopsies, are often helpful in establishing a diagnosis of Crohn's disease.

Nonsteroidal antiinflammatory drug ulcers may be multiple and deep, and chronic blood loss may lead to

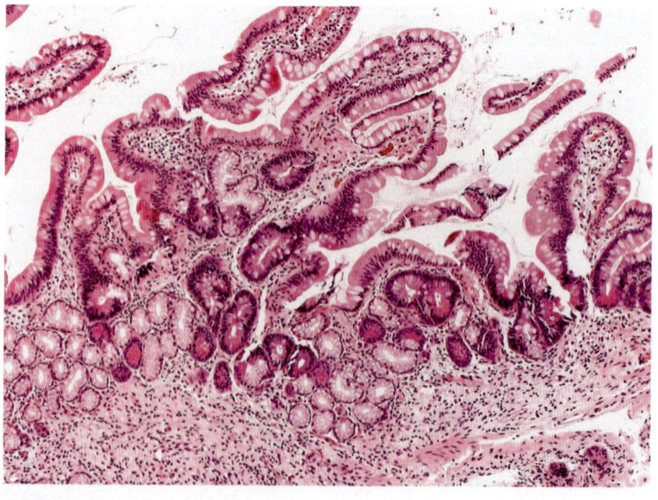

FIGURE 10.26

Chronic nonsteroidal antiinflammatory drug (NSAID) ileitis. This ileal biopsy demonstrates prominent pyloric gland metaplasia indicative of chronic mucosal injury. Active injury with neutrophilic inflammation is not seen in this particular example of chronic NSAID use.

a curative resection. These ulcers tend to be found on the top of mucosal folds and are circumferential rather than longitudinal. There is usually minimal inflammation away from the ulcers. Strictures may form in these cases and when circumferential, they appear like "diaphragms." *Yersinia* infection causes a granulomatous ileocolitis with preferential involvement of the right colon. Granulomas with central neutrophil-rich suppuration, marked mesenteric lymph node enlargement with a necrotizing lymphadenitis should favor *Yersinia* infection over Crohn's disease. Necrotizing granulomas predominate in tuberculosis and should be worked up with acid-fast bacilli stains or with more sensitive polymerase chain reaction techniques in cases in which clinical suspicion is high. Diverticular disease–associated colitis usually only involves the sigmoid colon, and the inflammation is confined to the area involved with diverticulosis.

Fulminant Crohn's colitis can be difficult or impossible to distinguish from ulcerative colitis in a mucosal biopsy specimen because many of the distinguishing features are deep to the mucosa. Furthermore, in fulminant ulcerative colitis, inflammation may be transmural but is composed of dispersed acute and chronic inflammatory cells without the characteristic lymphoid aggregates of Crohn's disease.

Prognosis and Therapy

Standard therapy includes antiinflammatory drugs, specifically the 5-ASA compounds (sulfasalazine and other salicylates), and steroids. Budesonide, a topical steroid that is taken orally, is effective in treating patients with ileal Crohn's disease. It is locally absorbed and metabolized in the liver minimizing the systemic side effects seen with other steroids. Infliximab, a monoclonal antibody against TNF-α, has been found to be helpful in treating acute episodes of Crohn's colitis, particularly fistulas and other complications. Vedolizumab, a monoclonal antibody against α4β7 integrin, is also approved for treatment of patients with Crohn's disease. Surgery is reserved for patients with refractory disease and those with obstruction, nonresponsive fistulas, sepsis, or carcinoma. Patients who have undergone surgical intervention are at increased risk for requiring additional surgery resulting from anastomotic complications such as strictures, anastomotic leaks, and fistulas.

There is a 4 to 20 times increased risk for adenocarcinoma in patients with Crohn's disease compared with the general population. Dysplasia occurs in patients with Crohn's disease similar to those with ulcerative colitis. Surveillance of patients with Crohn's colitis follows those with ulcerative colitis and depends on the extent and duration of disease. Adenocarcinomas may arise in a morphologically normal bowel, in areas of stricture, or within fistula tracts, making diagnosis difficult. Synchronous or metachronous adenocarcinomas may occur and involve the large or small intestine. Well-differentiated adenocarcinomas may arise in mucosa that has subtle low-grade dysplasia and infiltrate as deceptively bland glandular structures (Fig. 10.27). Well-differentiated mucinous adenocarcinomas that arise in chronic anal fistulas can be difficult to distinguish from non-neoplastic fistula lining.

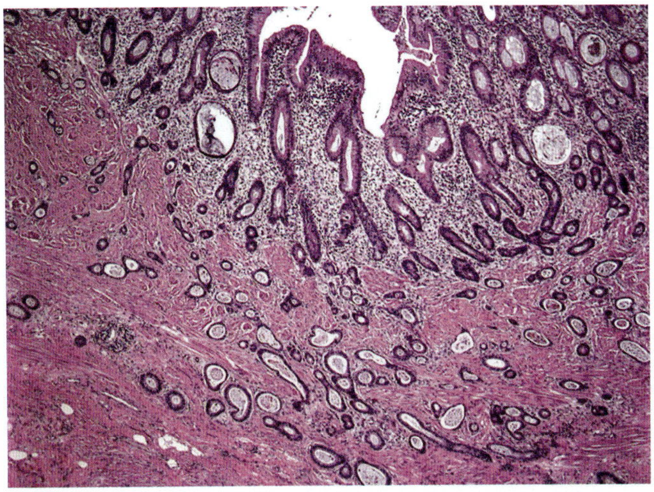

FIGURE 10.27

Well-differentiated adenocarcinoma arising in Crohn's disease extending into the bowel wall. The transition from low to high grade dysplasia to adenocarcinoma is not necessarily seen inflammatory bowel disease–associated carcinomas. The surface may look like low-grade dysplasia, and the carcinomas often show a low-grade tubuloglandular pattern.

CROHN'S DISEASE—FACT SHEET

Definition

- Idiopathic, chronic multifocal relapsing and remitting, inflammatory disorder of the gastrointestinal tract
- Small intestine, colon, or upper gastrointestinal tract may be involved
- Uncertainly etiology; combination of genetic and environmental factors
- Typically characterized by aphthous erosions or serpiginous ulcers, chronic colitis, transmural lymphoid aggregates, granulomas, strictures, fistula, and perianal disease

Incidence

- Uncommon (5–20 per 100,000 population annually)
- Higher incidence in North Americans and Northern Europeans

Gender, Race, and Age Distribution

- Incidence slightly higher in females than males
- Whites and Ashkenazi Jews with higher incidence than other ethnic groups
- Major peak at 20 to 30 years of age; minor peak at 60 to 70 years of age
- Familial association: approximately 10% have an affected relative

Clinical Features
- Cramping pain, nonbloody diarrhea, fever, malaise, and anorexia
- Hemorrhage and hematochezia uncommon
- Upper intestinal disease: dyspepsia, weight loss, hypoalbuminemia, and iron-deficiency anemia
- Inflammatory changes can also occur in the joints, eyes, liver, and skin

Endoscopic Features
- Aphthous erosions; longitudinal ulcers (train track or rake ulcers); cobblestone appearance
- Strictures, fistulas, anal and perianal disease
- Terminal ileal involvement
- Often rectal sparing; esophagus, stomach, and duodenum may be involved in a subset of cases

Prognosis and Therapy
- Low mortality, high morbidity
- Treatment: antiinflammatory, immunosuppressive drugs, and biologic therapy
- Surgery for refractory disease, strictures, fistulas
- Increased risk for dysplasia and adenocarcinoma
- Ileal pouch anal anastomosis (J-pouch) usually contraindicated

Crohn's Disease—Pathologic Features

Gross Findings
- Subserosal fat is firm and wraps around bowel wall in stenotic areas ("creeping fat")
- Firm, thick, and pipelike appearance with adhesions in some cases
- Aphthous erosions, longitudinal ulcers, cobblestone appearance, and inflammatory polyps
- Fissures, fistulas, and anal or perianal disease in distal resections

Microscopic Findings

Biopsy
- Chronic enteritis or colitis, aphthous erosions with underlying lymphoid aggregates
- Pyloric gland metaplasia in ileal biopsies
- Granulomas more common in pediatric age group and are seen in a minority of adult patients

Resection
- Chronic enteritis or colitis, sharp deep fissuring ulcers distinct from broad confluent ulcers seen in ulcerative colitis, fistula, or perianal disease
- Submucosal or mural fibrosis in areas of stricture
- Transmural lymphoid aggregates, granulomas, or both

Differential Diagnosis
- Infectious colitis
- Medication-associated colitis or enteritis
- Ulcerative colitis (including backwash ileitis)
- Ischemic colitis
- Diverticular disease–associated colitis

ILEAL POUCH ENTERITIS (POUCHITIS)

CLINICAL FEATURES

After total proctocolectomy, construction of an ileal pouch anal anastomosis (J-pouch) is often performed to restore continence and improve quality of life. This is often performed in the setting of ulcerative colitis, but a J-pouch may also be created in patients with other colonic disease, particularly hereditary colorectal cancer syndromes such as familial adenomatous polyposis. Inflammation of the pouch ("pouchitis") is a common complication that is diagnosed clinically based on symptoms of diarrhea, bleeding, urgency, low-grade fever, and occasionally abdominal pain. Although more than half of patients with a J-pouch experience at least one episode of pouchitis, pouch failure and excision are extremely rare. Pouchitis also decreases dramatically after the first 6 months of surgery and is likely related to an alteration in the small intestinal microbiome. Pouchitis is a clinical term that translates to histologic patterns of acute and/or chronic mucosal injury. First-line therapy for pouchitis is with antibiotics. Patients with chronic symptoms and refractory disease who do not respond to antibiotics are often treated with immunosuppression.

PATHOLOGIC FEATURES

The pouch is constructed from the ileum, and even healthy pouches demonstrate some abnormal histologic features in the ileal mucosa such as villous blunting, mild expansion of the lamina propria, increased eosinophils, and increased intraepithelial lymphocytes. These are part of the "adaptive response" as the small intestine transitions to functioning as a neorectum. Patients with clinically diagnosed pouchitis demonstrate neutrophilic inflammation in both the crypt and surface epithelium. Ulcers and erosions may be seen. Chronic pouchitis often demonstrates villous architectural distortion and pyloric gland metaplasia, but this should not be taken as evidence of Crohn's disease (Fig. 10.28).

DIFFERENTIAL DIAGNOSIS

Occasionally, patients may develop Crohn's disease of the pouch. This occurs mainly in patients with Crohn's disease who were mistakenly thought to have ulcerative colitis on the prior colectomy. Therefore, review of the prior colectomy specimen is very useful when a diagnosis of Crohn's disease of the pouch is being considered. It must be emphasized again that no histologic feature

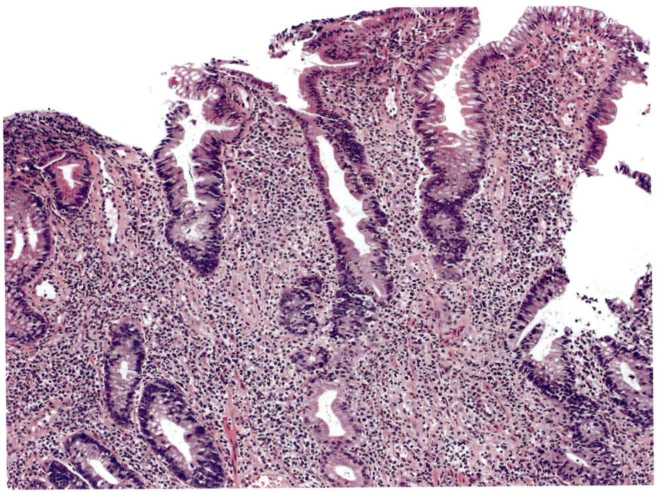

FIGURE 10.28

Pouchitis with marked architectural distortion, expanded lamina propria, and numerous foci of neutrophilic inflammation. Pyloric gland metaplasia is also seen.

in a pouch biopsy allows one to make a Crohn's disease diagnosis with certainty. Architectural alterations and pyloric gland metaplasia that suggest a chronic ileitis in a native ileum biopsy are not helpful in making this diagnosis when evaluating biopsies from the pouch. Granulomas may be helpful but are also not diagnostic of Crohn's disease in this setting. Inflammation of the prepouch ileum may be a risk factor for subsequent pouch failure but also does not qualify as definitive evidence of Crohn's disease. The diagnosis of Crohn's disease in this setting is entertained if definitive features of Crohn's disease, such as fistulas, perianal disease, or definite upper GI tract involvement, are present.

The pouch may also sustain ischemic injury as a result of surgical complications when the ileum is brought into the pelvis and the necessary lengthening procedures stretch the ileal mesentery. Chronic ischemia of the pouch is primarily an endoscopic diagnosis and often demonstrates an asymmetric distribution of inflammation, often with sharp demarcation between the inflamed and noninflamed parts of the pouch. The affected mucosa is mainly located in the distal pouch, along the staple line, or at the afferent limb side of the pouch body.

Prognosis and Therapy

Most patients respond to antibiotic therapy, and pouch excision is extremely rare. The risk of pouch failure rises with increasing number of episodes of pouchitis. Antibiotic refractory pouchitis is much more difficult to treat and may require immunosuppressive medications.

ILEAL POUCH INFLAMMATION (POUCHITIS)—FACT SHEET

Definition

- Inflammation of the ileal pouch following total proctocolectomy

Incidence and Location

- Common after total colectomy for ulcerative colitis; rare in noninflammatory bowel disease
- May involve any aspect of the pouch

Gender, Race, and Age Distribution

- No known predilection

Clinical Features

- Diarrhea, bleeding, low-grade fever, urgency

Prognosis and Therapy

- Incidence decreases over time
- First-line therapy with antibiotics and immunosuppression in refractory cases

Ileal Pouch Inflammation (Pouchitis)—Pathologic Features

Gross Findings

- Edema, granularity, exudates, ulcers

Microscopic Findings

- Neutrophilic infiltration of the crypt and surface epithelium
- Erosions and ulceration
- Chronic pouchitis may demonstrate architectural distortion and pyloric gland metaplasia

Differential Diagnosis

- Crohn's disease of the pouch
- Ischemia of the pouch

COLLAGENOUS COLITIS

Microscopic colitis is a term used to describe a distinctive constellation of clinical, endoscopic, and histologic findings. Patients with microscopic colitis typically present with watery diarrhea, colonoscopy is normal or shows subtle nonspecific alterations, and random biopsies from the colon show a colitis with increased intraepithelial lymphocytes (lymphocytic colitis [LC]) or an abnormal subepithelial collagen layer (CC). Both forms of microscopic colitis typically involve the entire colon, but there may be relative or absolute sparing of the distal sigmoid and rectum in a subset of cases. A full colonoscopy is, therefore, needed to establish the diagnosis.

CLINICAL FEATURES

Patients with CC present with chronic watery diarrhea. Females significantly outnumber males, and most patients are middle aged or older. Colonoscopy typically shows normal or near normal mucosa, with a few reports of linear mucosal tears that were thought to occur upon insufflation during endoscopy. In addition, there are rare reports of CC with pseudomembranes.

A luminal antigen or antigens may be important in the pathogenesis of CC because diversion of the fecal stream causes the histologic changes of CC to regress, while reestablishing the fecal stream induces a relapse. Studies have shown a strong association of CC with medications, including NSAIDs, selective serotonin reuptake inhibitors, proton pump inhibitors, simvastatin, ticlopidine, antihypertensive medications, and immune checkpoint receptor inhibitors. There is also a reported association with celiac disease.

Pathologic Features

At low power, biopsy specimens of CC often show a variably thick and irregular eosinophilic subepithelial "stripe" with an intact crypt architecture and an increase in lamina propria mononuclear cells (Fig. 10.29). At higher magnification, the lamina propria shows increased lymphocytes, plasma cells, and eosinophils, which may involve the full thickness of the mucosa, mimicking IBD, or may be confined to the upper half similar to the appearance in acute self-limited colitis. The surface epithelium has a patchy increase in intraepithelial lymphocytes with areas of surface damage. The surface epithelium is often stripped off from the thickened collagen table. The subepithelial collagen is irregular and usually blends imperceptibly with the basement membrane and often entraps small capillaries and inflammatory cells, which can be better visualized on a trichrome stain (Fig. 10.30). The thickness of the collagen often varies from site to site in individual patients and should be evaluated only in well-oriented sections. Whereas the normal basement membrane of the colon measures 2 to 5 μm, in CC, the collagen typically has a thickness of 10 to 30 μm. Biopsies from the rectum and sigmoid colon may show less thickening and may be within a normal range. When in doubt, a trichrome stain can be used to highlight the thick and irregular collagenous band. The irregular character of the subepithelial collagen rather than the absolute thickness is helpful in making a diagnosis of CC. Care should be taken not to overinterpret a

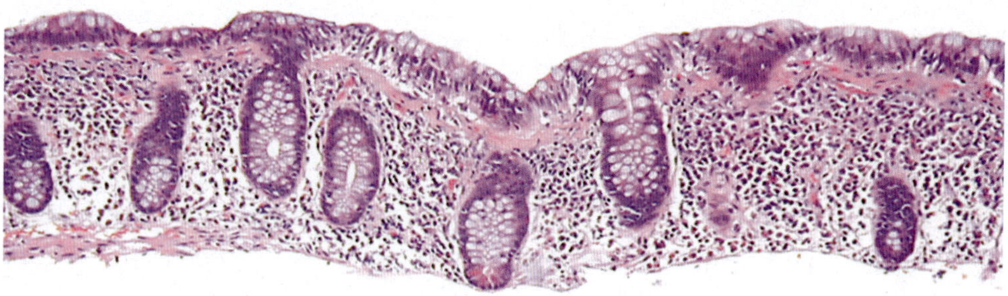

FIGURE 10.29

Collagenous colitis. This low-power view shows intact crypt architecture with a superficial plasmacytosis of the lamina propria. The thickened subepithelial collagen table appears as a pink stripe just beneath the surface epithelium. Even at this low magnification, increased intraepithelial lymphocytes are apparent.

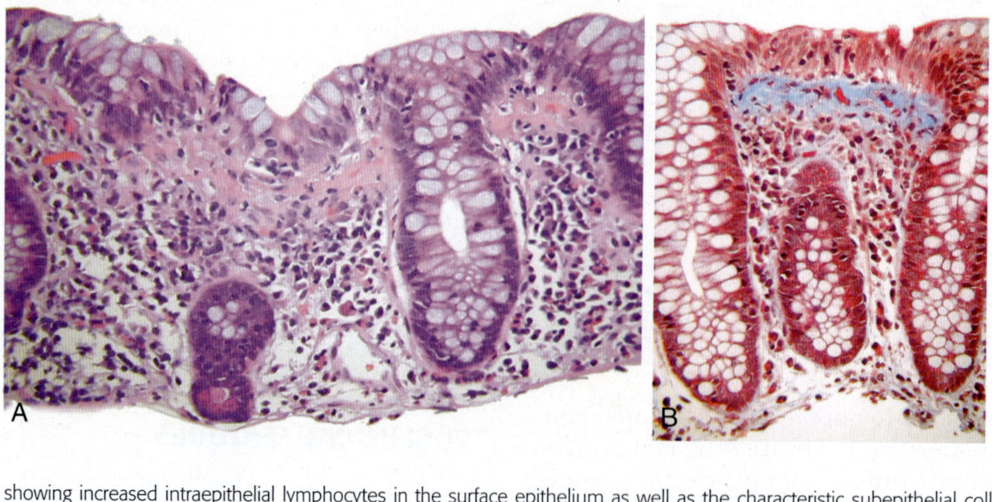

FIGURE 10.30

A, High-power view showing increased intraepithelial lymphocytes in the surface epithelium as well as the characteristic subepithelial collagenous thickening. There is Paneth cell metaplasia at the base of the mucosa, a marker of chronic colitis. **B**, A trichrome-stained section highlights the thick and irregular subepithelial collagen that entraps small capillaries and lymphocytes.

thickened basement membrane as CC because this may be a normal finding in the left colon. Surface epithelial damage with increased intraepithelial lymphocytes are always present in cases of CC. Intraepithelial neutrophils may be seen but are less prominent than the intraepithelial lymphocytes. Large numbers of crypt abscesses are probably indicative of either superimposed infection or another colitis. Paneth cell or pyloric gland metaplasia and mild crypt architectural distortion may also be present in a minority of cases because CC is a chronic colitis. The collagen layer abnormalities normalize in a significant proportion of patients on therapy, and recurrence of symptoms should not always be taken as a manifestation of relapsed CC. The terminal ileum may also be involved in a minor subset of cases with CC, and rare cases show a giant cell histiocytic response with multinucleated giant cells beneath the abnormal collagen layer.

Differential Diagnosis

Lymphocytic colitis is identical to CC except for the absence of abnormal subepithelial collagen. Eosinophils are typically less prominent in the lamina propria in LC. Chronic IBD typically shows more architectural distortion, and the clinical presentation is very different from that of CC. IBD patients present with bloody diarrhea and show mucosal abnormalities on colonoscopy. In extremely rare cases, features of both IBD and CC may be present in different part of the colon at the same procedure, and most such patients are clinically diagnosed and treated as having IBD. Mucosal prolapse shows fibromuscular proliferation in the lamina propria and architectural distortion, but the distinctive subepithelial band is not present in these cases. Enema effect may strip off the surface epithelium and make it difficult to evaluate the surface epithelium, but the lamina propria and collagen layer are both normal. Ischemia often has fibrosis and hyalinization of the lamina propria that may be misdiagnosed as CC but does not show the increased intraepithelial lymphocytosis seen in CC or the characteristic abnormal subepithelial abnormal collagen layer. Radiation colitis also shows hyalinization of the lamina propria, usually with telangiectatic blood vessels and atypical endothelial cells and fibroblasts. The hyaline material does not stain as intensely on the trichrome stain as the thick and irregular collagen layer in CC.

Prognosis and Therapy

Some patients with CC have a spontaneous remission, but others respond to simple over-the-counter antidiarrheal agents. Most patients, however, require some form of antiinflammatory therapy (steroids, 5-ASA compounds, or both). Rarely, patients with refractory disease may require a diverting ileostomy. The overall course of the disease tends to wax and wane, but it is generally not as severe as ulcerative colitis or Crohn's disease.

COLLAGENOUS COLITIS—FACT SHEET

Definition

- Colitis with characteristic abnormal subepithelial collagen deposition

Incidence and Location

- 1 to 2.3 per 100,000 population
- Generally involves the entire colon, but relative rectal or left-sided sparing can be seen

Gender, Race, and Age Distribution

- Female predominance (male-to-female ratio, 1 to 8)
- Primarily affects middle-aged to older adults
- Mean age is 59 years

Clinical Features

- Chronic watery diarrhea with normal or near-normal endoscopy results

Prognosis and Therapy

- Most patients respond to withdrawal of offending medication, antidiarrheal therapy, or budesonide

Collagenous Colitis—Pathologic Features

Gross Findings

- Usually normal endoscopic appearance or mild nonspecific alterations
- Rarely, linear ulcers or pseudomembranes

Microscopic Findings

- Abnormal thick (10–30 μm) and irregular subepithelial collagen deposition
- Collagen layer irregular and entraps capillaries and lymphocytes; better visualized on trichrome or Sirius red stains
- Rectum or left colon may be spared in about 20% cases; ileum may be involved in a small subset
- Surface epithelial damage with increased intraepithelial lymphocytes
- Increased lamina propria plasma infiltrate that may be full-thickness mimicking inflammatory bowel disease or in superficial half similar to acute self-limited colitis
- Occasional foci of cryptitis or neutrophils in surface epithelium may be present
- Crypt distortion and Paneth cell or pyloric gland metaplasia seen in a subset of cases

Differential Diagnosis

- Lymphocytic colitis
- Radiation colitis
- Ischemic colitis
- Mucosal prolapse or solitary rectal ulcer syndrome
- Inflammatory bowel disease
- Normal left colon with a thick basement membrane
- Enema effect

LYMPHOCYTIC COLITIS

CLINICAL FEATURES

There is considerable overlap of clinical and pathologic features between LC and CC. Patients have chronic watery diarrhea with normal or near-normal endoscopic findings. There tends to be less of a female predominance in LC than in CC, but the age range is quite similar.

Many medications known to cause CC, including ranitidine, sertraline, ticlopidine, NSAIDs, aspirin, immune checkpoint receptors, and proton pump inhibitors, have also been reported to cause LC. The association between LC and celiac disease is even stronger than the association between CC and celiac disease. These findings again support the notion that luminal antigens somehow induce this colitis. In addition, human leukocyte antigen (HLA) studies have shown an increased incidence of HLA A1, DQ2, DQ1, and DQ3 in patients with LC, as well as other autoimmune processes.

PATHOLOGIC FEATURES

In general, LC is similar to CC but lacks the thick and irregular abnormal subepithelial collagen layer. Eosinophils are usually less prominent in the lamina propria than in CC, and when increased, a careful look for subepithelial collagen irregularities is warranted because diagnostic changes can be mild and patchy. Special stains for collagen are also useful in this scenario to unmask subtle changes. The surface epithelial damage with increased intraepithelial lymphocytes is often more prominent in LC. Just as in CC, there is generally a superficial plasmacytosis without significant crypt distortion (Figs. 10.31 and 10.32). The pathologist must avoid evaluating the number of intraepithelial lymphocytes overlying a lymphoid follicle because numerous intraepithelial lymphocytes are normal in this location. One should also recognize that normally, there are more intraepithelial lymphocytes in the right colon than the left colon. A few foci of cryptitis or a rare crypt abscess may be seen in LC, but striking neutrophilic inflammation is usually suggestive of another diagnosis, such as infection or medication-induced colitis. Recently, it was recognized that some cases of LC have less surface damage and more intraepithelial lymphocytes in the deeper crypt epithelium. Another variation of LC has been described with collections of histiocytes and poorly formed granulomas underneath the surface epithelium.

DIFFERENTIAL DIAGNOSIS

The resolving phase of an infectious colitis can mimic LC because of surface damage and mild increase in intraepithelial lymphocytes. LC-like changes have also been described in outbreaks of chronic diarrhea linked to the water supply on a cruise ship. This so-called colonic epithelial lymphocytosis seemed to have less surface damage than LC. Reports have also been made of LC-like histology in patients with constipation as well as in patients with endoscopic abnormalities. Hence, it is important for the pathologist to make sure the clinical history is consistent with LC before making this diagnosis. Colon biopsies in patients with IBD may show an LC-like pattern either at initial presentation or in posttreatment biopsies. Patients in the latter scenario are asymptomatic, and this likely represents the resolving phase of inflammation similar to what is seen in those with infectious colitis. CC may be confused with lymphocytic cases when only rectal biopsy samples are obtained or when the subepithelial collagen

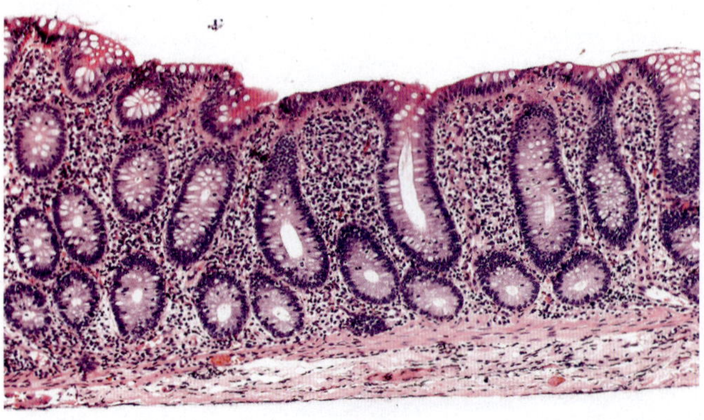

FIGURE 10.31

Lymphocytic colitis. This low-power view shows intact crypt architecture with a plasmacytosis of the lamina propria. Note the normal basement membrane and the increase in intraepithelial lymphocytes.

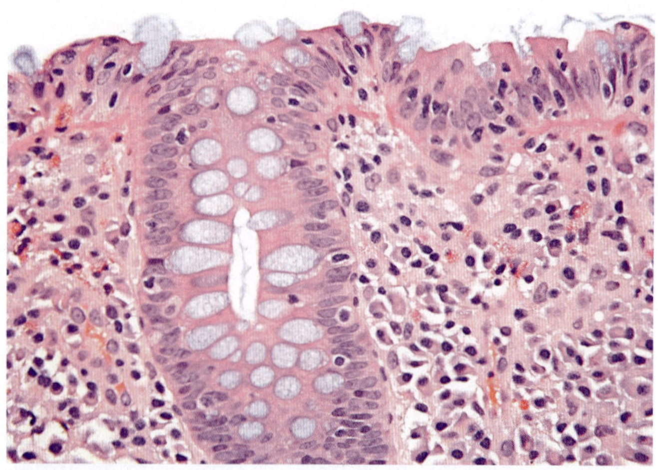

FIGURE 10.32

Lymphocytic colitis. This high-power view shows a marked increase in intraepithelial lymphocytes and a normal basement membrane. Note the increase in lamina propria plasma cells and lack of prominent eosinophils.

irregularities are mild and patchy. As mentioned earlier, prominent eosinophils in the lamina propria should prompt a closer look at the subepithelial collagen layer, and a trichrome stain should be performed in cases in which a subtle abnormality is suspected.

Prognosis and Therapy

Therapy for patients with LC is variable and is largely identical to that used for those with CC. Some patients' symptoms resolve spontaneously, but others may require over-the-counter antidiarrheal medications, bismuth subsalicylate, 5-ASA compounds, or immunosuppressants. Overall, the prognosis is good because most patients eventually respond to some form of therapy. However, there is a small subset of patients who have LC and spruelike changes in their small bowel biopsies that seem refractory to all therapy. These patients have been classified as having lymphocytic enterocolitis. Some patients with this finding may have autoimmune enteropathy, common variable immunodeficiency, or in rare instances a lymphoproliferative disorder.

LYMPHOCYTIC COLITIS—FACT SHEET

Definition
- Colitis characterized by increased intraepithelial lymphocytes and surface epithelial damage

Incidence and Location
- 3.1 per 100,000 population
- Generally involves the whole colon but may have distal sparing

Gender, Race, and Age Distribution
- Male-to-female ratio is 1 to 1
- Primarily affects middle-aged to older adults
- Mean age of onset is 51 years

Clinical Features
- Chronic watery diarrhea with normal or near normal endoscopy

Prognosis and Therapy
- Most patients respond to antidiarrheal or antiinflammatory therapy

LYMPHOCYTIC COLITIS—PATHOLOGIC FEATURES

Gross Findings
- Usually normal colonoscopic appearance

Microscopic Findings
- Surface damage with increased intraepithelial lymphocytes
- Increased lamina propria inflammation, often superficial, and less prominent eosinophils than collagenous colitis
- May have occasional foci of cryptitis or neutrophils in surface epithelium
- Minimal crypt distortion

Differential Diagnosis
- Collagenous colitis
- Resolving infectious colitis
- Crohn's disease
- Normal mucosa overlying a lymphoid aggregate
- Lymphocytic enterocolitis

ISCHEMIC COLITIS

CLINICAL FEATURES

Ischemia can give rise to a wide range of clinical presentations depending on the duration and severity of the underlying pathology. Although many cases of ischemia occur in older patients with known cardiovascular disease, ischemic colitis can also be seen in younger, seemingly healthy people secondary to endothelial toxin-mediated infections, hypercoagulable states, medications, vasculitis, or previous abdominal surgery. Drugs implicated in inducing an ischemic mucosal injury include antihypertensive and migraine medications, oral contraceptives and hormone replacement therapy, pseudoephedrine, NSAIDs, antibiotics, and chemotherapeutic agents. Symptoms may range from transient bloody diarrhea and abdominal pain to a surgical emergency resulting from an infarcted bowel. In some cases, usually in the right colon, marked submucosal edema may give rise to a masslike appearance that mimics malignancy.

A variety of disorders can lead to a lack of blood flow to the mucosa, which is the ultimate cause of ischemic colitis. Ischemic necrosis may be caused by thromboembolic disease secondary to atherosclerosis, low-flow states secondary to hypovolemia, vasculitis, adhesions, drugs, and even long-distance running. In some instances, the drug may induce vasospasm (catecholamines, cocaine), but in other cases, the medication may lead to thrombosis (estrogens). Enterohemorrhagic strains of *E. coli* (e.g., *E. coli* O157:H7) and *C. difficile* infection can also cause an ischemic-type colitis, presumably resulting from endothelial injury from the toxin-mediated infection.

Radiologic Features

The classic radiologic finding of ischemia on a barium enema study is that of "thumbprinting." This finding is produced by marked submucosal edema. CT findings of circumferential bowel wall thickening may also be a marker for ischemia. Rare cases, particularly in the right colon, may present as a mass lesion mimicking malignancy.

Pathologic Features

Gross Findings

In resection specimens, ischemic colitis typically shows geographic areas of ulceration that may have pseudomembranes. This is often accompanied by marked submucosal edema. Endoscopically, this submucosal edema can be prominent enough to mimic a tumor or mass lesion. The watershed areas around the splenic flexure are the most common sites for ischemia, but nearly any site can be involved, including the proximal rectum. Chronic or healed ischemic lesions may form isolated strictures that resemble Crohn's disease.

Microscopic Findings

In biopsies from symptomatic patients, acute ischemic lesions of the colon show superficial mucosal necrosis that often spares the deeper portions of the colonic crypts (Figs. 10.33 and 10.34). The remaining crypts typically have a withered and atrophic appearance. Ischemic colitis may show pseudomembranes, as well as hemorrhage and hyalinization of the lamina propria. A trichrome stain can be used to highlight the hyalinization of the lamina propria (Fig. 10.35). Cryptitis and crypt abscesses are usually not prominent. Depending on the severity of the decreased blood flow, these ischemic lesions may regress on their own or lead to perforation or stricture formation. There may be striking cytologic atypia, in some cases to the point at which they mimic dysplasia. The presence of mucin depletion, localization of the atypia to the basal crypts, and the associated hemorrhage and hyalinization of the lamina propria are helpful in excluding dysplasia. Degenerating epithelial cells can also mimic signet ring cells. Mesenteric vessels in resection specimens from patients with ischemic colitis caused by thromboembolic disease show atherosclerotic changes and intravascular thrombi in varying stages of organization may be detected. The chronic phase of ischemia is often more difficult to diagnose because the only histologic findings may be areas of submucosal fibrosis in the strictured segment. The presence of architectural changes of chronic injury in the mucosa or abnormal vasculature may be helpful in suggesting the correct diagnosis.

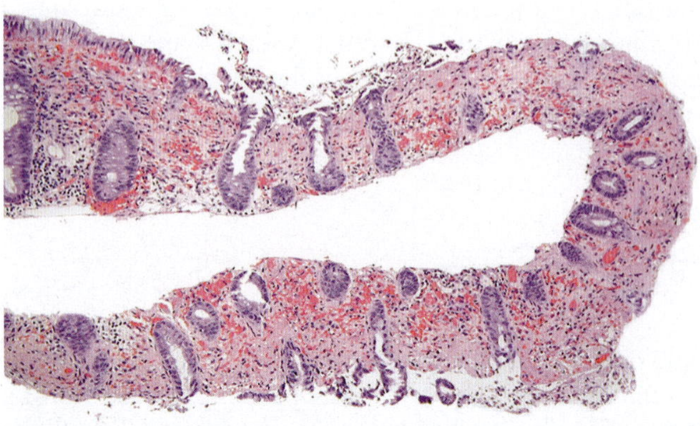

FIGURE 10.33

Ischemic colitis. This low-power view shows superficial mucosal necrosis with loss of surface epithelium and preservation of deep portions of colonic crypts. There is hyalinization of the lamina propria with a paucity of inflammation.

Differential Diagnosis

The differential diagnosis of ischemic colitis includes infectious such as *C. difficile* and enterohemorrhagic *E. coli*–associated colitis, NSAID-associated mucosal injury, CC, radiation colitis, and Crohn's disease. Ischemic and *C. difficile* colitis may be particularly difficult to differentiate because pseudomembranes may be present in both conditions. The presence of a hyalinized

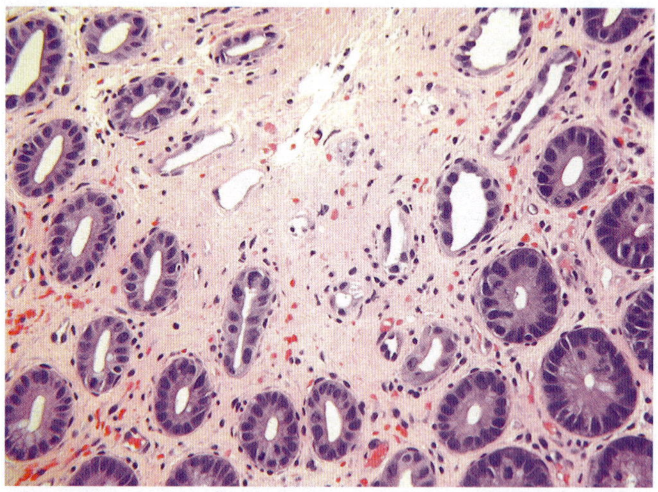

FIGURE 10.34

Ischemic colitis. This high-power view shows atrophic-appearing "micro crypts," which are typical of ischemia. There is also a prominently hyalinized lamina propria. Note the marked regenerative atypia, which can be mistaken for dysplasia.

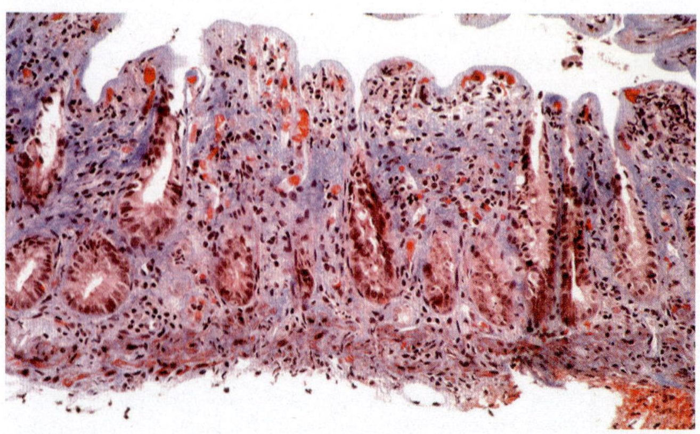

FIGURE 10.35

Ischemic colitis (trichrome stain). This trichrome-stained section shows blue staining of the lamina propria in areas of hyalinization.

lamina propria and withered, atrophic-appearing crypts are specific findings in ischemia that are not seen in *C. difficile* colitis. In addition, *C. difficile* colitis is typically a pancolitis, but ischemia is segmental. Even within involved segments, pseudomembranes tend to be more diffuse in *C. difficile* and patchy in ischemic colitis. The presence of an ischemic-appearing lesion in the right colon should also make one think of enterohemorrhagic *E. coli*, especially if fibrin thrombi are present.

Differentiating chronic ischemic ulcers from NSAID-induced damage or Crohn's disease may be impossible, especially on biopsy material. Chronic ischemic damage shows prominent architectural changes of chronicity without the marked inflammatory component typically seen in untreated IBD. Radiation exposure often causes arterial damage that can manifest itself as ischemia in the gut. In some instances, the hyalinized appearance of the lamina propria in radiation colitis and the subepithelial collagen in CC can mimic the hyalinized lamina propria seen in ischemic colitis. The presence of telangiectatic vessels and atypical endothelial cells and fibroblasts should help identify radiation colitis, and the inflammatory component and abnormal subepithelial collagen is diagnostic of CC. Last, the regenerative epithelial changes in ischemia may mimic dysplasia and recognition of the surrounding ischemic changes is key to avoiding this pitfall.

PROGNOSIS AND THERAPY

The prognosis for ischemic colitis depends entirely on the underlying etiology and severity. Ischemia in a long-distance runner is likely to be transient and self-limited, but severe thromboembolic disease may lead to a life-threatening bowel infarct with perforation and peritonitis. Overall, 35% of cases resolve with simple supportive care, and 15% to 20% may require surgery.

ISCHEMIC COLITIS—FACT SHEET

Definition

- Damage to the colon secondary to decreased blood flow

Incidence and Location

- 3 per 10,000 population
- The splenic flexure and descending and sigmoid colon are the most common sites of ischemia, but any site in the colon can be involved
- The rectum is the least common site for ischemia

Gender, Race, and Age Distribution

- Males and females affected equally
- Most patients are older than 50 years, but younger patients and even children can have ischemia, depending on the underlying disease process

Clinical Features

- Presentation is variable depending on the severity and underlying etiology
- Abdominal pain, bloody diarrhea, vomiting, and fever may be seen

Radiologic Features

- Barium enema shows "thumbprinting"
- Computed tomography shows "target lesions"
- Angiography can be used to identify vascular lesions
- Some cases may present as a masslike lesion mimicking malignancy

Prognosis and Therapy

- A majority of ischemic colitis cases resolve with supportive care, but 15% to 20% require surgical intervention
- Complications include perforation, peritonitis, and stricture formation

ISCHEMIC COLITIS—PATHOLOGIC FEATURES

Gross Findings

- Geographic ulcers or infarcts, pseudomembranes, submucosal edema, strictures

Microscopic Findings

- Superficial mucosal necrosis and withered or atrophic crypts
- Hyalinized lamina propria
- Pseudomembranes, strictures

Differential Diagnosis

- *Clostridium difficile* colitis
- Enterohemorrhagic *Escherichia coli*
- Nonsteroidal antiinflammatory drug damage
- Crohn's disease
- Radiation colitis
- Collagenous colitis
- Dysplasia

RADIATION COLITIS

CLINICAL FEATURES

Acute radiation damage is often subclinical, but patients with chronic radiation damage may complain of diarrhea, abdominal pain, or rectal bleeding. Patients receiving radiation therapy for cervical and prostate cancer have the highest risk for radiation colitis.

Acute radiation injury occurs within hours to days of radiation exposure and leads to epithelial injury that usually heals within 2 months. Chronic radiation colitis occurs secondary to damage to mesenchymal tissues of the gut. These changes may remain clinically silent for a long period or cause persistent symptoms for the life of the patient.

Pathologic Features

Gross Findings

Endoscopy may shows edema and a dusky mucosa in the early acute phase of injury. Much of the damage induced by radiation is caused by chronic ischemic damage to mesenteric vessels, and ulcers, strictures, fistulas, and adhesions may be seen in this stage. Endoscopically, there is typically patchy erythema secondary to telangiectasia of the mucosal capillaries.

Microscopic Findings

Acute radiation damage is rarely seen, but the changes are those of epithelial damage, including increased apoptosis, decreased mitoses, and regenerative atypia. Increased numbers of eosinophils may also be seen. In addition to telangiectasia of the mucosal capillaries, chronic radiation damage often has areas of hyalinization around these dilated vessels with atypical "radiation fibroblasts" (Fig. 10.36). The endothelial cells may also show similar radiation-induced atypia. Crypt distortion mimicking IBD may be seen.

Differential Diagnosis

An accurate history is paramount if one is to make a diagnosis of radiation colitis. Chronic radiation damage can be subtle in biopsy specimens because the vascular changes in the capillaries are easily overlooked. These vascular changes mimic the telangiectasia seen in portal colopathy or angiodysplasia. A hyalinized lamina propria or radiation fibroblasts is not present in these latter conditions. Occasionally, the hyalinized changes in the lamina propria can mimic CC, but the inflammatory changes in the lamina propria and the abnormal subepithelial collagen is absent. The presence of crypt distortion may mimic quiescent ulcerative colitis or proctitis. Many of the changes of radiation colitis are secondary to ischemia, which also enters the differential diagnosis of ischemic colitis. The regenerative atypia seen in acute radiation damage may mimic dysplasia, but a history of radiation exposure is imperative to make the correct diagnosis.

Prognosis and Therapy

The damage caused by radiation is permanent, and symptomatic patients may require surgical resection. Steroid therapy may be of some benefit. Laser therapy may be used to induce hemostasis in areas of active bleeding.

RADIATION COLITIS—FACT SHEET

Definition

- Colonic damage secondary to radiation exposure

Incidence and Location

- 5% to 15% of patients receiving radiation to the pelvis
- Most common in the rectum

Gender, Race, and Age Distribution

- Older men treated with radiation for prostate cancer
- Middle-aged to younger women treated with radiation for cervical cancer

Clinical Features

- Diarrhea, abdominal pain, rectal bleeding

Prognosis and Therapy

- Radiation damage is permanent
- May require surgery if steroids or laser coagulation do not work

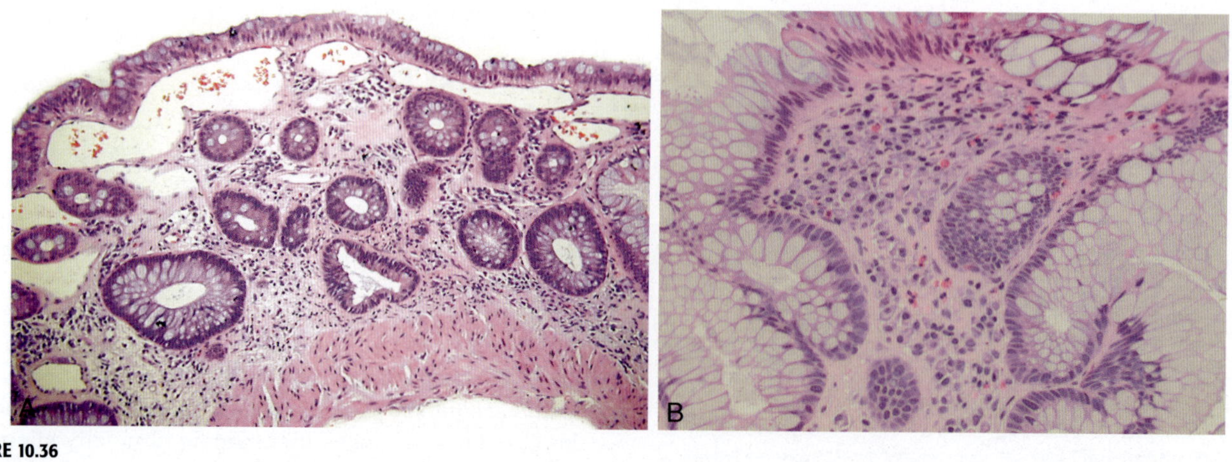

FIGURE 10.36

Radiation colitis. This medium-power photomicrograph shows telangiectatic blood vessels throughout the superficial lamina propria. There is also focal hyalinization of the lamina propria, similar to that seen in ischemia (**A**). Regenerative epithelial and stromal changes in radiation colitis may be mistaken for neoplasia (**B**).

Radiation Colitis—Pathologic Features

Gross Findings

- Acute: erythema, dusky mucosa
- Chronic: patchy erythema, ulcers, strictures, fistulas

Microscopic Findings

- Acute: increased apoptosis, decreased mitoses, abundant cytoplasm with vacuolation, and regenerative atypia; increased numbers of eosinophils
- Chronic: telangiectasia of mucosal capillaries, hyalinized lamina propria, radiation fibroblasts, atypical endothelial cells, crypt distortion

Differential Diagnosis

- Acute: dysplasia caused by nuclear enlargement and hyperchromasia
- Chronic: collagenous colitis, inflammatory bowel disease, portal colopathy, angiodysplasia, and ischemia

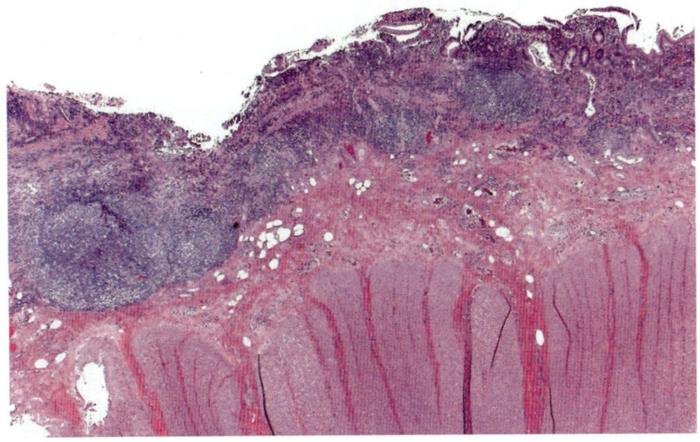

FIGURE 10.37

Diversion colitis. This low-power photomicrograph was taken from a patient with paraplegia with long-standing colonic diversion. There is marked lymphoid hyperplasia in addition to crypt architectural distortion and neutrophilic cryptitis. These features may mimic idiopathic inflammatory bowel disease.

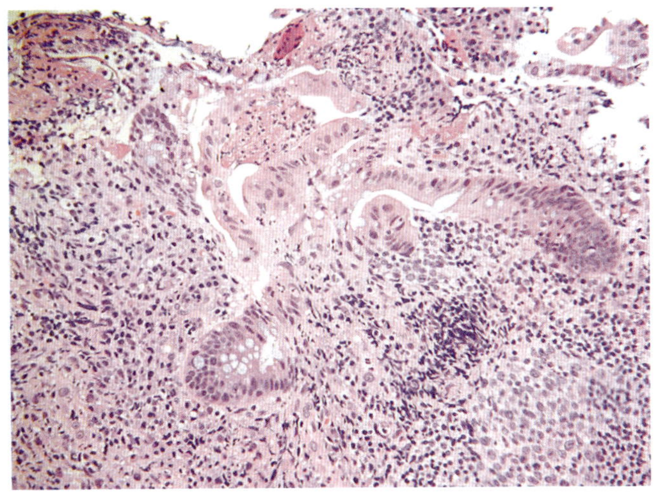

FIGURE 10.38

Diversion colitis. This high-power photomicrograph shows an aphthous lesion (erosion overlying a lymphoid aggregate). Note the neutrophils in the surface epithelium and luminal exudates.

DIVERSION COLITIS

CLINICAL FEATURES

Diversion colitis is usually a mild colitis that occurs in segments of the colon excluded from the fecal stream and is most often seen in a Hartmann's pouch. Although diversion colitis is often an incidental finding in asymptomatic patients, some patients may present with mucoid or bloody discharge or abdominal pain. The colitis occurs 3 to 36 months after the initial surgical bypass and completely regresses within 3 months of reestablishment of the fecal stream.

A deficiency of short-chain fatty acids is thought to be the cause of diversion colitis. Short-chain fatty acids are the main source of energy for colonocytes, and they are usually derived from fermentation of dietary starches by normal colonic bacterial flora. This lack of colonocyte nutrition leads to an inflammatory reaction. The inflammation can be reversed by giving short chain fatty acids via enemas several times a week or by reestablishing the fecal stream.

Pathologic Features

Gross Findings

The gross and endoscopic features of diversion colitis include erythema, friability, edema, and nodularity with aphthous ulcers.

Microscopic Findings

Histologically, the nodularity seen grossly corresponds to large lymphoid aggregates with prominent germinal centers (Fig. 10.37). The remaining features of diversion colitis are variable. In some instances, the inflammation may mimic severe ulcerative colitis with crypt distortion and marked chronic inflammation of the lamina propria (Fig. 10.38). In other cases, patchy cryptitis and aphthous lesions may mimic Crohn's disease. As a result of the nonspecific nature of these histologic changes, it is imperative that the pathologist be aware that the specimen is from a diverted segment of colon which, as mentioned earlier, is usually a Hartmann's pouch.

Differential Diagnosis

Many people with diverted segments of colon have IBD, and the main differential diagnosis of diversion colitis is generally with recurrent Crohn's disease or ulcerative colitis. The aphthous lesions may also mimic infectious colitis. Definitive diagnosis requires the knowledge of the clinical context that the pathologic changes are occurring in a diverted colonic segment.

Prognosis and Therapy

Prognosis is excellent because diversion colitis completely regresses after the fecal stream is reestablished. If this is not possible, then the inflammation can be reversed by giving short-chain fatty acid enemas. Therapy is often not necessary because diversion colitis is frequently asymptomatic,.

DIVERSION COLITIS–FACT SHEET

Definition

- Inflammation in a diverted segment of colon characterized by a diffuse colitis with lymphoid follicular hyperplasia

Incidence and Location

- Present (histologically) in 50% to 100% of patients with a diverted segment of colon
- Typically, the rectum or rectosigmoid in patients with a Hartmann's pouch is involved but can occur in any bypassed portion of colon

Gender, Race, and Age Distribution

- Equal in males and females
- Any age can be affected

Clinical Features

- Often asymptomatic but may have mucoid or bloody discharge or abdominal pain

Radiologic Features

- Double-contrast barium enemas show lymphoid follicular hyperplasia

Prognosis and Therapy

- Reestablishing the fecal stream is curative
- Short-chain fatty acid enemas also reverse the histologic changes

DIVERSION COLITIS–PATHOLOGIC FEATURES

Gross Findings

- Nodular mucosa with aphthous ulcers, erythema, and edema

Microscopic Findings

- Lymphoid follicular hyperplasia, aphthous ulcers, cryptitis, mild crypt distortion, and chronic inflammation of the lamina propria

Differential Diagnosis

- Crohn's disease
- Ulcerative colitis
- Infectious colitis

DIVERTICULAR DISEASE–ASSOCIATED COLITIS

CLINICAL FEATURES

Diverticular disease is common in patients older than age 60 years, particularly in the sigmoid colon, and patients often present with hematochezia. Diverticular disease–associated colitis is a chronic segmental colitis restricted to the colonic segment involved with diverticulosis that mimics IBD, particularly ulcerative colitis. There is also a form of diverticulitis that mimics Crohn's disease. This form of colitis occurs in patients with diverticulitis who do not have evidence of Crohn's disease elsewhere in the GI tract. The resection specimen demonstrates a Crohn's disease–like reaction to the diverticulitis.

Pathologic Features

Gross Findings

Colonoscopic evaluation generally reveals patchy or confluent hyperemia, often accentuated on the crests of mucosal folds. The mucosa may appear granular, and an exudate is variably present. The distribution is predominantly in the descending and sigmoid colon, the region most commonly involved with diverticular disease. The rectum is typically spared.

Microscopic Findings

Histologically, one can find a range of changes in the mucosa, from a mild plasmacytosis and mild crypt distortion to a full-blown ulcerative colitis–like appearance. Cryptitis and crypt abscesses are typically seen (Figs. 10.39 and 10.40).

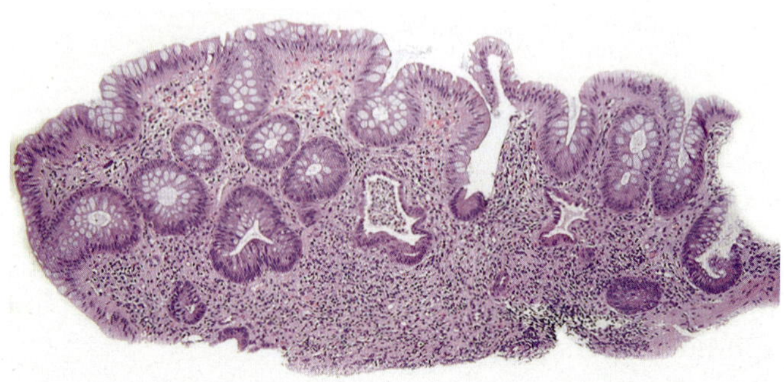

FIGURE 10.39

Diverticular disease–associated colitis. This low-power photomicrograph from the sigmoid colon shows crypt distortion and a chronically inflamed lamina propria. There is a crypt abscess in the center of the image. These changes resemble ulcerative colitis.

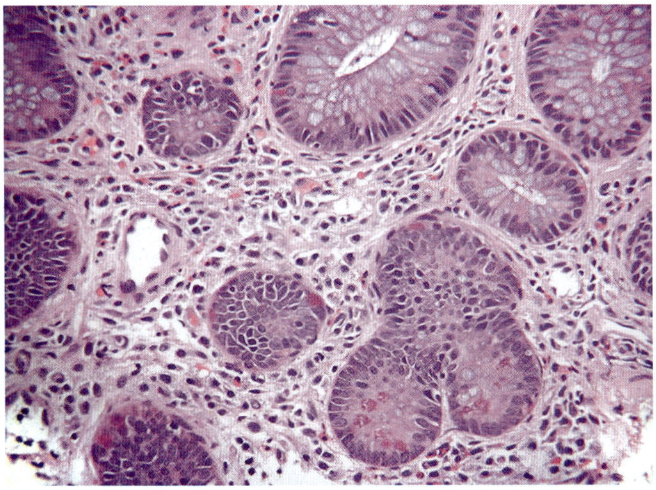

FIGURE 10.40

Diverticular disease–associated colitis. This high-power photomicrograph of the sigmoid colon shows a forked crypt with Paneth cell metaplasia and basal plasma cells, all features indicative of chronic colitis.

Differential Diagnosis

The main differential diagnosis is between diverticular disease–associated colitis and ulcerative colitis. The key to the correct diagnosis is to recognize that the distribution of disease is confined to the segment of diverticulosis coli. Crohn's disease is also in the differential diagnosis because of the usual rectal sparing in diverticular disease–associated colitis.

Prognosis and Therapy

The treatment of patients with diverticular disease–associated colitis varies from therapies aimed at diverticulitis, such as increased fiber intake and antibiotics, to antiinflammatory therapies similar to those used for ulcerative colitis. Some cases are refractory to medical management and require surgical resection.

DIVERTICULAR DISEASE–ASSOCIATED COLITIS–FACT SHEET

Definition

- Segmental colitis resembling ulcerative colitis confined to colonic segment involved with diverticulosis coli

Incidence and Location

- Sigmoid colon with rectal sparing

Gender, Race, and Age Distribution

- Men and women are affected equally
- Patients are generally 60 years of age or older

Clinical Features

- Patients typically present with hematochezia

Prognosis and Therapy

- Increased dietary fiber intake, antibiotics, antiinflammatory therapies used for ulcerative colitis

Diverticular Disease–Associated Colitis–Pathologic Features

Gross Findings

- Granular mucosa with exudates and crescentic hyperemia within the colonic segment involved with diverticulosis

Microscopic Findings

- Cryptitis and crypt abscesses with increased lamina propria chronic inflammation and crypt distortion

Differential Diagnosis

- Ulcerative colitis and Crohn's disease

MUCOSAL PROLAPSE OR SOLITARY RECTAL ULCER SYNDROME

CLINICAL FEATURES

Mucosal prolapse injury occurs in a variety of clinical scenarios such as solitary rectal ulcer syndrome (SRUS), in association with diverticular disease (polypoid prolapsing mucosal folds), and at ostomy sites. SRUS presents with alternating diarrhea and constipation, pain or difficulty defecating, and rectal bleeding. The cause is thought to be malfunction of the puborectalis muscle such that excessive straining on defecation leads to mucosal prolapse that may subsequently ulcerate and form polypoid masses.

Prolapse polyps also occur in association with diverticular disease, at ostomy sites, and adjacent to other mass lesions, the common denominator being an abnormality that causes mucosal prolapse and resultant injury. When this process occurs at the anal verge and forms a polyp, it has been described as *inflammatory cloacogenic polyp*, a term that is no longer used. These other forms of mucosal prolapse are typically asymptomatic but are important to recognize so as not to be confused with adenomas or chronic IBD.

Radiologic Features

Anal endosonography and defecography can be used to make the diagnosis, with the latter being the gold standard. Prolapse polyps throughout the GI tract may be picked up on barium enemas.

Pathologic Features

Gross Findings

Grossly, prolapse polyps are friable, ulcerated polyps with an irregular shape and a beefy red appearance. The surface may be granular and ulcerated, and occasionally, the polyps have an unusual brown color if they contain abundant hemosiderin. Endoscopically, these lesions can look quite threatening because the mass lesions mimic carcinoma, and the ulcerative lesions mimic Crohn's disease. Whereas SRUS is typically located on the anterior rectal wall between 4 and 10 cm from the anal verge, prolapse polyps associated with diverticular disease are typically found in the sigmoid colon at the mouths of diverticula. SRUS can have a varied gross appearance, including erythema, ulcer(s), and polypoid or mass lesions.

Microscopic Findings

The characteristic finding in mucosal prolapse at any site is the presence of fibromuscular hyperplasia of the lamina propria. The presence of strands of smooth muscle growing perpendicular to colonic crypts is diagnostic of prolapse. Occasionally, the amount of fibrosis can overshadow the smooth muscle proliferation. The epithelium is often inflamed and ulcerated, and in some cases, an ischemic appearance may be present with small pseudomembranes. There may be significant crypt architectural distortion. The lamina propria is often vascular, with numerous congested capillaries and hemosiderin deposition. The surface mucosa may be serrated and tufted with goblet cell hypertrophy. In polypoid cases, the mucosa often takes on a villiform configuration that can mimic a villous adenoma (Figs. 10.41 and 10.42). In some cases, glands may become trapped in the submucosa, forming what is known as *colitis cystica profunda*.

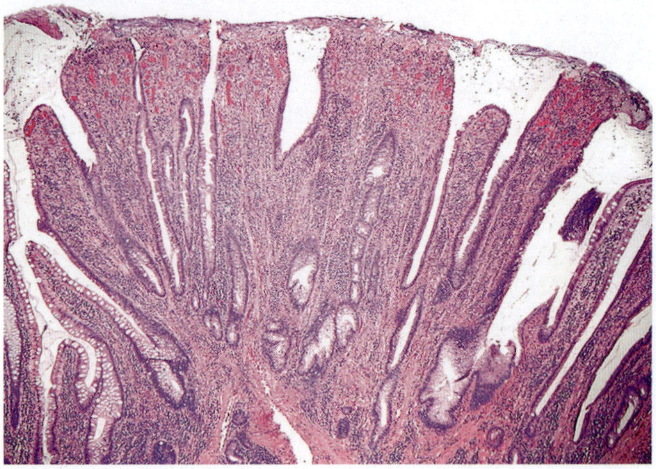

FIGURE 10.41
Mucosal prolapse or solitary rectal ulcer syndrome. This low-power photomicrograph of a solitary rectal ulcer shows villiform hyperplasia with surface ulceration. This villiform growth pattern can be mistaken for a villous adenoma. The base of the crypts is separated by proliferating smooth muscle.

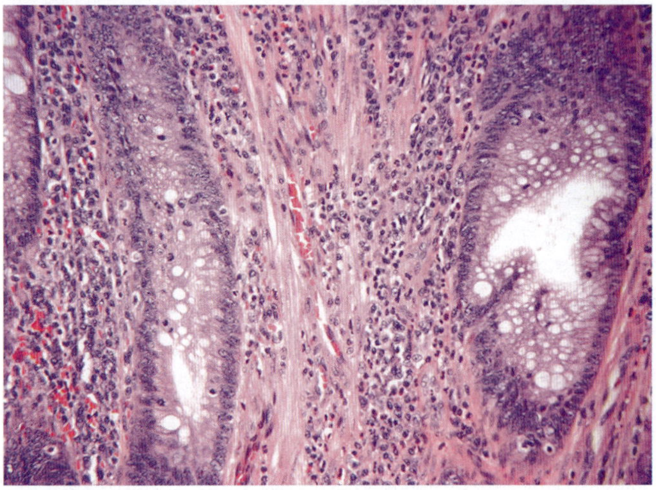

FIGURE 10.42
Mucosal prolapse or solitary rectal ulcer syndrome. This high-power view smooth muscle twigs growing parallel to the colonic crypts. This smooth muscle proliferation is the hallmark of mucosal prolapse and may be mistaken for Peutz-Jeghers polyps.

Differential Diagnosis

Perhaps the most crucial differential diagnosis is between mucosal prolapse and colorectal neoplasia. SRUS can easily be misinterpreted as a villous adenoma or even an invasive carcinoma, with disastrous consequences for the patient. It is important to evaluate the epithelium critically and notice that the changes are reactive or hyperplastic rather than dysplastic. Cases of SRUS with colitis cystica profunda may be mistaken for a well-differentiated mucinous carcinoma. Recognition that the lining epithelium in the cysts is not dysplastic is the key to an accurate diagnosis. Similarly, if the ulcerative component of SRUS is recognized without the characteristic fibromuscular hyperplasia of the lamina propria, an errant diagnosis of chronic IBD may be rendered.

Prolapsing polypoid mucosal folds may be confused with Peutz-Jeghers polyps caused by the increase in smooth muscle associated with prolapse. One can usually differentiate the two based on the lack of an arborizing architecture and lobular configuration of the glandular component in prolapse polyps.

Prognosis and Therapy

Prolapse changes are completely benign, and the patient outcome is determined by the underlying disorder.

If diverticular disease–associated polyps cause problematic bleeding, they may be excised. Patients with SRUS may respond to nonsurgical management such as bulk laxatives and stool softeners. Patients with severe rectal prolapse may require surgical intervention.

MUCOSAL PROLAPSE OR SOLITARY RECTAL ULCER SYNDROME—FACT SHEET

Definition

- Benign fibroinflammatory process secondary to mucosal prolapse

Incidence and Location

- Incidence of 1 in 100,000
- Solitary rectal ulcer syndrome (SRUS) in anterior rectum
- Prolapsing polypoid mucosal folds at mouths of diverticula (sigmoid colon) and near colostomy and ileostomy stomas
- Inflamed prolapse-type polyps at anal verge

Gender, Race, and Age Distribution

- Slight female predominance (SRUS)
- SRUS in young adults
- Prolapsing polypoid mucosal folds in older patients with diverticular disease (older than 60 years)

Clinical Features

- Alternating diarrhea and constipation, pain or difficulty defecating, and rectal bleeding

Radiologic Features

- Anal endosonography, defecography

Prognosis and Therapy

- Responds well to bulk laxatives and stool softeners
- May require rectopexy or resection

MUCOSAL PROLAPSE OR SOLITARY RECTAL ULCER SYNDROME—PATHOLOGIC FEATURES

Gross Findings

- Friable ulcerated polyps or masses on anterior rectal wall or at mouths of diverticula and stomas

Microscopic Findings

- Fibromuscular hyperplasia of the lamina propria
- Hyperplastic regenerative epithelium
- Crypt distortion
- Ulcers

Differential Diagnosis

- Adenoma or carcinoma
- Chronic inflammatory bowel disease
- Peutz-Jeghers polyp

EOSINOPHILIC PROCTOCOLITIS

CLINICAL FEATURES

Eosinophilic proctocolitis is a disease of infants in the first year of life who develop an allergy to formula or breast milk. Occasionally, the allergy is related to food ingested by the mother that is passed to the child via breast milk rather than the breast milk itself. These children present with blood-streaked stools, diarrhea, vomiting, or anemia.

PATHOLOGIC FEATURES

GROSS FINDINGS

Endoscopic features of eosinophilic proctocolitis include focal erythema and friability; ulcers and erosions are rare.

MICROSCOPIC FINDINGS

The histologic features of eosinophilic proctitis are often focal and may be subtle. The major finding is that of increased eosinophils, which can be in the lamina propria and within the epithelium and muscularis mucosae (Fig. 10.43). Studies from the northern United States have found that the presence of greater than 60 eosinophils per 10 hpf in the lamina propria correlates with an eosinophilic proctocolitis. Because the normal number of eosinophils in the lamina propria of the colon varies by geographic region, this number may be inappropriate in more southern climates, where eosinophil counts are higher. The distribution of eosinophils is also important because their presence in the epithelium and muscularis mucosae and at the periphery of lymphoid aggregates correlates with allergy. One may also find foci of cryptitis in eosinophilic proctocolitis.

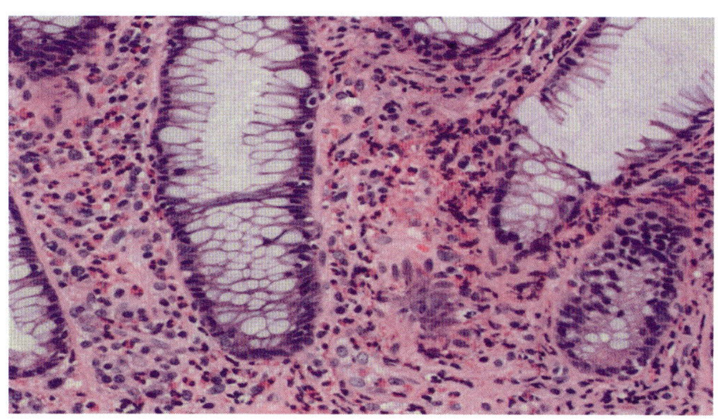

FIGURE 10.43

Eosinophilic colitis. This medium-power photomicrograph of the left colon shows dense eosinophilic infiltrate with clusters of eosinophils in the lamina propria, as well as several intraepithelial infiltration and crypt injury by eosinophils.

Differential Diagnosis

Eosinophilic proctocolitis needs to be distinguished from infectious colitis, necrotizing enterocolitis, medication-associated colitis, and colitis associated with Hirschsprung's disease. Because all of these conditions may show cryptitis, the diagnosis of allergy rests on finding abnormal numbers and distributions of eosinophils. Crohn's disease may show prominent eosinophils; however, eosinophilic proctocolitis lacks chronic mucosal injury.

Prognosis and Therapy

Treatment revolves around dietary manipulation to exclude whatever nutrient seems to be causing the symptoms. The prognosis is excellent because most children outgrow this condition.

EOSINOPHILIC PROCTOCOLITIS–FACT SHEET

Definition

- A disease of infants in the first year of life who develop an allergy to formula or breast milk

Incidence and Location

- 0.5% to 10% of pediatric population (lower in exclusively breastfed infants)
- Rectum most common site of involvement

Gender, Race, and Age Distribution

- Males equal to females
- Ages 1 month to 1 year

Clinical Features

- Blood-streaked stools, diarrhea, vomiting, and anemia

Prognosis and Therapy

- Change diet to eliminate allergen
- By age 3 years, most children outgrow the allergy

Eosinophilic Proctocolitis–Pathologic Features

Gross Findings

- Focal erythema and friability, as well as rare ulcers or erosions

Microscopic Findings

- Greater than 60 eosinophils per 10 hpf in the lamina propria
- Eosinophils in the epithelium, muscularis mucosae, and at the periphery of lymphoid aggregates
- Cryptitis

Differential Diagnosis

- Infectious colitis, necrotizing enterocolitis, and colitis associated with Hirschsprung's disease

SYSTEMIC MASTOCYTOSIS

CLINICAL FEATURES

Systemic mastocytosis is a neoplastic proliferation of mast cells within at least one extracutaneous organ. The GI tract is a common site of involvement and may be the first manifestation of the disease in a significant proportion of patients. Mast cells secrete multiple inflammatory mediators, including histamine, serotonin, and prostaglandins. These inflammatory mediators result in GI symptoms such as abdominal pain, diarrhea, nausea, and vomiting.

Pathologic Features

Gross Findings

The colonic mucosa usually appears erythematous, granular, or nodular.

Microscopic Findings

A major criterion for the diagnosis systemic mastocytosis involving the GI tract is the presence of multifocal dense aggregates of 15 or more mast cells within a mucosal biopsy. Minor criteria include (1) more than 25% of the mast cells with atypical morphology (often spindled), (2) aberrant expression of CD2 and/or CD25, (3) detection of *KIT* point mutation at codon 816, and (4) serum total tryptase persistently greater than 20 ng/mL. A definitive diagnosis of systemic mastocytosis may be rendered in the presence of one major plus one minor criterion or three minor criteria. The mast cell aggregates are often most prominent directly beneath the surface epithelium (Fig. 10.44). Involvement of the mucosa may be quite patchy and multiple biopsies may be needed to demonstrate the abnormal infiltrate. Subtle infiltration of abnormal mast cells may also be present, making the diagnosis quite difficult. Prominent eosinophilic infiltrates may be a clue that mast cell disease is present because increased eosinophils are seen in more than 40% of biopsies from patients with systemic mastocytosis. Given the patchy and subtle nature of mast cell infiltration, immunohistochemical stains for CD117 and CD25 should be performed on biopsies to rule out mast cell disease in patients in whom the clinical suspicion is high (Figs. 10.45 and 10.46).

More recently, there has been increased interest in mast cells as the cause of irritable bowel syndrome. Although mast cells may be involved in irritable bowel syndrome, immunohistochemical staining for CD117 and counting mast cells has no value in this setting because it is likely the increased secretion of inflammatory mediators from mast cells rather than mast cell

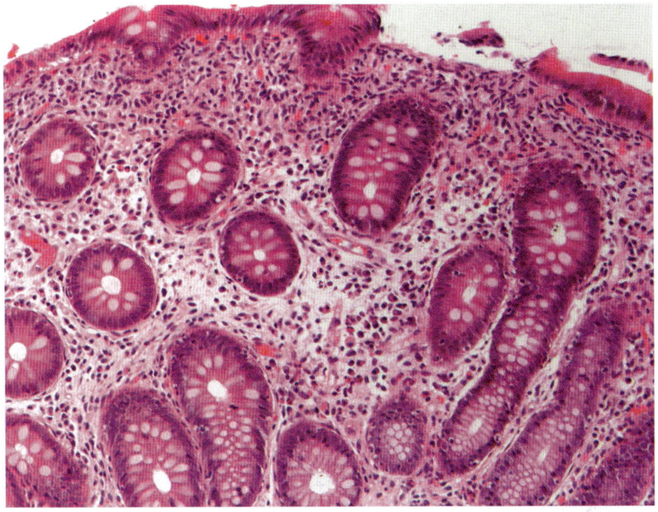

FIGURE 10.44

Systemic mastocytosis. Aggregates of ovoid to spindle cells present as a band underneath the surface epithelium associated with increased eosinophils.

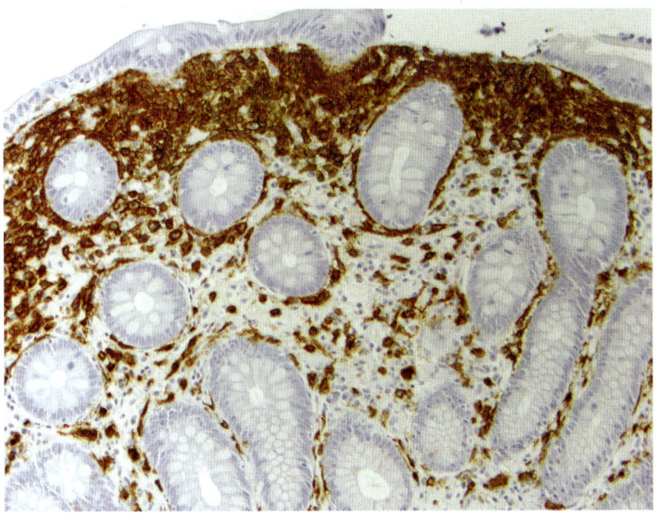

FIGURE 10.45

Immunohistochemical stain for CD117 highlights the band of mast cells in the lamina propria beneath the surface epithelium

number that contributes to the pathogenesis. Similarly, patients with mast cell activation syndrome often have normal number and distribution of mast cells.

Differential Diagnosis

If mast cell disease is suspected, immunohistochemical confirmation is recommended because histiocytes and spindle cell lesions can be mistaken for mast cells. Prominent eosinophilia should raise the possibility of mast cell disease, but other causes of mucosal eosinophilia (drug reaction, infection, idiopathic eosinophilic gastroenteritis) should be considered.

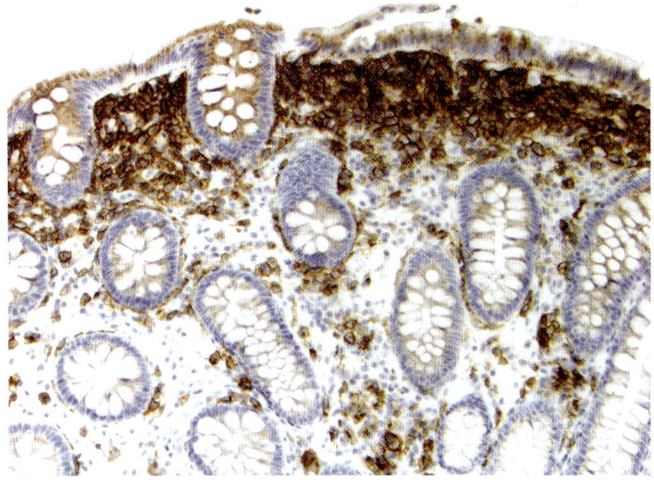

FIGURE 10.46

Aberrant expression of CD25 on CD117-positive mast cells is diagnostic of systemic mastocytosis.

Prognosis and Therapy

Systemic mastocytosis is not a curable disease. The prognosis is variable. Treatment is aimed at controlling symptoms.

SYSTEMIC MASTOCYTOSIS—FACT SHEET

Definition

- Clonal, neoplastic proliferation of mast cells that accumulates in one or more extracutaneous organs

Incidence and Location

- Rare disease; true incidence is unknown

Gender, Race, and Age Distribution

- Slight male predominance in childhood, slight female predominance in adulthood

Clinical Features

- Diarrhea, abdominal pain, nausea, vomiting

Prognosis and Therapy

- No cure; treatment is aimed at controlling symptoms
- Oral cromolyn, antihistamines, proton pump inhibitors

Systemic Mastocytosis—Pathologic Features

Gross Findings

- Erythema, nodularity, granular mucosa

Microscopic Findings

- Aggregates of mast cells (>15) within the mucosa often with ovoid or spindle morphology

- Most commonly subepithelial bandlike infiltrate
- Prominent eosinophilia characteristic
- CD117-positive mast cells with coexpression of CD25 and CD2

Differential Diagnosis

- If eosinophils are prominent, other causes of mucosal eosinophilia should be excluded

MYCOPHENOLATE MOFETIL COLITIS

CLINICAL FEATURES

Mycophenolate mofetil (MMF) is a drug used for immunosuppression, largely in patients who have undergone solid organ transplants. It is also used in bone marrow transplant patients to treat GVHD, and it may be used to help treat various autoimmune diseases. Patients taking MMF may present with a wide variety of GI complaints, including diarrhea, abdominal pain, malabsorption, weight loss, and bleeding. Symptoms are more likely to occur if MMF therapy is started later after transplantation or if the patient has an elevated creatinine measurement.

PATHOLOGIC FEATURES

GROSS FINDINGS

Ulcers, erosions, and granularity may be seen throughout the GI tract.

MICROSCOPIC FINDINGS

Mycophenolate mofetil damage in the colon is characterized by apoptosis similar to GVHD (Fig. 10.47). In addition, one may find dilated attenuated crypts containing a few eosinophils or neutrophils floating within the crypt lumen (Fig. 10.48). In severe cases, there may be crypt dropout with only small nests of residual neuroendocrine cells in the lamina propria. Over time, a fair amount of crypt distortion may develop such that the changes mimic chronic IBD. Often the lamina propria appears hypocellular resulting from the immunosuppressive effects of MMF.

DIFFERENTIAL DIAGNOSIS

Graft-versus-host disease can mimic MMF colitis to the point that they are indistinguishable. Prominence of an eosinophilic infiltrate has been reported to favor MMF colitis, whereas marked apoptosis and endocrine cell clusters are more in favor of a diagnosis of GVHD.

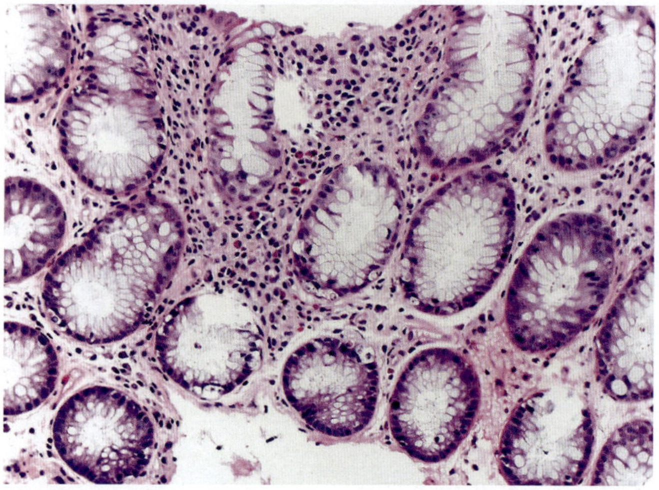

FIGURE 10.47
Mycophenolate mofetil colitis. This high-power photomicrograph shows a few apoptotic cells within the colonic crypts similar to the changes seen in mild graft-versus-host disease.

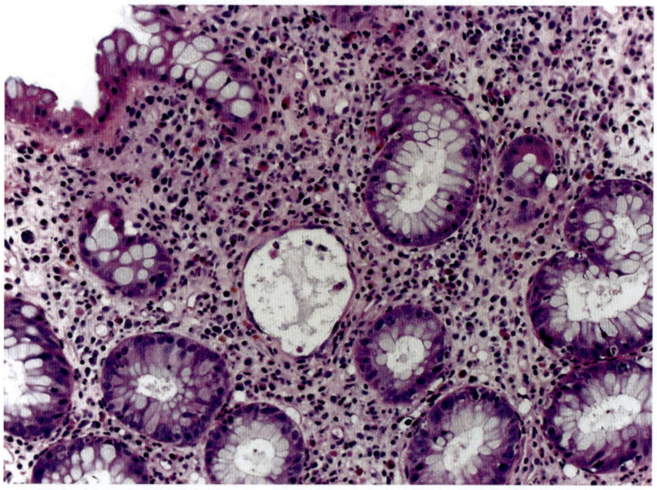

FIGURE 10.48
Mycophenolate mofetil colitis. This high-power photomicrograph shows a dilated crypt containing eosinophils and neutrophils. Such dilated crypts with attenuated epithelium are more typical of mycophenolate damage than graft-versus-host disease.

However, none of these features is entirely specific, and correlation with clinical findings, timeline of symptoms, and the presence of extraintestinal manifestations of GVHD are all useful in making this distinction. In some cases, the amount of crypt distortion can mimic quiescent ulcerative colitis. In addition, the amount of epithelial damage with minimal inflammation may also bring up the possibility of ischemia.

PROGNOSIS AND THERAPY

Discontinuing the drug or decreasing the dosage typically leads to rapid symptomatic improvement, often within 5 to 7 days.

MYCOPHENOLATE MOFETIL COLITIS—FACT SHEET

Definition
- Damage to the colon secondary to the drug mycophenolate mofetil (CellCept)

Incidence and Location
- Incidence is unknown, but more likely if patient's creatinine level is elevated or if drug is started later in the transplant course
- Location can be anywhere in the gastrointestinal tract

Gender, Race, and Age Distribution
- None known

Clinical Features
- Diarrhea, abdominal pain, weight loss, bleeding

Prognosis and Therapy
- Rapid response after drug is discontinued or dose is lowered

MYCOPHENOLATE MOFETIL COLITIS—PATHOLOGIC FEATURES

Gross Findings
- Ulcers, erosions, and granularity throughout gastrointestinal tract

Microscopic Findings
- Apoptosis, dilated crypts with eosinophils or neutrophils, crypt distortion

Differential Diagnosis
- Graft-versus-host disease, chronic inflammatory bowel disease, ischemia

IMMUNE CHECKPOINT RECEPTOR INHIBITOR–ASSOCIATED COLITIS

CLINICAL FEATURES

Ipilimumab, a monoclonal antibody against cytotoxic T lymphocyte–associated protein 4 (CTLA-4), is now used to treat patients with a wide variety of malignancies. Ipilimumab activates the immune system by disrupting negative regulation of T cells. Such immune activation can cause numerous side effects, of which GI side effects, particularly moderate to severe watery diarrhea, are quite common. Other immunotherapies such as pembrolizumab and nivolumab that activate the immune system by blocking the action of programmed cell death protein-1 (PD-1) may also produce similar GI symptoms. Additional immunotherapies are in development, and complications from this class of medications are likely to increase.

PATHOLOGIC FEATURES

GROSS FINDINGS

The colon may demonstrate an abnormal vascular pattern, exudates, granularity, and ulcers.

MICROSCOPIC FINDINGS

The lamina propria is hypercellular with increased lymphocytes and plasma cells. There are neutrophilic cryptitis, increased intraepithelial lymphocytes, and increased crypt apoptosis (Fig. 10.49). Erosions and ulcers may be seen. The crypt architecture is usually preserved, but some cases may show features of a chronic colitis with prominent basal lymphoplasmacytosis.

DIFFERENTIAL DIAGNOSIS

The main differential diagnosis is with an infectious colitis. Exclusion of CMV infection by immunohistochemistry may be warranted. Stool studies are often needed to exclude other infectious colitides. The lack of chronic mucosal injury such as crypt architectural distortion usually allows distinction from IBD. The combination of a moderate to severe active colitis with increased intraepithelial lymphocytes and prominent apoptosis should prompt consideration of an immunotherapy associated colitis.

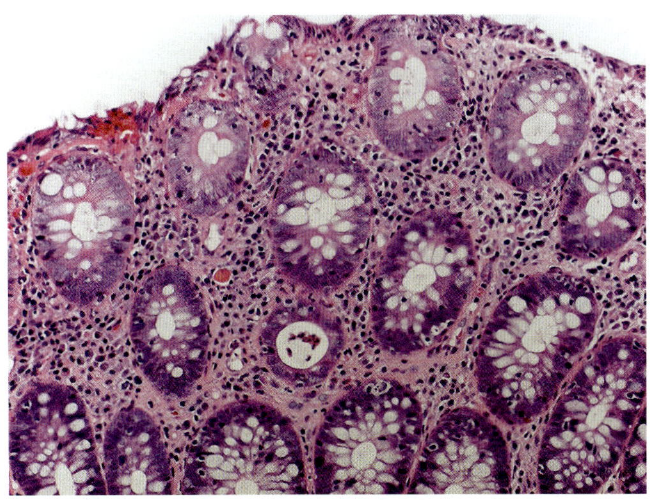

FIGURE 10.49

Ipilimumab colitis. This high-power photomicrograph shows a colonic mucosa with increased intraepithelial lymphocytes, increased crypt apoptosis, and focal neutrophilic cryptitis. This mixed pattern of injury is often seen with ipilimumab use.

Prognosis and Therapy

This condition usually improves after discontinuation of the medication. Immunosuppression with steroids or infliximab may be necessary in severe cases.

IPILIMUMAB COLITIS—FACT SHEET

Definition
- Colitis associated with administration of ipilimumab, nivolumab, or pembrolizumab

Incidence and Location
- Between 25% and 50% of patients treated with ipilimumab
- More commonly affects left colon

Gender, Race, and Age Distribution
- None known

Clinical Features
- Persistent watery diarrhea occurring within a few days to weeks of therapy

Prognosis and Therapy
- Generally responsive to discontinuation of medication
- Severe cases may require immunosuppression with steroids or infliximab or other anti–tumor necrosis factor agents

Ipilimumab Colitis—Pathologic Features

Gross Findings
- Mucosal erythema, edema, exudate, and ulcers

Microscopic Findings
- Neutrophilic cryptitis, increased intraepithelial lymphocytes, increased crypt apoptosis
- Increased lamina propria cellularity with increased lymphocytes and plasma cells

Differential Diagnosis
- Infectious colitis
- Inflammatory bowel disease

CORD COLITIS SYNDROME

CLINICAL FEATURES

Cord colitis syndrome occurs in about 10% of patients who undergo cord-blood hematopoietic stem cell transplant. Cord colitis syndrome presents with a persistent diarrheal illness not caused by GVHD, viral infection, or any other identifiable cause. More recent evidence suggests that this syndrome may be caused by the bacterium *Bradyrhizobium enterica*. Patients with cord colitis syndrome respond to antibiotics.

Pathologic Features

Gross Findings

The colon may demonstrate edema, erythema, and ulcers.

Microscopic Findings

Cord colitis syndrome is characterized by a chronic active colitis pattern of injury with crypt distortion, neutrophilic cryptitis, and increased lamina propria inflammatory cells (Fig. 10.50). There is often only a mild increase in crypt apoptosis. Crypt rupture granulomas and occasionally well-formed granulomas away from injured crypts may be seen.

Differential Diagnosis

The main differential diagnosis is with acute GVHD and IBD. GVHD usually lacks increased lamina propria lymphocytes and plasma cells and prominent neutrophilic cryptitis.

Prognosis and Therapy

Patients with cord colitis syndrome usually respond well to antibiotics, but prolonged therapy may be warranted to prevent relapse.

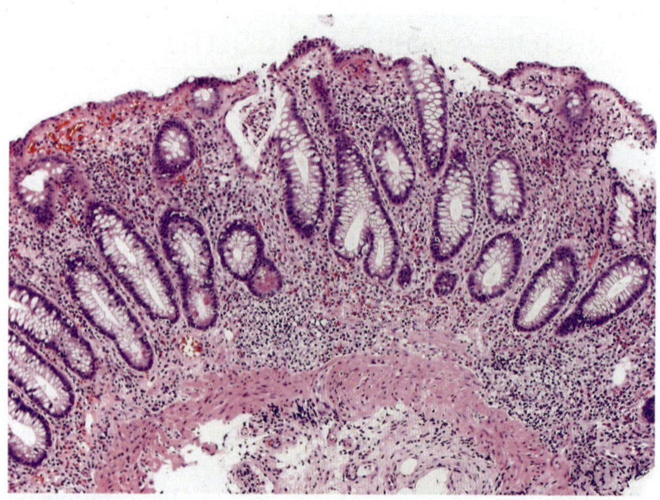

FIGURE 10.50

Cord colitis syndrome. The histologic features of this case are identical to those of inflammatory bowel disease with crypt architectural distortion, neutrophilic inflammation, and basal lymphoplasmacytosis.

CORD COLITIS SYNDROME—FACT SHEET

Definition
- Persistent diarrheal illness occurring in cord-blood hematopoietic stem cell transplant patients without identifiable cause

Incidence and Location
- Occurs in 10% of cord-blood hematopoietic stem cell transplant patients
- Location can be anywhere in the colon

Gender, Race, and Age Distribution
- None known

Clinical Features
- Persistent diarrheal illness (>7 days' duration)

Prognosis and Therapy
- Response to antibiotics (fluoroquinolone and metronidazole)

CORD-COLITIS SYNDROME—PATHOLOGIC FEATURES

Gross Findings
- Mucosal erythema, edema, and ulcers

Microscopic Findings
- Crypt architectural distortion with neutrophilic cryptitis
- Mixed lamina propria infiltrate with increased lymphocytes, plasma cells, histiocytes, and neutrophils

Differential Diagnosis
- Graft-versus-host disease
- Inflammatory bowel disease

NONSTEROIDAL ANTIINFLAMMATORY DRUG COLITIS

CLINICAL FEATURES

Nonsteroidal antiinflammatory drug use is ubiquitous, and doses as small as a baby aspirin a day can cause damage to the GI tract. Not only do these drugs have direct toxic effects on the mucosa, but they also inhibit prostaglandin synthesis, which helps protect the mucosa. Symptoms from mucosal injury include abdominal pain, bloody diarrhea, iron-deficiency anemia, and malabsorption. The risk of GI complications increases with dose, duration of therapy, age, and concurrent use of steroids or anticoagulants. It has been estimated that several thousand patients in the United States experience exsanguination from GI bleeding caused by NSAIDs each year. NSAIDs are also known to complicate or exacerbate ulcerative colitis and diverticular disease.

PATHOLOGIC FEATURES

GROSS FINDINGS

Ulcers and erosions may be seen throughout the GI tract. The terminal ileum and right colon, as well as the rectum (suppositories), are the most common sites of NSAID damage in the lower gut. Diaphragm disease is a rare complication most often seen in the small intestine, but this has also been reported in the colon.

MICROSCOPIC FINDINGS

A number of different patterns of mucosal damage in the colon have been reported with NSAIDs. Focal active colitis has been mentioned in several studies as being associated with NSAID use. Other articles have described a more mixed or lymphocytic infiltrate in the mucosa. Nonspecific ulcers or erosions are common, but crypt distortion like that seen in ulcerative colitis is generally not seen. There are also numerous reports of NSAIDs causing an injury identical to ischemic colitis as well. NSAIDs are also known to increase the amount of apoptosis seen in the gut or colon.

DIFFERENTIAL DIAGNOSIS

Whereas NSAID lesions in the terminal ileum and right colon can mimic Crohn's disease, the focal active colitis pattern mimics resolving infectious colitis. NSAIDs can also cause colonic lesions that are identical to ischemic colitis. History is of paramount importance in making the correct diagnosis.

PROGNOSIS AND THERAPY

Discontinuing the drug is the first line of defense, but patients may require surgical intervention for perforations, strictures, or bleeding ulcers. Metronidazole and sulfasalazine have been used as medical therapy. Misoprostol or proton pump inhibitors can be given with NSAIDs to protect the mucosal barrier (upper GI tract). Selective cyclooxygenase-2 inhibitors may cut down on NSAID damage in the gut.

NONSTEROIDAL ANTIINFLAMMATORY DRUG COLITIS—FACT SHEET

Definition
- Damage to the colon secondary to nonsteroidal antiinflammatory drugs (NSAIDs)

Incidence and Location

- Incidence is unknown, but 40% of those with NSAID damage have lower gastrointestinal (GI) tract involvement
- Location can be anywhere in the GI tract, but terminal ileum, right colon, and rectum more common

Gender, Race, and Age Distribution

- Age older than 60 years increases risk of GI damage from NSAIDs

Clinical Features

- Abdominal pain, bloody diarrhea, iron-deficiency anemia

Prognosis and Therapy

- May resolve with discontinuation of drug but may require medical or surgical intervention
- Thousands die every year from massive GI bleeding secondary to NSAIDs

Nonsteroidal Antiinflammatory Drug Colitis—Pathologic Features

Gross Findings

- Ulcers or erosions throughout the gastrointestinal tract
- Diaphragm disease

Microscopic Findings

- Focal active colitis, ischemic-type mucosal injury, increased apoptosis, nonspecific ulcers or erosions

Differential Diagnosis

- Crohn's disease, resolving infection, ischemia

CHEMOTHERAPY EFFECT OR MUCOSITIS

CLINICAL FEATURES

About 5% to 15% of patients on chemotherapy develop mucositis; this number jumps to 30% to 40% when radiation is added to the regimen. It has been theorized that chemotherapy generates reactive oxygen species that damage epithelial cell DNA, leading to apoptosis and clonal cell death. However, recent evidence suggests that cytokine activation may also play a role in causing mucositis. Even though chemotherapy damage is much more common in the small bowel, stomach, and esophagus, the colon can still be affected. Diarrhea and bleeding (rather than nausea and vomiting) are related to colonic injury. Overall mucositis is a major cause of morbidity that often leads to infection and causes delay or decreased dosing of chemotherapy.

PATHOLOGIC FEATURES

GROSS FINDINGS

Ulcers and erosions are endoscopic findings typical of chemotherapy damage.

MICROSCOPIC FINDINGS

Chemotherapy leads to epithelial damage with little, if any, inflammation. There are usually attenuated crypts with apoptosis, and the surviving cells have atypical hyperchromatic nuclei suggestive of CMV or herpes virus infection (Fig. 10.51). The atypia may also mimic dysplasia. In general, one can usually exclude viral infection, in that there are many cells with atypical nuclei but none with classic viral inclusions.

DIFFERENTIAL DIAGNOSIS

As previously mentioned, the nuclear changes induced by chemotherapy often resemble CMV inclusions; however, exhaustive searching will not yield any classic inclusions despite finding many atypical cells. Immunostains can also be helpful in excluding this possibility. In patients receiving bone marrow transplant, it generally takes 3 weeks for the apoptosis induced by conditioning chemotherapy to completely disappear. Therefore, extreme care should be taken in diagnosing GVHD before day 21 after transplantation. Chemotherapy effect can also mimic ischemia, in that both processes have epithelial damage with minimal inflammation. A hyalinized lamina propria favors the diagnosis of ischemia (as does a geographic distribution of disease).

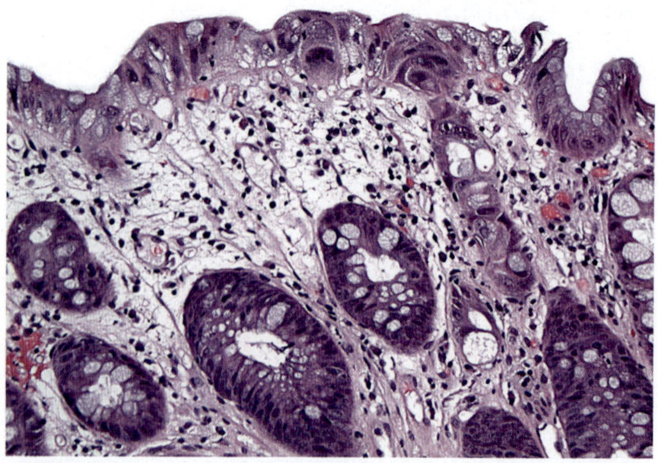

FIGURE 10.51

Chemotherapy effect. This medium-power photomicrograph shows reactive cytologic atypia, which raises the question of dysplasia, as well as viral infection.

Prognosis and Therapy

Overall mucositis is a major cause of morbidity that often causes delay or decreased dosing of chemotherapy. It is also a frequent cause of secondary infection. Although many treatment compounds are being studied, the only current therapy is supportive care and decreased or delayed dosing of chemotherapy.

CHEMOTHERAPY EFFECT OR MUCOSITIS—FACT SHEET

Definition

- Damage to the colon secondary to chemotherapy

Incidence and Location

- 5% to 15% of patients on chemotherapy
- More common in small intestine, stomach, and esophagus than colon

Gender, Race, and Age Distribution

- Female patients have more mucosal damage from 5-fluorouracil–based chemotherapy than male patients
- Mucositis is less common in African Americans than in whites

Clinical Features

- Diarrhea, hematochezia

Prognosis and Therapy

- Major cause of morbidity
- No therapy except delay or decreased dosing of chemotherapy

Chemotherapy Effect or Mucositis—Pathologic Features

Gross Findings

- Ulcers or erosions throughout the gastrointestinal tract

Microscopic Findings

- Attenuated crypts with apoptosis and little inflammation
- Marked regenerative changes with nuclei resembling cytomegalovirus (CMV) inclusions

Differential Diagnosis

- CMV, graft-versus-host disease , ischemia, dysplasia

SELECTED READINGS

1. Lazenby AJ, Yardley JH, Giardiello FM, et al. Lymphocytic ("microscopic") colitis: a comparative histopathologic study with particular reference to collagenous colitis. *Hum Pathol.* 1989;20:18–28.
2. Nostrant TT, Kumar NB, Appelman HD. Histopathology differentiates acute self-limited colitis from ulcerative colitis. *Gastroenterology.* 1987;92:318–328.
3. Noble C, Nimmo E, Gaya D, et al. Novel susceptibility genes in inflammatory bowel disease. *World J Gastroenterol.* 2006;12:1991–1999.
4. Shih DQ, Targan SR. Immunopathogenesis of inflammatory bowel disease. *World J Gastroenterol.* 2008;14:390–400.
5. Price AB, Morson BC. Inflammatory bowel disease: the surgical pathology of Crohn's disease and ulcerative colitis. *Hum Pathol.* 1975;6:7–29.
6. Kleer CG, Appelman HD. Ulcerative colitis: patterns of involvement in colorectal biopsies and changes with time. *Am J Surg Pathol.* 1998;22:983–989.
7. Kim B, Barnett JL, Kleer CG, et al. Endoscopic and histological patchiness in treated ulcerative colitis. *Am J Gastroenterol.* 1999;94:3258–3262.
8. D'Haens G, Geboes K, Peeters M, et al. Patchy cecal inflammation associated with distal ulcerative colitis: a prospective endoscopic study. *Am J Gastroenterol.* 1997;92:1275–1279.
9. Yantiss RK, Sapp HL, Farraye FA, et al. Histologic predictors of pouchitis in patients with chronic ulcerative colitis. *Am J Surg Pathol.* 2004;28:999–1006.
10. Glickman JN, Bousvaros A, Farraye FA, et al. Pediatric patients with untreated ulcerative colitis may present initially with unusual morphologic findings. *Am J Surg Pathol.* 2004;28:190–197.
11. Spiliadis CA, Lennard-Jones JE. Ulcerative colitis with relative sparing of the rectum: clinical features, histology, and prognosis. *Dis Colon Rectum.* 1987;30:334–336.
12. Haskell H, Andrews Jr CW, Reddy SI, et al. Pathologic features and clinical significance of "backwash" ileitis in ulcerative colitis. *Am J Surg Pathol.* 2005;29:1472–1481.
13. Terashima S, Hoshino Y, Kanzaki N, et al. Ulcerative duodenitis accompanying ulcerative colitis. *J Clin Gastroenterol.* 2001;32:172–175.
14. Lin J, McKenna BJ, Appelman HD. Morphologic findings in upper gastrointestinal biopsies of patients with ulcerative colitis: a controlled study. *Am J Surg Pathol.* 2010;34:1672–1677.
15. Mahadeva U, Martin JP, Patel NK, et al. Granulomatous ulcerative colitis: a re-appraisal of the mucosal granuloma in the distinction of Crohn's disease from ulcerative colitis. *Histopathology.* 2002;41:50–55.
16. Farmer RG, Hawk WA, Turnbull Jr RB. Clinical patterns in Crohn's disease: a statistical study of 615 cases. *Gastroenterology.* 1975;68:627–635.
17. Lamps LW, Madhusudhan KT, Havens JM, et al. Pathogenic Yersinia DNA is detected in bowel and mesenteric lymph nodes from patients with Crohn's disease. *Am J Surg Pathol.* 2003;27:220–227.
18. Loftus Jr EV, Schoenfeld P, Sandborn WJ. The epidemiology and natural history of Crohn's disease in population-based patient cohorts from North America: a systematic review. *Aliment Pharmacol Ther.* 2002;16:51–60.
19. Warren R, Barwick KW. Crohn's colitis with carcinoma and dysplasia: report of a case and review of 100 small and large bowel resections for Crohn's disease to detect incidence of dysplasia. *Am J Surg Pathol.* 1983;7:151–159.
20. Meucci G, Bortoli A, Riccioli FA, et al. Frequency and clinical evolution of indeterminate colitis: a retrospective multi-centre study in northern Italy. GSMII (Gruppo di Studio per le Malattie Infiammatorie Intestinali). *Eur J Gastroenterol Hepatol.* 1999;11:909–913.
21. Pezim ME, Pemberton JH, Beart Jr RW, et al. Outcome of "indeterminant" colitis following ileal pouch-anal anastomosis. *Dis Colon Rectum.* 1989;32:653–658.
22. Jess T, Loftus Jr EV, Velayos FS, et al. Risk of intestinal cancer in inflammatory bowel disease: a population-based study from Olmsted County, Minnesota. *Gastroenterology.* 2006;130:1039–1046.
23. Watanabe T, Konishi T, Kishimoto J, et al. Ulcerative colitis-associated colorectal cancer shows a poorer survival than sporadic colorectal cancer: a nationwide Japanese study. *Inflamm Bowel Dis.* 2011;17:802–808.
24. Riddell RH, Goldman H, Ransohoff DF, et al. Dysplasia in inflammatory bowel disease: standardized classification with provisional clinical applications. *Hum Pathol.* 1983;14:931–968.
25. Engelsgjerd M, Farraye FA, Odze RD. Polypectomy may be adequate treatment for adenoma-like dysplastic lesions in chronic ulcerative colitis. *Gastroenterology.* 1999;117:1288–1294.

26. Rubio CA, Befrits R, Jaramillo E, et al. Villous and serrated adenomatous growth bordering carcinomas in inflammatory bowel disease. *Anticancer Res*. 2000;20:4761–4764.
27. Srivastava A, Redston M, Farraye FA, et al. Hyperplastic/serrated polyposis in inflammatory bowel disease: a case series of a previously undescribed entity. *Am J Surg Pathol*. 2008;32:296–303.
28. Kisiel JB, Loftus Jr EV, Harmsen WS, et al. Outcome of sporadic adenomas and adenoma-like dysplasia in patients with ulcerative colitis undergoing polypectomy. *Inflamm Bowel Dis*. 2012;18:226–235.
29. Shetty S, Anjarwalla SM, Gupta J, et al. Focal active colitis: a prospective study of clinicopathological correlations in 90 patients. *Histopathology*. 2011;59:850–856.
30. Glauser PM, Wermuth P, Cathomas G, et al. Ischemic colitis: clinical presentation, localization in relation to risk factors, and long-term results. *World J Surg*. 2011;35:2549–2554.
31. Khor TS, Lauwers GY, Odze RD. "Mass-forming" ischemic colitis is a distinctive variant with predilection for the proximal colon: a clinicopathologic study of 16 cases. *Am J Surg Pathol*. 2015;39(9):1275–1281.
32. Berthrong M, Fajardo LF. Radiation injury in surgical pathology: part II. Alimentary tract. *Am J Surg Pathol*. 1981;5:153–178.
33. Odze RD, Bines J, Leichtner AM, et al. Allergic proctocolitis in infants: a prospective clinicopathologic biopsy study. *Hum Pathol*. 1993;24:668–674.
34. Olesen M, Eriksson S, Bohr J, et al. Microscopic colitis—a common diarrhoeal disease: an epidemiological study in Orebro, Sweden, 1993-1998. *Gut*. 2004;53:346–350.
35. Jarnerot G, Tysk C, Bohr J, et al. Collagenous colitis and fecal stream diversion. *Gastroenterology*. 1995;109:449–455.
36. Glotzer DJ, Glick ME, Goldman H. Proctitis and colitis following diversion of the fecal stream. *Gastroenterology*. 1981;80:438–441.
37. Geraghty JM, Talbot IC. Diversion colitis: histological features in the colon and rectum after defunctioning colostomy. *Gut*. 1991;32:1020–1023.
38. Parfitt JR, Driman DK. Pathological effects of drugs on the gastrointestinal tract: a review. *Hum Pathol*. 2007;38:527–536.
39. Papadimitriou JC, Drachenberg CB, Beskow CO, et al. Graft-versus-host disease-like features in mycophenolate mofetil-related colitis. *Transplant Proc*. 2001;33:2237–2238.
40. Selbst MK, Ahrens WA, Robert ME, et al. Spectrum of histologic changes in colonic biopsies in patients treated with mycophenolate mofetil. *Mod Pathol*. 2009;22:737–743.
41. Herrera AF, Soriano G, Bellizzi AM, et al. Cord colitis syndrome in cord-blood stem-cell transplantation. *N Engl J Med*. 2011;365:815–824.
42. Baert F, Schmit A, D'Haens G, et al. Budesonide in collagenous colitis: a double-blind placebo-controlled trial with histologic follow-up. *Gastroenterology*. 2002;122:20–25.
43. Beaugerie L, Luboinski J, Brousse N, et al. Drug induced lymphocytic colitis. *Gut*. 1994;35:426–428.
44. Libbrecht L, Croes R, Ectors N, et al. Microscopic colitis with giant cells. *Histopathology*. 2002;40:335–338.
45. Hahn HP, Hornick JL. Immunoreactivity for CD25 in gastrointestinal mucosal mast cells is specific for systemic mastocytosis. *Am J Surg Pathol*. 2007;31:1669–1676.
46. Goldstein NS, Leon-Armin C, Mani A. Crohn's colitis-like changes in sigmoid diverticulitis specimens is usually an idiosyncratic inflammatory response to the diverticulosis rather than Crohn's colitis. *Am J Surg Pathol*. 2000;24:668–675.
47. Makapugay LM, Dean PJ. Diverticular disease-associated chronic colitis. *Am J Surg Pathol*. 1996;20:94–102.
48. Saul SH. Inflammatory cloacogenic polyp: relationship to solitary rectal ulcer syndrome/mucosal prolapse and other bowel disorders. *Hum Pathol*. 1987;18:1120–1125.
49. Martin CJ, Parks TG, Biggart JD. Solitary rectal ulcer syndrome in Northern Ireland, 1971-1980. *Br J Surg*. 1981;68:744–747.

11

Gastrointestinal Polyposis Syndromes

Amitabh Srivastava, MD

Nearly every histologic type of polyp involving the gastrointestinal (GI) tract can occur in a sporadic or syndromic setting. In general, a syndromic diagnosis must be suspected when multiple polyps type are present concurrently or sequentially on surveillance colonoscopy; when the polyps occur at a very young age; when extraintestinal manifestations of particular syndromes are identified; and when there is a family history of similar polyps or cancer involving the GI tract or other organs known to be at risk in syndromic settings. The diagnosis is often challenging for multiple reasons. Very early age at presentation or an attenuated phenotype may not reveal the classic features of the syndrome, information regarding extraintestinal manifestations may be lacking, and relevant family history may be missing in patients with de novo germline mutations. It is therefore incumbent upon pathologists to flag any potential syndromic cases for further testing and genetic counseling that may prove beneficial not only to the index proband but also to the entire family.

Cancers arising in the setting of GI polyposis syndromes are rare and responsible for fewer than 1% of all lower GI tract malignancies. However, research into the pathogenesis and longitudinal outcome of polyposis syndromes has provided valuable insight into the genetic alterations that underlie neoplasia involving the GI tract. The most common polyposis syndromes are summarized in Table 11.1 and may be broadly categorized into those that result in numerous adenomas, multiple serrated polyps, in hamartomas with defined phenotype, or an admixture of polyps with different morphology. Syndromes that cause adenomatous polyps most commonly include familial adenomatous polyposis (FAP) and its phenotypic variants, whereas syndromes that cause hamartomatous polyps include Peutz-Jeghers syndrome (PJS), juvenile polyposis syndrome, and *PTEN* (phosphatase and tensin homolog) hamartoma syndrome (PTHS), which is often used synonymously with CS. It is also important to emphasize that although most polyposis syndromes are hereditary with well-defined germline genetic aberrations, a significant proportion of patients may be negative on germline testing, and for some syndromes, such as serrated polyposis syndrome (SPS), no germline defect has been identified thus far. The discussion in this chapter is restricted to the most common forms of polyposis syndromes and excludes lymphomatous polyposis, which is a peculiar macroscopic manifestation of lymphoproliferative disorders, and inflammatory polyposis, which is a non-neoplastic entity that most commonly occurs in the setting of inflammatory bowel disease (IBD). The organ-specific polyposis syndrome gastric adenocarcinoma with proximal polyposis syndrome (GAPPS) is discussed in the chapter on neoplastic gastric lesions (Chapter 4).

ADENOMATOUS POLYPOSIS SYNDROMES

Clinical Features

Numerous conventional adenomas occur in the colon and in the upper GI tract in three major familial settings: the classic and attenuated FAP syndrome and the *MUTYH*-associated polyposis (MAP) syndrome.

Classic FAP is an autosomal dominant syndrome caused by pathogenic germline mutations in the adenomatous polyposis coli (APC) gene, affecting approximately 1 in 8000 to 10,000 individuals. Males and females are equally affected, and fewer than 1% of all colorectal cancers occur in patients with FAP. The disorder is characterized by the development of adenomas at an early age along with characteristic extracolonic manifestations. Patients with classic FAP have more than 100 adenomas at presentation, and the colon may be completely carpeted with hundreds to thousands of adenomas in severe cases. The polyp burden can be lower in children because adenomas usually appear in the second decade of life. Colorectal cancers occur at an average of 39 years, and nearly all patients develop cancer by the time they are 45 to 50 years of age. However, cancer is

TABLE 11.1

Classification of Gastrointestinal Polyposis Syndromes

Hereditary Polyposis Syndromes
Adenomas
Familial adenomatous polyposis coli
Attenuated familial adenomatous polyposis coli
Gardner's syndrome
Turcot's syndrome
MUIYH-associated polyposis
Hamartomas
Peutz-Jeghers syndrome
Juvenile polyposis syndrome
Cowden's disease
Bannayan-Riley-Ruvalcaba syndrome
Devon family syndrome
OTHER SYNDROMES
Hereditary mixed polyposis syndrome
Neurofibromatosis type 1
Multiple endocrine neoplasia type 2
Nonhereditary polyposis syndromes
Serrated polyposis syndrome
Cronkhite-Canada syndrome
Lymphomatosis polyposis
Nodular lymphoid hyperplasia
Pneumatosis cystoides intestinalis
Colitis cystica profunda

exceedingly rare before 15 years of age, and prophylactic colectomy is typically performed around this age in most patients.

Duodenal adenomas occur in almost all patients with FAP and typically involve the periampullary region and the distal duodenum. Duodenal adenocarcinomas occur in 5% to 10% patients and are a common cause of death in patients who have undergone a prophylactic colectomy. Gastric involvement occurs in more than half of patients with FAP and typically manifests as numerous fundic gland polyps, some of which may show cytologic dysplasia. However, gastric cancer in the setting of FAP occurs in association with conventional or pyloric gland adenomas and not fundic gland polyps. A distinct FAP variant called GAPPS has been recently described and is discussed in greater detail in the chapter on gastric neoplasms (Chapter 4).

Extraintestinal manifestations in FAP are common and include osteomas, epidermoid cysts, fibromas, supernumerary teeth, odontomas, and congenital hypertrophy of the retinal pigment epithelium. These lesions are usually asymptomatic and are not associated with malignant potential. One exception, however, is desmoid tumor, occurring in 10% of patients with FAP. The small intestinal mesentery and the abdominal wall or the extremities are common sites of involvement with this tumor. FAP is also associated with an increased risk of extracolonic tumors, such as papillary thyroid carcinoma, childhood hepatoblastoma, benign and malignant adrenocortical tumors, and brain tumors, particularly medulloblastoma.

Gardner's and Turcot syndromes were terms used in the past to describe a subset of patients with FAP, but their use is no longer recommended; the former because nearly all patients with FAP have this constellation of findings and the latter because many of these patients ended up being eventually diagnosed as having Lynch syndrome rather than FAP.

An attenuated form of FAP (AFAP) is also recognized that shows autosomal dominant inheritance and is distinguished from classic FAP by the presence of fewer adenomas (<100), later onset of adenomas (35–45 years of age), later onset of colorectal cancer (mean age, 55 years), and a lower lifetime risk of colorectal cancer (80%). However, it must be recognized that colonoscopic methods using enhanced visualization may show more than 100 adenomas, which is an arbitrary threshold for distinguishing the classic and attenuated forms of the disease. Adenomas show preferential right colon involvement in AFAP, and the rectum may be relatively spared. Upper GI adenomas and fundic gland polyps occur similar to classic FAP but extracolonic manifestations may be limited. The diagnosis of AFAP can be excluded if any family member shows more than 100 adenomas before 30 years of age.

MUTYH- (formerly known as *MYH*-) associated polyposis (MAP) syndrome is an autosomal recessive syndrome caused by biallelic germline mutations in the *MUTYH* gene. Patients typically present in the fifth or sixth decade of life and show between 10 and 100 adenomas, but more than 100 adenomas may be seen in one-third of all patients. Germline *MUTYH* mutations are identified in roughly 30% of *APC*-negative patients with 10 to 100 adenomas and 14% of *APC*-negative patients with 100 to 1000 adenomas. Duodenal polyposis occurs in about 25% of patients and duodenal cancer in 4%. Sebaceous gland tumors and congenital hypertrophy of retinal pigmentary epithelium is uncommon, and the lifetime risks of extraintestinal manifestations, similar to FAP, is about 38%. Serrated polyps also occur in almost 50% of patients with MAP and are caused by *KRAS* gene mutations that are typically G:C to T:A transversions that are a consequence of defective DNA repair.

According to current screening guidelines for adenomatous polyposis syndromes, patients with a personal history of more than 10 cumulative colorectal adenomas or those with fewer than 10 adenomas but a positive family history or adenomas with FAP-type extracolonic manifestations (duodenal or ampullary adenoma, desmoids; papillary thyroid cancer, congenital hypertrophy of the retinal pigment epithelium [CHRPE]), epidermal cysts, and osteomas should be tested. Genetic testing should include *APC* and *MUTYH* gene mutation analysis.

ADENOMATOUS POLYPOSIS SYNDROMES—FACT SHEET

Definition

- Genetic syndromes associated with germline *APC* or *MUTYH* gene mutations that manifest as numerous adenomas involving the colon and upper gastrointestinal (GI) tract, an increased risk of cancer, and a variety of extracolonic manifestations

Incidence and Location

- Familial adenomatous polyposis (FAP) is the most common polyposis syndrome (1 in 8000–10,000)
- Inheritance is autosomal dominant for FAP and an attenuated form of FAP (AFAP) and autosomal recessive for *MUTYH*
- 1% to 2% of population carries monoallelic germline *MUTYH* pathogenic variant
- 80% to 100% patients develop colorectal cancer in AFAP and FAP, respectively
- 30% of patients with FAP have de novo mutations of the APC gene and may not have a positive family history

Morbidity and Mortality

- Average age of colorectal cancer diagnosis is 39 years in FAP; older in AFAP and *MUTYH*-associated polyposis (MAP)
- Vast majority of patients in all three syndromes have upper GI polyps, typically fundic gland polyps, and may also have conventional adenomas and pyloric gland adenomas
- Duodenal adenomas and carcinomas and desmoids are also major causes of morbidity and mortality in classic FAP

Gender, Race, and Age Distribution

- Males and females equally affected
- No racial or ethnic predominance
- Average ages of onset of adenomas are in second decade of life in classic FAP and a decade later in AFAP and MAP

Clinical Features

- Most patients asymptomatic; adenomas often present years before any symptoms occur
- The most common symptoms are rectal bleeding or diarrhea
- Synchronous cancers occur in 40% and metachronous cancers in 70% of patients with classic FAP
- Adenomas of variable size and number involve the colon, stomach, and duodenum in all three syndromes
- Serrated polyps may also be present in MAP
- Extraintestinal manifestations include desmoid tumors, epidermal cysts, osteomas, and congenital hypertrophy of retinal pigmentary epithelium and may be seen in FAP, AFAP, or MAP
- Risk of some extraintestinal cancers such as papillary thyroid cancer, hepatoblastoma, and brain tumors such as medulloblastoma is also increased in FAP and AFAP

Prognosis and Therapy

- 100% risk of colon cancer without prophylactic colectomy in classic FAP
- Most common cause of mortality after prophylactic colectomy is periampullary duodenal cancer

Pathologic Features

Gross Findings

Adenomas develop throughout the entire colorectum and appendix and macroscopically resemble their sporadic counterparts in classic FAP. The number, size, and shape of the adenomas can vary greatly between patients. Although they tend to be evenly dispersed, adenomas are relatively larger in the rectosigmoid, giving the appearance of a greater density of polyps in this region. In the classic and most dramatic form, the entire mucosa becomes carpeted with adenomatous polyps so that no intervening normal mucosa is recognizable (Figs. 11.1A–D). The size can vary from diminutive to large, and lesions may be sessile, pedunculated, or flat lateral spreading type. Colorectal carcinoma, when present, may be multifocal and shows a relative predilection for the left colon.

In AFAP, the polyp burden is much lower and typically less than 100, preferentially involving the right colon (Fig. 11.1E). Sparing of the rectum by adenomatous polyps may also be suggestive of a diagnosis of AFAP, as can the presence of numerous flat adenomas. The latter is not a specific feature and may be seen in patients with Lynch syndrome as well.

In addition to conventional adenomas, patients with MAP can also harbor a variable number of serrated polyps. The polyp burden is much lower than classic FAP in most patients, but a subset may present with severe polyposis similar to FAP.

Microscopic Findings

The adenomas and carcinomas that arise in FAP, AFAP, and MAP are morphologically indistinguishable from their sporadic counterparts (Fig. 11.2A). Similar to sporadic lesions, the incidence of malignancy is related to adenoma number, size, and histology. Single, double, or tricryptal adenomas are common in sections taken from grossly normal mucosa (Figs. 11.2B and C) in classic FAP and can be seen in AFAP as well. A variable number of serrated polyps can be seen in MAP, and they may resemble sporadic hyperplastic polyps or sessile serrated polyps. The predominance of adenomas is indicative of the correct diagnosis in such cases, but in patients with a low polyp burden and a combination of adenomas and serrated polyps, it may be virtually impossible to distinguish MAP from serrated polyposis syndrome (SPS; see later), and genetic testing is key to establishing the diagnosis. Carcinomas in MAP often show a high number of intratumoral lymphocytes and a mucinous adenocarcinoma phenotype, mimicking microsatellite instability high (MSI-H) colorectal carcinomas, but DNA mismatch repair immunohistochemistry (IHC) shows intact staining in the tumor cells.

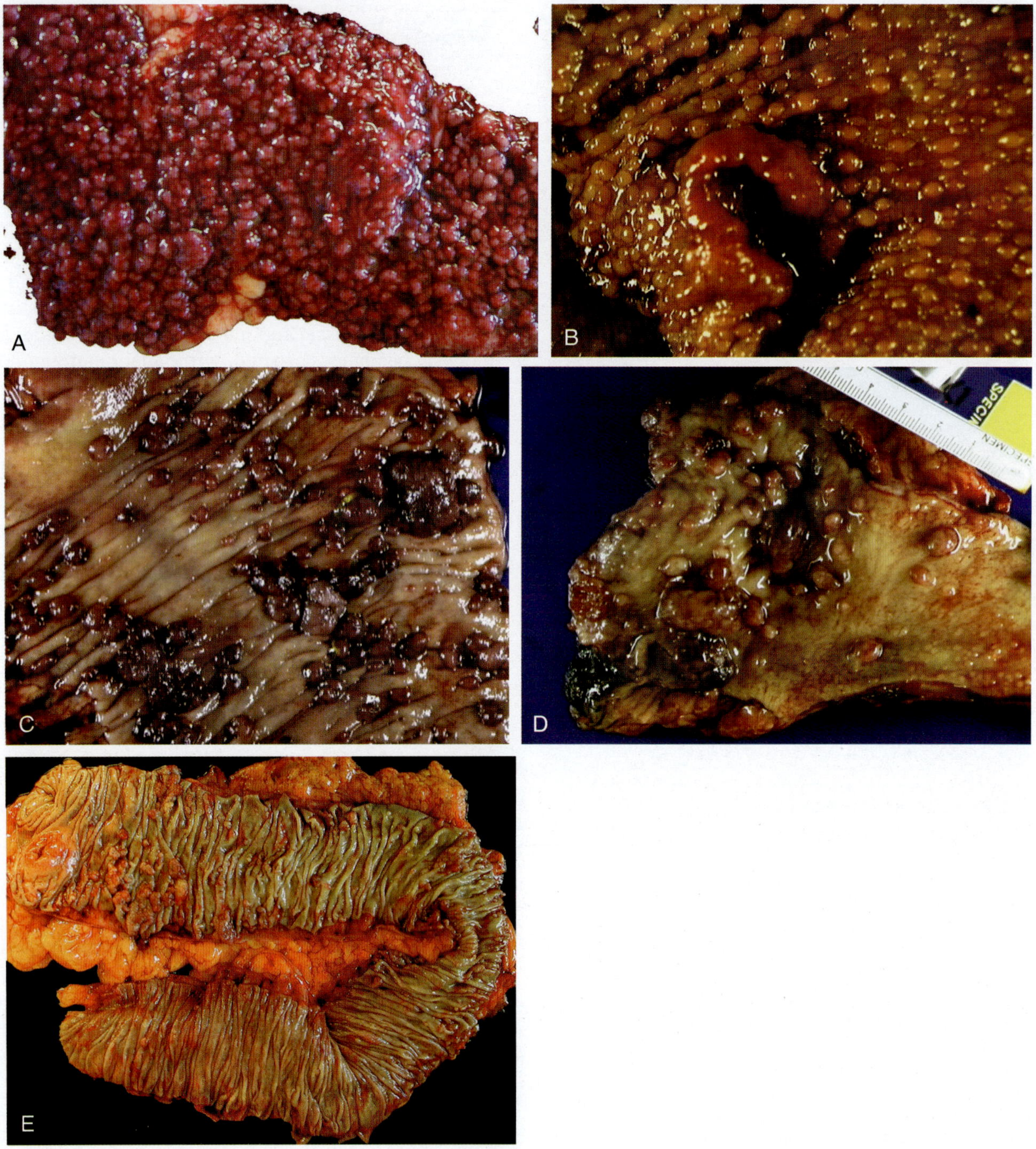

FIGURE 11.1

The number, size, and location of adenomas varies in familial adenomatous polyposis (FAP). The colon may be carpeted with lesions with barely visible normal colonic mucosa (**A**). Concurrent carcinoma may be present in some cases (**B**), and adenomas may cluster together (**C** and **D**). In attenuated FAP, the adenoma burden is lower than classic FAP, and preferential involvement of the right colon may be seen (**E**).

Upper GI polyps are found in virtually 100% of patients with FAP, most commonly fundic gland polyps and small bowel adenomas involving the ampulla and distal duodenum (Fig. 11.3). The histologic features of fundic gland polyps in FAP are similar to their sporadic counterparts, but dysplasia is more common in the syndromic setting and manifests as nuclear enlargement, hyperchromasia, and loss of polarity within dilated oxyntic glands that extends to the polyp surface. However, high-grade dysplasia or carcinoma arising in a fundic gland polyp in FAP is extremely rare. In addition to conventional adenomas, pyloric gland adenomas (Fig. 11.4), traditional serrated adenomas, and adenomas with hybrid features have also been described

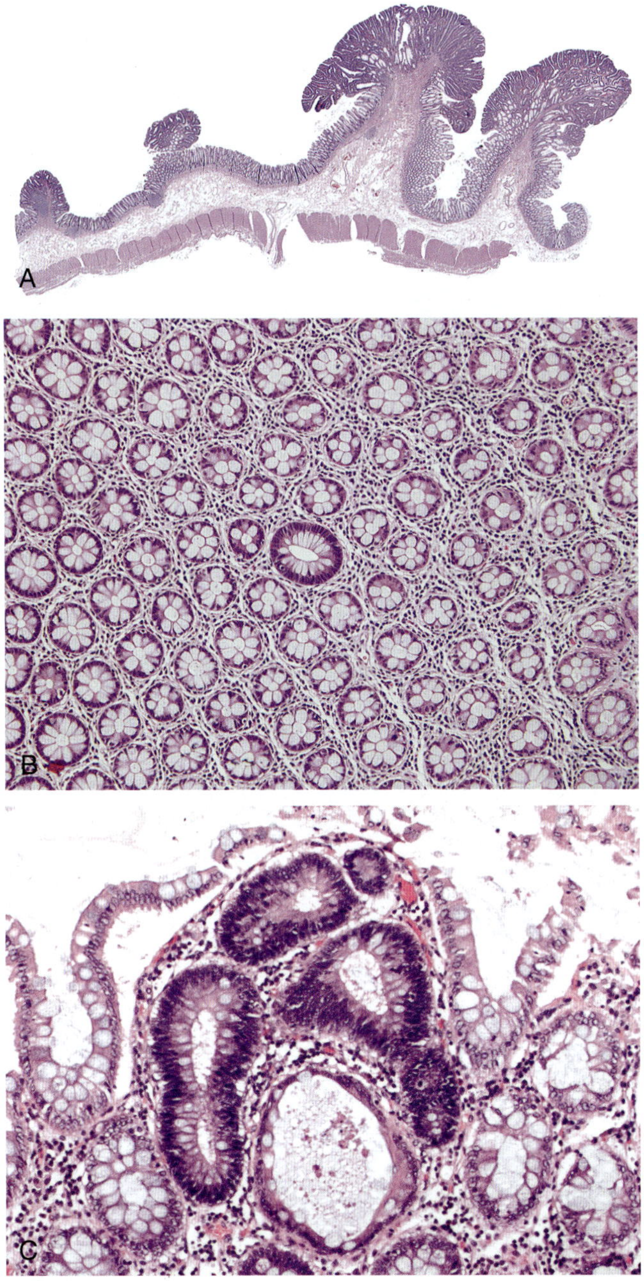

FIGURE 11.2

Scanning view of the colonic mucosa from a patient with familial adenomatous polyposis (FAP) reveals four different polypoid tubular adenomas (**A**). Single crypt adenomas (**B**) or adenomas involving two or three crypts (**C**) are commonly seen in FAP in random sections taken from macroscopically normal colonic mucosa.

Adenomatous Polyposis Syndromes—Pathologic Features

Gross Findings

- Hundreds to thousands of adenomas evenly distributed throughout colorectum and appendix in classic familial adenomatous polyposis (FAP); lower polyp burden in attenuated form of FAP (AFAP) and *MUTYH*-associated polyposis (MAP)
- Adenomas tend to be larger in the rectosigmoid in FAP; right-sided dominance, relative rectal sparing, and flat adenomas more common in AFAP; serrated polyps more common in MAP
- Adenomas range in size from microscopic (crypt adenomas) to pedunculated lesions greater than 1 cm in diameter
- Colorectal carcinomas may be multifocal

Microscopic Findings

- Adenomas in FAP, AFAP, and MAP are identical to sporadic adenomas
- Random sections of grossly normal mucosa may show early adenomas consisting of small tubules lined by adenomatous epithelium involving one or just a few crypts
- Adenomas may be tubular, tubulovillous, or villous
- Pyloric gland adenomas and traditional serrated adenomas can also occur
- Fundic gland polyps can be numerous and show dysplasia
- Carcinomas in MAP have high number of intratumoral lymphocytes and may be of a mucinous phenotype
- Gastric adenocarcinomas in FAP arise in adenomas and not in fundic gland polyps
- Duodenal adenoma and adenocarcinomas and desmoid tumors also resemble their sporadic counterparts
- Gardner fibroma is a distinctive mesenchymal tumor in children affected with FAP

Genetics

- Germline *APC* gene mutations in FAP and AFAP
- Mutations within the mutation cluster region in exon 15 is associated with classic FAP
- Mutations in the 5′ or 3′ region or exon 9 of the APC gene associated with AFAP
- Biallelic germline mutation involving the *MUTYH* gene in MAP

Differential Diagnosis

- Adenomatous polyposis related to other germline mutations (*NTHL-1, POLE, MSH-3, AXIN2*)
- Constitutional mismatch repair deficiency syndrome
- Immune deficiency–associated polyposis
- Serrated polyposis syndrome
- Hereditary mixed polyposis syndrome

in FAP. The spectrum of upper GI findings in AFAP and MAP is similar to classic FAP, but the polyp burden is much lower than in FAP. Mesenchymal tumors, such as desmoid and Gardner fibroma, that occur in association with adenomatous polyposis syndromes are discussed in Chapter 7.

Genetic testing for germline mutations in the *APC* gene identifies most patients with FAP and AFAP. As mentioned earlier, germline mutations in the *MUTYH* gene are detected in a subset of patients resembling FAP or AFAP who are negative for germline APC mutation. *MUTYH* gene is now universally included in the panels used for germline testing of patients with suspected hereditary polyposis syndromes.

Differential Diagnosis

Classic FAP is easy to recognize when the adenoma burden is massive. AFAP and MAP may be hard to distinguish from each other, but the presence of a significant

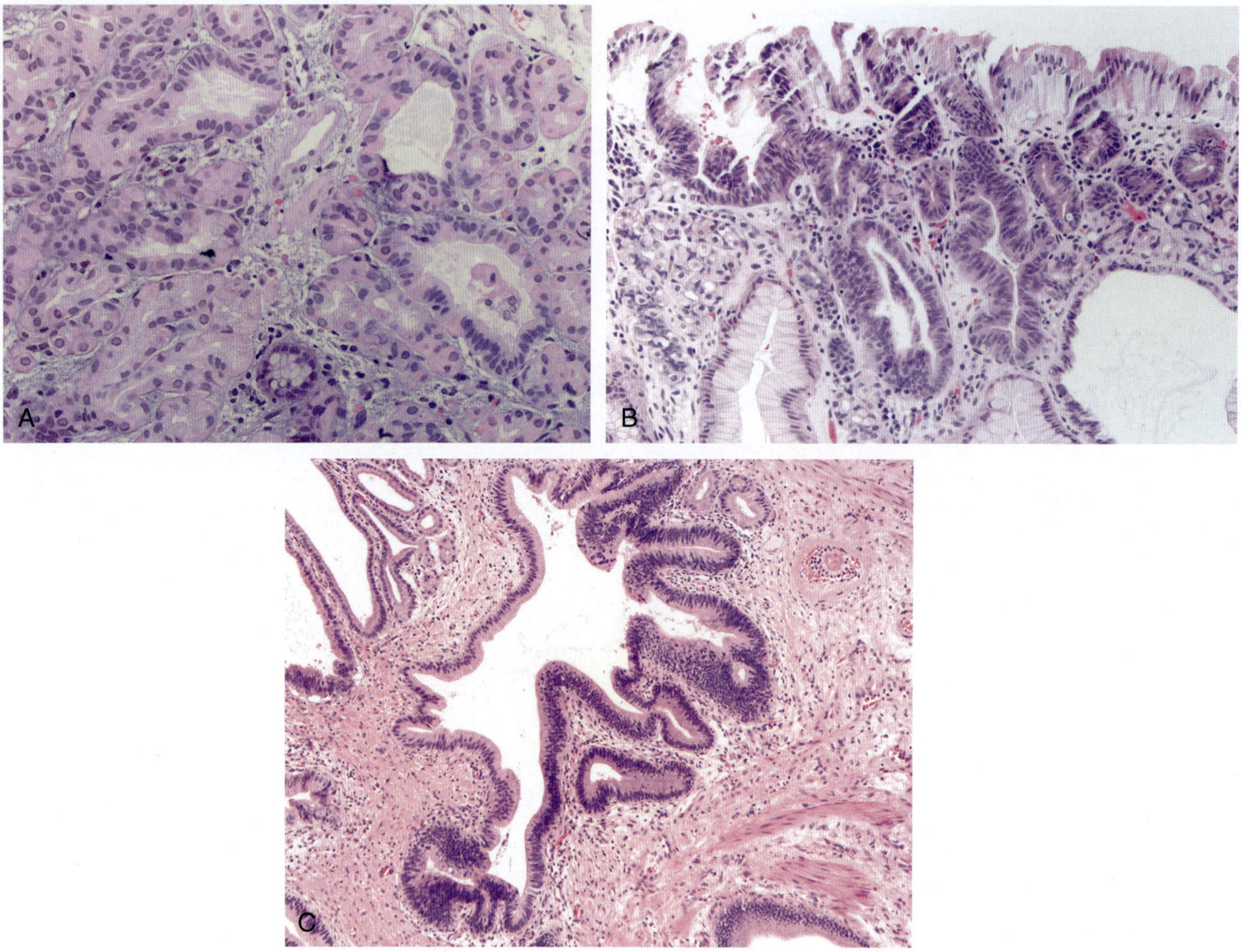

FIGURE 11.3

Upper gastrointestinal involvement in familial adenomatous polyposis (FAP) manifests as numerous fundic gland polyps (**A**) involving the stomach. Dysplastic fundic gland polyps are also quite common in patients with FAP (**B**). Duodenal and ampullary adenomas (**C**) are also prevalent; the latter may not be amenable to surveillance and necessitate a Whipple procedure for definite treatment.

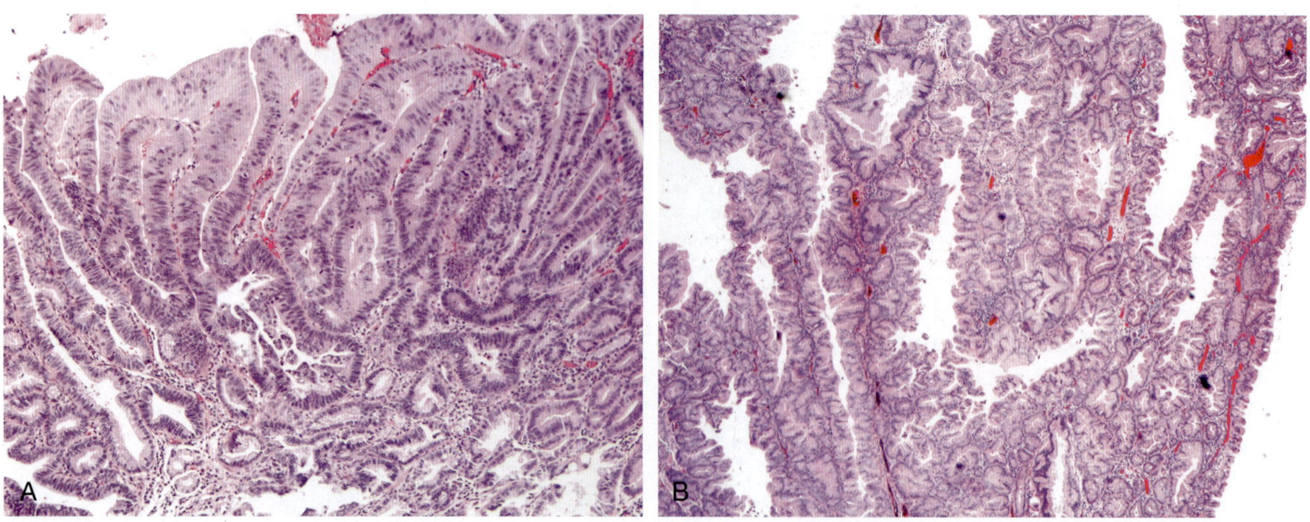

FIGURE 11.4

Although dysplastic fundic gland polyps are common in patients with familial adenomatous polyposis (FAP) gastric adenocarcinoma seldom arises in these lesions. Gastric cancer in FAP typically arises in conventional adenomas (**A**) or in pyloric gland adenomas (**B**).

number of serrated polyps is in favor of MAP. A combination of adenomas and serrated polyps can also be seen in SPS, discussed later, but the predominant polyp types in the latter entity are hyperplastic polyps and sessile serrated polyps, whereas MAP shows a predominance of adenomas.

NHTL1-associated polyposis (NAP) is an autosomal recessive base excision repair disorder that may resemble a Lynch-like syndrome or MAP because of the presence of sebaceous skin tumors and MSI-H phenotype of carcinomas. However, the tumors in the setting of NAP have a characteristic C→T somatic mutation spectrum. Polymerase proofreading–associated polyposis (PPAP) is an autosomal dominant disorder caused by mutations in *POLD1* and *POLE*. Adenomas occur in the colon as well as the upper GI tract, similar to classic FAP, but at a later age of onset. The morphology of adenomas and carcinomas resembles sporadic lesions, but a characteristic hypermutant somatic mutation genotype is typically seen. *MSH-3-* and *AXIN2*-associated polyposis syndromes have also been described and can result in multiple adenomas involving the colon similar to FAP. Constitutional mismatch repair deficiency syndrome is an autosomal recessive disorder caused by biallelic inactivation in one of the four DNA mismatch repair genes (*MLH1, MSH2, MSH6, PMS2*). This contrasts with the autosomal dominant inheritance in Lynch syndrome caused by germline mutation in the same DNA mismatch repair genes. Brain tumors, particularly glioblastomas, are present in nearly 50% of patients, and tumors of the GI tract and hematologic malignancies are commonly seen. Similar to FAP, patients are susceptible to developing multiple adenomas and carcinoma of the colon in childhood or young adulthood. Immunohistochemistry shows loss of the involved DNA mismatch repair protein in both the normal epithelium and the tumor cells. Hereditary mixed polyposis syndrome (HMPS) is a rare condition caused by abnormalities in the *GREM1* gene. Patients develop not just conventional adenomas but also inflammatory polyps, hyperplastic polyps, and mucosal prolapse-type polyps and have a high risk of colorectal cancer.

Prognosis and Therapy

The key to the management of FAP, AFAP, and MAP is to identify presymptomatic individuals, predominantly through screening of relatives of affected patients. The diagnosis can easily be made or excluded by sigmoidoscopy or barium enema examinations performed annually beginning at 10 to 12 years of age with histologic confirmation of an adenoma. Prophylactic colectomy is recommended in classic FAP even in asymptomatic individuals who may not have completed puberty. This may be delayed in AFAP given the later onset of adenomas and carcinomas. Apart from polyp burden in a patient, the youngest age for diagnosis of cancer in the family can also be a reasonable guide for timing a prophylactic colectomy. MAP shows an autosomal recessive inheritance, and no relevant family history of adenomas or cancer may be detected. In view of limited longitudinal data, the screening and surveillance recommendations for MAP are currently similar to those for AFAP. Patients with a prophylactic colectomy typically receive a small intestinal J-pouch reconstruction that serves as a neorectum. The remnant native rectum and the ileal J-pouch continue to be at risk, and periodic surveillance is recommended for early detection and removal of adenomas and cancer.

Patients who undergo prophylactic colectomy may still die of carcinomas arising in other sites, most commonly periampullary duodenal carcinomas or from desmoid tumors. Management of duodenal polyposis is often stratified using the Spiegelman classification that includes polyp number, size, histology, and degree of dysplasia. Surveillance may not be a viable option after adenomas develop or involve the ampulla, and a Whipple resection may be indicated for these patients. Gastrectomy is seldom indicated given the low risk of malignant transformation of gastric fundic gland polyps and adenomas. Endoscopic resections of any large lesions are the standard of care, and surgical resection is reserved for patients with deeply invasive adenocarcinomas.

SERRATED POLYPOSIS SYNDROME

Serrated polyposis syndrome is now the preferred designation for the entity previously described as hyperplastic polyposis and serrated adenomatous polyposis. It is characterized by the presence of multiple, large, proximal serrated polyps, and these patients are at high risk for synchronous or metachronous colorectal cancer and benefit from close surveillance.

Clinical Features

Serrated polyposis syndrome is an underrecognized entity characterized by the presence of multiple serrated polyps throughout the colorectum. Concurrent carcinoma may be present at initial diagnosis in a subset of patients. There is no sex predominance. Prevalence in screening colonoscopy patients may be as high as 0.1%, and the majority of patients are diagnosed in the sixth decade of life. However, the age range at first diagnosis is quite broad. A diagnosis of SPS may be rendered when one of two criteria is met: (1) five or more serrated polyps (any histological subtype) proximal to the rectum, with all being at least 5 mm in size and at least two being 10 mm or more in greatest dimension or (2) more than 20 serrated polyps of any size distributed throughout the colon with at least five being proximal to the rectum. The criteria are applied in a cumulative manner over several examinations and do not require all polyps to be present concurrently at the same colonoscopy. No germline mutation has been identified, although *RNF43* mutations have been reported in some families. Cigarette smoking and high body mass index are risk factors, and the risk of colorectal cancer is increased not just in the patient but also in first-degree relatives.

SERRATED POLYPOSIS SYNDROME—FACT SHEET

Definition

- Defined by the cumulative presence of either of these criteria:
  - ≥5 serrated polyps (any histological subtype: hyperplastic, sessile serrated polyp or traditional serrated adenoma) of which at least 2 are ≥10 mm in size and all polyps are ≥5 mm in size *OR*
  - >20 serrated polyps (any histologic subtype or size) distributed throughout the colon with at least 5 being proximal to the rectum

Incidence and Location

- Reported prevalence varies but as high as 0.1% in patients undergoing screening colonoscopy

Morbidity and Mortality

- Increased risk for colorectal cancer; first-degree relatives also have a five times greater risk of colorectal cancer compared with the general population

Gender, Race, and Age Distribution

- No gender predilection
- Most patients diagnosed between 50 and 60 years, but age at presentation varies widely

Clinical Features

- Family history of serrated polyposis or colorectal cancer may be present
- First presentation may be with carcinoma
- Underdiagnosed condition because flat serrated polyps may be missed during colonoscopy and gross examination of cancer resections
- Most patients (40%) fall into the second diagnostic criterion above, about a quarter into the first, and the rest fulfill both criteria
- Smoking and high body mass index are common risk factors

Prognosis and Therapy

- Close surveillance by colonoscopy
- Presence of concurrent adenomas is best predictor of cancer risk
- Colectomy may be indicated if number of polyps too numerous for adequate surveillance

PATHOLOGIC FEATURES

GROSS FINDINGS

The number of polyps is variable but usually reported to be within the 10 to 60 range. A more severe polyposis phenotype is rare which is why the disease often goes undiagnosed. The polyps show macroscopic appearance of a hyperplastic polyp or sessile serrated polyp. This is partly determined by the predominant location of the polyp burden. More proximal lesions are likely to be flat sessile polyps that blend into colonic mucosal folds and are easily missed. Distal lesions are more commonly sessile but elevated polyps that resemble sporadic hyperplastic polyps. Concurrent carcinoma may be present (Fig. 11.5) as a polypoid, flat, or depressed mass with ulceration.

MICROSCOPIC FINDINGS

Hyperplastic polyps, sessile serrated polyps with or without dysplasia, traditional serrated adenomas, or unclassified serrated polyps are included in the polyp count when rendering a diagnosis of SPS. The polyps in SPS resemble their sporadic counterparts. Hyperplastic polyps (Fig. 11.6A) show elongated colonic crypts with serrated architecture and a narrow base lined by cells with abundant microvesicular type mucin. Sessile serrated polyps are larger in size and show architectural distortion with dilated crypt bases and crypt disarray (Figs. 11.6B and C). Dysplastic change may be present and can resemble either traditional serrated adenoma or a conventional tubular adenoma (Fig. 11.7). Traditional serrated adenomas also resemble their sporadic counterparts and show serrated crypts with abundant eosinophilic cytoplasm and nuclear stratification and hyperchromasia similar to an adenoma. Conventional adenomas may also be present in SPS and are an independent predictor of high risk for progression to carcinoma. The histologic type of polyp or largest polyp size or distribution of polyps within the colon are not

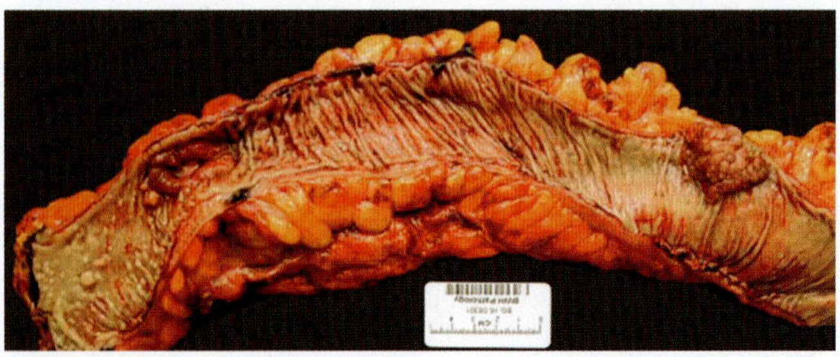

FIGURE 11.5

Serrated polyposis syndrome (SPS) is characterized by multiple, usually more than 20, or large (>10 mm) serrated polyps of any histologic subtype. These patients are at high risk for colon cancer and need close surveillance. Two synchronous adenocarcinomas are present, along with multiple serrated polyps, in this patient with SPS.

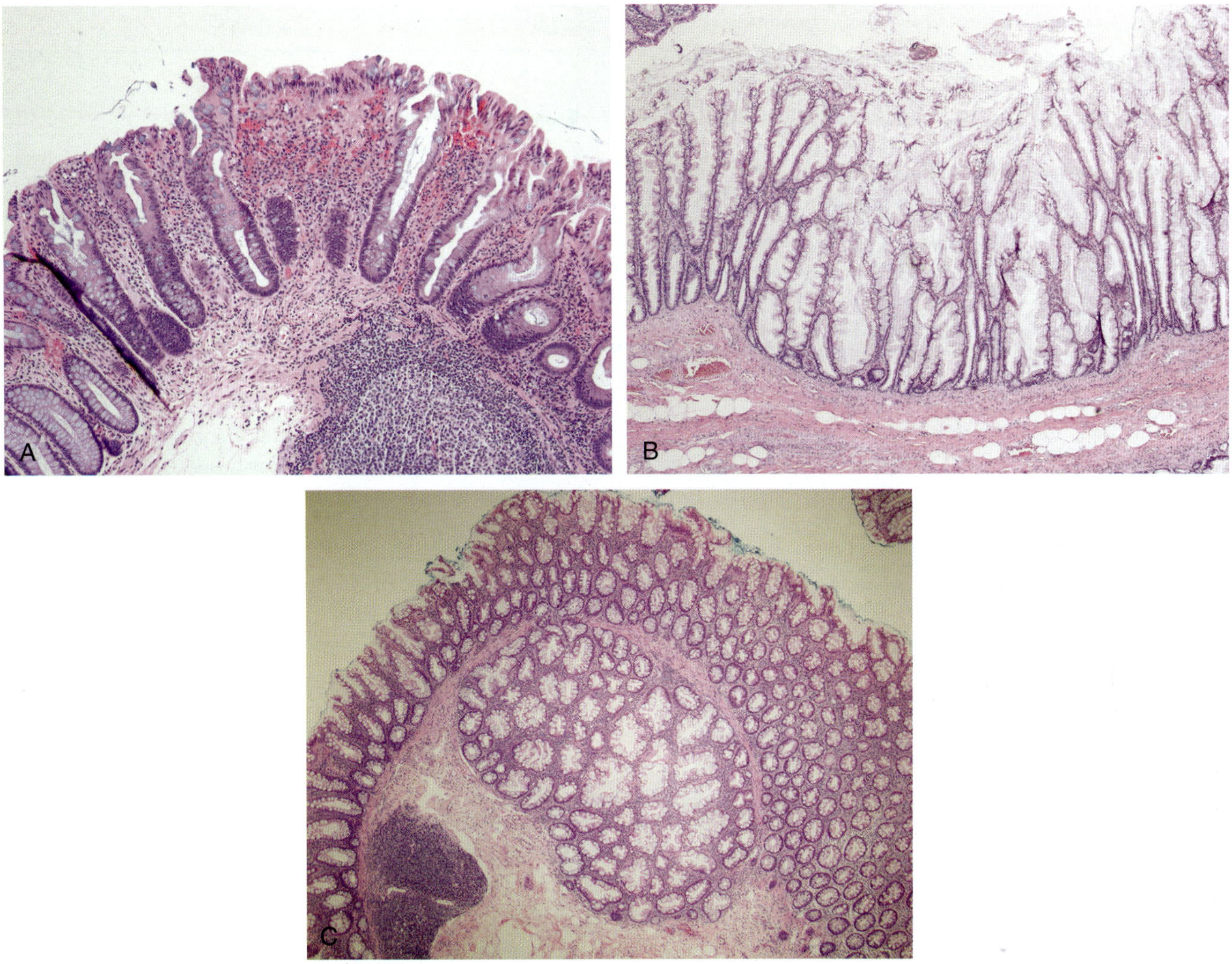

FIGURE 11.6

Serrated polyps in serrated polyposis syndrome resemble their sporadic counterparts. Hyperplastic polyps (**A**) show a narrow proliferative mucin depleted base with serrations in the upper half. Sessile serrated polyps show crypt disarray with mucin-rich, cystically dilated basal zone with boot- or anchor-shaped crypts (**B**). Submucosal misplacement (**C**) is also seen in some large sessile serrated polyps.

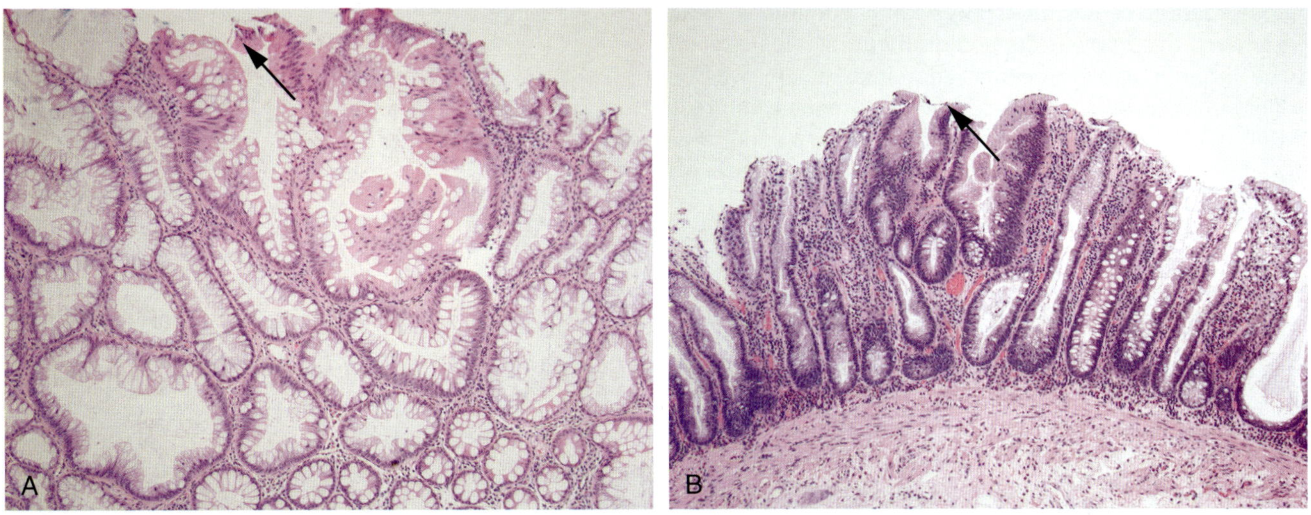

FIGURE 11.7

Dysplasia in serrated polyps in serrated polyposis syndrome (SPS) may show features similar to a traditional serrated adenoma (**A**) or a conventional tubular adenoma (**B**). The presence of concurrent adenomas is the best predictor of cancer risk in patients with SPS.

Serrated Polyposis Syndrome—Pathologic Features

Gross Findings

- Variable number and size of polyps, typically 10 to 60 in number
- Flat, sessile lesions more common proximally
- Distal small sessile elevated polyps resemble sporadic hyperplastic polyps
- Concurrent mass lesions may be present in cases with carcinoma

Microscopic Findings

- Serrated polyps in serrated polyposis syndrome (SPS) resemble sporadic hyperplastic polyps, sessile serrated polyps, and traditional serrated adenoma
- Sessile serrated polyps may show cytologic dysplasia
- Concurrent conventional adenomas can be seen and are predictive of a higher risk of cancer
- Adenocarcinoma in SPS may show features of microsatellite instability high phenotype, but half of all cancers are microsatellite stable

Genetics

- No high prevalence germline mutations identified so far
- *RNF43* germline mutations reported in some families
- Increased risk of colorectal cancer in first- and second-degree relatives is indicative of a familial predisposition

Differential Diagnosis

- *MUTYH* polyposis syndrome
- Hereditary mixed polyposis syndrome

predictive of cancer risk. Cancers in SPS may resemble MSI-H tumors, but nearly half of all cancers that occur in this setting are microsatellite stable with intact expression of DNA mismatch repair proteins.

Differential Diagnosis

A combination of serrated polyps and adenomas can also be seen in MAP but the predominant histologic type in the latter is a conventional adenoma, whereas SPS is characterized by a preponderance of serrated polyps. HMPS is characterized by presence of serrated polyps and adenomas in addition to juvenile-type hamartomatous polyps, some of which may be dysplastic.

Prognosis and Therapy

Up to 35% of patients with SPS have a synchronous colon cancer, indicating the increased malignant potential associated with this condition. Annual colonoscopic surveillance is typically recommended after complete removal of all large polyps. Colectomy is reserved for those with a high polyp burden that precludes complete polyp removal and close surveillance.

PEUTZ-JEGHERS SYNDROME

Clinical Features

Peutz-Jeghers syndrome is the second most common form of intestinal polyposis, with an incidence of 1 in 120,000. PJS is inherited in an autosomal dominant pattern and caused by germline mutations in the *LKB1 (STK11)* gene, which is detected in more than 90% of these patients. Unlike FAP, the disease shows an incomplete penetrance. Patient presentation is typically with abdominal pain, obstruction, or bleeding. Two major and characteristic components of the syndrome include hamartomatous PJ polyps involving the GI tract and pigmented macules involving the mucous membranes and skin.

The diagnosis of PJS can often be made in early childhood because mucocutaneous pigmentation is present at birth in 95% of patients, and small intestinal hamartomatous polyps are frequently symptomatic (Fig. 11.8). Common sites of mucocutaneous pigmentation include the lips, buccal mucosa, eyelids, and digits. The pigmentation of PJS can easily be distinguished from freckles because freckles are not present at birth, are sparse near the lips, and never involve the mucous membranes. Whereas the pigmentation of the skin may fade, the melanin deposits of the buccal mucosa persist throughout life.

Benign complications of PJS predominate in the pediatric population. Jejunal and ileal hamartomatous

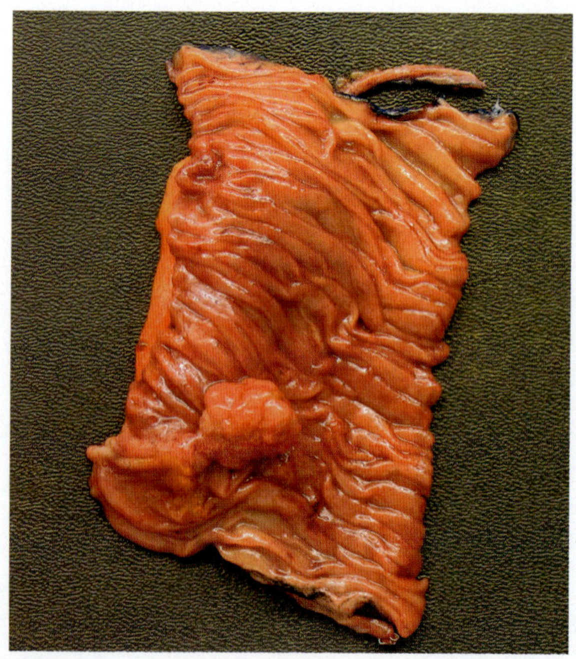

FIGURE 11.8

Peutz-Jeghers polyps most commonly occur in the small intestine. Large pedunculated lesions may cause intussusception and obstruction.

polyps can produce intussusception, leading to a partial or total bowel obstruction. When located within the rectum, hamartomatous polyps may prolapse, resulting in torsion, infarction, and GI bleeding. Tumors can develop in multiple organ sites in addition to the GI tract, including the breast, lung, pancreas, uterus, ovary, cervix, and Sertoli cells of the testis. Sex cord tumor with annular tubules is a unique ovarian neoplasm that may affect up to 12% of female patients with this syndrome, whereas hormonally active Sertoli cell testicular tumors may occur in males. Most common sites of cancer development are the GI tract, pancreas, breast, gynecologic tract, and lung, and the risk of malignancy increases with age. The diagnosis can be established by the presence of characteristic melanotic macules and one or more intestinal PJ-type polyp or the presence of two or more PJ-type polyps. In patients with a positive family history, the diagnosis can be made if either melanotic macules or one PJ-type polyp or an *LKB1* mutation is present.

PEUTZ-JEGHERS POLYPOSIS—FACT SHEET

Definition

- An autosomal dominant syndrome with incomplete penetrance characterized by Peutz-Jeghers (PJ)–type hamartomatous polyps involving the gastrointestinal (GI) tract and pigmented macules on the mucous membranes and skin

Incidence and Location

- 1 in 120,000 live births
- Second most common intestinal polyposis syndrome
- Jejunum and ileum commonly involved but any part of GI tract can be affected

Morbidity and Mortality

- Benign complications (intussusception and obstruction, torsion, infarction and bleeding) predominate in the pediatric population
- 85% cumulative lifetime risk of cancer, most often involving GI tract, pancreas, breast, lung, and gynecologic tract

Gender, Race, and Age Distribution

- No gender or ethnic predilection
- Symptoms can begin in infancy
- Average age at diagnosis of intestinal polyps is 25 years

Clinical Features

- Abdominal pain, obstruction, and bleeding are common presentations
- Pigmented lesions of the mucous membranes develop by 2 years of age and are present at birth in most patients
- Hamartomatous PJ-type polyps are present throughout the intestinal tract, most commonly the jejunum and ileum
- Polyp burden is typically low, and more than 20 polyps are rare in PJP

Prognosis and Therapy

- Increased lifetime risk of cancer in both intestinal and extraintestinal organs
- Periodic monitoring of high-risk organs for cancer should include the GI tract, breast, pancreas, and gynecologic tract
- Lung cancer risk is also increased, but no specific screening recommendations are available; annual chest radiography or computed tomography in smokers is often performed

PATHOLOGIC FEATURES

GROSS FINDINGS

Peutz-Jeghers–type hamartomatous polyps occur throughout the GI tract. In decreasing frequency, the most common sites affected are the jejunum, ileum, colon, stomach, duodenum, and appendix. Polyps may be sessile or pedunculated and often show a smooth, lobulated surface. The size of PJ-type polyps ranges from a few millimeters to several centimeters in diameter. Large polyps in the small intestine can cause obstruction with the polyp head forming the leading edge of the intussusception.

MICROSCOPIC FINDINGS

Peutz-Jeghers–type polyps have distinctive microscopic appearance characterized by lobulated epithelial compartments divided by broad bands of mature smooth muscle (Figs. 11.9 and 11.10). The epithelium is appropriate to the anatomic site, and the muscle fibers fan out from the center of the polyp to form a tree-like appearance. Absorptive enterocytes, Paneth cells, goblet cells, and endocrine cells are all present

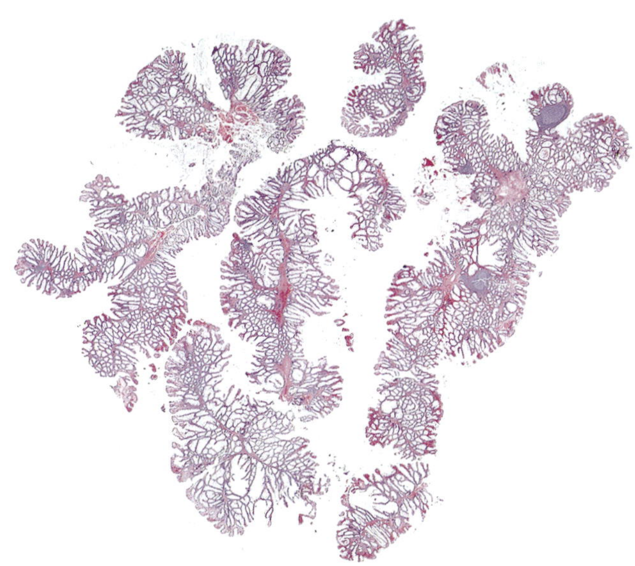

FIGURE 11.9

On low-power, Peutz-Jeghers polyps have a characteristic leaf-like appearance with smooth muscle bundles dividing the epithelial compartment into discrete lobules.

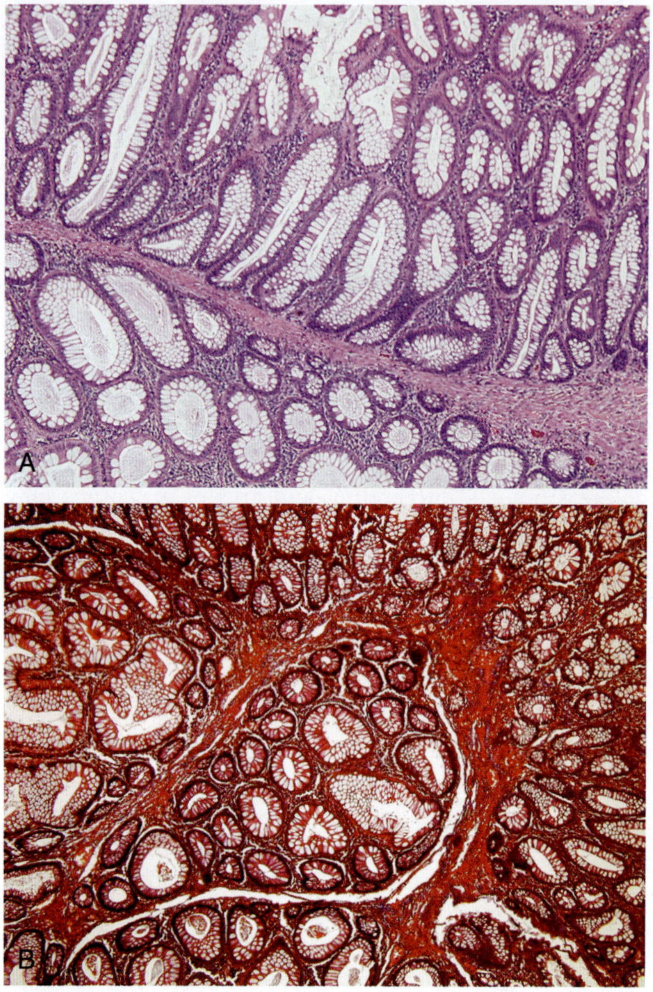

FIGURE 11.10

Histologic examination of the same polyp shown in Fig. 11.9 reveals regenerative epithelium separated by broad bands of smooth muscle (**A**). A trichrome stain highlights the bands of smooth muscle that are characteristic of these polyps (**B**).

within the epithelium of small intestinal PJ-type polyp (Figs. 11.11A–C). The lamina propria does not show significant edema or inflammation. Erosion of the surface epithelium is common, particularly for larger polyps, and may be associated with reactive and regenerative epithelium containing prominent mitoses. Intussusception may cause herniation of epithelium deep into the muscularis propria, which can be mistaken for an invasive carcinoma.

Colonic PJ-type polyps demonstrate similar histologic features but are less developed than those seen for their small bowel counterparts. Specifically, PJ polyps of the colon contain elongated, branched crypts that may simulate a villous architecture. Intussuscepted segments may show crypt architectural disarray that can be mistaken for sessile serrated polyps (Fig. 11.11D). Smooth muscle is not present in all polyps, particularly small lesions. The sharp demarcation of epithelial lobules by smooth muscle is in contrast to the more haphazard muscular proliferation in the lamina propria seen in colonic mucosal prolapse polyps (Fig. 11.11E).

Peutz-Jeghers Polyposis—Pathologic Features

Gross Findings

- Hamartomatous polyps present throughout the gastrointestinal (GI) tract
- Jejunum and ileum are the most common sites followed by the colon, stomach, duodenum, and appendix
- Sessile or pedunculated appearance
- Smooth, lobulated surface
- Wide size range (millimeters to several centimeters)

Microscopic Findings

- Regenerative epithelium appropriate to the site of origin divided into discrete lobules by arborizing bands of mature smooth muscle
- Cellular constituents of normal GI tract mucosa such as goblet cells, Paneth cells, absorptive cells, and endocrine cells are present within the polyp epithelium
- Lamina propria is not significantly edematous or inflamed
- Surface commonly eroded with underlying areas of reactive epithelial change
- Dysplastic change is rare, and cancers typically do not arise within the hamartomatous polyps in the GI tract

Genetics

- Inactivation of the *STK11/LKB1* gene identified in up to 90% of affected families

Differential Diagnosis

- Mucosal prolapse polyp
- Sporadic Peutz-Jeghers–type hamartomatous polyp
- Juvenile polyposis
- Cowden's syndrome
- Filiform polyp of inflammatory bowel disease

Gastric PJ-type polyps (Fig. 11.11F) can be difficult to distinguish from sporadic hyperplastic polyps (Fig. 11.11G) and other syndromic polyps, particularly when polyp size is small. Large, well-developed lesions show features similar to their small intestinal and colonic counterparts (Fig. 11.11H).

Differential Diagnosis

Sporadic mucosal prolapse polyps also have a prominent fibromuscular proliferation in the lamina propria and can be difficult to distinguish from PJ-type syndromic polyps. The smooth muscle proliferation in mucosal prolapse polyps is haphazard and does not divide the epithelial compartment into discrete lobules, unlike PJ-type polyps. Sporadic PJ-type polyps are incredibly rare, and limited data suggest these patients may also be at high risk for metachronous cancers. Small PJ-type polyps can be particularly difficult to differentiate from juvenile polyps and hamartomatous polyps in Cowden's syndrome (CS). However, in contrast to juvenile polyps,

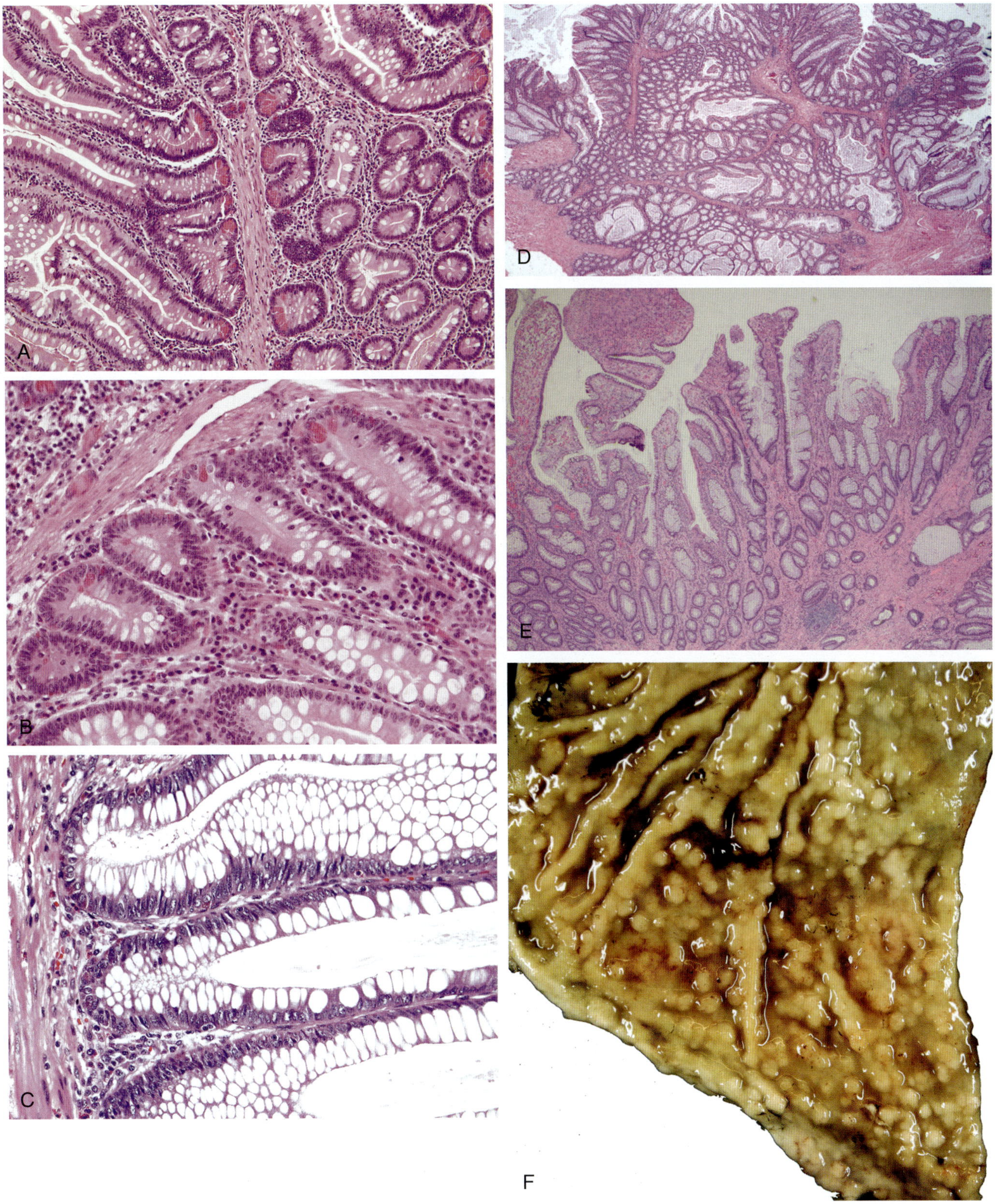

FIGURE 11.11

In Peutz-Jeghers (PJ) syndrome, polyps involving the small intestine show reactive epithelium (**A**) goblet cells, neuroendocrine cells, and Paneth cells within the bases of hyperplastic crypts (**B**). Polyps that arise within the colon contain predominantly goblet cells (**C**). Large colon PJ polyps often show crypt disarray with dilated crypt bases and boot-shaped crypts that should not be mistaken for sessile serrated polyps (**D**). Mucosal prolapse polyps are typically located in the rectosigmoid colon and may be mistaken for PJ polyps. The smooth muscle proliferation in prolapse-type polyps is more haphazard, and the epithelium is not divided into discrete well-demarcated lobules like a PJ polyp (**E**). Gastric involvement in PJ syndrome may occur as solitary or multiple polyps without a distinctive appearance (**F**). Small PJ polyps in the stomach are indistinguishable from sporadic hyperplastic polyps

Continued

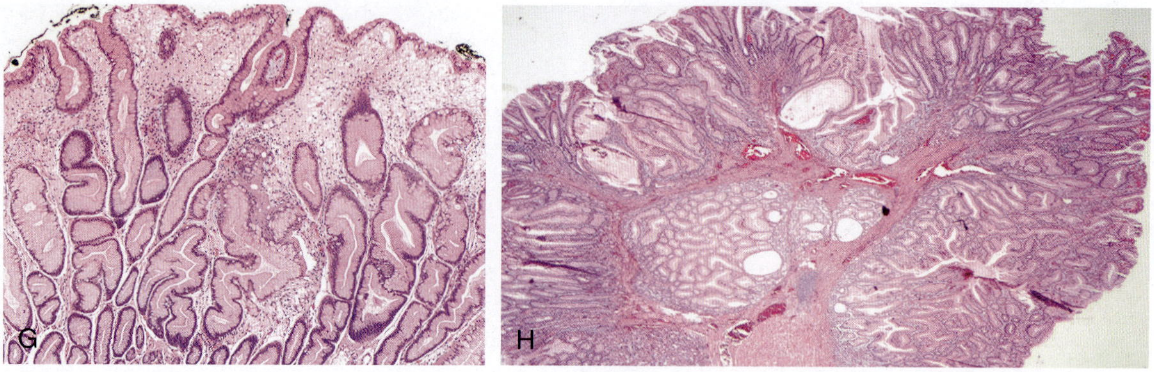

FIGURE 11.11 cont'd

(**G**), and knowledge of multiplicity or small intestinal or colonic involvement is necessary for definite diagnosis. Large gastric lesions, like this antral polyp, show characteristic smooth muscle arborization enclosing discrete epithelial lobules (**H**).

PJ polyps are more common within the small bowel and do not have an inflamed lamina propria. Granulation tissue may be seen in association with both PJ and juvenile polyps, but in PJ polyps, granulation tissue is typically present in association with surface erosion, and histologic examination of deeper regions of the polyp reveals the lack of inflammation. Hamartomas in CS do not have a distinctive appearance and resemble juvenile polyps. However, lamina propria inflammation is much less prominent in CS. Filiform polyps of IBD are inflammatory polyps with a slender finger-like gross appearance, the lamina propria is inflamed, the crypts show architectural disarray, and the adjacent mucosa shows features of a chronic colitis.

Prognosis and Therapy

The lifetime risk for developing cancer in individuals with PJS is estimated to be around 85%, with a mean age of 43 years at cancer diagnosis. Although a variety of neoplasms have been reported, the greatest risk for cancer in patients with PJS is in the GI tract, particularly the colorectum, stomach, and pancreas. At this time, management of patients with PJS involves periodic surveillance of high-risk organs for which early detection and screening are reasonable.

JUVENILE POLYPOSIS SYNDROME

Clinical Features

Juvenile polyps may occur in a sporadic or syndromic setting. Sporadic juvenile polyps are the most common type of polyp diagnosed in children and are estimated to be present in as many as 2% of asymptomatic children. They are first diagnosed in patients ranging from 1 to 10 years of age with a peak incidence between 2 and 4 years of age. Juvenile polyposis coli syndrome (JPS) is defined by more than five juvenile polyps in the colorectum or juvenile polyps throughout the GI tract or any number in a patient with a positive family history. Patients with JPS tend to present in the second or third decade of life. The incidence is 1 to 2 cases per 100,000 live births a year. Germline mutations in *SMAD4* or *BMPR1A* genes are identified in 25% and 20% patients, respectively. A family history can be elicited in up to 50% of affected patients.

Four clinical forms of juvenile polyposis are described: (1) juvenile polyposis coli with lesions restricted to the colorectum is the most common form with presentation typically in the first decade of life; (2) generalized polyposis coli with polyps distributed throughout the GI tract; (3) gastric juvenile polyposis associated with protein-losing enteropathy; (4) and juvenile polyposis of infancy, which is a rare lethal autosomal recessive disorder with death in infancy. Congenital birth defects are present in 15% of patients and include cardiac and cranial abnormalities, cleft palate and polydactyly, malrotation and Meckel's diverticulum, and undescended testes. Digital clubbing and failure to thrive are also considered to be extraintestinal manifestations of JPS.

Children with JPS usually present with painless rectal bleeding or anemia. Fewer than 10% have symptoms such as abdominal pain, rectal prolapse or polyp extrusion, anal pruritus, constipation, or diarrhea. Extensive and extracolonic polyposis in the small bowel or stomach may cause GI and systemic dysfunction such as intussusception, protein-losing enteropathy, malabsorption, diarrhea, or significant hemorrhage.

Pathologic Features

Gross Findings

The majority of juvenile polyps are solitary. Some series have reported that one-third to half of cases may be multiple, which likely reflects variable extent of

JUVENILE POLYPOSIS SYNDROME—FACT SHEET

Definition

- Defined by the presence of one of the following:
  - More than five juvenile polyps in the colorectum
  - Juvenile polyps throughout the gastrointestinal (GI) tract
  - Any juvenile polyp in a patient with a positive family history

Incidence and Location

- 1 in 100,000 live births
- Colon or any other part of the GI tract may be affected
- Gastric involvement more common in *SMAD4* mutant patients

Morbidity and Mortality

- Painless rectal bleeding and anemia are the most common presentations
- 10% of patients present with abdominal pain, rectal prolapse, anal pruritus, constipation, or diarrhea
- Extracolonic polyposis may present with intussusception, protein-losing enteropathy, or malabsorption
- Death from protein-losing enteropathy in infancy or cancer in adulthood

Gender, Race, and Age Distribution

- No gender, racial, or ethnic predilection
- Mean age at presentation is 9.5 years

Clinical Features

- Juvenile polyps in the colorectum or anywhere else in the GI tract
- Rare cases with polyps restricted to stomach have been described
- Congenital birth defects in 15% include cardiac and cranial abnormalities, cleft palate, polydactyly, intestinal malrotation or diverticulum, and undescended testis

Prognosis and Treatment

- Dysplasia reported in 8% to 31% of polyps
- Reported risk of colorectal cancer is 39% to 68%
- Screening and regular upper endoscopy and colonoscopy recommended for surveillance

colonoscopic evaluation. The vast majority are located in the rectum or rectosigmoid colon. Multiple juvenile polyps are usually discrete, but multilobular or clustered polyps may also occasionally be encountered. The macroscopic appearance ranges from relatively smooth homogeneous, pale, sessile polyps to large, pedunculated polyps with a coarsely nodular surface (Figs. 11.12A and B). These pedunculated polyps may rotate on their stalks, causing ischemia and hemorrhage leading to autoamputation or avulsion. Surface granulation tissue is common, often with visible capillaries and venules and occasionally coated with exudates. Patients with *SMAD4* mutations are more likely to have gastric polyps and hemorrhagic telangiectasia.

Microscopic Findings

The classic features of a juvenile polyp include a well-circumscribed contour with extensive surface ulceration (Figs. 11.12C and D). The smooth surface seen grossly corresponds to a cap of granulation tissue. The lamina propria is expanded with a mixed inflammatory infiltrate. In the colon, cystically dilated crypts with cryptitis and crypt abscess are often present. Bands of smooth muscle and thick-walled blood vessels may be present in large pedunculated juvenile polyps raising concern for PJ-type or mucosal prolapse–type polyps (Fig. 11.12E). Diminutive and small juvenile polyps can be virtually indistinguishable from sporadic inflammatory polyps and other hamartomatous polyps (Fig. 11.12F).

Extracolonic juvenile polyps also show a prominent cystic component that is lined by mature epithelium appropriate for the site involved. There are some data to suggest that whereas lamina propria expansion predominates in polyps with *BMPR1A* mutation, the epithelial compartment is predominant in those with *SMAD4* mutation. In addition, SMAD4 mutations are known to be more often associated with hereditary hemorrhagic telangiectasia and gastric polyposis.

Juvenile polyps in the stomach (Fig. 11.13) resemble sporadic hyperplastic polyps and show exuberant cystically dilated and inflamed foveolar epithelium separated by an edematous and inflamed lamina propria (Fig. 11.14). As in the colon, small juvenile polyps cannot be distinguished from sporadic hyperplastic polyps or other syndromic polyps involving the stomach, and correlation with patient history and findings elsewhere in in the GI tract is necessary for definite diagnosis.

The epithelium in juvenile polyps may show a range of cellular atypia varying from reactive changes to frank dysplasia (Fig. 11.15). Reactive changes are most prominent underneath the eroded surface epithelium and can mimic dysplasia caused by mucin-depletion and increased mitotic activity. True dysplastic change, on the other hand, shows abrupt transition from adjacent epithelium with crowded, large hyperchromatic nuclei with prominent nucleoli, pseudostratification, and mucin depletion. Patients with multiple polyps or generalized juvenile polyposis have an increased frequency of dysplastic change. Dysplasia in a juvenile polyp is found more frequently in polyps exceeding 1 cm in diameter, and thorough examination of large lesions is necessary to rule out neoplastic change.

Differential Diagnosis

The differential diagnosis of a syndromic juvenile polyp includes sporadic juvenile polyps and inflammatory polyps. The distinction between sporadic and syndromic juvenile polyps rests on the syndromic definition already mentioned. Inflammatory polyps that arise in IBD or any other form of colitis can mimic juvenile polyps. In these cases, examination of the surrounding nonpolypoid mucosa can identify the presence of colitis

Juvenile Polyposis Syndrome—Pathologic Features

Gross Findings

- More than 75% are pedunculated
- Average size is 1 to 1.5 cm (range, 0.2–4 cm)
- External surface is smooth or coarsely lobulated
- Cut surface shows grossly visible cystic spaces containing gray to yellow mucoid material

Microscopic Findings

- Prominent lamina propria with a mixed inflammatory infiltrate
- Cystically dilated crypts in colon with cryptitis and crypt abscesses
- Eroded surface lined by inflamed granulation tissue
- Reactive epithelium commonly present underneath surface ulceration and can mimic dysplasia
- Dysplastic change may be present, usually in large polyps, and shows abrupt transition from surrounding epithelium and is characterized by nuclear enlargement, hyperchromasia, pseudostratification, and mucin depletion

Genetics

- Germline mutation of either *SMAD4* or *BMPR1A* gene in 50% of cases

Differential Diagnosis

- Non-syndromic juvenile polyp
- Inflammatory polyp arising in inflammatory bowel disease
- Mucosal prolapse polyp
- Peutz-Jeghers polyposis
- Cowden syndrome

as the cause of the polyp formation. Inflammatory polyps usually lack the cystically dilated glandular component and the edematous character of lamina propria typically seen in juvenile polyps. Mucosal prolapse polyps also occur in the rectosigmoid region (a common site of involvement for juvenile polyps) but are usually seen in late adulthood. The lamina propria shows prominent fibromuscular hyperplasia, and a cystic glandular component is lacking. Differentiation from PJ polyps relies on recognition of the presence of an inflamed and prominent lamina propria and marked cystic change in juvenile polyps and presence of broad bands of smooth muscle dividing the epithelial component into discrete lobules in PJ polyps. Hamartomatous polyps in CS can mimic juvenile polyps very closely, but inflammation in the epithelium and stroma is less prominent in CS, and other GI and extraintestinal manifestations are necessary to make a distinction between these two conditions.

Prognosis and Therapy

Patients with JPS have a significant risk for adenocarcinoma of the colon, as well as increased risk for gastric, duodenal, and pancreatic cancer. Upper endoscopy and colonoscopy screening for affected patients begins in adolescence. Any polyps found are removed, and patients are followed up with annual surveillance. Polyps are submitted entirely for histological evaluation to rule out any dysplasia or carcinoma. If no polyps are identified, screening colonoscopy should be performed every 3 years. Colectomy is reserved for patients with significant polyp burden, dysplasia, or malignant transformation.

Cowden's Syndrome

Clinical Features

Cowden's syndrome, the most common subset of PTEN hamartoma tumor syndrome (PHTS), is an autosomal dominant syndrome caused by germline *PTEN* gene mutation. PHTS also includes Bannayan-Riley-Ruvalcaba syndrome, adult Lhermitte-Duclos disease, and autism spectrum disorders associated with macrocephaly. CS is the most common manifestation of PHTS, and the two terms are often used interchangeably. CS is a multiorgan disorder characterized by hamartomas involving not only the GI tract but also the skin, thyroid, and breast, and an increased risk of breast and thyroid malignancy. The facial lesions are trichilemmomas (lichenoid and verrucous papules); the oral mucosal lesions (gingiva and buccal mucosa) are often fibromas; and hyperkeratoses are seen on the hands and feet. Breast lesions occur in almost half of all adult patients, ranging from fibrocystic disease to cancer, commonly ductal carcinoma. Thyroid disease is the most common abnormality, occurring in up to 68% of patients. Recent studies have also shown an increased risk of colorectal cancer in patients with CS. The major and minor diagnostic criteria for CS are summarized in Table 11.2. Establishing a provisional diagnosis of CS requires presence of pathognomonic skin lesions, two or more major criteria, one major and at least three minor criteria, or four or more minor criteria. Positive germline mutations in *PTEN* gene confirm the diagnosis.

Pathologic Features

Gross Findings

Polyps associated with CS may occur anywhere from the esophagus to the rectum (Fig. 11.16A), but the distal large intestine is most commonly affected. The esophagus in patients with CS shows glycogen acanthosis, which is endoscopically visible as yellow-white nodules or plaques (Fig. 11.16B).

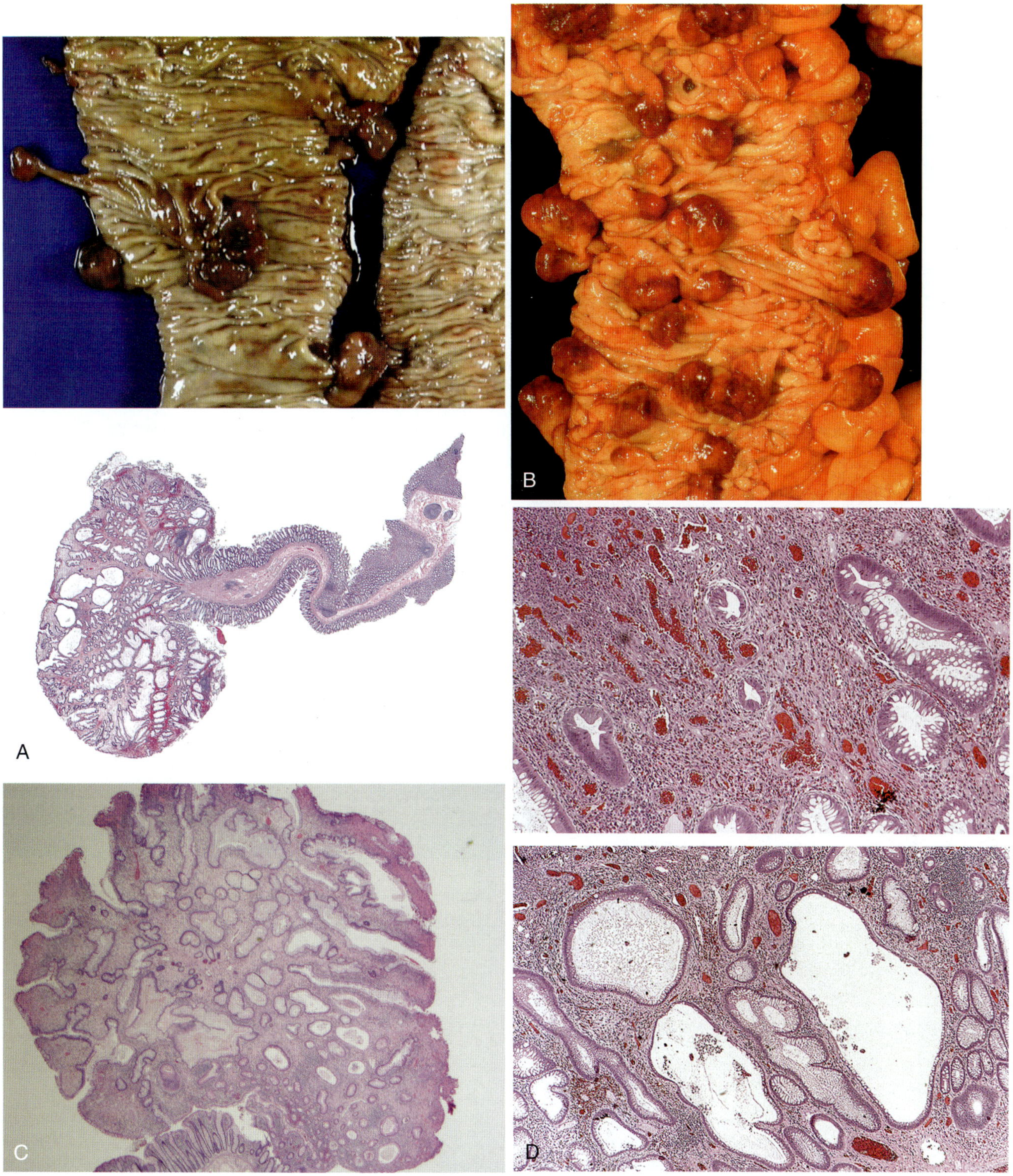

FIGURE 11.12

In this colectomy specimen from a young patient with juvenile polyposis syndrome, multiple polyps are present that range from large sessile multilobulated ones to small pedunculated ones on a slender stalk (**A**). Juvenile polyps have a rounded contour, and numerous cystically dilated glands can be appreciated below the polyp surface (**A**). Another resection from a patient with juvenile polyposis syndrome with multiple sessile and pedunculated polyps with smooth multilobulated surface (**B**). Some pedunculated lesions may undergo torsion and autoamputation. Typical juvenile polyps have expanded inflamed lamina propria and cystically dilated glandular component with cryptitis and crypt abscesses (**C**). The lamina propria contains acute and chronic inflammatory cells, congested vessels, and granulation tissue and cystically dilated glands (**D**). Large pedunculated juvenile polyps may mimic a mucosal prolapse polyp or a Peutz-Jeghers (PJ)–type hamartomatous polyp

Continued

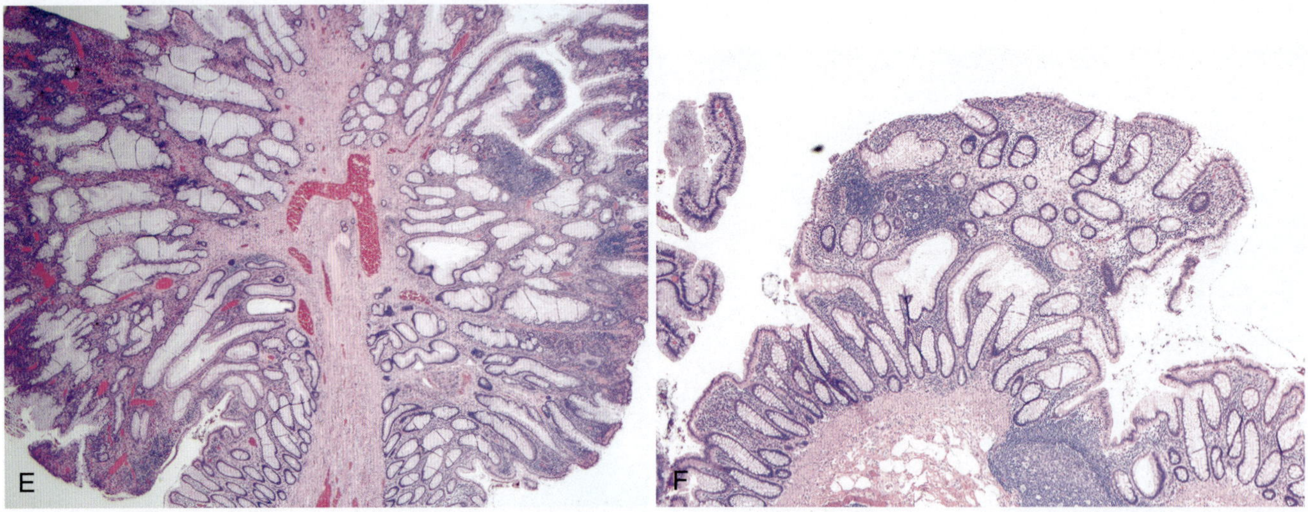

FIGURE 11.12 cont'd (**E**). Extensive surface ulceration, cystically dilated crypts, lack of distinct smooth muscle arborization typical of a PJ polyp, and multiplicity of polyps are useful features for diagnosis of juvenile polyp. The morphologically characteristic features of juvenile polyps are present in large lesions, but small polyps are virtually indistinguishable from sporadic inflammatory polyps (**F**).

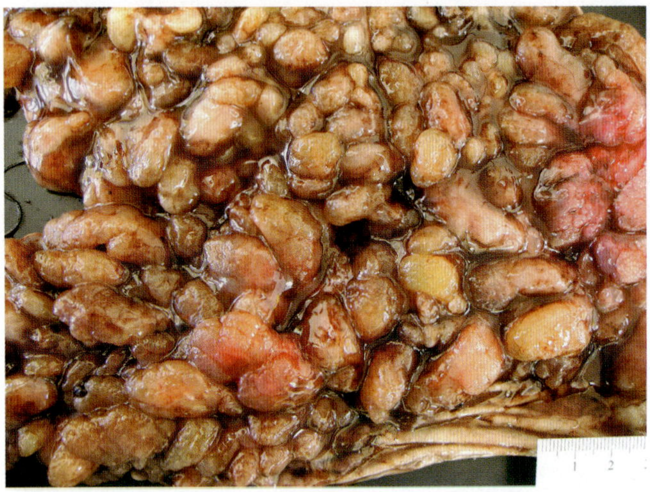

FIGURE 11.13

Gastric involvement in juvenile polyposis may be severe enough to warrant a resection, as in this example.

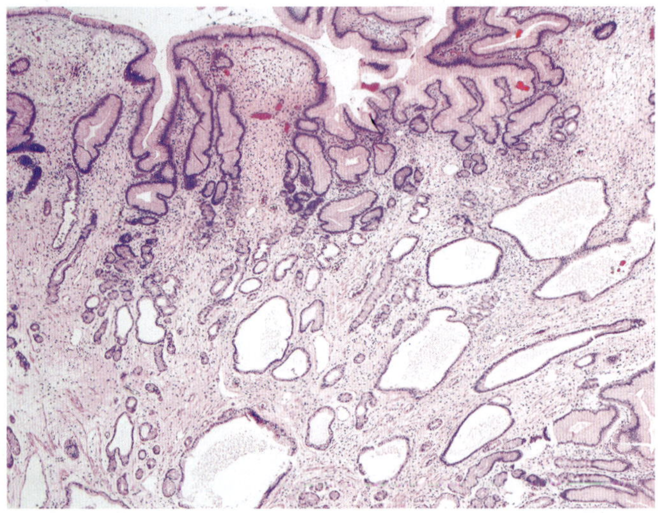

FIGURE 11.14

Microscopically, gastric syndromic juvenile polyps also resemble sporadic hyperplastic polyps, and knowledge of the endoscopic findings is essential for correct diagnosis. As in the colon, the lamina propria is expanded and inflamed, and the glandular compartment shows marked cystic dilation.

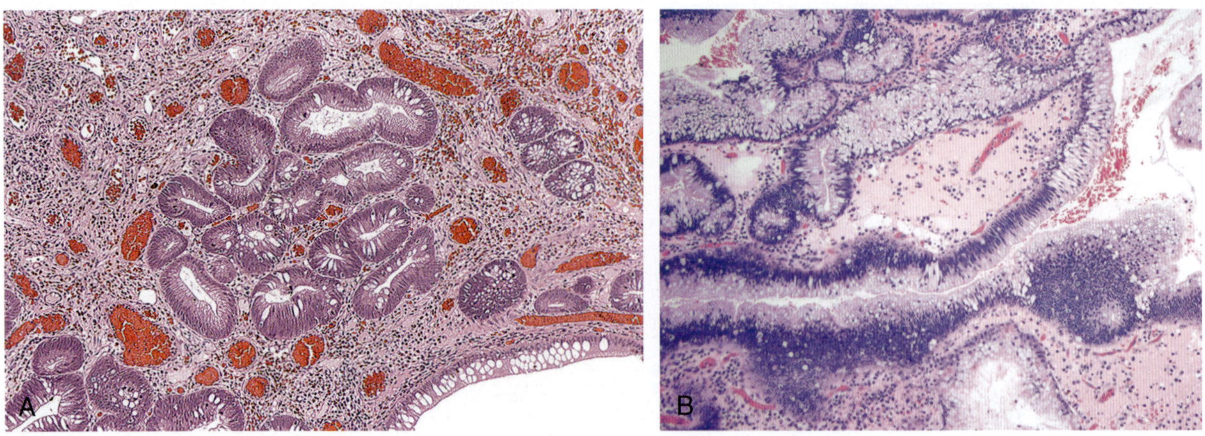

FIGURE 11.15

Reactive changes underneath the surface ulceration in juvenile polyps may be mistaken for dysplasia (**A**). True dysplastic change does occur in these lesions and is characterized by abrupt transition, nuclear hyperchromasia, stratification, and pleomorphism (**B**).

COWDEN'S SYNDROME—FACT SHEET

Definition

- Multiple hamartomas of ectodermal, mesodermal, and endodermal origin, including the gastrointestinal tract and associated with increased risk of breast, thyroid, and colon cancer

Incidence and Location

- Rare; approximately 1 in 200,000 individuals

Morbidity and Mortality

- Progressive macrocephaly and delayed mental development in children
- 50% incidence of breast cancer among adult patients
- 10% to 15% risk for papillary thyroid cancer

Gender, Race, and Age Distribution

- Males and females equally affected
- Mean age at diagnosis in the fourth decade of life

Clinical Features

- Hallmark of disease is multiple facial trichilemmomas around the mouth, nose, and eyes
- Café-au-lait spots, vitiligo, epidermoid cysts, skin carcinomas
- Benign soft tissue and visceral tumors also common

Prognosis and Therapy

- 50% lifetime risk for breast carcinoma
- 10% lifetime risk for thyroid cancer
- Ten times greater risk of colon cancer compared with the general population

TABLE 11.2
Criteria for Diagnosis of Cowden's syndrome

Criteria
Pathognomonic criteria
Characteristic mucocutaneous or mucosal lesions
Cerebellar tumors (Lhermitte-Duclos disease)
Autism spectrum disorder
Major criteria
Megalocephaly
Multiple gastrointestinal hamartomas or ganglioneuromas
Mucocutaneous lesions (multiple trichilemmomas, palmoplantar keratoses, cutaneous facial papules, or macular pigmentation of glans penis)
Thyroid (nonmedullary), breast, or endometrial cancer
Minor criteria
Solitary gastrointestinal hamartoma or ganglioneuroma
Lipomas, fibromas or uterine fibroids
Fibrocystic breast disease
Autism spectrum disorder or delayed mental development (IQ <75)
Genitourinary cysts or renal cell carcinoma

MICROSCOPIC FINDINGS

On microscopy, the esophageal squamous mucosa shows increased mucosal thickness and ballooned squamous cells with abundant clear cytoplasm (Fig. 11.16C), which is filled with glycogen that can be demonstrated by periodic acid–Schiff (PAS) and PAS with diastase histochemical stains. Gastric polyps in CS do not harbor any distinctive features and may resemble prolapse-type polyps with fibromuscular proliferation in the lamina propria (Fig. 11.17). Intestinal polyps in CS are also difficult to diagnose and may resemble juvenile polyps. The presence of multiple hamartomatous polyps without any distinctive features, mucosal lipomas or fibromas, ganglioneuromas, or benign lymphoid polyps should all raise suspicion for a diagnosis of CS (Fig. 11.18). Distinctive soft tissue vascular hamartomas (PTEN hamartoma of soft tissue) have also been described recently in CS. Colon adenomas and carcinomas may also occur at a young age in those with CS.

DIFFERENTIAL DIAGNOSIS

Ganglioneuromatous polyps of the colon can occur in CS and in a sporadic setting. Similar polyps are also known to occur in neurofibromatosis type 1. However, the distinctive extraintestinal manifestations of CS and neurofibromatosis allow correct classification of the patient's disease. Hamartomas in CS are not distinctive in appearance and are hard to distinguish from other hamartomatous polyps, such as juvenile and PJ polyps, particularly when the latter are small in size and diagnostically characteristic features are not fully developed. Correlation with upper GI tract findings and extraintestinal manifestations is necessary to establish the correct diagnosis.

COWDEN'S SYNDROME—PATHOLOGIC FEATURES

Gross Findings

- Polyps of variable size located throughout the gastrointestinal tract

Microscopic Findings

- Esophagus shows glycogen acanthosis
- Gastric polyps in Cowden's syndrome (CS) may resemble hyperplastic polyps or prolapse-type polyps
- Small intestinal and colon polyps in CS show a wide spectrum:
  - Hamartomas that may resemble juvenile polyps
  - Ganglioneuromatous polyps
  - Lipomas, fibromas
  - Benign lymphoid polyps
  - Soft tissue vascular malformations have also been described in CS

Genetics

- Autosomal dominant inheritance
- Germline *PTEN* gene mutation

Differential Diagnosis

- Sporadic polyps resembling hamartomas
- Other hamartomatous polyposis syndromes
- Neurofibromatosis

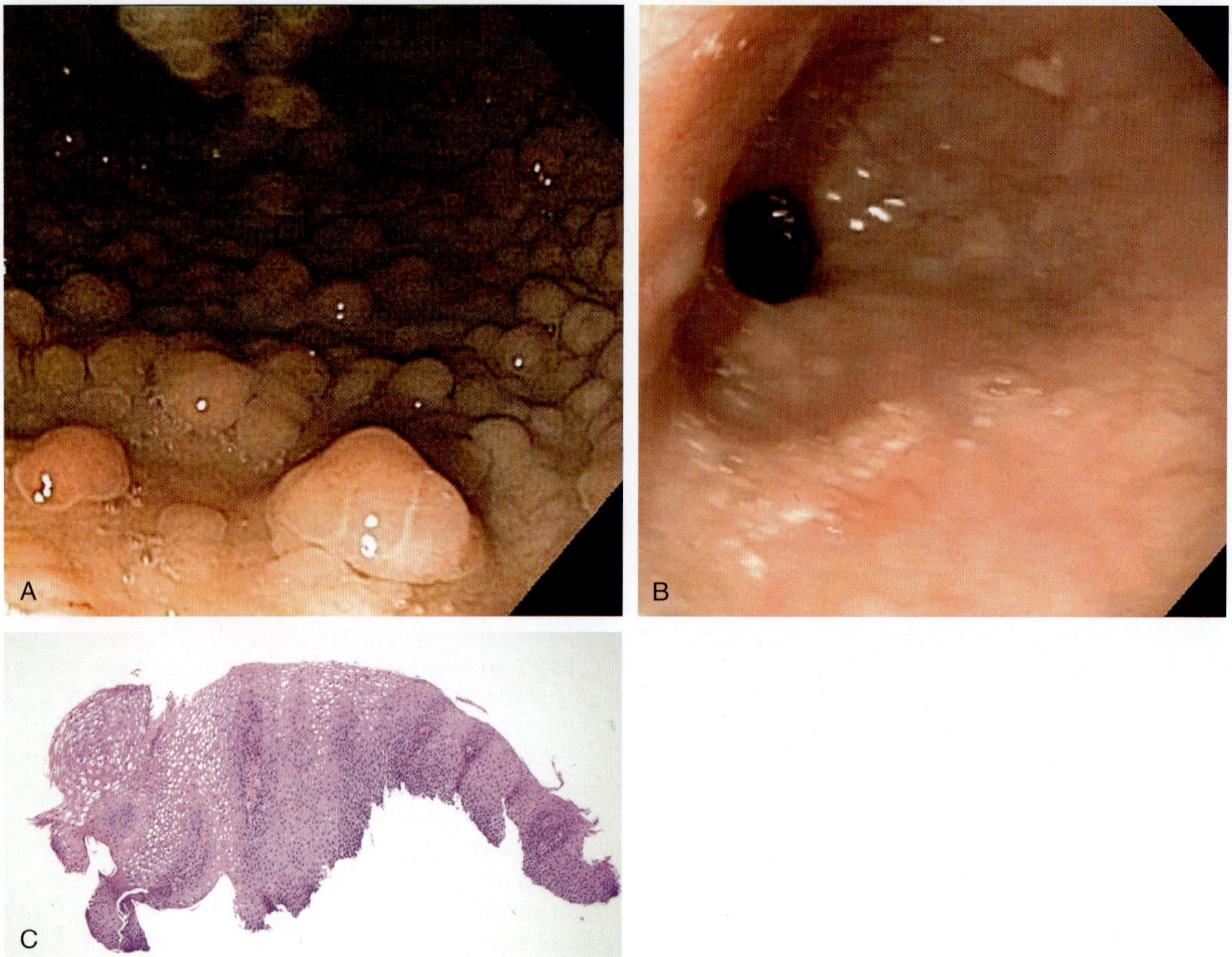

FIGURE 11.16

Upper gastrointestinal tract involvement is often seen in patients with Cowden's syndrome. This may manifest as numerous duodenal polyps (**A**) and glycogen acanthosis of the esophagus, which presents as white-yellow nodules or plaques (**B**). Microscopically, these foci in the esophagus show thickened squamous mucosa with large cells with abundant clear vacuolated cytoplasm filled with glycogen (**C**).

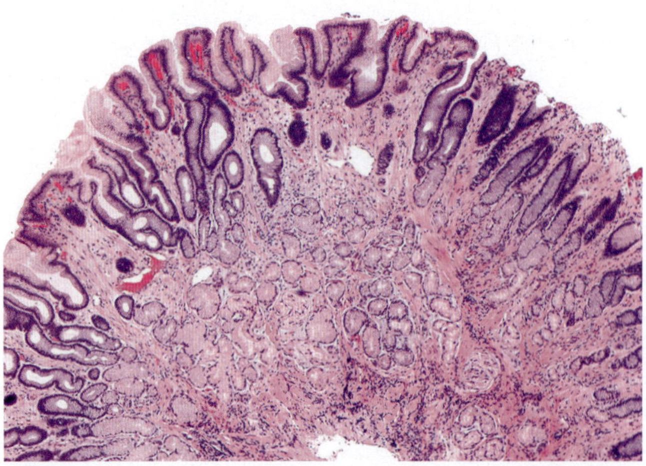

FIGURE 11.17

Gastric polyps in Cowden's syndrome do not have a distinctive appearance and may resemble mucosal prolapse polyps with haphazard proliferation of smooth muscle in the lamina propria.

Prognosis and Therapy

Patients with CS have a significantly higher risk for breast tumors, including fibroadenomas and lipomatosis. Breast carcinoma, the most common malignancy in CS, affects up to 50% of female patients. Male patients are also at increased risk for breast cancer, and regular surveillance for breast cancer is indicated in all patients. It was initially believed that CS does not confer an increased risk of GI cancer, but recent evidence suggests that the risk of colon cancer in CS is increased more than 10 times over the general population.

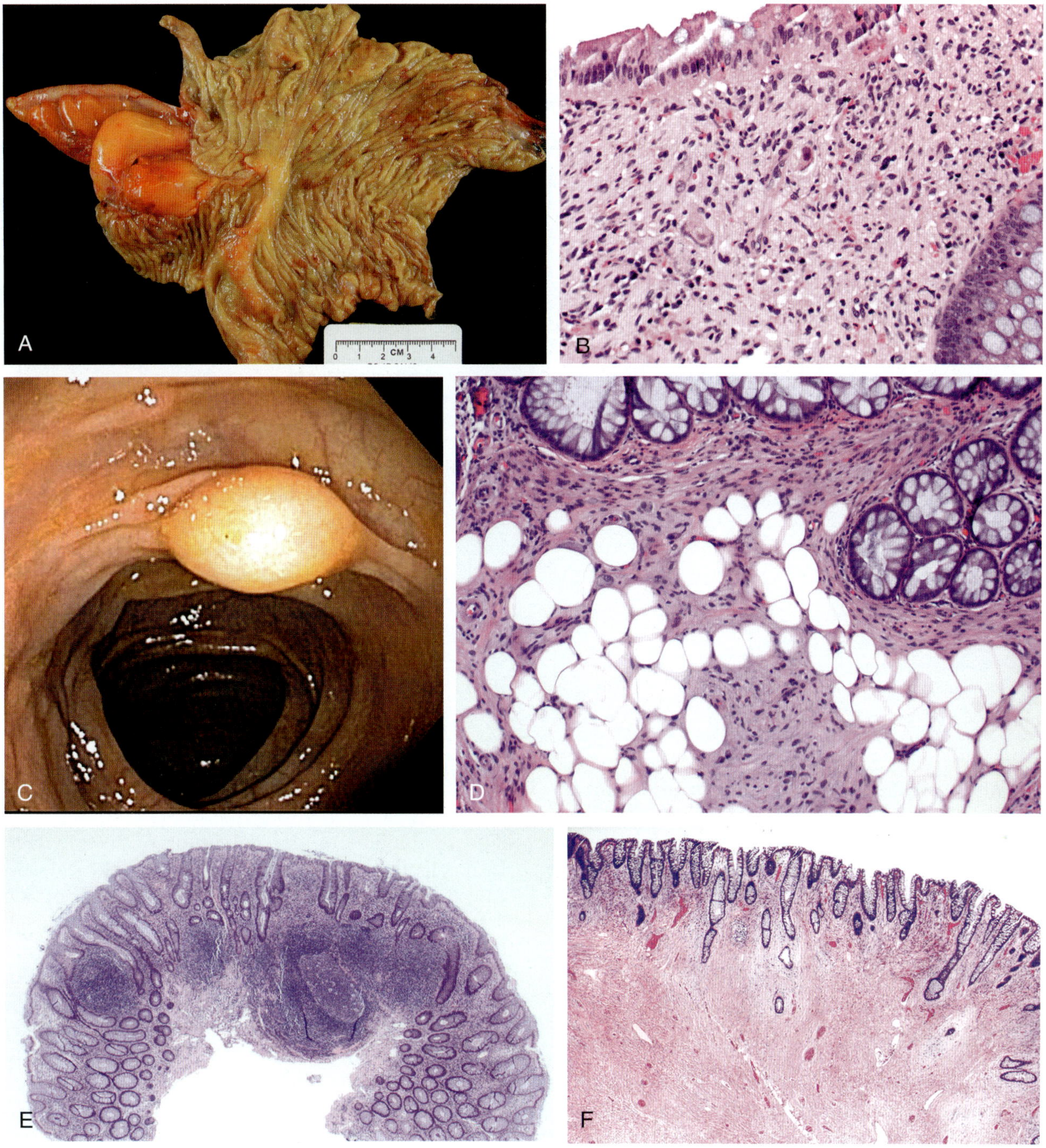

FIGURE 11.18

Colonic involvement in Cowden's syndrome (CS) may show multiple ganglioneuromatous polyps, which present as variably sized submucosal lesions (**A**) and consist of a spindle-shaped neural proliferation with admixed ganglion cells (**B**). Submucosal lipomas (**C**) appear as distinct smooth yellow lesions that are easily recognized on colonoscopy. Lipomatous tissue in the mucosa along with fibrous bands in a polyp should raise suspicion for involvement by CS (**D**). Multiple benign lymphoid polyps (**E**) and fibromas of the colon (**F**) are also lesions that should prompt evaluation for a possible diagnosis of CS.

CRONKHITE-CANADA SYNDROME

Clinical Features

Cronkhite-Canada syndrome (CCS) is a nonhereditary form of diffuse GI polyposis affecting adults and presenting with rapidly progressive diarrhea and malabsorption. In addition to GI polyposis, affected patients show changes of the integumentary system, including skin hyperpigmentation, vitiligo, alopecia, and dystrophic changes of the nails.

The average age of onset is in the fifth to sixth decade of life. A slight male predominance is found. All racial and ethnic groups are affected. The most common presenting symptoms are diarrhea, protein-losing

CRONKHITE-CANADA SYNDROME—FACT SHEET

Definition

- Diffuse gastrointestinal (GI) tract polyposis associated with protein-losing enteropathy, malabsorption, and cutaneous manifestations, including hyperpigmentation and nail dystrophy

Incidence and Location

- Rare disorder that can involve any part of the GI tract

Morbidity and Mortality

- 60% mortality rate if untreated

Gender, Race, and Age Distribution

- Male predominance
- Average age at diagnosis in sixth to seventh decades of life
- No racial predilection

Clinical Features

- Diarrhea, protein-losing enteropathy, weight loss, abdominal pain, and anorexia
- Laboratory findings notable for hypoalbuminemia, hypocalcemia, hypomagnesemia, and severe electrolyte deficiencies

Prognosis and Therapy

- Rapidly progressive and fatal if untreated
- Management is largely supportive with aggressive nutritional support or antibiotics

CRONKHITE-CANADA SYNDROME—PATHOLOGIC FEATURES

Gross Findings

- Diffuse polyposis affecting any portion of the gastrointestinal tract

Microscopic Findings

- Broad-based sessile polyp with prominent edema
- Epithelial component shows cystic change with inflammation and crypt abscesses reminiscent of juvenile polyps
- Nonpolypoid mucosa also shows similar changes which is helpful in making a diagnosis of Cronkhite-Canada syndrome

Differential Diagnosis

- Juvenile polyps
- Inflammatory polyps
- Ménétrier's disease

enteropathy, weight loss, abdominal pain, and anorexia. Laboratory findings are notable for hypoproteinemia, particularly hypoalbuminemia, hypocalcemia, hypomagnesemia, anemia, guaiac-positive stool, and severe electrolyte deficiency.

PATHOLOGIC FEATURES

GROSS FINDINGS

Polyps can be found anywhere in the GI tract but are most frequent in the stomach and colon. In severe cases, the entire mucosal surface of affected sites is involved. Grossly, the polyps of CCS vary from a subtle nodularity of the mucosal surface to large, edematous fronds of mucosa resulting from the presence of large cystically dilated glands within an edematous stroma (Fig. 11.19A).

MICROSCOPIC FINDINGS

In all sites, polyps are typically broad-based sessile lesions with no recognizable stalk. In the colon, CCS polyps are histologically similar to juvenile polyps with cystically dilated glands within an inflamed and edematous stroma (Figs. 11.19B and C). In the stomach, gastric CCS polyps resemble hyperplastic polyps and often show corkscrew-shaped glands, foveolar pits, and smooth muscle fibers extending into the lamina propria (Figs. 11.19D–F). In the small intestine, the lesions are similar, although the degree of inflammation and edema tends to be greater, and the lesions may involve the full thickness of the bowel wall. Sampling of adjacent nonpolypoid mucosa often shows early cystic changes and is helpful in establishing a morphologic diagnosis of CCS.

DIFFERENTIAL DIAGNOSIS

The distinction of the polyps of CCS from JPS can be difficult and often relies on the clinical history. Microscopic features that support a diagnosis of CCS are sessile appearance, abnormal intervening mucosa, and stromal edema that is typically much more severe than seen in juvenile polyps. In the stomach, the confluence of polyps may simulate the giant mucosal folds characteristic of Ménétrier's disease. The latter is restricted to the gastric corpus and shows diffuse enlargement of gastric rugal folds rather than discrete polypoid lesions seen in CCS.

PROGNOSIS AND THERAPY

The malabsorption syndrome is progressive and may be fatal without specific therapy. The mortality rate is 60% and results from severe protein and electrolyte losses from the intestinal tract. A variety of medical and surgical measures have been used to treat patients with this syndrome, including corticosteroids, antibiotics, and surgical resection. However, aggressive nutritional support in the form of calories, nitrogen, lipids, fluids, electrolytes, vitamins, and minerals appears the most important factor associated with a favorable outcome.

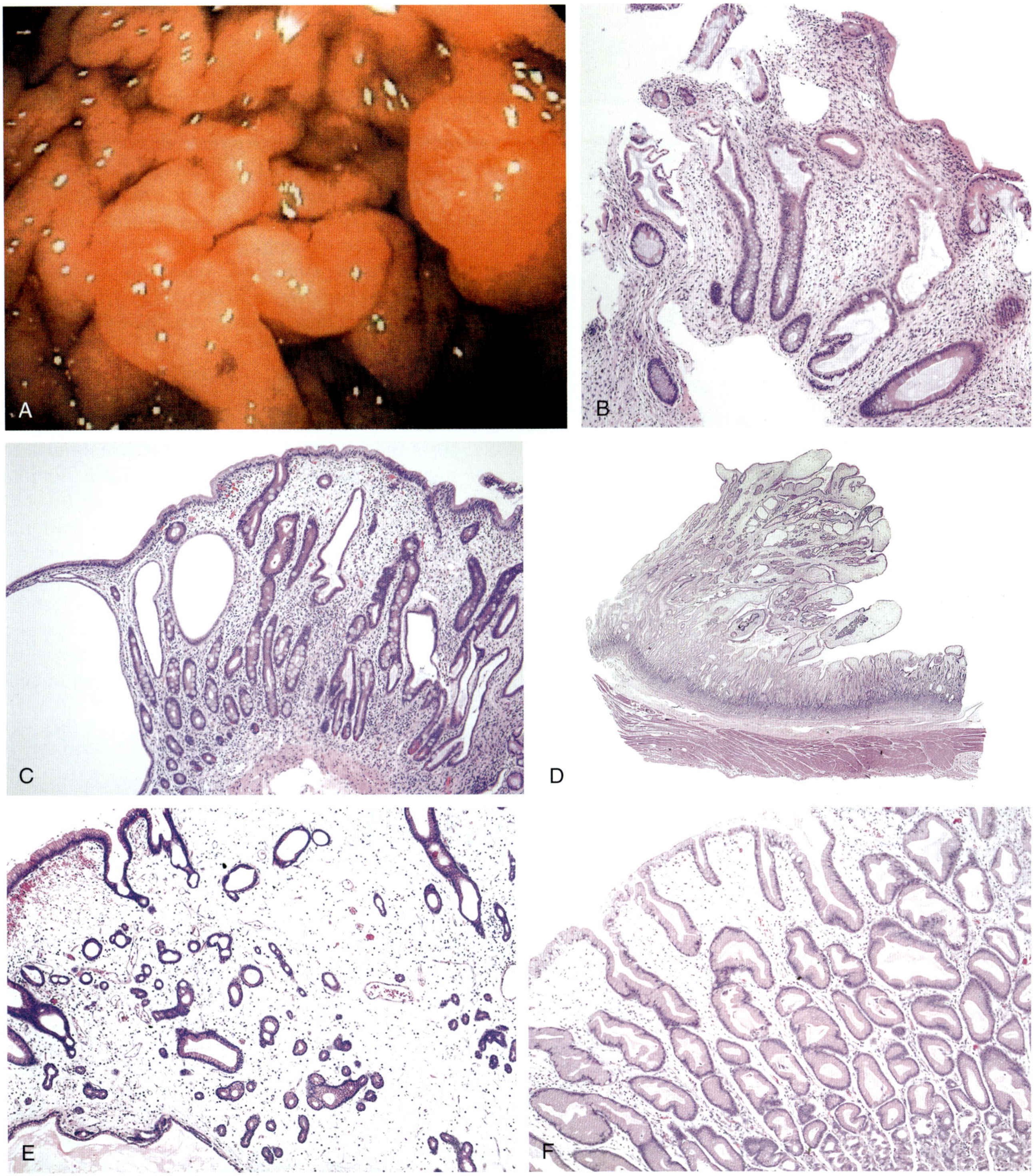

FIGURE 11.19

Cronkhite-Canada syndrome (CCS) shows diffuse nodularity of the colon (**A**), and the polypoid areas show an appearance resembling sporadic inflammatory polyps (**B**). Sections from intervening macroscopically normal mucosa also show cystically dilated crypts surrounded by an edematous lamina propria, a finding which is helpful in diagnosis (**C**). Gastric polyps in CCS are broad based and characterized by large, edematous fronds of mucosa (**D**). The lamina propria shows marked edema (**E**). The epithelial component shows hyperplastic and reactive changes, and the intervening nonpolypoid mucosa shows prominent lamina propria edema (**F**).

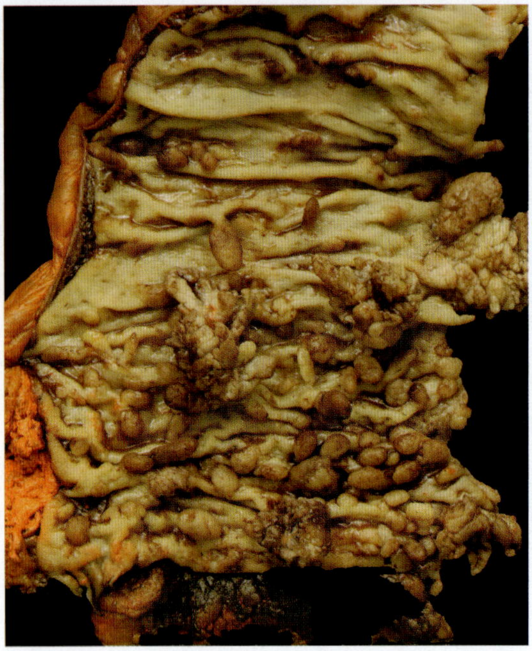

FIGURE 11.20

Hereditary mixed polyposis syndrome resembles juvenile polyposis on macroscopic examination. A spectrum of sessile, pedunculated, and multilobulated polyps is present in this colectomy specimen A germline *GREM1* gene mutation was present..

HEREDITARY MIXED POLYPOSIS SYNDROME

Hereditary mixed polyposis is characterized by a mixture of atypical juvenile, adenomatous, and serrated polyps, as well as polyps with mixed histology (Fig. 11.20). Patients in these families commonly present in the fifth decade of life with rectal bleeding, abdominal pain, change in bowel habits, anemia, or intestinal obstruction. Multiple polyps are seen at colonoscopy, and no extracolonic manifestations have been described. An increased risk for early-onset colorectal carcinoma has been noted. The disease is inherited in an autosomal dominant fashion and is now known to be associated with germline alterations in the *GREM1* gene.

MISCELLANEOUS SYNDROMES WITH ASSOCIATED GASTROINTESTINAL POLYPOSIS

Neurofibromatosis type 1, also known as von Recklinghausen's disease, is defined by the presence of more than five cutaneous café-au-lait spots together with numerous neurofibromas of the skin. This condition is autosomal dominantly inherited and arises from mutations of the NF1 gene on chromosome 17q. Approximately 25% of affected persons exhibit intestinal polypoid neurofibromas or ganglioneuromas. The small bowel is most commonly affected followed by the stomach and colon.

Multiple endocrine neoplasia (MEN) type 2, also called multiple neuroma syndrome, is characterized by the presence of medullary thyroid carcinoma, pheochromocytoma, parathyroid adenomas, a marfanoid habitus, and ganglioneuromatosis of the GI tract. The ganglioneuromas of MEN type 2 can occur anywhere throughout the GI tract from the lips to the anus but are most commonly found in the colon and rectum. This syndrome is a result of mutations of the *RET* protooncogene on chromosome 10q11.2.

Devon family syndrome refers to multiple and recurrent inflammatory fibroid polyps of the stomach and intestine. These lesions are histologically distinct from juvenile polyps. Patients within this family presented in their adult years, often with intestinal obstruction.

Lymphomatosis polyposis is used to describe the polyposis that results from malignant lymphomas that retain homing receptors for gut-associated lymphoid tissue. It can occur throughout the GI tract but tends to be more prominent in areas normally containing lymphoid follicles such as the terminal ileum and right colon. The intervening mucosa in areas of polyposis may be normal. Histologic examination of polypoid tissue indicates the presence of the abnormal lymphoid infiltrate, often with obliteration of the muscularis mucosa and involvement of mucosal and submucosal tissue.

SUGGESTED READINGS

1. Sieber OM, Segditsas S, Knudsen AL, et al. Disease severity and genetic pathways in attenuated familial adenomatous polyposis vary greatly but depend on the site of the germline mutation. *Gut*. 2006;55(10):1440–1448.
2. Sarre RG, Frost AG, Jagelman DG, et al. Gastric and duodenal polyps in familial adenomatous polyposis: a prospective study of the nature and prevalence of upper gastrointestinal polyps. *Gut*. 1987;28(3):306–314.
3. Vasen HF, Moslein G, Alonso A, et al. Guidelines for the clinical management of familial adenomatous polyposis (FAP). *Gut*. 2008;57(5):704–713.
4. Hernegger GS, Moore HG, Guillem JG. Attenuated familial adenomatous polyposis: an evolving and poorly understood entity. *Dis Colon Rectum*. 2002;45(1):127–134. [discussion134-6].
5. Knudsen AL, Bülow S, Tomlinson I, et al. Attenuated familial adenomatous polyposis: results from an international collaborative study. *Colorectal Dis*. 2010;12(10 Online):e243–e249.
6. Sieber OM, Segditsas S, Knudsen AL, et al. Disease severity and genetic pathways in attenuated familial adenomatous polyposis vary greatly but depend on the site of the germline mutation. *Gut*. 2006;55(10):1440–1448.
7. Cheadle JP, Sampson JR. MUTYH-associated polyposis—From defect in base excision repair to clinical genetic testing. *DNA Repair (Amst)*. 2007;6(3):274–279.
8. Weren RD, Ligtenberg MJ, Geurts van Kessel A, et al. NTHL1 and MUTYH polyposis syndromes: two sides of the same coin? *J Pathol*. 2018;244(2):135–142.
9. Belhadj S, Mur P, Navarro M, et al. Delineating the phenotypic spectrum of the NTHL1-associated polyposis. *Clin Gastroenterol Hepatol*. 2017;15(3):461–462.
10. Palles C, Cazier JB, Howarth KM, et al. Germline mutations affecting the proofreading domains of POLE and POLD1 predispose to colorectal adenomas and carcinomas. *Nat Genet*. 2013;45(2):136–144.

11. Spier I, Holzapfel S, Altmüller J, et al. Frequency and phenotypic spectrum of germline mutations in POLE and seven other polymerase genes in 266 patients with colorectal adenomas and carcinomas. *Int J Cancer*. 2015;137(2):320–331.
12. Wood LD, Salaria SN, Cruise MW, et al. Upper GI tract lesions in familial adenomatous polyposis (FAP): enrichment of pyloric gland adenomas and other gastric and duodenal neoplasms. *Am J Surg Pathol*. 2014;38(3):389–393.
13. Spigelman AD, Williams CB, Talbot IC, et al. Upper gastrointestinal cancer in patients with familial adenomatous polyposis. *Lancet*. 1989;2(8666):783–785.
14. Attard TM, Cuff\ari C, Tajouri T, et al. Multicenter experience with upper gastrointestinal polyps in pediatric patients with familial adenomatous polyposis. *Am J Gastroenterol*. 2004;99(4):681–686.
15. Arnason T, Liang WY, Alfaro E, et al. Morphology and natural history of familial adenomatous polyposis-associated dysplastic fundic gland polyps. *Histopathology*. 2014;65(3):353–362.
16. Bianchi LK, Burke CA, Bennett AE, et al. Fundic gland polyp dysplasia is common in familial adenomatous polyposis. *Clin Gastroenterol Hepatol*. 2008;6(2):180–185.
17. Nakamura S, Matsumoto T, Kobori Y, Iida M. Impact of Helicobacter pylori infection and mucosal atrophy on gastric lesions in patients with familial adenomatous polyposis. *Gut*. 2002;51(4):485–489.
18. Al-Tassan N, Chmiel NH, Maynard J, et al. Inherited variants of MYH associated with somatic G:C– > T:A mutations in colorectal tumors. *Nat Genet*. 2002;30(2):227–232.
19. Boparai KS, Dekker E, Van Eeden S, et al. Hyperplastic polyps and sessile serrated adenomas as a phenotypic expression of MYH-associated polyposis. *Gastroenterology*. 2008;135(6): 2014–2018.
20. Vogt S, Jones N, Christian D, et al. Expanded extracolonic tumor spectrum in MUTYH-associated polyposis. *Gastroenterology*. 2009;137(6):1976–1985. e1-10.
21. Walton SJ, Kallenberg FG, Clark SK, et al. Frequency and features of duodenal adenomas in patients with MUTYH-associated polyposis. *Clin Gastroenterol Hepatol*. 2016;14(7):986–992.
22. Nagase H, Miyoshi Y, Horii A, et al. Correlation between the location of germ-line mutations in the APC gene and the number of colorectal polyps in familial adenomatous polyposis patients. *Cancer Res*. 1992;52(14):4055–4057.
23. Enomoto M, Konishi M, Iwama T, et al. The relationship between frequencies of extracolonic manifestations and the position of APC germline mutation in patients with familial adenomatous polyposis. *Jpn J Clin Oncol*. 2000;30(2):82–88.
24. Spirio L, Olschwang S, Groden J, et al. Alleles of the APC gene: an attenuated form of familial polyposis. *Cell*. 1993;75(5): 951–957.
25. Slowik V, Attard T, Dai H, et al. Desmoid tumors complicating familial adenomatous polyposis: a meta-analysis mutation spectrum of affected individuals. *BMC Gastroenterol*. 2015;15:84.
26. Boparai KS, Dekker E, Polak MM, et al. A serrated colorectal cancer pathway predominates over the classic WNT pathway in patients with hyperplastic polyposis syndrome. *Am J Pathol*. 2011;178(6):2700–2707.
27. Boparai KS, Dekker E, Van Eeden S, et al. Hyperplastic polyps and sessile serrated adenomas as a phenotypic expression of MYH-associated polyposis. *Gastroenterology*. 2008;135(6): 2014–2018.
28. Buchanan DD, Clendenning M, Zhuoer L, et al. Lack of evidence for germline RNF43 mutations in patients with serrated polyposis syndrome from a large multinational study. *Gut*. 2017; 66(6):1170–1172.
29. Carballal S, Rodríguez-Alcalde D, Moreira L, et al. Colorectal cancer risk factors in patients with serrated polyposis syndrome: a large multicentre study. *Gut*. 2016;65(11):1829–1837.
30. Quintana I, Mejías-Luque R, Terradas M, et al. Evidence suggests that germline RNF43 mutations are a rare cause of serrated polyposis. *Gut*. 2018;67(12):2230–2232.
31. Rosty C, Walsh MD, Walters RJ, et al. Multiplicity and molecular heterogeneity of colorectal carcinomas in individuals with serrated polyposis. *Am J Surg Pathol*. 2013;37(3):434–442.
32. Rosty C, Buchanan DD, Walsh MD, et al. Phenotype and polyp landscape in serrated polyposis syndrome: a series of 100 patients from genetics clinics. *Am J Surg Pathol*. 2012;36(6):876–882.
33. Beggs AD, Latchford AR, Vasen HF, et al. Peutz-Jeghers syndrome: a systematic review and recommendations for management. *Gut*. 2010;59(7):975–986.
34. Schreibman IR, Baker M, Amos C, McGarrity TJ. The hamartomatous polyposis syndromes: a clinical and molecular review. *Am J Gastroenterol*. 2005;100(2):476–490.
35. Tse JY, Wu S, Shinagare SA, et al. Peutz-Jeghers syndrome: a critical look at colonic Peutz-Jeghers polyps. *Mod Pathol*. 2013;26 (9):1235–1240.
36. Shaco-Levy R, Jasperson KW, Martin K, et al. Morphologic characterization of hamartomatous gastrointestinal polyps in Cowden syndrome, Peutz-Jeghers syndrome, and juvenile polyposis syndrome. *Hum Pathol*. 2016;49:39–48.
37. Lam-Himlin D, Park JY, Cornish TC, et al. Morphologic characterization of syndromic gastric polyps. *Am J Surg Pathol*. 2010;34 (11):1656–1662.
38. Brosens LA, van Hattem A, Hylind LM, et al. Risk of colorectal cancer in juvenile polyposis. *Gut*. 2007;56(7):965–967.
39. van Hattem WA, Langeveld D, de Leng WW, et al. Histologic variations in juvenile polyp phenotype correlate with genetic defect underlying juvenile polyposis. *Am J Surg Pathol*. 2011;35(4): 530–536.
40. van Hattem WA, Brosens LA, de Leng WW, et al. Large genomic deletions of SMAD4, BMPR1A and PTEN in juvenile polyposis. *Gut*. 2008;57(5):623–627.
41. Sweet K, Willis J, Zhou XP, et al. Molecular classification of patients with unexplained hamartomatous and hyperplastic polyposis. *JAMA*. 2005;294(19):2465–2473.
42. Gonzalez RS, Adsay V, Graham RP, et al. Massive gastric juvenile-type polyposis: a clinicopathologic analysis of 22 cases. *Histopathology*. 2017;70(6):918–928.
43. Heald B, Mester J, Rybicki L, et al. Frequent gastrointestinal polyps and colorectal adenocarcinomas in a prospective series of PTEN mutation carriers. *Gastroenterology*. 2010;139(6): 1927–1933.
44. Borowsky J, Setia N, Lauwers G, et al. Gastrointestinal tract pathology in PTEN Hamartoma tumour syndrome: a review of 43 cases. *Mod Pathol*. 2015;28(S2):149A.
45. Syngal S, Brand RE, Church JM, et al. ACG clinical guideline: genetic testing and management of hereditary gastrointestinal cancer syndromes. *Am J Gastroenterol*. 2015;110(2):223–262.
46. Pilarski R, Burt R, Kohlman W, et al. Cowden syndrome and the PTEN hamartoma tumor syndrome: systematic review and revised diagnostic criteria. *J Natl Cancer Inst*. 2013;105(21):1607 –1616.
47. Jaeger E, Leedham S, Lewis A, et al. Hereditary mixed polyposis syndrome is caused by a 40-kb upstream duplication that leads to increased and ectopic expression of the BMP antagonist GREM1. *Nat Genet*. 2012;44(6):699–703.
48. Brosens LA, Offerhaus GJ, Canto MI, et al. Simultaneous juvenile polyposis syndrome and neurofibromatosis type 1. *Histopathology*. 2016;68(2):313–315.

12

Epithelial Neoplasms of the Colorectum

Deepa T. Patil, MD

A large variety of neoplasms may occur in the colorectum, reflecting the complexity of this organ and its cellular components. This chapter focuses primarily on those neoplasms arising from the epithelial and neuroendocrine cells of the colorectum. Epithelial neoplasms that arise as a component of a polyposis syndrome are discussed in Chapter 11.

COLORECTAL POLYPS

Given the widespread use of colonoscopy as a screening tool for detecting colorectal cancer (CRC), colorectal polyps constitute some of the most common types of specimens in gastrointestinal (GI) pathology practice. Colorectal polyps can be broadly classified into inflammatory polyps, hamartomatous polyps, mesenchymal polyps, and epithelial polyps. Inflammatory polyps usually occur in a background of mucosal injury, for example, idiopathic inflammatory bowel disease (IBD), drug-induced injury, or infections. Hamartomatous polyps are typically associated with GI polyposis syndromes (see Chapter 11). Occasionally, one may find mucosal polyps composed entirely of stromal elements. Most mesenchymal lesions that present as mucosal polyps tend to be benign in nature (leiomyoma, lipoma, ganglioneuroma, perineurioma or fibroblastic polyps, glomus tumor, and inflammatory fibroid polyps). Epithelial polyps are the most common types of polyps seen in daily practice. These can be categorized into adenomatous polyps and serrated polyps and are discussed in the following section.

ADENOMATOUS POLYPS

Clinical Features

The prevalence of adenomas varies in different parts of the world. Adenomas are common in Western countries and present in up to 60% of individuals in autopsy studies. The prevalence increases with age such that nearly 50% of the adult US population will develop an adenoma by age 50 years. Adenomas are of clinical importance because they can develop into an infiltrating adenocarcinoma, a notion supported by extensive epidemiologic data. The incidence of adenomas parallels the incidence of CRC, and countries with high rates of CRC also have high rates of colorectal adenoma. Clinical data in support of the neoplastic potential of adenomas relate to adenoma size, adenoma type, and the presence of high-grade dysplasia. Infiltrating carcinoma is found in 5% of all adenomas and is more commonly found in adenomas larger than 1.0 cm in diameter, with villous morphology, and with coexistent areas of high-grade dysplasia.

Four factors have been described in association with the formation of colorectal adenomas: environment, genetics, diet, and host factors. Colorectal adenomas show wide geographic variations in frequency among industrialized nations. They are most common in North America, Western Europe, New Zealand, and Australia. Variations in incidence are also found within industrialized nations. Patients with a high risk for developing CRC are those with an inherited predisposition to colorectal adenoma formation (i.e., familial adenomatous polyposis [FAP]), patients with chronic IBD (particularly ulcerative colitis), and patients with a family history of colon cancer (as in hereditary nonpolyposis colon cancer).

The relationship of diet to CRC risk is a topic of enormous interest and debate. Nonetheless, the role of dietary factors in the development of colorectal adenomas and carcinoma is generally accepted and thought to relate to diets that are high in animal fat and protein and low in fiber or vegetables.

A variety of host factors related to CRC risk include obesity, smoking history, and occupational exposures. Bile acid turnover in association with gut microflora metabolism is also related to tumor incidence. For example, fecapentaenes, a product of the gut microflora, are potent mutagenic compounds found in human feces that are correlated with colorectal carcinogenesis.

ADENOMATOUS POLYPS—FACT SHEET

Definition

- Dysplastic neoplasms of intestinal epithelium with the potential for transformation to invasive adenocarcinoma

Incidence And Location

- Common finding in patients living in industrialized countries

Morbidity And Mortality

- Related to risk for malignant progression
- Infiltrating adenocarcinoma more common in high-risk adenomas (adenomas >1 cm in diameter with villous morphology and high-grade dysplasia)

Gender, Race, And Age Distribution

- Males more than females
- More common in developed countries
- Average age at diagnosis in sixth decade of life

Clinical Features

- Associated with high-fat, low-fiber diet
- More common in patients with prior adenomas or positive family history

Prognosis And Therapy

- Left-sided adenomas are a biomarker for elevated colorectal cancer risk
- Routine surveillance is indicated to remove metachronous adenomas

Pathologic Features

Gross Findings

Adenomas smaller than 1 cm in diameter tend to be evenly distributed throughout the colorectum. In contrast, adenomas 1 cm or larger in diameter are more commonly found in the sigmoid colon and rectum. In general, the polyp size is correlated with the histologic type—tubular, tubulovillous, or villous. Among adenomas smaller than 1 cm in diameter, more than 90% are tubular adenomas, 7% are tubulovillous, and 2% are villous. In contrast, only 50% of adenomas larger than 2 cm are tubular, whereas 38% are tubulovillous and 12% villous. Grossly, colorectal adenomas may appear pedunculated, sessile, or flat. Tubular adenomas range in size from individual crypt adenomas to large exophytic lesions several centimeters in diameter. Larger tubular adenomas may become polypoid with a lobulated surface and a stalk at the base of the lesion. In addition to the surface lobulations, areas of hemorrhage may be present resulting from erosion of the surface epithelium. In contrast, villous adenomas are commonly sessile lesions with a broad base and grossly evident papillary architecture.

Flat adenomas are a morphologic type of adenoma that appear as flat or slightly raised plaques on the mucosal surface. By definition, they usually show a concave surface that does not exceed twice the thickness of the adjacent non-neoplastic mucosa.

Microscopic Findings

Similar to the rest of the GI tract, adenomas are graded using the two-tiered system—low-grade and high-grade dysplasia. By definition, adenomas harbor at least low-grade dysplasia. Low-grade dysplasia is characterized by atypical glands lined by cells with cigar-shaped or penicillate, pseudostratified, and hyperchromatic nuclei (Fig. 12.1). These cytologic changes involve both the crypts and the surface epithelium. The individual cells have increased nuclear-to-cytoplasmic ratio and frequent mitotic activity. High-grade dysplasia encompasses additional architectural and cytologic changes (Fig. 12.2). Architecturally, the crypts show irregular branching, gland crowding, and cribriform architecture.

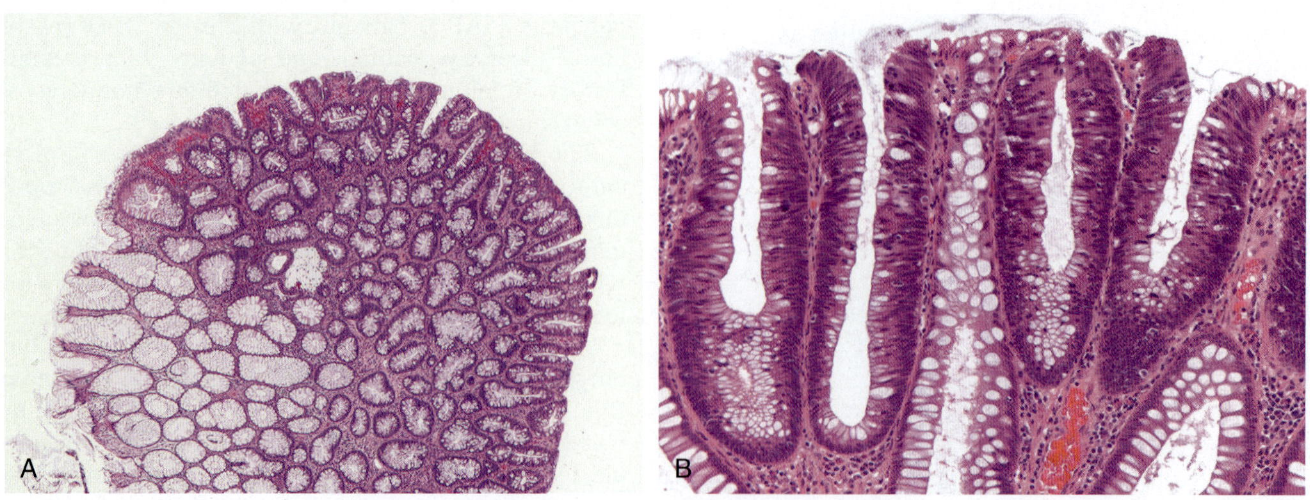

FIGURE 12.1

Adenomatous polyp: tubular adenoma. Low-grade dysplasia characterized by atypical glands lined by cells with cigar-shaped, pseudostratified, and hyperchromatic nuclei (**A**). The nuclei maintain their polarity (the long axis of the nuclei is perpendicular to the basement membrane) (**B**). These cytologic changes involve both the crypts and the surface epithelium.

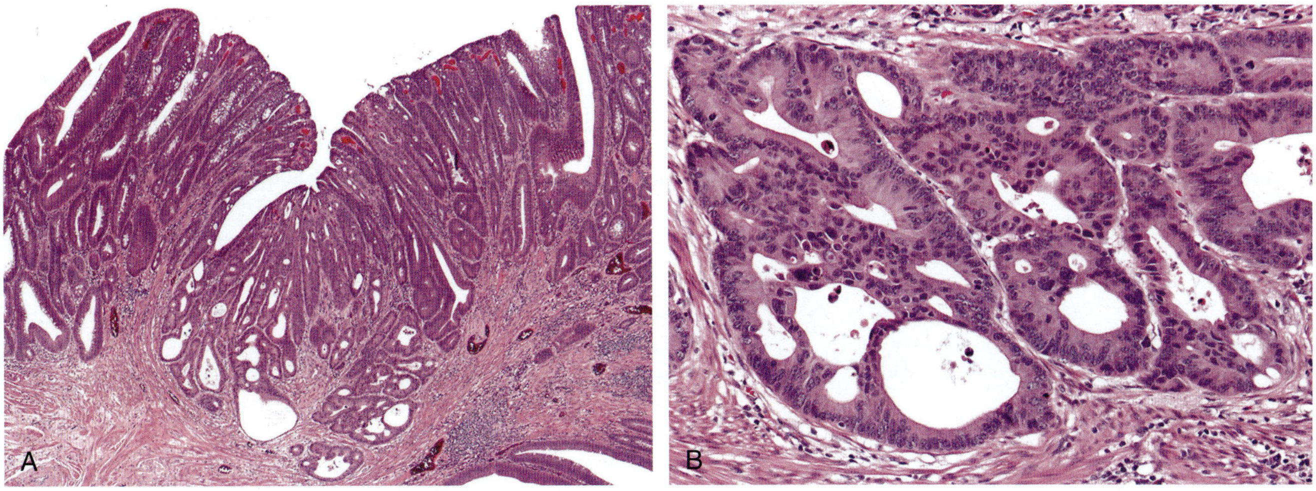

FIGURE 12.2

Tubulovillous adenoma with high-grade dysplasia. Adenomatous polyp with architectural atypia characterized by irregular branching, gland budding, and cribriform architecture (**A**). Cytologically, the nuclei show increased atypia with enlarged, hyperchromatic, vesicular nuclei; prominent nucleoli; and loss of nuclear polarity (the basement membrane of the cell is no longer perpendicular to the long axis of the nucleus) (**B**).

Cytologically, the nuclei show increased atypia with enlarged, hyperchromatic, vesicular nuclei; prominent nucleoli; and loss of nuclear polarity (basement membrane of the cell is no longer perpendicular to the long axis of the nucleus). Mitoses, including atypical mitotic figures, are prominent.

Flat adenomas are in essence tubular adenomas that lack a polypoid growth or an exophytic growth pattern. Rather than the complex branching of adenomatous glands, villous adenomas show tall, fingerlike projections of adenomatous epithelium with a central fibrovascular core that extends from the polyp base to the surface.

A variety of cell types may be encountered in adenomas, including Paneth cells, goblet cells, and endocrine cells. The finding of these cell types in an adenomatous polyp reflect the ability of the neoplastic cells to partially differentiate into a variety of cell types. Goblet cells within adenomatous polyps are often dystrophic, seen as cells or goblet cells with atypical nuclei oriented away from the basement membrane of the gland. Endocrine cells are present in at least half of adenomas and can best be discerned with the use of special stains. Paneth cells are present in 10% of adenomas, recognized for their characteristic eosinophilic granules. Excessive Paneth cells may be seen in patients with polyposis syndrome, especially FAP. Some adenomas may contain foci of squamous morular metaplasia (Fig. 12.3), osseous metaplasia, melanocytes, or even gastric type epithelium.

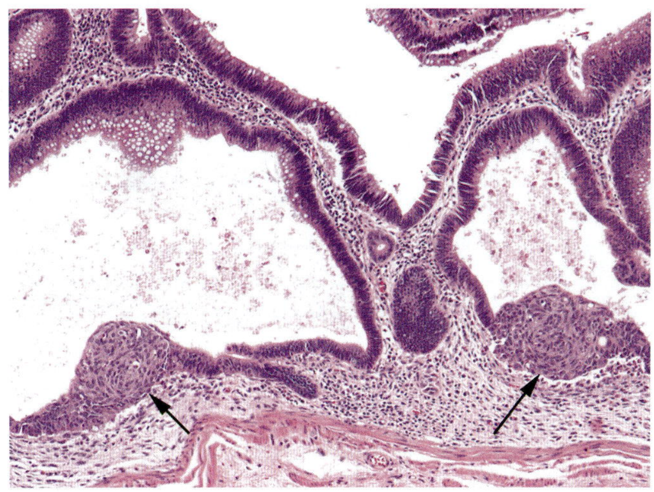

FIGURE 12.3

Adenomatous polyp with squamous morular metaplasia. The basal aspect of the polyp shows nests of cells with abundant eosinophilic cytoplasm and oval to spindle cells arranged in a whorled pattern *(arrows)*. These foci can be misinterpreted as high-grade dysplasia and have no clinical significance.

Neuroendocrine Proliferation In Adenomatous Polyps

In large adenomatous polyps, there may be small, multifocal clusters of neuroendocrine cells located at the base of the lamina propria (Fig. 12.4). There are various theories of histogenesis for this finding, including stem cells with divergent differentiation, collision tumor, or metaplastic phenomenon related to polyp trauma. These clusters are often surrounded by fibromyxoid stroma and mimic invasive adenocarcinoma. They are most common in adenomas that are 1 cm or larger in size, harbor high-grade dysplasia, and show villous morphology. They have been referred to as neuroendocrine proliferation or composite intestinal adenoma–microcarcinoid. The latter term is less preferred because the word *carcinoid* may result in unnecessary surgical treatment because of the implied malignant potential. In fact, studies have shown that these lesions are not associated with any lymph node or distant metastasis. Therefore, most pathologists do not report this finding in daily practice.

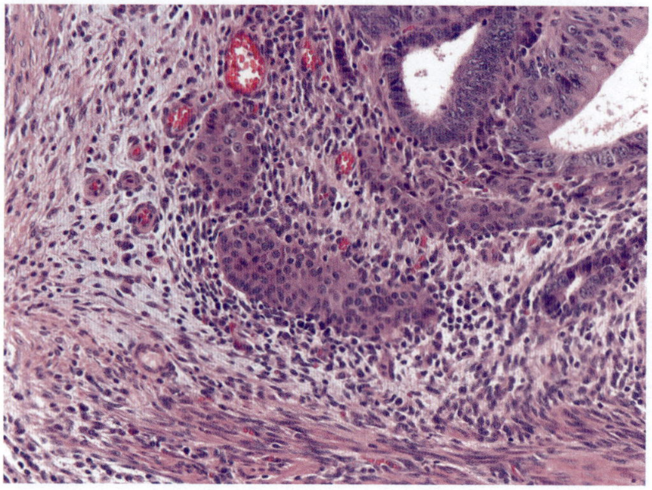

FIGURE 12.4

Neuroendocrine proliferation in an adenomatous polyp. The deep aspect of lamina propria shows nests and cords of uniform cells with abundant granular eosinophilic cytoplasm, centrally located round to oval nuclei, and stippled chromatin pattern. These nests are often surrounded by loose fibromyxoid stroma.

In contrast, the presence of high-grade neuroendocrine proliferation or high-grade neuroendocrine carcinoma (large cell or small cell type) is a significant finding that needs to be reported. These foci are often unifocal and associated with conventional invasive adenocarcinoma. However, rarely, the high-grade neuroendocrine component is seen in association with a tubular or tubulovillous adenoma.

Intramucosal Adenocarcinoma And "Carcinoma In Situ"

Adenomas that show invasion of the lamina propria or the muscularis mucosae (but not beyond) are considered intramucosal adenocarcinomas. The neoplastic proliferation may either show single-cell infiltration by atypical cells or marked expansion of the lamina propria or muscularis mucosae by closely packed glands without intervening lamina propria. However, compared with the other parts of the GI tract (esophagus, stomach, small bowel), which harbor a rich lymphatic plexus that facilitates metastatic spread, the colonic mucosa lacks lymphatic spaces, and therefore, in theory, intramucosal adenocarcinoma of the colon and rectum does not have any propensity to metastasize. Therefore, some authorities prefer not to use this term. Instead, these lesions are classified as adenoma with extensive high-grade dysplasia. The only situations when one might consider using this term is in the setting of biopsy obtained from a large mass or an incompletely resected polyp that shows the aforementioned cytoarchitectural features. However, when this term is used in a pathology report, it should be followed by a comment that clearly states the biologic potential of the lesion.

The use of the term *carcinoma in situ* is no longer recommended in the GI tract because the word *carcinoma* has the potential to be misinterpreted as malignancy and can result in unnecessary colectomy for a lesion that is confined to the basement membrane of the neoplastic glands. These lesions are therefore diagnosed as high-grade dysplasia.

Molecular Features Of Adenomatous Polyps

Most conventional adenomas progress toward carcinoma via the chromosomal instability pathway characterized by acquisition of several mutations during cancer development. Inactivation of *APC/β-catenin/Wnt* signaling pathway by germline or somatic mutation of one copy of the adenomatous polyposis coli *(APC)* gene is one of the early molecular events. Inactivation of the second allele and accumulation of additional mutations, such as in *KRAS, DCC*, and *p53*, drives carcinogenesis.

Adenomatous Polyps—Pathologic Features

Gross Findings

- Pedunculated or sessile growth pattern
- Pancolonic distribution
- Larger adenomas (>1 cm), more often left sided

Microscopic Findings

- Tubular adenomas consist of branching dysplastic glands
- Villous adenomas contain dysplastic glands growing in long, fingerlike projections
- Low-grade dysplasia
  - Nuclear hyperchromasia, enlargement, and pseudostratification involving crypts as well as surface epithelium
  - Individual nuclei show elongated or penicillate morphology but maintain their nuclear polarity (long axis of the nucleus is perpendicular to the basement membrane of the gland)
- High-grade dysplasia
  - Complex architecture composed of crowded glands with glandular budding and cribriform arrangement
  - Cytologic atypia consists of marked nuclear enlargement, pleomorphism, vesicular nuclei, prominent nucleoli, and loss of nuclear polarity
  - Mitotic figures are quite prominent

Genetics

- Complex genetic alterations
- Frequent alterations of *APC, KRAS*, and *p53*

Differential Diagnosis

- Reactive epithelial changes

Differential Diagnosis

Any pathologic entity in the colorectum in which the epithelium undergoes reactive changes can mimic adenomatous dysplasia, including hyperplastic polyp (HP), mucosal prolapse, and inflammatory polyp. Reactive epithelial changes are often associated with ongoing or resolving mucosal injury. The cells show slight nuclear hyperchromasia, enlargement, and mucin loss. However, these changes are often restricted to the epithelium adjacent to mucosal injury. The cells maintain their overall nuclear-to-cytoplasmic ratio, and there is surface epithelial maturation. All of these features indicate reactive atypia.

Prognosis and Therapy

Per consensus update by the United States Multi-Society Task Force on Colorectal Cancer, low-risk adenomas refer to one to adenomas smaller than 10 mm in diameter at baseline colonoscopy. High-risk adenomas are defined as adenomas that are 10 mm in size or larger, the presence of three or more adenomas, adenoma with villous histology, or adenomas with high-grade dysplasia (HGD). Advanced adenomas are adenomas that are large (>1 cm) and contain a villous architecture or at least HGD. Advanced adenomas are at a much higher risk for the development of HGD and invasive adenocarcinoma. In a meta-analysis, the relative risk for recurrent advanced adenomas was 1.84 times in advanced adenomas compared with patients with low-grade dysplasia at baseline colonoscopy. In the National Cancer Institute pooling project, patients with baseline polyps larger than 2 cm in size had a 19.3% risk of advanced neoplasia at follow-up. Whereas patients with adenomas that measured 1 to 2 cm in size had a 15.9% risk, those with adenomas smaller than 5 mm in size had a 7.7% risk of advanced neoplasia. These data support different surveillance intervals for adenomatous polyps based on the size and degree of dysplasia (Table 12.1). The appropriate treatment for all conventional adenomas (regardless of type, size, or degree of dysplasia) is complete removal. The current guidelines support the use of colonoscopy starting at age 45 years, given the rising incidence of CRC in young patients, or at a time 10 years earlier than the age of cancer development in a first-degree family member.

Malignant Polyps

A malignant polyp is defined as a polyp that shows neoplastic glands invading through the muscularis mucosae into the submucosa (pT1) (Fig. 12.5). These lesions represent the vast majority of early CRCs and carry a small risk of lymph node metastasis. Studies have suggested that the prevalence of invasive adenocarcinoma in an endoscopically resected adenoma is around 2% to 5%. In most cases, a good endoscopist recognizes the presence of a malignant polyp by the "non-lifting" sign in which the endoscopist is unable to elevate a sessile polyp following submucosal saline injection. Newer techniques such as endoscopic submucosal dissection (a technique similar to endoscopic mucosal resection) offer the advantage of en bloc resection with more accurate histologic assessment of large or sessile polyps that are more likely to harbor foci of invasive adenocarcinoma.

TABLE 12.1
Surveillance Guidelines for Colorectal Adenomas

Baseline Colonoscopy: Most Advanced Findings	Surveillance Interval (years)	Quality of Supporting evidence	New Evidence Stronger than 2006
No polyps	10	Moderate	Yes
1–2 small (<10 mm) tubular adenomas	5–10	Moderate	Yes
3–10 tubular adenomas	3	Moderate	Yes
>10 adenomas	<3	Moderate	No
Adenoma ≥10 mm	3	High	Yes
≥1 villous adenomas	3	Moderate	Yes
Adenoma with high-grade dysplasia	3	Moderate	No

Adapted from Lieberman DA, Rex DK, Winawer SJ, et al. Guidelines for colonoscopy surveillance after screening and polypectomy: a consensus update by the US Multi-Society Task Force on Colorectal Cancer. *Gastroenterology*. 2012;143:844-857.

Risk Assessment Of Malignant Polyps

Gross Evaluation

Gross description of a polyp should include size, presence or absence of a stalk, and intactness of specimen. Pathologists should avoid using the terms *pedunculated*, *sessile*, and *semi-pedunculated* because these terms refer to in vivo endoscopic assessment of these lesions. It is a common practice to ink the polyp base margin which is cauterized during polyp removal. The benefit of this process is that it allows for easy identification of margin on microscopic examination. However, improper identification of the polyp base and inaccurate inking can contribute to inaccuracy in assessment of the margin status. Therefore, cauterized tissue visualized under the microscope is the best guide for assessing the distance of invasive adenocarcinoma from the margin.

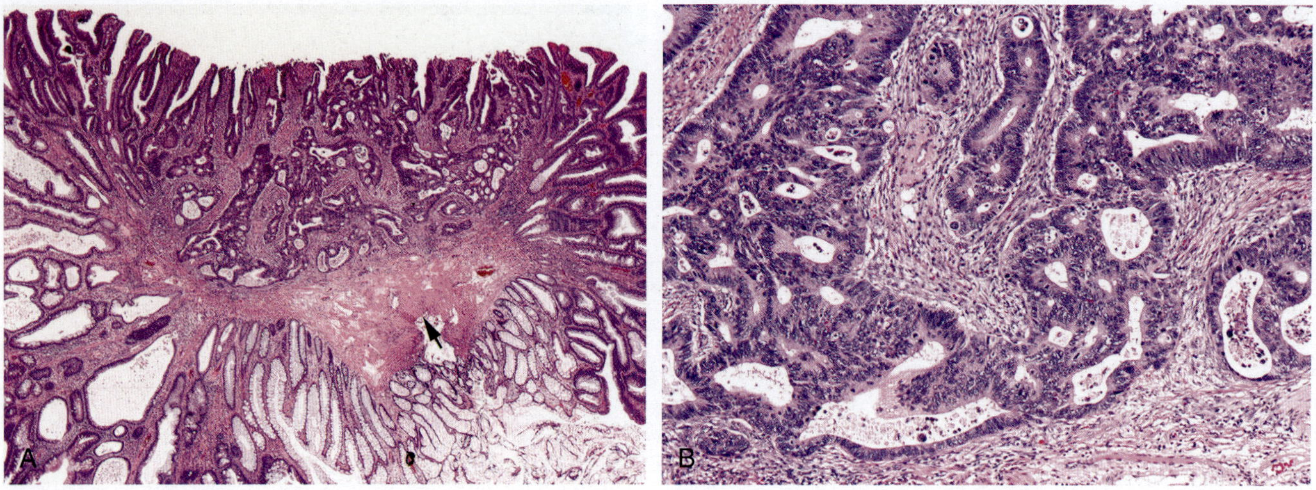

FIGURE 12.5

Invasive adenocarcinoma arising in a tubulovillous adenoma with high-grade dysplasia (malignant polyp). This sigmoid colon polyp shows a proliferation of neoplastic glands with irregular, angulated profiles infiltrating the muscularis mucosae and submucosa (A). The resection margin is indicated by the arrow. The neoplastic glands are surrounded by stromal desmoplasia that is diagnostic of submucosal invasion (B).

Histologic Reporting Parameters

Risk assessment of malignant polyp (low or high risk of adverse outcome) is performed using histologic parameters that include margin status, lymphovascular invasion, and tumor grade. Unfavorable histologic features that predict recurrent cancer or lymph node metastasis include tumor at or near the margin (≤1 mm), grade 3 (poorly differentiated adenocarcinoma), or lymphovascular invasion. In theory, the presence of any of these features is an indication for surgery. In the absence of these features, the polypectomy procedure is considered to be completely curative.

Tumor Grade

Similar to colorectal resection specimens, the grade of invasive adenocarcinoma is assessed using the American Joint Committee on Cancer (AJCC) eighth edition classification system. It is based on the degree of glandular differentiation:

Grade 1: well-differentiated adenocarcinoma, greater than 95% glandular differentiation or with well-formed glands with open lumina

Grade 2: moderately differentiated adenocarcinoma; 50% to 95% glandular differentiation

Grade 3: poorly differentiated adenocarcinoma, signet ring cell or mucinous adenocarcinoma, less than 50% glandular differentiation or solid sheets of neoplastic glands

Grade 4: undifferentiated; no gland formation or mucin; no squamous or neuroendocrine differentiation

Grade 1 and 2 are considered low-grade tumors.

Lymphovascular Invasion

Lymphatic space invasion requires the presence of tumor cells within endothelial-lined channels without significant red blood cells (Fig. 12.6A). Venous invasion is defined by the presence of tumor emboli within endothelial-lined channels surrounded by smooth muscle. There is a significant interobserver variability in assessing lymphovascular invasion. Lymphatic invasion should be distinguished from retraction artifact and micropapillary differentiation. Additional serial levels or ancillary stains such as D2-40 (Fig. 12.6B) and Movat stain may be used to confirm lymphovascular space invasion. Extramural venous invasion (tumor emboli within veins beyond the muscle layer), characterized by the "orphan artery sign" and "protruding tongue sign," represent a poor prognostic factor.

Margin Status

Cancer at or near the margin of resection is associated with an adverse outcome. The status of margin can only be assessed in intact polypectomy specimens. The resection margin is the actual free edge of submucosal connective tissue showing thermal artifact (see Fig. 12.5B, *black arrow*). There is no consensus as to the definition of what constitutes a positive margin of resection. The National Comprehensive Cancer Network 2018 Colon Cancer Guidelines define positive margin as follows: (1) tumor less than 1 mm from the transected margin, (2) tumor less than 2 mm from the transected margin, and (3) tumor cells present within the diathermy of the transected margin. It is therefore recommended that when the tumor is very close but not at the transected margin, the exact distance of the tumor from the cauterized margin be included in the report.

When invasive adenocarcinoma is present at or near the margin of resection (≤1 mm), the risk of relapse is between 21% and 33%. However, studies have shown that even in cases with "doubtfully complete" resections, the clinical outcome is favorable. This is because of the assumption that diathermy coagulation destroys

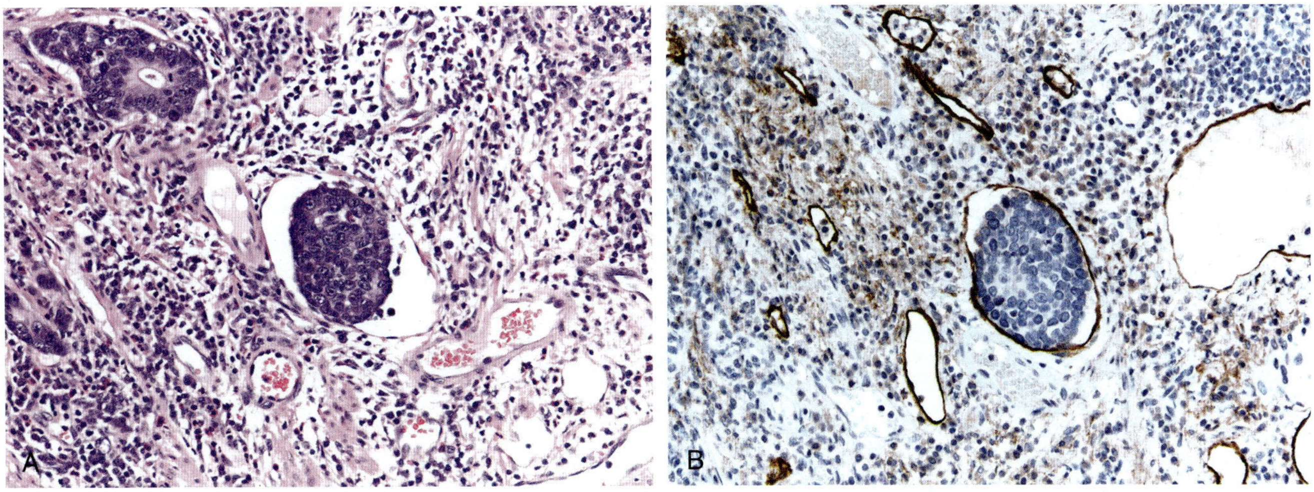

FIGURE 12.6

Lymphovascular invasion in a malignant colon polyp. **A**, Tumor cells within lymphatic space admixed with inflammatory cells. **B**, A D2-40 immunohistochemical stain highlights the lymphatic spaces and can be helpful in differentiating lymphatic invasion from retraction artifact.

an additional 3 to 5 mm of submucosal tissue beyond what is visualized by microscopy. Occasionally, the specimen orientation and processing make it difficult, if not impossible, to accurately assess the resection margin. In these cases, the report should clearly state the limitations of histologic assessment and encourage the clinician to assess completeness of excision by correlating with in vivo endoscopic findings of resection.

Tumor Budding

Tumor budding is considered as an independent adverse prognostic factor in CRC. It is associated with a higher TNM (tumor, node, metastasis) stage, high tumor grade, and presence of lymphovascular invasion and therefore, ultimately, with lymph node and distant metastasis. In malignant polyps, the presence of high tumor budding is associated with an increased risk of lymph node metastasis. Therefore, it has been suggested that the finding of high tumor budding may be an indication for surgical resection. A recent International Tumor Budding Consensus Conference (ITBCC) defined tumor budding as a single tumor cell or a cluster of up to four tumor cells (see section on tumor budding later). This finding is variably reported by pathologists.

Level or Depth of Invasion of Adenocarcinoma in a Polyp

It is not a routine practice to report depth of invasion in malignant polypectomy specimens. The Haggitt system is advocated for assessing depth of invasion in pedunculated malignant polyps. Per the Haggitt system for pedunculated malignant polyps, level 1 is defined as invasion into the polyp head, level 2 is invasion into the polyp neck, level 3 is carcinoma invading any part of polyp stalk, and level 4 is invasion beyond the stalk but above the muscularis propria. Specimen orientation, tissue shrinkage after fixation, interobserver disagreement between level 1 and level 2 invasion, and lack of muscularis propria in these specimens are some of the inherent issues that make it difficult to apply this system in routine practice. Therefore, many practices do not report Haggitt levels on pedunculated polyps.

The Kudo or Kikuchi method is used for assessing depth of invasion in sessile malignant colorectal polyps. Histologic assessment is performed by creating an imaginary division of the submucosal region into thirds (sm1, sm2, and sm3) and then determining the depth of invasion. However, accurate division of the submucosal space requires the presence of muscularis propria, and therefore this classification is most commonly employed only in transanal endoscopy microsurgery resections, which usually sample superficial layer of muscularis propria. Studies have shown that the incidence of lymph node metastasis increases from 1% to 3% in sm1 cancers to 8% and 23% in sm2 and sm3 cancers, respectively. Newer studies suggest that submucosal invasion greater than 1 mm represents an adverse prognostic factor and needs to be reported.

Invasive Adenocarcinoma Versus Misplaced Epithelium (Pseudoinvasion)

Pseudoinvasion or misplaced epithelium is a common phenomenon that occurs in large pedunculated colorectal polyps. It is most commonly observed in polyps located within the sigmoid or rectosigmoid colon. Repeated mucosal trauma related to the size of the polyp results in mechanical displacement of the adenomatous epithelium into deep lamina propria or submucosa of the polyp, mimicking invasive adenocarcinoma. Some features that can be helpful in identifying misplaced epithelium are listed in Table 12.2. Misplaced glands

TABLE 12.2

Pseudoinvasion (Misplaced Epithelium) versus Invasive Adenocarcinoma (Malignant Polyp)

Pseudoinvasion or Misplaced Epithelium	Invasive Adenocarcinoma in a Polyp
Rounded glandular contours	Infiltrative, angulated glands of variable size
Dysplastic glands invested by lamina propria	Dysplastic glands surrounded by stromal desmoplasia
Acellular mucin pools or mucin pools lined by attenuated epithelium	Clusters of dysplastic cells within mucin pools
Hemorrhage or hemosiderin-laden macrophages surrounding the dysplastic glands	Hemorrhage or hemosiderin-laden macrophages may be present
Degree of dysplasia usually resembles the overlying dysplastic epithelium	Degree of dysplasia usually exceeds that of the overlying dysplastic epithelium

are always accompanied by the surrounding lamina propria. In contrast, invasive adenocarcinoma is diagnosed in the presence of stromal desmoplastic response that surrounds the neoplastic glands. Misplaced glands retain their lobular arrangement, are often surrounded by hemorrhage or hemosiderin (related to trauma), and harbor the same degree of dysplasia as compared with the overlying dysplastic epithelium (Figs. 12.7 and 12.8). In some instances, misplaced epithelium may be associated with cystically dilated dysplastic glands, which may rupture and present as pools of acellular mucin within the stalk of the polyp. In these cases, the adenomatous epithelium may be seen partially lining the mucin pools. In contrast, the presence of free-floating clusters of dysplastic glands within the center of mucin pools is an ominous finding and indicates the presence of mucinous adenocarcinoma (Fig. 12.9).

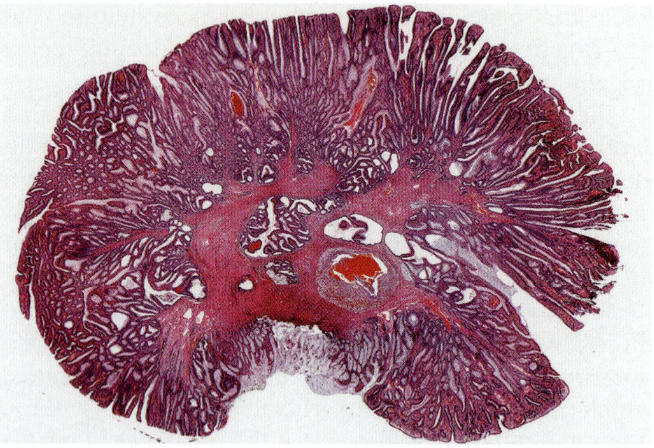

FIGURE 12.7

Polyp with pseudoinvasion or misplaced epithelium. A sigmoid colon polyp showing tubulovillous adenoma with aggregates of dysplastic glands within the stalk of the polyp.

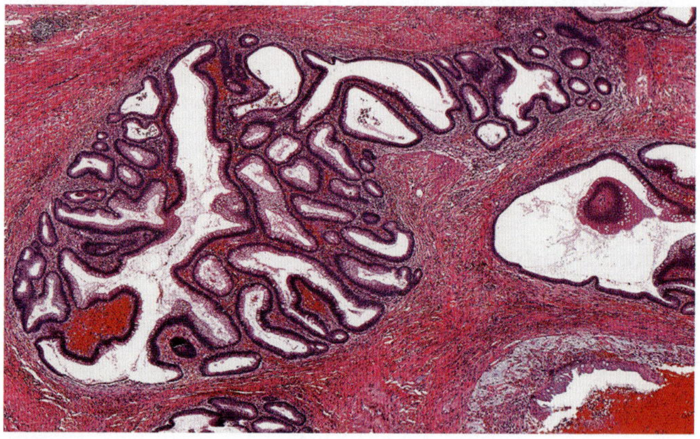

FIGURE 12.8

Polyp with pseudoinvasion or misplaced epithelium. Higher magnification shows that the glands maintain a rounded configuration and are surrounded by lamina propria and hemosiderin-laden histiocytes. Hemorrhage and mucin pools partially lined by epithelium are also present (lower right corner).

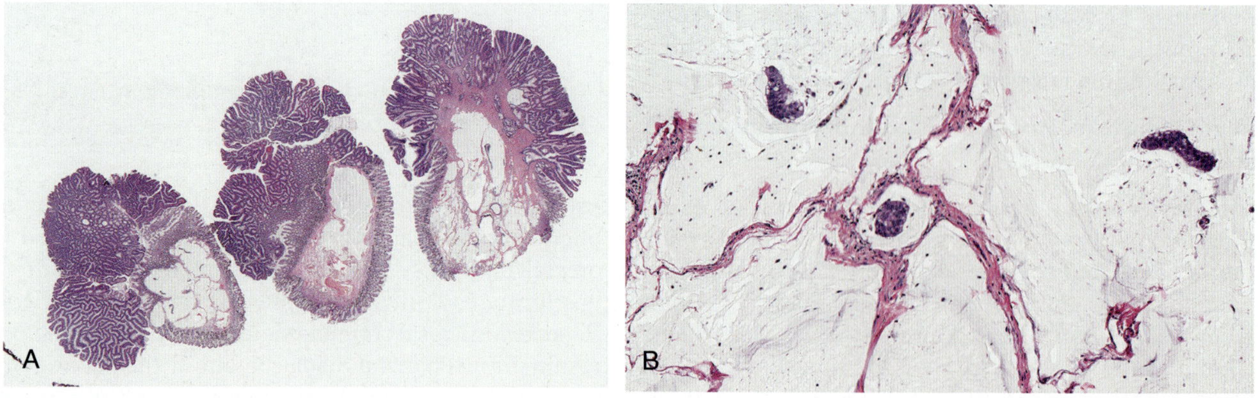

FIGURE 12.9

Invasive mucinous adenocarcinoma in a polyp. The trisected pedunculated polyp shows a tubulovillous adenoma with pools of mucin within the stalk of the polyp (**A**). In one of the three fragments (far right), the mucinous pools reach the cauterized base of excision. Higher magnification shows that these dissecting pools of mucin contain free-floating clusters of dysplastic cells, consistent with an invasive mucinous adenocarcinoma (**B**).

SERRATED POLYPS

Serrated colorectal polyps are characterized histologically by serrated appearance of the crypts. The current World Health Organization (WHO) edition classifies these polyps as

1. HP
2. Sessile serrated polyp/adenoma (SSP/A; also referred as sessile serrated lesion in the latest WHO edition)
3. Traditional serrated adenoma (TSA)

HYPERPLASTIC POLYPS

CLINICAL FEATURES

Hyperplastic polyps are the most commonly encountered polyps in the adult colorectum. They are found with increasing frequency in individuals older than 40 years of age and are more common in men than in women. HPs develop nearly a decade earlier than conventional adenomas and affect patients in the fifth and sixth decades of life but do not show a significant association with increasing age. They have an estimated prevalence of 10% to 15% among adult patients in Western populations and constitute approximately one-fourth of all endoscopically removed polyps but 80% to 90% of all serrated polyps. Because of their small size, HPs are asymptomatic and often detected incidentally at sigmoidoscopy or colonoscopy.

HYPERPLASTIC POLYPS—FACT SHEET

Definition
- Nondysplastic serrated polyp with low malignant potential

Incidence And Location
- Most common neoplastic polyp
- 10% to 20% of asymptomatic patients

Morbidity And Mortality
- Risk for neoplasia related to size and number

Gender, Race, And Age Distribution
- Usually affects individuals in fifth or sixth decade of life
- Incidence does not increase with age
- Male more than female
- No racial or ethnic associations

Clinical Features
- Asymptomatic
- Incidental finding at endoscopy

Prognosis And Therapy
- Polypectomy

PATHOLOGIC FEATURES

GROSS FINDINGS

Grossly, HPs are dome-shaped nodules that are usually smaller than 5 mm in diameter. They are often multiple and are most frequently found in the sigmoid colon and rectum. HPs are most commonly found on the crest of mucosal folds and are similar in color to the surrounding normal mucosa.

MICROSCOPIC FINDINGS

Hyperplastic polyps contain serrated colonic crypts lined by goblet and absorptive cells. The crypt serrations are usually restricted to the upper half or two-thirds of the crypt epithelium, resulting in the characteristic "saw-toothed" or serrated appearance (Fig. 12.10). The basal aspect of the crypts is normal. The number of absorptive cells lining the crypts is greater than the number of goblet cells. Mitoses are common but are confined to the bottom half of crypts (proliferative zone of the crypt). The basement membrane is often thickened, and this finding is best appreciated at the polyp surface (Fig. 12.11). The epithelial cells typically show basally located small and hyperchromatic nuclei with only slight enlargement. Scattered Paneth or endocrine cells may also be seen within the crypt bases. Larger HPs often show changes of mucosal prolapse. This is characterized by splaying of the muscularis mucosae fibers at the crypt bases, with extension of the smooth muscle fibers into the lamina propria and around individual crypts (Fig. 12.12). This often results in dilation of the crypt bases and can cause diagnostic confusion with SSP/A.

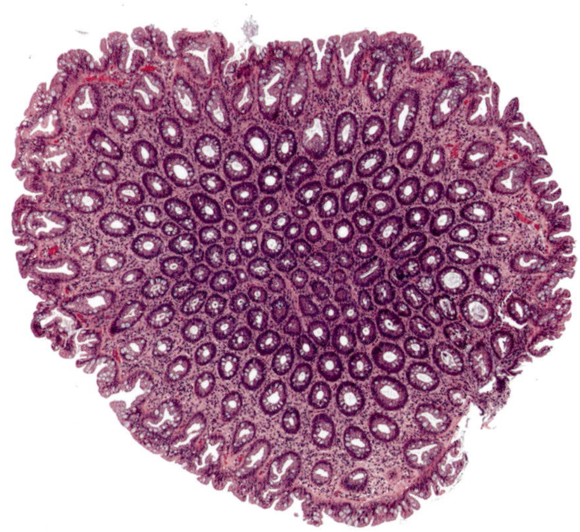

FIGURE 12.10

Hyperplastic polyp. A 0.5 mm diminutive polyp located in the sigmoid colon showing serrated crypts. The crypt serrations are restricted to the upper half to upper two-thirds of the crypt.

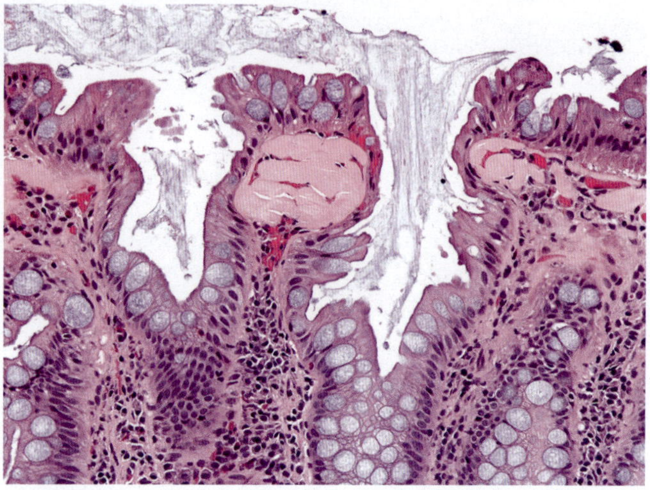

FIGURE 12.11

Hyperplastic polyp with thickened basement membrane. Hyperplastic polyp often shows variable thickening of the basement membrane. This finding is more commonly seen toward the surface of the polyp.

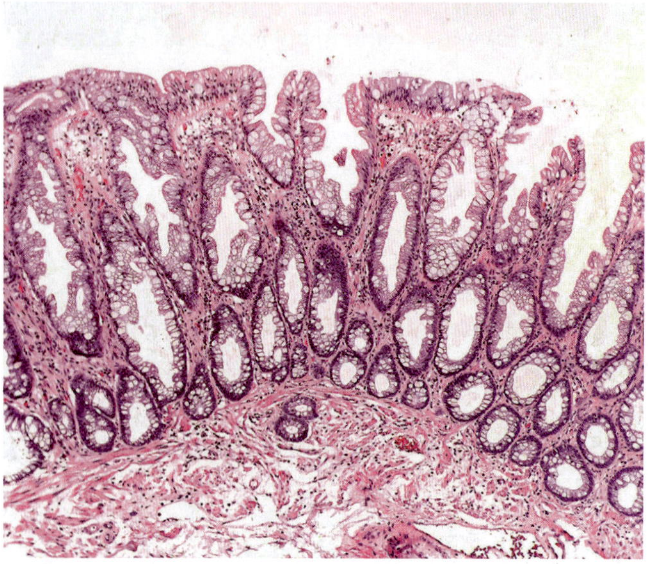

FIGURE 12.12

Hyperplastic polyp with prolapse changes. The image shows a hyperplastic polyp with basal dilation of some of the serrated crypts, mimicking a sessile serrated polyp/adenoma. However, the lamina propria shows splaying of the muscularis mucosae along with extension of the smooth muscle fibers into the lamina propria and around individual crypts, consistent with prolapse.

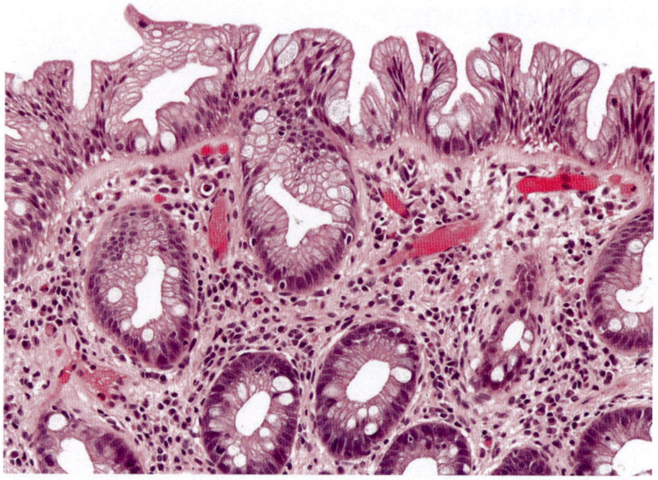

FIGURE 12.13

Microvesicular type hyperplastic polyp (HP). This variant of HP shows microvesicular mucin within the cytoplasm of the cells lining the serrated crypts. Goblet cells are interspersed between these cells.

Hyperplastic Polyps—Pathologic Features

Gross Findings

- Small (diminutive) sessile polyp (<5 mm)
- Rectosigmoid colon most common location

Microscopic Findings

- Crypt elongation with serrated crypt epithelium
- Crypt serrations are restricted to the upper third or two-thirds of the crypt epithelium
- Well-differentiated goblet and absorptive cells
- Mitoses restricted to crypt bases

Differential Diagnosis

- Mucosal prolapse polyp with hyperplastic epithelial changes
- Inflammatory polyp with hyperplastic epithelial changes
- Tubular adenoma

Hyperplastic polyps are composed of three histologic subtypes: microvesicular type, goblet cell–rich type, and mucin-depleted type. Microvesicular type HPs are the most common subtype and are characterized by microvesicular mucin with few goblet cells, including some dystrophic goblet cells (Fig. 12.13). Goblet cell–rich HPs show prominent goblet cells and subtle serrations of the crypts (Fig. 12.14). Mucin-depleted HPs are the least common subtype of HP and show reactive epithelial mucin loss with minimal cytoplasm (Fig. 12.15). Currently, there is no evidence to support subtyping HPs for prognostic purposes.

Differential Diagnosis

Other lesions with serrated epithelial features can mimic HP, including inflammatory cloacogenic polyps or polypoid mucosal prolapse, which often show prominent serrations of the crypt and surface epithelium. Features that are helpful in distinguishing mucosal prolapse or inflammatory cloacogenic polyps from HPs include the polyp location at the anal verge, presence of smooth muscle ingrowth between the dilated colonic crypts, and lamina propria hemorrhage and fibrosis (Fig. 12.16). In some instances, HPs may show reactive mucin loss, especially, the mucin-depleted variant. These lesions can mimic tubular adenoma. However, presence of surface

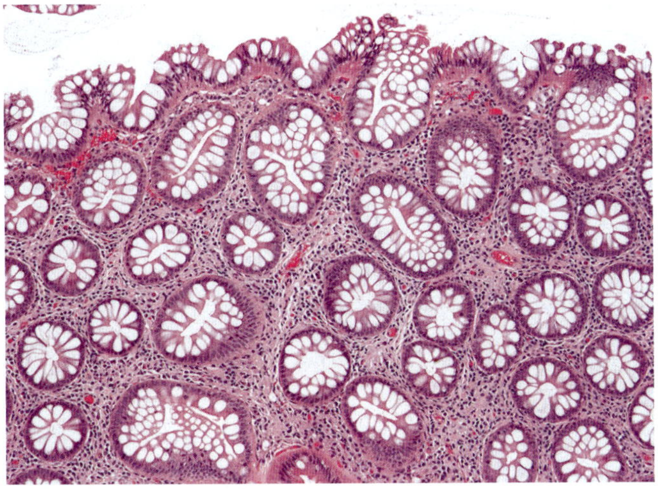

FIGURE 12.14

Goblet cell–rich hyperplastic polyp (HP). This variant of HP shows numerous goblet cells with subtle serrations within the crypts.

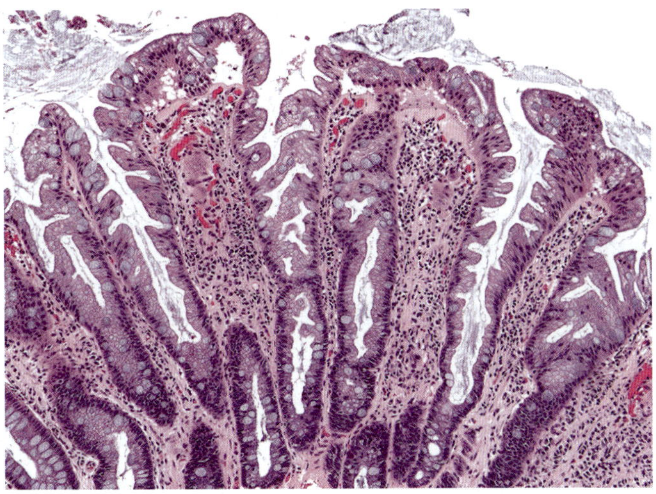

FIGURE 12.15

Mucin-depleted hyperplastic polyp. In this morphologic variant, the serrated epithelium lining the crypts is composed of cells with minimal intracytoplasmic mucin and rare goblet cells. Mild nuclear atypia is present. The epithelial changes are reminiscent of regenerative changes after mucosal injury.

epithelial maturation in HPs and lack of significant cytologic atypia help support a HP.

Prognosis and Therapy

Because they may be endoscopically similar in appearance to small adenomatous polyps, HPs are often removed by polypectomy solely to distinguish them on histologic grounds from adenomatous polyps. Based on the American College of Gastroenterology recommendations, surveillance for HPs ranges from 5 to 10 years and depends on the size, number, and location of the polyps (Table 12.3).

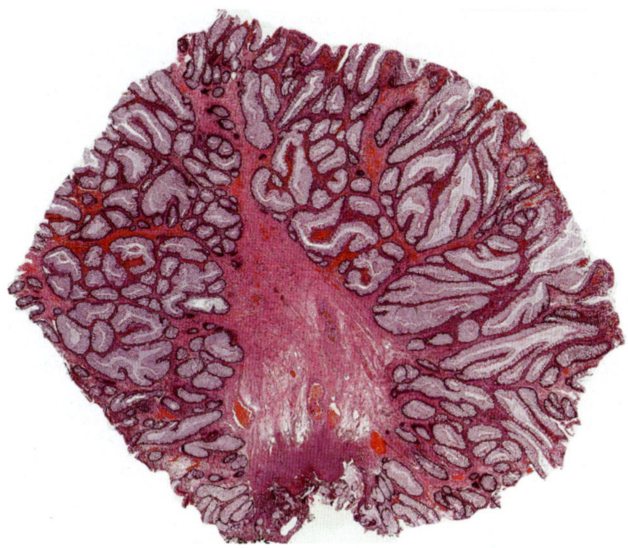

FIGURE 12.16

Polypoid mucosal prolapse. An example of a rectal polyp showing dilation and branching of the crypts. The crypts also show serrated architecture and are lined by cells with abundant mucinous cytoplasm. These findings can mimic a serrated polyp. However, there is fibromuscular replacement of the lamina propria along with extension of smooth muscle fibers alongside distorted crypts.

TABLE 12.3

Surveillance Guidelines for Serrated Polyps: Expert Panel Recommendations

Type of Polyp	Size	Number	Location	Interval (years)
HP	<10 mm	Any	Rectosigmoid colon	10
HP	≤5 mm	≤3	Proximal to sigmoid colon	10
HP	Any	≥4	Proximal to sigmoid colon	5
HP	>5 mm	≥1	Proximal to sigmoid colon	5
SSP/A or TSA	<10 mm	<3	Any	5
SSP/A or TSA	≥10 mm	1	Any	3
SSP/A or TSA	<10 mm	≥3	Any	3
SSP/A	≥10 mm	≥2	Any	1-3
SSP/A with dysplasia	Any	Any	Any	1-3

Adapted from Rex DK, Ahnen DJ, Baron JA, et al. Serrated lesions of the colorectum: review and recommendations from an expert panel. *Am J Gastroenterol.* 2012;107:1315-1329.

HP, Hyperplastic polyp; *SSP/A*, sessile serrated polyp/adenoma; *TSA*, traditional serrated adenoma.

SESSILE SERRATED POLYP/ADENOMA

CLINICAL FEATURES

Sessile serrated polyp/adenoma (also referred as sessile serrated lesion) constitute approximately 10 % of all serrated colorectal polyps. They are difficult to recognize endoscopically and therefore are often underreported. SSP/As are the precursor lesions that progress to colorectal carcinoma via the serrated pathway of carcinogenesis. Recognition of these lesions has largely stemmed from the observations that (1) patients with hyperplastic polyposis, a disorder characterized by numerous HPs, have an increased risk for colorectal neoplasia, and (2) sporadic right-sided HPs more commonly contain a variety of genetic alterations, including microsatellite instability (MSI) and increased gene methylation compared with their left-sided counterparts. Part of the reason for discrepancies in the literature is that these lesions have been called by a variety of names, including *serrated polyp with atypical proliferation, giant hyperplastic polyps, large hyperplastic polyps, mixed hyperplastic/adenomatous polyps, sessile serrated polyps, serrated adenomas*, and *inverted hyperplastic polyps.* Given the potential confusion with an adenomatous polyp, the 2017 British Society of Gastroenterology guidelines and the current WHO fifth edition recommend using the terminology sessile serrated lesions for SSA/Ps. The term has not been widely used. The most common age at diagnosis is in the sixth to seventh decade of life, similar to that for classic adenomatous polyps. Most patients are clinically asymptomatic, and the fecal occult test result is usually negative.

SESSILE SERRATED POLYP/ADENOMAS–FACT SHEET

Definition

- Epithelial neoplasms with distinctive serrated epithelial architecture and associated risk for colorectal neoplasia

Incidence And Location

- 10% of all serrated polyps encountered at endoscopy

Morbidity And Mortality

- Related to risk for progression to carcinoma
- 6% of colon cancers occur in association with a sessile serrated polyp/adenoma

Gender, Race, And Age Distribution

- Females more than males
- No known racial predominance
- Average age at diagnosis in seventh decade of life

Clinical Features

- Usually asymptomatic

Prognosis And Therapy

- Routine surveillance is indicated because of the risk for colorectal neoplasia

PATHOLOGIC FEATURES

GROSS FINDINGS

As their name indicates, SSP/As are generally sessile lesions. They can arise anywhere within the colorectum but are predominantly located in the proximal colon. They show a wide size range and may reach several centimeters in diameter, hence the former designation *giant hyperplastic polyps.* Most lesions resemble thickened mucosal folds with indiscrete borders that can be difficult to recognize endoscopically (Fig. 12.17). Adherent mucus or "mucin cap" is a frequent finding.

SESSILE SERRATED POLYP/ADENOMA–PATHOLOGIC FEATURES

Gross Findings

- Generally sessile
- Broad size range (millimeters to centimeters)
- Proximal distribution

Microscopic Findings

- Serrated crypts with serrations involving the entire length of the crypt
- Dilatation of crypt bases
- Horizontally arranged crypt bases with an L- or T- shaped configuration
- May have an inverted growth pattern
- Irregularly branching of crypts
- Individual cells show microvesicular cytoplasm
- May show prominent submucosal adipose tissue and perineurial-like stromal proliferation within the lamina propria
- Only one unequivocal abnormal shaped crypt is required to diagnose sessile serrated polyp/adenoma

Differential Diagnosis

- Hyperplastic polyp
- Traditional serrated adenoma
- Inflammatory polyp
- Polypoid mucosal prolapse

MICROSCOPIC FINDINGS

The two major morphologic features distinguish SSP/As from conventional HPs are architectural distortion and abnormal proliferation. Architectural features that are characteristic of SSP/As include crypt dilation, horizontal orientation of deep crypts, serrations extending to the crypt bases, and "boot-shaped", L- or inverted

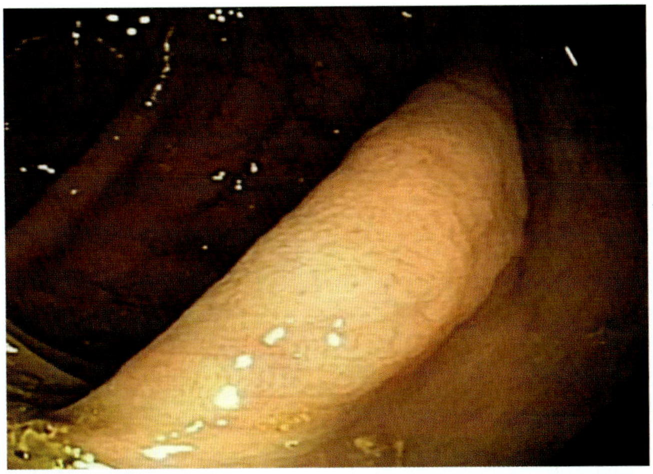

FIGURE 12.17

Endoscopic appearance of a sessile serrated polyp/adenoma. This ascending colon lesion consists of subtle thickening of the colonic mucosal fold with indiscrete borders. Saline-lift technique is often applied to delineate and resect sessile polyps.

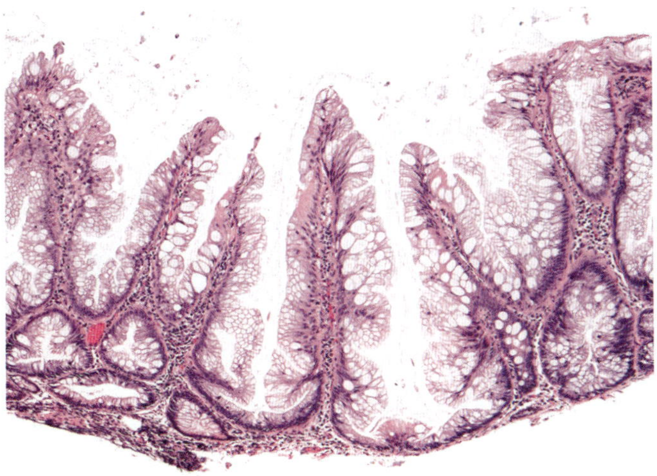

FIGURE 12.18

Sessile serrated polyp/adenoma (SSP/A). This 2-cm ascending colon polyp shows crypt dilation, horizontal orientation of deep crypts, and serrations extending to the crypt bases resulting in "boot-shaped" or "inverted T"–shaped crypts, characteristic of SSP/A.

T-shaped crypts (Fig. 12.18). Compared with conventional HPs in which atypia is confined to the crypt bases (proliferative zone of the crypt), in SSP/As, the proliferative zone of the crypt shifts to the midportion of the crypts. This results in epithelial proliferation toward the lumen as well as the crypts. As the neoplastic proliferation extends to the basal aspects of the crypts, the muscularis mucosae restricts further downward proliferation, and therefore, the crypts start proliferating laterally, resulting in dilation and branching as well as lateral extensions of the crypts. The basement membrane of the surface epithelial cells is not thickened. The serrated crypts show decreased to near-complete absence of neuroendocrine cells. The serrated crypts are lined by cells

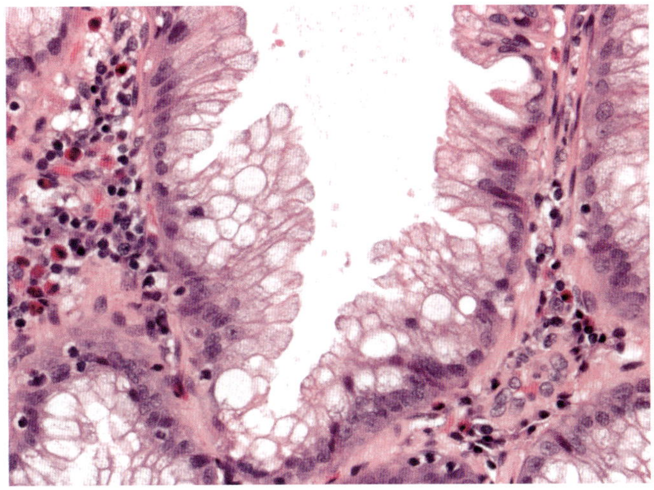

FIGURE 12.19

Sessile serrated polyp/adenoma (SSP/A). Higher magnification of the serrated crypts in a SSP/A shows that the individual cells harbor microvesicular mucin.

with distinct microvesicular mucin interspersed with goblet cells (Fig. 12.19). Dystrophic goblet cells are also common. Regardless of the size or location of the polyp, the presence of at least one unequivocal, architecturally distorted, dilated, or horizontally branched crypt is sufficient for a diagnosis of SSP/A.

Another unique histologic finding that may be seen in SSP/As is a bland spindle cell proliferation that surrounds the serrated crypts (Fig. 12.20). Studies have shown that these cells are of perineural origin, and these polyps harbor *BRAF* mutations similar to other serrated polyps and have no clinical significance with regards to neoplastic progression. An epithelial membrane antigen (EMA) immunohistochemical stain can be performed to highlight these cells. SSP/As can also show prominent submucosal adipose tissue that can be clinically mistaken for a lipoma (Fig. 12.21).

Sessile serrated polyps/adenomas may harbor foci of low- or high-grade dysplasia. In one large study, the incidence of dysplasia in SSP/As was reported to be 5%. These cases were previously diagnosed as mixed hyperplastic/adenomatous polyps. Although in most instances, the type of dysplasia resembles conventional adenomatous dysplasia (tubular or tubulovillous adenoma) characterized by nuclear enlargement, hyperchromasia, and pseudostratified nuclei, other morphologic variants of dysplasia, such as serrated and traditional serrated adenoma–like dysplasia have also been described. To diagnose dysplasia in an SSP/A, the dysplastic focus should be seen in continuity with the nondysplastic areas (Fig. 12.22). Because of the high interobserver variability, the current WHO edition does not specifically indicate classifying the grade of dysplasia in these lesions. However, most practices report the degree of dysplasia as either low- or high-grade dysplasia.

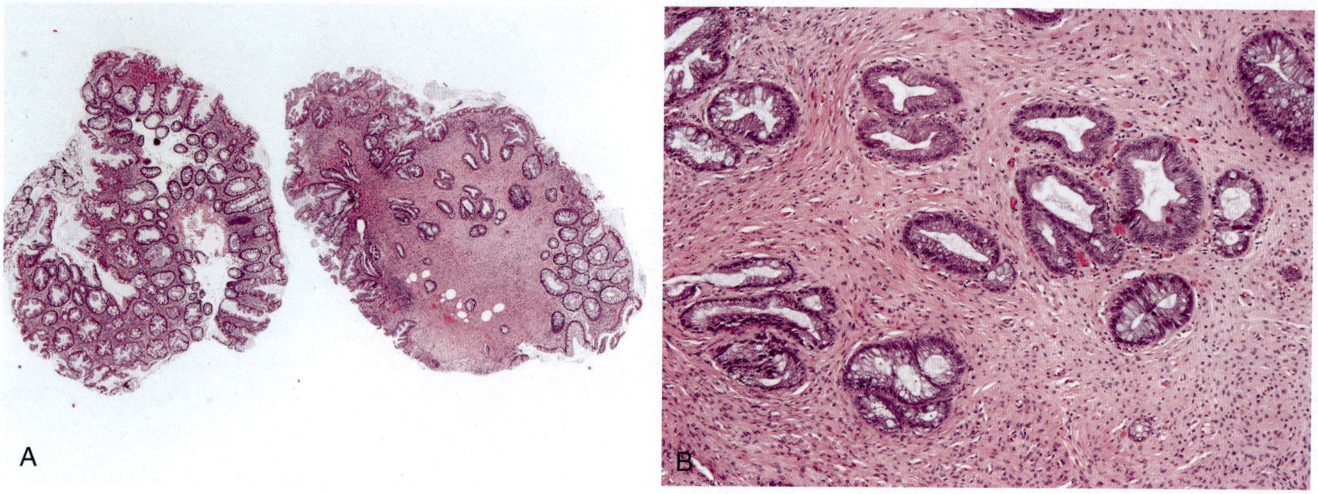

FIGURE 12.20

Sessile serrated polyp/adenoma (SSP/A) with perineurial-like stromal proliferation. A transverse colon sessile SSP/A showing two biopsy fragments (**A**). The fragment on the right shows expansion of the lamina propria by a bland spindle cell proliferation surrounding the crypts. This proliferation is a reactive process seen in serrated polyps. Higher magnification shows that the cells lack atypia or mitotic activity (**B**). Immunohistochemically, the cells express epithelial membrane antigen, a marker of perineurial differentiation.

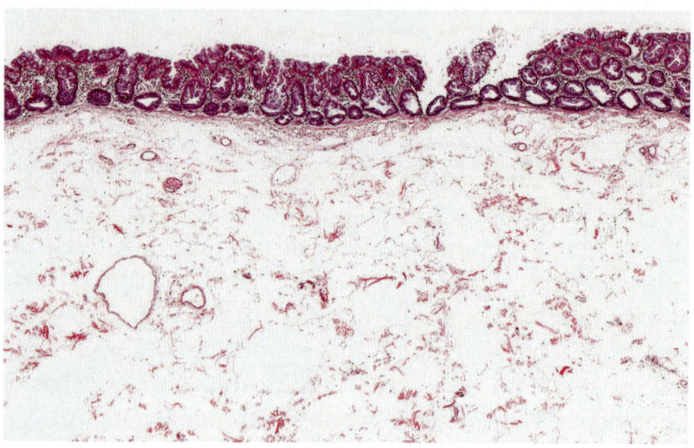

FIGURE 12.21

Sessile serrated polyp/adenoma (SSP/A) with prominent submucosal adipose tissue. An example of a cecal polypoid lesion that was clinically diagnosed as "lipoma." The image shows a SSP/A overlying submucosal adipose tissue, a finding that is frequently seen in large right-sided serrated polyps.

Ancillary Studies And Molecular Alterations

Because none of the markers have demonstrated appropriate sensitivity to discriminate small SSP/A from HPs, immunohistochemical labeling does not have a routine role in the diagnosis of SSP/As. Some markers, including MUC6, annexin A10, and MUC5AC, have been reported to be markers of SSP/As; however, these markers have not been validated by independent studies.

More recently, it was shown that some SSP/As show loss of hMLH1 protein expression, consistent with the increased rate of methylation-induced silencing of *MLH1* tumor suppressor genes with neoplastic progression. In about 70% of cases, loss of hMLH1 expression occurs in the setting of cytologic dysplasia.

The majority of SSP/As harbor a somatic *BRAF* mutation and show CpG island methylator phenotype.

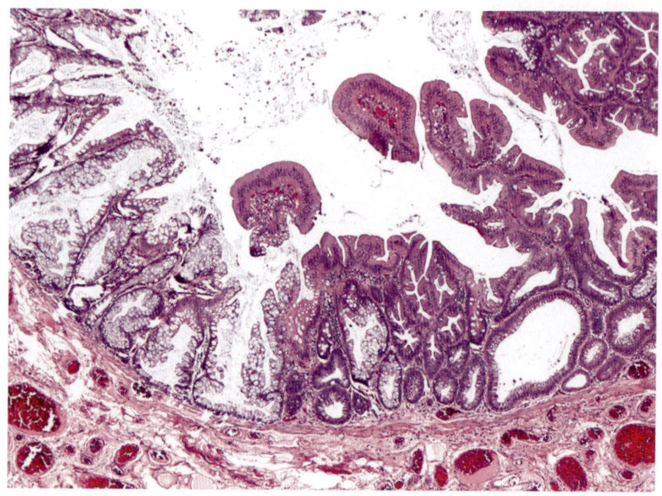

FIGURE 12.22

Sessile serrated polyp/adenoma (epithelial membrane antigen) with low-grade dysplasia. An example of a SSP/A that shows atypical glands lined by cells with enlarged, hyperchromatic, and stratified nuclei, consistent with low-grade dysplasia. The dysplastic foci are seen in continuity with the non-dysplastic SSP/A (left half of the image). In most cases, the dysplastic foci resemble conventional adenomatous polyps. In this case, there is cytoplasmic eosinophilia, resulting in a traditional serrated adenoma–like appearance.

As mentioned earlier, transition to dysplasia corresponds to methylation-induced silencing of tumor suppressor genes, of which *MLH1* is the most commonly gene.

Differential Diagnosis

Several interobserver agreement studies have highlighted the challenges in distinguishing SSP/As from HPs, especially when these polyps are smaller than 1 cm in size. The presence of abnormal crypt architecture and lack of thickened basement membrane are helpful in distinguishing SSP/A from HP. Mucosal prolapse in large HPs can lead to diagnostic confusion (see Fig. 12.12) and mimic SSP/A. Recognizing the features of prolapse, such as dilation of crypts, fibromuscular replacement of lamina propria, and vascular congestion, can be helpful to separate SSP/A from a large HP with prolapse.

Although traditional serrated adenoma is one of the subtypes of serrated polyps, the left-sided location, villiform growth pattern, distinct eosinophilic cytoplasm, and ectopic crypt formation are all helpful in distinguishing TSA from SSP/A.

Last, inflammatory polyps or polypoid mucosal prolapse can show serrated epithelial changes in some of the crypts (see Fig. 12.16), especially toward the surface of the polyp. However, the pedunculated nature of these lesions, an edematous and inflamed stroma, fibromuscular replacement of lamina propria in polypoid mucosal prolapse, and lack of the characteristic crypt architectural changes of an SSP/A are helpful in this distinction.

Prognosis and Therapy

Distinguishing SSP/A from HP is of clinical importance because SSP/As are associated with an increased risk for colorectal neoplasia, but HPs are not. The absolute risk for neoplastic transformation in an SSP/A remains unclear. However, an association is recognized between CRCs and serrated polyps, with up to 25% of CRCs found in association with the serrated neoplasia pathway (see details later). The surveillance guidelines for SSP/As are outlined in Table 12.3.

Patients with SSP/As are at an increased risk for development of adenomatous and metachronous serrated polyps. Studies have also shown that patients with SSP/As and synchronous high-risk adenomas (adenomas ≥1 cm in size, villous architecture, and high-grade dysplasia) are at an increased risk of developing metachronous high-risk adenomas, independent of the size of the lesion.

TRADITIONAL SERRATED ADENOMAS

Clinical Features

Traditional serrated adenomas are a subset of serrated colorectal polyps characterized histologically by the presence of a villiform growth pattern, ectopic crypt foci and tall columnar cells with distinct eosinophilic cytoplasm and minimal pseudostratification. TSAs are less prevalent than SSP/As, comprising approximately 2% to 5% of all serrated polyps and fewer than 1% of all colorectal polyps. The average age at diagnosis is during the seventh decade of life. They are slightly more common in men, and there is no racial predominance.

TRADITIONAL SERRATED ADENOMAS—FACT SHEET

Definition

- Epithelial neoplasms with serrated crypts, slitlike spaces; villiform growth pattern; ectopic crypt foci; and tall columnar cells with prominent eosinophilic cytoplasm and minimally pseudostratified nuclei
- Associated with an increased risk for colorectal neoplasia

Incidence And Location

- Approximately 2% to 5% of serrated polyps and fewer than 1% of all colorectal polyps

Morbidity And Mortality

- Actual risk for progression to carcinoma unknown

Gender, Race, And Age Distribution

- Slight male predominance
- No known racial predominance
- Average age at diagnosis is seventh decade of life

Clinical Features

- Usually asymptomatic
- Symptoms related to larger polyp size
- Associated with sporadic microsatellite instability

Prognosis And Therapy

- Routine surveillance (1–3 years depending on the size and number of polyps) because they have an increased risk for colorectal neoplasia

Pathologic Features

Gross Findings

Traditional serrated adenomas most commonly arise in the left colon. Their gross appearance is that of a polypoid growth that may or may not have villiform features. The lesions range in size from 0.5 to 2 cm in diameter. In some instances, TSAs may present as sessile lesions. These are usually located within the proximal colon. Grossly, small TSAs are indistinguishable from conventional HPs, and large TSAs may be difficult to distinguish from a classic adenomatous polyp.

Microscopic Findings

Traditional serrated adenomas show a complex polypoid or villiform growth pattern composed of glands with serrated architecture. They often harbor slitlike spaces within the proliferation. In many cases, the villi are elongated and may show bulbous tips (filiform TSAs). A characteristic feature of TSAs is the finding of ectopic crypt foci, which are proliferative crypts located perpendicular to the long axis of the villous structures (Fig. 12.23). The individual cells show prominent eosinophilic cytoplasm, basally located slightly elongated nuclei, and open chromatin pattern. There is minimal nuclear

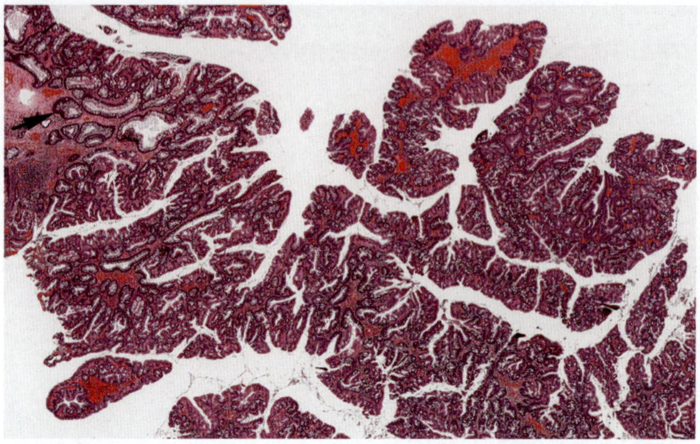

FIGURE 12.23

Traditional serrated adenoma. A rectosigmoid polyp showing polypoid or villiform growth pattern with slit-like spaces composed of glands with serrated crypts. The *arrow* highlights the native colonic crypts. Even at this magnification, the lesion is characterized by cytoplasmic eosinophilia.

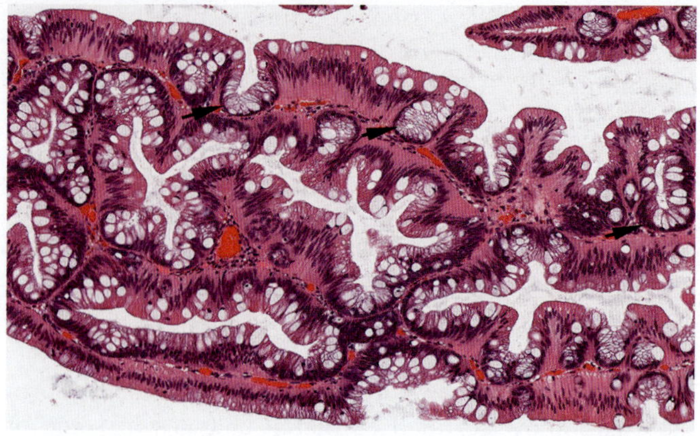

FIGURE 12.24

Traditional serrated adenoma. Higher magnification of traditional serrated adenoma showing prominent cytoplasmic eosinophilia, ectopic crypts *(black arrows)* and minimal nuclear atypia and pseudostratification. Mitotic activity and apoptotic activity is rare.

pseudostratification without significant mitotic or apoptotic activity (Fig. 12.24). Some examples may show an abundance of goblet cells. Up to 50% of TSAs may show a nondysplastic serrated precursor, either an HP or SSP/A in the background. A subset of TSAs may develop conventional adenomatous dysplasia (low or high grade). These foci resemble tubular or tubulovillous adenomas.

Molecular Alterations

At a molecular level, TSAs are far more diverse compared to SSP/As. They may either have *BRAF* or *KRAS* mutations and low or high levels of CpG island methylation. They do not show *MLH1* methylation or develop MSI. However, most cases show *MGMT* promoter methylation.

Traditional Serrated Adenomas—Pathologic Features

Gross Findings

- Polypoid or villiform growth; rarely sessile lesions
- Size ranges up to 2 cm
- Common in left colon

Microscopic Findings

- Villiform or polypoid growth
- Ectopic crypt foci
- Slitlike spaces
- Eosinophilic cytoplasm
- Minimal nuclear pseudostratification; rare mitotic or apoptotic activity
- May harbor foci of conventional low- or high-grade adenomatous dysplasia

Differential Diagnosis

- Sessile serrated polyp/adenoma
- Tubular or tubulovillous adenoma with serrated crypt architecture

Differential Diagnosis

The main entities in the differential diagnosis of a TSA are SSP/A and conventional tubular or tubulovillous adenomas. SSP/As can be recognized by their sessile growth pattern and the presence of crypt dilation, horizontal orientation of deep crypts, serrations of crypt epithelium extending to the crypt bases, and inverted crypts. SSP/As are also more commonly located in the right colon. Occasionally, large tubular or tubulovillous adenomas may harbor serrated crypts, raising the possibility of a TSA with conventional dysplasia. While there are no guidelines regarding the nomenclature for these large adenomatous polyps with serrated crypts, in most practices, if the predominant portion of the lesion is composed of a conventional tubular or tubulovillous adenoma, these lesions are designated as tubular or tubulovillous adenomas with serrated crypt architecture or with TSA-like areas. Regardless, in these cases, the lesions are clinically managed as conventional adenomatous polyps.

Prognosis and Therapy

The absolute risk for neoplastic transformation in a TSA is unknown. The AGA guidelines recommend routine surveillance at an interval of 1 to 3 years depending on the size and the number of polyps (see Table 12.3). In a large case-control study from Korea that consisted of 420 patients with TSA, it was shown that in comparison with patients with conventional adenomatous polyps, patients with TSAs have a higher metachronous occurrence rate of all polyp subtypes (adenomas, SSP/As, and HPs), and the presence of TSA was found to be an independent predictor of a high-risk polyp recurrence.

SERRATED POLYPOSIS SYNDROME

Serrated polyposis syndrome (SPS) (formerly "hyperplastic polyposis syndrome") is characterized by multiple serrated colorectal polyps (typically SSP/As and/or HPs) and is associated with a more than 50% cumulative risk for developing CRC. Because a definite genetic basis for SPS has not been established and patients cases do not have a family history of SPS or even CRC, endoscopic and histologic findings remain essential in establishing a diagnosis of SPS. Mutations in *MUTYH* have been documented in some patients with SPS, and therefore it has been suggested that genetic testing for *MUTYH* mutations may be performed in patients with SPS, especially if the patients is found to have concurrent adenomas. Another study proposed germline mutations in oncogene-induced senescence pathways as a predisposing factor.

The updated WHO criteria for SPS include (1) at least five serrated polyps proximal to the rectum, all at least 5 mm in size, with at least two more 10 mm or larger or 2) more than 20 serrated polyps of any size detected throughout the colon, with at least five being proximal to the rectum. All serrated polyp types—HP, SSP/A, and TSA—are included in the polyp counts when making this diagnosis. It is also important to remember that the counts can be cumulative over multiple examinations and do not have to be fulfilled at a single colonoscopy. In screening populations, prevalence rates of up to 1 in 127 have been reported. SPS is reported to occur more commonly in individuals with northern European ancestry and shows a positive correlation with smoking, specifically with regard to the number of serrated polyps. SPS occurs both in male and female patients with age at diagnosis ranging widely from 17 to 69 years (mean, 48 years).

It has been suggested that there are three phenotypes of SPS: (1) large SSP/As in the proximal colon with a high risk of CRC, (2) numerous small HPs throughout the colorectum with a lower risk of CRC, and (3) many small left-sided serrated polyps. In addition to serrated polyps, up to 80% of patients may show a concurrent conventional adenoma, which confers an increased risk for CRC. At present, patients diagnosed with SPS are subjected to colonoscopic surveillance every 1 to 3 years with attempted removal of all polyps larger than 5 mm in diameter. Indications for surgery include an inability to control the growth of serrated polyps or the development of cancer.

COLORECTAL ADENOCARCINOMA

Clinical Features

Colorectal carcinoma is among the most common neoplasms affecting industrialized nations. It is the fourth most frequently diagnosed cancer in the United States among both men and women, with an estimated 135,430 new cases of CRC diagnosed in the United States in 2017. Colorectal carcinoma is also the third most common cause of cancer deaths in the United States among men and women, with an estimated 50,260 patients dying of colorectal carcinoma in the year 2017.

The lifetime risk for developing CRC is approximately 6% and is greater for men than women. It is more common in individuals of African American descent. The risk for development of CRC increases significantly after the age of 40 years in both men and women, with the median age of diagnosis being 67 years. In contrast to the decreasing incidence rate among screening-aged individuals, CRC incidence rates in adults younger than 50 years rose by 1.6% from 2000 to 2013, for an overall increase of 22%. The cause of this increase is yet to be elucidated; however, factors such as excess body weight, unhealthy dietary patterns, and sedentary lifestyle have been implicated. CRC risk also varies by location within the colorectum. In low-risk countries, right-sided cancers are more common, whereas in high-risk countries, left-sided cancers are common. These statistics largely reflect the incidence of colon cancer because the incidence of rectal cancer is fairly constant among high- and low-risk countries. Right-sided cancers are more common in women, and the incidence increases with age.

The cause of CRC is multifactorial, with environment and inheritance playing variable roles. Approximately 70% to 80% of patients with CRC have sporadic disease; in the remaining 20% to 30% of patients, an inherited component, which may be identified, especially in patients younger than 50 years. The estimated time for development of an infiltrating carcinoma from a small adenoma is approximately 10 to 15 years. Thus, most patients do not have specific clinical symptoms to alert the clinician to the presence of a lesion. Initial symptoms may be vague and nonspecific, such as weight loss or malaise, whereas up to 12% of patients are entirely asymptomatic at the time of diagnosis. Of patients who are symptomatic, clinical presentation may be related to location of the carcinoma within the colorectum. Because the proximal bowel can accommodate large, bulky tumors, cancers of the cecum and right colon are often polypoid, may remain clinically silent, and rarely cause obstruction or bleeding. In contrast, left colon cancers may present with changes in bowel habits such as diarrhea, tenesmus, incontinence, or a decrease in stool caliber as the carcinoma grows and obstructs the lumen. Regardless of location, half of all patients present with rectal bleeding, which may be the result of frank hemorrhage or occult bleeding. Abdominal pain may be a presenting symptom in up to 50% of patients and appears to be more common in colon cancers than rectal cancers.

MOLECULAR PATHWAYS FOR COLORECTAL CARCINOGENESIS

Three molecular carcinogenesis pathways that have been identified for CRCs include (1) chromosomal instability (CIN), (2) microsatellite instability (MSI), and (3) CpG island methylator phenotype (CIMP) or epigenetic instability pathways. The CIN pathway is characterized by alterations in the number and structure of chromosomes and accompanying genetic mutations of proto-oncogenes and tumor suppressor genes. The MSI pathway features alterations in the number of nucleotide repeats (microsatellite sequences) located in the exons and subsequent frameshift mutations in tumor suppressor genes or tumor-related genes. The CIMP pathway is characterized by widespread hypermethylation of numerous promoter CpG island loci and consequent inactivation of tumor suppressor genes or tumor-related genes.

The morphologic multistep pathways include the classical pathway and the serrated neoplasia pathway. The classical adenoma–carcinoma sequence accounts for nearly 80% of sporadic CRCs. It is characterized by early *APC* mutation and subsequent mutations of *KRAS, SMAD2, SMAD4*, and *TP53* and can be driven by CIN or MSI. The precursor lesions consist of conventional adenomas. The serrated neoplasia pathway has epigenetic instability as its driving force and MSI as an optional event.

Microsatellite instability high (MSI-H) tumors can either result from sporadic or germline alterations (Lynch syndrome) of microsatellite sequences. However, the precursor lesions for sporadic MSI-H cancers are serrated in nature, but those in Lynch syndrome are tubular or tubulovillous adenomas. The Cancer Genome Atlas study results show that the CIN and MSI pathways are mutually exclusive. The CIMP pathway overlaps with the MSI pathway because of the presence of sporadic MSI-H CRCs, which are also usually CIMP-high (CIMP-H). However, the CIMP pathway does not appear to be in an exclusive relationship with the CIN pathway. CIMP-H or non–MSI-H CRCs show some copy number variations across the genome, although the degree of CIN is less pronounced than that of CIMP-negative or -low or non–MSI-H CRCs.

LYNCH SYNDROME

Lynch syndrome (formerly known as hereditary nonpolyposis CRC syndrome), the prototype of an autosomal dominant inherited colon cancer family syndrome, is the most common cause of inherited CRC, accounting for 3% of newly diagnosed cases of CRC. In contrast to GI polyposis syndromes in which risk of carcinoma is related to the development of innumerable adenomas, Lynch syndrome is not associated with increased colorectal adenoma formation. It is caused by a deleterious germline mutation in a DNA mismatch repair (MMR) gene, most commonly MLH1 and MSH2, and less commonly PMS2 and MSH6. The designation of Lynch syndrome is also applied to families and patients with loss of expression of the MSH2 gene caused by deletion in the *EPCAM* gene. These mutations result in deficient MMR function.

The Amsterdam II criteria for a diagnosis of Lynch syndrome have a 22% sensitivity and 98% specificity for diagnosis of Lynch syndrome (Table 12.4) Revised Bethesda guidelines are clinicopathologic criteria that have a sensitivity and specificity of 82% and 77%, respectively, for a diagnosis of Lynch syndrome (see Table 12.4). These guidelines work best in detecting patients with *MLH* and *MSH2* abnormalities compared

TABLE 12.4

Amsterdam Criteria and Revised Bethesda Guidelines for Diagnosis of Hereditary Nonpolyposis Colorectal Cancer (HNPCC)

AMSTERDAM I CRITERIA
1. Three or more relatives with histologically verified CRC, one of whom is a first-degree relative of the other two. FAP should be excluded.
2. Two or more generations with CRC
3. 3. One or more CRC cases diagnosed before the age of 50 years
AMSTERDAM II CRITERIA
1. Three or more relatives with histologically verified HNPCC-associated cancer (CRC or cancer of the endometrium, small bowel, ureter, or renal pelvis), one of whom is a first-degree relative of the other two. FAP should be excluded.
2. Cancer involving at least two generations
3. 3. One or more cancer cases diagnosed before the age of 50 years
REVISED BETHESDA GUIDELINES
1. CRC diagnosed at younger than 50 years
2. Presence of synchronous or metachronous colorectal cancer or other Lynch syndrome–associated tumors[a]
3. Colorectal cancer with MSI-H pathologic-associated features (Crohn's-like lymphocytic reaction, mucinous or signet cell differentiation, or medullary growth pattern) diagnosed in an individual younger than 60 years old
4. Patient with colorectal cancer and colorectal cancer or Lynch syndrome–associated tumor[a] diagnosed in at least one first-degree relative younger than 50 years old
5. 5. Patient with colorectal cancer and CRC or colorectal cancer or Lynch syndrome–associated tumor[a] diagnosed at any age in two first- or second-degree relatives

CRC, Colorectal cancer; *FAP*, familial adenomatous polyposis; *MSI-H*, microsatellite instability high.

[a]Lynch syndrome–associated tumors include tumors of the colorectum, endometrium, stomach, ovary, pancreas, ureter, renal pelvis, biliary tract, brain, small bowel, sebaceous glands, and keratoacanthomas.

with those with *MSH6* and *PMS2* abnormalities, which are likely to have low penetrant phenotypes and thus likely to be missed on family history. Lynch-like syndrome describes patients or families in which molecular testing demonstrates the presence of MSI or abnormalities in the expression of MMR gene proteins on immunohistochemistry (IHC) testing of tumor tissue but no pathogenic germline mutation can be found in the patient (e.g., in the absence of a *BRAF* mutation and/or *MLH1* promoter hypermethylation when there is loss of tumor expression of the MLH1 protein). More recently, it has been shown that about half of Lynch-like syndrome patients had biallelic somatic mutations of *MLH1* or *MSH2* to explain the MMR deficient tumors without having causal germline or promotor mutations.

Muir-Torre syndrome, a rare variant of Lynch syndrome, is diagnosed in patients or families with Lynch syndrome and skin sebaceous gland neoplasms (sebaceous adenomas and carcinomas) or neoplasms of the hair follicle (keratoacanthomas). *MSH2* mutation appears most common in these patients, and MSI can be identified in the skin neoplasms and colorectal tumors of affected patients.

Turcot's syndrome is defined as patients or families with colorectal neoplasia and brain tumors. However, these families can be cases of Lynch syndrome (associated with glioblastomas) or FAP (associated with medulloblastomas), so Turcot's syndrome is not an independent entity. Last, patients or families with biallelic mutations of the DNA MMR genes are categorized as having constitutional MMR deficiency syndrome. These patients are characterized by café au lait spots, early (in childhood and teenage years) onset of colorectal neoplasia or other Lynch syndrome cancers, oligopolyposis in the small bowel or colon, brain tumors, and hematologic malignancies.

The average age at diagnosis of cancer in patients with Lynch syndrome is 45 years, compared with 69 years for sporadic cases of CRC. Synchronous and metachronous colon cancers are common among patients with Lynch syndrome and affect up to 25 % of patients with this syndrome. About 60 % to 80 % of CRCs occur in the right colon. The number of adenomas in patients with Lynch syndrome is not more than those with attenuated polyposis syndrome, although the time for progression from adenoma to carcinoma appears to be accelerated in Lynch syndrome (estimated at 35 months compared with 10–15 years for sporadic cancer). These patients have an increased risk for a wide variety of extracolonic malignancies, most notably endometrial cancer; transitional cell carcinoma of the ureter, renal pelvis, and bladder,; adenocarcinomas of the ovary, stomach, hepatobiliary tract, and small bowel; brain cancer (glioblastoma); and cutaneous sebaceous neoplasms. Testing for Lynch syndrome is discussed in Chapter 13.

Other inherited syndromes associated with an increased risk of CRC include FAP, *MUTYH*-associated polyposis, serrated polyposis, hereditary mixed polyposis syndrome, Peutz-Jeghers syndrome, juvenile polyposis, and PTEN hamartoma syndrome (Cowden's syndrome). The polyposis disorders are discussed in Chapter 11. Chronic ulcerative colitis and Crohn's disease are also associated with an increased risk for colon cancer, typically beginning after 8 to 10 years of disease, especially in patients with pancolitis.

COLORECTAL ADENOCARCINOMA—FACT SHEET

Definition

- Malignant neoplasm of colorectal epithelium

Incidence And Location

- Fourth most common cancer in industrialized nations

Morbidity And Mortality

- Responsible for 8.4% of cancer deaths
- 5-year survival rate is 64.9%

Gender, Race, And Age Distribution

- Males more than females
- More common among African American populations
- Average age at diagnosis in sixth decade of life (fifth decade for hereditary nonpolyposis colorectal cancer)

Clinical Features

- High-risk populations include patients with positive family history, history of inflammatory bowel disease, polyposis syndromes
- 3% of colorectal cancers resulting from Lynch syndrome
- Proximal and mucinous carcinomas associated with younger age, female gender, and microsatellite instability (MSI)

Prognosis And Therapy

- Prognosis related to clinical stage, tumor differentiation, MSI status
- Adjuvant therapy recommended for advanced-stage carcinomas

Pathologic Features

Gross Findings

Grossly, CRCs may be polypoid, exophytic, ulcerative, diffusely infiltrating, or obstructing, producing a circumferential narrowing of the bowel lumen. Polypoid cancers that protrude into the lumen and are more common in the cecum and right colon (Fig. 12.25). In contrast, ulcerated carcinomas are more common in the left colon or rectum and show an edge that is barely discernable from the adjacent mucosa (Fig. 12.26). These tumors often involve the entire circumference of the bowel wall and result in constriction. Fungating tumors show a mixture of these two patterns, characteristically seen as a central ulcerated crater with raised edges.

On cut surface, infiltrating carcinomas are tan-white in color with indistinct edges, owing to the host

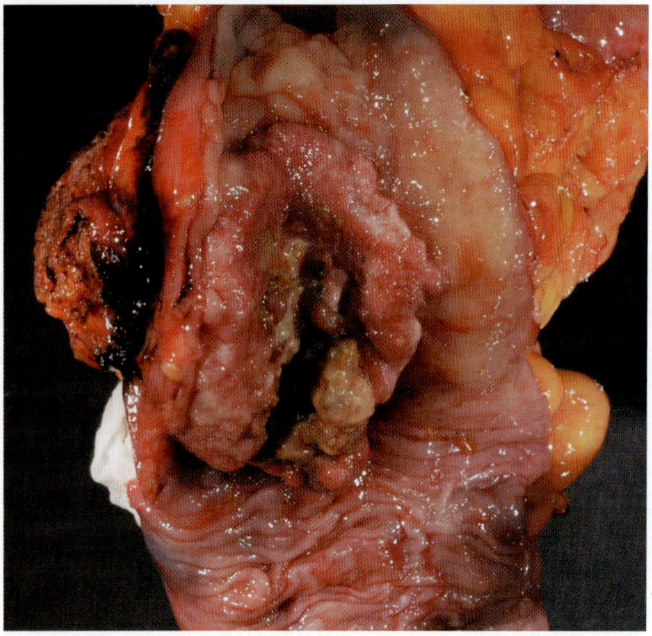

FIGURE 12.25

Gross appearance of an adenocarcinoma arising in the ascending colon showing an exophytic lesion with raised edges and central area of ulceration.

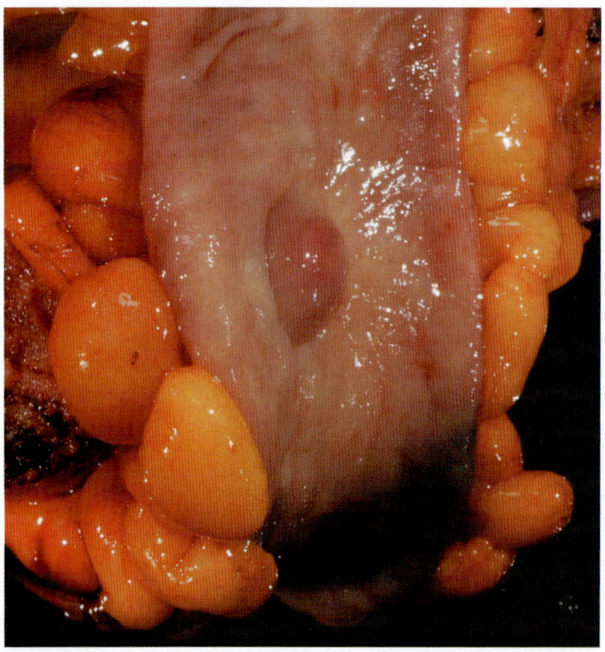

FIGURE 12.26

Gross appearance of an ulcerated adenocarcinoma arising in the sigmoid colon. The edges of the lesion blend with the surrounding mucosa.

desmoplastic response. Involvement of the muscularis propria usually results in thickening of the bowel wall. Invasion through the bowel wall may lead to perforation or foci of puckering on the serosal surface. These foci should be inked and thoroughly sampled for accurate staging. Continued invasion through the bowel wall may involve contiguous structures, including loops of small bowel, bladder, or stomach. Mucinous carcinomas are typically glistening as a result of the prominent extracellular mucin and may show a gelatinous cut surface.

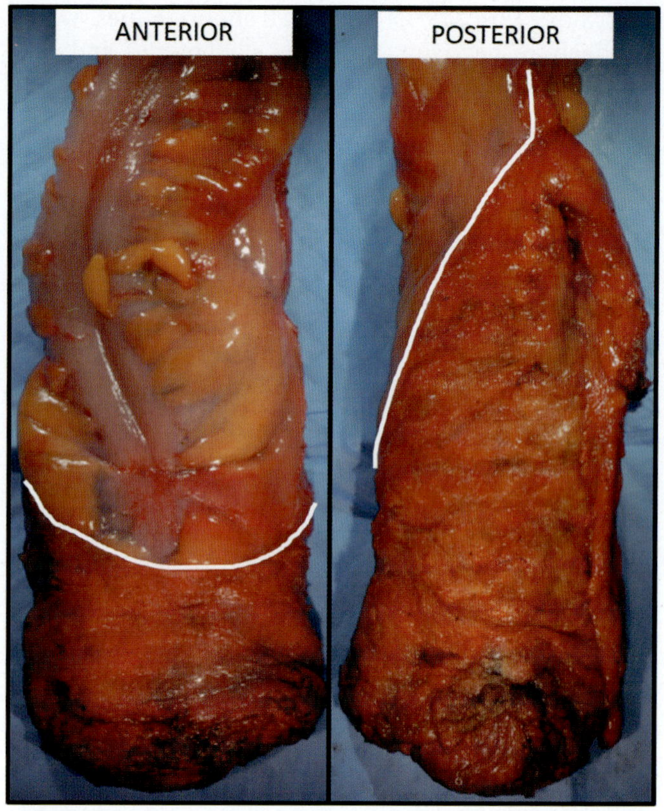

FIGURE 12.27

Low anterior resection specimen with total mesorectal excision for rectal cancer. Total mesorectal excision is a technique used for resecting rectal cancers. This procedure entails sharp dissection within the areolar plane outside (lateral to) the visceral mesorectal fascia to remove the rectum along with all regional nodes and mesorectal tissue. The image shows anterior and posterior view of a low anterior resection specimen with intact mesorectal surface. The peritonealized surface (shiny surface with taenia coli and fat) is demarcated from the nonperitonealized surface by a *white line*. The anterior peritoneal reflection is much lower on the anterior side than the posterior peritoneal reflection. The American Joint Committee on Cancer (AJCC) eighth edition and College of American Pathologists guidelines recommend assessing the mesorectal surface into three categories: incomplete, nearly complete, and complete.

Total mesorectal excision is a specific surgical technique used to resect rectal cancers. This technique entails precise sharp dissection within the areolar plane outside (lateral to) the visceral mesorectal fascia to remove the rectum along with all regional nodes (Fig. 12.27). This procedure prevents development of local recurrence and improves the corresponding survival rate by as much as 20%. Gross evaluation of the completeness of the mesorectum is critical in these specimens because this finding predicts both local recurrence and distant metastasis. The nonperitonealized surface of the fresh specimen is examined circumferentially, and the completeness of the mesorectum is scored as described in Table 12.5. Based on the AJCC eighth edition and CAP guidelines, the mesorectal surface is scored according to the worst area into three categories: incomplete, nearly complete, and complete mesorectum. In addition

TABLE 12.5

Scoring Intactness of Mesorectal Surface in Total Mesorectal Excision Specimens

Incomplete mesorectum
- Little bulk to the mesorectum
- Defects in the mesorectum down to the muscularis propria
- After transverse sectioning, the circumferential margin appears very irregular

Nearly complete mesorectum
- Moderate bulk to the mesorectum
- Irregularity of the mesorectal surface with defects greater than 5 mm, but none extending to the muscularis propria
- No areas of visibility of the muscularis propria except at the insertion site of the levator ani muscles

Complete mesorectum
- Intact bulky mesorectum with a smooth surface
- Only minor irregularities of the mesorectal surface
- No surface defects >5 mm in depth
- No coning towards the distal margin of the specimen
- After transverse sectioning, the circumferential margin appears smooth

to the proximal and distal margins of resection, the circumferential (radial) margin should be assessed in all rectal carcinomas as well as colonic segments with nonperitonealized surfaces.

The vast majority of rectal cancers are treated with adjuvant radiation therapy prior to resection, and depending on the response to therapy, the mucosal surface may show very minimal to no definite residual tumor. In these cases, any mucosal abnormality that potentially represents the tumor bed (ulcer, hemorrhage, tattoo site, puckering, or scarring) should be thoroughly sampled in addition to the adjacent colonic mucosa to ensure complete histologic assessment of the lesion.

Microscopic Findings

The vast majority of CRCs are adenocarcinomas. The current edition of AJCC recommends grading adenocarcinomas according to the degree of gland formation into 4 grades:

Grade 1: well-differentiated adenocarcinomas showing greater than 95 % gland formation

Grade 2: moderately differentiated adenocarcinomas showing 50 % to 95 % gland formation

Grade 3: poorly differentiated adenocarcinomas showing less than 50 % gland formation

Grade 4: undifferentiated adenocarcinomas that do not show any evidence of glands formation, mucin, squamous differentiation, or neuroendocrine differentiation

In well-differentiated adenocarcinomas, the tumor is usually composed of small glands or tubules that are lined by cells with cytologic atypia (Fig. 12.28A). Moderately differentiated adenocarcinomas retain the ability to make glands, but architecturally, they may be composed of a mixture of simple and complex glands with glandular fusion, budding, and cribriforming (Fig. 12.28B). Poorly differentiated adenocarcinomas show minimal gland formation, often seen as sheets of cytologically malignant cells (Fig. 12.28C). More than 80 % of colorectal adenocarcinomas are moderately differentiated and are associated with foci of partial to near complete destruction of the glandular walls and intraluminal necrosis, referred to as "dirty necrosis" (Fig. 12.29).

Mucinous (colloid) adenocarcinomas account for 10 % of all colon cancers and 30 % of rectal cancers and are characterized by abundant extracellular mucin pools (by definition >50 % of the tumor) (Fig. 12.30). Signet ring carcinomas are composed of diffuse, infiltrative nests, sheets of cells with abundant intracytoplasmic mucin, and eccentrically located hyperchromatic nuclei (Fig. 12.31). By definition, more than 50 % of the tumor should be composed of signet ring cells to be designated as a signet ring cell adenocarcinoma. Both mucinous and signet ring cell carcinomas commonly show neoplastic cells floating within pools of mucin. If the adenocarcinoma does not meet the requisite criteria for mucinous or signet ring cell adenocarcinoma, the presence of mucinous or signet ring cell component should be documented in the report because this histologic finding serves as prognostic and predictive marker of MSI.

Serrated adenocarcinomas represent 10 % to 15 % of all colorectal adenocarcinomas and are defined by glandular serration reminiscent of serrated polyps and can be accompanied by mucinous features. Adenoma-like adenocarcinomas (previously known as "villous adenocarcinoma" or "invasive papillary adenocarcinoma") represent fewer than 10 % of all CRCs and are characterized by minimal desmoplasia, pushing growth pattern and 50 % or less low-grade adenoma-like areas in the invasive component.

UNCOMMON VARIANTS OF COLORECTAL CARCINOMAS

Squamous carcinomas and adenosquamous carcinomas of the colorectum are exceedingly rare. A diagnosis of squamous cell carcinoma (SCC) is typically accomplished in the absence of a known primary SCC in any other organ, absence of squamous-lined fistula tracts, and a distinct demarcation of the tumor from the anal squamous epithelium. Chronic inflammation caused by ulcerative colitis or chronic infection, chronic schistosomiasis, pelvic radiation, smoking, human immunodeficiency virus, and human papillomavirus are factors associated with SCC. SCCs are associated with a higher mortality rate compared with conventional adenocarcinomas. Adenosquamous carcinoma consists of both squamous and glandular components. It is more commonly located in the cecum. Recent reports indicate that this morphology is associated with MSI-H status.

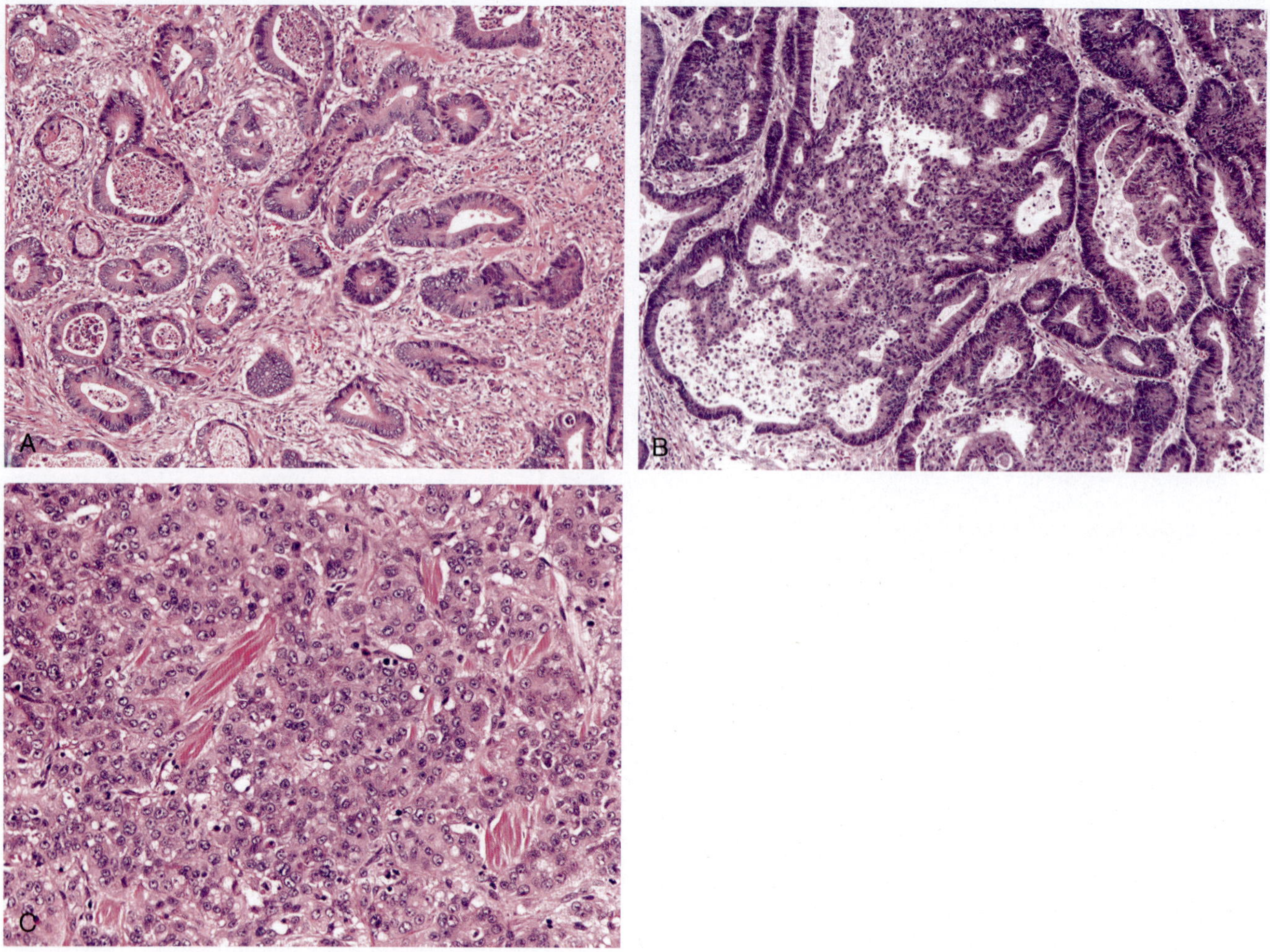

FIGURE 12.28

Colorectal adenocarcinoma. An example of a well-differentiated adenocarcinoma showing glands or tubules lined by atypical cells (**A**). The vast majority of the lesion (>95%) showed this morphology. An example of moderately differentiated adenocarcinoma showing architectural complexity with fusion, budding, and cribriform arrangement of the glands (**B**). Moderately differentiated adenocarcinoma account for majority of the colorectal adenocarcinoma, and gland formation is seen in 50% to 95% of the lesion. Poorly differentiated adenocarcinoma (**C**) showing sheets of atypical cells with abundant eosinophilic cytoplasm, pleomorphic nuclei, vesicular chromatin, and prominent nucleoli. By definition, there is minimal gland formation in these lesions.

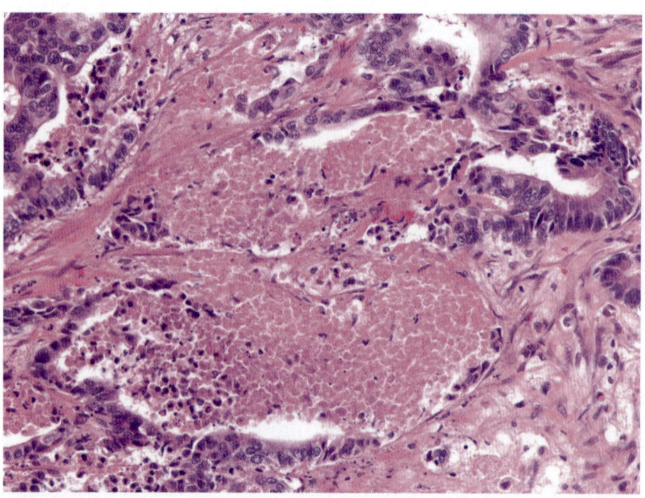

FIGURE 12.29

Colonic adenocarcinoma with "dirty necrosis." The image shows a colonic adenocarcinoma with characteristic "dirty necrosis" where there is partial to near complete destruction of the glandular lining and intraluminal eosinophilic necrotic debris.

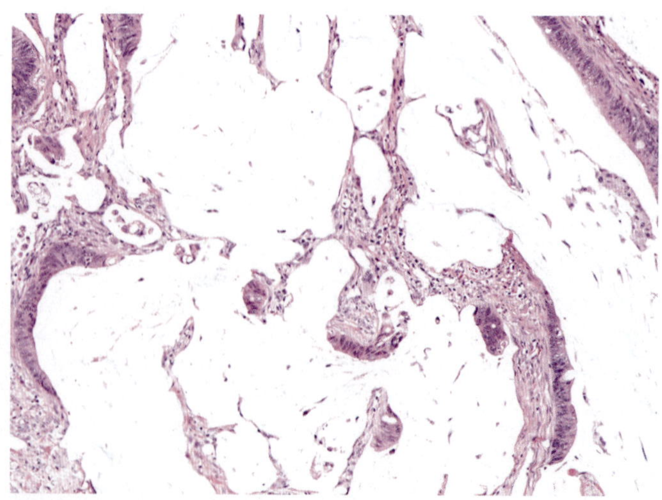

FIGURE 12.30

Mucinous adenocarcinoma. The neoplastic glands produce copious extracellular mucin that results in glandular rupture and extrusion into the surrounding stromal tissue. By definition, at least 50% of the tumor should show mucinous differentiation to be designated as a mucinous adenocarcinoma.

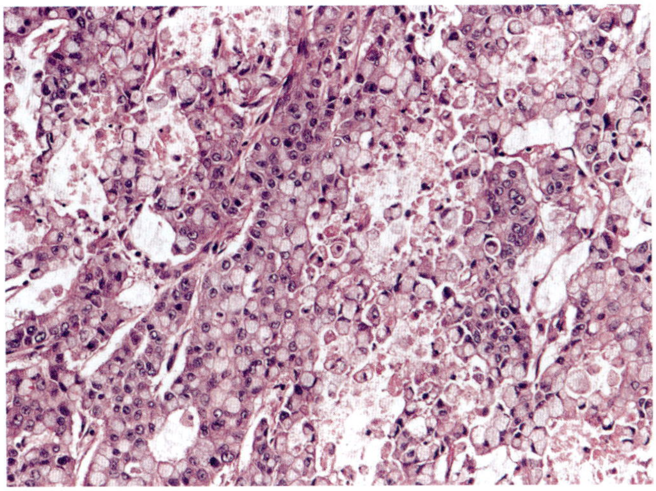

FIGURE 12.31

Signet ring cell adenocarcinoma. The image shows a neoplasm composed of diffuse, infiltrative nests and sheets of cells with abundant intracytoplasmic mucin and eccentrically located hyperchromatic nuclei. By definition, at least 50% of the tumor should show signet ring cell differentiation to be designated as a signet ring cell adenocarcinoma.

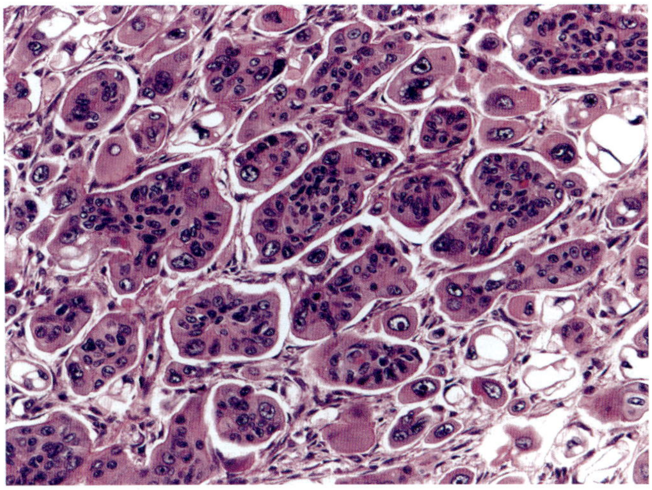

FIGURE 12.32

Micropapillary carcinoma. This is an uncommon variant of colorectal carcinoma with a poor prognosis. The image shows small clusters of tumor cells located within clear lacunar spaces lacking true fibrovascular cores. These spaces can be mistaken for lymphatic channels.

Rare cases of carcinosarcoma, spindle cell carcinoma, adenocarcinoma with areas of choriocarcinoma, hepatoid adenocarcinoma, and clear cell carcinoma have been reported in the colorectum.

Micropapillary carcinoma is an uncommon variant of colorectal carcinoma that is associated with aggressive histological features such as lymphovascular invasion, perineurial invasion, frequent lymph node and distant metastasis, and higher TNM stages. Histologically, it is characterized by small clusters of tumor cells located within clear lacunar spaces lacking true fibrovascular cores (Fig. 12.32). Given the poor clinical prognosis, the presence of a micropapillary component (at least 5% of the tumor) should be mentioned in pathology reports.

Small cell and large cell neuroendocrine carcinomas are categorized as high-grade neuroendocrine carcinomas and are now staged as CRCs instead of neuroendocrine tumors (NETs; see section on NETs later).

MORPHOLOGIC FEATURES ASSOCIATED WITH MICROSATELLITE INSTABILITY

Regardless of whether adenocarcinomas are sporadic in nature or associated with Lynch syndrome, those that show MSI are frequently right-sided, show a mucinous phenotype, and are either well-differentiated or poorly differentiated. In addition, the presence of signet ring cells and medullary phenotype is also a common phenotype. Tumors often show intratumoral heterogeneity characterized by an admixture of conventional, mucinous, and poorly differentiated carcinoma (Fig. 12.33). The "dirty necrosis" that is seen in association with microsatellite stable cancers is frequently absent.

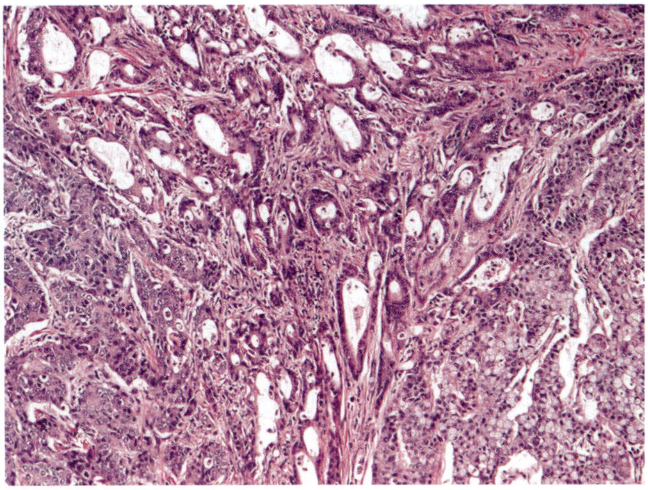

FIGURE 12.33

Colonic adenocarcinoma with microsatellite instability showing tumor heterogeneity. This cecal adenocarcinoma showed morphologic heterogeneity within the same lesion. The upper half of the image shows well-differentiated areas. In addition, there were areas of poorly differentiated (lower left) and signet ring cell phenotype (lower right). Some cases may show a combination of mucinous and well-differentiated morphology.

The individual tumor nests show increased density of intraepithelial lymphocytes, often referred to as tumor infiltrating lymphocytes (Fig. 12.34). The advancing edge of the tumor may show a prominent Crohn's-like reaction with lymphoid aggregates (Fig. 12.35). The molecular work-up of CRC is discussed in Chapter 13.

Undifferentiated carcinoma is another rare form of colorectal carcinoma, accounting for fewer than 1% of all colorectal neoplasms. They are characterized by the complete lack of glandular structures or other features (morphologic, immunohistochemical, or molecular) to indicate cellular differentiation. Only occasional are MSI-H. These cells are fairly round, with regular nuclei and

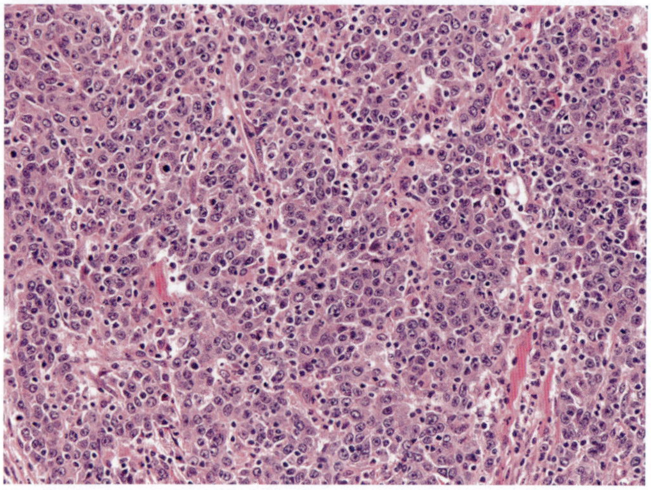

FIGURE 12.34

Tumor infiltrating lymphocytes in colonic adenocarcinoma with microsatellite instability. An example of an ascending colon adenocarcinoma showing sheets of neoplastic cells admixed with lymphocytes.

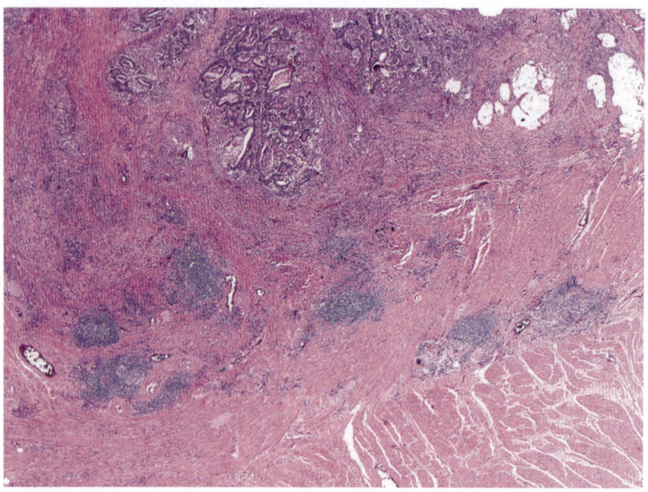

FIGURE 12.35

Crohn's-like lymphoid response in colonic adenocarcinoma with microsatellite instability (MSI). The image shows tumor heterogeneity with foci of well-differentiated and mucinous features (upper right). The advancing front of the tumor and the bowel wall is characterized by nodular lymphoid aggregates, a feature that is commonly associated with the MSI high phenotype.

abundant eosinophilic cytoplasm, raising the question of a neuroendocrine carcinoma. However, IHC stains for neuroendocrine markers are negative. Undifferentiated carcinomas are composed of solid sheets of tumor cells, but in contrast to medullary carcinomas (Fig. 12.36), they lack syncytial growth pattern, accompanying lymphoplasmacytic infiltrate, and pushing borders.

STAGING COLORECTAL CANCERS

Colorectal cancer staging is performed using AJCC staging system. Some of the challenges related to staging include assessment of serosal penetration (pT3 vs pT4a), distinguishing tumor deposits from lymph nodes, reporting isolated tumor cells (ITCs) and micrometastasis, assessment of tumor stage after neoadjuvant therapy, and tumor budding.

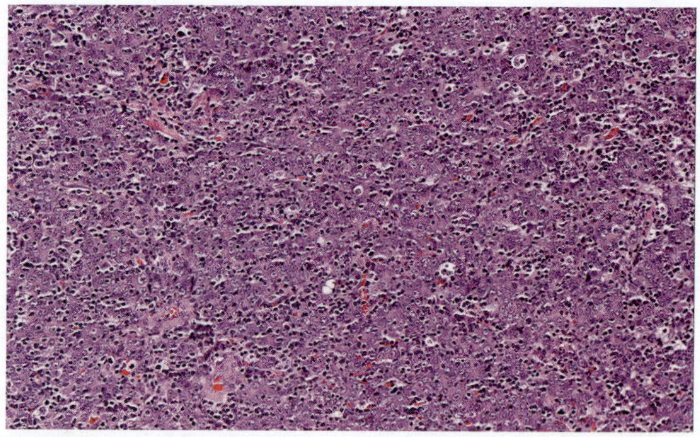

FIGURE 12.36

Medullary carcinoma. An example of a rare form of colorectal carcinoma that shows complete lack of glandular structures. The images shows a lesion composed of solid sheets of tumor cells with syncytial growth pattern with a lymphoplasmacytic infiltrate. These cells are round, with vesicular nuclei, prominent nucleoli, and abundant eosinophilic to amphophilic cytoplasm.

Assessing Serosal Penetration (pT3 vs pT4a)

pT4a classification only pertains to carcinomas that occur in close proximity to the peritoneal surface. The AJCC eighth edition defines invasion of the visceral peritoneum as gross perforation through the tumor; tumor cells at, or on, the peritoneal surface; or continuous invasion of tumor through areas of inflammation that extend to the peritoneal surface. Although it is easy to understand this definition, the practical application can be challenging and controversial because of the fibroinflammatory response that is often present when tumor is close to the serosal surface. Serosal penetration always induces a tissue reaction that may be in the form of fibrin plaques, fibrinous adhesions, creeping fat on serosal surface overlying tumor, mesothelial hyperplasia, mesothelial cells admixed with inflammation near serosa, inflamed septa in subserosal fat at the advancing edge of tumor, or peritumoral abscesses tracking to serosal surface. Because of these histologic changes, assessing cancers that are close to but not at the serosal surface can be problematic (Fig. 12.37). Although some pathologists classify these as pT4a, others stage them as pT3 with a comment indicating that the significance of tumors that are less than 1 mm from the serosal surface and accompanied by serosal reaction is unclear, with some but not all studies indicating a higher risk of peritoneal recurrence. Multiple level sections or additional section of the tumor (or both) should be examined in these cases. If the serosal involvement is not present after additional evaluation, the tumor should be assigned to the pT3 category.

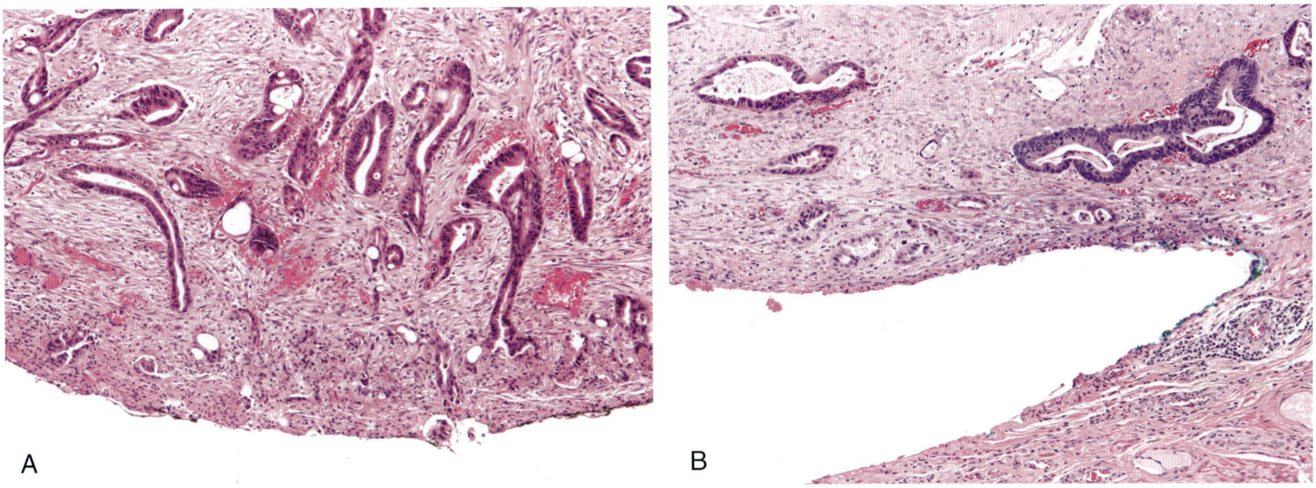

FIGURE 12.37

Serosal penetration in colon cancer (pT3 and pT4). The image shows transmural involvement of a colonic adenocarcinoma with penetration of the serosal surface (inked black). This tumor is staged as pT4a (**A**). In contrast, image **B** shows neoplastic glands that are very close to the serosal surface (inked green) and separated by fibroinflammatory debris. This constitutes serosal reaction to tumor. While some pathologists would interpret this as a pT3 cancer (because the neoplastic glands are not present at the inked serosal surface), others may interpret this as a pT4a cancer. In tumors that reach close to but are not at the serosal surface, a comment indicating that the significance of tumors that are less than 1 mm from the serosal surface and accompanied by serosal reaction is unclear, with some but not all studies indicating a higher risk of peritoneal recurrence, is helpful.

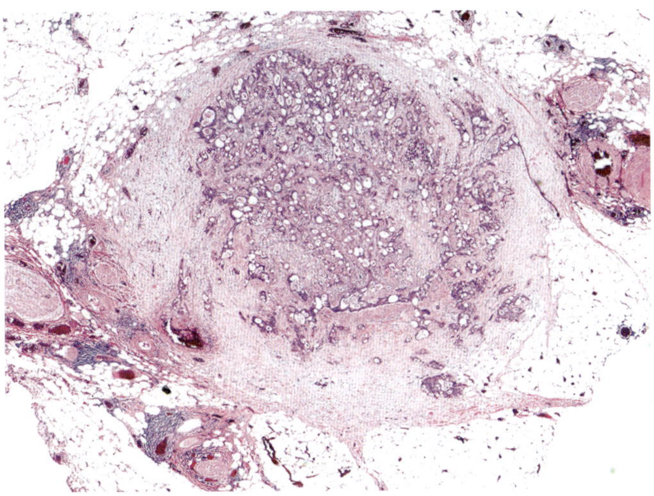

FIGURE 12.38

Tumor deposit. A discrete tumor nodules within the pericolonic adipose tissue without any identifiable lymph node tissue or vascular or neural structure. There is no distinct capsule or lymphoid cuff around this nodule.

Tumor Deposits

The AJCC eighth edition defines tumor deposits as discrete tumor nodules within the lymphatic drainage area of the primary carcinoma without identifiable lymph node tissue or identifiable vascular structure or neural structure (Fig. 12.38). It is important to distinguish them from foci of venous invasion or perineurial invasion. A Movat or elastic stain is very helpful to highlight vascular structures (Fig. 12.39). Tumor deposits tend to be irregular in contour and may have a thin rim of lymphocytes around the periphery. They do not show organized lymphoid tissue or a distinct capsule. An effaced lymph node usually retains its round shape and is surrounded by lymphocytes or lymphoid follicles. A capsule or subcapsular sinus is usually present.

Tumor deposits are associated with poor prognosis among patients with CRC even in the presence of numerous lymph node metastases. When they are noted in association with positive lymph nodes, they should be reported as a separate count in the synoptic summary and should not be counted as lymph nodes. In the absence of regional lymph node metastasis, they are categorized as pN1c.

Isolated Tumor Cells and Micrometastasis

The clinical outcome, especially in patients with stage II cancers, is directly linked to lymph node harvest. Although 12 lymph nodes is the minimum number of lymph nodes required for staging untreated carcinomas, all possible lymph nodes should be retrieved and examined.

In some cases, lymph nodes harbor individual tumor cells in the subcapsular or marginal sinus. These represent ITCs, the definition of which remains controversial. In some studies, clumps of up to 20 tumor cells are classified as ITCs. The most widely used definition includes presence of tumor cell clusters that are less than 0.2 mm in greatest dimension (Fig. 12.40). They are designated as "N0i+." Although one prospective trial showed that pN0i- patients are less likely to show disease recurrence compared with pN0i+ patients, its clinical significance remains unclear. These lymph nodes are staged as N0 with a note indicating the presence of ITCs. In cases in which there are other positive lymph nodes, there are no guidelines on how to report these cases. In our practice, we categorize them as positive lymph nodes. The ITC designation does not apply to treated CRCs. In a

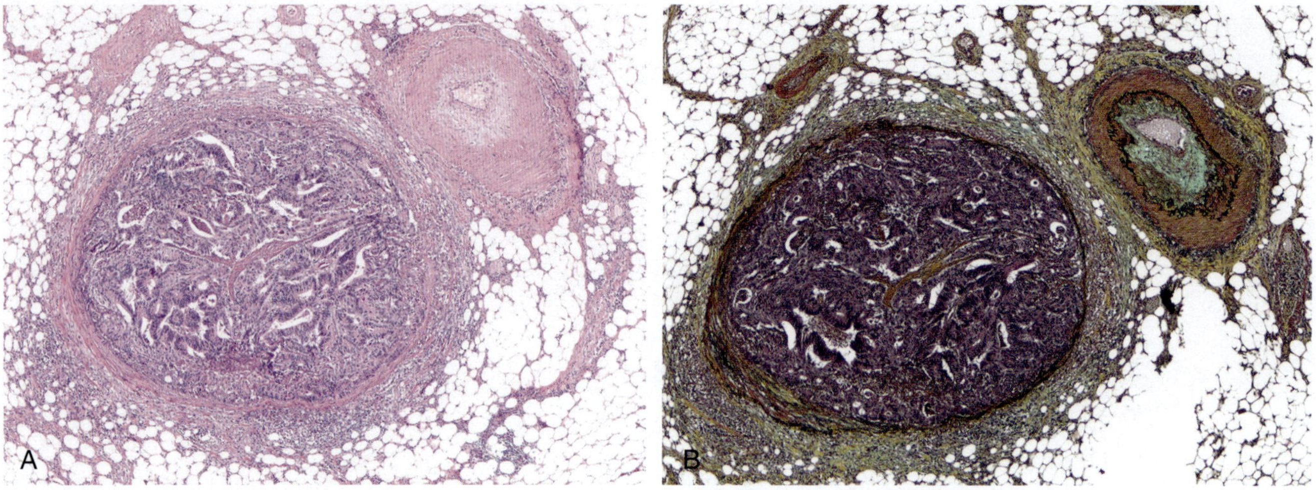

FIGURE 12.39

Venous invasion. An example of extramural venous invasion mimicking tumor deposit (**A**). This rounded aggregate of tumor nodule is present adjacent to an artery ("orphan artery" sign). A corresponding Movat stain (**B**) highlights the internal elastic lamina and media of the vein (left) and artery (right).

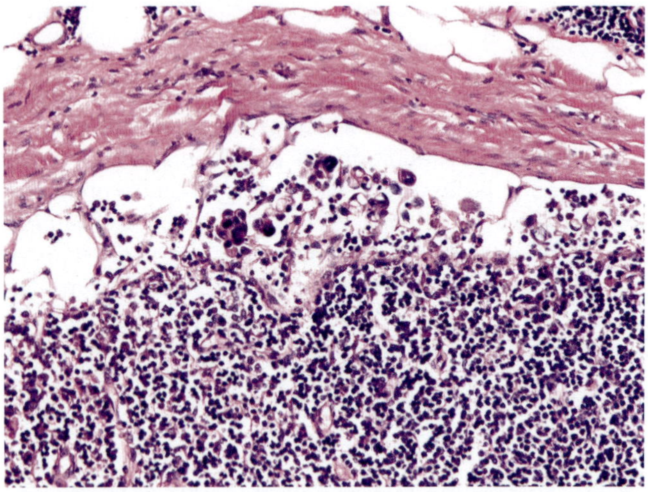

FIGURE 12.40

Lymph node with isolated tumor cells. This lymph nodes shows small clusters of tumor cells that measure less than 0.2 mm in greatest. Isolated tumor cells are designated as pN0i+, and the final nodal stage (in the absence of any other positive lymph nodes) is pN0.

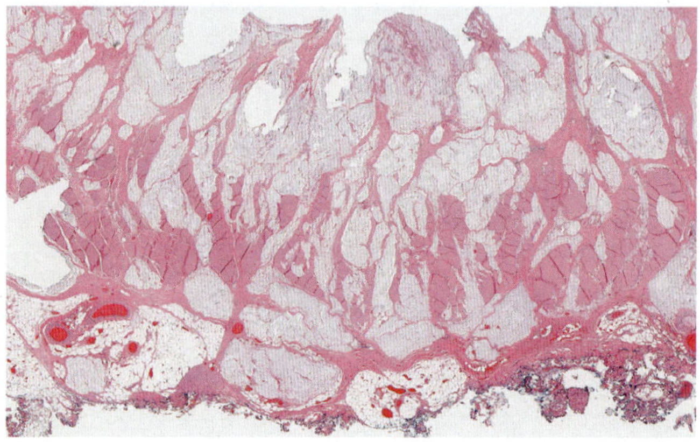

FIGURE 12.41

Treated rectal cancer with therapy effect. This image shows a full-thickness section of a tumor bed obtained from treated rectal cancer specimen. The entire wall shows pools of acellular mucin surrounded by fibrosis. Because no viable tumor cells are present in this section, the depth of acellular mucin or fibrosis does not contribute to the final stage of cancer. Similarly, acellular mucin in lymph nodes from treated cancers are considered as negative.

posttreatment setting, a lymph node is considered positive regardless of the size of the tumor cells.

Micrometastasis are defined as clumps of tumor measuring 0.2 mm or greater in diameter. Their presence indicates replication of tumor cells rather than mere presence of isolated dormant tumor cells. Because micrometastases are a significant poor prognostic factor, they are best considered as positive nodes.

Assessing Tumor Stage Following Neoadjuvant Therapy

Following therapy for rectal cancer, the tumor shows therapy-related changes that include tumor regression with fibrosis, pools of acellular mucin, and foci of dystrophic calcification (Fig. 12.41). Assessment of pT and pN stage is based on the extent of viable tumor. Acellular mucin or fibrosis does not change the stage of cancer. Similarly, lymph nodes with acellular mucin are considered as negative. The pathology report should include the extent of tumor regression because extensive therapeutic response with minimal residual tumor has been associated with a favorable clinical prognosis. Although there are numerous scoring systems, the AJCC and CAP recommend using the modified Ryan system (Table 12.6) for scoring the primary tumor.

Tumor Budding

Several studies have shown that tumor budding is a significant risk factor for nodal involvement in patients with malignant polyps and indicates an adverse prognosis in patients with stage II cancers. A recent ITBCC in

TABLE 12.6

Modified Ryan Scheme for Tumor Regression Score in Treated Rectal Cancers

Category	Description	Tumor Regression Score
Complete response	No viable cancer cells	0
Near complete response	Single cells or rare small groups of cancers cells	1
Partial response	Residual cancer with evident tumor response but more than single cells or rare small groups of cancer cells	2
Poor or no response	Extensive residual cancer with no evident tumor regression	3

TABLE 12.7

Conversion Table for Scoring Tumor Budding

Eyepiece Diameter (mm)	Specimen Area (mm^2)	Normalization Factor
18	0.636	0.810
19	0.709	0.903
20	0.785	1.000
21	0.866	1.103
22	0.950	1.210
23	1.039	1.323
24	1.131	1.440
25	1.227	1.563
26	1.327	1.690

2016 defined tumor budding as presence of single cells or small clusters of fewer than five cells at the advancing front of the tumor. They recommended the following criteria for evaluating tumor budding:

1. Tumor budding counts should be done on hematoxylin and eosin (H&E) sections.
2. Tumor budding should be reported by selecting a "hotspot" chosen after review of all available slides with invasive tumor. The total number of buds should be reported in an area measuring 0.785 mm^2, which corresponds to 20× field in some microscopes (use appropriate conversion for other microscopes; see Table 12.7)
3. Both the total number of buds and a three-tier score (based on 0.785 mm^2 field area) should be reported: low (0–4 buds), intermediate (5–9 buds) and high (≥10 buds) (Fig. 12.42). Although this is not a required element in CAP cancer staging template, it is recommended that this feature be reported for cancers arising in polyps as well as for stage I and II cancers.

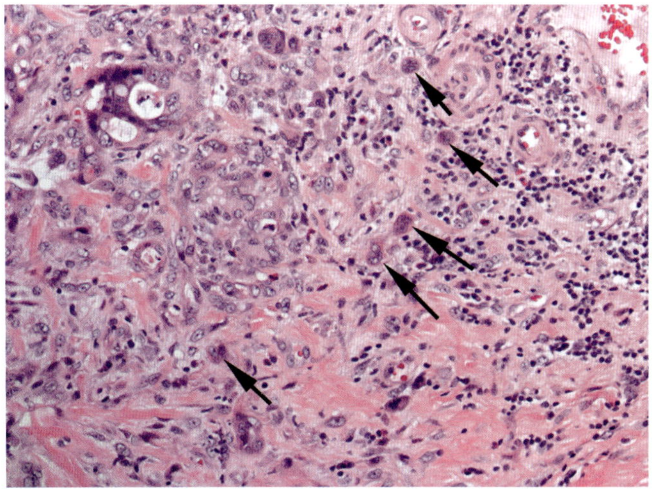

FIGURE 12.42

Tumor budding. The image shows advancing edge of colonic adenocarcinoma with tumor buds composed of single cells as well as small clusters of less than five cells *(arrows)*. Tumor buds count is performed on hematoxylin and eosin–stained sections and scored using recommendations from 2016 international Tumor Budding Consensus Conference.

In tumors that show prominent inflammation at their advancing edge, IHC for keratin can be obtained to identify tumor buds, but the scoring should be done on H&E sections. Tumor budding counts should not be reported in cases of treated rectal adenocarcinoma, mucinous or signet ring cell adenocarcinomas, medullary carcinoma, micropapillary carcinoma, or tumors that show glandular fragmentation secondary to inflammation.

COLORECTAL ADENOCARCINOMA—PATHOLOGIC FEATURES

Gross Findings

- Polypoid, fungating, or ulcerated appearance
- Larger tumors more common in proximal colon
- Circumferential growth (apple-core lesions) more common in left colon

Microscopic Findings

- Adenocarcinomas are graded as well-differentiated, moderately differentiated, poorly differentiated, or undifferentiated
- Abundant eosinophilic necrotic debris within gland lumens ("dirty necrosis")
- Mucinous carcinomas associated with extracellular mucin production and mucin pools comprising greater than 50% of tumor
- Other variants: signet ring cell adenocarcinoma, medullary, serrated, adenoma-like, carcinomas with sarcomatoid components, squamous, adenosquamous, micropapillary, undifferentiated
- Morphologic subtypes associated with an microsatellite instability high phenotype: mucinous, signet ring cell, medullary, tumors with morphologic heterogeneity (e.g., admixture of conventional, mucinous as well as poorly differentiated carcinoma)

Genetics

- Sporadic carcinomas associated with *APC, KRAS*, and *TP53* alterations
- 3% of carcinomas caused by Lynch syndrome

Immunohistochemistry

- Strong cytokeratin (AE1/AE3, CK20, and CAM5.2) positivity in sporadic carcinomas; variably positive for CK7
- Variable CK20 and CDX-2 positivity in MSI-high carcinomas
- SATB2 positive

Differential Diagnosis

- Metastatic carcinomas
- Endometriosis and carcinomas arising in endometriosis

Ancillary Studies

Immunohistochemically, colorectal adenocarcinomas are virtually always positive for broad-spectrum and low-molecular-weight cytokeratins (AE1/AE3, CAM5.2), EMA, and carcinoembryonic antigen (CEA). They are consistently positive for cytokeratin (CK) 20 and variably positive for CK7. CDX-2 and SATB2 are usually expressed by more than 90% of CRCs. In tumors that show MSI, there may be variable loss of both CK20 and CDX-2.

Differential Diagnosis

A variety of metastatic neoplasms may involve the colorectum, including prostate, breast, stomach, and ovarian cancers and melanoma. The lack of associated adenomatous epithelium combined with the gross findings and the growth pattern of the tumor (centered on the external or serosal aspect of the bowel wall) supports a metastatic lesion. Immunohistochemical stains for appropriate markers (prostatic-specific acid phosphatase [PSAP], NKX3.1 for prostate; CK7, GATA-3, estrogen receptor for breast; CK7, WT-1, or PAX8 for ovary; CK7 for stomach; S-100 or SOX-10 for melanoma) may also indicate the primary tumor of origin, whereas the vast majority of the colorectal carcinomas are positive for CK20, CDX-2, and SATB2.

Involvement of the colorectum by endometriosis is common among women of childbearing age (≤20% of patients with endometriosis). Endometriomas involving the colon form ill-defined masses involving the subserosal tissue and muscularis propria, although polypoid lesions have also been reported. Sigmoid colon and rectosigmoid region are the most common location within the GI tract. Histologic examination reveals the presence of normal mucosa overlying endometrial glands and stroma, which should be differentiated from adenocarcinoma glands with desmoplasia (Fig. 12.43).

Prognosis and Therapy

Pathologists play a major role in the management of colorectal carcinoma by proper staging, which provides the clinician with critical information regarding prognosis and choice of adjuvant therapy. In addition to the TNM stage, features that should be addressed in pathology reports include histologic type and grade, presence or absence of lymphovascular invasion, perineurial invasion, tumor deposits, and resection margins. Adjuvant therapy significantly improves survival of patients with stage III colon cancer, particularly adjuvant 5-fluorouracil (5-FU) and levamisole. However, adjuvant therapy can also be considered for patients with high-risk stage II disease, defined as those with poor prognostic features, including T4 tumors (stage IIB/IIC); poorly differentiated histology (exclusive of those cancers that are MSI-H); lymphovascular invasion; perineurial invasion; bowel obstruction; lesions with localized perforation or close, indeterminate, or positive margins; and cases with inadequately sampled lymph nodes (<12 lymph nodes).

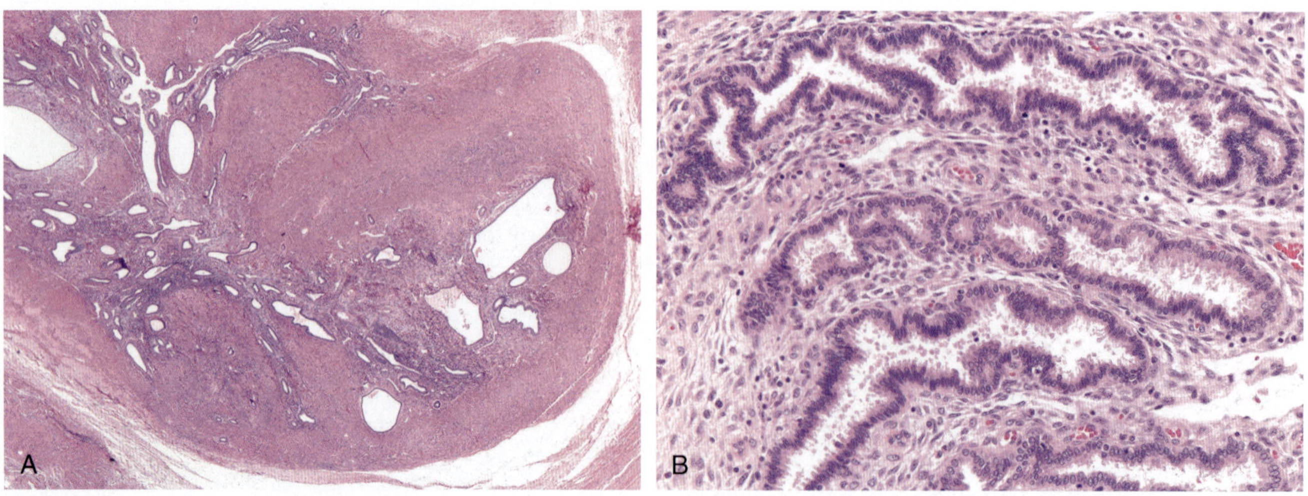

FIGURE 12.43

Colonic endometriosis. A section from thickened sigmoid colon wall showing numerous, variably sized cystically dilated glands surrounded by stromal cells (**A**). The angulated glandular profiles and mural thickening mimic colon cancer clinically and histologically. Higher magnification shows that the glands demonstrate endometrial phenotype with low columnar cells and are surrounded by endometrial stroma with spiral arterioles, diagnostic of endometriosis (**B**).

Radiation therapy may be used to treat rectal cancers preoperatively or postoperatively or to treat recurrent disease. Reductions in local recurrence and death have also been shown for stage II and III rectal cancers using a combination of 5-FU and radiation therapy.

In addition to TNM stage, MSI provides additional information when deciding about adjuvant chemotherapy in patients with stage II cancers. Studies have shown that MSI-H tumors show a favorable outcome among patients with stage II cancers. The favorable impact does not seem apply to stage III cancers and may vary with tumor location. MSI-H status also appears to be predictor of poor response to 5-FU–based therapy in stage II but not stage III cancers. Furthermore, it has been recently shown that MMR deficient tumors may be sensitive to programmed death-ligand 1 (PD-L1) inhibitors in patients with metastatic disease. Therefore, universal testing of MMR or MSI is recommended to identify individuals with Lynch syndrome, predict response to immune therapy, and select therapy for stage II cancers. Additional details on molecular testing and rationale for therapy are detailed in Chapter 13.

NEUROENDOCRINE NEOPLASMS

Clinical Features

Neuroendocrine neoplasms can arise anywhere throughout the colorectum. They constitute a range of clinicopathologic entities ranging from well-differentiated NETs ("carcinoid tumors") to aggressive neuroendocrine carcinomas. Because neuroendocrine neoplasms arise from cells of the diffuse neuroendocrine system, they are related to medullary carcinoma of the thyroid, pheochromocytoma, and pancreatic NETs. They occur in 9 % of patients with multiple endocrine neoplasia syndrome type 1.

Well-differentiated NETs of the GI tract account for up to 95 % of all NETs. Within the GI tract, well-differentiated NETs comprise 20 % of all GI neoplasms and 6 % of colorectal neoplasms. The incidence is estimated to be up to 8 per 100,000 individuals. The average age at diagnosis is in the sixth to seventh decade of life. They are more common in women than men and are more common in African Americans than other races.

At least half of all NETs are discovered as an incidental finding. The clinical presentation depends on the location of the tumor. Clinical symptoms associated with colonic NETs are usually vague (weight loss, abdominal pain) or related to the mass effect from bulky aggressive lesions. Symptoms related to rectal neoplasms include pain, rectal bleeding, and diarrhea, usually resulting from mechanical trauma associated with a polypoid lesion. Carcinoid syndrome is uncommon even in the presence of liver metastases.

NEUROENDOCRINE NEOPLASMS—FACT SHEET

Definition

- Neoplasms of the diffuse neuroendocrine system of the gastrointestinal tract

Incidence And Location

- Colorectal neuroendocrine tumors (NETs) represent 10% of all NETs

Morbidity And Mortality

- Overall survival rate is 42% to 72%
- One-third of patients have regional nodal or distant metastases at diagnosis

Gender, Race, And Age Distribution

- Female more than males
- Slight predominance in African American population
- Average age at diagnosis in sixth to seventh decades of life

Clinical Features

- Usually asymptomatic
- Symptoms such as obstruction, weight loss, and anorexia related to large bulky lesions
- Fecal occult blood test is usually negative because these are submucosal lesions

Prognosis And Therapy

- Surgical resection effective for small lesions
- Rectal NETs should be staged by endoscopic ultrasonography or magnetic resonance imaging
- Rectal neoplasms larger than 2 cm or with muscularis propria invasion are treated surgically with low anterior resection or abdominoperineal resection
- Neuroendocrine carcinomas
    - Aggressive clinical behavior; 85% show metastasis at presentation
    - Treated with platinum-based chemotherapy with or without radiation therapy

Pathologic Features

Gross Findings

Of the neuroendocrine neoplasms that occur in the large intestine, the most commonly affected site is the rectum followed by the cecum. This distribution parallels the distribution and density of endocrine cells in the large intestine. They usually occur singly, although in a minority of patients multiple tumors may occur, particularly within the rectum. Grossly, they present as a submucosal lesions with normal overlying mucosa. Their size can range from small nodules measuring 2 to 3 mm in diameter to large lesions in excess of 5 cm. Larger tumors are more commonly encountered in the proximal colon. On cut surface, they are yellow to tan-white in color with a homogeneous cut surface. Large lesions (especially neuroendocrine carcinomas) often show erosion and ulceration of the overlying mucosa.

Microscopic Findings

The morphologic features of large intestinal neuroendocrine neoplasms are similar to those arising in other locations. Well-differentiated NETs are composed of round or polygonal cells with uniform, round to oval nuclei, amphophilic or eosinophilic granular cytoplasm, and a speckled chromatin pattern ("salt and pepper" nuclei). Necrosis is absent. The tumor may show a variety of growth patterns, including a solid (Fig. 12.44A), nested, trabecular, ribbonlike (Fig. 12.44B), or acinar pattern.

Similar to rest of the NET in the GI tract, the CAP and AJCC eighth edition recommend the following grading system for well-differentiated NETs:

Well-differentiated NET (G1): mitotic rate less than 2 per 2 mm^2 and/or Ki-67 index less than 3%

Well-differentiated NET (G2): mitotic rate 2 to 20 per mm^2 and/or Ki-67 index 3% to 20%

Well-differentiated NET (G3): mitotic rate greater than 20 per 2 mm^2 and/or Ki-67 index less than 20%

Poorly differentiated neuroendocrine carcinomas (large cell and small cell type) are now staged as colorectal carcinomas (Fig. 12.45). Mixed neuroendocrine–non-neuroendocrine neoplasms (MiNENs, previously known as mixed adenoneuroendocrine carcinoma [MANEC]) comprise a neuroendocrine component ($\geq$30%) and a non-neuroendocrine component ($\geq$30%).

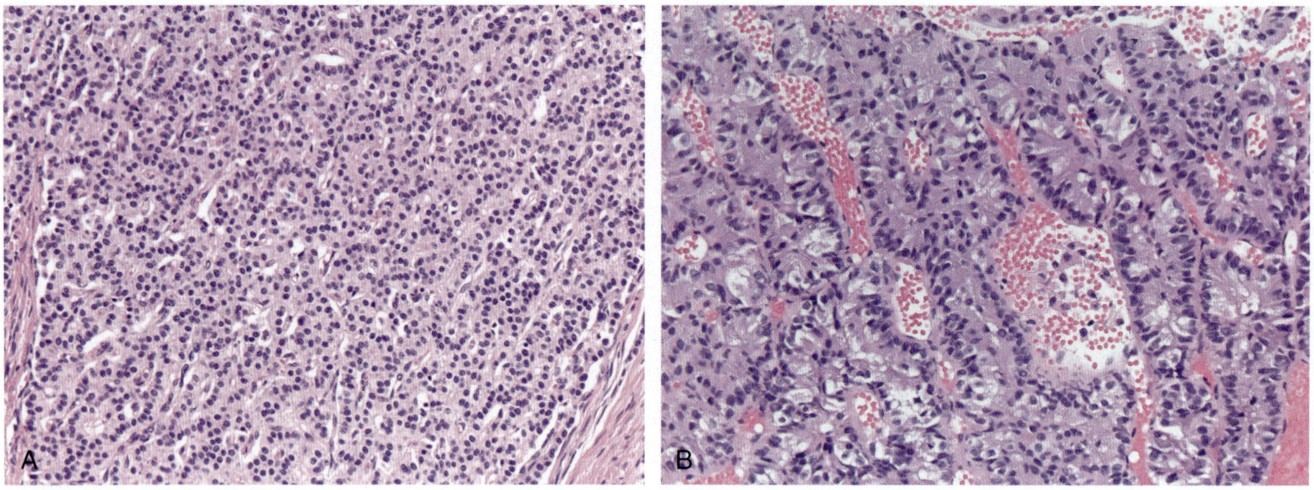

FIGURE 12.44

Well-differentiated neuroendocrine tumor. Well-differentiated neuroendocrine neoplasm with solid growth pattern (**A**). The tumor is composed of small uniform cells with abundant eosinophilic cytoplasm, centrally located round nuclei with finely dispersed chromatin. Delicate vessels are present within the tumor. These lesions may show a variety of growth patterns. An example of ribbonlike or trabecular pattern is shown in **B**.

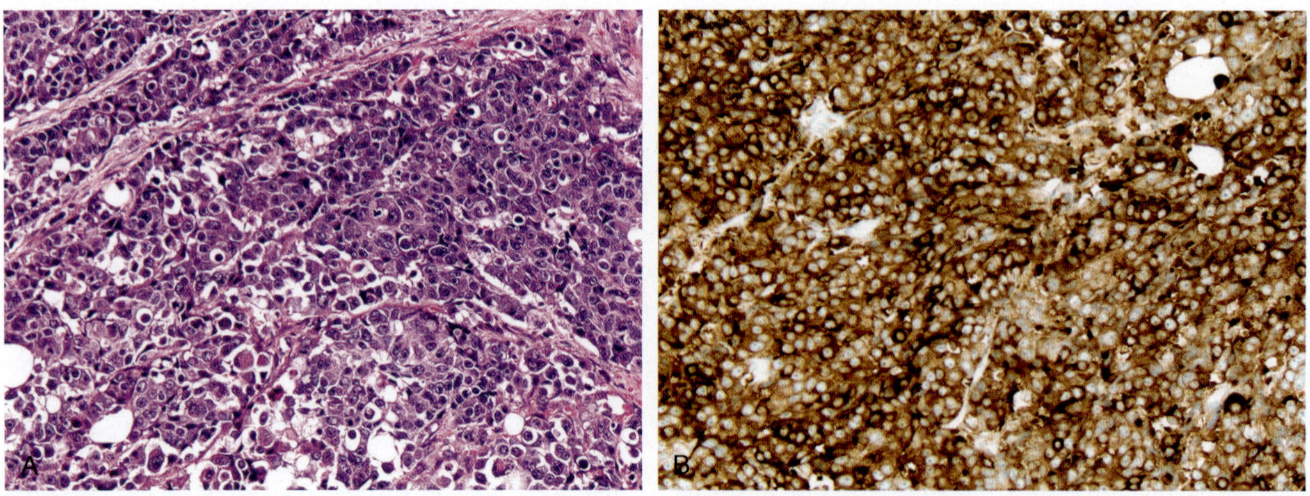

FIGURE 12.45

High-grade neuroendocrine carcinoma, large cell type. In this example, the tumor cells are arranged in solid sheets and show vesicular chromatin, prominent nucleoli, and marked atypia and pleomorphism (**A**). Mitoses and apoptotic debris are abundant. Immunohistochemical stain chromogranin shows diffuse cytoplasmic immunoreactivity, confirming the neuroendocrine origin (**B**).

Neuroendocrine Neoplasms—Pathologic Features

Gross Findings

- (Well-differentiated) neuroendocrine tumor (NET)
  - Submucosal mass with yellow-tan cut surface
  - Most commonly found in right colon or rectum
- (Poorly differentiated) neuroendocrine carcinoma (NEC)
  - Ulcerated mass-forming lesions

Microscopic Findings

- (Well-differentiated) NET
  - Uniform small round to oval cells with rare mitotic figures
  - Fine, speckled chromatin pattern and granular eosinophilic to amphophilic cytoplasm
  - Solid, ribbonlike, trabecular or nested growth patterns
- (Poorly differentiated) NEC
  - Small cell or large cell NEC
  - Sheets, nests, or trabecular growth
  - High mitotic activity

Immunohistochemistry

- Positive for synaptophysin, CD56 and variably positive for chromogranin
- Rectal lesions frequently positive for prostatic-specific acid phosphatase (>80%) and lack chromogranin expression
- Grading is performed based on mitotic activity (per 10 hpf) and Ki-67 index (per College of American Pathologists and American Joint Committee on Cancer (AJCC) eighth edition)
  - NET
    - Grade 1 (well-differentiated NET): <2 mitoses/10 hpf and/or <3% Ki-67 index
    - Grade 2 (well-differentiated NET): 2–20 mitoses/10 hpf and/or 3–20% Ki-67 index
    - Grade G3 (well-differentiated NET): >20 mitoses/10 hpf and/or >20% Ki-67 index
  - NEC
    - G3: >20 mitoses/10 hpf and/or >20% Ki-67 index

Differential Diagnosis

- Poorly differentiated colorectal carcinoma
- Lymphoid neoplasms (particularly in small biopsy specimens)
- Metastatic carcinomas
- Prostatic adenocarcinoma (especially in rectum)

Immunohistochemistry

Immunohistochemical stains are frequently positive for synaptophysin, CD56, and broad-spectrum cytokeratins (AE1/AE3) in colorectal neuroendocrine neoplasms, whereas chromogranin is variably positive in large intestinal tumors. Rectal NETs frequently express PSAP and may lack chromogranin expression.

Differential Diagnosis

Because NETs are typically submucosal in location, their identification within submucosal tissue in a rectal biopsy specimen may raise the possibility of prostatic adenocarcinoma. Immunohistochemical staining for prostate-specific antigen (PSA), NKX 3.1, and PSAP can be helpful, although 80% of rectal carcinoids express PSAP. Furthermore, rectal NET may lack chromogranin expression. Therefore, performing two neuroendocrine markers is helpful for rectal NETs. The uniform appearance of the neuroendocrine cells can mimic a lymphoid neoplasm, whereas the solid growth pattern can be suggestive of a poorly differentiated carcinoma. In all cases, performing neuroendocrine markers is very helpful in this differential diagnosis.

Prognosis and Therapy

Rectal NETs typically tend to be small and of lower grade than colonic NETs, which often present as masses and are associated with poor prognosis. For small (<1 cm) incidental lesions, complete endoscopic resection is usually considered sufficient. Rectal NETs should be staged with endoscopic ultrasonography or magnetic resonance imaging. Rectal tumors that are larger than 2 cm or those the demonstrate invasion of muscularis propria are treated with low anterior resection, or in rare cases, abdominoperineal resection. Although factors that would predict lymph node and distant metastasis are evolving, it appears that tumor size and depth are the strongest predictors of clinical behavior.

Neuroendocrine carcinomas have an aggressive clinical behavior. Approximately 85% of tumors have metastasis at the time of diagnosis. For localized disease, curative surgery is usually followed by platinum-based therapy with or without radiotherapy. Systemic chemotherapy is indicated for patients with advanced inoperable disease.

Suggested Readings

1. Imperiale TF, Wagner DR, Lin CY, et al. Results of screening colonoscopy among persons 40 to 49 years of age. *N Engl J Med.* 2002;346:1781–1785.
2. Kim EC, Lance P. Colorectal polyps and their relationship to cancer. *Gastroenterol Clin North Am.* 1997;26:1–17.
3. Kinzler KW, Vogelstein B. Lessons from hereditary colorectal cancer. *Cell.* 1996;87:159–170.
4. Winawer SJ, Zauber AG, Fletcher RH, et al. Guidelines for colonoscopy surveillance after polypectomy: a consensus update by the US Multi-Society Task Force on Colorectal Cancer and the American Cancer Society. *Gastroenterology.* 2006;130:1872–1885.
5. Lieberman DA, Rex DK, Winawer SJ, et al. Guidelines for colonoscopy surveillance after screening and polypectomy: a consensus update by the US Multi-Society Task Force on Colorectal Cancer. *Gastroenterology.* 2012;143:844–857.
6. Toll AD, Fabius D, Hyslop T, et al. Prognostic significance of high-grade dysplasia in colorectal adenomas. *Colorectal Dis.* 2011;13:370–373.
7. Vogelstein B, Fearon ER, Hamilton SR, et al. Genetic alterations during colorectal-tumor development. *N Engl J Med.* 1988;319:525–532.
8. Robert ME. The malignant colon polyp: diagnosis and therapeutic recommendations. *Clin Gastroenterol Hepatol.* 2007;5:662–667.

9. Coverlizza S, Risio M, Ferrari A, et al. Colorectal adenomas containing invasive carcinoma. *Pathologic assessment of lymph node metastatic potential. Cancer*. 1989;64:1937–1947.
10. Cooper HS, Deppisch LM, Gourley WK, et al. Endoscopically removed malignant colorectal polyps: clinicopathologic correlations. *Gastroenterology*. 1995;108:1657–1665.
11. Ueno H, Mochizuki H, Hashiguchi Y, et al. Risk factors for an adverse outcome in early invasive colorectal carcinoma. *Gastroenterology*. 2004;127:385–394.
12. Baatrup G, Endreseth BH, Isaksen V, et al. Preoperative staging and treatment options in T1 rectal adenocarcinoma. *Acta Oncol*. 2009;48:328–342.
13. National Comprehensive Cancer Network. https://www.nccn.org/professionals/physician_gls/pdf/colon.pdf
14. Bosch SL, Teerenstra S, de Wilt JH, Cunningham C, Nagtegaal ID. Predicting lymph node metastasis in pT1 colorectal cancer: a systematic review of risk factors providing rationale for therapy decisions. *Endoscopy*. 2013;45(10):827–834.
15. Brown IS, Bettington ML, Bettington A, et al. Adverse histological features in malignant colorectal polyps: a contemporary series of 239 cases. *J Clin Pathol*. 2016;69(4):292–299.
16. Rex DK, Ahnen DJ, Baron JA, et al. Serrated lesions of the colorectum: review and recommendations from an expert panel. *Am J Gastroenterol*. 2012;107:1315–1329. quiz 1314, 1330.
17. O'Brien MJ, Zhao Q, Yang S. Colorectal serrated pathway cancers and precursors. *Histopathology*. 2015;66:49–65.
18. Torlakovic EE, Gomez JD, Driman DK, et al. Sessile serrated adenoma (SSA) vs. traditional serrated adenoma (TSA). Am J Surg Pathol. 2008;32(1):21–29.
19. Anderson JC, Butterly LF, Robinson CM, et al. Risk of metachronous high-risk adenomas and large serrated polyps in individuals with serrated polyps on index colonoscopy: data from the New Hampshire Colonoscopy Registry. *Gastroenterology*. 2018;154(1):117–127.
20. Chetty R. Traditional serrated adenoma (TSA): morphological questions, queries and quandaries. *J Clin Pathol*. 2016; 69(1):6–11.
21. Wiland 4th HO, Shadrach B, Allende D, et al. Morphologic and molecular characterization of traditional serrated adenomas of the distal colon and rectum. *Am J Surg Pathol*. 2014; 38(9):1290–1297.
22. Spoto CPE, Gullo I, Carneiro F, et al. Hereditary gastrointestinal carcinomas and their precursors: an algorithm for genetic testing. *Semin Diagn Pathol*. 2018;S0740-2570(18). 30004-2.
23. National Cancer Institute Surveillance, Epidemiology, and End Results Program. Cancer stat facts: colorectal cancer. https://seer.cancer.gov/statfacts/html/colorect.html
24. Chen W, Swanson BJ, Frankel WL. Molecular genetics of microsatellite-unstable colorectal cancer for pathologists. Diagn Pathol. 2017;12(1):24.
25. Giardiello FM, Allen JI, Axilbund JE, et al. Guidelines on genetic evaluation and management of Lynch syndrome: a consensus statement by the US Multi-society Task Force on colorectal cancer. *Am J Gastroenterol*. 2014;109(8):1159–1179.
26. Vasen HF, Watson P, Mecklin JP, Lynch HT. New clinical criteria for hereditary nonpolyposis colorectal cancer (HNPCC, Lynch syndrome) proposed by the International Collaborative group on HNPCC. *Gastroenterology*. 1999;116(6):1453–1456.
27. Umar A, Boland CR, Terdiman JP, et al. Revised Bethesda Guidelines for hereditary nonpolyposis colorectal cancer (Lynch syndrome) and microsatellite instability. *J Natl Cancer Inst*. 2004;96(4):261–268.
28. Recommendations from the EGAPP Working Group genetic testing strategies in newly diagnosed individuals with colorectal cancer aimed at reducing morbidity and mortality from Lynch syndrome in relatives. *Genet Med*. 2009;11(1):35–41.
29. Greenson JK, Huang SC, Herron C, et al. Pathologic predictors of microsatellite instability in colorectal cancer. *Am J Surg Pathol*. 2009;33(1):126–133.
30. Frankel WL, Jin M. Serosal surfaces, mucin pools, and deposits, oh my: challenges in staging colorectal carcinoma. *Mod Pathol*. 2015;28(suppl 1):S95–S108.
31. Lugli A, Kirsch R, Ajioka Y, et al. Recommendations for reporting tumor budding in colorectal cancer based on the International Tumor Budding Consensus Conference (ITBCC) 2016. *Mod Pathol*. 2017;30(9):1299–1311.
32. Ryan R, Gibbons D, Hyland JMP, et al. Pathological response following long-course neoadjuvant chemoradiotherapy for locally advanced rectal cancer. *Histopathology*. 2005;47(2):141–146.
33. Arbman G, Nilsson E, Hallbook O, Sjodahl R. Local recurrence following total mesorectal excision for rectal cancer. *Br J Surg*. 1996;83(3):375–379.
34. Kapiteijn E, Marijnen CA, Nagtegaal ID, et al. Preoperative radiotherapy combined with total mesorectal excision for resectable rectal cancer. *N Engl J Med*. 2001;345(9):638–646.
35. Nagtegaal ID, Quirke P. What is the role for the circumferential margin in the modern treatment of rectal cancer? *J Clin Oncol*. 2008;26:303–312.

13

Molecular Testing of Gastrointestinal Neoplasms

Daniela S. Allende, MD, MBA and Amitabh Srivastava, MD

MOLECULAR TESTING OF COLORECTAL CARCINOMA

Although there are numerous esoteric tests that a molecular pathology laboratory may use on colorectal cancer (CRC) specimens, there are two tests that are the most common and important—assessment of mismatch repair (MMR) integrity and *RAS/RAF* mutational analysis (Tables 13.1 and 13.2). Assessment of MMR status serves two main functions. First, MMR testing is used to screen for Lynch syndrome. Second, it is used to aid oncologists in predicting response to certain chemotherapy drugs. MMR testing is accomplished in two complementary ways—microsatellite instability (MSI) testing by polymerase chain reaction (PCR) and immunohistochemistry (IHC) to assess protein expression of the key proteins involved in the MMR complex (MLH1, PMS2, MSH2, and MSH6). *RAS/RAF* mutational analysis is mainly used to help predict responsiveness to monoclonal anti–epidermal growth factor receptor (anti-EGFR) therapies (cetuximab and panitumumab) in the presence of distant metastases.

ASSESSMENT OF MISMATCH REPAIR FUNCTION

Lynch syndrome is the most common heritable CRC syndrome, accounting for 3% to 4% of colorectal carcinomas. In addition, patients with Lynch syndrome are at risk for an ever-expanding list of extracolonic malignancies, including endometrial, ovarian, urothelial, sebaceous, and upper gastrointestinal (GI), among others. So far, deleterious mutations have been identified in *MLH1, PMS2, MSH2*, and *MSH6* as well as deletion in *EPCAM*, which is upstream of *MSH2*. Rarely, Lynch syndrome is secondary to germline *MLH1* hypermethylation. All mutations are inherited in an autosomal dominant manner, and *MLH1* and *MSH2* mutations make up the vast majority of Lynch syndrome mutations. Consensus guidelines from organizations such as the National Comprehensive Cancer Network (NCCN), Evaluation of Genomic Applications in Practice and Prevention, and the US Multi-Society Task Force have, in an evidence-based manner, supported tissue-based screening methods (MSI testing by PCR or IHC for MMR protein expression) on a universal or near-universal basis.

Microsatellites are short, repetitive sequences of DNA, usually in noncoding regions of the genome, that are prone to mismatch errors during the process of DNA replication. A normally functioning MMR complex fixes these mismatches before they integrate into the genome. However, upon silencing of the MMR genes, usually through mutation or promoter methylation, these mismatches are not repaired and may perpetuate as mutations through DNA replication. In cells with high turnover, such as the gut epithelium, serial oncogenic mutations may occur, leading to neoplasia (i.e., the "mutator phenotype").

Polymerase Chain Reaction–Based Microsatellite Instability Testing

Microsatellite instability testing uses surrogate loci to identify the mutator phenotype, or high-frequency MSI (MSI-H), in a highly sensitive manner. An unstable locus is defined as one in which the tumor DNA contains a new, or mutant, allele compared with the host germline DNA. MSI testing is accomplished by performing the MSI assay on normal tissue and a relatively pure sample of tumor DNA (generally from formalin-fixed, paraffin-embedded tissue with ideally >50% tumor cellularity) and comparing the electropherograms of allele sizes (Fig. 13.1). The original "official" panel of microsatellites, known as the National Cancer Institute, or Bethesda, panel, recommended three dinucleotide repeats (D2S123, D5S346, and D17S250) and two mononucleotide repeats (BAT25 and BAT26); however, dinucleotide (e.g., CACACACACA…) repeats lead to a 5% to 10% rate of low-frequency MSI (MSI-L). MSI-L has been studied extensively, and currently, MSI-L CRCs have no different risk of Lynch syndrome and no different chemotherapy implications than microsatellite stable (MSS) tumors. A panel of mononucleotide repeats (e.g., poly-A) is preferred by most laboratories because it has virtually eliminated MSI-L phenotype and is likely more sensitive

TABLE 13.1
Mismatch Repair Function Terminology and Definitions

Mismatch Repair Function	Definition
MSI	Microsatellites are short, repetitive sequence of DNA, and MSI testing is typically reported as MSS, MSI-L, or MSI-H. Arbitrarily, MSI-H is defined as ≥30% of microsatellites tested showing instability, which is defined as generation of a new allele compared with normal.
MMR IHC	MMR IHC. Antibodies targeted at MLH1, MSH2, PMS2, and MSH6 are commercially available. Biologically, PMS2 expression requires intact MLH1 such that loss of PMS2 expression indicates either loss of PMS2 or, much more commonly, loss of MLH1. The same holds true for MSH6 expression depending on intact MSH2.
MLH1 promoter hypermethylation	The cause of the vast majority of sporadic (non-Lynch) MSI-H carcinomas. The *MLH1* gene is silenced by epigenetic methylation. Used as a test to exclude Lynch syndrome in patients with MSI-H MLH1 loss carcinoma; however, up to 5% of Lynch-associated colorectal cancers may harbor *MLH1* promoter hypermethylation.
BRAF V600E	Almost never mutated in Lynch syndrome–associated carcinomas and mutated in ≤75% of sporadic MLH1 loss MSI-H carcinomas. Therefore, finding *BRAF* mutation in MSI-H MLH1 loss carcinoma essentially excludes Lynch syndrome.
Lynch syndrome	Deleterious germline mutation in MMR genes *MLH1, MSH2, MSH6, PMS2*, or *EPCAM*. Rare cases of germline *MLH1* promoter hypermethylation also exist. Patients are most commonly affected by CRC and endometrial carcinoma (if female), but a minority also may have sebaceous (e.g., Muir-Torre), ovarian, upper, biliary, CNS, and genitourinary or urothelial neoplasia.
HNPCC	HNPCC is a clinical term for patients who fulfill Amsterdam criteria but germline mutation in Lynch syndrome gene is not detected.
Lynch-like syndrome	MMR-deficient tumors in which patients lack features of sporadic cancer (*MLH1* promoter hypermethylation or *BRAF* V600E mutation) and there is no demonstrable germline MMR mutation.
Familial colorectal cancer, type X	Patients fulfill Amsterdam criteria, but carcinomas are MMR proficient.

CNS, Central nervous system; *CRC*, colorectal cancer; *GI*, gastrointestinal; *HNPCC*, hereditary nonpolyposis colorectal carcinoma; *IHC*, immunohistochemistry; *MMR*, mismatch repair; *MSI*, microsatellite instability; *MSI-H*, high-frequency microsatellite instability; *MSI-L*, low-frequency microsatellite instability.

TABLE 13.2
Mismatch Repair Immunohistochemistry Interpretation

Protein Loss	Interpretation
MLH1	MLH1 loss; probably sporadic methylation; less likely germline mutation or somatic inactivation/mutation
PMS2	PMS2 or MLH1 loss; rule out MLH1 (even when isolated PMS2 loss)
MSH2	MSH2 loss; rule out germline *MSH2* mutation or somatic inactivation or mutation
MSH6	MSH6 or MSH2 loss; rule out MSH2 (even when isolated MSH6) or germline/somatic *MSH6* mutation

for detecting MSI-H, particularly those caused by *MSH6* mutations.

Microsatellite Instability High Carcinoma: Sporadic versus Lynch Syndrome

Microsatellite instability high almost always occurs as a result of one of three processes—Lynch syndrome (and constitutional MMR deficiency), *MLH1* promoter hypermethylation, or tumor-acquired somatic mutations in an *MMR* gene. Most commonly, an MSI-H carcinoma occurs because of epigenetic silencing of *MLH1* promoter. *MLH1* promoter hypermethylation is associated with the CpG island methylator phenotype (CIMP), the serrated pathway of colorectal carcinogenesis, and *BRAF* V600E mutations (~75% of cases), not Lynch syndrome. Therefore, assessment of *MLH1* promoter hypermethylation and/or *BRAF* mutation status is invaluable in helping determine whether a carcinoma with loss of MLH1 protein is sporadic or not. One must be aware, however, that *MLH1* promoter hypermethylation can occur in Lynch syndrome as the "second hit" of MMR gene silencing, more rarely, in the setting of germline *MLH1* methylation. *BRAF* V600E mutations are also reported in Lynch syndrome cancers but are about 1/10 as frequently as *MLH1* methylation. Thus, *BRAF* V600E mutations are more specific for sporadic carcinomas with MLH1 loss but less sensitive than *MLH1* promoter hypermethylation. Last, up to 50% of non-hypermethylated MSI-H carcinomas harbor tumor-acquired, rather than germline, MMR mutations. These "Lynch-like" or "tumor Lynch" carcinomas are difficult to identify. As few centers are testing tumors for somatic mutations in the *MMR* genes, Lynch-like carcinomas are usually a diagnosis of exclusion when no germline mutation is identified. However, a percentage of germline mutations are not detected with current methods.

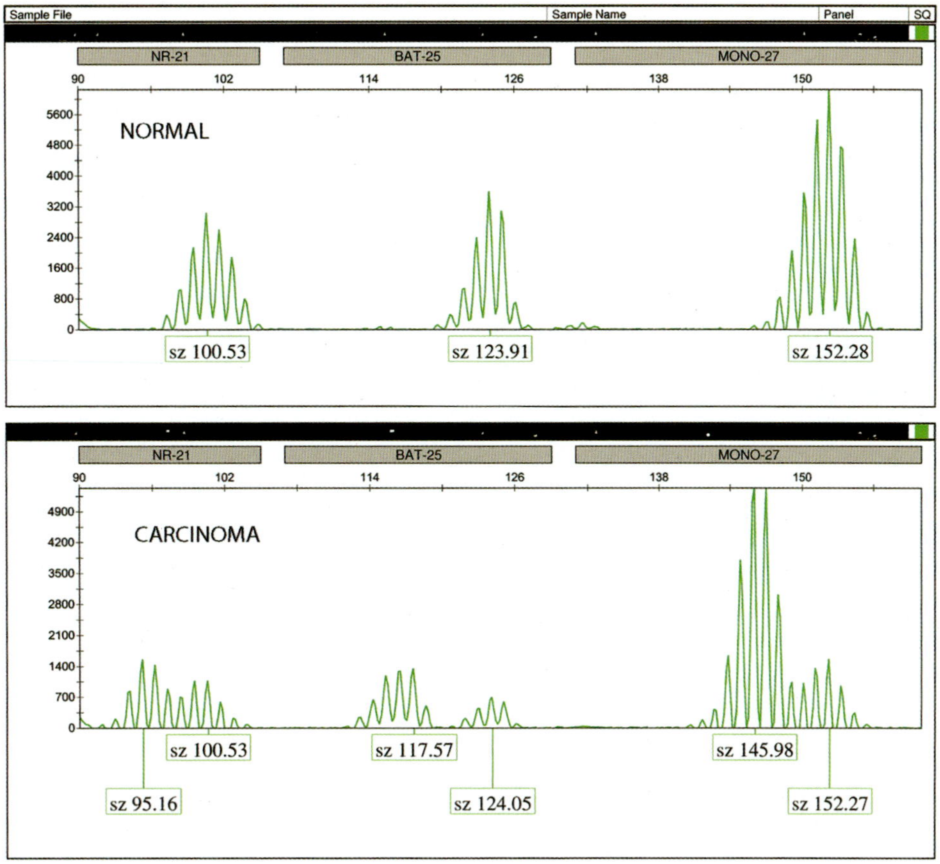

FIGURE 13.1

Electropherogram of a patient's three unstable alleles. An unstable allele is most readily recognized when comparing carcinoma microsatellite loci *(bottom)* with normal or non-neoplastic loci *(top)*. Mononucleotide microsatellites are characterized by groups of peaks, or stutter peaks, in which the tallest peak is assumed to be the patient's true allele size.

Therefore, these "Lynch-like" cases are almost certainly a mixture of undetected Lynch syndrome cancers and sporadic tumor-acquired mutations.

Mismatch Repair Immunohistochemistry

Most laboratories choose to screen for Lynch syndrome via IHC, mainly for logistical reasons: most have IHC capabilities, and most do not have PCR capabilities. Clinically, the tests are essentially equivalent such that an MSI-H by PCR is analogous to MMR protein loss of expression by IHC. In reality, the tests are complementary, and laboratories are best served when they can perform both assays because each has its strengths and weaknesses. In short, we prefer IHC when tissue is limited (e.g., biopsies, neoadjuvant therapy) and when rapid turnaround time is necessary. The immunostains are nuclear and essentially always have a built-in internal positive control. We prefer MSI testing on large, relatively pure samples of carcinoma (e.g., resections) because of its slightly better overall sensitivity and, counterintuitively, it is easier interpretation (see later). MSI-H results should be followed by IHC to determine the defected protein and help guide further testing.

The MMR stains may be difficult to interpret. Several studies have catalogued the relatively high observer variability in interpreting the DNA MMR immunostains. These studies usually conclude that some amount of experience is required to accurately interpret these stains or that all abnormal stains should be followed up by confirmatory MSI testing. In a perfect world, these IHC stains are "all or none," with no shades of gray, but the interpretation may be challenging in some cases. Some pearls to prevent misinterpreting DNA MMR IHC are as follows:

1. Gain experience and some background knowledge of the stains. Experience clearly plays a role in interpreting these stains such that "experts" are more reliable than those without experience. These are nuclear stains; no other cytologic location of immunoreactivity counts as positive (Figs. 13.2 and 13.3). Biopsies are easier to interpret than resection material, probably because of more consistent formalin fixation.
2. Understanding the protein pairings is quite helpful because the finding of one IHC stain may help confirm the result in its respective binding partner (Table 13.3). MMR proteins function as heterodimers. PMS2 requires

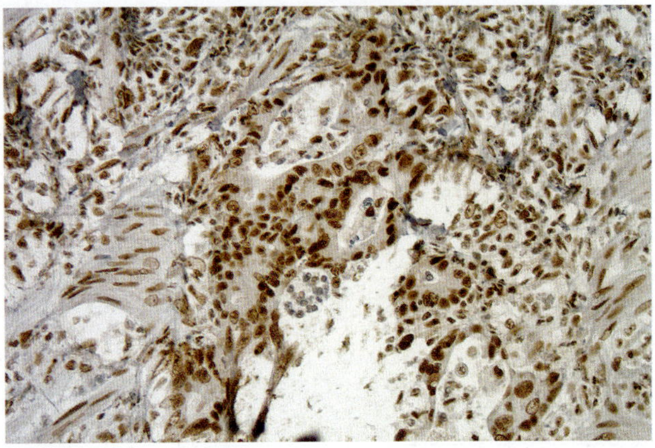

FIGURE 13.2

MLH1 immunostain that is positive in carcinoma and non-neoplastic nuclei.

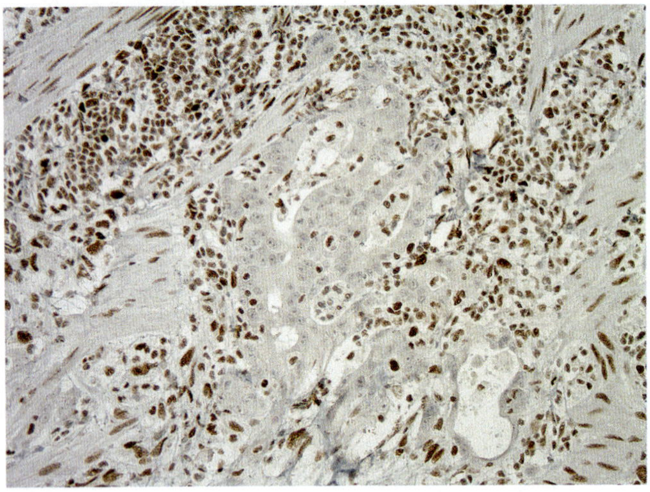

FIGURE 13.3

MSH2 immunostain that is lost in carcinoma nuclei but retained in tumor infiltrating lymphocytes as well as background non-neoplastic stromal cells.

binding by MLH1 for its stability within the nucleus, and MSH6 requires MSH2 as its binding partner such that loss of MLH1 shows concomitant loss of PMS2, and loss of MSH2 shows loss of MSH6. However, "isolated" loss of PMS2 and MSH6 are valid results. Thus, intact IHC results for PMS2 and MSH6 alone confirm that all four MMR proteins are intact in nearly all cases while reducing testing costs. We often screen with only these two IHC stains on small biopsies when MSI results would be of uncertain reliability.

3. Do not interpret the staining in tumor cells without adjacent positive internal control results. False interpretation of lost protein expression may occur if one examines areas without positive internal controls (e.g., stromal cells, lymphocytes, endothelial cells. A rare exception is constitutional MMR deficiency (discussed later).
4. Beware of overly aggressive antigen retrieval. Overstained slides may give the impression of falsely retained protein expression. In our hands and others', this often manifests as cytoplasmic staining with a perinuclear "rim" of staining (Fig. 13.4).

TABLE 13.3

Colorectal Cancer Biomarkers and Therapeutic Implications

	Actionable Result	Frequency (%)	Implication
MMR status	MSI-H or loss of IHC expression	15–20	Lack of benefit with 5-FU–based chemotherapy Benefit from PD-1 blockade
KRAS/ NRAS	Activating mutations in exon 2 (codons 12 and 13), exon 3 (codons 59 and 61), and exon 4 (codons 117 and 146)	50–60	Lack of benefit from anti-EGFR antibody therapy
BRAF	V600E mutation	8–10	Lack of benefit from anti-EGFR antibody therapy
CDX2	Loss of IHC expression	<5	Benefit from conventional chemotherapy

EGFR, epidermal growth factor receptor; *5-FU*, 5-Fluorouracil; *IHC*, immunohistochemistry; *MSI-H*, high-frequency microsatellite instability; *PD-1*, programmed death 1.

5. The stains may be patchy, especially MSH6 and after radiation therapy (Fig. 13.5). Remember, the vast majority of true loss of expression occurs in every tumor cell.
6. Do not interpret IHC stains as "positive" or "negative" because these terms can lead to confusion or misinterpretation. "Intact" expression and "loss" of expression are more clear and accurate terms.
7. Lynch syndrome–associated carcinomas, rarely, if ever, arise from sessile serrated polyps/adenomas; therefore, testing of these lesions is extremely low yield when screening for Lynch syndrome.

Much rarer than Lynch syndrome is so-called constitutional MMR deficiency in which an individual inherits two mutations in an *MMR* gene rather than one mutation in conventional Lynch syndrome. These patients are characterized by early-onset malignancies, including hematologic and central nervous system tumors as well as Lynch syndrome–associated neoplasms. Because both alleles of a particular MMR gene are affected, immunostains for the particular gene product protein are likely to be lost in both the neoplasm and the background non-neoplastic tissue, and one always should consider constitutional MMR deficiency before deciding that the immunostain was technically unsatisfactory (Fig. 13.6).

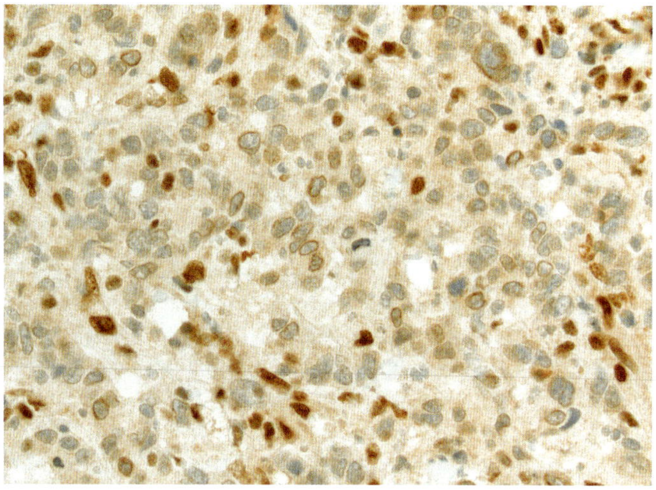

FIGURE 13.4

MLH1 immunostain with artifactual nuclear membrane staining in a cancer with MLH1 promoter hypermethylation. Intact protein expression is most reliably determined when diffuse nuclear staining is identified.

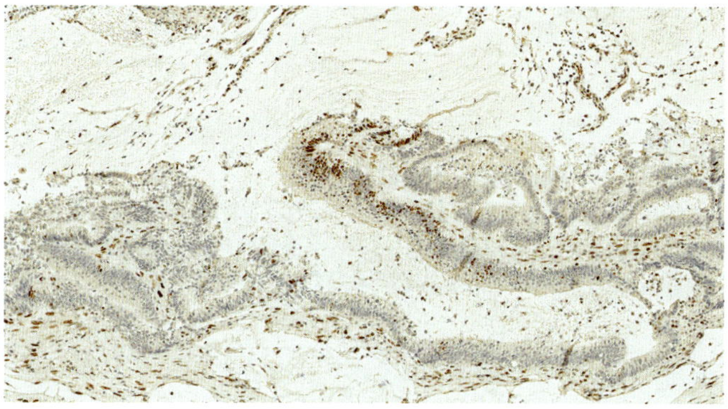

FIGURE 13.5

MSH6 immunostain is notoriously patchy, particularly after chemoradiotherapy. If there is even focal staining, as in this case, the mismatch repair expression should not be interpreted as lost.

Microsatellite instability testing also has clinical relevance in helping oncologists predict chemoresponsiveness. Initially, oncologists used MMR status to help with stage II carcinomas in which there is only a marginal (~5%) benefit with adjuvant chemotherapy. For years, it has been known that MSI-H carcinomas do not respond to 5-fluorouracil (5-FU) chemotherapy, and oncologists often forgo 5-FU–based chemotherapy in "high-risk" stage II colon cancers (i.e., those with poor differentiation, angiolymphatic invasion, perineural invasion, invasion of serosa or another organ, perforation) that are MMR deficient. More recently, in a phase 2 study of patients with metastatic carcinoma, led by researchers at Johns Hopkins University, it was reported that clinical benefit of pembrolizumab, an anti–programmed death 1 (anti–PD-1) immune checkpoint inhibitor, was predicted by the tumor's MMR status; the reported data supported the hypothesis that MMR deficient tumors are more responsive to PD-1 blockade than MMR proficient tumors. These results were followed-up in 2017 with a report of 86 patients with 12 different types of solid tumor malignancies that had progressed on conventional

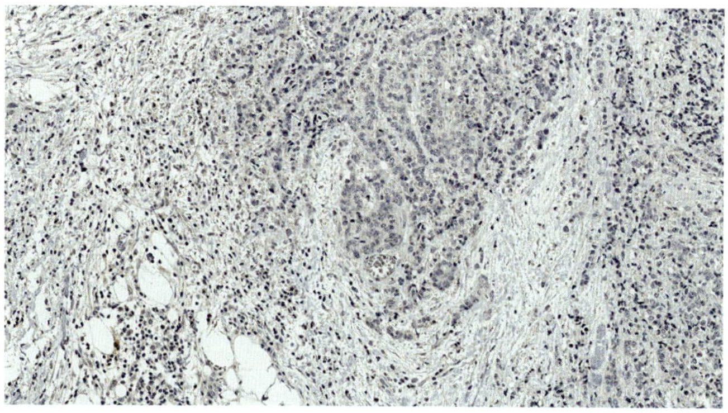

FIGURE 13.6

PMS2 immunostain that was originally interpreted as technically unsatisfactory because internal control tissue failed to stain. However, the patient had biallelic *PMS2* mutation such that internal control also did not express the protein product.

therapies, nearly half of whom had Lynch syndrome. Of these 86 patients, 46 (53%) had an objective response to pembrolizumab, including 18 (21%) with a complete response. These results, published in *Science*, led to the Food and Drug Administration (FDA) approval of pembrolizumab for MMR-deficient solid tumors (not just colorectal carcinoma) in May 2017. Type of testing—MSI versus IHC—is not specified by the FDA; therefore, the two methods should be viewed as equivalent, and principles in test selection and interpretation outlined in the preceding paragraphs still apply. Given that about 5% of solid tumors are MMR deficient, MMR testing is expected to play an expanded role in cancer care in the future. Last, preliminary data have shown that stage II CDX2-negative (by IHC) CRCs, although quite uncommon at about 5% of cases, may be another group of stage II carcinomas that would benefit from chemotherapy.

RAS, Extended *RAS*, and *BRAF* Testing

Anti-EGFR medications, cetuximab and panitumumab, are FDA approved for the treatment of patients with colorectal carcinoma with distant metastasis (i.e., stage IV). Although the original trials discovered that EGFR immunohistochemical detection did not predict response to therapy, the investigators quickly found that activating mutations in *KRAS* codons 12/13 (exon 2) were excellent predictors of nonresponse, prompting consensus recommendations that *KRAS* 12/13 should be tested and wild-type before initiating costly (~$80,000) and potentially toxic (skin rash) anti-EGFR therapies. Cetuximab and panitumumab work as competitive inhibitors of ligand binding and prevent receptor activation. It therefore stands to reason that activating mutations in *RAS* gene would not be affected by attempts at ligand-based inhibition. Interestingly, other EGFR inhibitors, aimed at the tyrosine kinase domain, are not effective against colorectal carcinoma, even those that are *RAS* wild type.

KRAS codon 12/13 mutations occur in about 40% of colorectal carcinomas. More recently, additional activating mutations in *KRAS* and *NRAS* have been shown to predict nonresponse to anti-EGFR monoclonal antibodies. These mutations, collectively known as extended *RAS* mutations, account for an additional 10% to 20% of patients. Current guidelines (American Society of Clinical Oncology, NCCN) call for extended *RAS* testing before anti-EGFR therapy with cetuximab or panitumumab. Codons 12, 13, 59, 61, 117, and 146 on both *KRAS* and *NRAS* genes are recommended on all stage IV tumors. Further, emerging data have suggested that patients with exon 2– or non–exon 2–activating mutations in *KRAS* or *NRAS* may be harmed by treatment with cetuximab or panitumumab, making timely extended *RAS* testing all the more important.

The utility of *BRAF* V600E mutation testing in terms of prediction of response to anti-EGFR therapy continues to evolve. *BRAF*-mutated tumors, particularly those that are MSS are difficult to study for two reasons: (1) *BRAF* mutations are uncommon in metastatic colorectal carcinoma, accounting for fewer than 10% of tumors, and (2) *BRAF* V600E mutation in combination with MSS phenotype engenders a significantly worse prognosis than *BRAF* wild-type tumors, so statistical survival benefit often translate to little or no clinical benefit. All that said, the pendulum appears to be swinging in the oncology community to use the identification of a *BRAF* V600E mutation in a similar manner as *RAS* testing (i.e., a *BRAF* mutation precludes anti-EGFR antibody therapy). For unknown reasons, BRAF inhibitor–based therapies are not effective against *BRAF*-mutated carcinomas.

Future Directions of Molecular Testing in Colorectal Carcinoma

Molecular oncology testing in colorectal carcinoma will become increasingly important in the future, particularly as cost per test decreases and throughput increases. Companion diagnostics (i.e., biomarker testing to predict response to chemotherapy) is expected to bear the brunt of the expanded testing focus. Next-generation sequencing (NGS), also known as deep sequencing or massive parallel sequencing, is the technology leading the charge. It allows for the relatively rapid and relatively low cost sequencing of multiple clinically relevant genes that may guide therapy or aid in diagnosis. For example, our institution performs NGS on all metastatic colorectal carcinomas to assess for *KRAS* and *NRAS* 12, 13, 61, 117, and 146 as well as *BRAF* codon 600 as a single multiplex assay rather than nine separate tests by Sanger sequencing, and this is just the tip of the iceberg. Similar technology is being applied to hereditary cancer syndrome diagnostics such as in patients with hereditary polyposis. A patient with a clinically determined polyposis can undergo testing for peripheral blood-based "polyposis" panel that searches for germline mutations in key polyposis genes such as *APC, MUTYH, PTEN, SMAD4, BMPR1A*, and *STK11*.

HER-2 IN COLORECTAL CARCINOMA

HER2 molecular alterations are observed in up 2 % of colorectal cancers and up to 5 % the *Kras* wild-type tumors (1). FDA has not yet approved anti-HER2 therapy for colorectal carcinoma and most cases pathologists order the test in the metastatic setting and at the request of the clinician. That said, NCCN guidelines (2021) colon cancer recommend testing all metastatic colon cancers for HER2 (with the exception of those that are known to be RAS/RAF Mutant) (2). Testing the primary tumor or metastases is appropriate. To keep in mind when interpreting the studies, landmark studies in the field (HERACLES, MyPathway and Destiny) have used different definitions of Her 2 positivity adding to the complexity of interpreting the stain (4–6).

HER2 TESTING IN UPPER GASTROINTESTINAL TRACT (ESOPHAGEAL, GASTRIC, AND GASTROESOPHAGEAL JUNCTION) ADENOCARCINOMA

Background and Rationale

Human epidermal growth factor receptor 2 (HER2), also known as *CerbB-2* and *ERBB2* is a proto-oncogene located on chromosome 17q21 that encodes for a transmembrane protein with tyrosine kinase activity. The receptor has an extracellular ligand-binding site, a transmembrane segment, and an intracellular domain. With binding of the ligands to the extracellular domains, HER2 protein undergoes dimerization and transphosphorylation of the intracellular domain. This initiates a variety of signaling pathways, especially mitogen-activated protein kinase (MAPK), phosphatidylinositol-4,5-biphosphate 3-kinase (PI3K), and protein kinase C (PKC) pathways, leading to cell proliferation, differentiation, angiogenesis, and invasion. Although amplification of *HER2* and overexpression of its product has been extensively investigated in breast cancer, many studies have now demonstrated role of HER2 in other malignancies, especially gastric and gastroesophageal junction (GEJ) cancers.

The frequency of HER2 overexpression in gastric and gastroesophageal adenocarcinoma ranges from 4.4% to 53.4%, with a mean of 17.9%. A recent meta-analysis confirmed that HER2-positive status is associated with decreased survival and adverse clinicopathologic features, such as serosal invasion, metastases, and higher stage of disease. As a result, analogous to HER2-positive breast cancer, upper GI adenocarcinomas can also be targeted with trastuzumab, a monoclonal antibody directed against HER2. Trastuzumab prevents dimerization of HER2, stimulates endocytosis, and cell-mediated immunity, and inhibits angiogenesis. In the trastuzumab for Gastric Cancer (ToGA) trial, 594 patients with HER2-positive (defined as 3+ expression by IHC or amplification by fluorescence in situ hybridization [FISH]) or *HER2 (ERBB2)*:CEP17 ratio ≥2) advanced gastric and GEJ adenocarcinoma were randomized to standard chemotherapy and trastuzumab or chemotherapy alone. Patients receiving trastuzumab had a significantly longer median overall survival (13.8 vs 11.1 months), progression-free survival (6.7 vs 5.5 months), and response rate (47% vs 35%), when the tumors were either 3+ by IHC or 2+ by IHC and positive FISH results (*HER2*:Chr17 ratio >2). Based on these results, the FDA has approved the use of trastuzumab for the treatment of patients with metastatic gastric, esophageal, and GEJ adenocarcinomas that meet the ToGA inclusion criteria. The European Medicines Agency has approved trastuzumab for HER2 overexpression as defined by IHC2+ and a confirmatory FISH result or by an IHC3+ result.

HER2 Testing Methods and Scoring

National Comprehensive Cancer Network Clinical Practice Guidelines in Oncology recommend assessment of HER2 expression by IHC and/or gene amplification using FISH or other in situ hybridization assays (silver-enhanced in situ hybridization or chromogenic in situ hybridization). FISH is considered as the gold standard; however, given the cost-effectiveness of IHC and high concordance between FISH and IHC-positive result, IHC is the preferred method in most laboratories. To standardize the testing methodology and scoring, the College of American Pathologists (CAP), American Society for Clinical Pathology, and American Society of Clinical Oncology recently published *HER2* testing guideline for gastroesophageal adenocarcinoma (see Fig. 13.7).

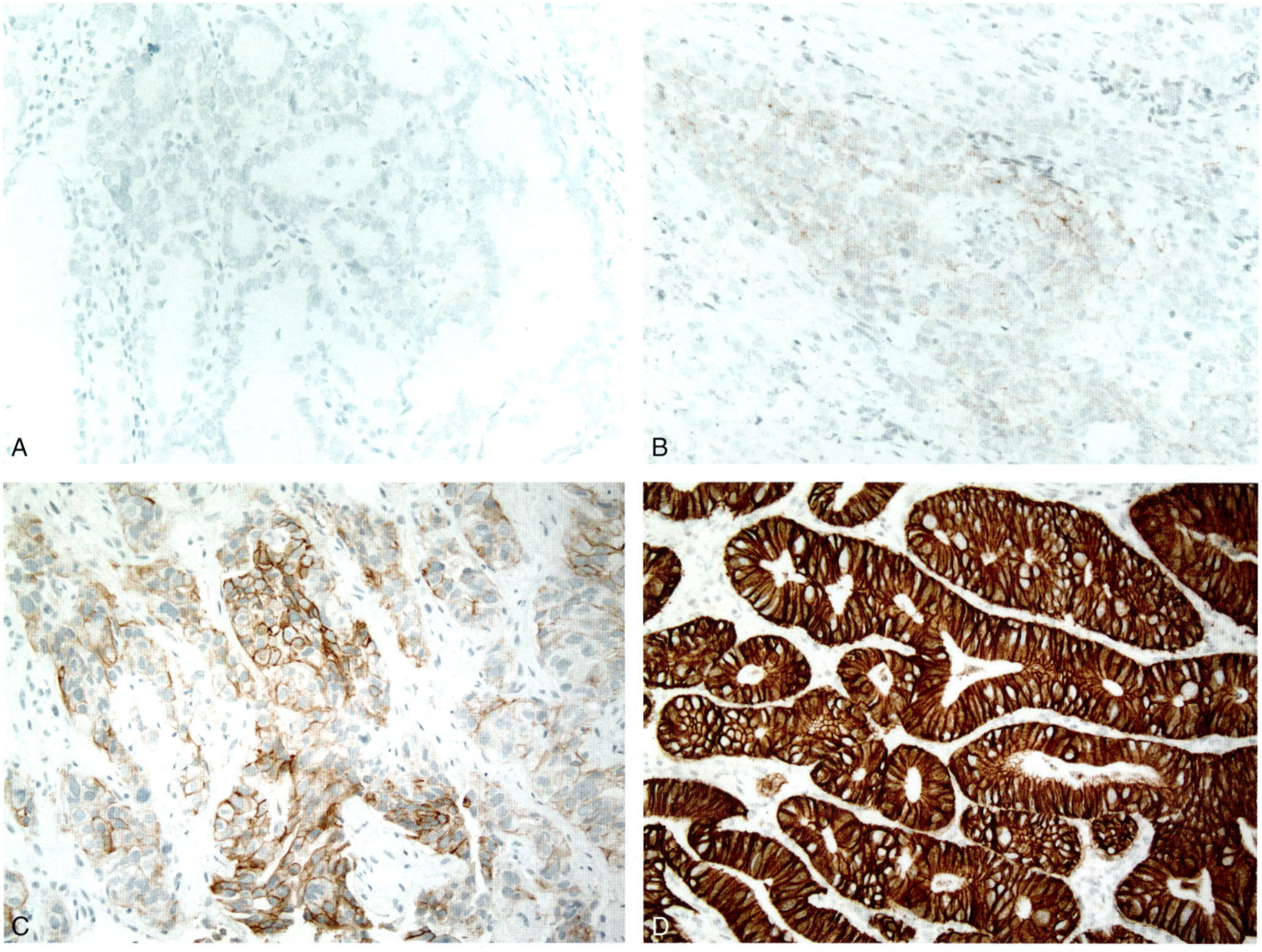

FIGURE 13.7

HER2 immunohistochemistry (IHC). **A**, HER2-negative (IHC 0) staining with complete lack of staining within the tumor cells. (400× magnification). **B**, HER2-negative (IHC 1+) staining wherein the tumor cells show faint or barely perceptible membranous reactivity (400× magnification). **C**, Equivocal HER2 (IHC 2+) staining with weak to moderate, complete, basolateral, and lateral membranous reactivity within the tumor cells (100× magnification). **D**, Positive (IHC 3+) IHC with strong, complete basolateral and lateral membranous reactivity in the tumor cells (100× magnification).

Specimen Type

The specimen of choice is formalin-fixed paraffin-embedded biopsy or resection specimen that has been obtained from the primary or metastatic site before initiation of therapy. In a series of 115 tumors tested for HER2, there was 92.9 % concordance between results of biopsy and resection specimens. Studies testing HER2 status in paired samples from primary tumor and metastatic organs and synchronous metastatic sites have reported concordance rates ranging from 87.5 % to 98.5 %, suggesting that tissue from metastatic tumor is an acceptable alternative for HER2 status evaluation.

Although there are no data on the impact of cold ischemia time (time between procurement of biopsy or resection and tissue fixation) and fixation time on HER2 status in GI cancers, based on information derived from breast cancer literature, it has been suggested that the specimen should be rapidly (ideally within 1 hour) placed in a fixative solution (10 % neutral buffered formalin), and the fixation time should be 6 to 72 hours. The thickness of the section can affect accurate interpretation. Thicker sections can lead to the presence of overlapping nuclei and difficulties in probe hybridization. Thinner sections can lead to fewer cells with adequate signals, thus resulting in undersampling of the tumor. Four-micron-thick paraffin sections are preferred unless specified differently by commercially available kits.

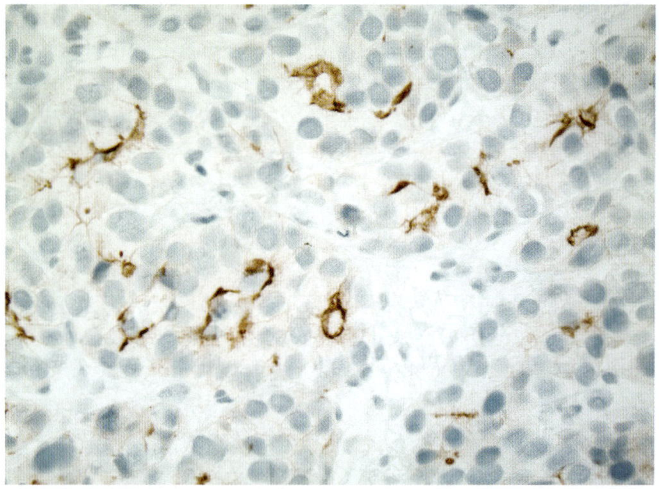

FIGURE 13.8

False-positive HER2 staining by immunohistochemistry. The tumor cells show luminal staining, which should not be interpreted for HER2 scoring.

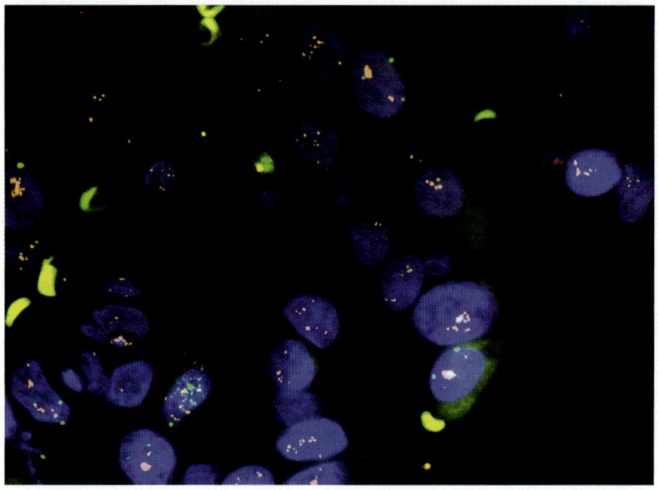

FIGURE 13.9

HER2 fluorescence in situ hybridization. An example of amplified HER2 with *HER2*:CEP17 ratio of 2.9. HER2 signals are represented in red, and CEP17 signals are represented in *green*.

Immunohistochemistry

The two FDA-approved kits that are routinely used in most laboratories include HercepTest kit (Dako) and PATHWAY anti-HER2/neu rabbit monoclonal antibody (clone 4B5, Ventana Medical Systems). Both these antibodies target the intracellular domain of HER2 protein.

The scoring system proposed by Hofmann et al has been approved by the CAPs and FDA. Figure 13.7 outlines the HER2 IHC scoring criteria for upper GI cancers. Cases with membranous staining in fewer than 10 % of tumor cells (resection), weak or barely discernible staining requiring high magnification (40× objective) to visualize the staining (IHC 1+), or complete lack of staining (IHC 0), are scored as HER2 negative (Figs. 13.8A and 13.8B). Cases with weak to moderate complete, basolateral to lateral membranous staining in at least 10 % of cells (resections) or in at least a single tumor cluster (biopsies) are scored as IHC 2+ or equivocal (Fig. 13.8C). In most instances, these cases require an intermediate magnification (10× or 20× objective) to confirm membranous immunoreactivity.

Positive staining (IHC 3+) is usually readily visible at low magnification (2× to 4× objective) and requires strong, complete basolateral or lateral membranous staining in at least 10 % of invasive adenocarcinoma cells in resection specimens (Fig. 13.8D). This is in contrast to breast carcinoma in which HER2 positivity is in the form of complete, circumferential membranous staining. In a biopsy specimen, strong staining in at least a single tumor cluster (defined as five or more cells) is scored as positive. The prevalence of IHC-positive HER2 cases is quite variable and depends on the morphologic subtype and location of adenocarcinoma. The rate of HER2 positivity is higher for intestinal-type adenocarcinomas (3 %–23.5 %) than diffuse type gastric cancers (0 %–6 %). GEJ adenocarcinomas are more frequently positive than distal gastric cancers.

False-positive staining can be seen in areas with intestinal metaplasia, adjacent to mucosal ulcers, and in dysplastic foci. Luminal surface staining in the absence of lateral or basal staining should be interpreted as negative (IHC 0). Care should be taken when interpreting tissue with thermal or crush artifact, areas of necrosis, and staining restricted to the edges of biopsy fragments (edge artifact; Fig. 13.9).

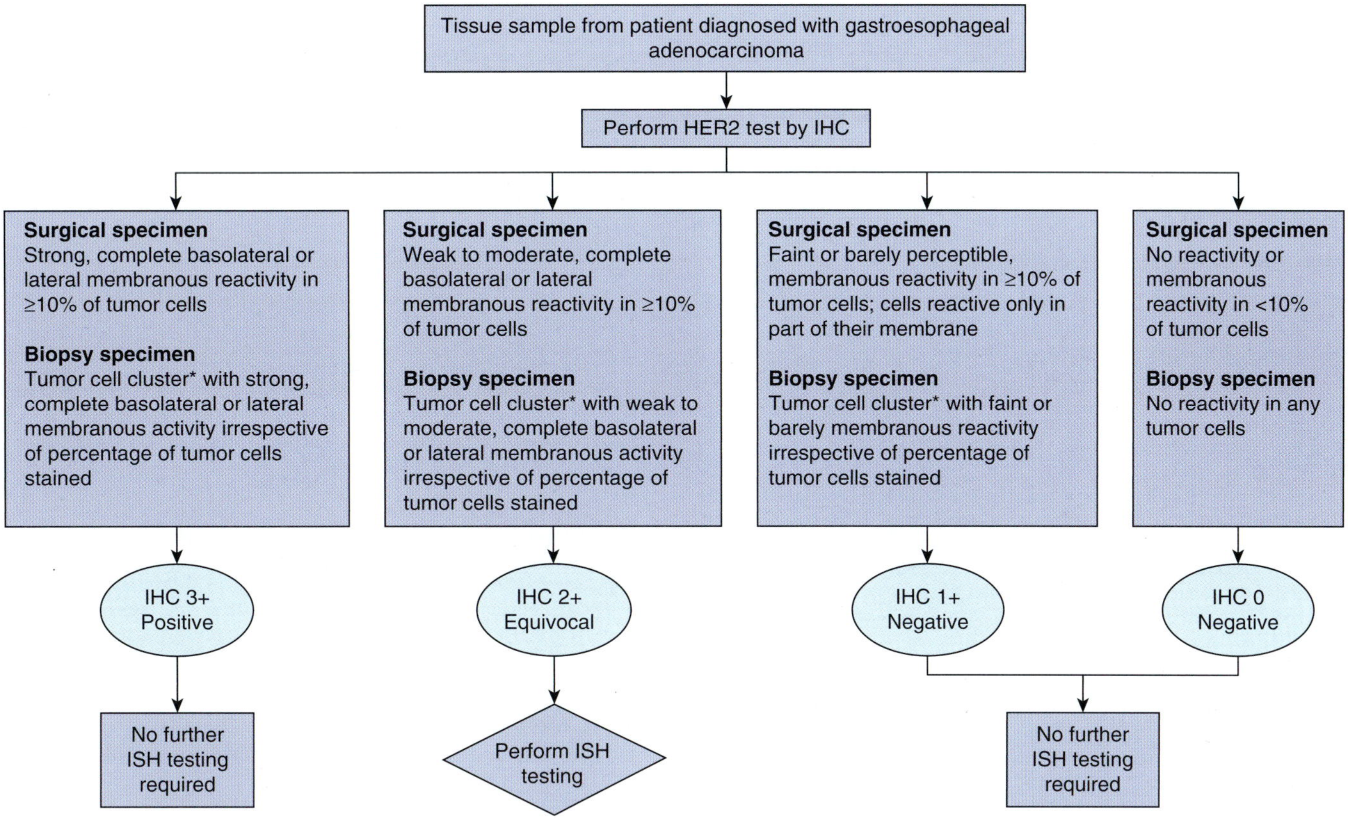

FIGURE 13.10

HER2 testing algorithm based on recommendations by College of American Pathologists (CAP), American Society for Clinical Pathology (ASCP), and American Society of Clinical Oncology (ASCO). * Tumor cell clusters is defined as ≥ 5 neoplastic cells. *IHC*, Immunohistochemistry; *ISH*, in situ hybridization. (Adapted with permission from CAP, ASCP, and ASCO guidelines.)

In Situ Hybridization

Fluorescence in situ hybridization is considered as the gold standard test for evaluating *HER2* amplification. It is indicated in all cases with a 2+ HER2 IHC score. The test can be performed either by using a *HER2* probe or dual *HER2* and centromere (CEP17) probes. At least 20 nonoverlapping tumor cell nuclei are evaluated at 20× magnification for *HER2* and CEP17 probe signal enumeration. A ratio of *HER2* signal to CEP17 of 2.0 or greater is considered positive (Fig. 13.10), and a ratio of *HER2* signal to CEP17 less than 2.0 is considered negative.

Other in situ hybridization techniques that use bright-field microscopy include chromogenic in situ hybridization and silver-enhanced in situ hybridization. These techniques allow for better visualization of tumor morphology and easy enumeration in cases with tumor heterogeneity.

One of the pitfalls regarding FISH interpretation is that chromosome 17 polysomy (defined in ToGA trial as three or more signals per nuclei) or amplification of the centromeric region of chromosome 17 can lead to increased CEP17 signals. In patients who have increased *HER2* signals, this phenomenon can result in a *HER2*:CEP17 ratio of less than 2 and misclassification of *HER2* status as nonamplified. In the ToGA trial, chromosome 17 polysomy was observed in 4.1% cases, but other investigators have found this in up to 16% of gastric cancers. In these cases, *HER2* gene copy number can be used to determine trastuzumab eligibility: presence of more than 6 *HER2* signals/nuclei is interpreted as positive for HER2 amplification, fewer than four *HER2* signals/nuclei is interpreted as negative for *HER2* amplification, and four to six *HER2* signals/nuclei are interpreted as an equivocal result.

PD-1/PDL-1 In Esophageal And Gastric Carcinomas

Bases on published data (1), FDA granted approval for the use of Pembrolizumab in patients with locally advanced, recurrent or metastatic squamous cell carcinoma of the esophagus or adenocarcinoma of the gastroesophageal junction or gastric. Subsequent KEYNOTE studies also supported this practice. The drug is indicated if the tumors expresses PDL-1 on immunohistochemistry (clone 22C3) with a combine positive score (CPS) equal or greater than 10 for squamous carcinoma and equal or greater than 1 for adenocarcinomas (2). The CPS is calculated based on the number of PDL-1 positive cells (tumor, lymphocytes, histiocytes) divided by total number of viable tumor cells, then multiplied by 100%. Studies have shown conflicting results on the concordance between biopsy and resection results when using different clones (3–5). Recent publications suggest that EBV+ or MSI gastric cancers are more likely to express PD-L1 (6). Pathologists should be aware that chemotherapy and radiation may decrease PDL-1 immunohistochemical expression (7).

SUGGESTED READINGS

Molecular Testing of Colorectal Carcinoma

1. Pai RK, Pai RK. A practical approach to the evaluation of gastrointestinal tract carcinomas for Lynch syndrome. *Am J Surg Pathol*. 2016;40:e17–e34.
2. Vasen HF, Watson P, Mecklin JP, et al. New clinical criteria for hereditary nonpolyposis colorectal cancer (HNPCC, Lynch syndrome) proposed by the International Collaborative group on HNPCC. *Gastroenterology*. 1999;116:1453–1456.
3. Umar A, Boland CR, Terdiman JP, et al. Revised Bethesda Guidelines for hereditary nonpolyposis colorectal cancer (Lynch syndrome) and microsatellite instability. *J Natl Cancer Inst*. 2004;96:261–268.
4. Vasen HFA, Blanco I, Aktan-Collan K, et al. Revised guidelines for the clinical management of Lynch syndrome (HNPCC): recommendations by a group of European experts. *Gut*. 2013;62:812–823.
5. Evaluation of Genomic Applications in Practice and Prevention (EGAPP) Working Group. Recommendations from the EGAPP Working Group: genetic testing strategies in newly diagnosed individuals with colorectal cancer aimed at reducing morbidity and mortality from Lynch syndrome in relatives. *Genet Med*. 2009;11:35–41.
6. Palomaki GE, McClain MR, Melillo S, et al. EGAPP supplementary evidence review: DNA testing strategies aimed at reducing morbidity and mortality from Lynch syndrome. *Genet Med*. 2009;11:42–65.
7. Parsons MT, Buchanan DD, Thompson B, et al. Correlation of tumour BRAF mutations and MLH1 methylation with germline mismatch repair (MMR) gene mutation status: a literature review assessing utility of tumour features for MMR variant classification. *J Med Genet*. 2012;49:151–157.
8. Allegra CJ, Jessup JM, Somerfield MR, et al. American Society of Clinical Oncology provisional clinical opinion: testing for KRAS gene mutations in patients with metastatic colorectal carcinoma to predict response to anti-epidermal growth factor receptor monoclonal antibody therapy. *J Clin Oncol*. 2009;27:2091–2096.
9. Allegra CJ, Rumble RB, Hamilton SR, et al. Extended RAS gene mutation testing in metastatic colorectal carcinoma to predict response to anti-epidermal growth factor receptor monoclonal antibody therapy: American Society of Clinical Oncology Provisional Clinical Opinion Update 2015. *J Clin Oncol*. 2016;34:179–185.
10. Dalerba P, Sahoo D, Paik S, et al. CDX2 as a prognostic biomarker in stage II and stage III colon cancer. *N Engl J Med*. 2016;374:211–222.
11. Le DT, Uram JN, Wang H, et al. PD-1 Blockade in tumors with mismatch-repair deficiency. *N Engl J Med*. 2015;372:2509–2520.
12. Hampel H, Frankel WL, Martin E, et al. Feasibility of screening for Lynch syndrome among patients with colorectal cancer. *J Clin Oncol*. 2008;26:5783–5788.
13. Hampel H, Frankel WL, Martin E, et al. Screening for the Lynch syndrome (hereditary nonpolyposis colorectal cancer). *N Engl J Med*. 2005;352:1851–1860.
14. Giardiello FM, Allen JI, Axilbund JE, et al. Guidelines on genetic evaluation and management of Lynch syndrome: a consensus statement by the US Multi-society Task Force on colorectal cancer. *Am J Gastroenterol*. 2014;109:1159–1179.
15. Haraldsdottir S, Hampel H, Tomsic J, et al. Colon and endometrial cancers with mismatch repair deficiency can arise from somatic, rather than germline, mutations. *Gastroenterology*. 2014;147 1308–1316.e1.
16. Pritchard CC, Smith C, Salipante SJ, et al. ColoSeq provides comprehensive lynch and polyposis syndrome mutational analysis using massively parallel sequencing. *J Mol Diagn*. 2012;14:357–366.
17. Douillard J-Y, Oliner KS, Siena S, et al. Panitumumab-FOLFOX4 treatment and RAS mutations in colorectal cancer. *N Engl J Med*. 2013;369:1023–1034.
18. National Comprehensive Cancer Network. Colon Cancer (version 2. 2016). https://www.nccn.org/professionals/physician_gls/pdf/colon.pdf
19. Le DT, Durham J, Smith KN, et al. Mismatch-repair deficiency predicts response of solid tumors to PD-1 blockade. *Science*. 2017 28;357(6349):409–413.

HER-2 in Colorectal Carcinoma

20. Richman SD, Southward K, Chambers P, et al. HER2 overexpression and amplification as a potential therapeutic target in colorectal cancer: analysis of 3256 patients enrolled in the QUASAR, FOCUS and PICCOLO colorectal cancer trials. *J Pathol*. 2016;238 (4):562–570.
21. NCCN Clinical Practice Guidelines in Oncology: Colon Cancer (Version 2.2021). Available at: https://www.nccn.org/professionals/physician_gls/pdf/colon.pdf.
22. Valtorta E, Martino C, Sartore-Bianchi A, et al. Assessment of a HER2 scoring system for colorectal cancer: results from a validation study. *Mod Pathol*. 2015;28(11):1481–1491.
23. Sartore-Bianchi A, Trusolino L, Martino C, et al. Dual-targeted therapy with trastuzumab and lapatinib in treatment-refractory, KRAS codon 12/13 wild-type, HER2-positive metastatic colorectal cancer (HERACLES): a proof-of-concept, multicentre, open-label, phase 2 trial. *The Lancet Oncology*. 2016;17:738–746.
24. Meric-Bernstam F, Hurwitz H, Raghav KPS, et al. Pertuzumab plus trastuzumab for HER2-amplified metastatic colorectal cancer (MyPathway): an updated report from a multicentre, openlabel, phase 2a, multiple basket study. *The Lancet Oncology*. 2019;20: 518–530.
25. Siena S, Di Bartolomeo M, Raghav K, et al. Trastuzumab deruxtecan (DS-8201) in patients with HER2-expressing metastatic colorectal cancer (DESTINY-CRC01): a multicentre, open-label, phase 2 trial. *Lancet Oncol*. 2021 Jun;22(6):779–789.

HER2 Testing in Upper Gastrointestinal Tract (Esophageal, Gastric, and Gastroesophageal junction) Adenocarcinoma

26. Abrahao-Machado LF, Scapulatempo-Neto C. HER2 testing in gastric cancer: an update. *World J Gastroenterol*. 2016;22: 4619–4625.
27. Bang Y-J, Van Cutsem E, Feyereislova A, et al. Trastuzumab in combination with chemotherapy versus chemotherapy alone for treatment of HER2-positive advanced gastric or gastro-oesophageal junction cancer (ToGA): a phase 3, open-label, randomised controlled trial. *Lancet*. 2010;376:687–697.
28. Bozzetti C, Negri FV, Lagrasta CA, et al. Comparison of HER2 status in primary and paired metastatic sites of gastric carcinoma. *Br J Cancer*. 2011;104:1372–1376.
29. Hayes DF, Thor AD, Dressler LG, et al. HER2 and response to paclitaxel in node-positive breast cancer. *N Engl J Med*. 2007;357:1496–1506.
30. Jørgensen JT, Hersom M. HER2 as a prognostic marker in gastric cancer—a systematic analysis of data from the literature. *J Cancer*. 2012;3:137–144.
31. Moasser MM. Targeting the function of the HER2 oncogene in human cancer therapeutics. *Oncogene*. 2007;26:6577–6592.
32. Okines AFC, Thompson LC, Cunningham D, et al. Effect of HER2 on prognosis and benefit from peri-operative chemotherapy in early oesophago-gastric adenocarcinoma in the MAGIC trial. *Ann Oncol*. 2013;24:1253–1261.
33. Qiu Z, Sun W, Zhou C, et al. HER2 expression variability between primary gastric cancers and corresponding lymph node metastases. *Hepatogastroenterology*. 2015;62:231–233.
34. Yan M, Schwaederle M, Arguello D, et al. HER2 expression status in diverse cancers: review of results from 37,992 patients. *Cancer Metastasis Rev*. 2015;34:157–164.
35. European Medicines Agency. Herceptin. http://www.ema.europa.eu/ema/index.jsp?curl=pages/medicines/human/medicines/000278/human_med_000818.jsp&mid=WC0b01ac058001d124
36. Bartley AN, Washington K, Ventura CB, et al. HER2 testing and clinical decision making in gastroesophageal adenocarcinoma: guideline from the College of American Pathologists, American

Society for Clinical Pathology and the American Society of Clinical Oncology [published online ahead of print November 14, 2016]. *Arch Pathol Lab Med*. 2016;146(6):647–669.

37. Hofmann M, Stoss O, Shi D, et al. Assessment of a HER2 scoring system for gastric cancer: results from a validation study. *Histopathology*. 2008;52(7):797–805.

PD-1/PDL-1 in Esophageal and Gastric Carcinomas

38. Kojima T, Shah MA, Muro K, et al. KEYNOTE-181 Investigators. Randomized Phase III KEYNOTE-181 Study of Pembrolizumab Versus Chemotherapy in Advanced Esophageal Cancer. *J Clin Oncol*. 2020;38(35):4138–4148.
39. Paver EC, Cooper WA, Colebatch AJ, et al. Programmed death ligand-1 (PD-L1) as a predictive marker for immunotherapy in solid tumours: a guide to immunohistochemistry implementation and interpretation. *Pathology*. 2021;53(2):141–156.
40. Heo YJ, Kim B, Kim H, Kim S, Jang MS, Kim KM. PD-L1 expression in paired biopsies and surgical specimens in gastric adenocarcinoma: A digital image analysis study. *Pathol Res Pract*. 2021;218:153338.
41. Kim SW, Jeong G, Ryu MH, Park YS. Comparison of PD-L1 immunohistochemical assays in advanced gastric adenocarcinomas using endoscopic biopsy and paired resected specimens. *Pathology*. 2021;53(5):586–594.
42. Ahn S, Kim KM. PD-L1 expression in gastric cancer: interchangeability of 22C3 and 28-8 pharmDx assays for responses to immunotherapy. *Mod Pathol*. 2021;34(9):1719–1727.
43. Ma C, Patel K, Singhi AD, Ren B, Zhu B, Shaikh F, Sun W. Programmed Death-Ligand 1 Expression Is Common in Gastric Cancer Associated With Epstein-Barr Virus or Microsatellite Instability. *Am J Surg Pathol*. 2016;40(11):1496–1506.
44. Sheng J, Fang W, Yu J, et al. Expression of programmed death ligand-1 on tumor cells varies pre and post chemotherapy in non-small cell lung cancer. *Sci Rep*. 2016;6:20090. Erratum in: *Sci Rep*. 2016;6:23850. Yanhuang, [corrected to Huang, Yan].

14

Pathology of the Anal Canal

■ **Mikhail Lisovsky, MD**

■ ANAL ANATOMIC AND HISTOLOGIC LANDMARKS

The anal canal encompasses the distal most 3 to 4 cm of the most distal intestinal tract. It is defined proximally by the palpable upper border of the internal sphincter muscle, which is a continuation of the muscularis propria of the rectum. Distally, the anal canal is limited by the anal verge, an imaginary line where the squamous mucosa of the anal canal meets the perianal skin. The perianus extends 5 cm laterally from the anal verge and is characterized by the presence of adnexal structures, such as hair and sebaceous glands. The horizontal circular dentate line, located equidistant from the anal canal borders, is the main anal canal landmark and is formed by the bases of vertical mucosal folds called anal columns and by anal valves that connect the bases of anal columns. Behind the valves are small spaces called anal sinuses. Anal papillae are seen as small excrescences of squamous mucosa at the dentate line starting from the base of anal columns or valves. Below the dentate line, the anal canal is lined by nonkeratinizing squamous mucosa. Above the dentate line lies the anal transition zone, measuring a few millimeters to 1 cm in width and lined by stratified epithelium similar to the urothelial mucosa of the bladder. The anal transition zone may be covered by squamous epithelium in some cases and may have islands of colorectal crypts. The most proximal part of the anal canal has colorectal mucosa. Melanocytes are an integral part of the transition zone mucosa and of the squamous zone of the anal canal. The anal sinuses of the transition zone serve as openings for anal glands, which are formed by simple or branching ducts, ramifying in the submucosa. Anal glands may extend into or through the internal anal sphincter and are lined by urothelium-like epithelium at the point of origin and by two cell thick epithelium distally. In both locations, the luminal cell layer is cytokeratin (CK) 7–positive and mucin-producing cells. The basal and intermediate cell layers are p63 and CK5/6 positive, similar to squamous epithelium.

The anal canal is the source of multiple types of primary malignant neoplasms. Whereas the colorectal zone or islands of colorectal mucosa in the transition zone can give rise to adenocarcinoma of colorectal type, intramural adenocarcinoma without a luminal component may originate in anal glands or fistulae. Anal transition zone and the squamous zone are the source of several histologic subtypes of squamous cell carcinoma (SCC) and of melanoma.

■ INFLAMMATORY AND NON-NEOPLASTIC

A number of inflammatory and infectious processes may affect the anal canal; however, the histologic findings of anal fissures, ulcers, abscesses, and fistulas are nonspecific and are discussed only briefly. Infectious agents that can affect the anal canal include human papillomavirus (HPV), herpes simplex virus, *Treponema pallidum*, *Chlamydia* spp., *Neisseria* spp., and *Enterobius vermicularis*. These infections are described in detail in Chapter 9.

Anal fissure is a vertical tear or defect in the squamous mucosa of the anal canal distal to the dentate line. The vast majority of fissures are primary, with 90 % located in the posterior midline and 10 % in the anterior midline. The tear is thought to result from local trauma caused by passage of hard stools, prolonged diarrhea, vaginal delivery, and other injuries, that trigger spasm of the internal anal sphincter, leading to ischemia, necrosis, and poor healing. Secondary fissures are seen in fewer than 1 % of patients and are located laterally or are multiple. They are seen in patients with Crohn's disease other granulomatous diseases, such as tuberculosis and sarcoidosis, infections and malignancy. The typical symptoms of anal fissure include severe pain during defecation and passage of small amount of bright red blood. An acute anal fissure is a fresh laceration, which usually heals within 6 to 8 weeks of conservative treatment with sitz baths and diet modification to increase fiber consumption. Some fissures persist and progress to chronic stage, sometimes called anal ulcer. Typical features of chronic anal fissure include exposure of the internal anal sphincter muscle, indurated and raised fissure edges, and development of an external skin tag (sentinel pile) at the distal end of the fissure and of a hypertrophied anal papilla (fibroepithelial polyp) at the proximal end. The treatment of patients with chronic fissure is surgical and is aimed at reducing spasm of the internal anal sphincter. This may be accomplished by lateral internal sphincterotomy or pneumatic balloon dilation.

Biopsies are rarely used in the assessment of acute anal fissures; however, in chronic lesions to exclude inflammatory bowel disease (IBD) or underlying malignancy. Histopathology of a chronic fissure is poorly studied. Scarce studies paucicellular scar at the base of the ulcer and surprisingly minimal inflammation. Secondary fissures warrant a high degree of suspicion of associated.

Suppurative disease of the anal canal is thought to derive from nonspecific infection of an anal duct or gland, beginning as an abscess, with infection following the least resistant path, determining the location of the abscess (perianal, ischiorectal, or intersphincteric). Less frequently, perianal abscess is associated with Crohn's disease; or with infections such as actinomycosis, tuberculosis, or lymphogranuloma venereum; and in other instances with incontinence, chronic diarrhea, irradiation, and malignancy. The formation of fistula tract leading to the surface of the perianal skin is the chronic phase of suppurative disease. Histologic features of the perianal abscess and fistula are nonspecific and include acute and chronic inflammation, granulation tissue, fibrosis, and foreign body giant cell granulomas (Fig. 14.1). The latter should be distinguished from the compact epithelioid granulomas of Crohn's disease. The presence of multiple lymphoid aggregates and more typical sarcoid-type granulomas should raise suspicion for Crohn's disease.

The treatment of patients with the suppurative disease is surgical and focuses on curing the fistula, preventing or minimizing recurrence, and retaining continence. Long-standing (decades) fistulas are associated with an increased risk of perianal mucinous adenocarcinomas.

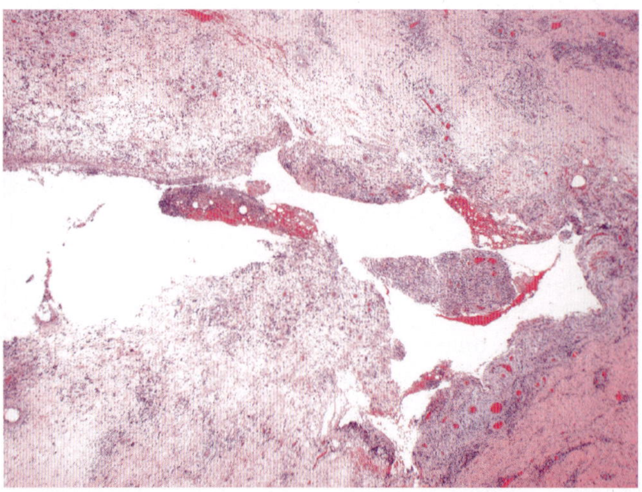

FIGURE 14.1

Anal fistula tract. Necrosis, acute and chronic inflammation, and granulation tissue are present.

CROHN'S DISEASE

Inflammatory bowel disease is discussed in detail in Chapter 10. However, anal involvement by Crohn's disease is described in more detail next.

CLINICAL FEATURES

Perianal Crohn's disease may manifest at any age, but most patients are diagnosed in the third or fourth decade of life. Anal involvement in Crohn's disease is seen in 14% to 38% of the patients. It is present in approximately 15% of patients with ileocolic disease and in 90% of patients with Crohn's disease involving the colon

CROHN'S DISEASE—FACT SHEET

Definition

- A chronic idiopathic inflammatory process that may involve any portion of the gastrointestinal tract, along with extraintestinal manifestations

Incidence and Location

- Anal involvement in 14% to 38% of patients with Crohn's disease
  - In 15% of patients with ileocolic disease
  - In 92% of patients with Crohn's disease involving the colon and rectum
- Location in anal canal and perianal skin

Morbidity and Mortality

- High morbidity with high relapse rate after therapy

Gender, Race, and Age Distribution

- No gender predominance
- Whites of Anglo-Saxon descent most often affected
- Most common in third and fourth decades of life, but individuals of any age may be affected

Clinical Features

- Perianal pain, blood in stool, sepsis, incontinence

Prognosis and Therapy

- Anal lesions are poorly responsive to usual medical therapy for intestinal Crohn's disease, such as steroids and aminosalicylates
- Antibiotics and immunomodulators (e.g., cyclosporin A, azathioprine) are useful in managing fistulas
- Surgery: drainage of abscesses, fistulotomy, flap or graft repair of fistulas, proctectomy
- Prognosis is guarded; high relapse rate regardless of therapeutic modality

CROHN'S DISEASE—PATHOLOGIC FEATURES

Gross Findings

- Spectrum of lesions include fissure, ulcer, abscess, fistula, stricture
- Thickened perianal skin; may have fistulous openings
- Anal tag (a fibroepithelial polyp)

Microscopic Findings

- Abscesses and fistulas show acute and chronic inflammation with granulation tissue
- Sarcoid-like granuloma are characteristic

Differential Diagnosis

- Idiopathic abscess and fistula
- Tuberculosis
- Granuloma inguinale
- Sarcoidosis

and rectum. Although intestinal inflammation precedes perianal involvement in the majority of cases, perianal disease maybe the first manifestation of Crohn's disease. The lesions in perianal Crohn's disease include fissures, deep anal ulcers, abscesses, fistulas, anal tags, strictures, SCC, and adenocarcinoma. The clinical presentation depends on the type of perianal lesion and may include perianal pain, blood admixed with stool, incontinence, and sepsis. Patients with perianal disease also have more extraintestinal manifestations and increased resistance to steroids.

Pathologic Features

Gross Findings

Gross findings include ulcers and fissures, fistulous openings in or around the anal canal, thickened and discolored perianal skin, and prominent anal tags. Multiplicity of lesions is common (Fig. 14.2A).

Microscopic Findings

Acute and chronic inflammation, necrosis, presence of granulation tissue, and fibrosis are usually present, but are nonspecific. However, the presence of well-defined sarcoid-like granulomas with associated multinucleated giant cells, particularly in close proximity to the anal mucosa, is suggestive of Crohn's disease (Figs. 14.2B and C). In many patients with perianal Crohn's disease, the histologic findings are nonspecific.

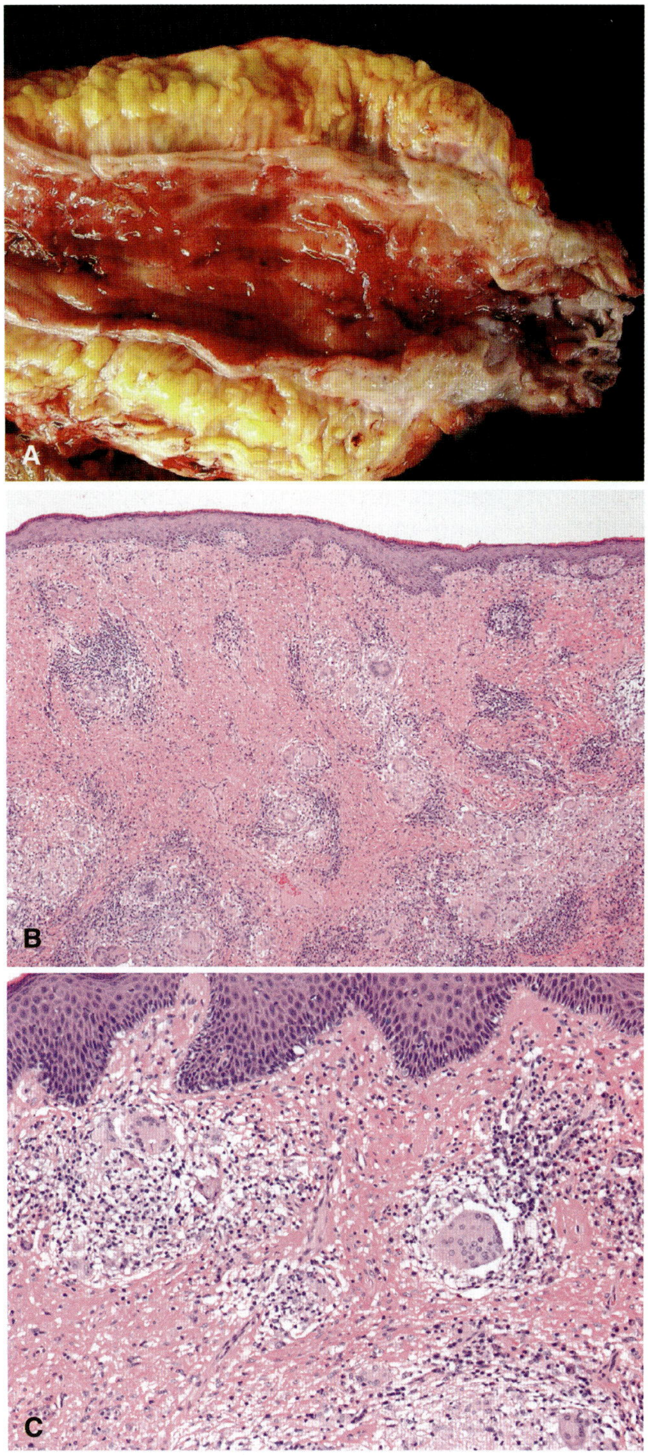

FIGURE 14.2
Anal Crohn's disease. **A**, Gross photograph of the inflamed anal canal and rectum. Mucosal inflammation, edema, and ulcers are present in the anal canal. Rectum is involved by the same process. **B**, At low power, multiple granulomas are seen in the anal wall. **C**, At high power, granulomas with multinucleated giant cells are located in close proximity to the surface epithelium, which is typical of Crohn's disease.

Differential Diagnosis

Idiopathic anal abscesses, fistulas, and primary fissures may be difficult to distinguish from anal Crohn's disease if granulomas are not present and the diagnosis of IBD is not established. The differential diagnosis of granulomatous inflammation includes foreign body reaction, tuberculosis, sarcoidosis, and granuloma inguinale. Perianal tuberculosis is rare but should be suspected in high-risk populations, such as HIV-infected individuals, low-income patients, homeless people, and people with alcoholism. Tuberculous granulomas are usually characterized by caseation, acid-fast bacilli, and positive mycobacterial cultures. The diagnosis of granuloma inguinale is supported by identification of intracellular Donovan bodies using silver-based stains (e.g., Warthin-Starry stain). Sarcoidosis is another potential cause of perianal granulomatous inflammation, but is extremely rare.

Prognosis and Therapy

Medical treatment of patients with perianal Crohn's disease includes antibiotics; steroids and immunomodulators, such as mercaptopurine, azathioprine, or methotrexate; anti–tumor necrosis factor-α agents; and cyclosporin A. Relapse is common after cessation of therapy. Fistulas may require placement of drains or diversion of the fecal stream to allow clearing of the underlying infection. Operative procedures include fistulotomy, placement of flaps or grafts to repair the defect, resection of proximal intestinal disease, a permanent diverting colostomy, and as a measure of last resort, proctectomy. The prognosis for patients with perianal Crohn's disease is guarded because of the high incidence of recurrence. Approximately 20% of patients eventually require proctectomy. In addition, the incidence of anal SCC and adenocarcinoma is significantly increased in patients with perianal Crohn's disease.

HEMORRHOIDS AND ANAL TAGS

Symptomatic hemorrhoids have a prevalence of 4.4% to 12.8% in the general population. In a recent study of screening colonoscopy, weighted toward individuals older than 50 years of age, hemorrhoids were found in 39% with approximately half having symptoms. In both sexes, peak prevalence of symptomatic hemorrhoids appears to be between the ages of 45 and 65 years. Whites are affected more frequently than Blacks, and increased prevalence rates are associated with higher socioeconomic status. Pregnancy is also associated with an increased risk of hemorrhoids. There is no established association between hemorrhoids and chronic constipation or portal hypertension.

Current evidence suggests that hemorrhoids represent "sagging" or "slippage" of the thickened submucosal tissue of the anal canal called cushions. The cushions carry the superior (above the dentate line) and inferior (below the dentate line) hemorrhoidal vascular plexus that have direct arteriovenous communication. With aging, the supportive connective tissue of the cushions may weaken, causing distal displacement of the cushions, which in turn leads to venous distention, erosion, bleeding, and thrombosis. "Internal" hemorrhoids arise above the dentate line and are subclassified on the basis of whether they prolapse out of the canal and on the persistence of the prolapse. Hemorrhoids that are permanently prolapsed are prone to thrombosis and infarction. External hemorrhoids, arising below the dentate line, are prone to thrombosis.

CLINICAL FEATURES

The main complaint is minor painless bleeding, which is associated mostly with internal hemorrhoids. They rarely show thrombosis and are not painful. In contrast, pain is usually associated with thrombosed external hemorrhoids.

Pathologic Features

Gross Findings

Hemorrhoids are fragments of dark purple connective tissue covered by mucosa. They may be firm when thrombosed, and sectioning typically reveals dilated vascular spaces.

Microscopic Findings

The overlying mucosa of hemorrhoid specimens may be columnar, transitional, or nonkeratinizing squamous. The submucosa contains dilated thick-walled vessels and thin sinusoidal spaces in a loose and often edematous fibrous tissue, which may show variable chronic inflammation (Fig. 14.3A). Thrombosis is common, and hemosiderin deposits indicate previous trauma and hemorrhage. Organization of intravascular thrombi may produce cellular masses of granulation tissue that may obliterate the vascular lumen. Excised hemorrhoidal tissue should always be carefully examined microscopically to exclude an inflammatory or infectious condition, or associated squamous neoplasia or melanoma.

Differential Diagnosis

The most common differential diagnosis is with an anal skin tag. If an organizing thrombus results in florid intravascular granulation tissue, a question of a vascular neoplasm can be raised, but the intravascular distribution and residual thrombus with recanalization allow easy distinction in most cases.

HEMORRHOIDS—FACT SHEET

Definition

- Enlarged and edematous soft tissue lesions associated with the anal mucosa that result from slippage or sagging of the normal soft tissue in this region

Incidence and Location

- Reported incidence varies from 4.4% to 12.8%
- Location above and below the dentate line

Morbidity and Mortality

- Not a significant cause of mortality but a common cause of discomfort and morbidity

Gender, Race, and Age Distribution

- Males equal to females; males more likely to seek medical attention
- Wide age and ethnicity range, peaking in middle age and declining thereafter

Clinical Features

- Painless bleeding most common symptom; also anal discomfort on defecation
- Acute pain exacerbations with thrombosis and infarction
- Commonly symptomatic during pregnancy

Prognosis and Therapy

- Medical therapy is mainstay of therapy: increases in dietary fiber, injection sclerotherapy, banding, ablative photocoagulation, electrocoagulation, laser ablation, and cryotherapy
- Surgical therapy is reserved for the 5% to 10% of those who fail conservative measures
- Surgical excision should include only symptomatic hemorrhoidal tissue to protect continence
- Recurrence rate is high

HEMORRHOIDS—PATHOLOGIC FEATURES

Gross Findings

- Usually 1 to 3 cm in diameter
- Pale connective tissue covered by thin gray to tan mucosa
- Infarcted or thrombosed hemorrhoids are dark purple and firm
- Cut surface with dilated vascular spaces, some with thrombi

Microscopic Findings

- Epithelium: columnar, transitional, or squamous
- Submucosa with edematous stroma and dilated vessels
- Vessels may contain thrombi, with intravascular and perivascular hemosiderin deposits, often with marked reactive changes

Differential Diagnosis

- Gross differential diagnosis includes melanoma and carcinoma
- Histologic differential diagnosis of a thrombosed hemorrhoid with organization includes angiosarcoma and Kaposi's sarcoma

Prognosis and Therapy

Treatment options for patients with mild symptoms include analgesics, sitz baths, increased dietary fiber, and stool softeners. In those with more severe symptoms or failed therapy, sclerotherapy and banding to induce fibrosis and fixation of the sagging tissue is used. Surgical excision or ablative techniques such as photocoagulation, electrocoagulation, laser ablation, and cryotherapy are also widely used in patient management.

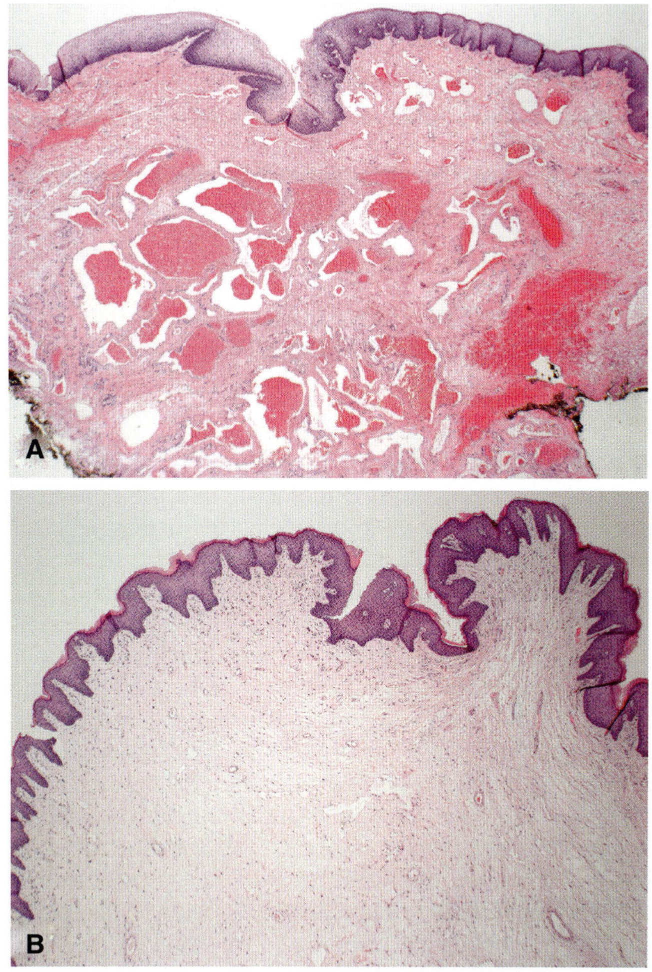

FIGURE 14.3

A, Low-power view demonstrating a typical hemorrhoid, in this case covered by squamous epithelium. The submucosa contains thick-walled dilated blood vessels in a loose fibroconnective tissue. **B**, Anal fibroepithelial polyp or tag demonstrating loose fibrovascular stroma covered by squamous epithelium. The fibroblastic cells are widely spaced and have no mitotic activity. The vasculature is delicate.

ANAL TAGS

Anal tag, also known as hypertrophied anal papilla or anal fibroepithelial polyp, is a polypoid excrescence of anal squamous mucosa and underlying tissue caused by enlargement of an anal papilla. Anal tags can be idiopathic, associated with fissures or fistulas, or associated with Crohn's disease. The gross appearance may be similar to hemorrhoids, but the dilated blood vessels of hemorrhoidal tissue are lacking. Anal tags resemble cutaneous fibroepithelial polyps, with a squamous epithelial lining over loose fibrovascular tissue (Fig. 14.3B). The stroma contains a variably cellular fibroblastic proliferation, which may show small spindle cells or, if the tissue was traumatized, enlarged stellate multinucleated cells with bizarre nuclei. Such stellate cells are evenly distributed within the collagenous stroma and are of no clinical significance. Anal tags are easily removed by a snare or snip excision.

ANAL AND PERIANAL SQUAMOUS NEOPLASIA TERMINOLOGY

A unified lower anogenital squamous terminology (LAST) for HPV-associated lesions was proposed by the College of American Pathologists and the American Society for Colposcopy and Cervical Pathology in 2012 and includes updated nomenclature for squamous neoplasia of both the anal canal and perianal skin. LAST is based on the assumption of similar biology and morphologic equivalence of HPV-related squamous lesions across lower anogenital sites is an attempt to standardize diagnostic categories to improve interdisciplinary communication and patient management. The recommended nomenclature uses a two-tiered system for premalignant squamous lesions: low-grade squamous intraepithelial lesion (LSIL) and high-grade SIL (HSIL). Reported reproducibility is superior to prior three-tiered systems, and in addition, a two-tiered classification system is supported by our current understanding of the biology of HPV infection. LSIL is usually associated with transient extrachromosomal HPV replication, whereas HSIL is associated with genomically integrated HPV DNA. Because LSIL and HSIL terminology does not distinguish between different anogenital sites, a site-specific classification using two-tiered intraepithelial neoplasia (IN) terminology (e.g., AIN; see later) has been proposed for clarity of communication. It was acknowledged, however, that currently used clinical guidelines may stratify management of HPV-related lesion according to a three-tiered (AIN1–3) classification. The latter can therefore be used in parenthesis when necessary. Comparison of the LAST terminology with the three- and two-tiered anal and perianal IN terminology is presented in Table 14.1.

TABLE 14.1

Terminology for Intraepithelial Neoplasia (Dysplasia) of the Anal Canal and Perianal Skin

AIN (Three-Tiered System)	ASIN (Two-Tiered System, WHO)	Anal SIL (LAST)
I	ASIN-L	LSIL (AIN 1 or ASIN-L)
II	ASIN-H	HSIL (AIN 2 or ASIN-H)
III	ASIN-H	HSIL (AIN 3 or ASIN-H)
Condyloma acuminatum	Condyloma acuminatum	LSIL (condyloma acuminatum)
Bowen's disease	Bowen's disease/ PSIN	HSIL (PAIN 3, PSIN-H)

AIN, anal intraepithelial neoplasia; *ASIN-H*, high-grade anal squamous intraepithelial neoplasia; *ASIN-L*, low-grade anal squamous intraepithelial neoplasia; *LSIL*, low-grade squamous intraepithelial lesion; *PAIN*, perianal intraepithelial neoplasia; *PSIN-H*, high-grade perianal squamous intraepithelial neoplasia.

TUMORS AND PRECURSOR LESIONS OF THE ANAL CANAL

Low-Grade Squamous Intraepithelial Lesion (Condyloma Acuminatum) of the Anal Canal

Condyloma acuminatum is more common in the perianal skin and is associated with low-risk HPV genotypes 6 and 11. This is described in greater detail in the section on perianal lesions.

ANAL CANAL SQUAMOUS INTRAEPITHELIAL LESION

Clinical Features

Anal canal SIL (ASIL) has been also termed anal (canal) intraepithelial neoplasia (AIN), anal squamous intraepithelial neoplasia, and anal squamous dysplasia. It is considered to be a precursor of SCC of the anal canal and frequently accompanies SIL of the perianal skin, cervix, and vulvar and other lower genital sites. There is a strong association of ASIL with HPV infection. Low-grade lesions, in general, are associated with low-risk HPV genotypes, whereas high-grade lesions occur in association with high-risk HPV genotypes, particularly 16 and 18. ASIL is most common in HIV-positive homosexual men and is rare in heterosexual men. About 5% to 20% of ASIL cases occur in HIV-negative homosexual men. In women, ASIL is also linked to anal intercourse and HIV-positive status. Immunosuppression from causes other than HIV, such as solid organ transplantation, also increases the risk for high-grade ASIL. ASIL is more likely to occur in the transition zone and can be identified as acetowhite epithelium similar to lesions of cervical SIL.

Pathologic Features

Gross Findings

Anal precursor lesions may be macroscopically invisible or present as plaque-like or warty lesions or as mass lesions mimicking malignancy.

ANAL SQUAMOUS INTRAEPITHELIAL LESION–FACT SHEET

Definition

- A precursor of invasive squamous cell carcinoma, also known as anal intraepithelial neoplasia

Incidence and Location

- True incidence of anal squamous intraepithelial lesion in the general public is unknown because only high-risk populations are screened for dysplasia
- The incidence of high-grade squamous intraepithelial lesion (HSIL)in HIV-negative men who have sex with men (MSM) is 17% to 21%, whereas HIV-infected MSM have a rate of 29% to 52%
- The prevalences of anal HSIL are 0% to 3% and 0% to 9% in HIV-negative women without and with known HPV-related pathology of the lower genital tract, respectively, and in 3% to 26% of HIV-positive women

Morbidity and Mortality

- Little or no morbidity and no mortality

Gender, Race, and Age Distribution

- Males more than females
- Men who have sex with men (MSM) have a higher incidence of anal SIL
- The rate of anal SIL does not decrease with age in MSM

Clinical Features

- Anal SIL is asymptomatic
- Detection by anal cytology and by anoscopy with biopsy

Prognosis and Therapy

- Progression rates of HSIL to anal cancer are 0.17% per year for HIV-positive MSM and 0.03% for HIV-negative MSM
- Topical treatment: fluorouracil, imiquimod, cidofovir, trichloroacetic acid and lopinavir
- Ablative treatment: laser, infrared coagulation, and electrocautery
- High recurrence rate in high-risk populations

ANAL SQUAMOUS INTRAEPITHELIAL LESION–PATHOLOGIC FEATURES

Gross Findings

- No distinctive features

Microscopic Findings

- Nuclear atypia, delayed maturation, and abrupt transition from uninvolved epithelium to squamous intraepithelial lesion
- Low-grade squamous intraepithelial lesion (LSIL): lack of maturation involves the lower third of the epithelium
- High-grade squamous intraepithelial lesion (HSIL): lack of maturation in at least the lower two-thirds or the epithelium; prominent nuclear atypia
- Koilocytotic change is common in upper epithelial layers, especially in LSIL but can also be seen in HSIL
- Mitotic figures are limited to basal layers in LSIL and throughout the full thickness of the epithelium in HSIL

Molecular Studies

- Polymerase chain reaction and fluorescent in situ hybridization are frequently positive for human papillomavirus (HPV) types 6 and 11 in LSIL and 16 and 18 in HSIL
- Risk for developing invasive carcinoma is higher with HPV 16 and 18

Immunohistochemistry

- p16 immunohistochemistry is helpful in selected situations

Differential Diagnosis

- Reactive epithelial proliferation

Microscopic Findings

ASIL is characterized by nuclear atypia, abnormal maturation, and abrupt transition from uninvolved epithelium to SIL. Nuclear atypia is characterized by hyperchromasia, pleomorphism, irregular nuclear borders, coarse chromatin, and loss of nuclear polarity. *Abnormal maturation* refers to a delay in cytoplasm accumulation, which normally begins from the second or third basal cell layer. LSIL is defined by mild cytologic atypia and minimal maturation in the lower third of the epithelium. Cells appear basaloid and immature because of high nuclear-to-cytoplasmic ratio, and mitotic figures are increased but limited to the lower third of the epithelium. Koilocytic change may be seen in the superficial epithelial layers and is diagnostic of HPV cytopathic effect. Koilocytes characteristically have enlarged hyperchromatic nuclei with irregular nuclear borders and perinuclear clear halo and may show binucleation (Fig. 14.4A). HSIL is characterized by prominent nuclear atypia and lack of maturation involving more than one-third of the epithelium. Mitotic figures, including atypical forms, may be present (Figs. 14.4B and C). In the previous three-tiered grading system, AIN I (mild dysplasia) is characterized by nuclear atypia and lack of maturation in the lower third of the epithelium; AIN II (moderate dysplasia) involves the lower two-thirds of the epithelium; and AIN III (severe dysplasia) is diagnosed when dysmaturation involves the full thickness of the epithelium.

ANCILLARY STUDIES

Immunohistochemistry

A broad array of biomarkers that includes p16, Ki-67 (Mib1), ProEx C, telomerase/TERC, HPV genotyping, and HPV16/18 mRNA levels is available for ancillary testing in anal neoplasia. However, LAST guidelines recommend only p16 immunohistochemistry (IHC) as a surrogate assay for HPV infection in biopsies. Positive p16 IHC is defined as continuous

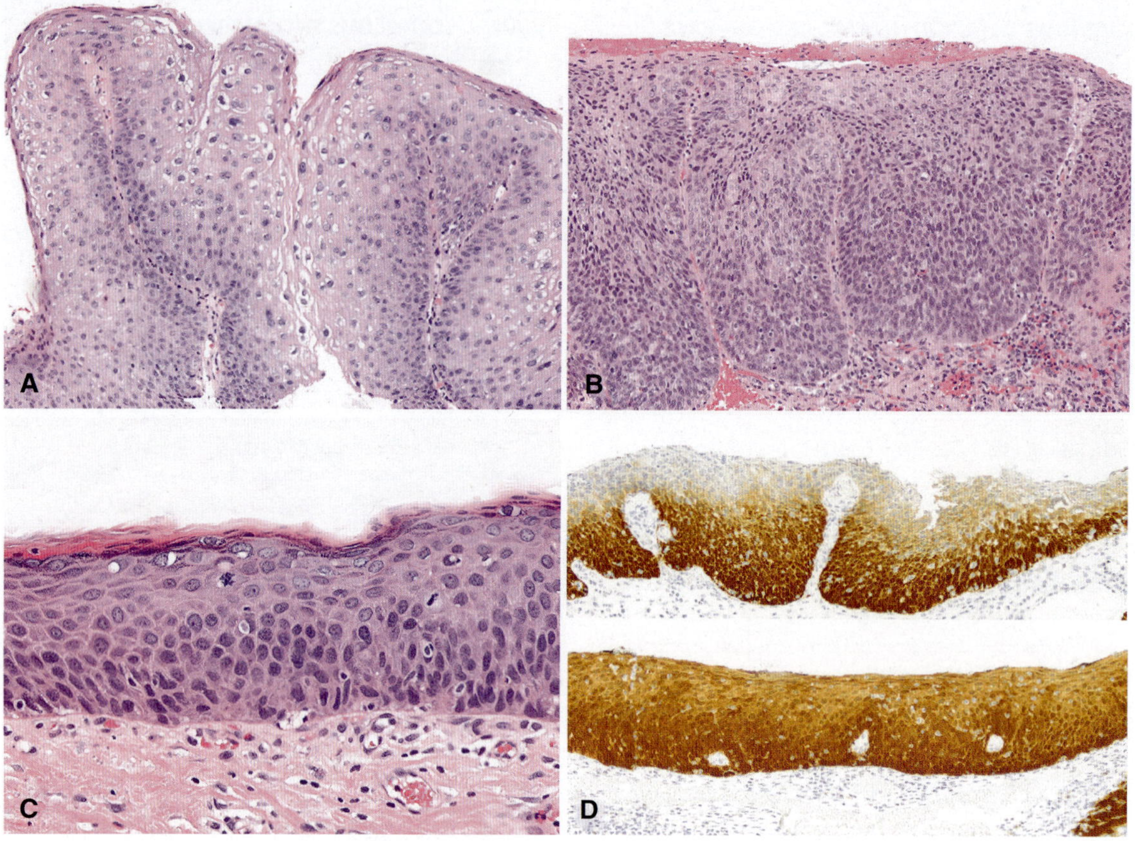

FIGURE 14.4

A, Anal low-grade squamous intraepithelial lesion (anal intraepithelial neoplasia AIN I) has expansion of the basal layer with delayed maturation in the lower third of the epithelial thickness. Cell crowding and some loss of cellular polarity are present in the basal layers. Note the koilocytotic change in the superficial layers of the epithelium consisting of irregular, enlarged, and hyperchromatic nuclei, binucleation, and perinuclear halo. Mitoses are limited to the lower third of the epithelium. **B** and **C**, Anal high-grade squamous intraepithelial lesion (AIN II and AIN III) is characterized by nuclear crowding and lack of maturation in the lower two-thirds (AIN II) or greater (AIN III) of the epithelial thickness. There is prominent nuclear crowding and atypia. Mitotic figures may extend to the very top. Atypical mitoses may be present (**C**). **D**, Two examples of positive p16 immunohistochemistry showing continuous and strong nuclear and cytoplasmic staining that involves at least the basal third of the epithelial thickness.

and strong nuclear or nuclear and cytoplasmic staining involving at least the basal third of the epithelial thickness (Fig. 14.4D). Focal or patchy nuclear staining can be seen in both reactive squamous metaplasia and in LSIL and is therefore nonspecific. Other staining patterns, such as cytoplasmic only, single cell, and blob-like positivity, are considered negative. LAST guidelines propose to limit p16 IHC to the following scenarios: (1) differential diagnosis between HSIL and a neoplastic mimic, such as immature squamous metaplasia, atrophy, reparative change, or tangential cutting; (2) differentiation of HSIL from LSIL when it is not clear whether hematoxylin and eosin morphology is that of AIN 2 or AIN 1 in the older three-tiered nomenclature. (block-positive strong staining supports the diagnosis of HSIL); or (3) there is a difference of opinion regarding the presence of HSIL. P16 IHC is currently not recommended for the diagnosis of LSIL, which should be definitely established morphologically, or for the differential diagnosis of LSIL versus non-HPV-associated abnormalities.

Molecular Pathology

Although not necessary for histologic diagnosis of ASIL, in situ hybridization and polymerase chain reaction (PCR) techniques have been used in epidemiologic studies. In one systematic meta-analysis, crude prevalences of HPV in LSIL and HSIL were 88% and 91%, respectively. In order of prevalence, HPV genotypes 11, 6, 16, 70, and 31 were detected in LSIL and genotypes 16, 18, 6, 33, 31, and 11 in HSIL. The combined prevalences of genotypes 16 and 18 were 27% in LSIL and 69% in HSIL, supporting the view that LSIL and HSIL are associated with different HPV subtypes.

Differential Diagnosis

One of the main challenges in the diagnosis of ASIL is its distinction from reactive squamous proliferation. There is significant interobserver variability in the diagnosis of LSIL because of mild cytologic abnormalities and because delayed maturation in regenerative epithelium is difficult to distinguish from the dysmaturation seen in LSIL. An abrupt transition from normal epithelium to an atypical area and koilocytes in the upper epithelium are the hallmarks of LSIL. Even though a subset of LSIL cases show strong diffuse p16 immunostaining, the use of p16 IHC is not recommended for diagnosis. Positive staining may lead to overinterpretation and inappropriate upgrade to HSIL. Similarly, negative p16 in an otherwise unequivocal HSIL should not be used to downgrade the lesion to LSIL. ASIL can be encountered in specimens from benign anal disease, such as hemorrhoids, fissures, and fistulas. The prevalence of incidental HSIL in surgical specimens varies from 0.25 % to 2.5 %.

Prognosis and Therapy

Low-grade squamous intraepithelial lesion is mainly caused by transient HPV infection and is self-limited. The estimates from a meta-analysis showed that progression rate from HSIL to anal cancer in men who have sex with men (MSM) is 0.17 % per year for HIV-positive MSM and 0.03 % for HIV-negative MSM, suggesting that immunologic status plays an important role in progression to cancer.

Cytopathologic techniques similar to those used for the cervix have been used for screening high-risk populations for anal SIL. Reflex testing for HPV is often performed on specimens with atypical cytology, and patients with positive results are referred for high-resolution anoscopy and biopsy.

The quadrivalent HPV vaccine, now administered to prevent cervical cancer, offers protection against HPV 6, 11, 16, and 18 and has demonstrated high efficacy against anogenital warts and may also prevent anal SIL.

Options available for treatment of anal SIL can be divided into topical and ablative. Topically applied agents include fluorouracil, imiquimod, cidofovir, trichloroacetic acid, and lopinavir. Ablation methods include laser, infrared coagulation, and electrocautery. Ablative methods are more effective than self-applied topical treatments, but the recurrence rates are high. One recent study of HSIL ablation in MSM demonstrated recurrence rate of 68 % at 2 years for HIV-positive patients and 57 % for HIV-negative patients.

SQUAMOUS CELL CARCINOMA

Clinical Features

Squamous cell carcinoma comprises 75 % to 80 % of all malignant tumors of the anal canal. The overall incidence of the disease, although still rare at 0.2 to 4.4 per 100,000, has increased dramatically in recent decades. There has been also a demographic shift of the affected individuals with an increase in young adults, particularly in patients with HIV and other immune deficiencies, and in transplant patients on immunosuppression. The average age of diagnosis in HIV-infected individuals is in the fourth decade of life. The risk is higher in urban populations and in Blacks. In contrast, the risk is particularly low among Asians and Pacific Islanders. The incidence in MSM is 35 per 100,000, which doubles in those infected with HIV to approximately 70 per 100,000. Other associated risk factors include multiple sexual partners, receptive anal intercourse, and presence of other sexually transmitted diseases. HPV is detected in the majority of anal SCCs. A strong link to tobacco smoking has been noted in women but is less definitive in men. Hemorrhoids, fissures, fistulas, abscesses, and IBD are not associated with increased incidence of SCC.

The initial presentation of SCC may be nonspecific, resulting in delayed diagnosis. Minor anal bleeding, pain, discharge, altered bowel habits, pelvic pain, discomfort in the sitting position, anal fissure or fistula, and incontinence from the involvement of the anal sphincter may be noted. A mass lesion is often evident on digital examination. Clinical evaluation typically includes rigid proctoscopy for biopsy, assessment for inguinal lymphadenopathy, computed tomography or magnetic resonance imaging to evaluate other lymph node groups (inferior mesenteric, inferior rectal, and internal iliac), colonoscopy to exclude extension from a primary rectal tumor, and ultrasonography to assess depth of invasion.

Pathologic Features

Gross Findings

Anal canal SCCs are typically ulcerated, with raised borders and may extend into the distal rectum and perianal skin (Fig. 14.5A). It is uncommon to see an intact lesion from the anal canal because most patients are treated with neoadjuvant therapy. In such specimens, the tumor may not be grossly evident. Careful and extensive sampling may be necessary to demonstrate the lesion; areas of induration or mucosal thickening are of particular concern and should be selected for histologic examination.

Microscopic Findings

Although SCC of the anal canal may demonstrate one predominant pattern, the majority of tumors are characterized by a varied histologic appearance. The tumors above the dentate line often show basaloid pattern, characterized by small cells with high nuclear-to-cytoplasmic ratio and nuclear palisading at the periphery of tumor islands. The tumor islands may have necrotic centers

SQUAMOUS CELL CARCINOMA OF THE ANAL CANAL—FACT SHEET

Definition

- Invasive malignant neoplasm demonstrating squamous differentiation

Incidence and Location

- 75% to 80% of anal cancers
- Incidence: 3400 new cases annually
- Worldwide incidence is increasing, especially among HIV-positive individuals

Morbidity and Mortality

- Anal canal lesions: 5-year survival rate is 60% to 86%
- Survival has increased with the advent of combined chemoradiation, eliminating the need for abdominoperineal resection

Gender, Race, and Age Distribution

- Females more than males, 2 to 1
- Increase in young males over past two decades, especially HIV-positive men who have sex with men
- Higher incidence among urban populations
- More common in Blacks than in Whites; very low incidence in Asians and Pacific Islanders
- Demographic shift in progress from older women to young men

Clinical Features

- Symptoms include pain, itching, bleeding, nonhealing ulcer, anal discharge, altered bowel habits, anal fissure, fistula, and incontinence
- Risk factors: multiple sexual partners, anal-receptive intercourse, presence of other sexually transmitted diseases, tobacco smoking in women, immunosuppression, HIV seropositivity

Prognosis and Therapy

- May metastasize to perirectal, iliac, or inguinal lymph nodes
- Chemoradiation therapy usually eliminates the need for radical resection and yields 5-year survival rates of 60% to 86%
- Abdominoperineal resection is used as salvage procedure for recurrence or persistence after chemoradiation therapy; the 3– to 5-year survival rates are 44% to 100%

SQUAMOUS CELL CARCINOMA OF THE ANAL CANAL—PATHOLOGIC FEATURES

Gross Findings

- Mass, ulcer, or stricture may be seen
- In salvage surgery cases, carcinoma may not be grossly evident; diagnosed by biopsy of the area of induration or mucosal thickening

Microscopic Findings

- Varied histologic patterns and two predominant cell types: (1) large cells with or without evidence of keratinization and (2) basaloid cells. One cell type may predominate, or an admixture of patterns may be seen
- Irregular infiltration with desmoplasia or rounded pushing margin
- Two more aggressive patterns: small cell (anaplastic) carcinoma and squamous cell carcinoma with mucinous microcysts

Molecular Studies

- Human papillomavirus (HPV) DNA is identified in most anal squamous cell carcinomas
- Polymerase chain reaction is most sensitive; HPV types 16 and 18 are most often identified
- Gains in chromosomes 3q, 17, and 19; losses in 4p, 11q, and 18q
- Expression of p53, RB, and HER2 has no prognostic significance

Differential Diagnosis

- Basal cell carcinoma: a basaloid-predominant pattern may require immunohistochemistry to exclude melanoma, undifferentiated carcinoma and lymphoma

and small mucinous microcysts (Figs. 14.5B and C). The tumors below the dentate line may have predominance of large cells with pale eosinophilic cytoplasm without keratinization or keratinization of lamellar or single-cell type or (Figs. 14.5D and E). There is frequently a transition from one pattern to another with a spectrum of intermediate variations.

In the past, anal canal tumors were subclassified into large-cell keratinizing, large-cell nonkeratinizing, and basaloid types. However, the majority of tumors demonstrate a mixture of histologic patterns, and no definite association between histologic patterns and prognosis has been established. In addition, the diagnosis is usually based on a small biopsy specimen that may not be representative of the entire tumor. Therapy has also shifted from radical surgery to combined modality chemoradiation, which is not dependent on the histologic subtype. Therefore, the current World Health Organization (WHO) classification suggests that the broader term SCC be used for these tumors. It may be accompanied by a comment describing additional histologic features, such as basaloid features, degree of keratinization, presence of mucinous microcysts, or adjacent SIL.

The LAST guidelines also define a category of superficially invasive SCC of the anal canal, which can be managed by local surgical excision with lower morbidity than chemoradiation. SCC with an invasive depth of 3 mm or less from the basement membrane at the point of origin and horizontal spread of 7 mm or less in maximal extent can be safely treated with surgical excision alone.

Verrucous SCCs are considered a subtype of SCC and represent bulky exophytic tumors with a bulbous acanthotic basal component with a pushing interface. HPV-associated cytopathic changes are absent, and these tumors show only mild atypia. Diagnosing these lesions on a small biopsy is challenging.

ANCILLARY STUDIES

IMMUNOHISTOCHEMISTRY

Immunohistochemical stains are usually not needed, except in poorly differentiated cases. Coexpression of a

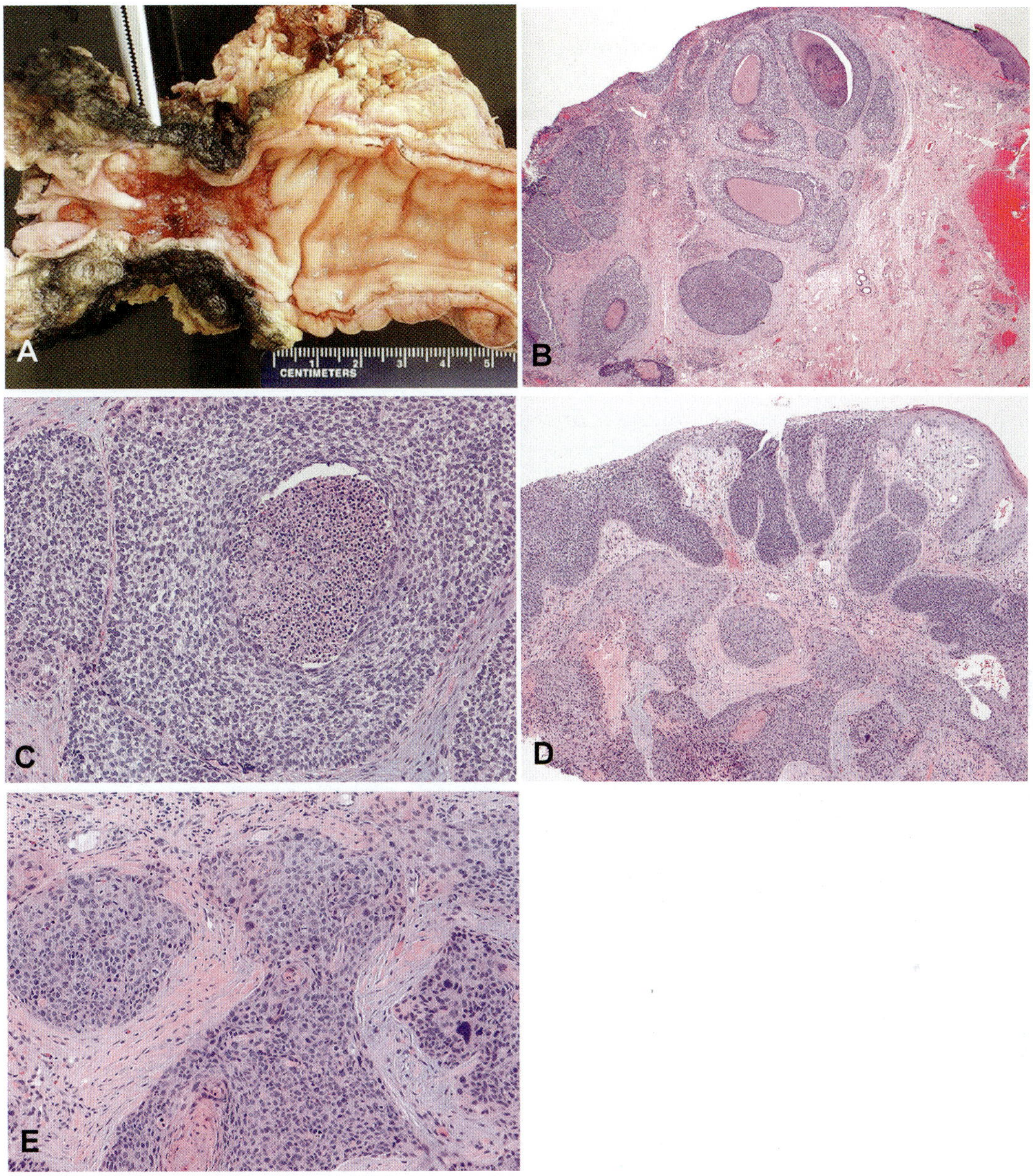

FIGURE 14.5

A, Squamous cell carcinoma (SCC) arising above the dentate line, with the typical ulcerated appearance. **B**, A low-power view of SCC with basaloid features showing large lobulated nests of cells with central necrosis. **C**, At higher power, cells are small, with a high nuclear-to-cytoplasmic ratio and scant amphophilic to clear cytoplasm. **D**, A low-power view of keratinizing SCC producing a prominent desmoplastic reaction. **E**, At higher power, the polygonal cells have pale eosinophilic cytoplasm; markedly atypical nuclei, scattered dyskeratotic cells; and lamellar keratinization. A brisk mitotic rate is noted.

high-molecular-weight keratin CK5 and of p63 or p40 supports the diagnosis of SCC. The surrogate marker p16 may be used to suggest association with high-risk types of HPV. Chromogranin and synaptophysin immunostains are also helpful in poorly differentiated tumors to rule out the possibility of a poorly differentiated (small or large cell) neuroendocrine carcinoma.

Molecular Pathology

Human papillomavirus DNA is identified in the vast majority of anal canal SCCs, and high-risk HPV genotypes 16 and 18 are most frequently found. HPV increases the risk of anal carcinoma by inactivating the tumor suppressor gene *P53*. Genetic alterations include point mutations or deletions in chromosome 17p, which harbors the *P53* gene. Another pathway of *P53* inactivation involves viral protein E6, produced by high-risk types of HPV. E6, when bound to a specific cellular protein, causes proteolytic degradation of p53. In addition to alterations in p53 activity, the E7 protein of high-risk HPV binds to the product of retinoblastoma gene *Rb*, which normally restricts proliferative activity in the basal layers of squamous epithelium, leading to increased epithelial proliferation. The increased proliferation and decreased apoptosis in response to DNA injury are important in HPV-related squamous carcinogenesis. Mutations in the *PIK3CA* are quite prevalent, and *c-myc* amplification has been reported in one-third of anal SCCs. Genomic hybridization studies have also demonstrated gains in chromosomes 3q, 17, and 19 and losses in chromosomes 4p, 11q, and 18q. Expression of the p53, Rb, and HER2 proteins does not appear to have prognostic significance.

Differential Diagnosis

A small biopsy specimen with tumor exhibiting a predominantly basaloid pattern may require further investigation to exclude neuroendocrine carcinoma of small cell type, melanoma, lymphoma, or basal cell carcinoma (BCC) of the perianal skin. In such cases, neuroendocrine markers (e.g., chromogranin and synaptophysin), markers of melanocytic differentiation (e.g., S-100 protein, Melan-A, human melanoma black [HMB-45], and microphthalmia transcription factor [MiTF]), or lymphoid markers are helpful. Poorly differentiated metastatic tumors from the prostate or colorectal primary can also mimic a primary anal SCC but can easily be distinguished based on clinical history, imaging findings, and immunostaining with PSA (prostate-specific antigen) and CDX2 (caudal type homeobox 2), respectively. The giant condyloma of Buschke-Lowenstein was thought to be synonymous with verrucous carcinoma, but it is actually associated with low-risk HPV genotypes and shows viral cytopathic changes and is now regarded as a separate entity. Pseudoepitheliomatous hyperplasia may also mimic an invasive SCC, but is typically associated either with an underlying granular cell tumor or with syphilis. BCC of the perianal skin may also enter the differential diagnosis with basaloid SCC but is seldom a challenging distinction. Basaloid SCC present as bulky anal tumors with large nests of tumor cells with central necrosis and peripheral palisading, marked nuclear atypia, and proliferative activity. An in situ component is usually discernable. In contrast, BCCs present as nodular lesions involving perianal skin and show nests of monomorphic basaloid cells with peripheral palisading and a characteristic retraction artifact, along with myxoid stroma. Central necrosis, atypical mitoses, and an in situ squamous neoplasia component are not characteristic of BCC of the skin (Fig. 14.6A). The diagnosis of BCC of the skin may be supported by diffuse Ber-EP4 (Fig. 14.6B) and Bcl2 staining.

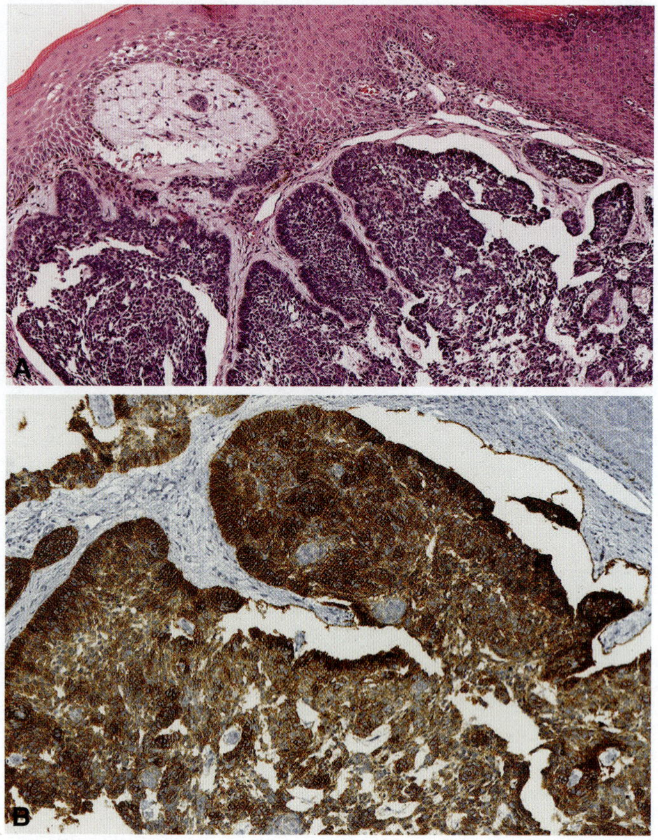

FIGURE 14.6

Basal cell carcinoma of perianal skin. **A**, Tumor nests with peripheral palisading, the classic retraction artifact and myxoid stroma that help differentiate this tumor from basaloid squamous cell carcinoma. **B**, Diffuse Ber-EP 4 expression within the tumor supports this diagnosis.

Prognosis and Therapy

The tumor spreads by direct invasion into the anal sphincter muscle and adjacent soft tissue, and metastasizes to the perirectal, iliac, and inguinal lymph nodes. The current therapy of choice is combined modality therapy (radiation + 5-flouracil [5-FU] + mitomycin C or cisplatin), which achieves complete pathologic response in the majority of patients. For local disease, 5-year survival rates range from approximately 40% to 70% depending on the stage. Up to 25% of patients relapse and undergo salvage abdominoperineal resection, which is also performed in patients with persistent disease after chemoradiation. Abdominoperineal resection results in 5-year survival rate in the range of 40% to 60%. The primary prognostic factors are tumor stage, which is based on size rather than depth of invasion, and nodal status. Small tumors that conform to the definition of superficially invasive SCC ($\leq$3 mm depth of invasion and $\leq$7 mm horizontal spread) are treated with local excision. Verrucous carcinomas recur locally but do not metastasize, and surgical excision is the treatment of choice. Recent studies have also shown PD-L1 expression in nearly 50% of SCCs, raising hopes that a significant proportion of advanced staged tumors may respond well to anti–programmed cell death protein-1(PD-1)–targeted therapy.

ADENOCARCINOMA

Adenocarcinomas of the anal canal are uncommon, constituting up to 10 % of all anal canal cancers. The WHO classification recognizes two groups of adenocarcinomas. A majority involving the anal rectal-type mucosa with features essentially identical to colorectal adenocarcinoma and a second rare extramucosal (intramural) group of adenocarcinomas, also called perianal adenocarcinomas, defined by the lack of a luminal component. Extramucosal adenocarcinomas include tumors arising in anal glands or anal fistulas and those arising in malformations or embryologic remnants.

CLINICAL FEATURES

The clinical features of adenocarcinomas of the anal canal include bleeding, pain, a palpable mass, incontinence, and change in bowel habits. Anal adenocarcinomas characteristically grow slowly, and their diagnosis may be delayed because of the lack of luminal component. Adenocarcinomas arise in fistulas of typically of 20 and more years of duration. The average age at diagnosis is approximately 60 years with a male predominance.

PATHOLOGIC FEATURES

GROSS FINDINGS

Adenocarcinomas of the colorectal type arise in the uppermost mucosa of the anal canal. More often, they are an extension of a low rectal adenocarcinomas. Anal extramucosal adenocarcinomas present as a submucosal mass; the surface mucosa may be ulcerated. The cut surface is tan and firm or may demonstrate abundant mucinous material. There may be evidence of a fistula in the vicinity of the tumor.

MICROSCOPIC FINDINGS

Adenocarcinomas arising in anal colorectal mucosa are histologically identical to adenocarcinomas elsewhere in the colorectum. Adenocarcinomas associated with fistulas are usually of the mucinous type, with abundant extracellular mucin containing islands of atypical glandular epithelium; these tumors have also been referred to as colloid carcinoma. Historically, the diagnosis of anal gland carcinoma was made when continuity of the tumor with normal anal glands could be demonstrated. However, the continuity can be rarely established. The currently favored definition describes anal gland carcinoma as haphazardly dispersed small glands with cuboidal epithelium and scant mucin production invading the wall of the anorectal area without an intraluminal component (Fig. 14.7). Some carcinomas have mucinous phenotype in the absence of an identifiable fistula and have been tracked to normal anal glands, suggesting that anal gland carcinomas may also have a mucinous phenotype.

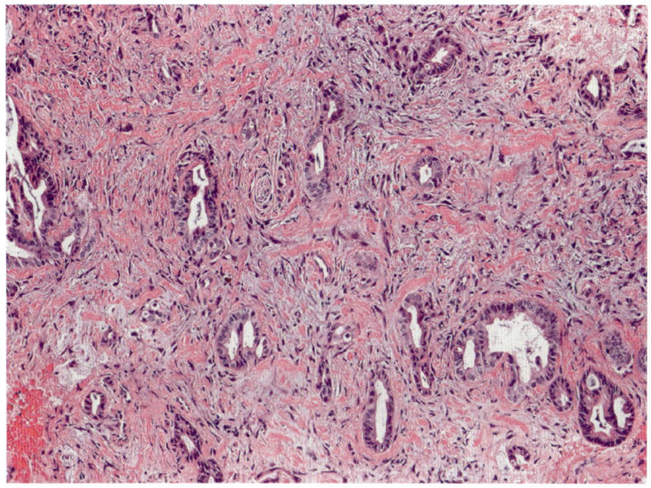

FIGURE 14.7

Anal gland adenocarcinoma. This perianal adenocarcinoma lacks surface mucosal abnormalities grossly and histologically. The tumor is characterized by haphazardly arranged small glands with scant mucin production in the perianal stroma.

ANCILLARY STUDIES

IMMUNOHISTOCHEMISTRY

The adenocarcinoma of the colorectal-type is typically CK7−/CK20+/CDX2+, whereas the mucinous adenocarcinomas are generally CK7+/CK20+, and the anal gland carcinomas are CK7+/CK20−. In addition, anal gland carcinomas lose basal cell layer with associated CK5/6 and p63 expression of normal anal glands and are negative for CDX2. The reported immunophenotype of fistula tract-associated and nonanal gland, non–fistula-associated anal adenocarcinomas is heterogeneous and cannot be used to define a specific subtype.

DIFFERENTIAL DIAGNOSIS

Adenocarcinoma of colorectal type cannot be separated from its lower rectal counterpart based on microscopic features alone. Differential diagnosis of poorly differentiated carcinoma of the anal canal includes adenocarcinoma, SCC, and neuroendocrine carcinoma. IHC is helpful, and the algorithm is summarized in Table 14.2. Melanoma can be distinguished using melanocytic markers S100, Sox10, Melan-A, and HMB-45. Anal gland carcinoma is a diagnosis of exclusion, and the origin of a carcinoma in anal luminal mucosa or a fistula

TABLE 14.2
Immunohistochemical Panel for Discrimination Between Poorly Differentiated Anal Carcinomas

	CK7	CK20	Synaptophysin	Chromogranin	CK5/6	P63/p40
Squamous cell carcinoma	+	−	−	−	+	+
Adenocarcinoma	+/−	+/−	−	−	−	−
Neuroendocrine carcinoma	+/−	−	+	+	−	−

CK, Cytokeratin.

ADENOCARCINOMA—FACT SHEET

Definition

- Malignant neoplasm with glandular differentiation
- May arise either in the anal colorectal-type mucosa or extramucosally in deeper anal structures with no involvement of luminal mucosa
- Extramucosal adenocarcinomas include anal gland carcinoma and adenocarcinoma arising in a fistula

Incidence and Location

- 3% to 4% of all anal carcinomas
- The majority of adenocarcinomas are extensions from a rectal primary cancer
- Colorectal-type adenocarcinomas localize to the upper anal canal; anal gland carcinomas localize to the transitional zone

Morbidity and Mortality

- High level of morbidity because of locally destructive disease
- Stage is primary prognostic indicator; prognosis is less favorable than in squamous cell carcinoma of the anal canal

Gender, Race, and Age Distribution

- Perianal adenocarcinomas are male predominant
- No clear racial or geographic predominance
- Average age is approximately 60 years

Clinical Features

- Symptoms include bleeding, pain, a palpable mass, incontinence, and other changes in bowel habits
- Perianal adenocarcinomas may grow slowly and present with a soft tissue mass in the buttock

Prognosis and Therapy

- The rarity of perianal adenocarcinomas makes prognostication difficult
- Treatment includes abdominoperineal resection with preoperative or postoperative combined chemotherapy and radiation
- The prognosis is highly stage dependent

ADENOCARCINOMA—PATHOLOGIC FEATURES

Gross Findings

- Adenocarcinoma arising in the anal mucosa is an exophytic or ulcerated mass similar to usual colorectal adenocarcinoma
- Extramucosal perianal adenocarcinoma is a submucosal mass with no surface epithelial involvement. Mucosal ulceration may be present

Microscopic Findings

- Adenocarcinoma arising in anal mucosa: epithelial dysplasia adjacent to invasive component. Tubulovillous pattern with "dirty necrosis" is common, similar to colorectal adenocarcinoma
- Extramucosal perianal adenocarcinomas
  - Anal gland carcinoma: haphazardly arranged small tubular glands with scant mucin production and no surface mucosal component
  - Adenocarcinoma associated with anal fistula: mucinous type, with no surface mucosal component

Immunohistochemistry

- Adenocarcinomas of colorectal type are usually cytokeratin (CK) 7-/CK20+, CDX2+
- Anal gland carcinomas are CK7+/CK20-, CDX2-
- Mucinous adenocarcinomas associated with anal fistula are most often CK7-/CK20+, CDX2+

Differential Diagnosis

- Colorectal adenocarcinoma extending from the lower rectum; adenocarcinoma arising in the duplication of terminal hindgut; adenocarcinoma of the prostate; metastasis

and a metastatic tumor should be excluded. Negative staining of anal gland carcinoma for CDX2 is helpful in differentiation from a colorectal adenocarcinoma. Secondary involvement of anal squamous mucosa may mimic Paget's disease. Primary Paget's disease typically arises in perianal skin as a plaque-like lesion, shows CK7 and GCDFP-15 positivity, and is negative for CK20 and CDX2.

Prognosis and Therapy

The rarity of perianal adenocarcinomas makes generalizations with regard to prognosis and optimal therapy of patients with these cancers difficult. Tumor stage, lymph node status, and the degree of differentiation are primary prognostic indicators. Stage for stage, adenocarcinoma of the anal canal has a less favorable prognosis than SCC with a 5-year survival rate of approximately 30%. Treatment may include abdominoperineal resection with preoperative or postoperative radiation and chemotherapy, depending on stage at presentation.

MELANOMA

CLINICAL FEATURES

Anal melanoma is a rare mucosal malignancy accounting for 0.05 % of all colorectal tumors. The median age at diagnosis is 71 years. It is 1.6 times more common in women than men and 1.7 times more common among Whites than Blacks. The most common presenting symptoms are rectal bleeding and anal discomfort, and patients are often misdiagnosed as having hemorrhoidal disease. Others may present with inguinal lymphadenopathy, and up to 26 % of patients have metastatic disease at the time of diagnosis.

PATHOLOGIC FEATURES

GROSS FINDINGS

Anal melanomas are polypoid lesions arising in the vicinity of the dentate line and thus may be mistaken for anal tags or hemorrhoids. The presence of brown or black tumor discoloration may point to a melanoma. Small lesions may be covered by intact mucosa, and larger lesions are often ulcerated.

MICROSCOPIC FINDINGS

Microscopically, anal melanomas are similar to cutaneous melanomas (Fig. 14.8A). An in situ component demonstrating junctional nests indicates an anal primary (Fig. 14.8B). Pagetoid spread is common. The invasive component may contain epithelioid, polygonal cells, spindle cells, or an admixture of both. The epithelioid cells often have eosinophilic granular cytoplasm, variably pleomorphic nuclei, frequent mitotic figures, and prominent nucleoli. Pigmented tumors may demonstrate intracellular brown-to-black melanin (Fig. 14.8C). Approximately 30 % of tumors are amelanotic. Tumor depth or thickness (Breslow's level) is measured from the top of overlying mucosa or ulcer using an ocular micrometer. A depth of more than 2 mm is associated with significantly more aggressive disease.

ANCILLARY STUDIES

IMMUNOHISTOCHEMISTRY

S-100, Sox10, HMB-45, Melan-A, and MiTF are useful markers of melanocytic differentiation. Even though S-100 is the least specific, it is the most sensitive marker, making it a mainstay in the differential diagnostic workup of a potential anal melanoma. HMB-45 and

ANAL MELANOMA—FACT SHEET

Definition

- Primary anal malignant tumor of melanocytic origin

Incidence and Location

- Fewer than 0.1% of colorectal malignancies
- Vicinity of the dentate line

Morbidity and Mortality

- Death usually caused by disseminated disease rather than local recurrence

Gender, Race, and Age Distribution

- Women more than men, 1.6 to 1
- Median age at diagnosis is 71 years
- 1.7-fold higher among Whites than Blacks

Clinical Features

- Most common symptom is rectal bleeding
- Other symptoms include pain, change in bowel habits, and inguinal lymphadenopathy

Prognosis and Therapy

- Virtually uniformly fatal, with few long-term survivors
- 26% of patients have metastatic disease at the time of presentation
- Wide local excision is the treatment of choice
- Abdominoperineal resection is reserved for those in whom transanal excision is not technically feasible
- Tyrosine kinase inhibitors have provided symptomatic relief in a subset of patients with mucosal melanoma and *KIT* mutations

ANAL MELANOMA—PATHOLOGIC FEATURES

Gross Findings

- Frequently polypoid; can be mistaken for hemorrhoids or anal tags
- Presence of brown or black pigment suggests melanoma

Microscopic Findings

- Similar to cutaneous counterpart
- In situ component with junctional nests and pagetoid intraepithelial spread is common
- Cell types: epithelioid, with eosinophilic granular cytoplasm and large nuclei with prominent nucleoli; spindle cell type, or mixed
- Intracellular melanin may be visible in tumor cells

Immunohistochemistry

- S-100 and SOX10 positive in most cases
- Melan-A is positive, sensitive, and specific
- HMB-45 (human melanoma black) is positive but often very focal

Differential Diagnosis

- Poorly differentiated carcinoma
- Lymphoma
- Metastatic melanoma

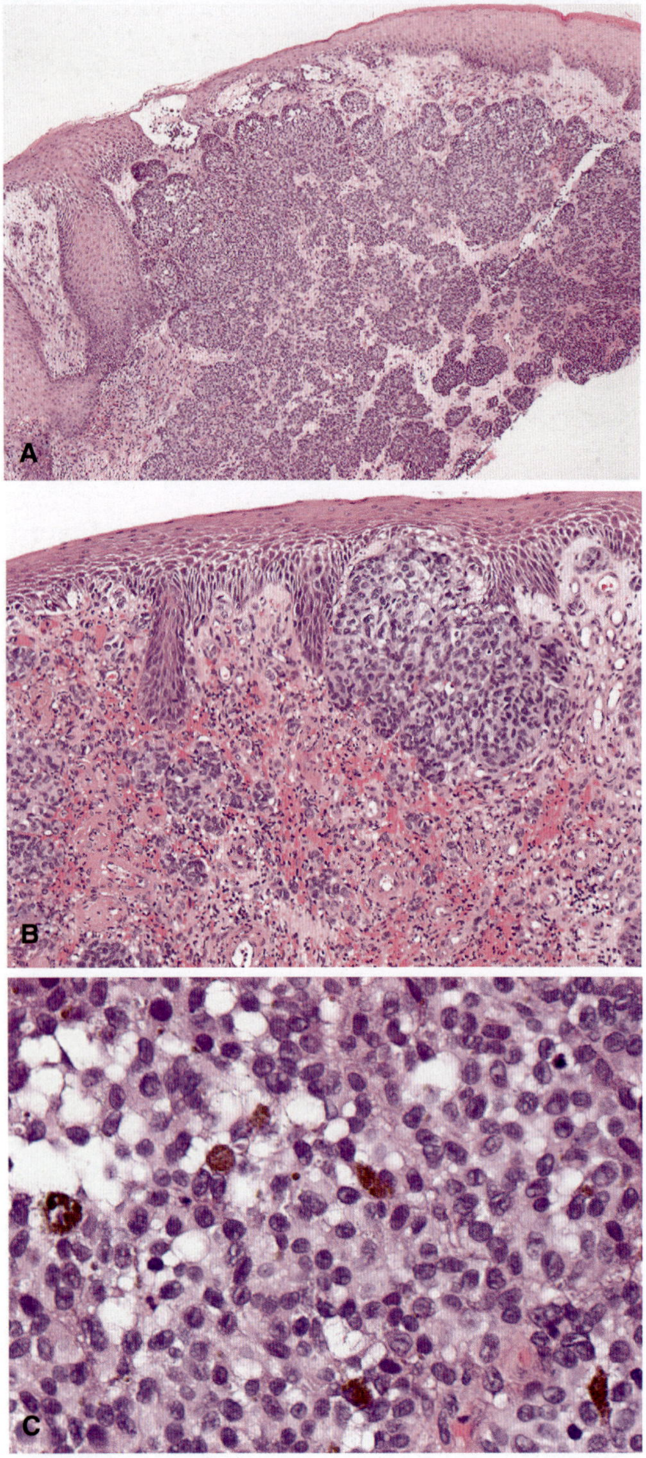

FIGURE 14.8

A, Anal melanoma growing in a nested pattern. **B**, Junctional nest of in situ melanoma indicating primary site in the anal canal. **C**, Higher power view illustrates epithelioid-type cells with abundant pale eosinophilic or clear cytoplasm and large nuclei with prominent nucleoli. Deposits of fine brown melanin pigment are seen.

MiTF are specific, but less sensitive markers, and the staining may be focal. Melan-A generally provides more diffuse staining of tumor cells.

Molecular Pathology

A recent targeted exon sequencing analysis of 467 cancer-related genes demonstrated that oncogenic mutational driver events could be identified in 14 of 15 anal melanomas. Among the most common were activating mutations in C-KIT, accounting for 30% of cases. Forty percent of tumors had mutations suggestive of mitogen-activated protein kinase (MAPK) pathway activation, which included loss-of-function *NF1* mutations in 20% of all cases, a novel finding in mucosal melanomas. Activating mutations of *BRAF* or *RAS* isoforms are rare in primary anal malignant melanomas.

Differential Diagnosis

Differentiation of anal melanoma from poorly differentiated carcinoma and lymphoma is straightforward with use of ancillary immunostains when the diagnosis is suspected. Absence of junctional component raises the possibility of a metastatic melanoma. However, junctional component may be destroyed by the invasive tumor, making distinction between primary and secondary melanoma difficult. A prior history of cutaneous melanoma is helpful in establishing the diagnosis.

Prognosis and Therapy

The prognosis of anal melanoma is poor. The 5-year survival rate for stage I (clinically localized) disease is approximately 27%; for stage II (regional lymph node metastasis) disease is 10%; and for stage III (distant metastases) disease, the rate is 0%. Patients with anal melanoma are treated surgically, but the extent of surgical intervention does not correlate with survival. Therefore, the surgery of choice is transanal wide local excision. Abdominoperineal resection is reserved for cases in which transanal excision is not technically feasible.

Several studies have shown survival benefit from the use of tyrosine kinase inhibitor imatinib in a subset of patients with metastatic mucosal melanoma and activating *KIT* mutations. Molecular testing to determine the site of activating mutation is required to identify the patients likely to respond to treatment with imatinib. Patients carrying mutations in exons 11 or 13 are usually sensitive. Eventual development of resistance to imatinib is common. The utility of chemotherapy, radiation therapy, and immunotherapy has not been demonstrated in the treatment of patients with anal melanoma.

TUMORS AND PRECURSOR LESIONS OF THE PERIANAL SKIN

HIDRADENOMA PAPILLIFERUM

Hidradenoma papilliferum is an uncommon benign cutaneous neoplasm that is almost exclusively seen in the vulvar and perianal regions. Although traditionally considered a tumor of adnexal apocrine glands, convincing morphologic and immunohistochemical evidence supports its development from mammary-like glands, a recently described normal adnexal structure previously thought to represent ectopic mammary tissue. Mammary-like glands are found in both sexes and are believed to be a source of a spectrum of neoplastic and reactive lesions with striking resemblance to tumors of the breast.

CLINICAL FEATURES

Hidradenoma papilliferum occurs predominantly in the anogenital skin of white women in the fourth to seventh decades of life. The most commonly involved sites are the vulva and perineum. Perianal tumors are rare. The typical lesion manifests as a painless mass of a few millimeters in diameter. Rare cases of up to 2 cm in greatest dimension have been described. Surface erosion or ulceration may sometimes be present. Malignant transformation to adenocarcinoma or adenosquamous carcinoma is exceedingly rare.

PATHOLOGIC FEATURES

GROSS FINDINGS

A typical excisional biopsy specimen demonstrates a small well-circumscribed dermal nodule without a capsule, and the overlying skin may be ulcerated. The cut surface of the lesion is usually tan to brown and may have a papillary appearance in larger tumors.

MICROSCOPIC FINDINGS

Microscopically, the lesion has a complex papillary pattern of growth (Fig. 14.9) The papillae have a fibrovascular core and are lined by a double layer of luminal cuboidal to low columnar cells with pale eosinophilic cytoplasm and occasional apical snouts (decapitation secretion) and a deeper layer of myoepithelial cells. The luminal cells may be slightly pleomorphic and stratified. Lymphoplasmacytic infiltration within stroma is common.

HIDRADENOMA PAPILLIFERUM—FACT SHEET

Definition

- Benign cutaneous neoplasm originating in adnexal mammary-like glands

Incidence and Location

- Incidence uncertain; uncommon at any site
- Occur in vulvar, perineum, and perianal skin

Morbidity and Mortality

- Benign lesion with limited morbidity

Gender, Race, and Age Distribution

- Exclusively in women
- Fourth to seventh decades of life
- Most occur in whites

Clinical Features

- Dermal nodule covered by intact skin in most cases
- Occasionally skin is eroded or ulcerated

Prognosis and Therapy

- Benign lesion; conservative excision is usually curative
- Extremely rare reports of possible malignant change

HIDRADENOMA PAPILLIFERUM—PATHOLOGIC FEATURES

Gross Findings

- Firm, ill-defined mass within dermis, with normal or ulcerated overlying skin
- Cut surface yellow-tan to brown
- Size ranges from a few millimeters (typical) to 2 cm (rare)

Microscopic Findings

- Complex papillary pattern with arborizing fibrovascular cores
- Double epithelial cell layer with outer layer of low columnar cells with apocrine snouts; inner layer consists of flattened myoepithelial cells
- Chronic inflammation with prominent plasma cells is common/
- No connection with overlying epidermis

Differential Diagnosis

- Gross differential diagnosis includes cutaneous cyst, hemorrhoids, polyps, carcinoma
- Histologic differential diagnosis includes adenocarcinoma

DIFFERENTIAL DIAGNOSIS

An erroneous diagnosis of SCC may be made on a small biopsy. The presence of a distinctive double epithelial–myoepithelial cell layer favors the diagnosis of hidradenoma papilliferum. Other adnexal tumors, such as apocrine gland adenoma and trichoepithelioma should also be considered.

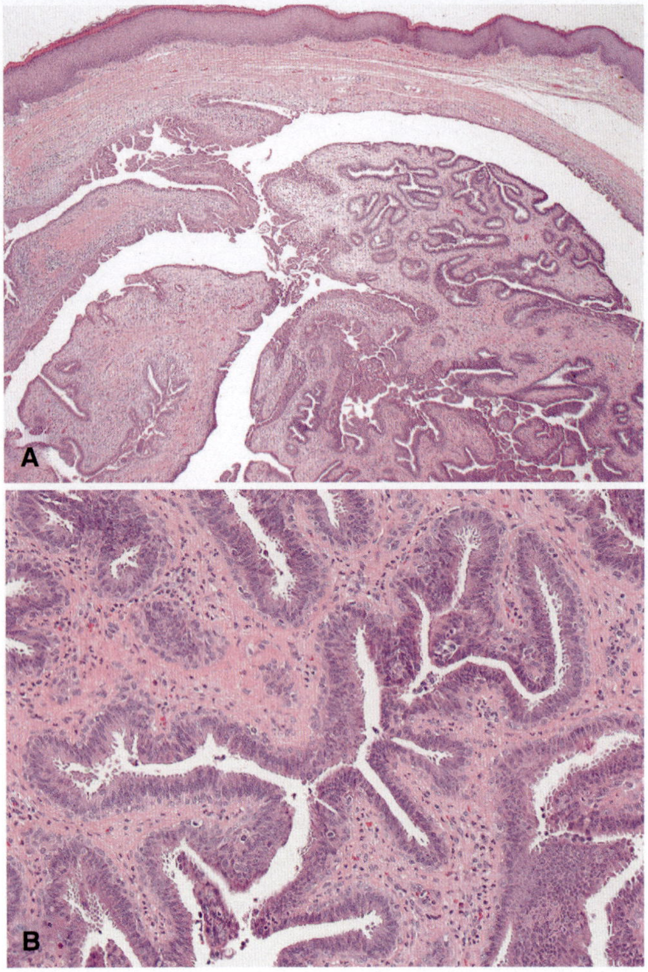

FIGURE 14.9

Hidradenoma papilliferum. **A**, A low-power view demonstrates an intracystic complex papillary proliferation with a lobulated appearance. **B**, The lesion is characterized by fibrovascular cores with two-cell layers. The luminal secretory cells are columnar, with eosinophilic cytoplasm and apical snouts. The layer of flattened myoepithelial cells is visible between the secretory cells and the fibrovascular cores.

Prognosis and Therapy

Hidradenoma papilliferum is a benign lesion treated by surgical excision with no risk of local recurrence.

CONDYLOMA ACUMINATUM

Condyloma acuminatum is a papillary epithelial proliferation of the anogenital skin and, more rarely, of the squamous mucosa of the anal canal. It is usually caused by low-risk HPV types 6 and 11. In previous classifications, condyloma acuminatum was not equivalent to low-grade intraepithelial dysplasia or neoplasia; however, LAST recommends to designate this lesion as LSIL with an optional designation of condyloma within parentheses.

Clinical Features

Condyloma acuminatum is the most common manifestation of sexually transmitted HPV infection occurring both in women and men. It affects the perianal skin more commonly than the anal canal and can also involve other genital organs. The incidence and demographics of anal condyloma parallel the recent increase in anal cancers, particularly among young men who practice anal intercourse.

Other conditions associated with increased incidence of anal condyloma include HIV-affected individuals, other sexually transmitted diseases, organ transplantation, cigarette smoking, alcohol use, and low socioeconomic status. Most patients present with visible or palpable polypoid perianal lesions.

Pathologic Features

Gross Findings

Condyloma acuminatum is a tan to gray lobulated polypoid mass ranging in size from a few millimeters to several centimeters. It commonly grows in clusters and is reminiscent of cauliflower florets (Fig. 14.10A). Large lesions should prompt a thorough assessment to exclude verrucous carcinoma.

Microscopic Findings

The lesion typically shows epidermal papillomatous architecture with prominent acanthosis and variable surface parakeratosis (Fig. 14.10B). Koilocytes, a marker of HPV infection, can be present in the superficial epithelial layers. Expansion of basal layers with delayed maturation in the lower third of the epithelium is common (Fig. 14.10C). Mitotic figures, if present, are restricted to the basal zone. These features are essentially those of LSIL. In lesions treated with podophyllin, there may be more atypia, along with individual cell keratinization and mitotic figures above the basal zone. These features do not imply a more aggressive lesion and are a response to the topical treatment.

Foci of HSIL (Fig.14.11) or even of microinvasive carcinoma may be seen in up to 15 % of condylomatas smaller than 5 cm in size. These lesions tend to harbor high-risk HPV genotypes 16 and 18. High-grade dysplasia arising within a condyloma should be reported as "perianal HSIL (condyloma with high-grade dysplasia)."

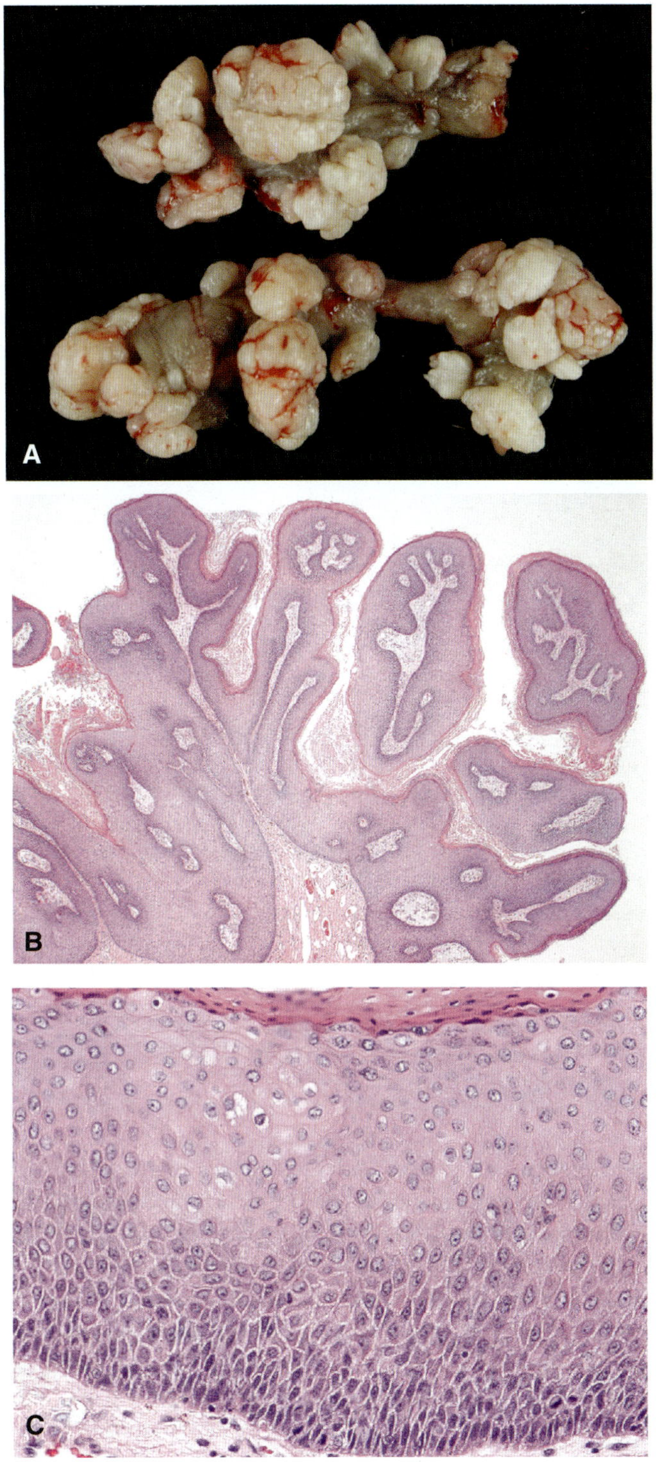

FIGURE 14.10

Condyloma acuminatum. **A**, Exophytic rubbery to firm lobulated or warty cutaneous nodules. They are often light gray to white, bearing a striking resemblance to cauliflower florets. **B**, At low power, the warty papillomatous pattern of condyloma is readily apparent. Note the overlying hyperkeratosis. **C**, A high-power view reveals low-grade squamous intraepithelial lesion (anal intraepithelial neoplasia I) in the lower third of the epithelium.

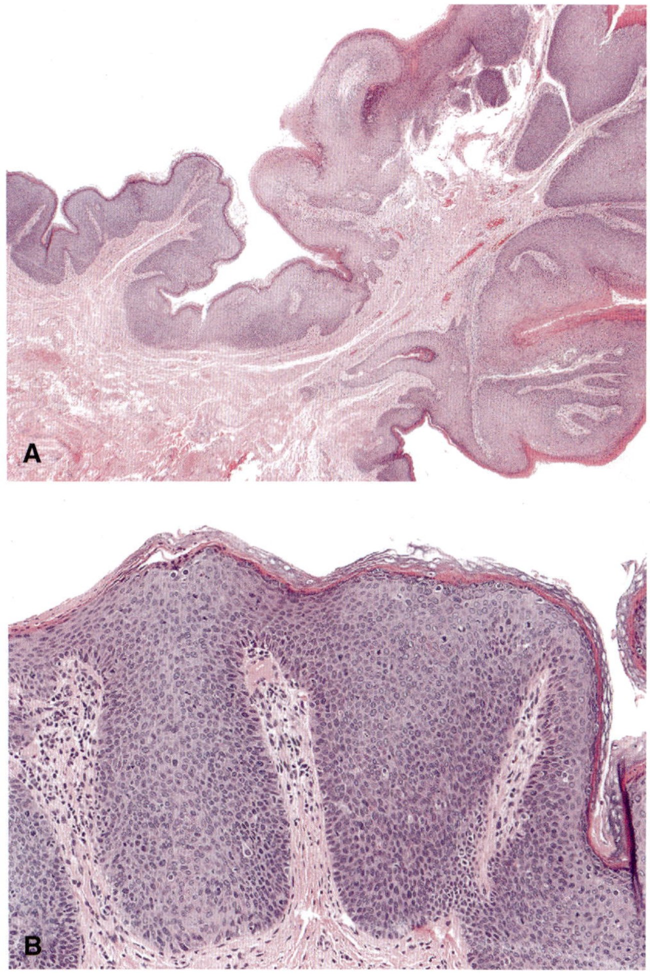

FIGURE 14.11

A, Low power view of a condyloma acuminatum with high-grade dysplasia. **B**, High-power view demonstrating high-grade squamous intraepithelial lesion in the left part of the condyloma.

ANCILLARY STUDIES

IMMUNOHISTOCHEMISTRY

Routine use of p16 immunostain is not recommended for diagnosis. Block positivity for p16 is usually seen in foci of HSIL arising within a condyloma but is not necessary for diagnosis. Serial sections to rule out foci of HSIL and invasive tumor are more useful than ancillary stains.

MOLECULAR PATHOLOGY

The detection of HPV DNA is currently performed using either real-time PCR-based techniques (for genotypes 16 and 18) or multiplex PCR with line-probe hybridization (all genotypes). Whereas the majority of condyloma harbor HPV types 6 and 11, those with high-grade dysplasia demonstrate genotypes 16 and 18, underscoring the link between HPV types 16 and 18 and malignancy.

CONDYLOMA—FACT SHEET

Definition

- Exophytic papillomatous human papillomavirus–related lesion of squamous epithelium with low propensity for progression to malignancy

Incidence and Location

- High incidence in general population; particularly common in men who have sex with men (MSM)
- Most commonly develop in the perianal skin; may be also seen in the anal canal

Morbidity and Mortality

- Most are benign; some may progress to cancer

Gender, Race, and Age Distribution

- Formerly more prevalent in females; now more in MSM
- Low socioeconomic status is linked to a higher incidence
- The age range is broad, encompassing sexually active men and women

Clinical Features

- Most patients present with visible or palpable polypoid lesions
- Coexisting lesions of the vulva are common in women; penile lesions are frequently encountered in men

Prognosis and Therapy

- Most pursue a benign clinical course
- Immunosuppressed individuals, including organ transplant patients, HIV-positive patients, particularly those with a low CD4 count, have a higher risk for recurrence and progression to high-grade squamous intraepithelial lesion
- Treatment includes topical agents, such as podophyllin and ablative procedures, such as local excision, cryotherapy, and electrocoagulation

CONDYLOMA—PATHOLOGIC FEATURES

Gross Findings

- Polypoid, exophytic, cauliflower-like lesions
- Frequently multiple
- Few millimeters to 2 cm or larger in size

Microscopic Findings

- Papillomatous proliferation of squamous epithelium with acanthosis and parakeratosis
- Koilocytes with perinuclear halo and enlarged, hyperchromatic, irregularly shaped nuclei in the upper epithelial layers
- Binucleated koilocytes are common
- Epithelium demonstrates orderly maturation, with possible atypia in the basal two to three layers
- Mitoses limited to the basal zone
- High-grade squamous intraepithelial lesion (HSIL) within a condyloma should be reported

Molecular Pathology

- Low-risk human papillomavirus (HPV) types 6 and 11 are found in the majority of condyloma cases
- High-risk HPV types 16 and 18 may be found in condyloma with HSIL

Differential Diagnosis

- Verrucous carcinoma
- Hemorrhoid, fibroepithelial polyp, mucosal prolapse polyp

DIFFERENTIAL DIAGNOSIS

Condyloma acuminatum should be distinguished from a verrucous carcinoma. Any large condylomatous lesion should be scrutinized for subtle evidence of invasion, which may manifest as endophytic growth with "pushing" border extending into the underlying stroma. The histologic similarity between a condyloma and verrucous carcinoma can make distinction virtually impossible on a biopsy. Benign lesions to be distinguished from condyloma include fibroepithelial polyp, hemorrhoids, and mucosal prolapse polyps.

PROGNOSIS AND THERAPY

Treatment of anal condyloma includes topical agents such as podophyllin or ablative techniques, including local excision, electrocautery, or cryotherapy. The recurrence rate is high because of field effect of HPV infection and is further increased because of immunosuppression related to multiple causes including HIV and organ transplantation.

PERIANAL HIGH-GRADE SQUAMOUS INTRAEPITHELIAL LESION (BOWEN'S DISEASE)

Perianal SIL is similarly subdivided into LSIL and HSIL by LAST terminology. The term *Bowen's disease* is typically applied to high-grade squamous intraepithelial neoplasia occurring in the perianal (marginal) skin, similar to Bowen's disease in other cutaneous sites, where it is synonymous with SCC in situ. Bowen's disease is similar to anal HSIL (AIN-3), being associated with high-risk HPV genotypes 16 and 18. However, the treatment and prognosis of these two conditions are different, making the distinction important.

CLINICAL FEATURES

Bowen's disease occurs in middle-aged and older individuals with female predominance. It is roughly four times more common in whites than in African Americans. The dominant complaint is perianal itching; other symptoms include slight bleeding or induration. Other synchronous HPV-associated lesions, such as condyloma acuminatum, vulvar SIL, and cervical SIL, are also commonly present.

PAGET'S DISEASE—FACT SHEET

Definition

- Intraepithelial form of adenocarcinoma that may or may not have an underlying component of invasive adenocarcinoma

Incidence and Location

- Most cases of primary perianal Paget's disease represent extension of Paget's disease of the vulva
- Secondary perianal Paget's disease is associated with internal malignancy, most commonly rectal adenocarcinoma
- Secondary Paget's disease constitutes approximately 50% of all cases

Morbidity and Mortality

- Significant morbidity because of wide local excision for primary Paget's disease and by the complications of radical surgery for the underlying rectal adenocarcinoma

Gender, Race, and Age Distribution

- Majority of cases of primary Paget's disease occur in postmenopausal white women
- Men and women are affected equally in secondary Paget's disease

Clinical Features

- Pruritic erythematous, scaly patches; lesion may extend beyond visible borders
- Vulvar lesions often present

Prognosis and Therapy

- For primary Paget's disease, wide local excision is indicated
- Recurrences are frequent and are addressed by reexcision
- Primary Paget's disease with dermal invasion may metastasize and has a less favorable prognosis
- If Paget's disease is associated with distal rectal adenocarcinoma, the stage of the rectal tumor determines the prognosis
- Paget's disease is often a marker of soft tissue extension of rectal adenocarcinoma. The prognosis is often poor

PATHOLOGIC FEATURES

Grossly, a reddish scaly patch or plaque can be seen on the skin surface (Fig. 14.12A). Microscopically, there are features of HSIL with lack of maturation and nuclear atypia involving the full epithelial thickness. Mitotic figures, sometimes atypical, are seen in the middle or upper third of the epidermis (Figs. 14.12B and C).

DIFFERENTIAL DIAGNOSIS

Differential diagnosis includes bowenoid papulosis, Paget's disease, and malignant melanoma. Whereas Paget's disease can be distinguished by mucicarmine or periodic acid–Schiff (PAS) positivity, melanoma shows positive immunostaining for S-100, Sox10, HMB-45, MiTF, and Melan-A.

PAGET'S DISEASE—PATHOLOGIC FEATURES

Gross Findings

- Erythematous patches, irregular in shape and variable in extent
- If invasive component is present, the dermis may be indurated or may contain pools of mucin

Microscopic Findings

- The squamous epithelium is infiltrated by large cells with pale cytoplasm, a central vesicular nucleus, and prominent nucleolus
- Secondary Paget cells may have signet ring morphology
- Paget cells may form clusters or intraepithelial glands
- Paget cells may infiltrate the dermis and may extend into the cutaneous adnexal structures
- Mucin stains such as mucicarmine, Alcian blue, and periodic acid–Schiff–diastase are helpful

Immunohistochemistry

- Cytokeratin (CK) 7-/CK20+/GCDFP-/CDX2+: secondary Paget's disease with associated colorectal adenocarcinoma
- CK7+/CK20-/GCDFP+/CDX2-: primary Paget's disease

Differential Diagnosis

- Squamous hyperplasia with koilocytes
- Pagetoid high-grade squamous intraepithelial lesion or Bowen's disease
- Melanoma

PROGNOSIS AND THERAPY

The rate of progression of Bowen's disease to invasive SCC is approximately 2% to 5% per year. Wide local excision remains the gold standard for therapy. Other modalities used in the management of perianal Bowen's disease include cryotherapy, CO_2 laser ablation, topical 5-FU, argon laser therapy, and photodynamic therapy.

BOWENOID PAPULOSIS

Bowenoid papulosis, also an HPV-associated lesion, is seen primarily in young adults and is characterized by red-violaceous skin papules. It is more common in the penis or scrotum but can occur in the perianal region and can be seen synchronously with condyloma acuminatum. The natural history of bowenoid papulosis is usually innocuous, with resolution spontaneously or a benign outcome after local excision. The histologic features of bowenoid papulosis resemble those of anal HSIL (Fig. 14.13) and Bowen's disease, with highly atypical nuclei scattered throughout the epithelial thickness. Closer examination, however, reveals orderly background maturation in contrast to crowded distribution of nuclei in anal HSIL and Bowen's disease. Sparing of the pilosebaceous units and involvement of

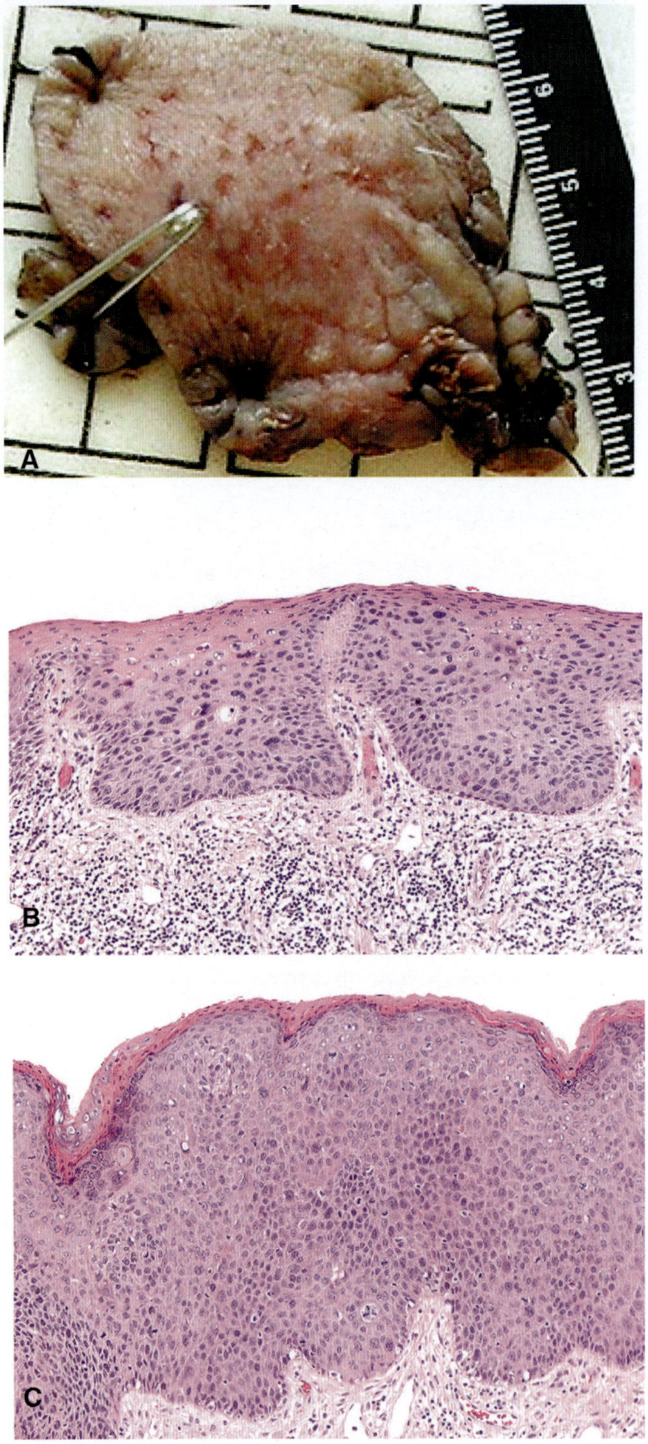

FIGURE 14.12

Perianal high-grade squamous intraepithelial lesion (HSIL) or Bowen's disease. **A**, Excisional specimen showing thin reddish patches on the perianal skin; these represent areas of HSIL microscopically. **B** and **C**, High-power view of two different examples of Bowen's disease. Note the lack of epithelial maturation with nuclear pleiomorphism (**B**) and multiple, including atypical, mitoses (**C**).

the upper zone of the eccrine glands by dysplastic cells is typical of bowenoid papulosis, whereas the opposite pattern is generally seen in anal HSIL and Bowen's disease.

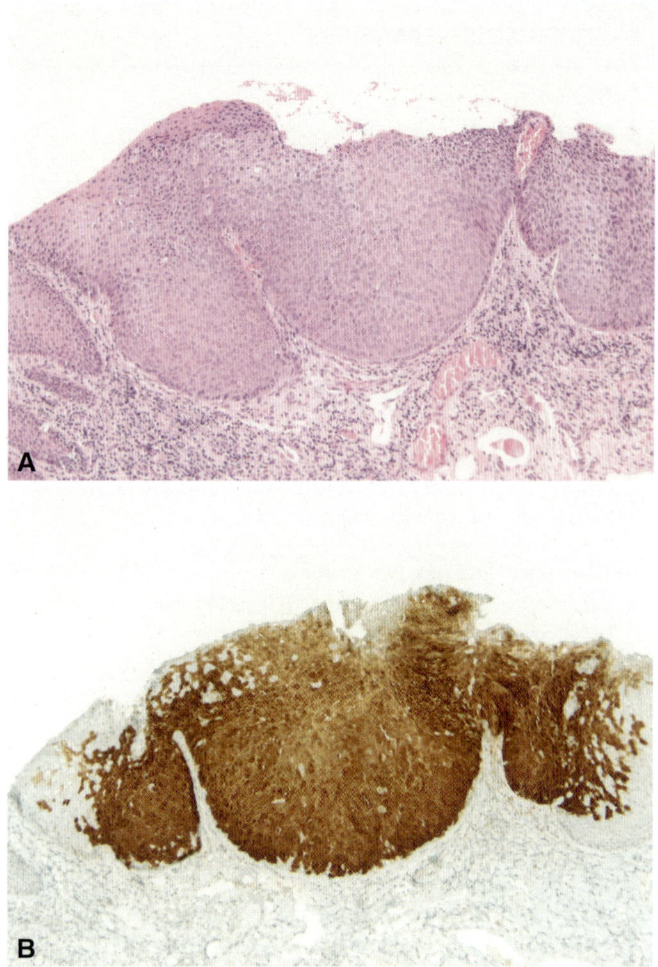

FIGURE 14.13

Bowenoid papulosis is similar to anal intraepithelial neoplasia (anal intraepithelial neoplasia), grade III (**A**), with positive immunostaining for p16, a surrogate marker for high-risk human papillomavirus infection (**B**).

SQUAMOUS CELL CARCINOMA OF THE PERIANAL SKIN

Tumors that cannot be visualized on gentle traction to the buttocks and are within 5 cm of the mucocutaneous junction are categorized as perianal. The distinction between anal and perianal tumors has therapeutic implications. SCC of the perianal skin is less common than SCC of the anal canal and has a better prognosis. It usually occurs in the sixth and seventh decade of life, has no clear gender predominance, and is associated with high-risk genotypes of HPV, similar to SCC of the anal canal. Perianal SCC may present with a painful mass, itching, tenesmus, or bleeding and usually has raised rolled borders with central ulceration (Fig. 14.14A). Advanced tumors may invade anal canal. Any nonhealing ulcer of the perianal skin should be examined via biopsy to exclude malignancy.

The typical histology is that of well- or moderately differentiated keratinizing SCC (Figs. 14.14B and C).

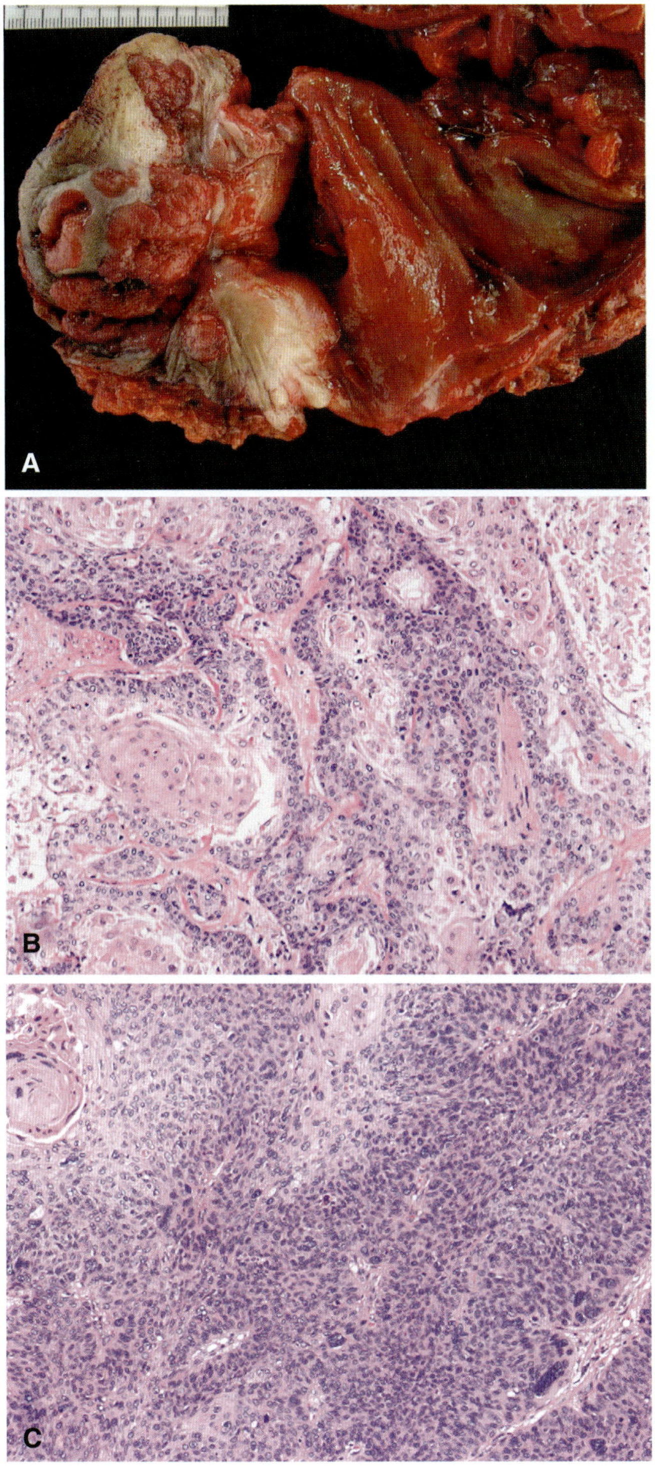

FIGURE 14.14

Squamous cell carcinoma (SCC) of the perianal skin (anal margin). Tumors in this location are usually of the keratinizing type, identical to cutaneous SCC. **B**, A well-differentiated area of SCC. **C**, An area of poor differentiation in the same tumor.

Tumor staging follows the criteria used in other cutaneous SCCs. The tumor may metastasize to inguinal lymph nodes, which is an adverse prognostic factor.

Differential diagnosis includes cutaneous BCC and melanoma. BCC of perianal skin is rare and presents as pearly nodules with raised borders, central ulceration, and occasional bleeding and crusting. Nodular growth of basophilic basaloid cells and distinct palisading of the peripheral row of cells is typical for BCC. Strong immunoreactivity for Ber-EP4 is seen in BCCs and is absent in SCC.

The preferred treatment is surgery, contrasting sharply with combined modality chemoradiation used for SCC of the anal canal, which underscores the importance of correct site designation for these tumors. Small lesions (<3 cm) are managed by local excision with wide (1-cm) negative margins. Larger and more invasive lesions may require abdominoperineal resection and radiation with or without chemotherapy. The tumor may metastasize to inguinal lymph nodes; therefore, prophylactic radiation to the nodal region is given for T2 to T4 lesions. The 5-year survival rate ranges from 70% to 89%. Local control for the same period is between 69% and 87%.

VERRUCOUS CARCINOMA

Verrucous carcinoma differs from a usual condyloma acuminatum by larger size and distinctive endophytic growth. Cases harboring areas of infiltrative or destructive invasion and/or marked cytologic atypia are classified as a subtype of SCC.

CLINICAL FEATURES

Verrucous carcinoma is more common in men, with a male-to-female ratio of 2.7 to 1. The average age of presentation is approximately 44 years. The most common symptom is perianal mass; other complaints include pain, abscess, fistula, bleeding, weight loss, and pruritus. The tumor presents as a slowly growing lesion, poorly responsive to topical therapy. When fully formed, it is a large fungating mass that deeply invades perirectal tissue with fistula formation.

PATHOLOGIC FEATURES

GROSS FINDINGS

Verrucous carcinomas are firm, warty, white to gray cauliflower-like masses, measuring up to 30 cm in size. Although the exophytic nature of the lesion is most obvious, the endophytic component may also be appreciated grossly.

MICROSCOPIC FINDINGS

The epithelium shows prominent acanthosis and papillomatosis with blunt, broad epithelial extensions

VERRUCOUS CARCINOMA—FACT SHEET

Definition

- A well-differentiated, locally aggressive squamous cell carcinoma with no potential for metastasis

Incidence and Location

- Rare
- Perianal skin but may involve any part of the anogenital region

Morbidity and Mortality

- High morbidity and 20% mortality rate

Gender, Race, and Age Distribution

- Males more than females, 2.7 to 1
- Average age of presentation is 44 years
- No racial predominance

Clinical Features

- Cauliflower-like exophytic mass
- Resembles condyloma; large size suspicious
- Complaints include mass lesion, pain, bleeding, abscess, fistula, pruritus, and weight loss

Prognosis and Therapy

- Treatment of choice is wide local excision, which is potentially curative
- Larger lesions with extensive locally destructive growth are treated with abdominoperineal resection or combined radiation and chemotherapy

VERRUCOUS CARCINOMA— PATHOLOGIC FEATURES

Gross Findings

- Firm, tan-white, cauliflower-like polypoid mass; also shows an endophytic component on sectioning

Microscopic Findings

- Squamous mucosa shows acanthosis, papillomatosis and virtually no cytologic atypia
- Blunt epithelial extensions push into underlying stroma, with no desmoplastic reaction
- Lymphoplasmacytic inflammation is common at the base of lesion

Molecular Pathology

- Limited utility in diagnosis

Immunohistochemistry

- Not required for diagnosis

Differential Diagnosis

- Condyloma, particularly Giant condyloma of Buschke-Lowenstein (which is associated with low-risk human papillomavirus and does not show an endophytic components)
- Squamous cell carcinoma

"pushing" downward into the underlying stroma (Fig. 14.15A). The epithelial–stromal interface may correspond to an area of destruction of native structures and often shows a lymphoplasmacytic inflammation. Keratin-filled cysts may be present in the endophytic portion of the lesion, and surface keratinization may be prominent. The cytologic atypia is minimal, if any, and neoplastic epithelium appears benign, with orderly maturation, basal mitoses, and retention of cellular polarity (Fig. 14.15B). The diagnosis may be difficult because of limited sampling, especially in biopsies, and requires awareness of a possibility of verrucous carcinoma. As mentioned earlier under the discussion of anal tumors, verrucous carcinoma is distinct from the giant condyloma of Buschke-Lowenstein. The latter is associated with low-risk HPV DNA genotypes, shows viral cytopathic changes, and only has an exophytic component.

ANCILLARY STUDIES

Ancillary testing is of limited value in the diagnosis of anal or perianal verrucous carcinoma.

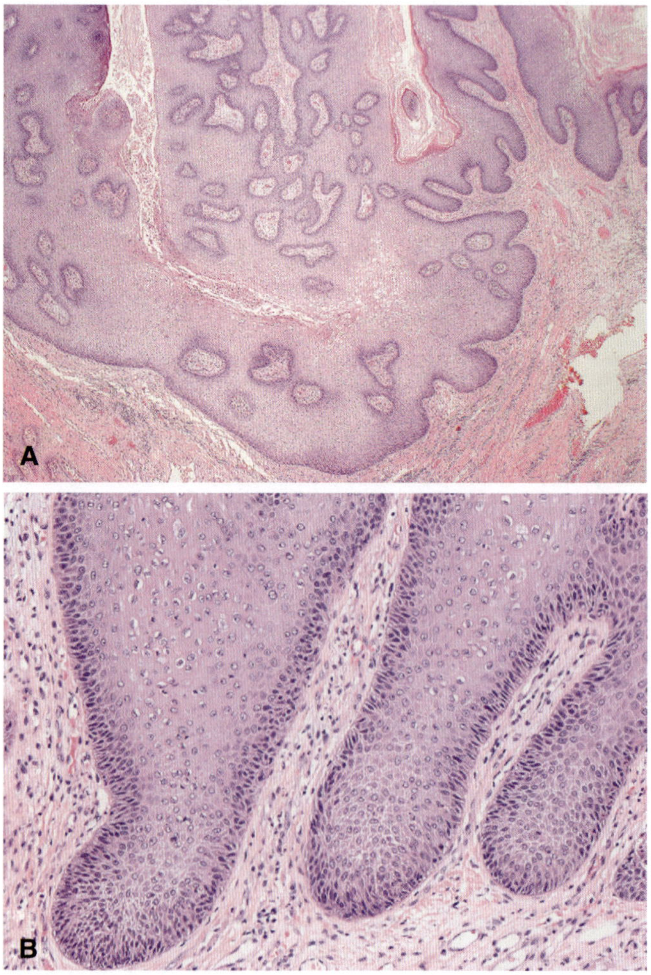

FIGURE 14.15

Verrucous carcinoma. **A**, At low power, the papillomatous pattern with abundant surface keratinization and innocuous-appearing cytologic features are evident. Note the downward projections of the neoplasm into the submucosal connective tissue. **B**, Typical "pushing" invasion of verrucous carcinoma without desmoplastic reaction. There is no significant nuclear atypia or dysmaturation in this tumor. Mitotic activity is not present above this basal zone.

MOLECULAR PATHOLOGY

The diagnosis of verrucous carcinoma is based on histology and molecular testing has limited utility. The presence of high-risk HPV genotype in biopsy samples from perianal mass lesions should raise suspicion against a diagnosis of verrucous carcinoma.

Differential Diagnosis

Verrucous carcinoma can be distinguished from condyloma acuminatum by larger size (>10 cm), presence of endophytic growth with a broad pushing interface, a thicker keratinized layer, and more prominent papillomatosis. If a lesion contains areas with irregular infiltrating tumor interface, desmoplastic stromal response, or areas with marked cytologic atypia, it should be classified as SCC.

Prognosis and Therapy

Perianal verrucous carcinomas are locally destructive but do not metastasize. The treatment of choice is wide local excision, which is curative in early phases of the disease. For particularly large and destructive lesions, more aggressive surgery, such as abdominoperineal resection and (neo)adjuvant radiation and chemotherapy, may be necessary. Local recurrences are common, and approximately 20% of patients eventually succumb to the disease.

PAGET'S DISEASE

Paget's disease of the perianal region is a form of adenocarcinoma localized within the squamous epithelium. In the primary form of the disease, Paget cells are thought to originate from the apocrine glands of cutaneous adnexal structures. The secondary form of the disease represents approximately half of all cases and is caused by pagetoid extension of the primary colorectal or anal adenocarcinoma into the overlying squamous epithelium.

CLINICAL FEATURES

The majority of cases of primary perianal Paget's disease occur in postmenopausal white women with Paget's disease of the vulva extending to the perianal skin. Secondary Paget's disease equally affects men and women, and the majority of cases are diagnosed in the sixth to eighth decades of life. Early Paget's lesions appear as erythematous, scaly patches and are typically pruritic; erosions or ulcers may also develop. The lesions may look small; however, neoplastic cells expand far beyond the visible abnormality within the epithelium and may involve the anal canal. The rarity of the disease and its resemblance to a variety of benign dermatologic disorders may result in delayed diagnosis and treatment.

Pathologic Features

Gross Findings

A typical specimen is a punch biopsy. Excision specimens may demonstrate scaly, erythematous patches or plaques or, less commonly, erosion or ulcer. If an invasive component is present, the dermal or submucosal tissue may appear indurated or nodular or may contain mucinous material.

Microscopic Findings

The squamous epithelium is infiltrated by scattered large cells with abundant pale or amphophilic mucin-containing cytoplasm, a centrally placed nucleus, vesicular chromatin, and a conspicuous nucleolus (Fig. 14.16A). In addition to the classic Paget cell, a signet ring cell–type cell may also be seen in secondary Paget's disease. Paget cells may infiltrate the epithelium as single cells or as clusters or even form intraepithelial glandular structures with intraluminal necrosis. Paget cells may also involve cutaneous adnexal pilosebaceous units and eccrine and apocrine ducts. Rarely, Paget cells appear to directly infiltrate the perianal stromal tissue, a condition called invasive Paget's disease. In some cases, an underlying eccrine or apocrine adenocarcinoma of the skin or synchronous anorectal adenocarcinoma may be identified. In addition, the epidermis may demonstrate a spectrum of proliferative changes, such as simple hyperplasia or papillomatous hyperplasia. Parakeratosis, hyperkeratosis, erosion, or ulceration may be also seen.

ANCILLARY STUDIES

Histochemistry

Because Paget cells contain acid mucopolysaccharides, they stain with mucicarmine, Alcian blue (pH, 2.5), and PAS–diastase.

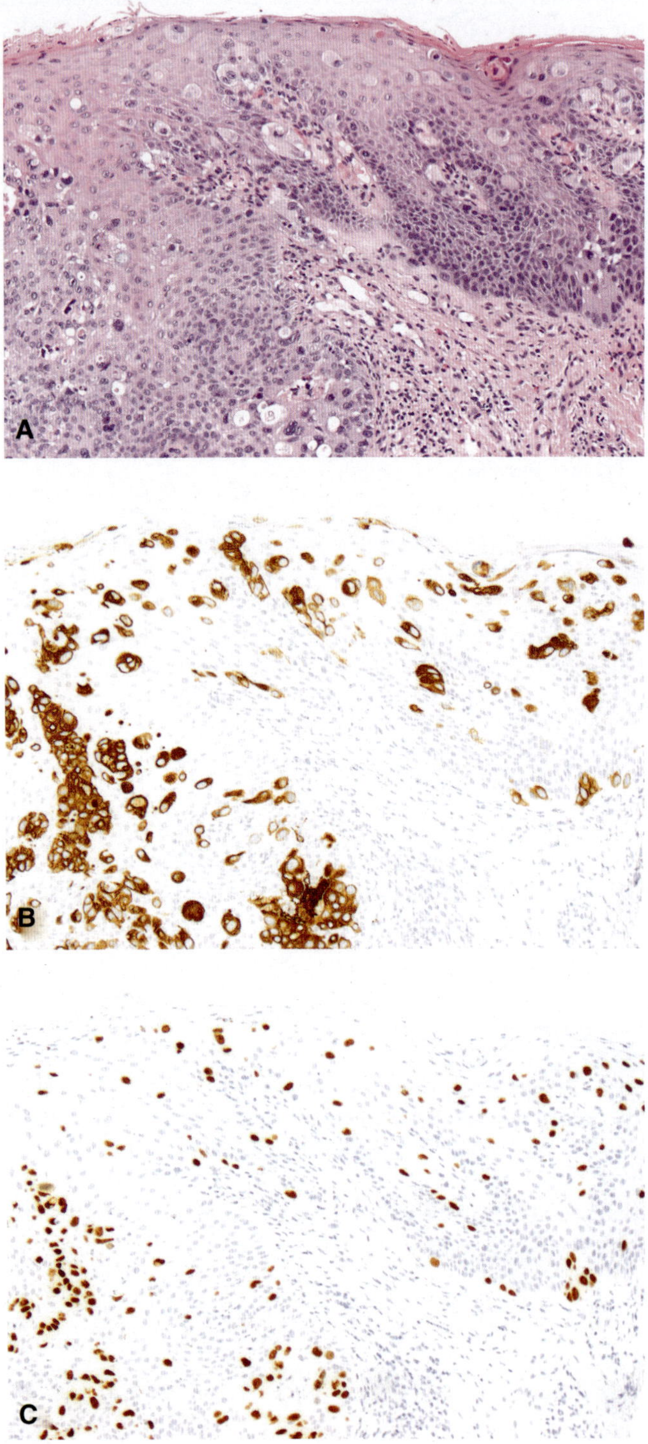

FIGURE 14.16

Secondary Paget's disease associated with rectal adenocarcinoma. **A**, Paget cells have abundant pale to amphophilic cytoplasm and a centrally located vesicular nucleus with conspicuous nucleolus. They are scattered singly and in small clusters throughout the squamous epithelium. The Paget cells are positive for cytokeratin 20 (**B**) and CDX2 (**C**) and negative for cytokeratin 7 (not shown), suggestive of colorectal origin of Paget cells.

IMMUNOHISTOCHEMISTRY

Two major patterns of immunostaining have been described. Paget cells of the primary Paget's disease are positive for CK7 and gross cystic disease fluid protein (GCDFP) and are negative for CK20, consistent with apocrine gland differentiation. In secondary Paget's disease, Paget cells are most commonly CK7−/CK20+/CDX2+, consistent with the origin from a colorectal adenocarcinoma (Fig. 14.16B and C). A CK7+/CK20+/GCDFP− profile may be seen in secondary Paget's disease associated with a urothelial carcinoma.

Differential Diagnosis

When perianal Paget's disease is associated with papillomatous squamous hyperplasia, Paget cells can show small, pyknotic nuclei and perinuclear halo mimicking koilocytes. Pagetoid Bowen disease may also exhibit a nested growth pattern mimicking Paget's disease. However, mucin stains and immunopositivity for CK7, as well as negativity for p63 and CK5/6 are helpful in confirming the diagnosis of Paget's disease. The presence of melanin in neoplastic cells is not a proof of melanoma because both Paget cells and dysplastic cells of Bowen's disease may contain melanin pigment. Melanocytic immunomarkers, such as S-100, SOX10, HMB-45, and MART-1 (melanoma antigen recognized by T cells 1), are positive in melanoma and negative in Paget's disease.

Prognosis and Therapy

Patients with primary perianal Paget's disease are treated with wide local excision. Local recurrence is frequent and is treated with reexcision. The prognosis is favorable with normal life expectancy. If Paget cells invade the dermis, which may occur in primary Paget's disease, the risk of metastasis adversely affects the prognosis. Secondary Paget's disease has a poor prognosis, defined by the primary visceral tumor, most commonly a distal rectal adenocarcinoma.

SUGGESTED READINGS

Inflammatory Processes and Non-Neoplastic Lesions

1. Brown AC, Sumfest JM, Rozwadowski JV. Histopathology of the internal anal sphincter in chronic anal fissure. *Dis Colon Rectum*. 1989;32:680–683.
2. Steele SR, Kumar R, Feingold DL, et al. Practice parameters for the management of perianal abscess and fistula-in-ano. *Dis Colon Rectum*. 2011;54:1465–1474.

Crohn's Disease

3. Gecse KB, Bemelman W, Kamm MA, et al. A global consensus on the classification, diagnosis and multidisciplinary treatment of perianal fistulising Crohn's disease. *Gut*. 2014;63:1381–1392.
4. Lewis RT, Bleier JI. Surgical treatment of anorectal Crohn's disease. *Clin Colon Rectal Surg*. 2013;26:90–99.

5. Zabana Y, Van Domselaar M, Garcia-Planella E, et al. Perianal disease in patients with ulcerative colitis: a case-control study. *J Crohns Colitis*. 2011;5:338–341.

Hemorrhoids and Anal Tags

6. Ganz RA. The evaluation and treatment of hemorrhoids: a guide for the gastroenterologist. *Clin Gastroenterol Hepatol*. 2013;11:593–603.
7. Johanson JF, Sonnenberg A. The prevalence of hemorrhoids and chronic constipation. *An epidemiologic study. Gastroenterology*. 1990;98:380–386.
8. Lemarchand N, Tanne F, Aubert M, et al. Is routine pathologic evaluation of hemorrhoidectomy specimens necessary? *Gastroenterol Clin Biol*. 2004;28:659–661.
9. Riss S, Weiser FA, Schwameis K, et al. The prevalence of hemorrhoids in adults. *Int J Colorectal Dis*. 2012;27:215–220.

Anal Squamous Intraepithelial Lesion

10. Berry JM, Jay N, Cranston RD, et al. Progression of anal high-grade squamous intraepithelial lesions to invasive anal cancer among HIV-infected men who have sex with men International journal of cancer. *Int J Cancer*. 2014;134:1147–1155.
11. Etienney I, Fléjou J, Si-Mohamed A, et al. Five-year single-center prospective search for anal intraepithelial neoplasia and human papillomavirus infection in all hemorrhoidectomy and fissurectomy surgical samples. *Dis Colon Rectum*. 2014;57:e152.
12. Fenger C, Nielsen VT. Dysplastic changes in the anal canal epithelium in minor surgical specimens. *Acta Pathol Microbiol Scand A*. 1981;89:463–465.
13. Fox PA. Treatment options for anal intraepithelial neoplasia and evidence for their effectiveness. *Sex Health*. 2012;9: 587–592.
14. Machalek DA, Poynten M, Jin F, et al. Anal human papillomavirus infection and associated neoplastic lesions in men who have sex with men: a systematic review and meta-analysis. *Lancet Oncol*. 2012;13:487–500.

Squamous Cell Carcinoma of the Anal Canal

15. Bernardi MP, Ngan SY, Michael M, et al. Molecular biology of anal squamous cell carcinoma: implications for future research and clinical intervention. *Lancet Oncol*. 2015;16:e611–e621.
16. Hoots BE, Palefsky JM, Pimenta JM, et al. Human papillomavirus type distribution in anal cancer and anal intraepithelial lesions. *Int J Cancer*. 2009;124:2375–2383.
17. Steele SR, Varma MG, Melton GB, et al. Practice parameters for anal squamous neoplasms. *Dis Colon Rectum*. 2012;55: 735–749.

Adenocarcinoma

18. Hobbs CM, Lowry MA, Owen D, et al. Anal gland carcinoma. *Cancer*. 2001;92:2045–2049.
19. Lisovsky M, Patel K, Cymes K, et al. Immunophenotypic characterization of anal gland carcinoma: loss of p63 and cytokeratin 5/6. *Arch Pathol Lab Med*. 2007;131:1304–1311.
20. Nishigami T, Kataoka TR, Ikeuchi H, et al. Adenocarcinomas associated with perianal fistulae in Crohn's disease have a rectal, not an anal immunophenotype. *Pathology*. 2011;43:36–39.
21. Ramalingam P, Hart WR, Goldblum JR. Cytokeratin subset immunostaining in rectal adenocarcinoma and normal anal glands. *Arch Pathol Lab Med*. 2001;125:1074–1077.
22. Tarazi R, Nelson RL. Anal adenocarcinoma: a comprehensive review. *Semin Surg Oncol*. 1994;10:235–240.

Melanoma

23. Knowles J, Lynch AC, Warrier SK, et al. A case series of anal melanoma including the results of treatment with imatinib in selected patients. *Colorectal Dis*. 2016;18:877–882.
24. Santi R, Simi L, Fucci R, et al. KIT genetic alterations in anorectal melanomas. *J Clin Pathol*. 2015;68:130–134.
25. Yang HM, Hsiao SJ, Schaeffer DF, et al. Identification of recurrent mutational events in anorectal melanoma. *Mod Pathol*. 2017;30(2):286–296.

Hidradenoma Papilliferum

26. Kazakov DV, Spagnolo DV, Kacerovska D, et al. Lesions of anogenital mammary-like glands: an update. *Adv Anat Pathol*. 2011;18:1–28.

Condyloma

27. Oon SF, Winter DC. Perianal condylomas, anal squamous intraepithelial neoplasms and screening: a review of the literature. *J Med Screen*. 2010;17:44–49.
28. Pirog EC, Quint KD, Yantiss RK. P16/CDKN2A and Ki-67 enhance the detection of anal intraepithelial neoplasia and condyloma and correlate with human papillomavirus detection by polymerase chain reaction. *Am J Surg Path*. 2010;34:1449–1455.

Perianal Squamous Intraepithelial Lesion, Bowen Disease, and Bowenoid Papillosis

29. Cleary RK, Schaldenbrand JD, Fowler JJ, et al. Perianal Bowen's disease and anal intraepithelial neoplasia: review of the literature. *Dis Colon Rectum*. 1999;42:945–951.
30. Marchesa P, Fazio VW, Oliart S, et al. Perianal Bowen's disease: a clinicopathologic study of 47 patients. *Dis Colon Rectum*. 1997;40:1286–1293.
31. Sah SP, Kelly PJ, McManus DT, et al. Diffuse CK7, CAM5.2 and BerEP4 positivity in pagetoid squamous cell carcinoma in situ (pagetoid Bowen's disease) of the perianal region: a mimic of extramammary Paget's disease. *Histopathology*. 2013;62:511–514.

Perianal Squamous Cell Carcinoma

32. Swanson PE, Fitzpatrick MM, Ritter JH, et al. Immunohistologic differential diagnosis of basal cell carcinoma, squamous cell carcinoma, and trichoepithelioma in small cutaneous biopsy specimens. *J Cutan Pathol*. 1998;25:153–159.
33. Tellechea O, Reis JP, Domingues JC, et al. Monoclonal antibody Ber EP4 distinguishes basal-cell carcinoma from squamous-cell carcinoma of the skin. *Am J Dermatopathol*. 1993;15:452–455.

Verrucous Carcinoma or Giant Condyloma of Buschke

34. Chu QD, Vezeridis MP, Libbey NP, et al. Giant condyloma acuminatum (Buschke-Lowenstein tumor) of the anorectal and perianal regions. Analysis of 42 cases. *Dis Colon Rectum*. 1994;37:950–957.
35. del Pino M, Bleeker MC, Quint WG, et al. Comprehensive analysis of human papillomavirus prevalence and the potential role of low-risk types in verrucous carcinoma. *Mod Pathol*. 2012;25:1354–1363.

Paget's Disease

36. Kim NR, Cho HY, Baek JH, et al. Rare case of anal canal signet ring cell carcinoma associated with perianal and vulvar pagetoid spread. *J Pathol Transl Med*. 2016;50:231–237.
37. Wong AY, Rahilly MA, Adams W, et al. Mucinous anal gland carcinoma with perianal Pagetoid spread. *Pathology*. 1998;30:1–3.

15

Pathology of the Gallbladder and Extrahepatic Bile Ducts

James Conner, MD, PhD and Amitabh Srivastava, MD

The gallbladder and extrahepatic bile ducts show a limited spectrum of inflammatory and neoplastic disorders, but these disorders are significant because they affect a large proportion of the world's population. The most common (>95%) is cholelithiasis. Inflammation in the gallbladder secondary to stones presents either as acute or chronic cholecystitis and may lead to significant complications such as empyema, perforation, or fistula. Carcinomas of the gallbladder are uncommon and arise from flat, polypoid or cystic precursor lesions and may sometimes be detected incidentally in patients undergoing a routine cholecystectomy. The recent World Health Organization (WHO) classification has proposed a new nomenclature for these precursor lesions to align them with precursors seen elsewhere in the pancreaticobiliary tree. Stage is the most important prognostic factor, and the 5-year survival rate is dismal because most cases are at an advanced stage at initial presentation or have multifocal biliary dysplasia.

GALLBLADDER

CHOLECYSTITIS

Clinical Features

Cholecystitis presents with intermittent postprandial epigastric or right upper quadrant pain. By far the most common underlying cause is cholelithiasis, which in some cases may also lead to obstruction of the bile duct (choledocholithiasis). Acute cholecystitis is also associated with fever and leukocytosis. Clinical examination is supported by a positive "Murphy sign" in which pain is elicited when the inflamed gallbladder descends during inspiration. The clinical impression may be confirmed by ultrasound, which demonstrates choleliths, gallbladder wall thickening, and pericholecystic fluid. Xanthogranulomatous cholecystitis may show mural nodularity and dense adhesions to adjacent organs, which may cause clinical concern for malignancy.

In 0.5% to 1% of cases, a porcelain gallbladder, characterized by diffuse calcification of the wall, is seen radiographically and intraoperatively. This finding correlates with the pathologic diagnosis of hyalinizing cholecystitis (HC) and has classically been associated with an increased risk of gallbladder carcinoma. This risk has traditionally been considered sufficient to warrant prophylactic cholecystectomy, but recent studies have shown the risk to be lower than previously reported.

Sterile acalculous cholecystitis is much less common, and most patients present with multiple other comorbidities, especially in the hospital setting. It is most commonly associated with ischemia and dysmotility. Infectious cholecystitis is rare, occurring predominantly in immunocompromised patients. The most common infections are *Cryptosporidium parvum* and cytomegalovirus. Rare cases of cholecystitis represent manifestations of systemic diseases, including eosinophilic cholecystitis, presenting as a component of eosinophilic gastroenteritis, primary sclerosing cholangitis (PSC)–associated cholecystitis, and immunoglobulin (Ig) G4–associated sclerosing cholecystitis, which is present in almost all patients with IgG4 sclerosing cholangitis of the bile duct.

Pathologic Features

Gross Findings

Acute cholecystitis is characterized by mucosal erythema, friability, and ulceration. The gallbladder wall may be thickened and edematous. In severe cases, serositis may be present with a fibrinous exudate on the serosal surface. Chronic cholecystitis most often exhibits mural fibrosis with a thick and firm gallbladder wall. Extensive hyalinization and calcification (>80% of the circumferential wall) is classified as porcelain gallbladder. Xanthogranulomatous cholecystitis may be associated with mural nodules that can grossly mimic malignancy (Fig. 15.1A). Cholesterolosis, which is found in approximately 20% of cholecystectomy specimens, results in a

Cholecystitis—Fact Sheet

Definition

- Acute or chronic inflammatory injury to the gallbladder, usually as a consequence of cholelithiasis

Incidence and Location

- 10% to 20% of adult population in the United States and Western Europe with cholelithiasis
- 80% to 90% are calculous cholecystitis; rest are acalculous
- 1000 to 4000 per 100,000 individuals present with symptomatic disease

Morbidity and Mortality

- Complications include sepsis, abscess, perforation, peritonitis, and fistulas

Gender, Race, and Age Distribution

- Risk increases with age
- Female predominance for calculous cholecystitis
- Males affected more frequently for acalculous cholecystitis
- North American Indians affected more commonly than White Americans, African Americans, and Asians

Clinical Features

- Right upper quadrant or epigastric pain with tenderness ("Murphy sign")
- Fever, nausea, vomiting
- Mild jaundice may be present

Differential Diagnosis

- Peptic ulcer, pancreatitis, kidney stones
- Appendicitis or intestinal obstruction

stippled mucosal surface, often described as "strawberry gallbladder" (Figs. 15.1B and C). Choleliths or choledocholiths may be present. Cholesterol gallstones, the most common type, are yellow-green, whereas gallstones composed of abundant bilirubin ("pigment stones") are black or brown. Black pigment stones are sometimes associated with hereditary hemolytic conditions, although the majority of cases are sporadic.

Microscopic Findings

Features of acute cholecystitis include neutrophilic or eosinophilic infiltration, mucosal erosion or ulceration, hemorrhage, gangrenous necrosis, and reactive epithelial changes (Fig. 15.2). The predominant findings in chronic cholecystitis are mural fibrosis, muscular hypertrophy, and a variable degree of mononuclear cell infiltration (Fig. 15.3). Mucosal invaginations through the muscularis propria, known as Rokitansky-Aschoff sinuses, are frequently seen in chronic cholecystitis and are usually associated with muscular hypertrophy. The sinuses may undergo striking cystic change because of outflow obstruction and can mimic a neoplastic process (Fig. 15.4). Inflammatory polyps may also be present. In cases of both acute and chronic cholecystitis, these polyps may have associated reactive epithelial changes and must be distinguished from the polypoid dysplastic lesions. Pyloric gland and intestinal metaplasia may also be present as a consequence of chronic injury and repair (Fig. 15.5). Less frequently, squamous metaplasia may be seen. Xanthogranulomatous cholecystitis is caused by extravasation of bile into the gallbladder wall, eliciting a florid histiocytic response (Fig. 15.6). Reactive fibroblasts are present, which can be so cellular as to mimic a mesenchymal neoplasm. Clues to a benign diagnosis include bland histology, abundant foamy macrophages, and admixed cholesterol clefts and bile pigment. Cholesterolosis is characterized by clusters of cholesterol-laden macrophages that accumulate under the epithelial surface. It is generally considered an incidental finding and does not necessitate further work-up.

Hyalinizing cholecystitis is defined by paucicellular hyaline sclerosis that obliterates all of the layers of the gallbladder wall (Fig. 15.7). It is typically seen, on average, in patients one decade older than other variants of cholecystitis and in those with long-standing gallbladder inflammation. Focal or diffuse dystrophic calcification may be present in the gallbladder wall. HC cases with diffuse (>80%) calcification correlate with porcelain gallbladder, but all cases of radiographically identified porcelain gallbladder show HC histologically. However, the converse is not always true. Paucicellular hyalinizing sclerosis of HC may be present in some patients with only minimal or no mural calcification. HC, and in particular cases with minimal or no calcification, is associated with an increased (10%–20%) risk for gallbladder carcinoma. Given this risk, complete histologic

Cholecystitis—Pathologic Features

Gross Findings

- Acute cholecystitis: mucosal erythema, friability, and ulceration or frank necrosis
- Chronic cholecystitis: mural fibrosis with thick, firm wall
- Xanthogranulomatous cholecystitis: mural nodules and extension into adjacent organs may mimic malignancy
- Choleliths may be present
- Thick wall with calcification in porcelain gallbladder

Microscopic Findings

- Mucosal erosion, ulcer, or hemorrhage with neutrophilic infiltrate in acute cholecystitis
- Transmural necrosis in gangrenous cholecystitis
- Chronic inflammation with mural thickening, pyloric gland, and intestinal metaplasia in chronic cholecystitis
- Foamy histiocytes with a reactive spindle cell proliferation in xanthogranulomatous cholecystitis
- Hyalinized wall with calcification in porcelain gallbladder

Genetics

- Not relevant

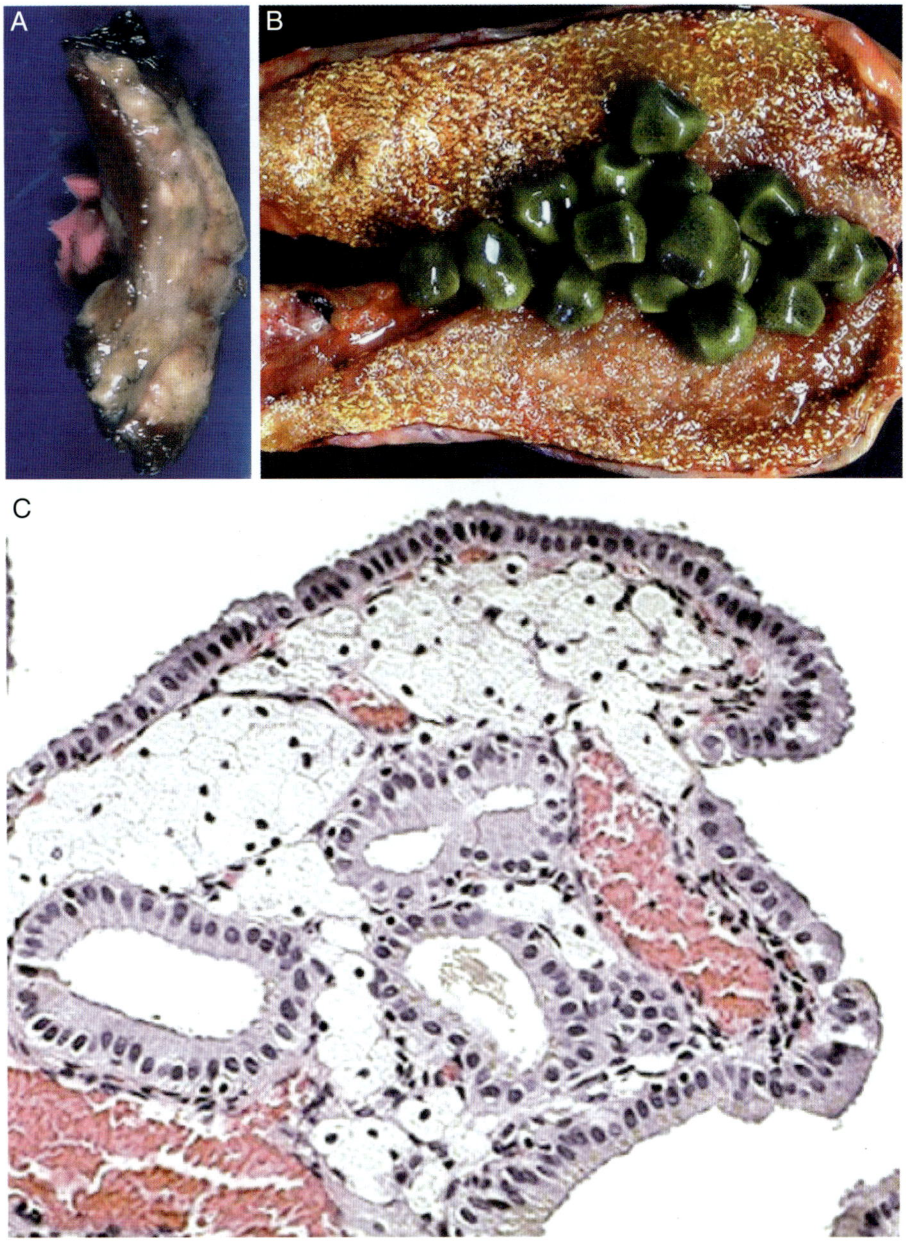

FIGURE 15.1

Xanthogranulomatous cholecystitis with a thickened gallbladder wall and gray-yellow nodules (**A**), which can mimic malignancy on radiologic examination. Cholesterolosis is a frequent finding in cholecystectomy specimens and shows a yellow stippled mucosal appearance (**B**), which corresponds to foamy lipid-laden macrophages in lamina propria on microscopy (**C**). At times, this deposition may be exuberant and form a discrete polypoid lesion ("cholesterol polyp").

examination of gallbladder specimens with HC is warranted. Carcinomas associated with HC are generally very well differentiated and may be paucicellular with only scattered neoplastic glands present in the wall. An overt desmoplastic response is not always present.

Gallbladder Dysplasia and Carcinoma

Neoplasia involving the gallbladder is diagnosed in two distinct clinical scenarios. Dysplasia or early carcinoma may be an incidental diagnosis in a gallbladder removed for acute or chronic cholecystitis. In other instances, cholecystectomy is performed for a preoperative finding of a mass lesion suspicious for cancer. Not surprisingly, the clinical presentation and morphologic differential diagnosis are quite different in these two situations. For this reason, early and advanced gallbladder carcinomas are discussed under separate headers later. However, it must be emphasized that early and advanced cancers are not distinct entities and represent two stages of the same neoplastic process.

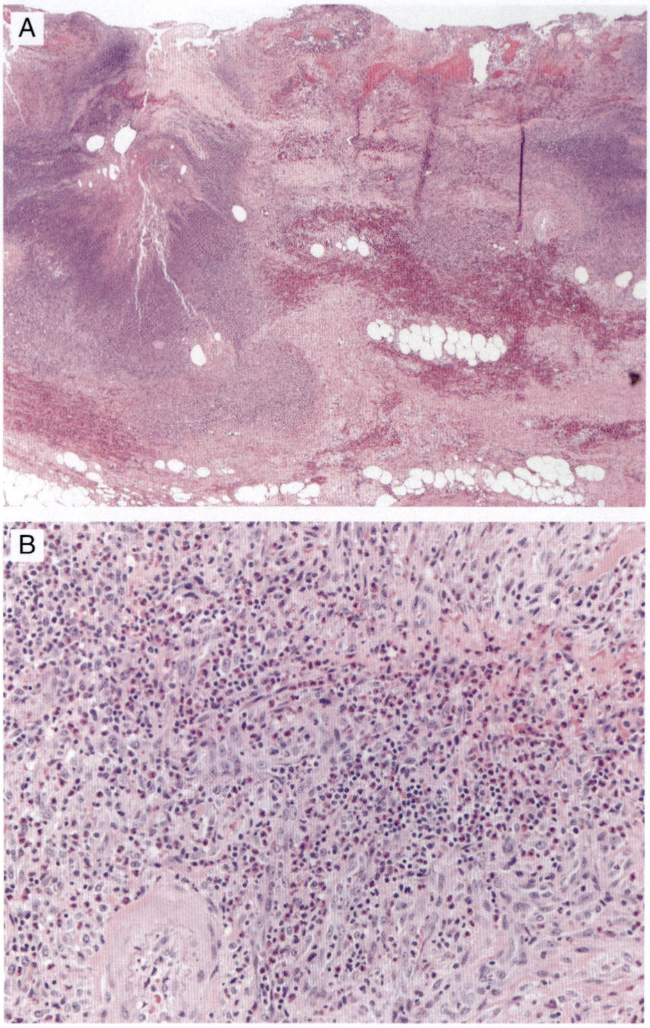

FIGURE 15.2

Acute cholecystitis presents microscopically with marked acute inflammation, edema, hemorrhage, or necrosis and any one of these features can predominate. Acute gangrenous cholecystitis shows striking transmural necrosis (**A**), but in other examples, a marked acute inflammatory infiltrate composed of neutrophils and eosinophils may be present (**B**).

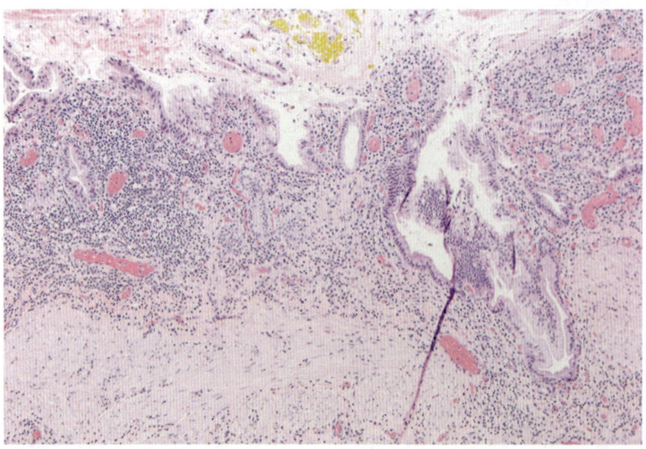

FIGURE 15.3

The typical features of chronic cholecystitis include marked expansion of the lamina propria by a lymphoplasmacytic inflammatory infiltrate or metaplastic features of chronicity such as pyloric gland and intestinal metaplasia. Deep invaginations of the mucosa into and beyond the muscularis propria (Rokitansky-Aschoff sinuses) are often present.

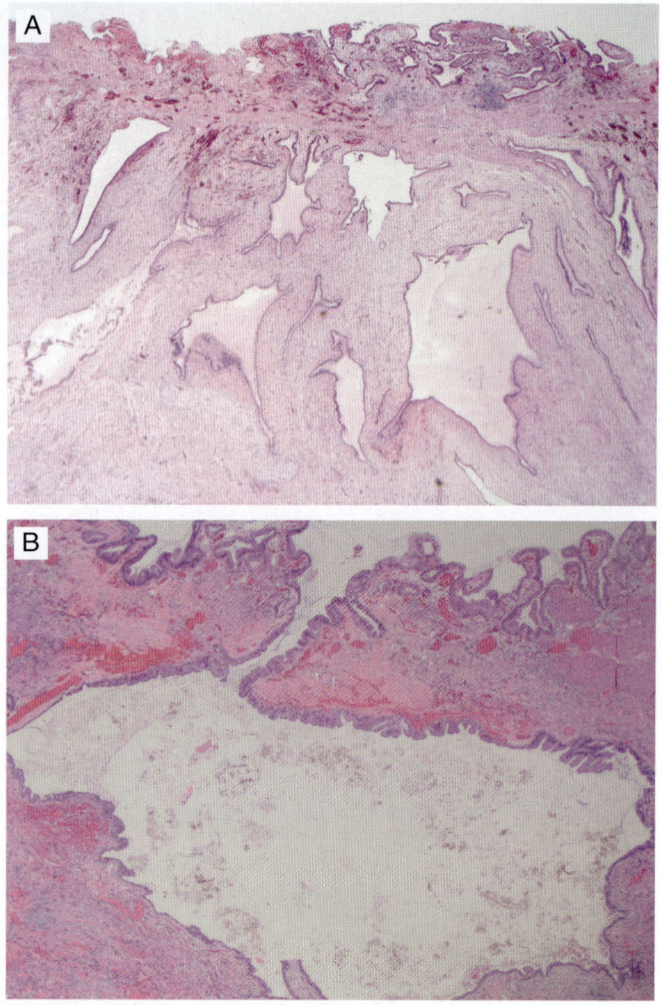

FIGURE 15.4

Adenomyoma. **A**, At low power, the presence of epithelium in the perimuscular connective tissue raises the possibility of invasive carcinoma, but the lining epithelium is benign and does not show any atypia. **B**, In some cases, deeper levels can demonstrate communication with the surface mucosa. Note the marked cystic dilation that may appear radiologically as a mass worrisome for neoplasia.

DYSPLASIA AND EARLY GALLBLADDER CARCINOMA

CLINICAL FEATURES

Many cases of early gallbladder neoplasia are found unexpectedly at the time of pathologic evaluation of a routine cholecystectomy rather than by symptomatic presentation or radiographic imaging. Gallbladder dysplasia can be divided into flat (or micropapillary) lesions (biliary intraepithelial neoplasia [BilIN]) and exophytic lesions (intracholecystic papillary neoplasm [ICPN]). Exophytic lesions may be suspected on preoperative imaging, but BilIN is usually clinically occult. Early invasive gallbladder carcinoma with invasion into the lamina propria (T1a) or into the muscular layer (T1b)

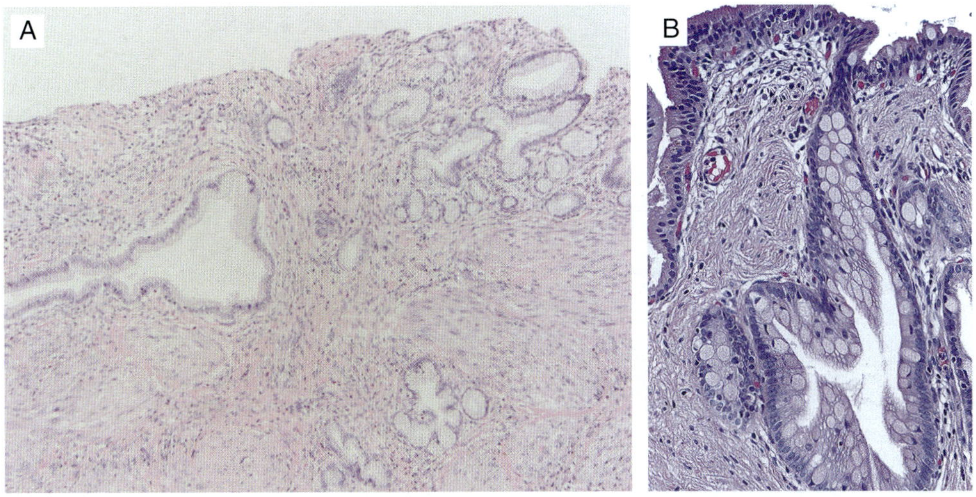

FIGURE 15.5

Common forms of metaplasia in the gallbladder include pyloric gland metaplasia (**A**), where small tubular gastric-type pyloric glands replace the native pancreaticobiliary type epithelium. These foci are MUC6 positive, similar to glandular epithelium in the gastric antrum. Intestinal metaplasia is often present adjacent to neoplasia in the gallbladder and is characterized by goblet cells (**B**). Paneth cells or intestinal-type neuroendocrine cells with basal red granules may also be seen in some cases as part of the metaplastic process.

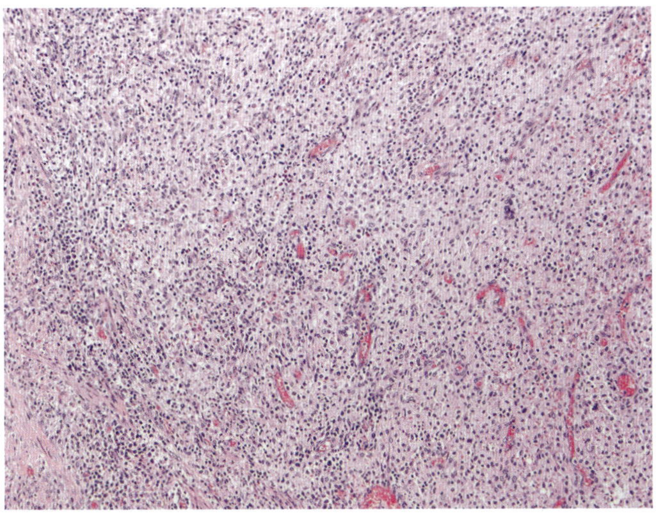

FIGURE 15.6

Xanthogranulomatous cholecystitis can mimic malignancy on imaging and extend into adjacent hepatic parenchyma. The inflammatory infiltrate is characterized by foamy histiocytes, often around extruded bile; variable acute inflammation; and dense fibrosis.

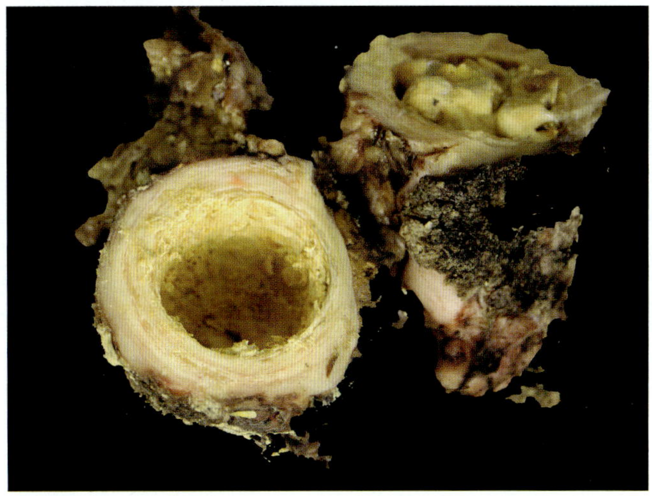

FIGURE 15.7

Hyalinizing chronic cholecystitis, also known as "porcelain gallbladder," shows massive thickening of the gallbladder wall with fibrosis and calcification. A meticulous gross and microscopic examination is essential to rule out the possibility of malignancy in these cases.

arising from BilIN cannot be identified preoperatively with certainty. ICPNs are present in 0.5 % of all cholecystectomies and about 6 % of all gallbladder carcinomas arising in an ICPN.

Risk factors for BilIN and early gallbladder carcinomas include cholelithiasis, chronic cholecystitis, history of gallbladder polyps, PSC, anomalous union of pancreatobiliary ducts, and familial adenomatous polyposis. In contrast to flat dysplasia, ICPN is not strongly associated with cholelithiasis. Both types of dysplasia are associated with advanced age. There appears to be geographic variance in the incidence of early gallbladder carcinoma. Asia and South America have two to three times the incidence in North America and Europe.

Pathologic Features

Gross Findings

As expected, flat dysplasia or BilIN is invisible on gross examination and is detected in random sections from a cholecystectomy. However, ICPN, by definition, is a grossly visible lesion, typically 1 cm or larger, with a median size around 2 cm. Some ICPNs are friable and may be present as detached fragments within the gallbladder lumen. They can be mistaken for luminal debris if this possibility is not considered. Mild thickening of the gallbladder wall may be seen in early invasive carcinomas, but this is often too subtle to be of practical

Dysplasia and Early Gallbladder Carcinoma—Fact Sheet

Definition

- Neoplasia confined to the gallbladder epithelium (dysplasia) or carcinoma confined to the lamina propria (T1a) or the muscular wall (T1b)

Incidence and Location

- Approximately 2% to 5% of patients undergoing cholecystectomy in North America and Europe
- Higher incidence in South America and Asia
- Risk factors: cholelithiasis, primary sclerosing cholangitis, advanced age, gallbladder polyps, familial adenomatous polyposis, anomalous union of pancreatobiliary ducts
- 6% of all cancers arise in an intracholecystic papillary neoplasm

Morbidity and Mortality

- Dysplasia: cholecystectomy with negative margins is curative
- Early carcinoma: favorable prognosis (~90% 5-year survival) if gallbladder is examined entirely to exclude deeply invasive tumor

Gender, Race, and Age Distribution

- Female predominance
- Mostly affects adults

Clinical Features

- Often asymptomatic
- Cholecystitis and cholelithiasis are usual indications for cholecystectomy

Differential Diagnosis

- Reactive epithelial atypia
- Dysplasia involving Rokitansky-Aschoff sinuses versus invasive carcinoma

utility, especially because most inflamed gallbladders are edematous. Adequate sampling is key to ensure an accurate diagnosis. Although there is some variation in "optimal practice" based on expert opinion, most agree on the general principle that more sections should be taken with increasing degrees of atypia or dysplasia. The cystic duct margin and one to three sections of representative mucosa are sampled routinely in all cholecystectomy specimens. When low-grade dysplasia or epithelial atypia insufficient for a definite diagnosis of dysplasia is found, submission of extra random sections is useful to exclude high-grade dysplasia or to detect more easily diagnosed foci of neoplasia, respectively. When high-grade dysplasia is seen, thorough sampling is mandatory to rule out an invasive carcinoma. Similarly, multiple additional sections should be submitted in T1a or T1b carcinomas to exclude a more advanced tumor. Areas grossly suspicious for invasive carcinoma should be entirely examined. ICPNs should be submitted entirely along with generous sampling of adjacent mucosa because they are commonly associated with high-grade dysplasia or invasive carcinoma away from the grossly apparent lesion.

Microscopic Findings

Biliary intraepithelial neoplasia used to be graded using a three-tiered system (BilIN 1–3), but a two-tiered scheme is now preferred. BilIN 1–2 is now classified as low grade and BilIN-3 as high grade. Low-grade BilIN is characterized by mild to moderate cytologic atypia characterized by nuclear enlargement, hyperchromasia, and mildly irregular contours (Fig. 15.8). Nuclear polarity toward the basement membrane is maintained. Architecturally, the epithelium may be completely flat or form small simple papillae, but complex architectural abnormalities are not seen. In contrast, high-grade BilIN is characterized by marked nuclear atypia, pleomorphism, and loss of polarity. Significant architectural complexity is often present with papillary fronds, cribriforming, tufting, and intraluminal bridging (Fig. 15.9).

Because architectural complexity, including formation of papillae, may also be seen in BilIN, a macroscopic criterion of a grossly visible lesion, typically 1 cm or larger, is required for a diagnosis of ICPN (Fig. 15.10). Gland architecture in ICPN may be papillary or tubular but is most commonly a mixture of both. Extensive papillary architecture is associated with a higher risk for invasive carcinoma. ICPNs are also subclassified according to the predominant cytologic type: biliary, gastric, intestinal, and oncocytic. Gastric-type ICPNs may be further subdivided into foveolar and pyloric subtypes,

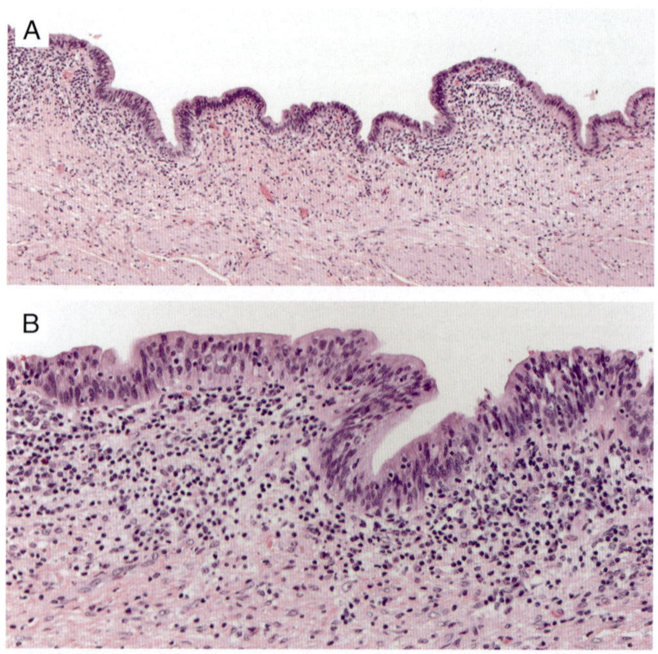

FIGURE 15.8

Low-grade dysplasia (biliary intraepithelial neoplasia) of the gallbladder. The dysplastic epithelium's cytology is identical to that of a colonic adenoma and shows abrupt transition from the normal epithelium on the right (**A**). Higher magnification (**B**) shows typical features with hyperchromatic penicillate nuclei with stratification, dense chromatin, and inconspicuous nucleoli. The architecture is still tubular and does not show complex branching or papillary fronds.

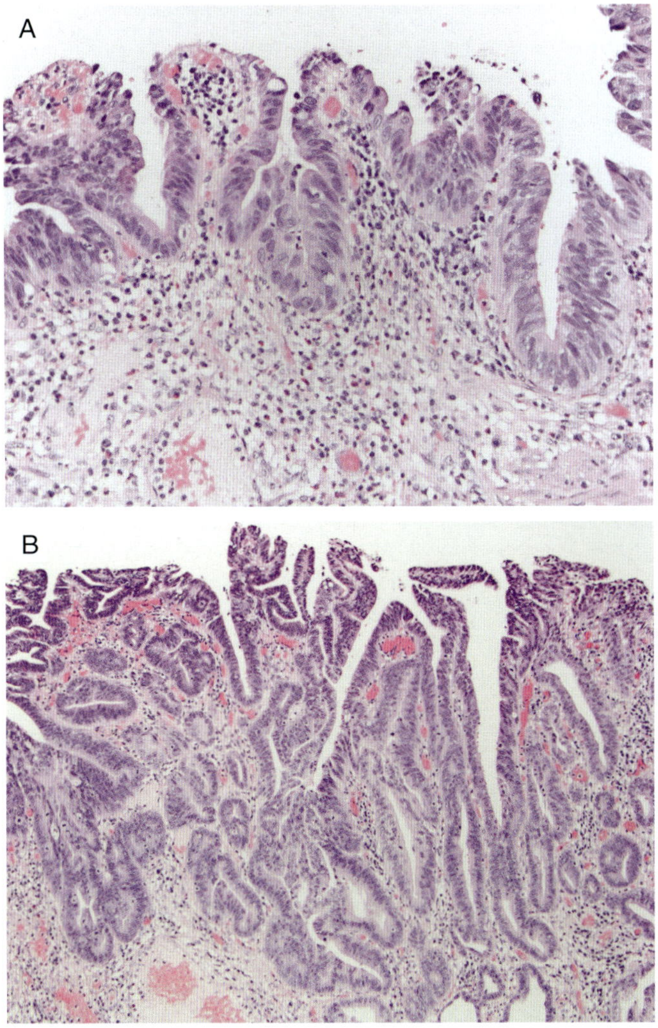

FIGURE 15.9

High-grade dysplasia (biliary intraepithelial neoplasia) of the gallbladder. **A**, Markedly hyperchromatic pleomorphic round nuclei with loss of polarity, vesicular chromatin, and prominent nucleoli. **B**, Another example with similar nuclear features, which also shows marked architectural complexity. When this is an incidental finding in a cholecystectomy, deeper levels and examination of the entire gallbladder may be necessary to rule out an invasive adenocarcinoma depending on the multifocality of the lesion.

the latter often resembling pyloric gland adenomas of the gastrointestinal (GI) tract. MUC5 lines the surface epithelium in these lesions, and the glandular component is strongly MUC6 positive (Fig. 15.11).

Invasive adenocarcinoma is defined by the presence of small, tubular glands with an infiltrating pattern surrounded by desmoplastic stroma. Approximately half of gallbladder carcinomas are either well or moderately differentiated, are incidentally diagnosed, and present at late stages.

Molecular Findings

There is a wide range of reported frequencies of *KRAS* alterations in gallbladder dysplasia and carcinoma.

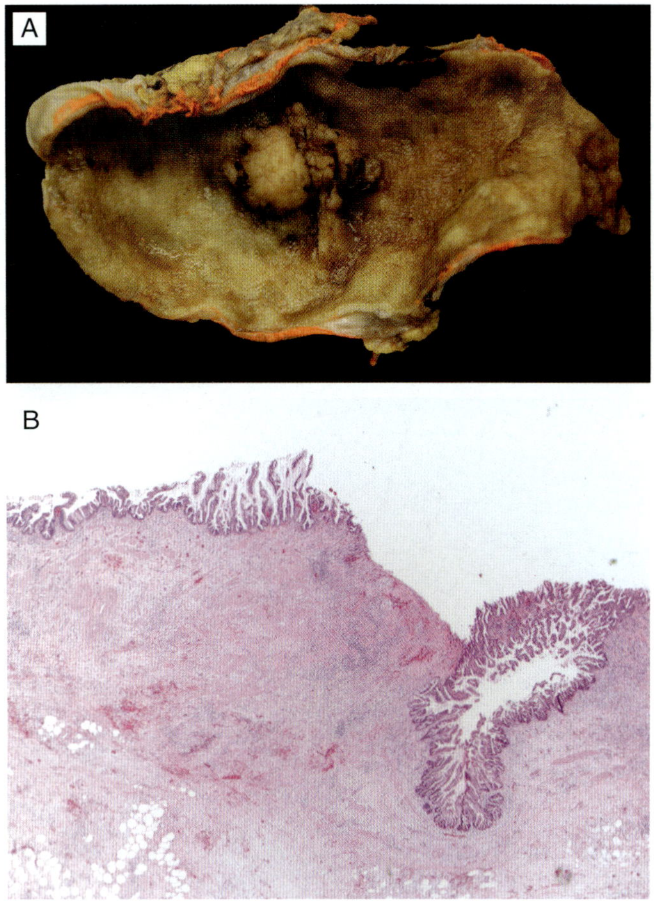

FIGURE 15.10

Intracholecystic papillary tubular neoplasm of the gallbladder is defined as a grossly visible neoplastic mass (**A**). The microscopic spectrum of these lesions is broad and most commonly resembles colonic-type tubular, tubulovillous, and villous adenomas (**B**). Rarely, gastric pyloric gland adenoma–type lesions may also occur in the gallbladder.

Overall, *KRAS* mutations are likely present in approximately one-third of cases of preinvasive gallbladder neoplasia. Carcinomas arising in patients with anomalous union of pancreatobiliary ducts are consistently reported to have a higher frequency of *KRAS* alterations. More advanced neoplasia (BilIN3 and invasive carcinoma) is associated with *TP53, CDKN2A/B*, and *PIK3CA* alterations. Unlike intraductal papillary mucinous neoplasms of the pancreas, ICPN is not classically associated with *GNAS* alterations. *EGFR, ERBB3, PTEN, ARID2*, and *TERT* promoter mutations are more prevalent in the gallbladder than in the intra- and extrahepatic bile ducts.

Differential Diagnosis

Awareness of the spectrum of reactive epithelial changes is critical because severe changes may closely mimic dysplasia or invasive carcinoma.

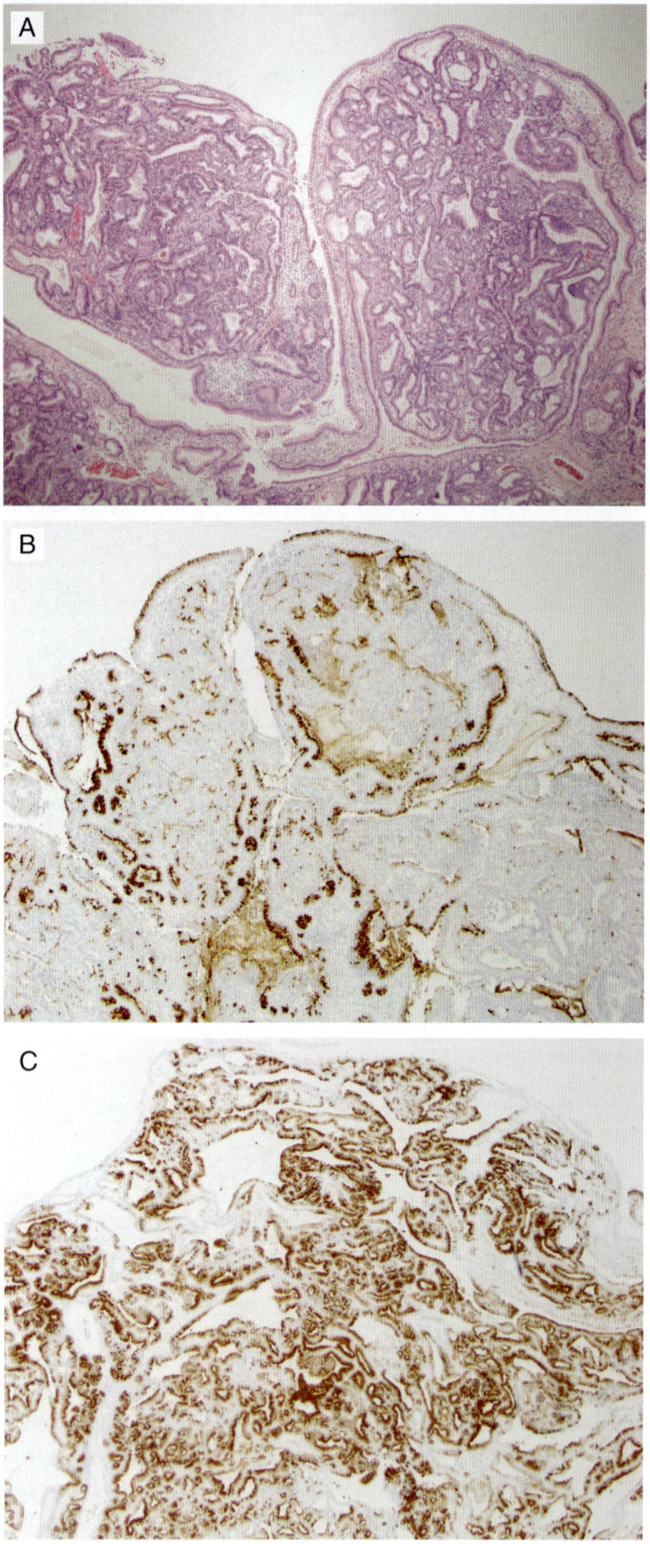

FIGURE 15.11

Pyloric gland adenoma of gallbladder with crowded small tubular glands with abundant mucin and mild nuclear atypia (**A**). Similar to their more common gastric counterparts, these lesions show positive MUC5 staining in the surface epithelium (**B**) and diffuse strong MUC6 positivity (**C**) in the small tubular glands that make up bulk of the lesion.

Dysplasia and Early Gallbladder Carcinoma – Pathologic Features

Gross Findings

- Biliary intraepithelial neoplasia (BilIN) and early invasive carcinomas may be grossly normal
- Intracholecystic papillary neoplasm (ICPN) is a grossly visible lesion, usually 1 cm or larger
- Invasive carcinoma may be associated with wall thickening and mimic chronic cholecystitis

Microscopic Findings

- Low-grade (previously BilIN 1 and 2) have relatively simple architecture with mild to moderate cytologic atypia
- High-grade BilIN (previously BilIN 3) has an in situ carcinoma-like appearance with marked cytologic atypia and complex architecture
- ICPNs may be classified as biliary, gastric (foveolar or pyloric), intestinal, and oncocytic types; architecture may be tubular, papillary, or usually mixed
- Early invasive carcinoma has an infiltrative pattern and often desmoplastic stroma
- Dysplasia extending into Rokitansky-Aschoff sinuses may mimic invasive adenocarcinoma

Genetics

- *KRAS* alterations occur in approximately one-third of BilIN lesions and carcinomas; there is a higher frequency in patients with anomalous union of pancreatobiliary ducts
- Alterations in *TP53*, *SMAD4*, *PIK3CA*, and p16 inactivation occur in high-grade BilIN and invasive carcinoma
- *GNAS* mutations are not frequent

Although there is substantial morphologic overlap, several useful histologic features distinguish between benign reactive changes and neoplastic atypia, and these are summarized in Table 15.1. Unfortunately, none of these features are entirely sensitive or specific. They must be considered in combination and in context of the clinical and radiographic features. In general, reactive cytologic atypia often shows vesicular nuclei with mild to moderate enlargement, smooth nuclear contours, and at most mild pleomorphism and hyperchromasia (Fig. 15.12). Surface maturation and the presence of an adjacent ulcer, often with mucin-depleted "restituting" epithelium, are helpful features when present. Architectural complexity, such as simple papillary growth at the mucosal surface, is acceptable within the realm of reactive changes. However, complex papillary architecture, cribriforming, or copious tufting should prompt consideration of dysplasia or malignancy.

Early invasive lesions in the gallbladder can be extremely difficult to distinguish from dysplasia involving Rokitansky-Aschoff sinuses (Fig. 15.13). In extremely well-differentiated cases, non-neoplastic Rokitansky-Aschoff sinuses may also enter the differential diagnosis. The distinction is often best made at low

TABLE 15.1
Features of Benign Reactive Atypia and Dysplasia and Malignancy in Gallbladder and Biliary Epithelium

Feature	Benign or Reactive	Dysplasia or Malignancy
Chromatin	Vesicular, less commonly hyperchromatic	Coarse, hyperchromatic
Nuclear size	Increased, sometimes with accompanying increase in cytoplasm	Increased with increased nuclear-to-cytoplasmic ratios
Nuclear contours	Smooth	Smooth or irregular
Nucleoli	Small to moderately sized	Absent to very large "cherry nucleoli"
Pleomorphism	Not marked	Mild to marked, depending on grade
Surface maturation	Usually present	Usually absent
Background inflammation, ulceration, and restituting epithelium	Often present	Occasionally present
Surface architecture	Flat, simple papillary	Flat, complex papillary, cribiforming, tufting
Mural architecture	Lobulated, perpendicular orientation to surface (Rokitansky-Aschoff sinuses)	Irregular or infiltrative, parallel orientation to surface

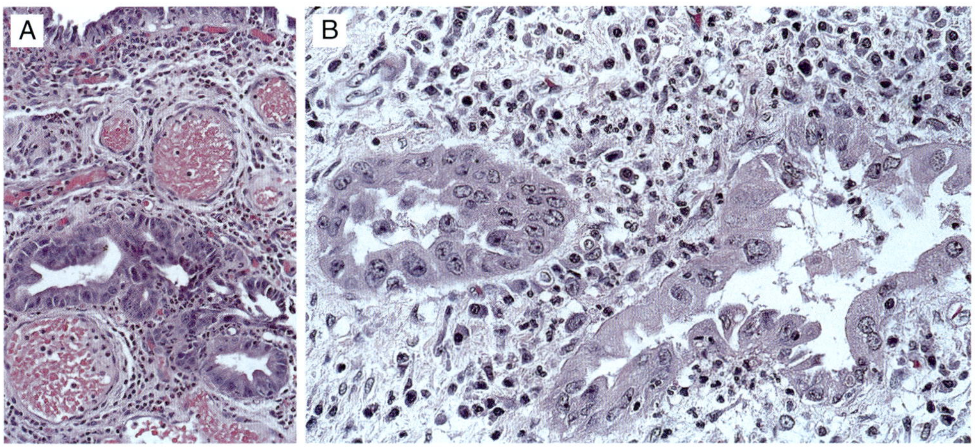

FIGURE 15.12

Reactive changes in the gallbladder and extrahepatic bile ducts can mimic neoplasia. The nuclei may be round with prominent nucleoli, similar to neoplastic glands, but the contours are smooth, and the background mucosa shows acute or chronic inflammation (**A**) or erosions and ulcers, which are all helpful in making the correct diagnosis. A history of stented bile duct is also useful in this differential diagnosis and should raise the threshold for a neoplastic diagnosis. Dense chronic inflammatory infiltrate and patchy acute inflammation in the setting of primary sclerosing cholangitis, in another example, suggests that the epithelial changes seen here are best considered reactive (**B**).

power, where native sinuses appear as organized, flask-shaped invaginations with a long axis perpendicular to the epithelial surface. Invasive carcinomas have an infiltrative, disorganized appearance, with glands invading both perpendicular and parallel to the surface.

Prognosis and Therapy

Like other preneoplastic lesions of the GI tract, gallbladder dysplasia, of either low or high grade, is cured by cholecystectomy with negative margins. Although some studies have reported the 5-year survival rate as low as 50% for early invasive carcinoma, more recent data restricted to patients with tumors considered T1a or T1b after histologic examination of the entire cholecystectomy specimen have shown 5-year survival rates in the order of 90%. The lower survival rates from earlier studies are likely due to pathologic understaging when the entire gallbladder was not submitted for evaluation. Pathologic stage is critical for predicting risk of residual disease and to guide subsequent therapy in incidentally detected gallbladder adenocarcinomas. Tumors invading into the lamina propria (T1a) are considered appropriately treated by cholecystectomy alone. Invasion into the muscular wall (T1b) is associated with a higher risk of recurrence. Although management of T1b gallbladder carcinoma remains somewhat controversial, most data suggest that en bloc resection of the adjacent liver parenchyma is associated with better outcomes. Other important pathologic prognostic parameters include the status of cystic duct resection margin and nodal metastasis.

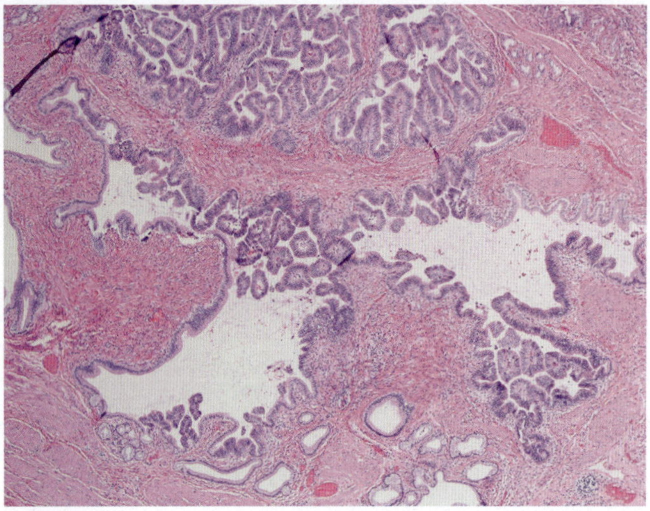

FIGURE 15.13

Biliary intraepithelial neoplasia–type changes extending into preexisting Rokitansky-Aschoff sinuses can mimic an invasive adenocarcinoma. These foci are cystically dilated and sharply circumscribed, and the typical architecture of an invasive adenocarcinoma with small, angulated glands in a haphazard distribution is not present in these cases. A desmoplastic stromal response is also missing.

Advanced Gallbladder Carcinoma—Fact Sheet

Definition

- Carcinoma invading through the muscular wall of the gallbladder

Epidemiology

- Rare: fewer than 5000 new cases each year in the United States
- Constitutes majority of biliary tract malignancies
- Higher incidence in South America and Asia
- Females > males; increasing incidence with age
- Risk factors: cholelithiasis, anomalous union of the pancreatobiliary ducts, hyalinizing cholecystitis
- Five-year survival rates are approximately 5%

Clinical Features

- Vague presenting symptoms: abdominal pain, anorexia, and weight loss
- Some cases may be asymptomatic
- Ultrasound can detect some case preoperatively

ADVANCED GALLBLADDER CARCINOMA

CLINICAL FEATURES

Advanced gallbladder carcinoma, defined as tumor invasion beyond the muscular wall, is relatively rare, with fewer than 5000 new cases reported in the United States each year. However, it is by far the most common advanced malignancy of the biliary tract, constituting at least 80% of these lesions. The risk factors are generally the same as those for early neoplasia, in particular gallstones, long-standing chronic inflammation, hyalinizing cholecystitis, PSC, and anomalous union of the pancreatobiliary ducts. The geographic distribution is also similar, with increased incidence in South America and Asia compared with North America and Europe. Women are at slightly higher risk than men, likely because of an increased incidence of gallstones. The incidence of advanced gallbladder carcinomas increases with increasing age. Most series report median ages in the seventh or eighth decades.

Gallbladder carcinomas are often high stage at presentation, which is a major contributor to the overall poor outcomes. Symptoms, when present, are typically vague and include abdominal pain, anorexia, and occasionally weight loss. Many cases, especially those associated with polypoid dysplasia, can be suspected by ultrasound. If the diagnosis can be made preoperatively, endoscopic ultrasound is considered the modality of choice for clinical staging.

PATHOLOGIC FEATURES

GROSS FINDINGS

Unlike early gallbladder neoplasia, advanced carcinomas most often present with mass lesions on gross examination. In most cases, a fibrotic, infiltrative mass is present in the gallbladder wall. Occasionally, mural involvement by carcinoma can be difficult to distinguish from the inflammatory changes and fibrosis of acute and chronic cholecystitis. Less commonly, a polypoid lesion may protrude into the lumen. The fundus is the most common site of involvement, followed by the body and neck regions. Carcinomas arising in the setting of hyalinizing cholecystitis are not grossly apparent. Areas of serosal puckering or distortion and induration around adherent hepatic parenchyma should raise suspicion for an advanced stage tumor. Tumor location should be specified as either on the hepatic side of the gallbladder or the serosal side of the gallbladder. Carcinomas located on the hepatic side of the gallbladder are associated with worse prognosis than those on the serosal side. The eighth edition of the American Joint Commission on Cancer (AJCC) staging guidelines subclassifies T2 lesions as T2a (serosal side of the gallbladder) or T2b (hepatic side of the gallbladder).

MICROSCOPIC FINDINGS

Most invasive gallbladder carcinomas arise in a background of high-grade dysplasia and are of the pancreatobiliary type with small tubular glands that are lined by cuboidal cells with eosinophilic or amphophilic cytoplasm (Fig. 15.14). Although the degree of differentiation is variable, most cases have well-formed glandular architecture and abundant desmoplastic stroma.

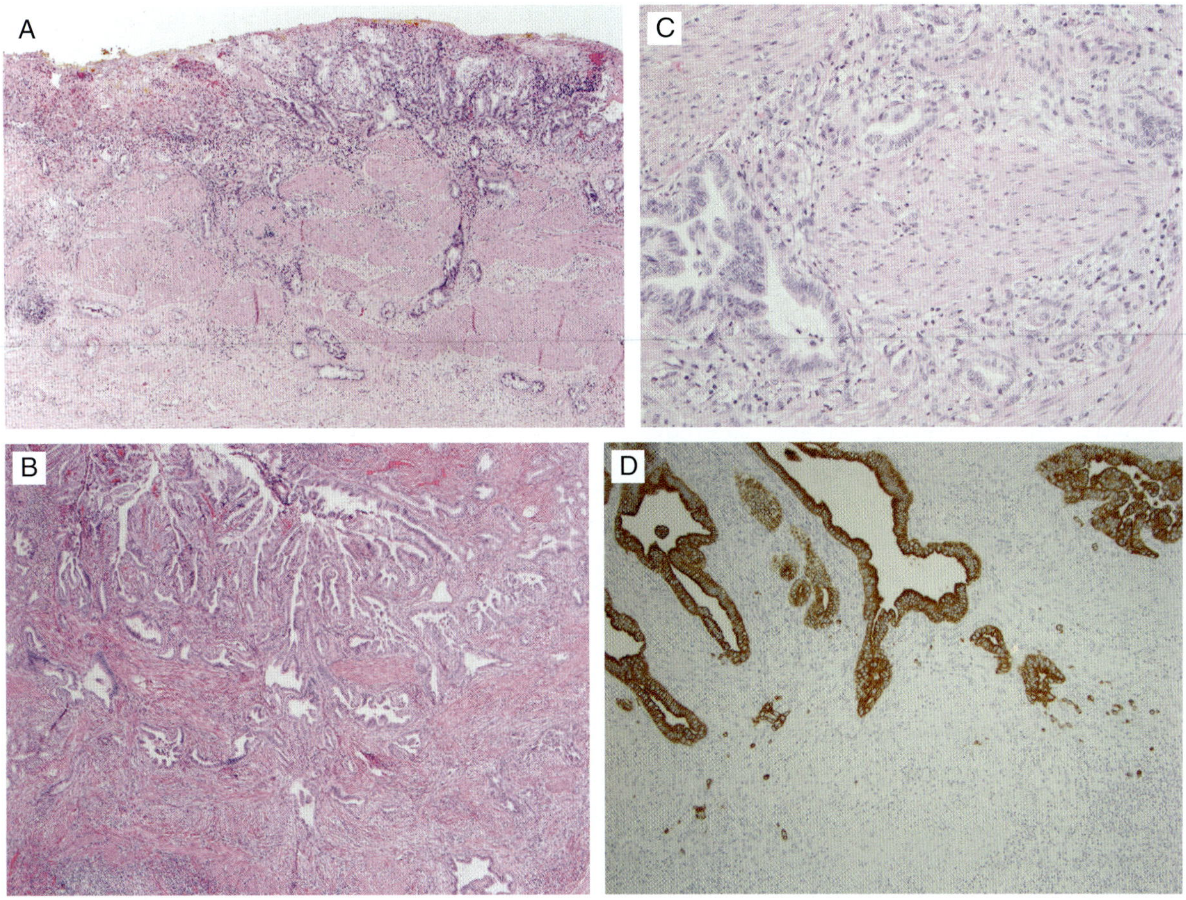

FIGURE 15.14

Invasive adenocarcinoma of the gallbladder arising in the background of extensive high-grade dysplasia (**A**). The neoplastic glands are small and show an irregular infiltrative pattern that is in sharp contrast to the changes seen in Fig. 15.13. Well-differentiated adenocarcinoma can be difficult to diagnose because glandular atypia may be minimal in some cases. The haphazard architecture of infiltrating glands and the surrounding desmoplastic stroma is helpful in this example (**B**) to establish the diagnosis. Identification of small clusters of neoplastic cells adjacent to well-formed neoplastic glands (**C**), perineural or vascular invasion, or single cell infiltration deep into the perimuscular tissue on a pankeratin immunostain (**D**) can also be helpful in making a diagnosis of invasive adenocarcinoma in challenging cases.

Intestinal and/or gastric differentiation, either focally or diffusely, is fairly common. Unusual subtypes of carcinoma include mucinous (>50% extracellular mucin), colloid (predominantly mucin with occasional strips or clusters of tumor cells), poorly cohesive carcinoma with or without signet ring cells, adenosquamous or squamous cell, clear cell, sarcomatoid, hepatoid, and undifferentiated. The latter may resemble medullary carcinomas of the GI tract or lymphoepithelioma-like carcinoma (Fig. 15.15) of the aerodigestive tract but are not positive for Epstein-Barr virus (EBV). Poorly differentiated neuroendocrine carcinomas (small cell or large cell) comprise approximately 5% of cases.

Pathologic stage is the most important prognostic feature in the evaluation of malignant cholecystectomy specimens. Extensive fibrosis and distortion of the gallbladder wall often precludes precise identification of the point of deepest invasion grossly, and extensive microscopic evaluation is warranted to determine the T stage accurately. Important prognostic features include degree of differentiation, lymphovascular invasion, and nodal status.

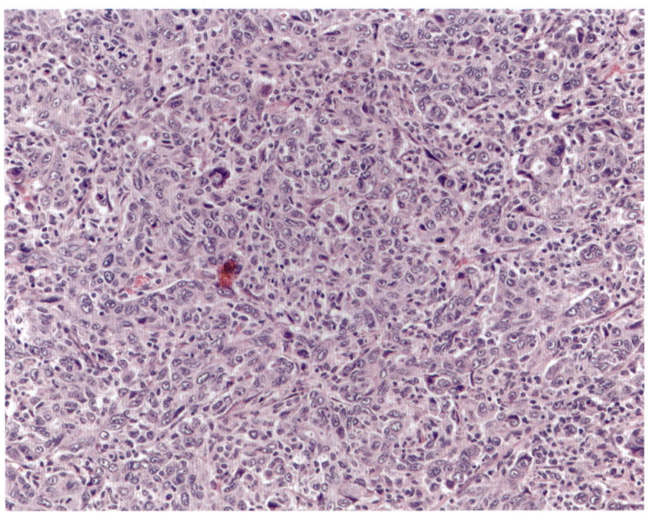

FIGURE 15.15

Undifferentiated gallbladder carcinoma with abundant intratumoral lymphocytes resembles lymphoepithelioma-like carcinoma of the head and neck region but does not show any association with Epstein-Barr virus. Programmed death-ligand 1 can be positive in such cases and offer a therapeutic option to these patients, who otherwise have a dismal prognosis.

Immunohistochemistry (IHC) has a limited role in gallbladder carcinoma because there are no reliable markers to distinguish a benign from malignant proliferation. It may be useful when the differential diagnosis includes a metastasis. Primary gallbladder carcinomas are usually positive for cytokeratin (CK) 7 with patchy CK20 and CDX2 reactivity. However, because this profile is not entirely specific for the gallbladder, the overall morphology is more often helpful in excluding metastases, which are usually centered around the serosa or the middle of the wall rather than the mucosa. The presence of flat or polypoid dysplasia in the background epithelium favors a gallbladder primary.

The genetic landscape of gallbladder carcinomas appears complex and is more heterogenous than that of pancreatic ductal adenocarcinoma. Common molecular alterations typically associated with advanced gallbladder carcinoma include mutations in MAP kinase genes, *KRAS*, *TP53*, *CDKN2A/B*, and *PIK3CA*. Loss of *SMAD4* occasionally occurs, but like *KRAS* alterations, this is not as frequent as in pancreatic ductal adenocarcinoma.

Gallbladder Carcinoma—Pathologic Features

Gross Findings

- Most often fibrotic, infiltrative mass in the gallbladder wall
- Can be difficult to distinguish from fibrosis secondary to chronic cholecystitis
- The most frequent location is the fundus followed by the body

Microscopic Findings

- The most common phenotype is pancreatobiliary with well-spaced glands separated by abundant desmoplastic stroma
- Intestinal and gastric differentiation is common
- Other variants include mucinous, colloid, adenosquamous, squamous, clear cell, sarcomatoid, poorly cohesive carcinoma with or without signet ring cells, hepatoid and undifferentiated carcinoma (including medullary and lymphoepithelioma-like carcinomas)

Genetics

- Genetic landscape is complex and heterogeneous
- *KRAS, TP53, CDKN2A/B, PIK3CA* mutations

Immunohistochemistry

- Typically cytokeratin (CK) 7 positive; CK20 and CDX2 variable

Differential Diagnosis

Unlike early neoplasia, most advanced invasive gallbladder carcinomas are overtly malignant and are not often confused with reactive changes. One exception is the extension of Rokitansky-Aschoff sinuses deep into the muscular layer, which can sometimes be difficult to distinguish from invasive carcinoma, especially when the sinus is involved by dysplastic epithelium. Rokitansky-Aschoff sinuses are typically oriented in a perpendicular fashion relative to the surface epithelium and have a lobulated rather than an infiltrative advancing front. Occasionally, ducts of Luschka, native subserosal or subhepatic ducts, can mimic well-differentiated carcinoma. However, they lack cytologic atypia or infiltrative growth. The absence of carcinoma in the mucosa or muscular wall usually prevents any confusion with malignancy.

Treatment and Prognosis

The extent of resection depends on the depth of invasion. T2 carcinomas are often managed by radical cholecystectomy with resection of liver segments IVb and V. T3 lesions usually require more radical resections that can include extended right hepatectomy, lobectomy, and regional lymph node dissection. The prognosis is poor with overall 5-year survival rates of around 5%.

EXTRAHEPATIC BILE DUCTS

INFLAMMATORY DISORDERS OF EXTRAHEPATIC BILE DUCTS

Clinical Features

Choledocholithiasis, the presence of entrapped gallstones in the common bile duct (CBD), is the most common cause of benign bile duct obstruction. Stones may be classified as primary, arising within the CBD or intrahepatic bile ducts, or secondary, migrating from the gallbladder. Secondary stones are far more common than primary stones, especially in Western countries. Primary stones occur more frequently in Asian patients and are thought to be related to biliary stasis and chronic bacterial infection (recurrent pyogenic cholangitis). Choledocholithiasis secondary to cholelithiasis occurs in up to 10% of patients who undergo cholecystectomy. Risk factors include a cystic duct diameter larger than 4 mm, female gender, age older than 40 years, and obesity. Imaging modalities that may detect choledocholithiasis include abdominal ultrasound, computed tomography, endoscopic retrograde cholangiopancreatography (ERCP), and magnetic resonance cholangiopancreatography (MRCP). A large majority of patients are successfully treated by ERCP.

Primary sclerosing cholangitis may involve the extrahepatic bile ducts with or without concurrent involvement of smaller intrahepatic ducts. The diagnosis of extrahepatic PSC is most often radiographic. MRCP is the preferred modality. ERCP is also highly sensitive and specific but has a higher rate of complications. In most cases, a diffuse, strictured, and beaded appearance is characteristic. The pathogenesis of PSC is not well understood, although it is clearly an immune-mediated disease given its association with specific human leukocyte antigen haplotypes (B8, DR3, and DQ2) and its close relationship with inflammatory bowel disease (IBD). Approximately 50% of patients have IBD at the time of presentation with PSC, and another roughly 30% develop IBD within 10 years of diagnosis. Although patients with PSC are at increased risk for both ulcerative colitis and Crohn's disease, most patients have ulcerative colitis. Patients with PSC are at high risk for both biliary and colorectal dysplasia and malignancy. The cumulative 30-year risk of cholangiocarcinoma (CC) is approximately 20% and of colorectal carcinoma is 10% to 15%. In addition to malignancy, benign bile duct strictures are a common complication. Treatment options for PSC are quite limited and are mostly targeted toward alleviating or preventing complications rather than cure. Endoscopic dilation and stenting are used to treat benign strictures. Liver transplantation may be indicated in patients with advanced disease. All patients with PSC should be screened for IBD and colorectal carcinoma.

IgG4 sclerosing cholangitis is part of the emerging class of IgG4-related diseases and is now considered an important consideration in the differential diagnosis of benign bile duct strictures. It is critical to distinguish IgG4-related sclerosing cholangitis from PSC because the former often responds to steroid therapy. Imaging of the bile ducts shows stricturing, either single or multiple, which may mimic PSC or CC. The disease is most common in older men, although any age group may be affected. Most patients with IgG4 sclerosing cholangitis also have IgG4-related (type 1) autoimmune pancreatitis. Accordingly, IgG4 sclerosing disease should be strongly considered in patients with bile duct strictures who have associated findings suggestive of autoimmune pancreatitis. An increase in serum IgG4 is often sufficient for diagnosis, and biopsy is not generally required to initiate therapy. However, because of the increased awareness and implications for therapy, bile duct biopsy is often performed in cases with equivocal imaging and laboratory features to evaluate for IgG4 sclerosing cholangitis.

Pathologic Features

Pathologic examination of extrahepatic bile ducts involved by PSC may be performed on segmental bile duct excisions for obstruction, resection specimens performed for an associated CC, or liver explant specimens in patients with end-stage disease. Biopsies of the extrahepatic ducts are generally not specific for PSC and are usually only performed to rule out a CC in a stricture or less commonly to exclude IgG4 sclerosing cholangitis. Most cases of PSC show some degree of chronic inflammation and fibrosis (Fig. 15.16) along with foci of duct stenosis and dilation. The inflammation is predominantly lymphocytic with some admixed plasma cells. Neutrophils may be seen but are usually not prominent. The overlying epithelium is often ulcerated. Dense fibrosis, usually circumferential around the duct ("onion-skin" appearance), is a hallmark feature. The fibrosis results in luminal narrowing, and in advanced cases, the lumen may appear slitlike or contain inspissated bile. The lining epithelium shows evidence of injury with cytoplasmic eosinophilia, nuclear disarray, and attenuation.

In characteristic cases, IgG4 sclerosing cholangitis consists of increased numbers of IgG4-positive plasma cells, storiform fibrosis of the bile duct, and obliterative phlebitis. Unlike PSC, in which the inflammation primarily targets the bile duct mucosa, in IgG4 sclerosing cholangitis, the inflammation is more often transmural. Although plasma cell inflammation is usually prominent on hematoxylin and eosin morphology, demonstration of an elevated ratio of IgG4-positive plasma cells to total IgG-positive plasma cells (>40%) and finding at least 10 IgG4-positive plasma cells per high-power field by IHC is needed for histologic diagnosis.

Inflammatory Disorders Of Extrahepatic Bile Ducts—Fact Sheet

Definition

- Primary sclerosing cholangitis (PSC): autoimmune disease targeting intrahepatic and extrahepatic bile ducts
- Immunoglobulin (Ig) G4 sclerosing cholangitis: part of a systemic disease of increased IgG4 production

Epidemiology

- PSC typically associated with younger age (males > females) and is strongly associated with inflammatory bowel disease
- IgG4 sclerosing cholangitis is associated with older age (males > females), and most patients have manifestations of systemic IgG4 disease in other organs
- Both diseases are associated with increased risk for cholangiocarcinoma, though the risk appears to be higher in PSC

Clinical Features

- Patients with PSC may be asymptomatic at presentation or present with abdominal pain, fatigue, pruritis, or jaundice
- IgG4 sclerosing cholangitis patients may be asymptomatic or present with obstructive symptoms (jaundice, pruritis)
- Diagnostic imaging includes endoscopic retrograde cholangiopancreatography and magnetic resonance cholangiopancreatography, which most often show stricture; some cases of IgG4 sclerosing cholangitis may present with a mass
- Systemic IgG4 levels are typically increased in patients with IgG4 sclerosing cholangitis

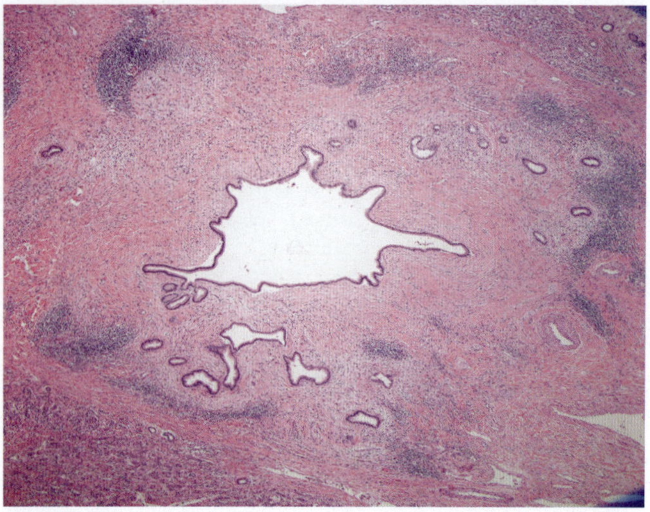

FIGURE 15.16

Primary sclerosing cholangitis with duct ectasia and tortuosity, periductal scarring, and marked chronic inflammation. Correlation with clinical and imaging findings is often necessary to render a definite diagnosis.

Inflammatory Disorders of Extrahepatic Bile Ducts—Pathologic Features

Gross Findings

- Primary sclerosing cholangitis (PSC) shows multiple strictures separated by segments of bile duct of normal or dilated caliber ("beads on a string" appearance)
- Immunoglobulin (Ig) G4 sclerosing cholangitis most commonly shows strictures, but some cases present as a mass

Microscopic Findings

- PSC invariably shows dense hyaline fibrosis, often concentric around bile duct
- PSC consists of a predominantly mucosal infiltrate of mononuclear cells with great variability in degree
- Ulceration of epithelium and hyperplasia of intramural glands is common
- IgG4 sclerosing cholangitis has three hallmarks:
  - Increased IgG4-positive plasma cells
- >10 IgG4 positive cells in a single high-power field
- IgG4 to IgG positive plasma cell ratio >40%
  - Storiform fibrosis
  - Obliterative phlebitis
- In contrast to PSC, IgG4 sclerosing cholangitis is more often transmural; occasionally, there is relative sparing of the bile duct mucosa

Differential Diagnosis

- Cholangiocarcinoma, which typically shows irregular, infiltrative glands in desmoplastic stroma in contrast to the lobulated configuration of hyperplastic intramural glands

As noted earlier biopsies to rule out IgG4 sclerosing cholangitis are becoming increasingly common because of the steroid-responsive nature of this disease in contrast to PSC. Small biopsies have limited sensitivity, and even when some diagnostic features are present, a definitive diagnosis can be difficult. All three diagnostic features (increased IgG4 plasma cells, storiform fibrosis, and obliterative phlebitis) are rarely sampled in a single biopsy sample, so distinction from PSC can be difficult. In these cases, documenting some of these histologic features in a patient with increased serum IgG4 levels may be helpful even if a definitive diagnosis is not possible. Caution is especially warranted in the setting of a mass lesion. Although IgG4 sclerosing cholangitis can cause mass formation, CCs may also be associated with increased IgG4-to-IgG ratios. Accordingly, demonstration of increased IgG4-positive plasma cells alone is not sufficient to entirely exclude malignancy.

CARCINOMA OF EXTRAHEPATIC BILE DUCTS

CLINICAL FEATURES

Cholangiocarcinoma is by far the most common malignancy of the extrahepatic bile ducts, but it remains a relatively rare tumor. The incidence in the United States is estimated to be 0.6 to 1.0 per 100,000 persons yearly. By some estimates, the rate is higher in Asia, although the data to suggest significant geographic variation are less clear for CC than for adenocarcinoma of the gallbladder. PSC is the best-known risk factor for CC. Other associations include choledochal cysts and parasite infections, such as *Clonorchis sinensis* or *Opisthorchis viverrine*. The mean age at presentation in most Western series is around 70 years. There appears to be a slight male predominance.

The most common symptoms are caused by duct obstruction and include jaundice, pruritis, pale stools, and dark urine. Imaging modalities (ultrasonography, computed tomography, ERCP, MRCP) overall have high sensitivity and specificity but malignant strictures may occasionally be difficult to distinguish on imaging from benign ones in the absence of a mass lesion. CC is classified into three subtypes according to anatomic location: intrahepatic (proximal to secondary branches of left and right hepatic ducts), perihilar (proximal to the origin of the cystic duct and distal to the secondary branches of left and right hepatic ducts), and distal extrahepatic (distal to the cystic duct origin and proximal to the ampulla). Perihilar CC, also commonly referred to as Klatskin tumor, may be further subdivided into one of five categories based on the precise anatomic location (Bismuth-Corlette classification).

Carcinoma of Extrahepatic Bile Ducts—Fact Sheet

Definition

- Carcinoma arising from the epithelial lining of the bile ducts

Incidence and Location

- Rare: incidence fewer than 1 per 100,000 persons per year in the United States
- Risk factors include primary sclerosing cholangitis, choledochal cyst, and parasite infection *(Clonorchis sinensis, Opisthorchis viverrine)*
- Subclassified based on location. Extrahepatic carcinomas include perihilar (Klatskin tumors) and distal extrahepatic lesions (distal to the insertion of the cystic duct)
- Males slightly more affected than females (male-to-female ratio, ~1.5 to 1)
- Predominantly affects older adults (average age ~70 years)

Morbidity and Mortality

- Poor prognosis: overall 5-year survival less than 10%
- Better outcomes in patients who have curative surgical resection (5-year survival rate, 30%–67%)

Clinical Features

- Obstructive symptoms common at presentation: jaundice, pruritis, pale stools, and dark urine

Therapy

- Surgery is the only curative treatment
- Procedure is highly location dependent:
  - Perihilar tumors treated with bile duct resection or right or left partial hepatectomy
  - Distal tumors treated with pancreaticoduodenectomy

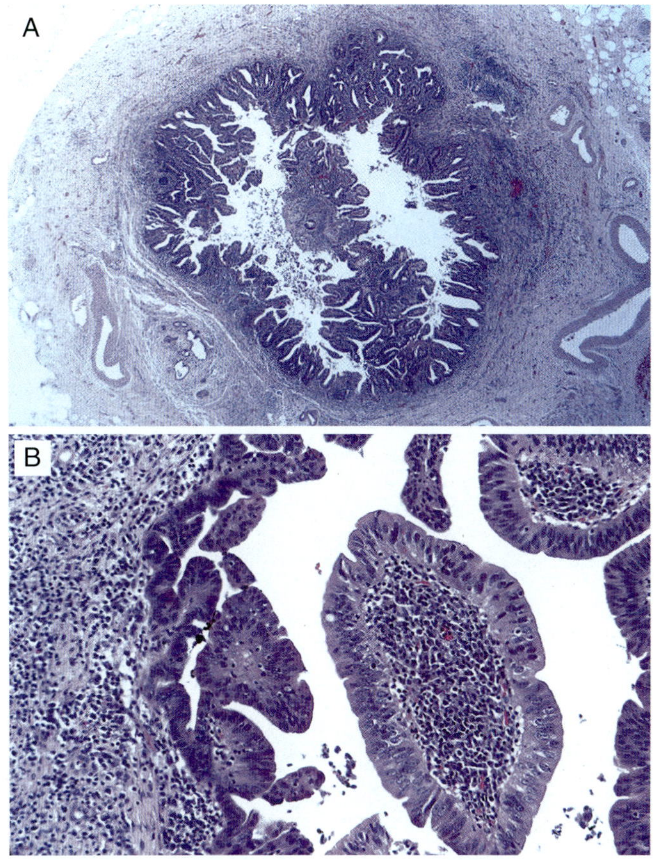

FIGURE 15.17

Intraductal papillary neoplasm of the bile duct (IPNB). IPNBs show a morphologic spectrum similar to their more common pancreatic counterparts, and gastric, intestinal, pancreaticobiliary, or oncocytic differentiation may be seen in the lining epithelium. This IPNB, at low power, shows circumferential involvement by an intraductal neoplastic papillary proliferation (**A**). The nuclear atypia is striking, consistent with high-grade IPNB, but there is no invasion into adjacent stroma (**B**).

Pathologic Features

Gross Findings

Cholangiocarcinoma may present grossly in one of three ways: mass forming, periductal, or intraductal. The most common finding is an ill-defined sclerotic mass or stricture. Some periductal cases may be extremely subtle, with a thickened bile duct being the only notable finding on gross examination. Exophytic intraductal cases are less common. They are typically associated with intraductal papillary neoplasms of the bile ducts, similar to their more common pancreatic counterparts.

Microscopic Findings

Precursor Neoplasia

The same preinvasive neoplastic lesions that occur in the gallbladder can be found in the extrahepatic biliary tree. Isolated cases of flat dysplasia (low- and high-grade BilIN) are rare because they are asymptomatic and, unlike with the gallbladder, bile duct resection is rarely performed for benign indications. However, BilIN may be found in association with invasive carcinoma or in patients with strictures (often in the setting of PSC) that are undergoing examination.

Intraductal papillary neoplasm of the bile duct (IPNB; Figs. 15.17 and 15.18) and the related lesion intraductal tubulopapillary neoplasm of the bile duct are similar to their counterparts in the gallbladder and pancreas. These tumors are, by definition, grossly and radiographically visible and usually larger than 1 cm in size, although size is not a mandatory feature. Resection is indicated given their premalignant potential and frequent association with invasive carcinoma. IPNBs, similar to ICPN (and IPMN of the pancreas), can be classified based on predominant cell type as biliary, intestinal, gastric, or oncocytic. The criteria for grade of dysplasia are the same as those described in the gallbladder. Intraductal tubulopapillary neoplasm are often high grade and distinguished from IPNB based on the presence of greater than 70% nonmucinous tubular architecture and negative MUC5AC. Extensive microscopic evaluation is appropriate for both because these lesions

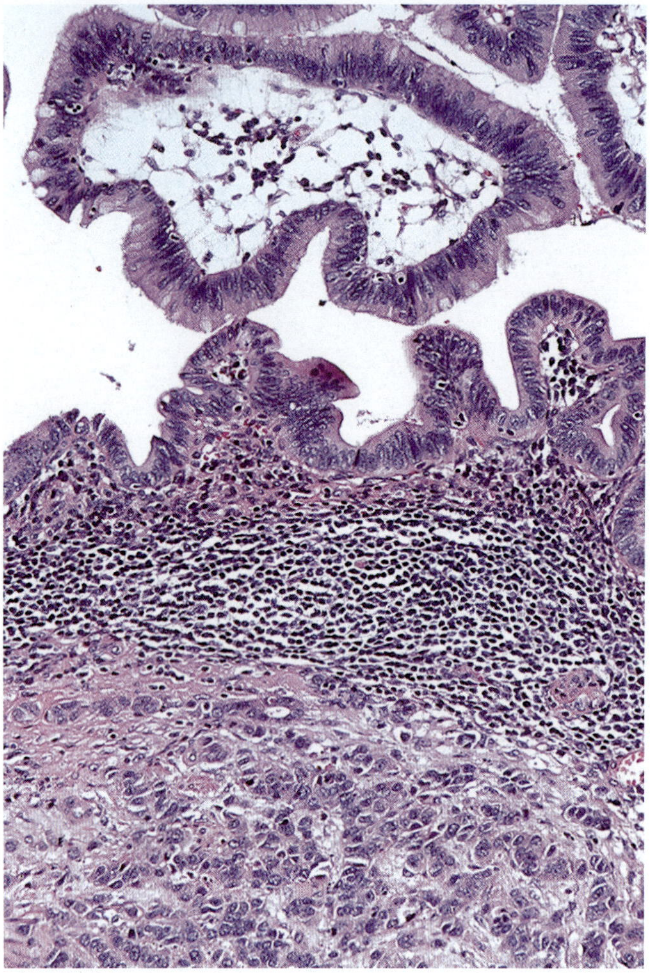

FIGURE 15.18

Intraductal papillary neoplasms of the bile duct are precursor lesions that can give rise to invasive cholangiocarcinomas and must be examined in their entirety to rule out this possibility. The exophytic intraductal papillary component projects into the lumen, in this case, and the invasive carcinoma forms cords within the underlying stroma.

are often associated with small, grossly invisible areas of invasive carcinoma.

Invasive Carcinoma

Cholangiocarcinoma is an adenocarcinoma with the same spectrum of morphologic features as the gallbladder (Fig. 15.19). Marked stromal desmoplasia is a characteristic finding that surrounds infiltrating well to moderately differentiated neoplastic glands. Cytologic features are variable. Most cases consist of biliary-type cuboidal epithelium, although intestinal, gastric (foveolar or pyloric gland), and oncocytic variants occur. In some poorly differentiated cases, marked nuclear atypia and pleomorphism can be present. Less common subtypes include mucinous (colloid), signet ring cell, clear cell, adenosquamous, squamous, lymphoepithelioma-like (which may be EBV associated), hepatoid, micropapillary, undifferentiated, and sarcomatoid carcinoma. Neuroendocrine differentiation may be present in some poorly differentiated carcinomas.

Distinction of distal CBD carcinomas arising within the intrapancreatic portion of the duct from a pancreatic ductal adenocarcinoma in the head of the pancreas or ampullary adenocarcinoma can be challenging in some cases. Generally, carcinomas of the bile duct are circumferential around the duct, which is more or less centered in the middle of the lesion. Presence of an in situ component facilitates the diagnosis, but this helpful feature is not always present.

Pathologic risk factors associated with prognosis that are considered while deciding on the need for adjuvant therapy include T stage, lymph node and margin status, small vessel invasion, portal vein invasion, and perineural invasion.

The molecular genetics of extrahepatic bile duct carcinomas is complex. Alterations in *KRAS* occur in approximately 20% to 30% of extrahepatic CCs, which is significantly lower than pancreatic ductal adenocarcinoma. MDM2 amplifications occur in roughly 10% of perihilar CC but are rare in distal CC. Other commonly altered genes include *TP53*, *CDKN2A*, *SMAD4*, *ARID1A*, and *GNAS*. Genetic aberrations specific for extrahepatic CCs include *PRKACA/PRKACB* fusion,

Carcinoma of Extrahepatic Bile Ducts—Pathologic Features

Gross Findings

- Most often an ill-defined fibrous mass
- In some cases, subtle bile duct thickening is the only abnormality
- Intraductal papillary neoplasm of the bile duct is (IPNB) characterized by an exophytic intraluminal mass

Microscopic Findings

- Most tumors are composed of infiltrative, well0 to moderately differentiated biliary-type glands surrounded by a desmoplastic stroma. Less commonly, intestinal type or gastric type
- Other types include mucinous (colloid), signet ring cell, clear cell, adenosquamous, squamous, lymphoepithelioma-like, hepatoid, micropapillary, undifferentiated, and sarcomatoid carcinoma
- Dysplasia of background epithelium is often present in association with invasive tumors
- Flat dysplasia graded as low- and high-grade biliary intraepithelial neoplasia
- IPNB and intraductal tubulopapillary neoplasms are grossly visible dysplastic lesions, frequently associated with invasive carcinoma

Genetics

- *KRAS* alterations occur in approximately 20% to 30% of cases
- Other recurring alterations include *TP53, SMAD4, ARID1A, GNAS,* and *CDKN2A/B*

Immunohistochemistry

- Usually cytokeratin (CK) 7 positive; CK20 and CDX-2 variable

Differential Diagnosis

- Reactive atypia caused by a bile duct stent, stricture, or primary sclerosing cholangitis

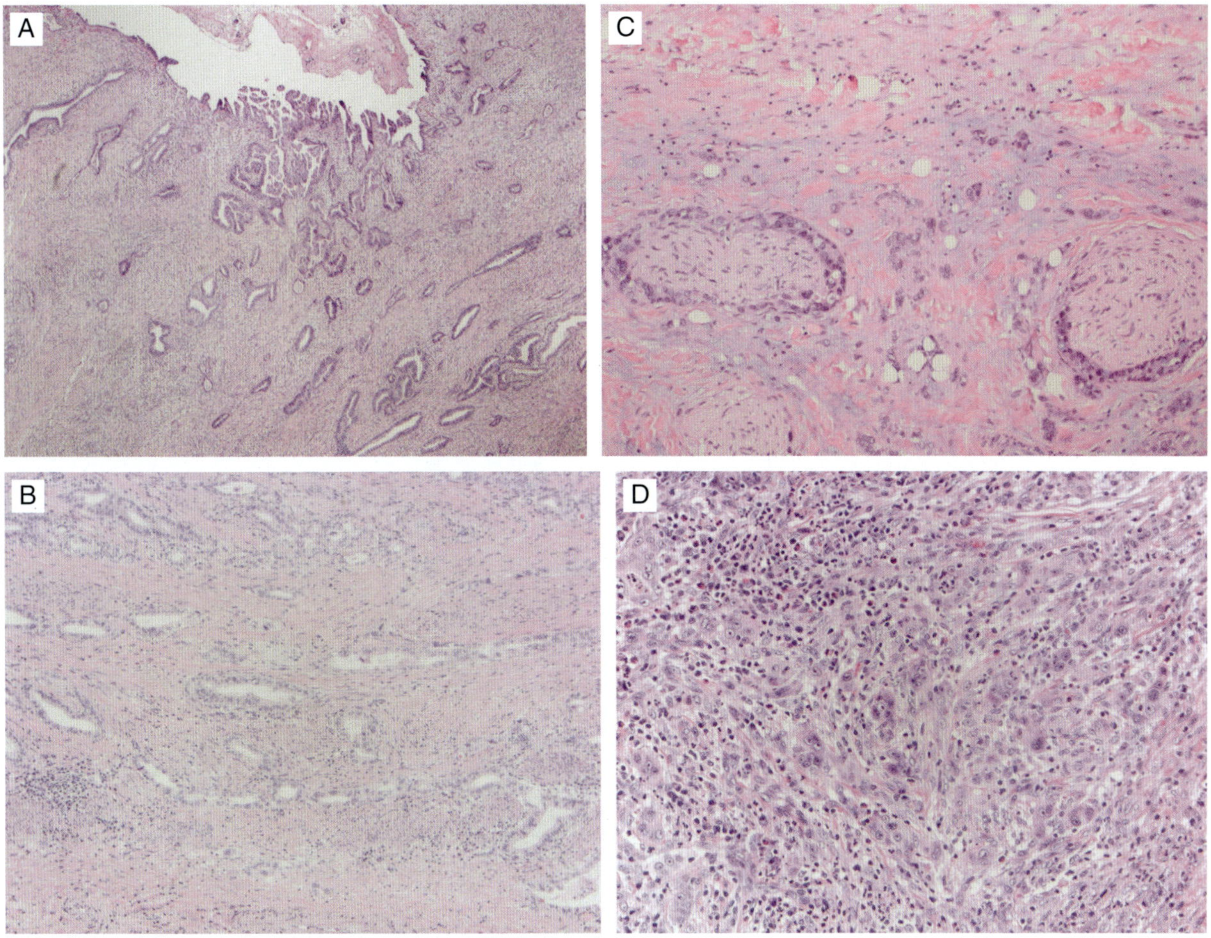

FIGURE 15.19

Cholangiocarcinomas can also arise from grossly invisible (flat) precursor lesions. A distal extrahepatic invasive cholangiocarcinoma with an intestinal phenotype arising from high-grade biliary intraepithelial neoplasia (**A**). Invasive adenocarcinoma involving the extrahepatic bile ducts can also show a bland pancreaticobiliary phenotype (**B**), striking perineural invasion (**C**), or an undifferentiated morphology with hardly any gland formation (**D**).

ELF3 and *ARID1B* mutation. *FGFR2* fusion and *IDH1/2* and *BAP1* mutations are specific for intrahepatic CC and are not detected in extrahepatic tumors.

Differential Diagnosis

Inflammation of any cause, either acute or chronic, may lead to marked reactive epithelial changes. Cholecystitis, extrahepatic primary sclerosing cholangitis, and IgG4 sclerosing cholangitis are the most common underlying causes of florid reactive atypia in the setting of severe inflammation. Choledocholithiasis and iatrogenic causes for reactive biliary atypia should also be considered, especially in patients who have had biliary stents or those who had a recent ERCP. Acute conditions such as cholecystitis and bacterial cholangitis present with fever, leukocytosis, and abdominal pain. More chronic conditions such as PSC are typically associated with strictures and, less commonly, obstructive symptoms. The morphologic features that allow distinction of reactive changes from true neoplasia are similar to those described in the gallbladder neoplasia section earlier.

Treatment and Prognosis

Extrahepatic CC (both perihilar and distal subtypes) is associated with a poor prognosis. The overall 5-year survival rate is less than 10%. However, this is because most patients present at an advanced stage, preventing curative-intent surgical resection. Five-year survival rates between 30% and 67% have been reported in patients after an R0 resection. The surgical approach depends on the tumor location. Some patients of perihilar CC can be treated with cholecystectomy combined with extrahepatic bile duct resection and regional lymph node dissection, whereas others require right or left hepatectomy with an en bloc caudate lobectomy. Patients with PSC and perihilar CC are sometimes considered for liver transplantation because of the high risk of subsequent PSC-associated carcinomas throughout the intrahepatic and extrahepatic biliary tree. Patients with distal CC are typically treated with standard pancreaticoduodenectomy.

OTHER LESIONS OF THE GALLBLADDER AND EXTRAHEPATIC BILE DUCTS

Unilocular cystic dilations of the bile duct, known as choledochal cysts, are rare lesions occurring most often in female infants and children, though they have been reported in adults as well. They are more common in East Asia than in Western populations. Although they are generally considered to be congenital, their close association with anomalous pancreatobiliary duct union has led some to hypothesize that many choledochal cysts are secondary reactive lesions arising because of bile and pancreatic juice reflux. They are classified into five types based on anatomic location. Histologically, they consist of a fibrous wall with variable amounts of chronic inflammation often lined by simple or papillary biliary epithelium with reactive changes. Choledochal cysts are benign, but patients with these lesions are at increased risk for extrahepatic CC.

Primary well-differentiated neuroendocrine ("carcinoid") tumors of the gallbladder and extrahepatic bile ducts are exceptionally rare. They most likely originate from intestinal metaplasia because normal biliary mucosa lacks endocrine cells. Typically, these tumors are composed of nests of endocrine cells with round nuclei, stippled chromatin, and moderately abundant cytoplasm (Fig. 15.20). Expression of a wide variety of peptide hormones, including gastrin, serotonin, pancreatic polypeptide, and somatostatin, has been reported. The WHO grading system is the same as that used in other GI neuroendocrine tumors. Because of their rarity, the AJCC eighth edition guidelines do not have a specific category for staging neuroendocrine neoplasms of the gallbladder and bile duct, so in clinical practice, such cases are often staged using the respective carcinoma templates. The morphologic differential diagnosis includes metastasis from another primary site and paragangliomas, which may occur in the gallbladder or in close anatomic vicinity to the bile ducts. Poorly differentiated neuroendocrine carcinomas, with either small cell or large cell morphology, may also rarely arise as primary lesions of the gallbladder or extrahepatic bile ducts. Like neuroendocrine carcinomas of other sites, these tumors are associated with aggressive behavior and poor prognosis. Although some are "pure" neuroendocrine carcinomas, others arise as divergent differentiation in poorly differentiated adenocarcinomas.

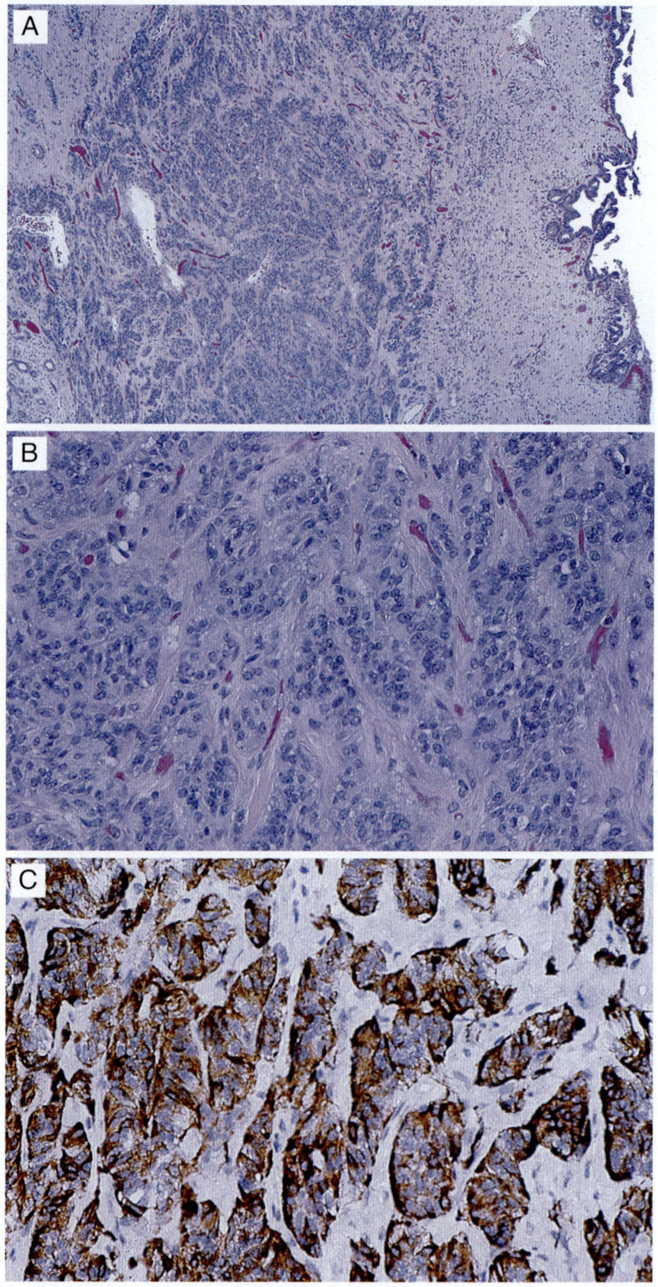

FIGURE 15.20

Well-differentiated neuroendocrine tumor involving the bile duct. Tumor cells arranged in a trabecular pattern within the bile duct wall (**A**) with uniform round nuclei (**B**) and diffuse positivity for chromogranin (**C**).

Mucinous cystic neoplasms, referred to as hepatobiliary cystadenomas in the past, may also occur in either the gallbladder or the extrahepatic biliary system, though most cases outside of the pancreas are intrahepatic. The clinical and pathologic features of these lesions are similar to their counterparts in the pancreas. Specifically, they are found almost exclusively in women. Most patients are between 30 and 60 years old. These lesions are often multiloculated and lined by mucinous epithelium. Characteristic ovarian-type stroma is required for the diagnosis (Fig. 15.21). The epithelial lining is, by definition, dysplastic and usually consists of low-grade simple mucinous columnar cells with minimal cytologic

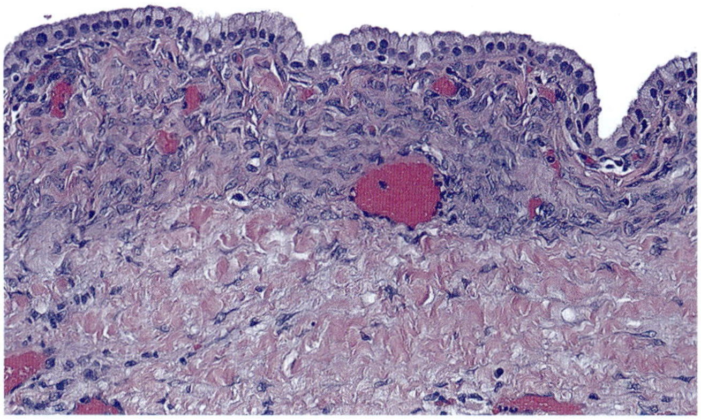

FIGURE 15.21

Mucinous cystic neoplasm of the bile duct is characterized by a pancreatico-biliary-type lining and surrounding cellular ovarian-type stroma. These lesions can also show a spectrum of histologic differentiation and tumor grade similar to their pancreatic counterparts and may be associated with an invasive adenocarcinoma.

atypia. However, high-grade dysplasia and invasive carcinoma can occur in some lesions. Malignant transformation in intrahepatic mucinous cystic neoplasms occurs at a lower frequency compared with their more common pancreatic counterparts.

Mesenchymal tumors of the gallbladder and extrahepatic bile ducts are extremely rare. Based on its higher incidence, sarcomatoid carcinoma should be considered in the differential diagnosis of high-grade spindle cell malignancies. Of note, these tumors often show only focal keratin immunoreactivity. Granular cell tumors are among the more common mesenchymal neoplasms in this location and can clinically mimic carcinoma by causing bile duct strictures. Approximately 90% of cases occur in young and middle-aged women. Histologically, they are characterized by nests and sheets of cells with abundant eosinophilic granular cytoplasm. The overlying epithelium is often hyperplastic, which in extreme cases may mimic carcinoma. The tumor cells are periodic acid–Schiff positive and diastase resistant and strongly immunoreactive for S-100.

Botryoid embryonal rhabdomyosarcoma is the most common malignant tumor of the extrahepatic biliary tree in children, typically presenting in patients younger than 5 years of age. The tumors characteristically project into the bile duct lumen, and patients often present with obstructive symptoms. Grossly, they often have a "grape-like" botryoid appearance and in some cases can reach more than 10 cm in size. Sampling of hypocellular areas of the lesion is a known pitfall in biopsy specimens that can be misinterpreted as the wall of a choledochal cyst. One characteristic feature is the presence of a cambium layer, consisting of condensed primitive rhabdomyoblasts immediately subjacent to the epithelium. The tumor cells are positive by IHC for desmin and myogenin.

SUGGESTED READINGS

1. Adsay V, Jang KT, Roa JC, et al. Intracholecystic papillary-tubular neoplasms (ICPN) of the gallbladder (neoplastic polyps, adenomas, and papillary neoplasms that are; 1.0 em): clinicopathologic and immunohistochemical analysis of 123 cases. *Am J Surg Pathol.* 2012;36(9):1279–1301.
2. Albores-Saa vedra J, Batich K, Hossain S, et al. Carcinoid tumors and small-cell carcinomas of the gallbladder and extrahepatic bile ducts: a comparative study based on 221 cases from the Surveillance, Epidemiology, and End Results Program. *Ann Diagn Pathol.* 2009;13(6):378–383.
3. Albores-Saave dra J, Chable-Montero F, Angeles-Aibores O, et al. Early gallbladder carcinoma: a clinicopathologic study of 13 cases of intramucosal carcinoma. *Am J Clin Pathol.* 2011;135(4):637–642.
4. Albores-Saavedra J, Chable-Montero F, Gonzalez-Romo MA, et al. Adenomas of the gallbladder. Morphologic features, expression of gastric and intestinal mucins, and incidence of high-grade dysplasia/carcinoma in situ and invasive carcinoma. *Hum Pathol.* 2012;43(9):1506–1513.
5. Albores-Saavedra J, Henson DE, Klimstra OS. *Tumors of the gallbladder, extrahepatic bile ducts and ampulla of Vater. AFIP Atlas of Tumor Pathology, series 3; fascicle 27. : Armed Forces Institute of Pathology*; 2000.
6. Albores-Saavedra J, Melberg K, Henson DE. Unusual malignant epithelial tumors of the gallbladder. *Semin Diagn Pathol.* 1996;13(4):326–338.
7. Albores-Saavedra J, Shukla O, Carrick K, et al. In situ and invasive adenocarcinomas of the gallbladder extending into or arising from Rokitansky-Aschoff sinuses: a clinicopathologic study of 49 cases. *Am J Surg Pathol.* 2004;28(5):621–628.
8. Chang HJ, Jee CD, Kim WH. Mutation and altered expression of beta-catenin during gallbladder carcinogenesis. *Am J Surg Pathol.* 2002;26(6):758–766.
9. Chen C, Wang L, Liu X, et al. Gallbladder neuroendocrine carcinoma: report of 10 cases and comparison of clinicopathologic features with gallbladder adenocarcinoma. *Int J Clin Exp Pathol.* 2015;8(7):8218–8226.
10. Foster DR, Foster DB. Gallbladder polyps in Peutz-Jeghers syndrome. *Postgrad Med J.* 1980;56(655):373–376.
11. Guo KJ, Yamaguchi K, Enjoji M. Undifferentiated carcinoma of the gallbladder. A clinicopathologic, histochemical, and immunohistochemical study of 21 patients with a poor prognosis. *Cancer.* 1988;61(9):1872–1879.
12. Honda M, Furuta Y, Naoe H, et al. Primary mucosa-associated lymphoid tissue (MALT) lymphoma of the gallbladder and review of the literature. *BMJ Case Rep.* 2017;2017: bcr2017220161.
13. Kamboj M, Gandhi JS, Gupta G, et al. Neuroendocrine carcinoma of gallbladder: a series of 19 cases with review of literature. *J Gastrointest Cancer.* 2015;46(4):356–364.
14. Kushima R, Remmele W, Stolte M, et al. Pyloric gland type adenoma of the gallbladder with squamoid spindle cell metaplasia. *Pathol Res Pract.* 1996;192(9):963–969, Discussion 970–971.
15. Lazcano-Ponce EC, Miquel JF, Muiioz N, et al. Epidemiology and molecular pathology of gallbladder cancer. *CA Cancer J Clin.* 2001;51(6):349–364.
16. Lewis JT, Talwalkar JA, Rosen CB, et al. Prevalence and risk factors for gallbladder neoplasia in patients with primary sclerosing cholangitis: evidence for a metaplasia-dysplasia-carcinoma sequence. *Am J Surg Pathol.* 2007;31(6):907–913.
17. Maitra A, Tascilar M, Hruban RH, et al. Small cell carcinoma of the gallbladder: a clinicopathologic, immunohistochemical, and molecular pathology study of 12 cases. *Am J Surg Pathol.* 2001;25(5):595–601.
18. Mani H, Climent F, Coloma L, et al. Gall bladder and extrahepatic bile duct lymphomas: clinicopathological observations and biological implications. *Am J Surg Pathol.* 2010;34(9):1277–1286.
19. Matsumoto T, Imai Y, Inokuma T. Neuroendocrine carcinoma of the gallbladder accompanied by pancreaticobiliary maljunction. *Clin Gastroenterol Hepatol.* 2016;14(3):e29–e30.
20. Mclean CA, Pedersen JS. Endocrine cell carcinoma of the gallbladder. *Histopathology.* 1991;19(2):173–176.
21. Morikawa T, Okabayashi T, Shima Y, et al. Adenomyomatosis concomitant with primary gallbladder carcinoma. *Acta Med Okayama.* 2017;71(2):113–118.

22. Muraki T, Memis B, Reid MD, et al. Reflux-associated cholecystopathy: analysis of 76 gallbladders from patients with Supra-Oddi union of the pancreatic duct and common bile duct (pancreatobiliary maljunction) elucidates a specific diagnostic pattern of mucosal hyperplasia as a prelude to carcinoma. *Am J Surg Pathol.* 2017;41(9):1167–1177.
23. Nishihara K, Tsuneyoshi M. Undifferentiated spindle cell carcinoma of the gallbladder: a clinicopathologic, immunohistochemical, and flow cytometric study of 11 cases. *Hum Pathol.* 1993;24(12):1298–1305.
24. Nishihara K, Yamaguchi K, Hashimoto H, et al. Tubular adenoma of the gallbladder with squamoid spindle cell metaplasia. Report of three cases with immunohistochemical study. *Acta Pathol Jpn.* 1991;41(1):41–45.
25. Pai RK, Mojtahed K, Pai RK. Mutations in the RAS/RAF/MAP kinase pathway commonly occur in gallbladder adenomas but are uncommon in gallbladder adenocarcinomas. *Appl Immunohistochem Mol Morphol.* 2011;19(2):133–140.
26. Parwani AV, Geradts J, Caspers E, et al. Immunohistochemical and genetic analysis of non-small cell and small cell gallbladder carcinoma and their precursor lesions. *Mod Pathol.* 2003;16(4):299–308.
27. Roa I, Ibacache G, Munoz S, et al. Gallbladder cancer in Chile: pathologic characteristics of survival and prognostic factors: analysis of 1,366 cases. *Am J Clin Pathol.* 2014;141(5):675–682.
28. Roa JC, Roa I, Correa P, et al. Microsatellite instability in preneoplastic and neoplastic lesions of the gallbladder. *J Gastroenterol.* 2005;40(1):79–86.
29. Roa JC, Tapia O, Cakir A, et al. Squamous cell and adenosquamous carcinomas of the gallbladder: clinicopathological analysis of 34 cases identified in 606 carcinomas. *Mod Pathol.* 2011;24(8):1069–1078.
30. Roa JC, Tapia O, Manterola C, et al. Early gallbladder carcinoma has a favorable outcome but Rokitansky-Aschoff sinus involvement is an adverse prognostic factor. *Virchows Arch.* 2013;463(5):651–661.
31. Shindoh J, de Aretxabala X, Aloia TA, et al. Tumor location is a strong predictor of tumor progression and survival in T2 gallbladder cancer: an international multicenter study. *Ann Surg.* 2015;261(4):733–739.
32. Singhi AD, Adsay NV, Swierczynski SL, et al. Hyperplastic Luschka ducts: a mimic of adenocarcinoma in the gallbladder fossa. *Am J Surg Pathol.* 2011;35(6):883–890.
33. Sinkre PA, Murakata L, Rabin L, et al. Clear cell carcinoid tumor of the gallbladder: another distinctive manifestation of von Hippel-Lindau disease. *Am J Surg Pathol.* 2001;25(10):1334–1339.
34. Stephen AE, Berger DL. Carcinoma in the porcelain gallbladder: a relationship revisited. *Surgery.* 2001;129(6):699–703.
35. Sugawara S, Hirai I, Watanabe T, et al. A case of mucinous cystic neoplasm of the gallbladder. *Clin J Gastroenterol.* 2018;11(5):428–432.
36. Suster S, Huszar M, Herczeg E, et al. Adenosquamous carcinoma of the gallbladder with spindle cell features. A light microscopic and immunocytochemical study of a case. *Histopathology.* 1987;11(2):209–214.
37. Tuncel D, Roa JC, Araya JC, et al. Poorly cohesive cell (diffuse-infiltrative/signet ring cell) carcinomas of the gallbladder: clinicopathological analysis of 24 cases identified in 628 gallbladder carcinomas. *Hum Pathol.* 2017;60:24–31.
38. Vardaman C, Albores-Saavedra J. Clear cell carcinomas of the gallbladder and extrahepatic bile ducts. *Am J Surg Pathol.* 1995;19(1):91–99.
39. Wistuba II, Gazdar AF, Roa I, et al. p53 protein overexpression in gallbladder carcinoma and its precursor lesions: an immunohistochemical study. *Hum Pathol.* 1996;27(4):360–365.
40. Wistuba II, Miquel JF, Gazdar AF, et al. Gallbladder adenomas have molecular abnormalities different from those present in gallbladder carcinomas. *Hum Pathol.* 1999;30(1):21–25.
41. Yanagisawa N, Mikami T, Saegusa M, et al. More frequent beta-catenin exon 3 mutations in gallbladder adenomas than in carcinomas indicate different lineages. *Cancer Res.* 2001;61(1):19–22.
42. Zevallos Quiroz JC, Jimenez Aguero R, Garmendi Irizar M, et al. Mucinous cystic neoplasm of the gallbladder obstructing the common bile duct, a rare entity with a new name. *Cir Esp.* 2014;92(8):567–569.

16

Non-Neoplastic and Neoplastic Pathology of the Pancreas

Lodewijk A.A. Brosens, MD, PhD, Mari Mino-Kenudson, MD and Laura D. Wood, MD, PhD

NON-NEOPLASTIC DISEASES

Developmental Anomalies

The three most commonly encountered developmental anomalies of the pancreas in routine surgical pathology practice are pancreas divisum, annular pancreas, and ectopic pancreas.

Pancreas Divisum

Pancreas divisum occurs in 3% to 7% of the population as a result of failure of the embryonic dorsal and ventral pancreatic buds to fuse properly. The duct of Santorini becomes the major ductal system of the pancreas, and it drains into the duodenum through the diminutive minor papilla. The small size of the minor papilla relative to the substantial flow through the major duct impedes the flow of pancreatic secretions and, in some patients, produces pancreatitis. Endoscopic retrograde cholangiopancreatography can be used to demonstrate the abnormal ductal anatomy and to exclude other causes of the patient's symptoms.

Pancreas divisum is best appreciated through careful gross dissection of the duct system. Imaging of a resected pancreas after the injection of a radiopaque dye into the duct system can also be used to establish the diagnosis. It is often associated with chronic pancreatitis, but the microscopic appearance is etiologically nonspecific. The differential diagnosis includes other causes of pancreatitis. Sphincterotomy of the minor papilla has been used to treat some patients with mixed results. The prognosis is dependent on the severity of pancreatitis.

Annular Pancreas

Annular pancreas is a rare malformation in which the dorsal and ventral buds of the pancreas abnormally fuse, forming a ring of pancreatic parenchyma around the duodenum. This ring can cause duodenal obstruction later in life. Most patients present clinically at a young age (~1 year), but some do not develop symptoms until adulthood. Children with annular pancreas can present with vomiting after meals and abdominal distention. Abdominal radiographs may show a classic "double-bubble" sign of intestinal obstruction.

A careful dissection of the resected specimen and clinical correlation with preoperative imaging studies and findings at surgery is the best way to establish the diagnosis. The differential diagnosis includes other causes of obstruction such as pyloric stenosis, ectopic pancreas, and duodenal atresia. Surgical resection of the obstruction is the treatment of choice, with an excellent prognosis after surgery.

Ectopic Pancreas

Pancreatic parenchyma located outside of the normal pancreas is referred to as ectopic pancreas. Ectopic pancreas is found in 2% of the population. Although ectopic pancreas is usually an incidental finding, it can cause bleeding and, in rare instances, intestinal obstruction. Ectopic pancreas only rarely forms a mass large enough to be detected radiographically. The upper gastrointestinal tract (stomach, duodenum, jejunum) is the most common location of ectopic pancreas. Other sites include ileum and Meckel's diverticulum (Fig. 16.1). These foci are composed of collections of normal acini and ducts and frequently islets of Langerhans. Surgical resection is the treatment of choice in symptomatic patients and is usually curative.

Pancreatic Hamartoma

Pancreatic hamartoma presents at a mean age of 60 years, and men and women are equally affected.

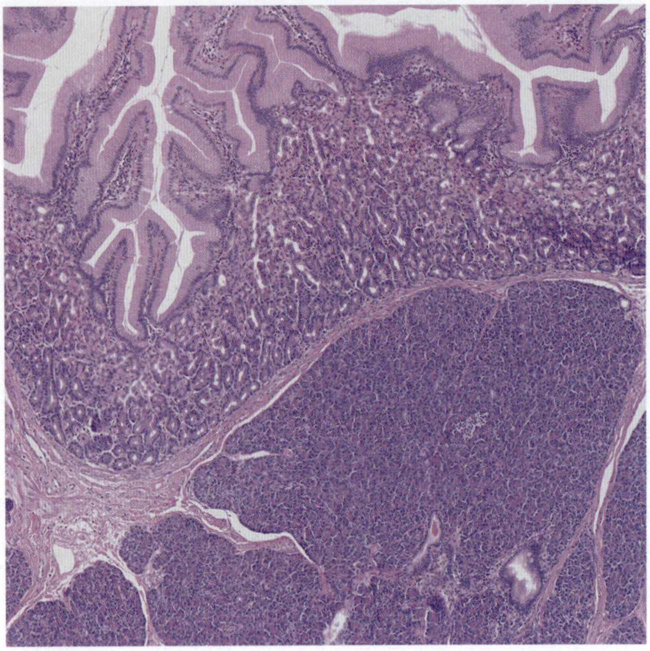

FIGURE 16.1

Ectopic pancreatic tissue in Meckel's diverticulum showing collections of normal acini and ducts and islets of Langerhans underneath gastric-type mucosa (hematoxylin and eosin).

Most patients are asymptomatic, but some may complain of abdominal pain and weight loss. Preoperative diagnosis is based on imaging, and in most cases, a pancreatic neoplasm such as pancreatic ductal adenocarcinoma (PDAC) or neuroendocrine tumor (NET) is suspected. Endoscopic ultrasound-guided fine-needle aspiration typically contains normal-looking pancreatic tissue and does not help to make a definite preoperative diagnosis. These lesions show nonspecific heterogeneous contrast enhancement on computed tomography (CT) and magnetic resonance imaging (MRI), and the radiologic differential diagnosis is broad.

Pancreatic hamartoma forms a well-demarcated lesion composed of mature acini and ducts with distorted architecture embedded in fibroblastic and collagenized stroma. There are no discrete islets of Langerhans, but scattered neuroendocrine cells are seen when immunohistochemistry (IHC) is applied. Ducts show variable amount of cystic dilation, which may be prominent in some cases. Adjacent pancreatic parenchyma is usually normal (Fig. 16.2). Localized chronic pancreatitis is the main histopathologic differential diagnosis, but this typically is not as well demarcated as a pancreatic hamartoma and contains islets of Langerhans. Pancreatic hamartoma is a benign lesion with an excellent prognosis.

Lymphoepithelial Cyst

Lymphoepithelial cysts account for approximately 0.5 % of pancreatic cysts, predominantly occurring in men between 60 and 70 years of age. It is usually asymptomatic and detected incidentally on imaging studies performed for other reasons. Lymphoepithelial cyst is typically a uni- or multiloculated cyst that is commonly located within the pancreas. Rarely, it may present as a cyst protruding over the pancreatic surface. The mean size of these cysts is about 5 cm, and they are lined by squamous epithelium with or without prominent keratinization. The cyst wall also contains abundant mature T lymphocytes and lymphoid aggregates with germinal centers (Fig. 16.3). Cyst content varies from serous to caseous, depending on the degree of keratin formation.

The differential diagnosis includes other cystic lesions such as mucinous cystic neoplasm (MCN), intraductal papillary mucinous neoplasm (IPMN), pseudocyst, dermoid cyst, and epidermoid cyst in intrapancreatic accessory spleen. Both dermoid cyst and epidermoid cyst in intrapancreatic accessory spleen occur in a younger age group. The large amount of organized lymphoid tissue and the lack of adnexal structures help to distinguish these lesions from dermoid cyst.

Intrapancreatic Spleen and Epidermoid Cyst

Accessory spleens exist in up to 10 % of the general population. Presence of an epidermoid cyst in an intrapancreatic accessory spleen (ECIPAS) is remarkably rare. Intrapancreatic spleen is usually asymptomatic and an incidental finding, although it may cause vague abdominal pain. On imaging studies, intrapancreatic spleen forms a well-demarcated mass that may resemble a small solid or cystic pancreatic neoplasm. The density of the tumor's solid component matches splenic tissue on postcontrast CT and MRI.

Grossly, intrapancreatic spleen forms a well-circumscribed dark red mass. In the case of ECIPAS, a unilocular cyst with serous or keratinaceous contents is present and is surrounded by splenic tissue. ECIPAS is lined by a benign multilayered squamous or urothelial-like epithelium surrounded by splenic tissue. The differential diagnosis includes solid-pseudopapillary neoplasm (SPN), NET, lymphoepithelial cyst, and other cystic lesions. When the diagnosis can be made preoperatively using fine-needle aspiration cytology and the patient is asymptomatic, no further treatment or follow-up is needed. In all other instances, conservative resection is curative.

Other Benign Cystic Lesions in the Pancreas

Simple Mucinous Cyst

Simple mucinous cysts are larger than 1 cm in size, lined by flat mucinous gastric type epithelium with minimal

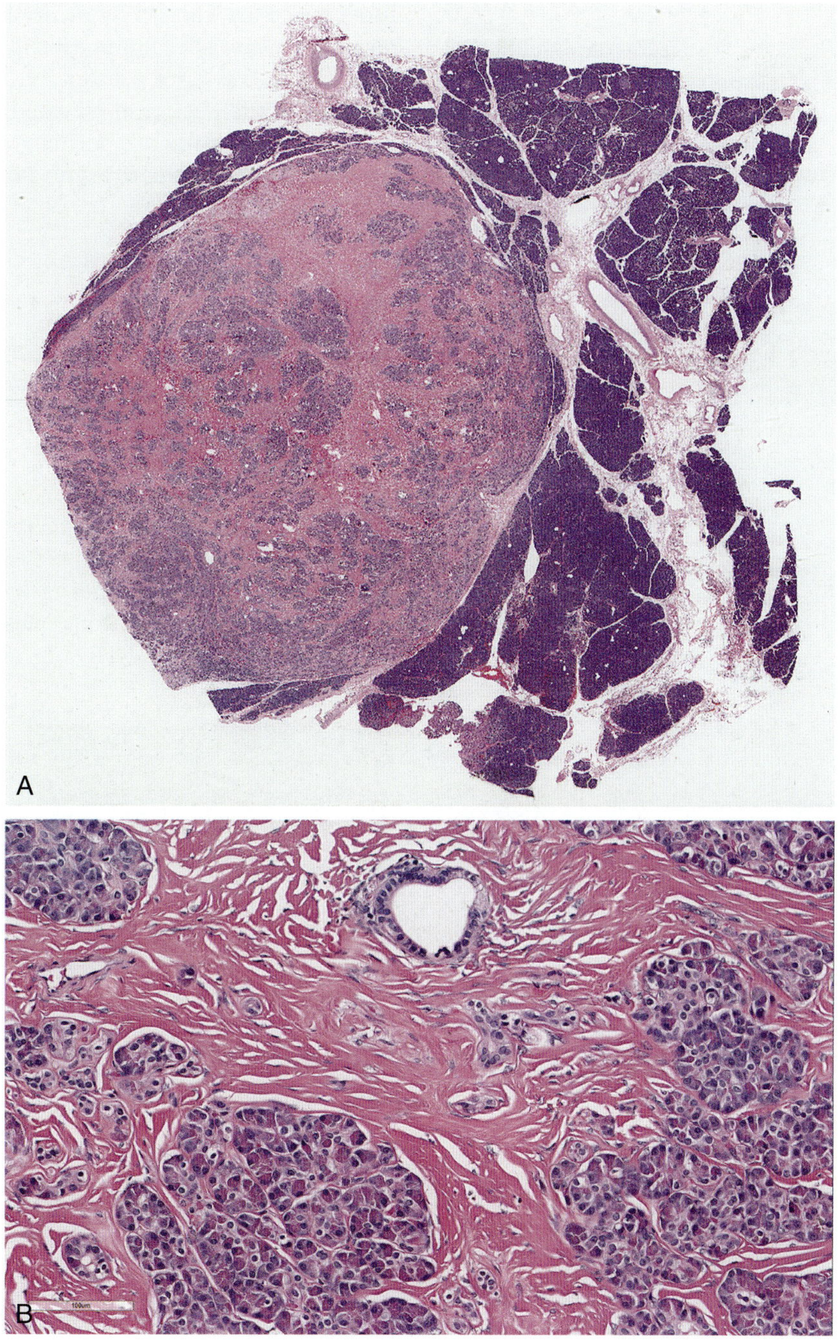

FIGURE 16.2

A, Pancreatic hamartoma showing a well-demarcated lesion surrounded by normal pancreatic parenchyma (hematoxylin and eosin [H&E]). **B**, Microscopically, pancreatic hamartoma is composed of mature acini and ducts with distorted architecture embedded in fibroblastic and collagenized stroma (H&E).

atypia, and lack ovarian-type stroma (Fig. 16.4). Depending on the features of the surrounding pancreatic tissue, different terms have been used to address these cysts. In case of an obstruction of the pancreatic duct, these cysts have been interpreted as retention cysts with partial pancreatic intraepithelial neoplasia 1 (PanIN-1) lining. Terms such as *mucinous non-neoplastic cyst* and *cystic mucinous duct lesion* have been used for lesions not associated with an obstructive process. Simple mucinous cysts can carry Kras mutations and even high-grade dysplasia in keeping with a neoplastic process.

Congenital Cyst

Congenital cysts are usually 1 to 2 cm in diameter and do not communicate with the duct system. These cysts have a paucicellular fibrous wall and are lined by cuboidal epithelium resembling the lining of normal ducts. The epithelium can be flattened and atrophic, and squamous epithelium is sometimes present. These cysts are mostly solitary but may be multiple when associated with cysts of the kidney and liver. Congenital cysts are most often found in children. In adults, congenital cysts are indistinguishable from retention cysts.

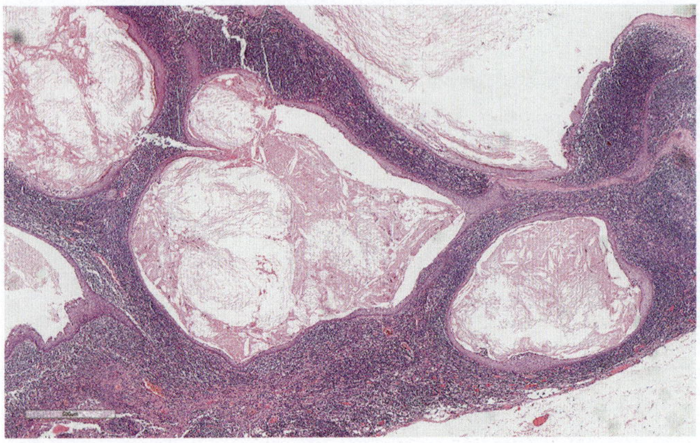

FIGURE 16.3

Multilocular lymphoepithelial cyst composed of lymphoid stroma and a cyst wall lined by squamous epithelium with some keratinization (hematoxylin and eosin).

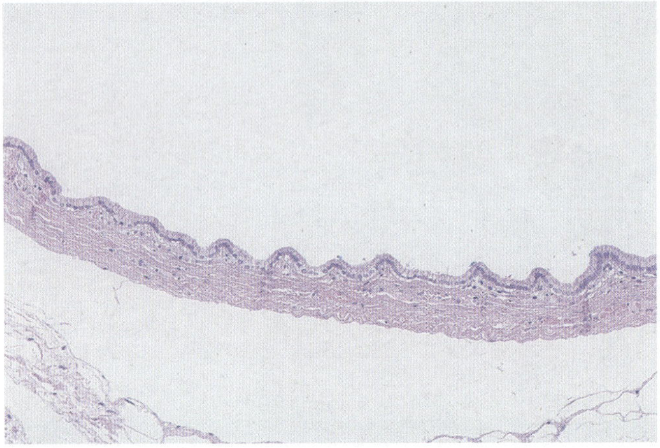

FIGURE 16.4

Simple mucinous cyst lined by flat nonpapillary mucinous gastric-type epithelium without and without ovarian-type stroma (hematoxylin and eosin).

Duodenal Diverticulum

A duodenal diverticulum on the pancreatic side of the duodenum can appear as a unilocular intrapancreatic or peripancreatic cyst and mimic a pancreatic cyst. Duodenal diverticula communicate with the duodenal lumen, in contrast to enteric duplication cysts, which do not communicate with the duodenal lumen and are most often lined by gastric mucosa. Duodenal diverticula are composed of small intestinal mucosa, which may cause confusion with intestinal-type IPMN (Fig. 16.5).

PANCREATITIS

Acute Pancreatitis

Clinical Features

Acute pancreatitis affects approximately 20 individuals per 100,000 population each year in Western nations. Most cases are caused by alcohol abuse or biliary tract disease. Other risk factors are smoking and genetic predisposition. Patients present with epigastric pain that radiates to the back and elevated serum amylase levels. Local complications are peripancreatic fluid collections, pancreatic and peripancreatic necrosis, infections, and pseudocyst.

Radiologic Features

Ultrasonography and CT reveal diffuse enlargement of the gland.

Pathologic Features

The pancreas is usually enlarged and soft, and the pancreatic and peripancreatic fat contains chalky white foci of fat necrosis. Severe cases may show hemorrhage into the gland. Microscopic findings range from mild edema with scattered inflammatory cells to extensive necrosis and hemorrhage (Fig. 16.6).

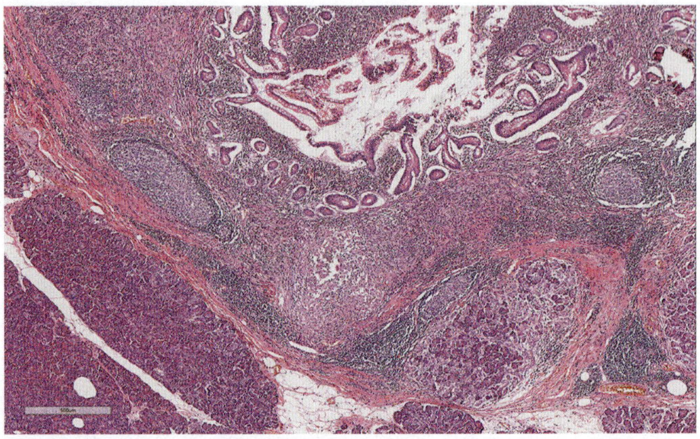

FIGURE 16.5

Duodenal diverticula showing intestinal mucosa with reactive changes surrounded by pancreatic tissue (hematoxylin and eosin).

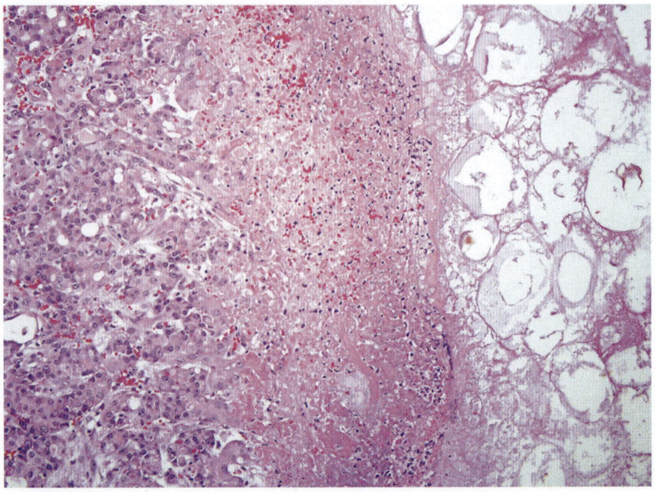

FIGURE 16.6

Acute pancreatitis with associated fat necrosis (hematoxylin and eosin).

Ancillary Studies

Elevated serum amylase levels support the diagnosis.

Differential Diagnosis

The differential diagnosis for acute pancreatitis is narrow and includes recurrent chronic pancreatitis. Clinical history is essential for making this distinction.

Prognosis and Therapy

Acute pancreatitis has an overall low mortality rate of approximately 1%, but this varies with the severity. Several scoring systems (Ranson's criteria, APACHE-II, BiSAP, Marshall score) are used to predict the prognosis of patients with pancreatitis. The treatment of patients with acute pancreatitis primarily consists of "resting" the pancreas and supportive care. Approximately 20% to 30% of patients with acute pancreatitis have a recurrence, and approximately 10% develop chronic pancreatitis. Progression from acute to chronic pancreatitis occurs more frequently in patients with continued alcohol and tobacco use and in patients with hereditary pancreatitis.

Chronic Pancreatitis

Clinical Features

Patients with chronic pancreatitis present with abdominal pain; exocrine and endocrine insufficiency, including diabetes mellitus and malabsorption with steatorrhea; and weight loss. Most cases in Western countries are caused by chronic alcohol abuse. In addition, obstruction of the pancreatic duct from ductal stones, tumors, strictures, or anatomical anomalies such as pancreas divisum can also cause chronic pancreatitis. A minority of patients have an inherited syndrome, including familial pancreatitis caused by mutations in *PRSS1* or *SPINK1* or cystic fibrosis.

Radiologic Features

Calcifications within the pancreas can be visualized on plain abdominal radiographs. Ultrasonography demonstrates ductal dilation; CT shows an atrophic pancreas with calcifications and small cysts.

Pathologic Features

Chronic pancreatitis is characterized by an inflammatory cell infiltrate associated with replacement of the normal pancreatic parenchyma with fibrous connective tissue (Fig. 16.7). This loss of acinar tissue can be

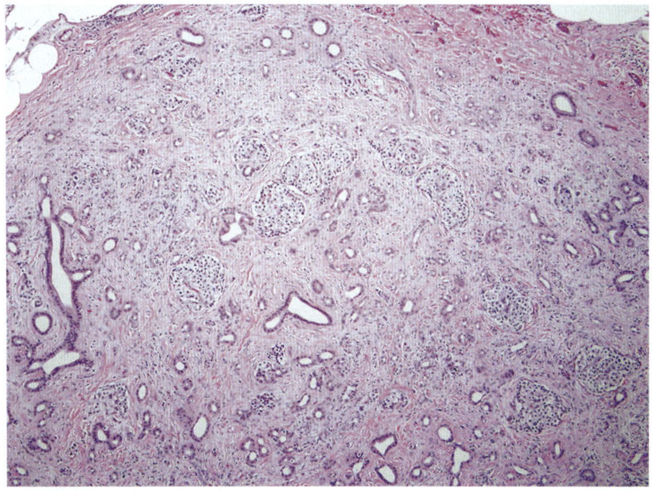

FIGURE 16.7

Chronic pancreatitis. Fibrosis, loss of exocrine parenchyma, and a relative enlargement of residual islets of Langerhans are seen (hematoxylin and eosin).

associated with dilation of the pancreatic ducts and intraductal inspissated secretions. The islets of Langerhans are relatively spared, with evidence of islet cell aggregation in some cases. The inflammatory cell infiltrate is usually composed of a mixture of lymphocytes, plasma cells, and scattered neutrophils.

Ancillary Studies

None are needed.

Differential Diagnosis

The atrophic glands of chronic pancreatitis can mimic a well-differentiated infiltrating adenocarcinoma. Features that favor a reactive process over a neoplastic process include retention of normal lobular architecture of the acini, glands with complete lumina, absence of luminal necrosis, and only mild nuclear pleomorphism. Perineural and vascular invasion, when present, are diagnostic of invasive adenocarcinoma.

Prognosis and Therapy

Patients with chronic pancreatitis have shorter survival times than the general population, but most die from non-pancreatic causes, such as other chronic diseases, cancers, or infections. Chronic pancreatitis, particularly young onset and hereditary pancreatitis, also increases risk of pancreatic cancer. Treatment is mostly supportive, with pancreatic exocrine enzyme replacement and careful management of diabetes and pain. Endoscopic intervention is indicated for ductal stones, main pancreatic duct strictures, and symptomatic pseudocysts. Indications for surgical intervention include poorly controlled pain, symptomatic pseudocysts, and suspicion of malignancy.

CHRONIC PANCREATITIS—FACT SHEET

Definition

- An inflammatory process of the pancreas characterized by an irreversible loss of exocrine and endocrine function

Incidence and Location

- 4–12 cases per 100,000 per year

Gender, Race, and Age Distribution

- Males > females
- 30–50 years of age
- Alcoholism most common cause in Western countries

Clinical Features

- Abdominal pain
- Diabetes mellitus
- Malabsorption with steatorrhea
- Weight loss

Radiologic Features

- Calcifications within the pancreas
- Ductal dilation
- Small cysts

Prognosis and Therapy

- Shorter survival than the general population
- Increased risk of pancreatic cancer
- Mostly supportive therapy; management of pain, exocrine and endocrine enzyme insufficiency, and complications

CHRONIC PANCREATITIS—PATHOLOGIC FEATURES

Gross Findings

- Firm, atrophic gland
- Calcifications
- Ductal dilation

Microscopic Findings

- Inflammatory infiltrate (predominantly chronic inflammation)
- Scattered foci of acute neutrophilic infiltrate may be present
- Fibrosis
- Loss of acinar tissue
- Relative sparing of the islets of Langerhans

Differential Diagnosis

- Well-differentiated ductal adenocarcinoma
- Retention of lobular architecture favors reactive proliferation
- Marked atypia or perineural or vascular invasion favors malignancy

AUTOIMMUNE PANCREATITIS

CLINICAL FEATURES

Autoimmune pancreatitis (AIP) is a rare form of chronic pancreatitis in which patients present with obstructive jaundice, imaging findings mimic pancreatic cancer, and conventional risk factors for pancreatitis such as alcoholism are lacking. Two subtypes of AIP with different histopathologic and clinical characteristics are recognized. Type 1 AIP, also called lymphoplasmacytic sclerosing pancreatitis, is a disorder in the spectrum of immunoglobulin (Ig) G4–related diseases. Type 1 AIP most often affects men, with a male-to-female ratio of approximately 3 to 1. The mean age of diagnosis is 60 years or older. Serum IgG4 levels are elevated in most patients, and extrapancreatic involvement, such as proximal bile duct strictures, retroperitoneal fibrosis, or bilateral salivary gland enlargement, is seen in about half of these patients. IgG4 elevation is variably defined depending on the laboratory, and levels greater than 135 mg/dL, greater than 121 mg/dL, or greater than 86 mg/dL have all been reported as cutoffs in the literature. Type 2 AIP, also called *idiopathic duct-centric chronic pancreatitis*, occurs in patients between 40 and 50 years of age. Men and women are equally affected. About 25% of patients have concurrent inflammatory bowel disease, and patients typically do not have elevated serum IgG4 levels.

RADIOLOGIC FEATURES

Type 1 and type 2 AIP are radiologically indistinguishable. About 30% to 50% of patients show the classic radiologic appearance of a diffuse enlargement of the gland with loss of the normal lobulated contour, the so-called "sausage-shaped pancreas." Alternatively, focal or multifocal enlargement of the pancreas can be seen.

PATHOLOGIC FEATURES

Type 1 and type 2 AIP are indistinguishable on gross examination. Most cases show diffuse enlargement of the pancreas, although localized "pseudotumor" or discrete nodules can also be seen (Fig. 16.8). International consensus histopathologic diagnostic criteria have been formulated that distinguish AIP from other forms of chronic pancreatitis and distinguish type 1 AIP from type 2. Periductal lymphoplasmacytic infiltrate and an inflammatory cellular stroma are the key diagnostic features of both types of AIP that distinguish AIP from other types of chronic pancreatitis. Storiform fibrosis, obliterative phlebitis, and lymphoid follicles are also typically seen in type 1 AIP. Obliterative phlebitis is often best seen at the interface between diseased and normal tissues (Fig. 16.9A). Marked pancreatic acinar atrophy is often associated with a brisk myofibroblastic proliferation in a storiform pattern (Fig. 16.9B). Importantly, although type 1 AIP typically shows marked infiltration by IgG4+ plasma cells of greater than 10 per hpf, this is not a specific finding for type 1 AIP and should only be used as an adjunct to support the diagnosis (Fig. 16.9C). Granulocytic epithelial lesions are pathognomonic for

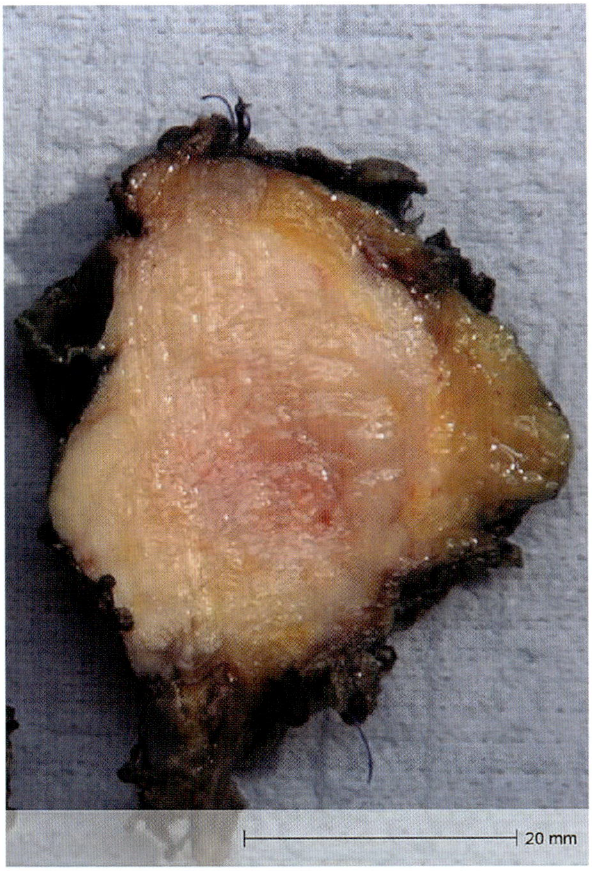

FIGURE 16.8

Autoimmune pancreatitis showing diffuse enlargement of the pancreas with effacement of the normal pancreatic lobular architecture.

type 2 AIP and are characterized by aggregates of neutrophils within the ductal epithelium and lumen (Fig. 16.10). In addition, neutrophilic infiltration in surrounding acinar tissue may be present.

Ancillary Studies

International consensus diagnostic criteria for AIP and to differentiate between type 1 and type 2 include five cardinal features of AIP, which are imaging, serology, other organ involvement, histology of the pancreas, and response to steroid therapy. A diagnostic steroid trial can be considered to confirm a strong suspicion of AIP. Serum IgG4 levels are elevated in most patients with type 1 AIP, and this finding can be used to support a preoperative diagnosis.

Differential Diagnosis

The differential diagnosis includes other forms of pancreatitis and pancreatic cancer in cases of focal mass on imaging. Duct-centric lymphoplasmacytic infiltrates, with or without granulocytic lesions, increased IgG4 positive plasma cells, inflamed stroma with storiform fibrosis, and obliterative phlebitis are features that favor a diagnosis of AIP. In contrast, ectatic ducts with inspissated secretions, marked acute inflammation within acinar or interlobular stroma, fat necrosis, and dense hyaline fibrosis involving intra- and interlobular stroma are suggestive of chronic obstructive pancreatitis rather than AIP. Differentiating type 2 AIP from acute on chronic pancreatitis not otherwise specified can be challenging and should be done in correlation with clinical findings.

Prognosis and Therapy

Autoimmune pancreatitis is important to recognize because it can clinically mimic pancreatic cancer. Both type 1 and type 2 AIP respond well to steroid therapy, and type 1 AIP also responds to rituximab. Type 1 AIP frequently relapses, whereas relapses are uncommon in type 2. Both types of AIP have excellent long-term survival rates.

AUTOIMMUNE PANCREATITIS—FACT SHEET

Definition

- Type 1: disorder in the spectrum of IgG4-related diseases characterized by a dense periductal lymphoplasmacytic infiltrate, storiform fibrosis, and marked immunoglobulin (Ig) G4–positive plasma cell infiltration
- Type 2: characterized by granulocyte epithelial lesions without prominence of IgG4-positive plasma cells

Incidence and Location

- Estimated prevalence of fewer than 1 per 100,000
- Recognized with increasing frequency

Gender, Race, and Age Distribution

- Type 1: more common in men than in women. Most patients are 60 years of age or older
- Type 2: affects men and women equally. Most patients between 40 and 50 years of age

Clinical Features

- Can mimic pancreatic cancer with abdominal pain, weight loss, and jaundice
- Type 1 is a disorder in spectrum of immunoglobulin (Ig) G-related disease, and 50% have extrapancreatic involvement and elevated serum IgG4 levels
- Type 2 is associated with inflammatory bowel disease in 25% of patients

Radiologic Features

- Similar for type 1 and type 2: diffuse, focal, or multifocal enlargement of the pancreas

Prognosis and Therapy

- Steroid therapy
- Type 1 frequently relapses, whereas type 2 does not
- Both types have excellent long-term survival

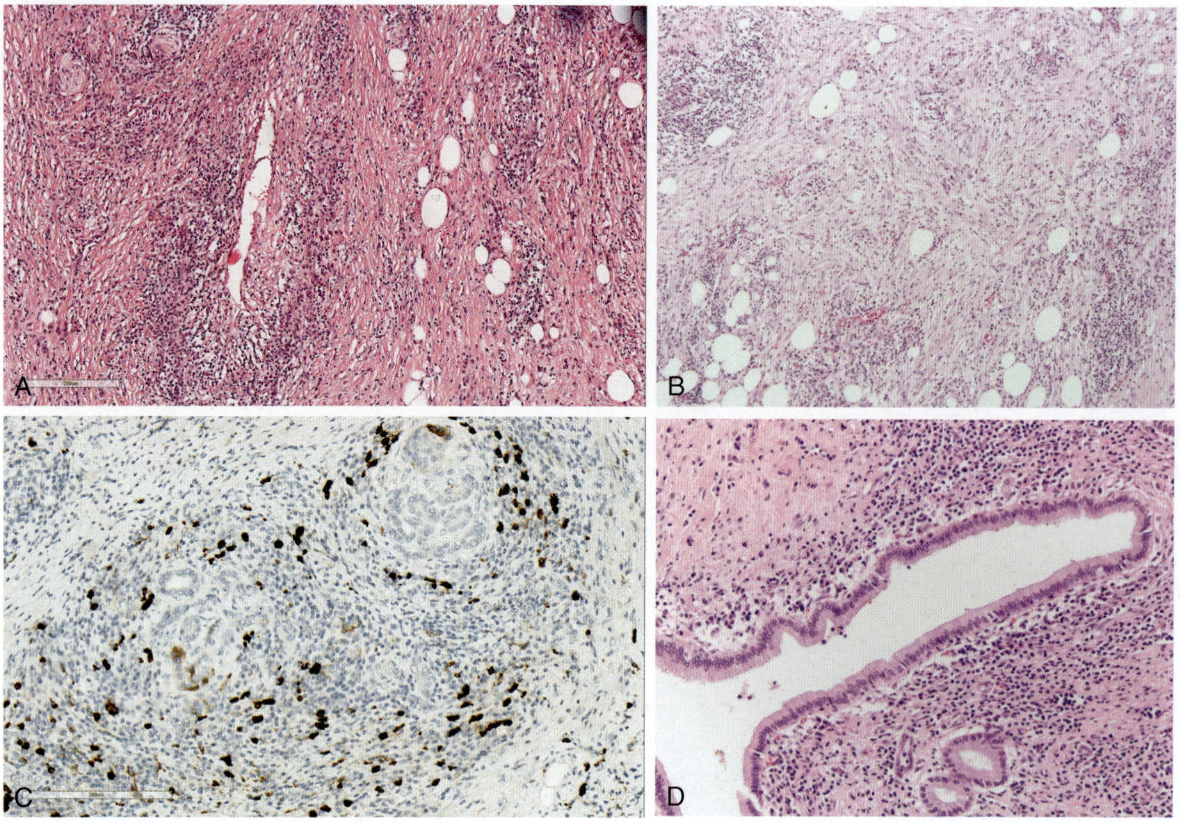

FIGURE 16.9

A, Type 1 autoimmune pancreatitis (AIP) showing inflammatory cellular stroma, storiform fibrosis, and obliterative phlebitis (hematoxylin and eosin [H&E]). **B**, Brisk myofibroblastic proliferation in a storiform pattern seen in a case of AIP (H&E). **C**, Type 1 AIP showing many immunoglobulin G4+ plasma cells **D**, Periductal mononuclear cell infiltrate, rich in plasma cells, is characteristic of type 1 AIP.

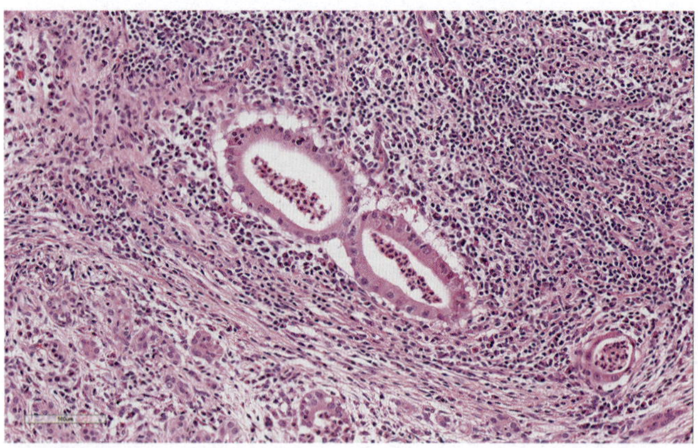

FIGURE 16.10

Granulocytic epithelial lesion in type 2 autoimmune pancreatitis, characterized by periductal lymphoplasmacytic infiltrate and neutrophils in the ductal epithelium and lumen (hematoxylin and eosin).

Autoimmune Pancreatitis—Pathologic Features

Gross Findings

- Diffuse or segmental enlargement of the pancreas ("pseudotumor")

Microscopic Findings

- Both types: periductal lymphoplasmacytic infiltrate and an inflammatory cellular stroma
- Type 1: storiform fibrosis, obliterative phlebitis, lymphoid follicles, and infiltration by immunoglobulin (Ig) G4+ plasma cells
- Type 2: granulocytic epithelial lesions

Immunohistochemistry

- Type 1: increased numbers of IgG4-positive plasma cells (>10 IgG4-positive plasma cells per hpf)
- Type 2: scant to absent IgG4-positive plasma cells

Differential Diagnosis

- Other forms of chronic pancreatitis
- Pancreatic adenocarcinoma

Paraduodenal (Groove) Pancreatitis

Clinical Features. Paraduodenal or "groove" pancreatitis is a distinctive form of pancreatitis that occurs in the "groove" region demarcated by the superior aspect of the pancreas, the common bile duct, and the minor papilla. Alternative names that have been used for this lesion are cystic *dystrophy of heterotopic pancreas*, *paraduodenal wall cyst*, *pancreatic hamartoma of duodenum*, and *myoadenomatosis*. Most patients are young to middle-aged men with a history of alcohol abuse.

Radiologic Features. Computed tomography usually reveals a thickened duodenum associated with cyst formation in the duodenal wall or subjacent pancreas.

Pathologic Features. Paraduodenal pancreatitis, in addition to arising in a very specific region, has a characteristic microscopic appearance. The cysts, which may contain inspissated secretions and degenerated polymorphonuclear cells, are lined by partially or completely denuded ductal epithelium and are often surrounded by granulation tissue (Fig. 16.11). In addition, pseudocysts can be present. A reactive spindle cell proliferation is often present, which may be very prominent, raising suspicion of leiomyoma or gastrointestinal stromal tumor. Almost all cases show Brunner's gland hyperplasia, which is largely responsible for the thickening and polypoid appearance of the duodenal mucosa.

Differential Diagnosis. The differential diagnosis includes cystic neoplasms of the pancreas, as well as mesenchymal neoplasms in cases that show marked reactive myofibroblastic proliferation. The characteristic location of the lesion, and the presence of a partially denuded but otherwise unremarkable epithelium lining the cyst helps establish the diagnosis.

Prognosis and Therapy. These are benign lesions that have an excellent outcome but may need surgical intervention.

PARADUODENAL (GROOVE) PANCREATITIS—FACT SHEET

Definition

- Distinctive form of pancreatitis, often with cystic changes, occurring in the "groove region" demarcated by the superior aspect of the pancreatic head, the common bile duct, and the duodenum

Incidence and Location

- Rare
- By definition, located in the "groove" region

Gender, Race, and Age Distribution

- Strong male predominance
- Most patients are in their 50s

Clinical Features

- A history of alcohol abuse is common
- Common symptoms include abdominal pain and weight loss

Radiologic Features

- May produce a solid or a cystic mass lesion in the head of the pancreas or duodenum

Prognosis and Therapy

- Prognosis is excellent because these are non-neoplastic lesions; they may require surgery

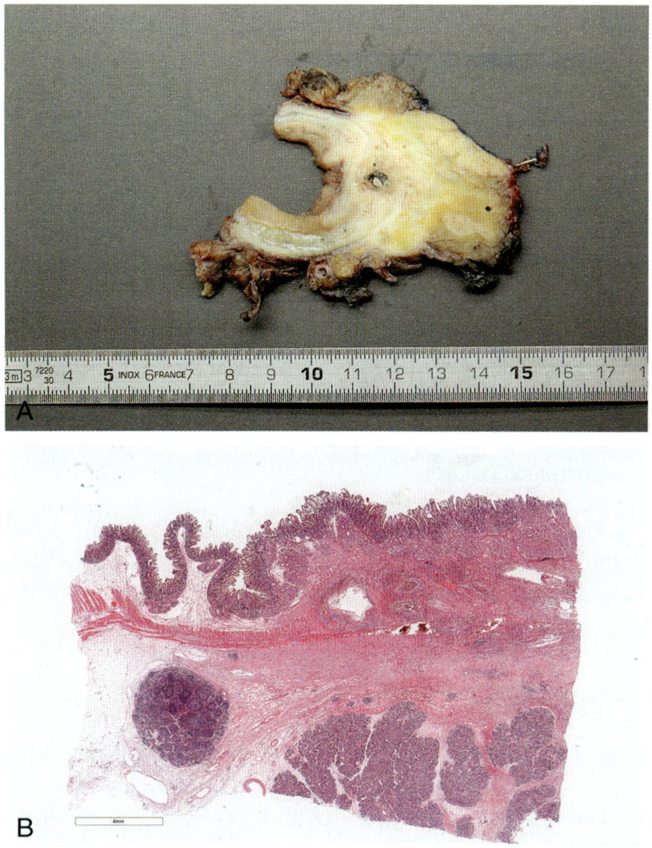

FIGURE 16.11

A, Paraduodenal pancreatitis showing a solid and cystic mass in the groove region of the pancreas. **B**, Microscopically, paraduodenal pancreatitis is characterized by cysts, which may contain inspissated secretions and degenerated polymorphonuclear cells, are lined by partially or completely denuded ductal epithelium, and are often surrounded by granulation tissue (hematoxylin and eosin).

GROOVE PANCREATITIS OR PARADUODENAL WALL CYST—PATHOLOGIC FEATURES

Gross Findings

- Cystic or solid mass lesion located in the groove region of the pancreas

Microscopic Findings

- Cysts lined by partially or completely denuded ductal epithelium and pseudocysts
- Associated inflammatory cell infiltrate
- A prominent reactive spindle cell proliferation is present in some cases

Differential Diagnosis

- Cystic neoplasms of the pancreas
- Leiomyoma or gastrointestinal stromal tumor

PSEUDOCYSTS

CLINICAL FEATURES

Pseudocysts are localized collections, usually extrapancreatic, of necrotic material rich in pancreatic enzymes that account for 75% of all pancreatic "cysts." They usually develop after an episode of acute pancreatitis or after trauma to the pancreas. Patients often have a severe epigastric pain that radiates to the back. In the United

States, most patients have a history of heavy alcohol consumption.

Radiologic Features

Abdominal imaging shows a unilocular cystic mass.

Pathologic Features

Pseudocysts are usually solitary and extrapancreatic and filled with necrotic or hemorrhagic material. They do not have an epithelial lining and are lined by variably inflamed granulation tissue and necrotic debris (Fig. 16.12).

Ancillary Studies

Aspirates of pseudocysts show abundant thin and watery, turbid, and sometimes hemorrhagic fluid, which is rich in lipase and amylase and low in carcinoembryonic antigen (CEA) levels.

Differential Diagnosis

The differential diagnosis of a pseudocyst includes retention cyst, serous cystadenomas (SCAs), MCN, IPMN, SPN, and cystic change in a usually solid pancreatic neoplasm. The absence of an epithelial lining combined with necrotic or hemorrhagic cyst contents rich in lipase and amylase establish the diagnosis of a pseudocyst.

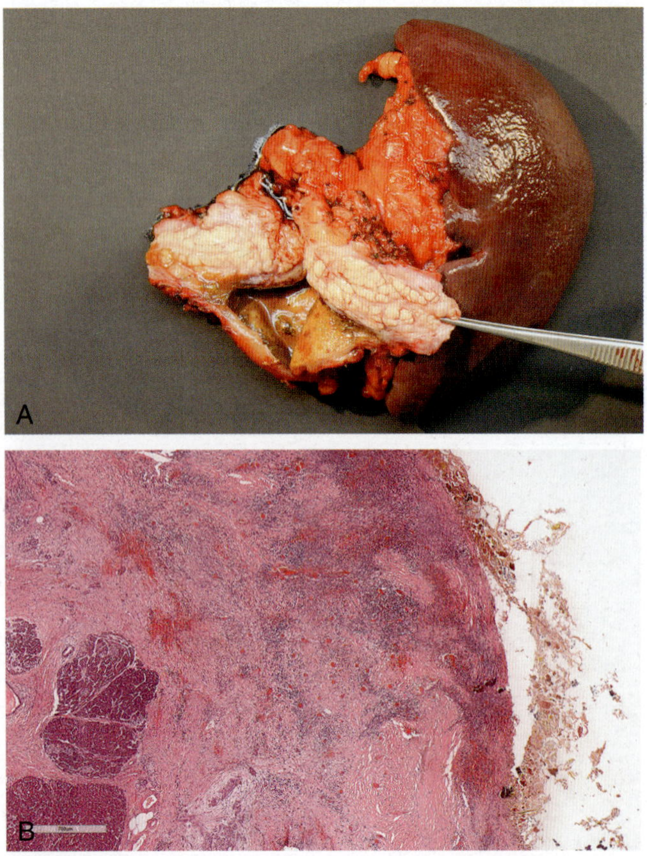

FIGURE 16.12

A, Pseudocyst filled with necrotic or hemorrhagic material rich in pancreatic exocrine enzymes. **B**, Pseudocyst lined by granulation and fibrous tissue (hematoxylin and eosin).

Prognosis and Therapy

Most pseudocysts resolve with supportive care, but some require surgical drainage. Superinfection of a pseudocyst is a serious complication.

NEOPLASTIC DISEASES

Ductal Neoplasms

Neoplastic pancreatic ductal lesions may present as a solid or cystic mass. In the latter scenario, the neoplastic proliferation can be confined within the duct (intraductal) or infiltrate into periductal tissues (invasive). The lining epithelium of neoplastic glands may resemble gastric, intestinal, or pancreaticobiliary type epithelium. Ductal neoplasms are therefore categorized into distinct groups based on their macroscopic appearance (invisible, cystic, solid), type of lining epithelium, presence or absence of an invasive component, and predominant genetic alterations found in each group.

Precursor Lesions

The following lesions are currently considered to be precursors to ductal carcinoma of the pancreas and its variants: PanIN, IPMN, intraductal oncocytic papillary neoplasm, MCN, and intraductal tubulopapillary neoplasm (ITPN).

Pancreatic Intraepithelial Neoplasia

Clinical Features. Most ductal carcinomas of the pancreas are associated with noninvasive epithelial proliferations within the smaller pancreatic ducts, called PanIN, which are classified into low and high grade. Low-grade PanIN lesions are quite common, and their prevalence correlates with age, increasing sharply after the age of 40 years. Whereas low-grade PanIN has a low malignant potential, high-grade PanIN is associated with a significant risk of progression to PCAC and is rarely (<5%) seen in resections for benign cysts or chronic pancreatitis.

Radiologic Features. PanIN lesions are microscopic and undetectable radiologically.

Pathological Features. Pancreatic intraepithelial neoplasia typically involves the epithelium of intra- and interlobular ducts that are smaller than 5 mm in diameter, but the main pancreatic duct may also be involved in some cases. By definition, the lesions are not visible grossly unless the ducts get dilated because of obstruction or some other mechanisms. PanIN is classified into low (previous PanIN-1 and PanIN-2 categories) and high grade (previous PanIN-3 category). Low-grade PanIN is characterized by a flat or papillary or micropapillary proliferation of tall columnar epithelial cells with abundant intracytoplasmic mucin and basally located round to oval nuclei. Nuclear atypia varies from none to mild nuclear crowding, enlargement, pseudostratification, and hyperchromasia. Mitoses are rare, and when present, they are not atypical (Fig. 16.13A). Conversely, high-grade PanIN is usually papillary/micropapillary and is characterized by cribriforming, budding, luminal necrosis, and irregular nuclei with visible nucleoli and frequent mitoses (Fig. 16.13B).

Importantly, PanIN harbors many of the same genetic alterations seen in PDAC. Although the genetic alterations do not occur in a specific sequence, their prevalence tends to increase from low to high grade. Whereas telomere shortening and activating mutations in codon 12 of the *KRAS* gene occur early in low-grade PanIN, inactivating mutations in the *p16/CDKN2A* gene tend to be seen in low-grade PanIN with more significant cytomorphologic atypia. *SMAD4* and *TP53* mutations usually occur in high-grade lesions. In addition, hypermethylation of several genes, including *p16*, has been reported, and the prevalence of hypermethylation increases from low- to high-grade PanIN.

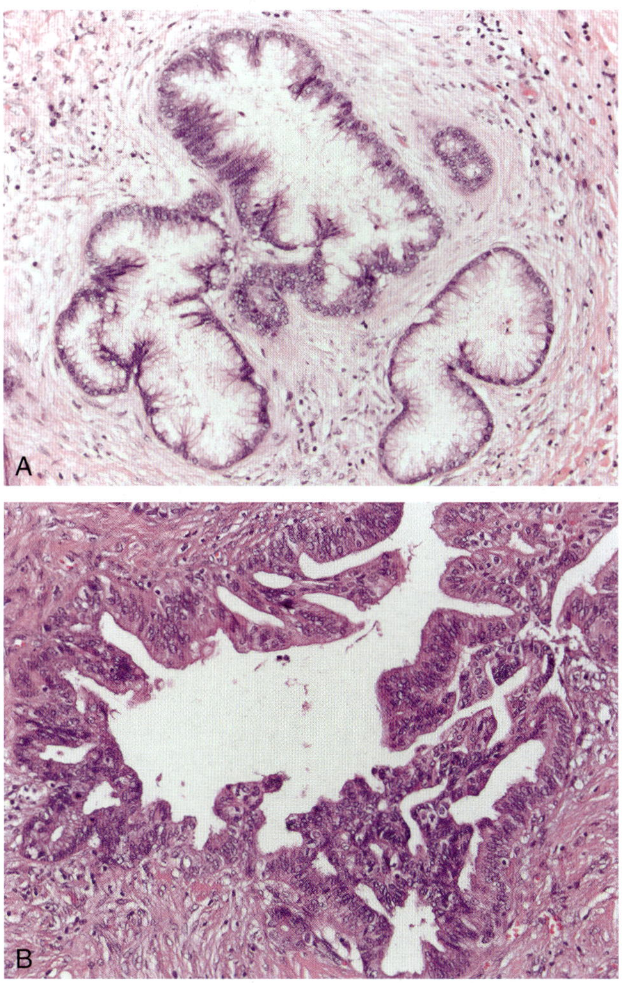

FIGURE 16.13

A, Low-grade pancreatic intraepithelial neoplasia (PanIN) lesion exhibiting papillary proliferation of tall columnar epithelial cells with abundant intracytoplasmic mucin, basally located round to oval nuclei, and no mitosis (hematoxylin and eosin [H&E]). **B**, High-grade PanIN demonstrating micropapillary proliferation of unequivocally atypical cells with irregular nuclei, visible nucleoli, and frequent and often abnormal mitoses (H&E).

Ancillary Studies. Ancillary studies are usually not required for the diagnosis of PanIN. PanIN exhibits a gastric type immunoprofile including positive MUC5AC, +/− MUC6, and negative MUC2 and CDX2. Although MUC1 is negative in low-grade PanIN, high-grade PanIN may express MUC1.

Differential Diagnosis. The differential diagnosis includes IPMN, in particular the branch-duct type. The latter is usually larger than 1.0 cm in diameter and grossly visible. Other lesions that may mimic PanIN include reactive ductal epithelial changes associated with inflammation and cancerization of ducts. The latter is spread of invasive carcinoma along preexisting ducts and may be difficult to distinguish from high-grade PanIN. Abrupt transition from normal to markedly atypical epithelium or the close proximity of invasive carcinoma with the involved duct favors cancerization.

Prognosis and Therapy. Although some PanIN lesions progress to invasive adenocarcinoma, it is not known how often and how rapidly they progress. The presence of even high-grade PanIN at a surgical resection margin does not appear to affect survival in patients who undergo complete (R0) resection for PDAC, although anecdotal case reports have described high-grade PanIN lesions progressing to invasive adenocarcinoma. However, in the setting of hereditary pancreatic cancer, the presence of high-grade PanIN in a distal pancreatectomy specimen obtained as part of a surveillance protocol is an indication for total pancreatectomy.

PANCREATIC INTRAEPITHELIAL NEOPLASIA—FACT SHEET

Definition

- Noninvasive neoplastic pancreatic ductal epithelial proliferations that typically involve smaller pancreatic ducts

Incidence and Location

- The incidence is unknown
- Low-grade pancreatic intraepithelial neoplasia (PanIN) often seen in pancreatic resections for benign cysts or chronic pancreatitis
- High-grade PanIN rarely (<5%) seen rarely in surgical resections without cancer; can occur throughout the pancreas

Gender, Race, and Age Distribution

- Increasing frequency of low-grade PanIN with age; common after age 40 years

Clinical Features

- No association with clinical symptoms

Radiologic Features

- Typically not detectable by imaging studies

Prognosis and Therapy

- The frequency and rate of progression to invasive ductal carcinoma are unknown
- The presence of high-grade PanIN may be an indication for further intervention depending on the clinical scenario

Pancreatic Intraepithelial Neoplasia—Pathologic Features

Gross Findings

- Typically invisible on gross examination

Microscopic Findings

- Ductal epithelial proliferations typically seen in smaller pancreatic ducts with various degrees of cytologic and architectural atypia; classified into low and high grade

Immunohistochemistry

- Positive for gastric-type markers (MUC5AC and MUC6)

Differential Diagnosis

- Other epithelial proliferation involving smaller pancreatic ducts: branch-duct intraductal papillary mucinous neoplasm, reactive ductal epithelial changes, cancerization of ducts

Intraductal Papillary Mucinous Neoplasm

Clinical Features. Intraductal papillary mucinous neoplasm is a grossly visible, mucin-producing epithelial neoplasm that predominantly grows within the main pancreatic duct or its major branches and exhibits a papillary architecture (Fig. 16.14). IPMNs make up 3% to 5% of all pancreatic neoplasms and are usually diagnosed in the sixth to seventh decade of life with a mean age of 63 years. They are slightly more common in men (male-to-female ratio, 3 to 2). The majority are found incidentally in asymptomatic patients during imaging for another indication. Symptoms are typically caused by intermittent pancreatic duct obstruction and manifest as abdominal pain, back pain, anorexia and weight loss, and recurrent symptoms of pancreatitis. Jaundice often indicates the presence of more advanced lesions, including invasive carcinoma arising in IPMN.

Radiologic Features. Intraductal papillary mucinous neoplasm lesions are classified into main-duct, mixed, and branch-duct types based on the pattern of involvement of the pancreatic duct system. Whereas main-duct and mixed-type IPMNs are characterized by a markedly dilated main pancreatic duct, often with concurrently dilated branch ducts, branch-duct IPMNs exhibit single or numerous cysts that represent dilated branch ducts.

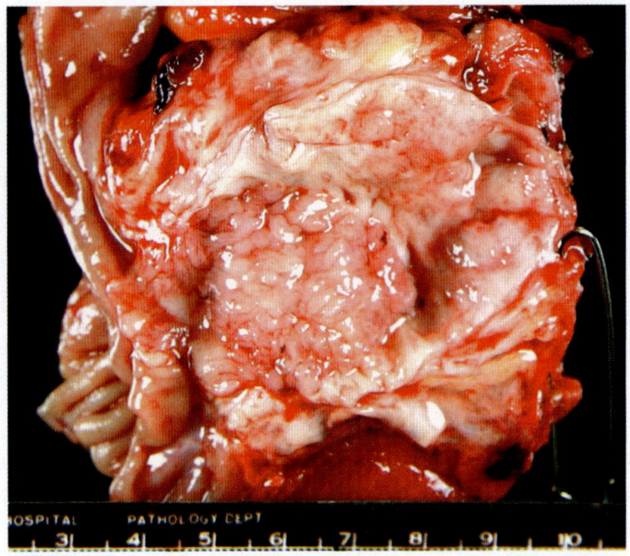

FIGURE 16.14

A gross photograph of intraductal papillary mucinous neoplasm, main-duct type.

Pathological Features. The majority of IPMNs arise in the head of the pancreas. Duct involvement may be unifocal, multifocal, or diffuse. IPMNs are usually localized on gross examination but can involve the entire length of the main duct. Histologically, IPMNs are characterized by cysts of variable size lined by tall columnar mucinous cells with a flat, undulating or papillary architecture. IPMNs exhibit varying degrees of epithelial atypia and are classified accordingly into low-grade dysplasia, high-grade dysplasia, and invasive carcinoma. They are also classified into various subtypes based on the epithelial morphology of the intraductal components: gastric, intestinal, pancreato-biliary, or oncocytic. The gastric type IPMN is typically low grade and characterized by abundant, slightly eosinophilic cytoplasmic mucin and basally located nuclei (Fig. 16.15A). Whereas most branch-duct IPMNs are of gastric type, main-duct and mixed-type IPMN often contain epithelia of multiple subtypes. The intestinal type exhibits villous papillae with basophilic cytoplasm and enlarged, oval, hyperchromatic nuclei with pseudostratification (Fig. 16.15B). The pancreatobiliary type consists of thin, branching papillae with amphophilic cytoplasm and enlarged hyperchromatic nuclei (Fig. 16.15C). The oncocytic type is characterized by thick branching papillae with intracellular and/or intercellular lumina, abundant eosinophilic cytoplasm, and large round nuclei with prominent nucleoli (Fig. 16.15D). The oncocytic subtype is genetically distinct from the remaining three subtypes and is now regarded as a separate entity (intraductal oncocytic papillary neoplasm) in the latest World Health Organization (WHO) classification (fifth edition). Various grades of dysplasia are often mixed in a single IPMN, and multiple epithelial subtypes may also be seen in a single

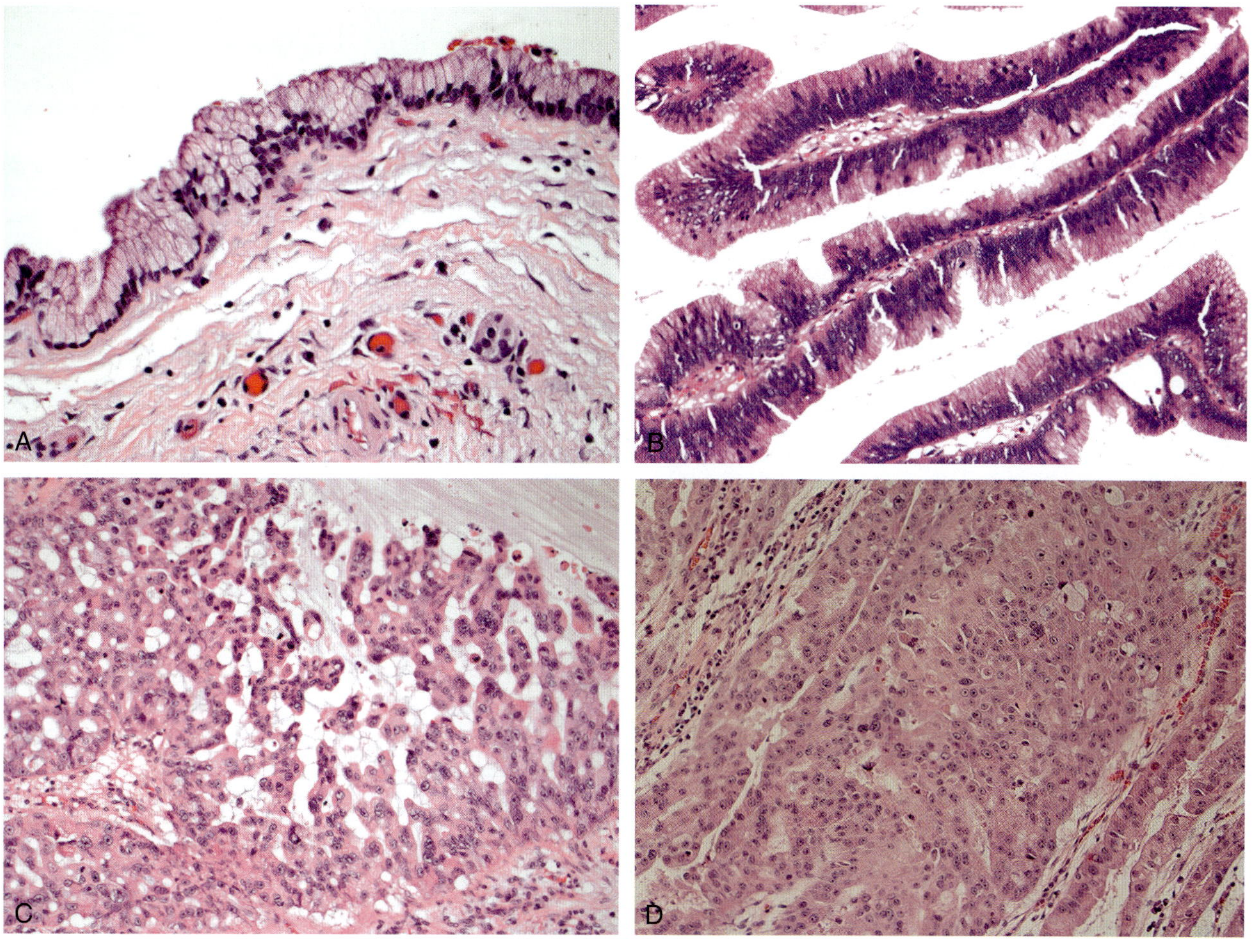

FIGURE 16.15

A, Gastric-type intraductal papillary mucinous neoplasm (IPMN) characterized by gastric foveolar-type epithelium with basally located nuclei and abundant apical cytoplasmic mucin (hematoxylin and eosin [H&E]). **B**, Intestinal-type IPMN exhibiting villous papillae with basophilic cytoplasm and enlarged, oval, hyperchromatic nuclei with pseudostratification (H&E). **C**, Pancreatobiliary-type IPMN consisting of thin, branching papillae and/or micropapillae with large nuclei (H&E). **D**, Oncocytic-type IPMN characterized by thick branching papillae with intracellular and/or intercellular lumina, abundant eosinophilic cytoplasm, and large round nuclei with prominent nucleoli (H&E).

lesion. Invasive carcinoma is found up to one-third of cases and is often small (<2 cm) and can be multifocal. The histology of invasive carcinoma is classified into three types: tubular adenocarcinoma that resembles conventional PDAC (Fig. 16.16A), colloid carcinoma (Fig. 16.16B), and oncocytic carcinoma. Interestingly, the histology of invasive components usually correlates with the epithelial morphology of intraductal components. Gastric- and pancreatobiliary-type IPMNs are associated with tubular adenocarcinoma, intestinal-type IPMN with colloid carcinoma, and the oncocytic type with oncocytic carcinoma.

The vast majority (80%) of IPMNs harbor activating mutations in codon 12 of the *KRAS* gene. In addition, hotspot *GNAS* codon 201 mutations are found in two-thirds of the lesions, irrespective of grade of dysplasia. Inactivating mutations in the tumor suppressor gene *RNF43* are also common in IPMNs. Mutations in other genes such as *TP53*, *SMAD4*, *p16*, and *BRAF* are seen only in IPMNs with high-grade dysplasia and/or carcinoma. As mentioned earlier, the oncocytic subtype is genetically distinct from other subtypes and does not show mutations in *KRAS*, *GNAS*, and *RNF43*.

Ancillary Studies. Expression of MUC5AC is a hallmark of IPMN. Other immunomarkers are variably expressed based on the epithelial morphology: the gastric type are MUC6+/MUC1−/MUC2−/CDX2−, intestinal type are MUC6−/MUC1−/MUC2+/CDX2+, pancreatobiliary type are MUC6+ (weak)/MUC1+/MUC2−/CDX2−, and oncocytic type are MUC6+/MUC1 variable/MUC2 variable/CDX2 variable. Loss of SMAD4 and aberrant TP53 expression can be seen in high-grade lesions.

Differential Diagnosis. The differential diagnosis is mainly with other cystic lesions of the pancreas, including MCN, simple mucinous cyst (cystic mucinous duct lesion), PanIN, and SCA (oligocystic variant), retention cyst, cancerization of ducts, and large duct-type invasive adenocarcinoma. IPMNs can usually be differentiated from these entities based on clinical features and cytomorphology. Differentiation of branch-duct IPMN from PanIN is dependent on the size of the lesion but could be subjective in lesions between 0.5 cm and

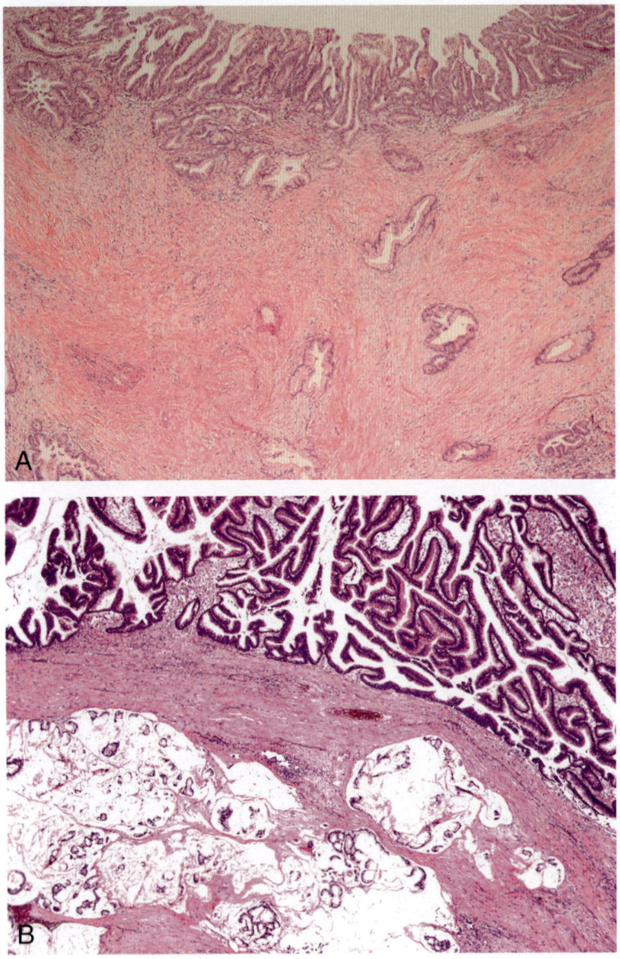

FIGURE 16.16

A, Tubular adenocarcinoma arising in a high-grade gastric-type intraductal papillary mucinous neoplasm (IPMN) that resembles conventional pancreatic ductal adenocarcinoma (hematoxylin and eosin [H&E]). **B**, Colloid carcinoma arising in the background of an intestinal-type IPMN exhibiting mucin pools with atypical glands (H&E).

1.0 cm in diameter. Similarly, discrimination of IPMN with invasive carcinoma from conventional PDAC with cancerization of ducts and/or retention cysts with mucinous epithelial changes may be challenging and requires correlation with imaging findings.

Prognosis and Therapy. The prognosis is excellent in noninvasive tumors, and the 5-year survival rate is close to 100%, provided that appropriate sampling to rule out invasive carcinoma has been performed. However, at least 10% of patients with completely resected noninvasive IPMN experience a recurrence of IPMN. The 5-year survival rate of invasive carcinoma arising in IPMN is significantly worse (40%) than that of noninvasive IPMN, although it is better than that of conventional ductal adenocarcinoma (5%). Thus, curative resection preferably at the preinvasive stage (high-grade dysplasia) is the most appropriate therapy. To identify high-risk lesions, the international consensus guidelines for the management of IPMN and MCN of the pancreas have introduced high-risk stigmata and worrisome features.

INTRADUCTAL PAPILLARY MUCINOUS NEOPLASM—FACT SHEET

Definition

- Grossly visible, mucin-producing epithelial neoplasm that primarily grows within the main pancreatic duct and/or its branches

Incidence and Location

- Most common cystic neoplasm of the pancreas; comprises 8% to 20% of all resected pancreatectomy specimens
- Most common in the pancreatic head

Gender, Race, and Age Distribution

- Slightly more common in men
- Mean age is 63 years (range, 25–94 years)

Clinical Features

- The majority found incidentally
- Can present with abdominal or back pain, anorexia, weight loss, and recurrent episodes of pancreatitis
- The presence of jaundice is suggestive for high-grade lesions or invasive carcinoma

Radiologic Features

- Markedly dilated main pancreatic duct with or without cysts (main-duct or mixed type) and single or numerous cysts (branch-duct type)

Prognosis and Therapy

- Excellent prognosis for noninvasive intraductal papillary mucinous neoplasm (IPMN)
- 40% 5-year survival rate for invasive carcinomas arising in IPMN
- Curative resection at the preinvasive stage has best prognosis

INTRADUCTAL PAPILLARY MUCINOUS NEOPLASM—PATHOLOGIC FEATURES

Gross Findings

- Dilated main or branch ducts with peripheral cysts often connecting to the main pancreatic duct; cyst lining smooth or with florid papillary projections
- Solid areas in cases associated with invasive carcinoma

Microscopic Findings

- Intraductal proliferation of mucin producing epithelium often with papillary architecture and no ovarian-type stroma
- Four epithelial types of mucinous epithelium
- Varying degrees of dysplasia (low-grade and high-grade) with or without invasive carcinoma
- Oncocytic subtype now regarded as a separate entity

Immunohistochemistry

- MUC5AC expression seen in all intraductal papillary mucinous neoplasm subtypes and various expressions of other markers (MUC6, MUC1, MUC2, and CDX2) depending on the epithelial subtypes

Differential Diagnosis

- Other cystic lesions of the pancreas such as mucinous cystic neoplasm, simple mucinous cyst, and serous cystadenoma, as well as pancreatic intraepithelial neoplasia, retention cyst, cancerization of ducts, and large duct-type invasive adenocarcinoma

Mucinous Cystic Neoplasm

Clinical Features. Mucinous cystic neoplasms comprise 10% of cystic lesions of the pancreas and are almost exclusively diagnosed in women (average age at diagnosis, 40–50 years). Tumors may reach a large size and rarely communicate with the pancreatic duct system. MCN has a propensity to involve the body and/or tail of the pancreas. Patients with MCN typically present with epigastric pain and/or abdominal fullness secondary to compression of adjacent organs and tissues.

Radiologic Features. Mucinous cystic neoplasm is characterized by a large, well-demarcated, thick-walled multilocular cystic mass. Peripheral calcification may be present (in 20% of cases). The main pancreatic duct and interlobular ducts typically do not communicate with the cyst. Mural nodules may be seen but are more common in MCN with invasive carcinoma.

Pathological Features. Mucinous cystic neoplasms are usually solitary and large (mean diameter, 7–10 cm) cystic tumors located in the body or tail of the pancreas. They can be multiloculated and filled with viscous mucoid material. Intracystic papillary excrescences and/or mural nodules, when present, are indicative of high-grade dysplasia or invasive carcinoma. The cyst wall lining is composed of tall or cuboidal mucin-secreting epithelium surrounded by a cellular ovarian-type stroma. The presence of ovarian-type stroma is a hallmark of MCN (Fig. 16.17). Similar to IPMNs, MCNs exhibit a varying degree of epithelial atypia and are classified into low-grade dysplasia, high-grade dysplasia, and invasive carcinoma. The epithelium may be focally denuded or consist of intact pancreaticobiliary type epithelium, and the ovarian-type stroma may be replaced by broad areas of hyalinization, making the diagnosis challenging. Multiple sections may be required to appropriately determine the grade of dysplasia or to demonstrate the ovarian-type stroma. The prevalence of invasive carcinoma arising in the background of MCN is less than that of IPMN. Several distinct histologic types of invasive carcinoma may arise in MCNs, including undifferentiated carcinoma with osteoclast-like giant cells. Importantly, invasive components can be very focal, so submission of the entire lesion is recommended.

Molecularly, activating mutations in codon 12 of the *KRAS* gene have been reported in up to 75% of MCNs, but *RNF43* mutations are found in up to 50% of the lesions. *GNAS* mutations are specific for IPMNs and do not occur in MCNs. *TP53* and *SMAD4* mutations are seen only in high-grade dysplasia and/or associated invasive carcinoma.

Ancillary Studies. The ovarian-type stroma can be highlighted by estrogen receptor (ER) and/or progesterone receptor (PR), and calretinin and inhibin expressions are seen in luteinized cells in the ovarian-like stroma. CD10, ER, and PR immunostains may be useful in highlighting the findings in cases of more hyalinized and hypocellular ovarian-type stroma.

Differential Diagnosis. The differential diagnosis is mainly with other cystic lesions of the pancreas including pseudocyst, simple mucinous cyst, branch-duct type IPMN, SCA (oligocystic variant), and SPN. MCN can usually be differentiated from those entities based on clinical features and the morphology on hematoxylin and eosin (H&E), in particular the presence of ovarian-type stroma.

Prognosis and Therapy. The prognosis of MCN is excellent if it is noninvasive and completely removed. The 5-year survival rate of MCNs with invasive carcinoma is approximately 50% and correlates with the extent of invasion and patient's age (lower survival rate in those older than 50 years of age). The current standard clinical care is resection for all MCNs, given the relatively young age at presentation and potential progression to invasive carcinoma.

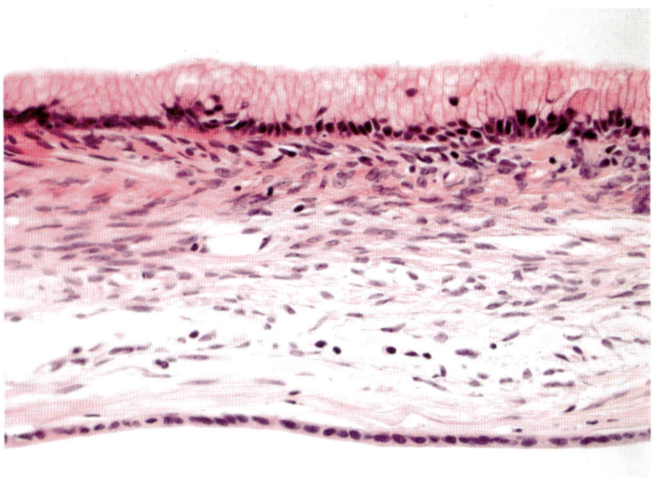

FIGURE 16.17

Mucinous cystic neoplasm demonstrating tall or cuboidal mucin-secreting epithelium supported by a cellular ovarian-like stroma (hematoxylin and eosin).

MUCINOUS CYSTIC NEOPLASM—FACT SHEET

Definition

- Cystic neoplasm composed at least focally of mucin-producing epithelial cells associated with ovarian-type stroma, typically without communication with the pancreatic duct system

Incidence and Location

- 10% of cystic lesions of the pancreas; usually involves body or tail of the pancreas (90%)

Gender, Race, and Age Distribution

- Almost exclusively in women (average age, 40–50 years)

Clinical Features

- Vague abdominal symptoms associated with compression of adjacent organs and tissues

Radiologic Features

- Large, well-demarcated thick-walled multilocular cystic mass without communication with the pancreatic duct system; peripheral calcification in 20%; the presence of mural nodule indicative of an invasive component

Prognosis and Therapy

- Excellent prognosis for noninvasive, completely removed lesions, and 50% 5-year survival rate for invasive carcinomas arising in mucinous cystic neoplasm (MCN)
- Complete resection is the current standard of care for all MCN lesions

Mucinous Cystic Neoplasm—Pathologic Features

Gross Findings

- Usually solitary and large (mean diameter, 7–10 cm) cystic lesions in the pancreatic body or tail of the pancreas
- Often multiloculated and filled with viscous mucoid material
- Mural nodules indicative of high-grade dysplasia or invasive carcinoma

Microscopic Findings

- Lined by tall columnar or cuboidal mucin-producing epithelium surrounded by cellular ovarian-type stroma
- The cyst lining may be focally denuded in large tumors, or intact pancreatic epithelium may partially line the cyst, and the ovarian-type stroma may be replaced by hyalinized tissue in some areas

Immunohistochemistry

- Expression of estrogen and progesterone receptors is seen in the ovarian-like stroma
- Luteinized cells in the ovarian-like stroma are positive for calretinin and inhibin

Differential Diagnosis

- Other cystic lesions of the pancreas: pseudocyst, simple mucinous cyst, branch-duct type intraductal papillary mucinous neoplasm, oligocystic serous cystadenoma, and solid-pseudopapillary neoplasm

Intraductal Tubulopapillary Neoplasm

Clinical Features. Intraductal tubulopapillary neoplasm is rare, accounting for only 3% of intraductal neoplasms of the pancreas. A limited number of reported cases indicate that ITPN occurs in both genders equally, and the age ranges from 35 to 84 years. Clinical presentations are similar to those of IPMN.

Radiologic Features. Most ITPNs resemble IPMNs on imaging studies. About half of ITPNs develop in the pancreatic head, one-third diffusely involve the pancreas, and 15% are limited to the tail.

Pathological Features. Grossly, ITPNs form solid, large, nodular masses within dilated pancreatic ducts, and the surrounding pancreatic parenchyma often shows marked sclerosis. Cyst formation is less evident compared with IPMNs, and mucinous secretions are not present in the dilated ducts. The intraductal location of the tumor may need to be confirmed by a careful dissection of the pancreatic duct system. Histologically, ITPNs are characterized by back-to-back tubular glands, resulting in a large cribriform pattern. The majority is predominantly or exclusively tubular, but papillae or solid areas may be present. Each neoplastic nodule appears relatively homogeneous and consists of tightly packed small acinar glands lined by cuboidal cells with modest amounts of eosinophilic or amphophilic cytoplasm and round to oval, moderately to markedly atypical nuclei. Mitotic figures are often evident, and necrosis may be seen in some cases. Because of the architectural complexity and cytologic atypia, ITPNs are essentially classified as high-grade dysplasia (Fig. 16.18). Invasive carcinoma is found in 40% of reported cases. The invasive component is usually limited and is characterized by thin strands of tubules extending into the stroma surrounding the neoplastic nodules. The cytology of the invasive tubules is essentially the same as that of the intraductal component, leading to difficulty in identifying the invasive component. At the molecular level, ITPNs are distinct from IPMNs. *PIK3CA* mutations have been identified in one-fifth of ITPNs opposed to none of IPMNs; *GNAS* mutations have not been identified, and *KRAS* mutations are rare in ITPNs. In addition, the protein expression of phosphorylated-AKT, a marker for PI3K-AKT pathway activation, is significantly more prominent in ITPNs than in IPMNs.

Ancillary Studies. Intraductal tubulopapillary neoplasms commonly label for keratins 7 and 19, markers of pancreatic duct epithelium. Neither MUC5AC (a consistent marker for IPMN) nor MUC2 (a marker for intestinal-type IPMN) is expressed in ITPNs, but MUC1 is expressed in 90% and MUC6 in 60%. ITPNs are

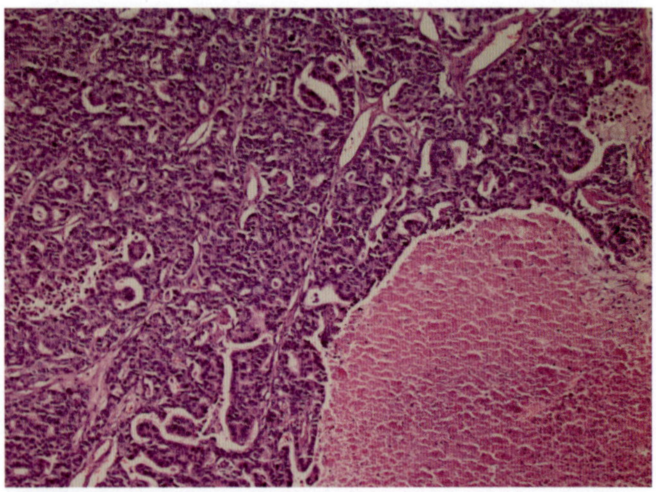

FIGURE 16.18

Intraductal tubulopapillary neoplasm characterized by back-to-back tubular glands resulting in a large cribriform pattern. The glands are lined by predominantly cuboidal cells with cytologic atypia and no intracytoplasmic mucin. A large area of necrosis is also seen (hematoxylin and eosin).

essentially negative for markers of pancreatic exocrine enzymes, and β-catenin nuclear expression has been reported in fewer than 10% of cases.

Differential Diagnosis. The main differential diagnosis of ITPNs is with IPMNs. Gastric- and intestinal-type IPMNs can be easily distinguished from ITPNs on microscopic examination, but some pancreatobiliary-type IPMNs may resemble ITPNs. Discernible mucin, the presence of gastric-type epithelium in the background, and the expression of MUC5AC favor a diagnosis of IPMN. ITPNs, in particular those with predominantly tubular areas, may be difficult to distinguish from acinar cell carcinomas (ACCs) with an intraductal growth. The presence of apical acidophilic granules that can be highlighted by periodic acid–Schiff (PAS) stain and immunohistochemical labeling for trypsin and/or chymotrypsin are consistent with the diagnosis of ACC.

Prognosis and Therapy. Given that ITPNs are essentially high-grade dysplastic lesions with or without invasive components, resection is considered to be the most appropriate therapy for all ITPNs. ITPNs appear to follow an indolent clinical course, although only limited clinical data are currently available. Recurrence and metastases to lymph nodes and/or to the liver have been reported in one-third of cases, but even these patients may survive for more than 2 years.

Pancreatic Ductal Adenocarcinoma

Clinical Features. Pancreatic ductal adenocarcinoma is a disease of older adults, with most patients being older than 60 years at presentation. Men are affected slightly more frequently than women, and in the United States, African Americans more often than Whites. Common presenting signs and symptoms include painless jaundice, unexplained weight loss, and epigastric pain radiating to the back. New-onset diabetes mellitus may be the first manifestation of the disease.

Radiologic Features. Pancreatic ductal adenocarcinomas typically produce a hypodense mass lesion that distorts normal gland architecture. The pancreatic duct is often dilated secondary to duct obstruction by the infiltrating tumor.

Pathologic Features. Grossly, most tumors form poorly defined, firm, white-yellow masses (Fig. 16.19). Most arise in the head of the pancreas, but they can also involve the body, the tail, or even the entire gland. Focal cystic degeneration and areas of necrosis are common. The pancreatic duct is often dilated upstream from the neoplasm. Microscopically, varying degrees of differentiation can be seen based on extent of gland formation, extracellular mucin pools, cytologic atypia, and mitotic activity. Well-differentiated adenocarcinoma is characterized by clearly formed neoplastic glands with an infiltrating, haphazard growth pattern. This growth pattern, more than any other feature, helps distinguish well-differentiated adenocarcinomas from non-neoplastic reactive glands that retain the circumscribed architecture of normal acini. Perineural and vascular invasion, when present, can help establish the diagnosis. Moderately differentiated adenocarcinomas show the same haphazard growth pattern but, in addition, are characterized by greater architectural complexity and increased cytologic atypia (Fig. 16.20). The neoplastic cells may form incomplete glands, cribriform structures, or papillae without fibrovascular cores. Significant nuclear pleomorphism can be appreciated, and the nuclei in a single gland often vary in size by more than 4 to 1. Nucleoli may be quite prominent, and mitoses, including abnormal mitoses, can be seen. Poorly differentiated adenocarcinoma is characterized by solid sheets of neoplastic cells with very rare gland formation as well as single-cell infiltration. Significant nuclear pleomorphism with brisk mitotic activity and atypical mitotic figures are common.

Several variants of ductal adenocarcinoma have been described. *Adenosquamous carcinoma* is characterized by the presence of both glandular and squamous differentiation and is associated with a poor prognosis (Fig. 16.21). *Hepatoid carcinoma* shows morphologic and immunophenotypic

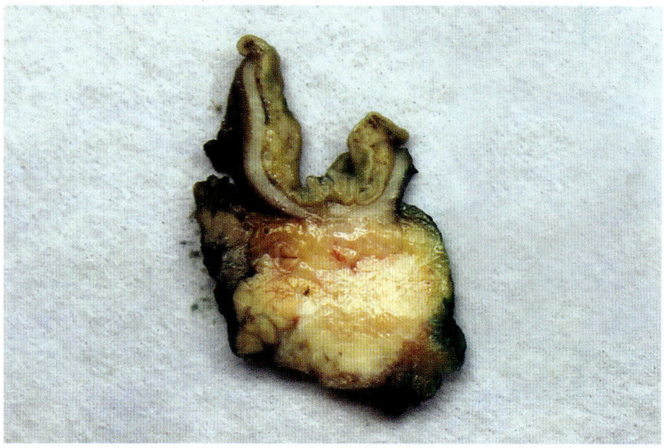

FIGURE 16.19

Infiltrating adenocarcinoma of the pancreas. An irregular firm white mass is present in the head of the pancreas (hematoxylin and eosin).

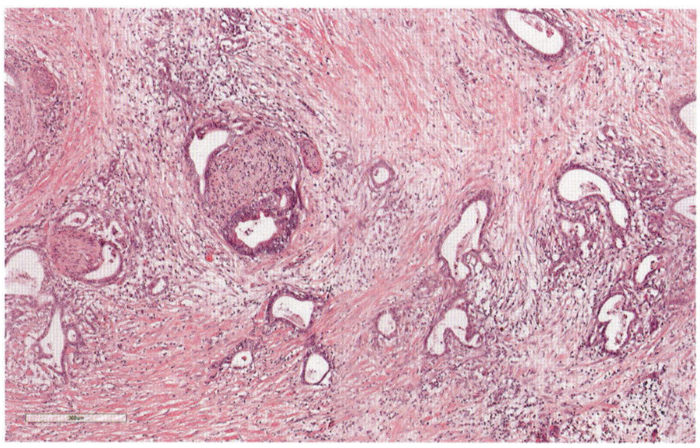

FIGURE 16.20

Pancreatic ductal adenocarcinoma showing neoplastic glands arranged haphazardly and surrounded by desmoplastic stroma. Note the perineural growth (hematoxylin and eosin).

features of hepatocellular differentiation, and metastasis from a liver primary cancer should be ruled out clinically before making this diagnosis. *Colloid carcinoma* is also known as the mucinous noncystic adenocarcinoma and is characterized by well-differentiated, neoplastic, mucin-producing epithelial cells "floating" in large pools of extracellular mucin (see Fig. 16.16B). This variant may have a slightly better prognosis than PDAC and almost always arises in association with an IPMN, which may explain the better prognosis. *Signet ring cell carcinoma* is composed of noncohesive neoplastic cells with abundant cytoplasmic mucin that indents the nuclei pushing them toward the periphery. Infiltration as single cells, small clusters, or cords is characteristic. Metastases from a breast or gastric primary cancer should be considered before making this diagnosis. *Medullary carcinoma* is characterized by poor differentiation, syncytial growth pattern, tumor-infiltrating lymphocytes, pushing borders, and microsatellite instability. Medullary carcinoma can occur sporadically or in patients with Lynch syndrome and has a better prognosis than ordinary PDAC. (Fig. 16.22) *Undifferentiated (anaplastic) carcinoma*, as the name suggests, is an extremely aggressive neoplasm composed of highly atypical cells, with significant pleomorphism and frequent, often bizarre, mitoses. These carcinomas can have a significant spindle cell component, or they can be composed of large polygonal cells. *Undifferentiated carcinoma with osteoclast-like giant cells (UCOGC)* is composed of mononuclear cells with severe cytologic atypia, admixed with large multinucleated osteoclast-like giant cells with uniform nuclei (Fig. 16.23). Whereas the mononuclear cells are malignant, the osteoclast-like giant cells are reactive. An in situ or invasive adenocarcinoma is also frequently present. The prognosis for UCOGCs is better than that of PDAC. Undifferentiated carcinomas with a rhabdoid morphology and loss of SMARCA4 or INI-1 may also arise in the pancreas but are extremely rare.

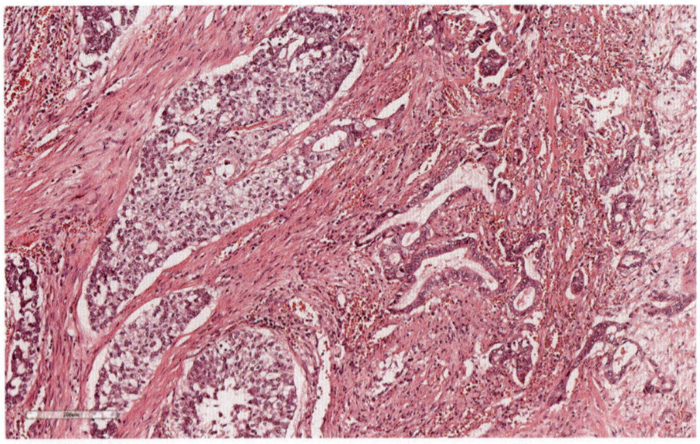

FIGURE 16.21

Adenosquamous carcinoma showing both glandular and squamous differentiation (hematoxylin and eosin).

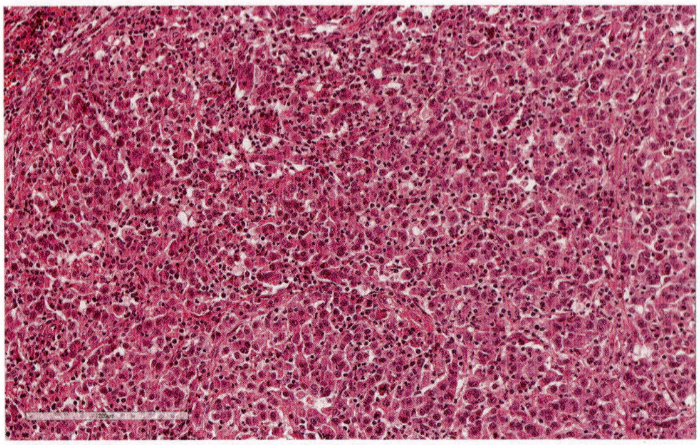

FIGURE 16.22

Medullary carcinoma showing poor differentiation, a syncytial growth pattern, and tumor-infiltrating lymphocytes (hematoxylin and eosin).

Pancreatic adenocarcinomas are genetically very complex, with widespread chromosomal abnormalities, numerous losses and gains of large segments of DNA, and on an average more than 60 exomic alterations per cancer. *KRAS, CDKN2A, TP53*, and *SMAD4* are the most frequently altered genes in PDAC. In addition, a number of less commonly mutated genes have been identified, including *MLL3, ARID1A*, and *TGFBR2*. Approximately 10 % of pancreatic cancers are familial. Germline mutations in *BRCA2* and *CDKN2A* and less frequently in *BRCA1, PALB2*, and *ATM* have been identified in a small subset of patients with familial PDAC. In addition, patients with Lynch syndrome, Peutz-Jeghers syndrome, and hereditary chronic pancreatitis are also at increased risk of PDAC. The genetic basis for the majority of familial pancreatic cancers still remains unknown.

Ancillary Studies. Immunohistochemical labeling can be used to highlight epithelial and glandular differentiation of ductal adenocarcinomas, as well as to demonstrate some of the molecular alterations present

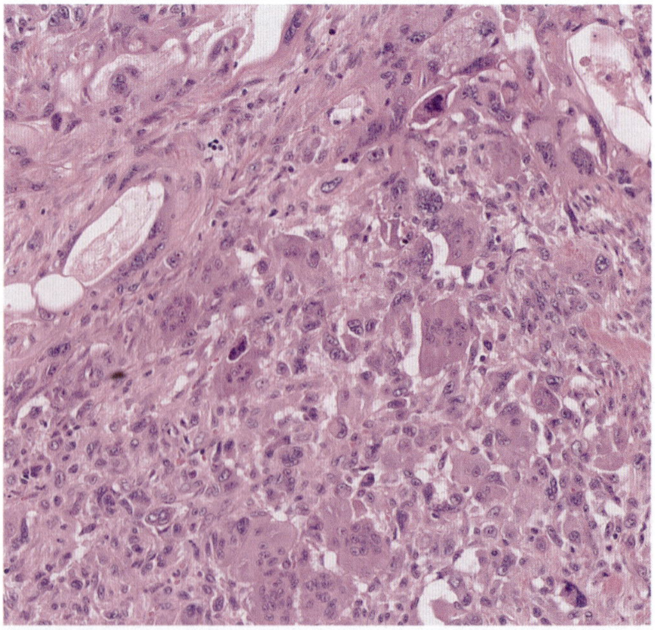

FIGURE 16.23

Undifferentiated carcinoma with osteoclast-like giant cells composed of atypical mononuclear cells admixed with non-neoplastic multinucleated giant cells. The nuclei in the giant cells are uniform (hematoxylin and eosin).

in the neoplastic cells. Immunolabeling for cytokeratin (CK) 7, CK8, CK18, and CK19 is positive, as is immunolabeling for CEA, CA19-9, Dupan-2, MUC1, MUC4, and MUC5AC. The vast majority of adenocarcinomas of the pancreas also label for mesothelin, claudin 18, and fascin. Colloid carcinomas label for MUC2; the squamous component of adenosquamous carcinomas with antibodies to p63. Aberrant p53 expression and loss of expression of Smad4 is seen in 60% to 80% and 50% to 60% of the cases, respectively, and correlates with *TP53* and *SMAD4* mutational status. (Fig. 16.24). Of all these markers, the most commonly one used in routine practice is SMAD4 for work-up of metastatic carcinomas of unknown primary origin. Loss of nuclear SMAD4 staining is often used to favor a pancreaticobiliary origin.

Differential Diagnosis. Reactive non-neoplastic glands of chronic pancreatitis top the differential diagnosis. Features useful in establishing a diagnosis of infiltrating adenocarcinomas in histologic sections are (1) haphazard infiltrative growth pattern; (2) variation in the size of nuclei by more than 4:1 in a single gland; (3) incomplete lumen formation; (4) glands adjacent to muscular vessels; (5) perineural or vascular invasion; (6) mitoses, especially abnormal mitoses; (7) glandular luminal necrotic debris; and (8) aberrant p53 or Smad4 immunolabeling. The distinction of a pancreatic from an ampullary primary cancer can be challenging in some instances and is discussed in greater detail in the section on ampullary tumors in Chapter 6. A careful gross examination to assess bulk of tumor localization and a thorough microscopic evaluation to determine presence of any precursor lesions (ampullary adenoma or high-grade PanIN) can usually resolve this differential diagnosis in most cases.

Prognosis and Therapy. The prognosis of patients with an infiltrating adenocarcinoma of the pancreas is extremely poor. Most patients die of their disease, often within months of diagnosis. Even though surgery is the treatment of choice, most patients (~80%) have metastatic disease at diagnosis and are not candidates for surgery. Radiation and chemotherapy have a small impact on survival. Colloid carcinoma and UCOGC have been associated with a slightly better prognosis, whereas the adenosquamous and undifferentiated variants have a worse prognosis.

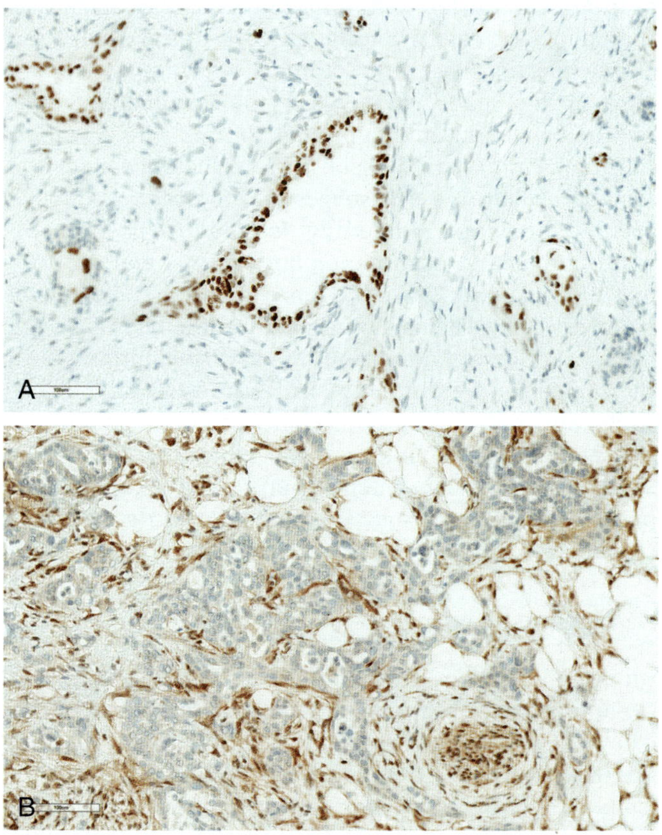

FIGURE 16.24

A, Strong and diffuse p53 immunolabeling in pancreatic ductal adenocarcinoma (PDA). **B**, Loss of immunolabeling for the *SMAD4/DPC4* gene product in PDA. Note the positivity of the stromal cells.

PANCREATIC DUCTAL ADENOCARCINOMA—FACT SHEET

Definition

- A malignant infiltrative epithelial neoplasm with ductal differentiation

Incidence and Location

- 85% to 90% of all pancreatic neoplasms
- Pancreatic head (>60%)

Gender, Race, and Age Distribution

- More often in men (male-to-female ratio, 2 to 1)
- Increased risk with smoking and family history of pancreatic cancer
- Older age group; usually older than 60 years

Clinical Features

- Epigastric pain, often radiating to the back
- Weight loss
- Painless jaundice
- Less often, migratory thrombophlebitis, pancreatitis, new-onset diabetes mellitus

Radiologic Features

- Ill-defined infiltrative nonenhancing pancreatic mass

Prognosis and Therapy

- Surgical resection
- Palliative bypass procedures
- Radiation and chemotherapy
- Prognosis extremely poor (slightly better for colloid carcinoma)
- 5-year survival rate around 5%

PANCREATIC DUCTAL ADENOCARCINOMA—PATHOLOGIC FEATURES

Gross Findings

- Poorly defined, firm mass with irregular borders
- Cut surface: yellow-white microcystic areas, hemorrhage, and necrosis

Microscopic Findings

- Neoplastic glands in a haphazard infiltrative growth pattern
- Architectural atypia with incomplete glands and luminal necrosis
- Cytologic atypia with nuclei in a single gland varying by more than 4 to 1
- Vascular and perineural invasion
- Glands adjacent to muscular vessels
- Brisk mitoses and necrosis
- Solid sheets or single cell infiltration (poorly differentiated tumors)
- Glandular and squamous differentiation (adenosquamous carcinoma)
- Hepatocellular differentiation (hepatoid carcinoma)
- Mucin-producing cells floating in pools of mucin (colloid carcinoma)
- Individual cells with eccentric mucin vacuoles (signet ring cell carcinoma)
- Undifferentiated spindle cell component (undifferentiated or anaplastic carcinoma)
- Mixture of malignant mononuclear cells and reactive osteoclast-like giant cells

Immunohistochemistry

- Positive for cytokeratin (CK) 7, CK8, CK18, and CK19
- Positive for carcinoembryonic antigen, CA19-9, Dupan-2, MUC1, MUC4, and MUC5AC
- Most tumors also positive for mesothelin, claudin 18, prostate stem cell antigen, and fascin
- Aberrant p53 expression (60%–80%)
- Loss of Smad4 protein expression (50%–60%)

Differential Diagnosis

- Chronic pancreatitis
- Ampullary carcinoma
- Other primary and metastatic pancreatic neoplasms

NEUROENDOCRINE TUMORS

Well-Differentiated Neuroendocrine Tumors (Grades 1–3)

Clinical Features

Pancreatic neuroendocrine tumors (PanNETs) are uncommon primary pancreatic neoplasms, accounting for only 1% to 2% of all pancreatic neoplasms that present mostly in adults. The clinical presentation of PanNETs depends largely on whether the tumor secretes a hormone that causes clinical symptoms (functional PanNETs) or does not secrete hormones (nonfunctional PanNETs). Patients with functional NETs often present with symptoms caused by hormone hypersecretion; characteristic clinical syndromes have been described for the commonly secreted hormones, such as insulin and glucagon. Because of clinical symptoms, functional PanNETs are often diagnosed at smaller size than nonfunctional PanNETs. However, with the increased use of abdominal imaging, incidental nonfunctional PanNETs are being increasingly identified. Large nonfunctional tumors can present with vague abdominal symptoms caused by compression of adjacent structures.

Pancreatic neuroendocrine tumors also occur as key features of multiple inherited syndromes. PanNETs, often multicentric, occur in 60% to 70% of patients with multiple endocrine neoplasia syndrome type 1. Pancreatic manifestations of von Hippel-Lindau (VHL) syndrome include SCA, PanNETs with or without clear cell features, and mixed serous neuroendocrine lesions. In addition, PanNETs may be associated with other genetic syndromes, including tuberous sclerosis complex and neurofibromatosis type 1.

Radiologic Features

Pancreatic neuroendocrine tumors present as well-circumscribed masses on CT scans.

Pathological Features

Grossly, PanNETs are typically solitary, well-demarcated tumors with a tan-white to yellow cut surface (Fig. 16.25A). They can be fleshy or fibrotic, and larger tumors may show hemorrhage or necrosis. Cystic degeneration can occur but is not common. Microscopically, PanNETs can show multiple growth patterns, including nesting, trabecular, glandular, or pseudorosetting (Figs. 16.25B and C). Tumors showing any of these growth patterns are classified as "well-differentiated." In contrast, "poorly differentiated" PanNETs typically show confluent aggregates or sheets of tumor cells, often with tumor necrosis. Cytologically, the neoplastic cells are uniform with round nuclei and characteristic coarsely clumped "salt-and-pepper" chromatin (Fig. 16.25D). The cytoplasm can be amphophilic or eosinophilic and may contain fine granules. Luminal mucin can be seen in rare instances. Several histologic features are suggestive of production of a specific hormone, including amyloid deposition in insulinomas and psammoma bodies in somatostatinomas. Molecularly, PanNETs are distinct from ductal pancreatic neoplasms. Somatic mutations in *MEN1* are the most common alteration. Inactivating mutations in the tumor suppressor genes *ATRX* and *DAXX*, leading to the alternative lengthening of telomeres (ALT) phenotype, are also common, as are mutations in components of the mTOR (mammalian target of rapamycin) pathway. The latter may be important in determining response to targeted therapy.

Ancillary Studies

Immunohistochemical staining for chromogranin and synaptophysin is typically diffusely positive in PanNETs. They usually express cytokeratins, though CK7 is often negative. PanNETs frequently label immunohistochemically with antibodies to hormones, but hormone expression as defined by immunolabeling is insufficient to classify a PanNET as functional in the absence of clinical symptoms. Only PanNETs in patients with symptoms associated with hormone hypersecretion are

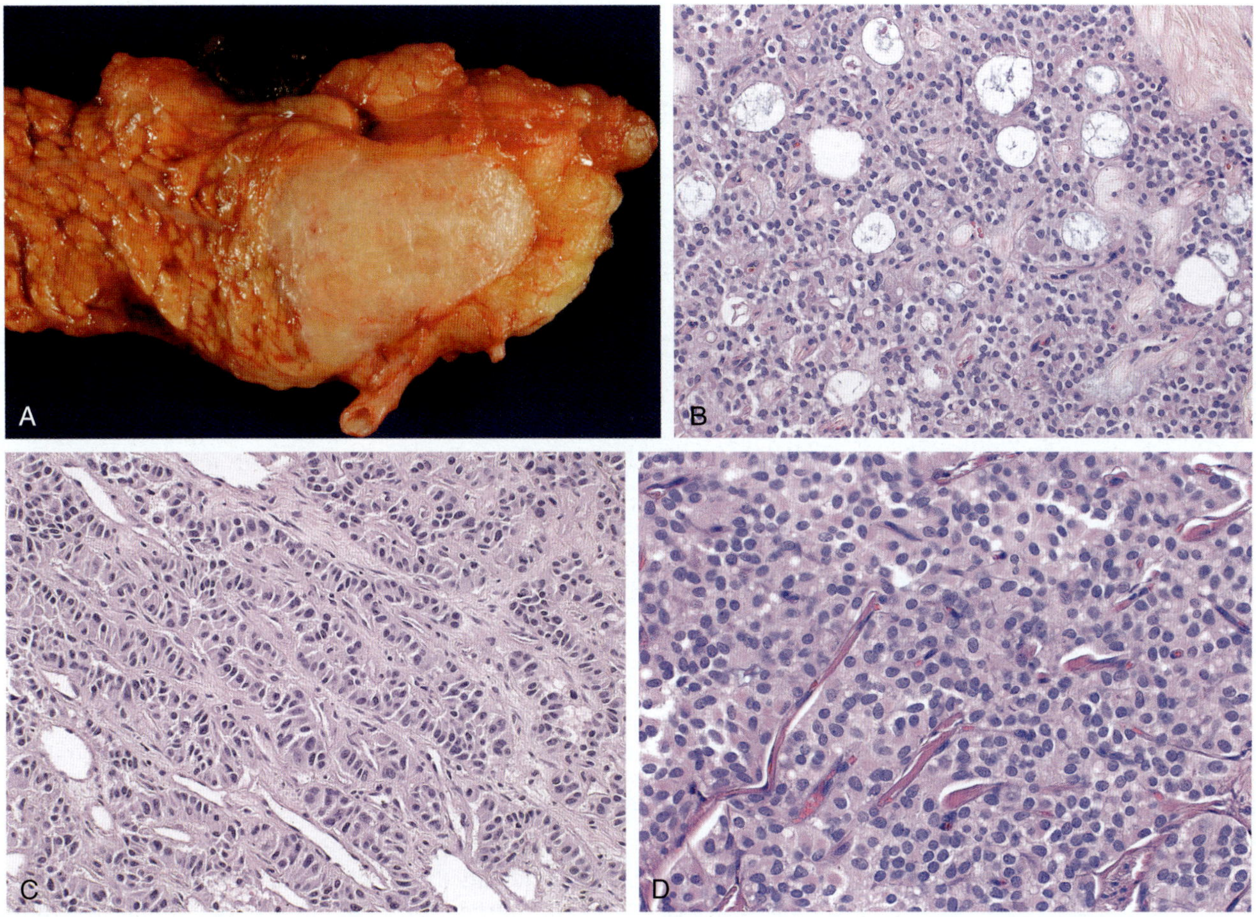

FIGURE 16.25

Well-differentiated pancreatic neuroendocrine tumor (PanNET). **A**, Grossly, PanNETs are solid, well-circumscribed, fleshy masses. Multiple growth patterns can occur, including glandular (**B**) and trabecular (**C**). **D**, PanNETs have characteristic neuroendocrine cytologic features, including round nuclei with "salt-and-pepper" chromatin.

classified as functional and labeled as an "-oma" of their hormone (e.g., insulinoma, gastrinoma).

Differential Diagnosis

The differential diagnosis is chiefly with other solid cellular neoplasms of the pancreas, including ACC, pancreatoblastoma, and SPN. Although morphology on H&E can be strongly suggestive of PanNET, there is also considerable morphologic overlap between these entities, and IHC is often required for definitive diagnosis. Importantly, PanNETs do not express pancreatic exocrine enzymes (e.g., trypsin, chymotrypsin), and β-catenin is not nuclear.

Prognosis and Therapy

Pancreatic neuroendocrine tumors are graded based on mitotic rate, as determined by mitotic count or Ki67 labeling index, and tumor grade is the most significant prognostic factor. Low-grade (G1) PanNET have a mitotic count of 0 to 1 per $2 mm^2$ and/or a nuclear Ki-67 labeling index of 0% to 2%. Intermediate-grade (G2) PanNET are those with 2 to 20 mitoses per 2 mm^2 or a nuclear Ki-67 labeling index of 3% to 20%. Rarely, architecturally well-differentiated PanNET may show a mitotic count greater than 20 per 2 mm^2 or a Ki-67 proliferative index greater than 20%. These tumors are now classified as grade 3 PanNET in the 2017 WHO classification, and although they do not respond well to platinum based chemotherapy, the outcome is better than small cell or large cell pancreatic neuroendocrine carcinomas (NECs). Well-differentiated grade 3 PanNET typically show a proliferative index in the 30% to 60% range, although no upper limit is currently defined for excluding tumors from this group. In contrast, small cell or large cell PanNECs are poorly differentiated, and the proliferative index on a Ki-67 immunostain is typically greater than 60%. Loss of Rb protein and abnormal p53 expression is almost never seen in grade 3 well-differentiated PanNET but is quite prevalent in poorly differentiated NEC. Surgery is the treatment of choice for PanNET. Although the prognosis is better than that for patients with PDAC, tumor recurrence after resection is common. Targeted therapies with mTOR inhibitors have shown promise in ongoing clinical trials.

WELL-DIFFERENTIATED NEUROENDOCRINE TUMOR—FACT SHEET

Definition
- Primary pancreatic epithelial neoplasm with neuroendocrine differentiation and well-differentiated architectural growth pattern (nested, trabecular, glandular)

Incidence and Location
- 1% to 2% of all primary pancreatic neoplasms; more common in the pancreatic head but can occur throughout the pancreas

Gender, Race, and Age Distribution
- Men and women are equally affected
- No racial predilection
- Peak incidence between 30 and 60 years of age

Clinical Features
- Functional pancreatic neuroendocrine tumors (PanNETs) present with defined clinical syndromes because of hormone hypersecretion. Nonfunctional PanNETs can be discovered incidentally on abdominal imaging or present with vague abdominal symptoms caused by compression of adjacent structures

Radiologic Features
- Well-demarcated mass

Prognosis and Therapy
- Prognosis largely defined by tumor grade, determined by proliferation rate defined by mitotic count or proliferation index on Ki67 immunostain
- Surgery is treatment of choice
- mTOR (mammalian target of rapamycin) inhibitors are promising for patients in whom surgery is not curative

WELL-DIFFERENTIATED NEUROENDOCRINE TUMOR—PATHOLOGIC FEATURES

Gross Findings
- Well-circumscribed, solitary, fleshy or fibrotic mass

Microscopic Findings
- Variety of architectural patterns (trabecular, nested, pseudorosetting, glandular); round uniform nuclei with "salt-and-pepper" chromatin; granular cytoplasm

Ultrastructural Findings
- Neurosecretory granules are common

Immunohistochemistry
- Positive for chromogranin and synaptophysin
- Frequently express pancreatic hormones
- Clinical syndrome with defined symptoms and signs is required to classify tumors as "functional"

Differential Diagnosis
- Other solid pancreatic neoplasms: acinar cell carcinoma, pancreatoblastoma, solid-pseudopapillary tumor

NEUROENDOCRINE CARCINOMAS

Pancreatic neuroendocrine tumors that are poorly differentiated with greater than 20 mitoses per 2 mm^2 and/or a Ki67 proliferation index of greater than 20% are classified as NEC. Overall, these are considered to be aggressive neoplasms with poor prognosis. Tumors may show a small cell or large cell NEC phenotype. Whereas small cell carcinoma, as at other sites, shows tumor cells with minimal cytoplasm and molded nuclei, large cell carcinomas show abundant cytoplasm, prominent nucleoli, and marked pleomorphism. The latter appear to be more common than small cell carcinomas in the pancreas. PanNEC are genetically similar to ductal adenocarcinomas and harbor *KRAS* mutations.

TUMORS WITH ACINAR DIFFERENTIATION

ACINAR CELL CYSTADENOMA

Acinar cell cystadenoma, also known as acinar cystic transformation in the new WHO classification, is a rare benign cystic lesion of the pancreas that may involve any portion of the pancreas but is most commonly found in the pancreatic head. They can be detected because of clinical symptoms, most commonly abdominal pain, or found incidentally on abdominal imaging studies. Grossly, acinar cell cystadenomas can range in size from smaller than 1 cm to larger than 10 cm and can be uni- or multilocular. The cysts contain watery fluid, and the cyst lining is usually smooth. Microscopically, the cysts are lined by a combination of well-differentiated, benign-appearing acinar and ductal epithelium (Fig. 16.26). Whereas the acinar-type cells have uniform basally oriented nuclei and apical cytoplasmic granules, the ductal-type cells lack cytoplasmic granules; these two cell types have been confirmed by IHC studies of acinar cell cystadenomas by dual labeling with chymotrypsin and BCL10 (acinar) and CK19 (ductal). The neoplastic nature of these lesions remains controversial, but current data suggest that acinar cell cystadenomas represent non-neoplastic cystic transformation rather than true neoplasms. Perhaps most important, these lesions are clinically benign because there has never been a reported case of malignant transformation or association with ACC.

ACINAR CELL CARCINOMA

CLINICAL FEATURES

Acinar cell carcinoma is a rare pancreatic malignancy, accounting for fewer than 2% of all exocrine pancreatic

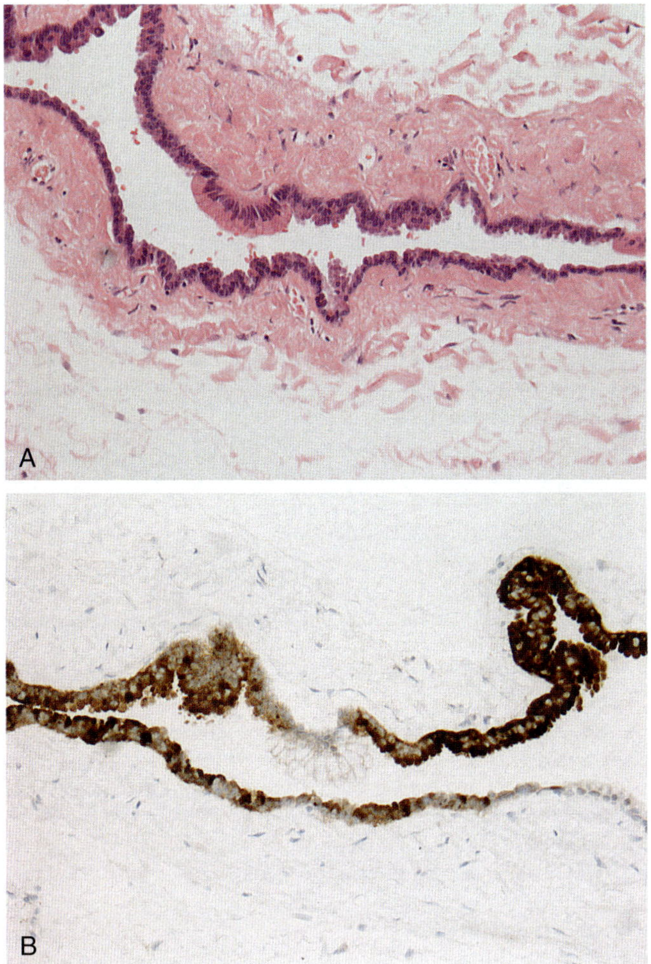

FIG 16.26

Acinar cell cystadenoma. **A**, The cyst is lined by cuboidal acinar cells and patches of mucin-containing ductal cells. **B**, BCL10 is positive in the cuboidal acinar cells but negative in the mucin-containing ductal cells.

neoplasms. Most occur in older adults, but up to 10% occur in children. They are more common in men (male-to-female ratio, 3.6 to 1) and present with nonspecific symptoms caused by compression of adjacent structures, including abdominal and back pain, nausea, and diarrhea. Jaundice is rare because of the growth pattern of the tumor. A minority of patients present with a constellation of symptoms caused by hypersecretion of lipase by the neoplastic cells, including subcutaneous fat necrosis, polyarthralgia, and eosinophilia.

Radiologic Features

Acinar cell carcinomas are large, circumscribed, homogeneously enhancing masses on CT scan.

Pathological Features

Acinar cell carcinomas form solitary, well-circumscribed masses with soft, fleshy, red-tan cut surfaces. They are large tumors, with an average size of 10 cm, and can have central necrosis or cystic degeneration. ACCs can occur throughout the pancreas but are slightly more common in the pancreatic head. Microscopically, they are composed of neoplastic cells with architectural, cytologic, and immunohistochemical evidence of acinar differentiation. The most common architectural patterns are acinar structures with pyramidal-shaped cells forming small lumina (Fig. 16.27A) or solid with sheets of tumor cells without any well-defined structures. Less commonly, glandular and trabecular patterns can also occur. Extensive intraductal growth can also occur but is uncommon. The cytoplasm typically contains amphophilic or eosinophilic zymogen granules. However, these granules are also not a diagnostic requirement because they can be poorly developed and difficult to appreciate on routine stains. The nuclei are round to oval, and there is usually a single prominent nucleolus (Fig. 16.27B). Molecularly, ACCs are characterized by striking genomic instability, either at the base pair or chromosomal level. There are no mutations prevalent in a majority of ACCs, but *SMAD4, CDKN2A*, and *CDKN2B* mutations have been described in a minor subset of cases.

Ancillary Studies

Immunolabeling for pancreatic exocrine enzymes is typically positive in ACC, including trypsin (Fig. 16.27C), chymotrypsin, lipase, and elastase. In addition, a relatively new marker BCL10 is strongly and diffusely positive in ACC. Chromogranin and synaptophysin can be focally positive, but if positive in more than 25% of the cells, a diagnosis of mixed tumor should be considered. Immunolabeling for β-catenin can be aberrantly nuclear in a minority of ACCs because these tumors can have mutations in *APC* or *CTNNB1*, leading to aberrant nuclear localization of the β-catenin protein.

Differential Diagnosis

The histologic differential diagnosis lies chiefly between other solid cellular neoplasms of the pancreas, including PanNET or PanNEC, SPN, and pancreatoblastoma. Metastasis to the pancreas, although uncommon, should always be considered. ACCs with extensive intraductal and papillary growth patterns can mimic an intraductal neoplasm, such as ITPN or IPMN. Acinar architecture, cytoplasmic granules, and single prominent nucleoli favor a diagnosis of ACC, though there is considerable morphological overlap with other entities on routine morphology. Pancreatoblastomas typically have a significant component with acinar differentiation, but squamoid nests are diagnostic of pancreatoblastoma and are absent in ACC. As described earlier, IHC can confirm a diagnosis of ACC through demonstration of expression of BCL10 or pancreatic exocrine enzymes. When interpreting β-catenin immunohistochemistry, it is important to remember that a subset of ACCs can also have aberrant nuclear staining.

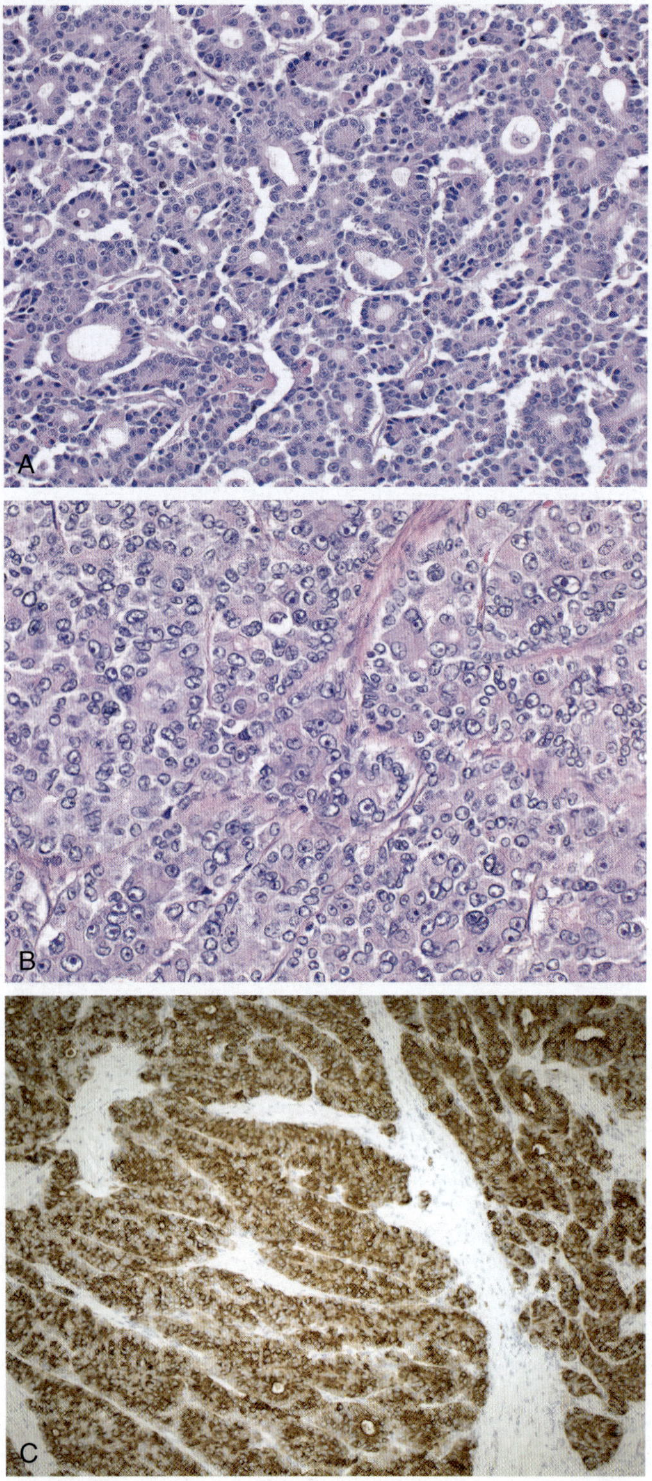

FIGURE 16.27

Acinar cell carcinoma (ACC). **A**, Acinar architecture, with pyramidal-shaped cells polarized around small lumina, is characteristic but not required for the diagnosis. **B**, Cytoplasmic granules are common, and single prominent nucleoli are a characteristic feature. **C**, Trypsin is diffusely and strongly positive in ACC.

PROGNOSIS AND THERAPY

Acinar cell carcinomas are aggressive cancers, with a 5-year survival rate of only 25%. Stage is the best predictor of outcome, which is better than stage-matched PDAC. There is currently no accepted system for grading ACCs. Surgery is the treatment of choice for patients with organ-confined tumors. Chemotherapy is typically used for patients with metastatic disease, but there are no prospective randomized clinical trials to guide treatment for this rare malignancy. Typical regimens are similar to those used in PDAC or colorectal cancer because of molecular similarities.

ACINAR CELL CARCINOMA—FACT SHEET

Definition

- Malignant epithelial neoplasm with acinar differentiation similar to pancreatic acinar cells

Incidence and Location

- Rare (<2% of all pancreatic malignancies); can occur throughout pancreas but more common in head

Gender, Race, and Age Distribution

- More common in men (male-to-female ratio, 3.6 to 1)
- No racial predilection
- Most common in older adults, but a significant minority may occur in children

Clinical Features

- Usually presents with nonspecific abdominal symptoms
- Minority of patients may show subcutaneous fat necrosis, polyarthralgia, and eosinophilia caused by lipase hypersecretion

Radiologic Features

- Large, circumscribed, homogeneously enhancing mass

Prognosis and Therapy

- Poor prognosis with 5-year-survival of about 25%; treatment is surgery for localized disease and chemotherapy for systemic disease

ACINAR CELL CARCINOMA—PATHOLOGIC FEATURES

Gross Findings

- Solitary, circumscribed fleshy mass

Microscopic Findings

- Architecture: most commonly acinar but can also be solid, glandular, or trabecular
- Cytology: cytoplasm with zymogen granules, round polarized nuclei with prominent nucleoli

Ultrastructural Findings

- Electron-dense zymogen granules in cytoplasm

Immunohistochemistry

- Diffuse expression of BCL10 and pancreatic exocrine enzymes (trypsin, chymotrypsin, lipase, elastase)
- Can have focal (<25%) expression of chromogranin and synaptophysin
- Subset of cases can have nuclear β-catenin

Differential Diagnosis

- Other solid cellular pancreatic neoplasms: pancreatic neuroendocrine tumor or carcinoma, solid-pseudopapillary tumor, pancreatoblastoma; metastasis from another site

Acinar Cell Cystadenocarcinoma

Acinar cell cystadenocarcinoma is a very rare grossly cystic, malignant neoplasm with acinar differentiation. Most cases are very large with variably sized cysts lined by cytologically malignant cells with acinar differentiation as demonstrated by morphology and IHC. Although few cases have been described in the literature, the clinical behavior does not seem to be significantly different from that of ACC.

Pancreatoblastoma

Clinical Features

Pancreatoblastoma is a very rare pancreatic malignancy that accounts for a very small proportion of adult malignancies but for approximately 25% of pancreatic neoplasms in the first decade of life. The majority occur in children younger than 10 years of age. There is a slight male predominance. In young patients, pancreatoblastoma can be diagnosed because of a palpable abdominal mass, or patients can present with nonspecific symptoms such as abdominal pain and nausea. As with ACC, jaundice is uncommon. Approximately one-third of patients with pancreatoblastoma have elevated serum levels of alpha-fetoprotein caused by production by the tumor. Pancreatoblastoma has been reported in patients with Beckwith-Wiedemann syndrome, a disorder associated with imprinting dysregulation on chromosome 11p, as well as in patients with familial adenomatous polyposis.

Radiologic Features

Pancreatoblastomas form large, circumscribed, heterogeneous masses, which may have calcifications.

Pathological Features

Pancreatoblastomas are not associated with a specific location in the pancreas and are evenly distributed throughout the head, body, and tail. Grossly, they typically form solitary well-circumscribed fleshy masses and can be encapsulated. There is a wide size range, but on average, pancreatoblastomas are large tumors (>10 cm in size). Microscopically, they can consist of multiple components, but a combination of cells with acinar differentiation with round nuclei and prominent nucleoli, granular cytoplasm, and architecturally polarized around small lumina (Fig. 16.28A) and squamoid nests with whorled groups of plump squamoid cells with eosinophilic cytoplasm and clear nuclei (Fig. 16.28B) must be present for diagnosis. The squamoid nests are a diagnostic requirement and can distinguish pancreatoblastoma from ACC. Other possible components include neuroendocrine cells; ductal cells, which can produce mucin; and immature small round blue cells. These components are typically arranged in well-defined islands separated by stromal bands. The stroma can rarely have heterologous elements such as bone or cartilage. Because of the rarity of these tumors, they have not been as well characterized at the genetic level, though loss of chromosome 11p and mutations in the *APC/CTNNB1* pathway have been reported.

Ancillary Studies

The cells in each component have immunohistochemical profiles in keeping with their line of differentiation. The acinar component expresses pancreatic exocrine enzymes (trypsin, chymotrypsin, lipase), the neuroendocrine component expresses chromogranin and synaptophysin, and the ductal component expresses CK7 and CK19. Of note, the squamoid nests are negative for most markers, but the nuclei contain biotin and thus label

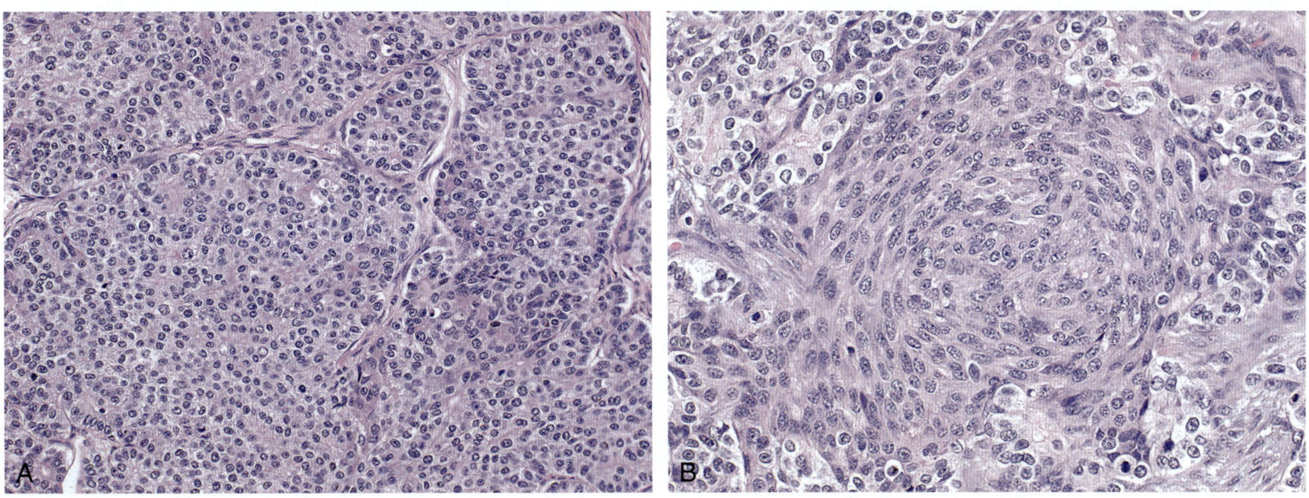

FIGURE 16.28

Pancreatoblastoma. These tumors consist of multiple components. **A**, Most tumors show predominantly acinar differentiation. **B**, Squamoid nests are specific for pancreatoblastoma and required to establish a diagnosis.

nonspecifically with a variety of antibodies. Nuclear β -catenin labeling is typically restricted to the squamoid nests and is a useful feature for diagnosis.

Differential Diagnosis

The differential diagnosis lies mostly with the other solid cellular neoplasms of the pancreas. Squamoid nests are a truly unique feature of pancreatoblastoma and can be used to establish this diagnosis. ACC similarly consists of cells with acinar differentiation but does not have squamoid nests. Importantly, *CTNNB1* mutations have been reported in pancreatoblastoma, and thus they can have nuclear β-catenin immunolabeling, which is characteristically restricted to the squamoid nests. As such, this antibody cannot be used to distinguish pancreatoblastoma from SPN, which uniformly shows aberrant nuclear labeling for β-catenin throughout the tumor. The presence of acinar cell differentiation on IHC and squamoid nests is helpful in distinguishing these two tumors. Although uncommon, metastasis to the pancreas should always be considered in the differential diagnosis.

Prognosis and Therapy

The overall survival rate is approximately 50%. Surgery is the treatment of choice in localized disease, and chemotherapy is often used for metastatic tumors. Even in patients with resectable disease, local recurrence and metachronous metastasis are common. Pancreatoblastoma is staged using the same system as PDAC, and stage is the best predictor of outcome.

PANCREATOBLASTOMA—FACT SHEET

Definition

- Malignant epithelial neoplasm with pancreatic acinar differentiation and squamoid nests

Incidence and Location

- Rare primary pancreatic tumor; extremely rare in adults, but about 25% of pancreatic neoplasms are in children younger than 10 years old

Gender, Race, and Age Distribution

- Slight male predominance
- No racial predilection
- Most common in children younger than 10 years old but can occur in adults

Clinical Features

- Usually diagnosed because of a palpable abdominal mass in children or nonspecific abdominal symptoms

Radiologic Features

- Large, circumscribed, heterogeneous mass

Prognosis and Therapy

- Treated with surgery (localized disease) or chemotherapy (systemic disease)
- Overall survival rate is about 50%
- Recurrence common even in patients with complete resection

Pancreatoblastoma—Pathologic Features

Gross Findings

- Large, circumscribed, fleshy mass

Microscopic Findings

- Multiple components arranged in islands separated by stromal bands
- Must have at least acinar component and squamoid nests but can also have neuroendocrine, ductal, and primitive components

Ultrastructural Findings

- Findings vary by differentiation of components: electron-dense granules in acinar and endocrine components; desmosomes in squamoid nests

Immunohistochemistry

- Each component has labeling typical of its line of differentiation: acinar (trypsin, chymotrypsin, BCL10), neuroendocrine (chromogranin, synaptophysin), ductal (CK7, CK19)
- Squamoid nests have nuclear biotin and thus show nonspecific nuclear labeling, but nuclear β-catenin in these nests is characteristic

Differential Diagnosis

- Other solid cellular pancreatic neoplasms: acinar cell carcinoma, pancreatic neuroendocrine tumor or carcinoma, solid-pseudopapillary tumor; metastasis from another site

Serous Cystadenoma

Clinical Features

Serous cystadenomas are uncommon but account for almost one-third of all cystic pancreatic neoplasms. They occur primarily in adults and have a female predominance (male-to-female ratio, 3 to 7). SCAs are frequently discovered incidentally on abdominal imaging but can also present with nonspecific abdominal symptoms. SCAs are frequently found in patients with VHL syndrome, an autosomal dominant tumor predisposition syndrome characterized by clear cell neoplasms in multiple organs. In patients with VHL syndrome, the pancreas can be diffusely involved by SCAs, and patients can have combined serous neuroendocrine neoplasms in addition to typical SCAs.

Radiologic Features

Serous cystadenomas present as well-circumscribed, multilocular cystic masses, often with central stellate scars.

Pathological Features

Grossly, SCAs are well-circumscribed round lesions with an average size of 6 cm. On cut section, the most common appearance is a spongelike aggregation of tiny cysts with a central stellate scar (Fig. 16.29A). SCAs do not communicate with the pancreatic duct system. Microscopically, the cysts are lined by a single layer of cuboidal cells with uniform round nuclei and clear cytoplasm (Fig. 16.29B). These findings are characteristic of a microcystic SCA, which is the most common growth pattern. SCA variants include macrocystic or oligocystic SCAs, which are composed of a few large cysts and can even be unilocular, and solid SCA, which has a solid gross appearance and is microscopically composed of small acinar structures with minute central lumina. The cytology in these variants is similar to typical microcystic SCA. Rarely, intracystic epithelial papillae can also occur. Genetically, SCAs can be distinguished from other cystic neoplasms by frequent mutation and loss of the *VHL* locus on chromosome 3, as well as a lack of mutations in the key driver genes of ductal neoplasia, such as *KRAS* and *GNAS*.

Ancillary Studies

The cytoplasm of the neoplastic cells is positive on PAS stain because of abundant glycogen. On immunohistochemical stains, SCAs are positive for cytokeratin, including CK7 and CK19, and negative for neuroendocrine markers and pancreatic exocrine enzymes.

Differential Diagnosis

The differential diagnosis includes other cystic pancreatic neoplasms, such as IPMN and MCN. Unlike these entities, SCAs do not produce mucin, do not have ovarian-type stroma, and do not communicate with the pancreatic duct system. Other entities on the differential diagnosis include lymphangiomas and hemangiomas, which, unlike SCAs, are lined by flattened endothelial cells that are positive for CD31, CD34, or ERG. Metastatic renal cell carcinoma (RCC) is in the differential diagnosis, particularly of solid SCA, but this can be resolved by IHC for PAX8, which is positive in RCC and negative in SCA. This differential diagnosis is particularly important in patients with VHL syndrome, who are at increased risk for both neoplasms.

Prognosis and Therapy

Serous cystadenomas are benign neoplasms. Surgical resection is curative but is only necessary when SCA causes symptoms because of compression of adjacent structures. Otherwise, SCAs are resected when they cannot be distinguished preoperatively from IPMNs and MCNs.

SEROUS CYSTADENOMA—FACT SHEET

Definition

- Benign cystic pancreatic neoplasm

Incidence and Location

- Rare cystic neoplasm; more common in body and tail of pancreas

Gender, Race, and Age Distribution

- Female predominance
- No racial predilection
- Usually occurs in adults with an average age of 65 years

Clinical Features

- Can be incidental findings on imaging or present with nonspecific abdominal symptoms

Radiologic Features

- Well-circumscribed multilocular cystic mass, sometimes with a central scar

Prognosis and Therapy

- Surgical resection is curative

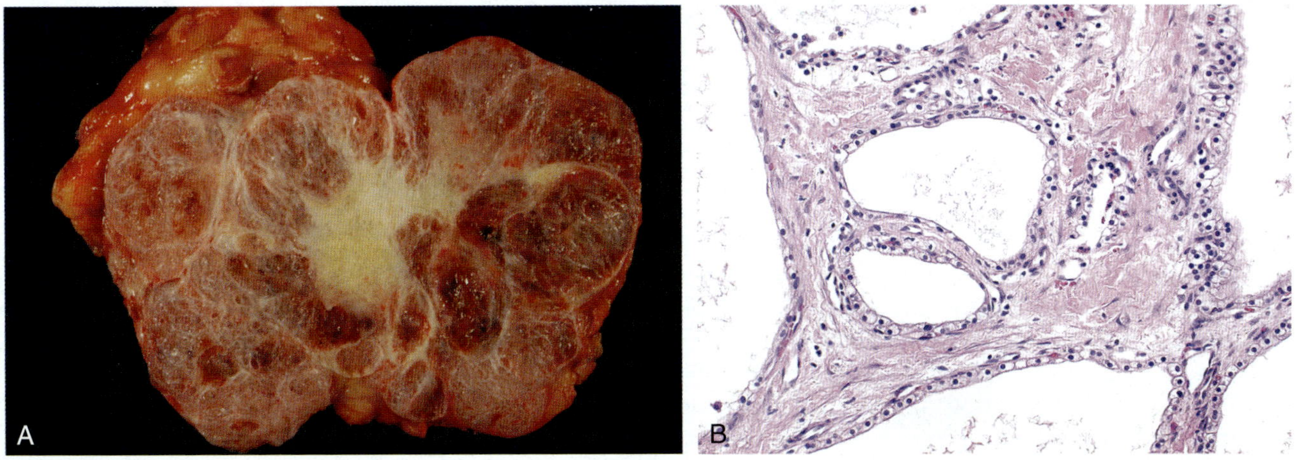

FIGURE 16.29

Serous cystadenoma (SCA). **A**, The characteristic gross appearance is of a spongelike aggregation of small cysts with a central stellate scar. **B**, The cuboidal cells of SCA have small, round nuclei and clear cytoplasm.

Serous Cystadenoma—Pathologic Features

Gross Findings

- Classic microcystic type shows a spongelike mass composed of tiny cysts with central stellate scar
- Macrocystic and oligocystic variants show a small number of smooth-walled cysts
- Solid variant shows a fleshy solid mass

Microscopic Findings

- Single layer of uniform cuboidal cells lining the cyst wall
- Cells with clear cytoplasm and uniform central round monomorphic nuclei

Ultrastructural Findings

- Abundant cytoplasmic glycogen
- Lack of zymogen or neurosecretory granules

Immunohistochemistry

- Periodic acid–Schiff positive cytoplasm because of abundant glycogen
- Cytokeratin positive; negative for chromogranin, synaptophysin, pancreatic exocrine enzymes, and endothelial markers

Differential Diagnosis

- Intraductal papillary mucinous neoplasm, mucinous cystic neoplasm, lymphangioma/hemangioma, metastatic renal cell carcinoma can mimic solid serous cystadenoma

Serous Cystadenocarcinoma

Serous cystadenocarcinoma is an extremely rare malignant pancreatic neoplasm composed of cuboidal epithelial cells with clear cytoplasm. Grossly and microscopically, they are remarkably similar to benign SCAs: they typically do not exhibit cytologic atypia or an elevated mitotic rate. Metastatic disease is the only way to establish a diagnosis of malignancy. Although only a small number of cases have been reported, the prognosis seems good, with most patients still alive at a mean follow-up period of 36 months.

Solid-Pseudopapillary Neoplasm

Clinical Features

Solid-pseudopapillary neoplasm (SPN) is a rare pancreatic malignancy, accounting for fewer than 5% of all pancreatic cancers. They occur predominantly in young women, with a mean age of 28 years and a male-to-female ratio of 1 to 9. SPNs can be found incidentally on abdominal imaging or can present with symptoms caused by compression of adjacent structures, including abdominal pain, nausea, and early satiety. Jaundice is very rare.

Radiologic Features

Solid-pseudopapillary neoplasms are circumscribed, are often solid and cystic, and demonstrate heterogeneous enhancing on imaging.

Pathological Features

Grossly, SPNs are large, solitary, well-circumscribed or even encapsulated tumors. On cut section, most have a combination of soft yellow-brown solid areas and cystic degenerative areas with friable material and hemorrhage (Fig. 16.30A). Microscopically, SPNs are cellular neoplasms consisting of poorly cohesive cells supported by delicate small vessels. The architecture is a mixture of solid and cystic areas with characteristic pseudopapillae consisting of thin layers of neoplastic cells clinging to small blood vessels (Fig. 16.30B). Although grossly well circumscribed, the neoplastic cells often infiltrate into the adjacent non-neoplastic pancreas. The cytoplasm is usually eosinophilic, sometimes with vacuoles or hyaline globules, which are characteristic but not entirely specific (Fig. 16.30C). Nuclei are round to oval and frequently have prominent nuclear grooves. Additional typical features include foamy macrophages, cholesterol clefts, and hemorrhage. SPNs are characterized by almost universal mutation of *CTNNB1*, leading to aberrant nuclear localization of the β-catenin protein, which is diagnostically useful.

Ancillary Studies

The most characteristic immunohistochemical finding in SPN is aberrant nuclear accumulation of β-catenin caused by somatic mutations in the *CTNNB1* gene, which are present in more than 95% of SPNs. SPNs also express CD10, LEF1, transcription factor enhancer 3, androgen receptor, vimentin, PR, and α-1 antitrypsin. Depending on the antibody used, E-cadherin IHC can show complete loss of expression (antibodies to extracellular domain) or abnormal nuclear/cytoplasmic staining (antibodies to intracellular domain). Cytokeratin expression is variable. SPNs do not express pancreatic exocrine enzymes, and although synaptophysin can be focally positive, chromogranin is typically negative.

Differential Diagnosis

The differential diagnosis lies chiefly with the other solid cellular neoplasms of the pancreas, including PanNET or PanNEC, ACC, and pancreatoblastoma. Although uncommon, metastases to the pancreas should also be considered. Aberrant nuclear localization of β-catenin is very helpful in establishing a diagnosis of SPN. However, it is important to note that nuclear β-catenin is not specific for SPN because this aberrant staining can occur uncommonly in both ACC and within squamoid morules in pancreatoblastoma. Because SPNs do not express pancreatic

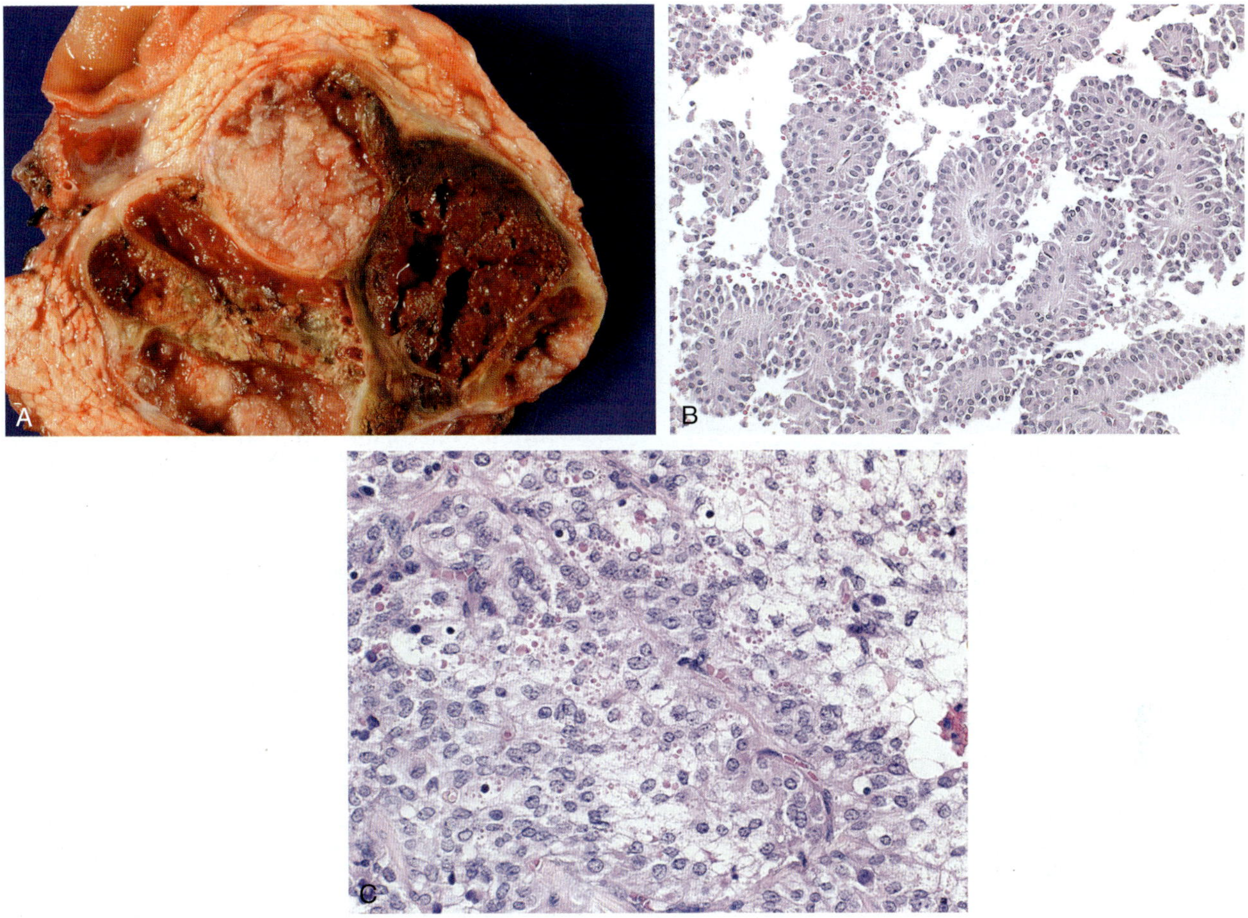

FIGURE 16.30

Solid-pseudopapillary neoplasm (SPN). **A**, Grossly, SPNs are solid masses but frequently show areas of hemorrhage and cystic degeneration. **B**, Microscopically, SPNs frequently have a solid component, but areas of degeneration in which the neoplastic cells cling to delicate blood vessels are also common. **C**, At high power, the nuclei frequently contain grooves, and cytoplasmic hyaline globules are characteristic but not entirely specific.

exocrine enzymes, IHC for these proteins can exclude ACC or pancreatoblastoma in difficult cases.

Prognosis and Therapy

Although SPNs are considered low-grade malignant neoplasms that can metastasize, the prognosis is quite good compared with other pancreatic malignancies. Approximately 90% of patients can be cured with complete surgical resection. Even recurrences and metastases can often be surgically resected, with only a few patients reportedly dying of this disease. Stage is the best predictor of outcome, and the current staging scheme is the same as that for PDAC.

Mixed Tumors

Neoplasms containing cells with multiple lines of differentiation have been increasingly recognized in the pancreas. These carcinomas are rare, so there are insufficient data to rigorously define the biology and clinical course. However, in reported cases, the clinical course is highly

SOLID-PSEUDOPAPILLARY NEOPLASM—FACT SHEET

Definition

- Low-grade malignant epithelial neoplasm with uncertain line of differentiation

Incidence and Location

- Uncommon primary pancreatic tumor; occurs throughout the pancreas

Gender, Race, and Age Distribution

- Much more common in women
- No racial predilection
- Most common in the third decade of life

Clinical Features

- Can be found incidentally on imaging or diagnosed because of vague abdominal symptoms

Radiologic Features

- Well-circumscribed heterogeneous mass with solid and cystic components

Prognosis and Therapy

- Excellent prognosis; surgery usually curative

Solid-Pseudopapillary Neoplasm—Pathologic Features

Gross Findings

- Well-circumscribed and often encapsulated; mixture of solid areas and necrosis or cystic degeneration

Microscopic Findings

- Tumor shows a mixture of solid and discohesive areas with pseudopapillae
- Cytoplasm can be eosinophilic or vacuolated and display characteristic hyaline globules
- Nuclei are round to oval with prominent nuclear grooves
- Foam cells and cholesterol clefts within the tips of papillae are common

Ultrastructural Findings

- Abundant mitochondria and zymogen-like granules
- Neurosecretory granules present less frequently

Immunohistochemistry

- Nuclear localization of β-catenin is characteristic
- Also positive for CD10, LEF1, transcription factor enhancer 3, androgen receptor, vimentin, progesterone receptor, and α-1 antitrypsin
- Cytokeratin and synaptophysin variably positive
- Negative for chromogranin and pancreatic exocrine enzymes

Differential Diagnosis

- Acinar cell carcinoma, pancreatic neuroendocrine tumor or carcinoma, pancreatoblastoma, metastasis from another site

aggressive, and the prognosis is poor. These tumors are now designated mixed neuroendocrine and non-neuroendocrine neoplasms in the new WHO classification. The non-neuroendocrine component may be ductal or acinar and must constitute at least 30% of the entire tumor.

Mixed Ductal–Neuroendocrine Carcinoma

Mixed ductal–neuroendocrine carcinoma consist of a mixture of neoplastic ductal and neoplastic neuroendocrine cells, each including at least 30% of the neoplastic cells. Two growth patterns are recognized: (1) intermingled ductal and neuroendocrine cells forming glandular and solid structures and (2) neoplastic ductal elements embedded in a background of solid neoplastic neuroendocrine cells. Whereas the ductal cells express CEA and mucins, the neuroendocrine cells express chromogranin and synaptophysin. A key feature of this diagnosis is that both the ductal and neuroendocrine components are neoplastic. As such, it must be distinguished morphologically from NETs that entrap normal non-neoplastic ducts as well as ductal adenocarcinomas with adjacent reactive non-neoplastic islets. Both of these mimics are much more common than true mixed ductal–neuroendocrine carcinomas.

Mixed Acinar–Neuroendocrine Carcinoma

Mixed acinar–neuroendocrine carcinomas are composed of malignant epithelial cells with both acinar and neuroendocrine differentiation. Although the different components can sometimes be appreciated on H&E-stained sections, in many cases, the divergent directions of differentiation are most easily appreciated on immunohistochemical stains, which can show two different components, one labeling with neuroendocrine markers and the other with acinar markers. A subset of cells that label with markers for both lineages may also be present. Typically, the majority of the tumor shows acinar differentiation, but the neuroendocrine component must account for at least 30% of the neoplastic cells to diagnose a mixed carcinoma.

Mixed Acinar–Ductal and Mixed Acinar–Ductal–Neuroendocrine Carcinoma

Mixed acinar–ductal carcinoma is a malignant epithelial neoplasm with components of both acinar and ductal differentiation. Each component must account for at least 30% of the neoplasm to make a diagnosis of mixed acinar-ductal carcinoma. Typically, the acinar component is more prominent. In addition to the acinar component, which resembles ACC, some tumors contain a component morphologically similar to PDAC, but others show intracellular and sometimes extracellular mucin in cells that cytologically resemble ACC. Rare tumors also have a neuroendocrine component and are best classified as mixed acinar–endocrine–ductal carcinoma.

Other Neoplasms

Although much less common than the epithelial neoplasms described in this chapter, a variety of mesenchymal and hematopoietic neoplasms can involve the pancreas either primarily or secondarily. The diagnostic criteria and clinical features of these mesenchymal and hematopoietic neoplasms parallel those in other organs. In addition, carcinomas originally in other sites can also metastasize to the pancreas; thus, metastatic carcinoma from another organ should always be considered in the differential diagnosis, particularly of a morphologically unusual tumor.

FROZEN SECTION EVALUATION AND DIAGNOSIS

The reasons for intraoperative consultations for pancreatic lesions are twofold: (1) to determine if a pancreatic mass is a PDAC or a benign inflammatory process and

(2) to evaluate pancreatic parenchymal and bile duct margins for tumor. The uncinate margin is not usually examined by frozen section because additional tissue cannot be resected; however, in the institution that has capability of intraoperative radiation therapy, frozen section consultation on the uncinate margin status for PDAC may be requested. Similarly, in the setting of post–neoadjuvant therapy resection, tissue adjacent to the superior mesenteric artery (SMA) or hepatic artery may be submitted to determine the resectability of the carcinoma.

Diagnosis of Pancreatic Ductal Adenocarcinoma on Frozen Section

Definitive diagnosis of pancreatic adenocarcinoma usually depends on one of two features: (1) architectural and/or cytologic features of infiltrating ducts that are unequivocal for carcinoma and (2) evidence of invasion into other structures such as nerves, lymphatics, blood vessels, extrapancreatic soft tissue, duodenum, or lymph nodes. The infiltrative haphazard growth pattern, glands adjacent to muscular vessels, four-to-one nuclear size variation within one gland rule, huge irregular nucleoli, glandular necrotic debris, and mitoses (in particular atypical mitoses) favor a diagnosis of carcinoma. Importantly, benign lobular atrophy with acinar–ductal metaplasia often results in an aggregate of small ducts in an infiltrating pattern (Fig. 16.31); thus, judgments based on constellation of features are warranted. When tumor morphology is well differentiated, it mimics reactive ducts or low-grade PanIN. In this context, architectural criteria for malignancy, such as loss of lobular configuration of proliferating ducts, angulated and fused glands, and the presence of desmoplastic stroma and close proximity of ducts to medium-sized arteries or large vessels are helpful features for the diagnosis of carcinoma (Fig. 16.32). Other key features to keep in mind are islet cell proliferation and juxtaposition of benign glands to nerves secondary to marked parenchymal atrophy in chronic pancreatitis because the former may mimic solid foci of carcinoma and the latter may be mistaken for perineural invasion.

The differential diagnosis includes chronic alcoholic or obstructive pancreatitis, AIP, or paraduodenal or groove pancreatitis. PDAC can usually be differentiated from these entities based on the aforementioned features.

Evaluation of Resection Margins

Intraoperative consultation of the pancreatic parenchymal margin and/or bile duct margin may be requested in a variety of entities of the pancreas. Understanding the morphology of the tumor in question is necessary to render an appropriate interpretation. Several issues are worth discussing in this context.

Parenchymal Margin

1. Gross evidence of tumor, in particular IPMN, at the pancreatic parenchymal margin leads to additional resections, if feasible, regardless of the diagnosis and grade of dysplasia.
2. If invasive carcinoma is present at the margin, it should be reported.
3. If a high-grade intraductal lesion (either IPMN of PanIN) is present at the margin, it should be reported. In addition, PDAC may exhibit cancerization

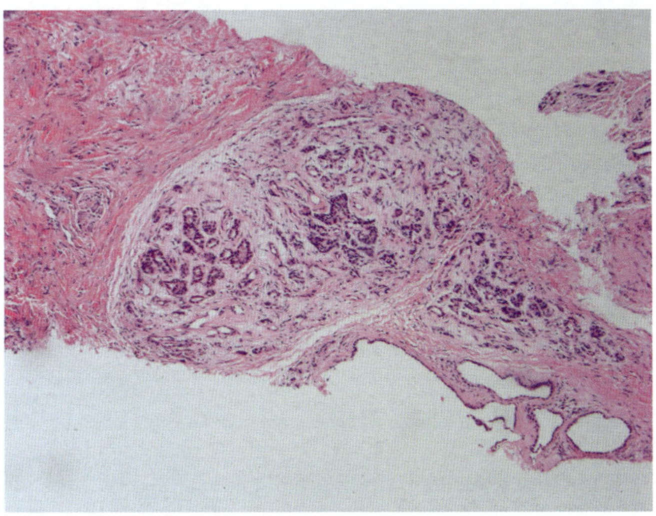

FIGURE 16.31

Benign lobular atrophy with acinar–ductal metaplasia exhibiting an infiltrating pattern (hematoxylin and eosin, frozen section).

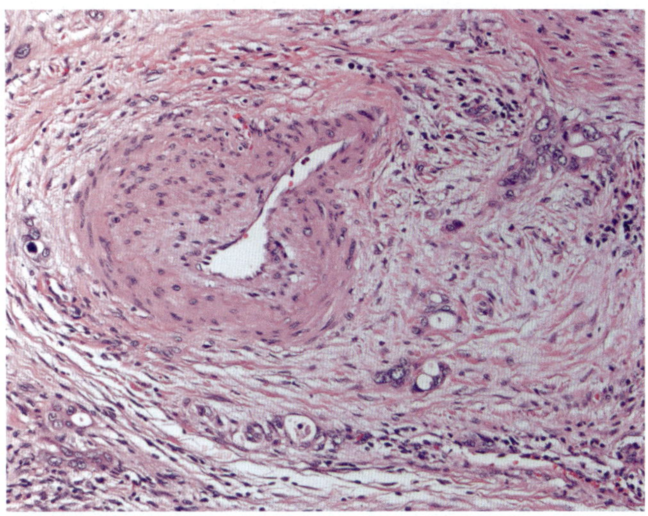

FIGURE 16.32

Close proximity of benign-appearing ducts to medium-sized arteries or large vessels are helpful features for the diagnosis of carcinoma (hematoxylin and eosin, frozen section).

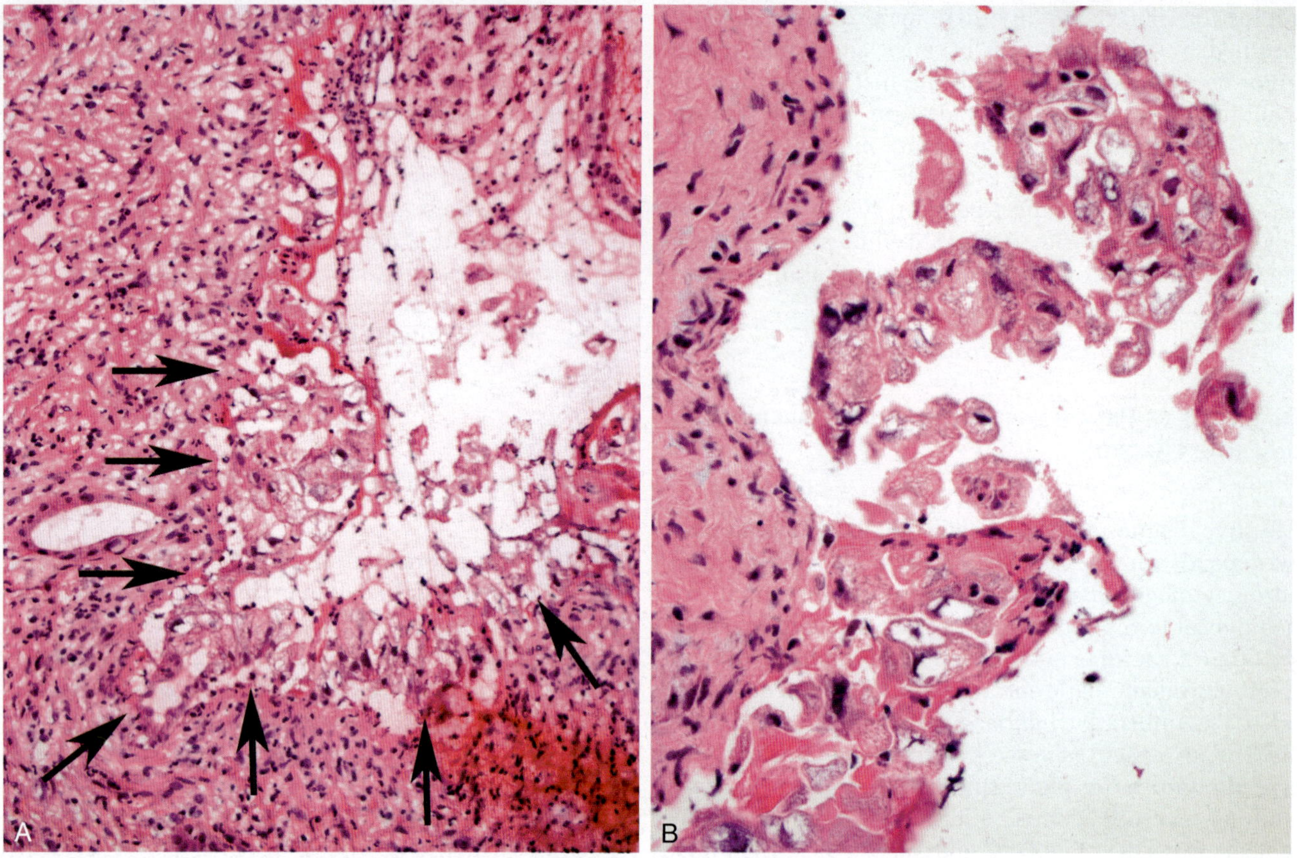

FIGURE 16.33

A frozen section of the pancreatic transection margin (**A**, hematoxylin and eosin H&E]) demonstrating the main pancreatic duct involved by cancerization *(arrows)*, confirmed by the corresponding permanent section (**B**, H&E).

involving the main pancreatic duct and/or interlobular ducts at the margin (Fig. 16.33) and resemble a high-grade intraductal lesion. Thus, the presence of high-grade intraductal lesion may sometimes lead to additional surgery to achieve negative margin status.

4. If only a low-grade intraductal lesion (either IPMN or PanIN) is present at the margin, the report of intraoperative consultation should indicate that no invasive or in situ carcinoma is identified and that only intraductal/intraepithelial neoplasm of low-grade dysplasia, either IPMN or PanIN, is present. Low-grade dysplasia at the margin is usually not an indication for additional tissue resection. However, if intraductal intestinal-type IPMN is identified at the margin, it may be a consideration for additional tissue removal, regardless of the grade of dysplasia, because of a high risk of recurrence. The significance and management of low-grade IPMN at the margin is an area of considerable controversy.
5. If the main pancreatic duct is denuded because of inflammation at the margin, it may be indicative of close proximity to the lesion, in particular IPMN. The report of intraoperative consultation should add the possibility that subsequent evaluation on permanent sections may reveal dysplasia.

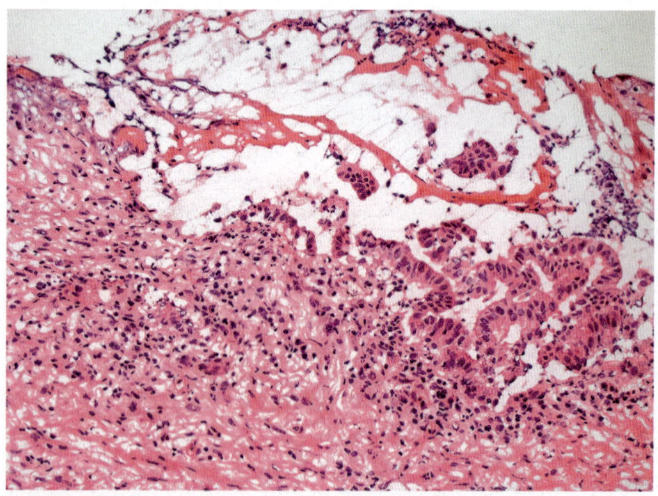

FIGURE 16.34

A frozen section of the bile duct at the margin (hematoxylin and eosin). Reactive changes secondary to stent insertion characterized by micropapillary architecture, cytologic atypia, and disruption of epithelial lining can mimic high-grade dysplasia of the biliary epithelium and/or invasive carcinoma.

Bile Duct Margin

1. In the setting of bile duct obstruction caused by pancreatic cancer, a stent may be placed in the bile duct, which can cause severe inflammation, mucosal

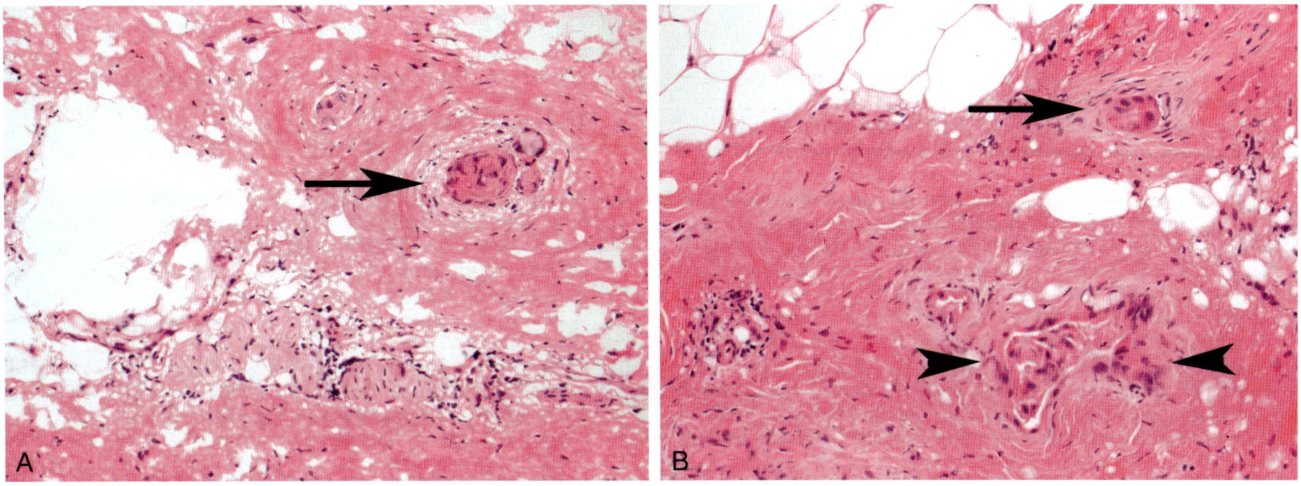

FIG 16.35

A frozen section (**A**, hematoxylin and eosin [H&E]) demonstrates residual carcinoma after neoadjuvant therapy involving a perineural space in tissue adjacent the superior mesenteric artery *(arrow)*. Because of the degenerative appearance of the gland secondary to therapeutic effects, it may be difficult to confirm the presence of carcinoma. The corresponding permanent section (**B**, H&E) reveals unequivocal gland formation *(arrow)* and additional degenerated glands in the region *(arrowheads)*.

ulceration, and marked reactive changes that may be difficult to distinguish from dysplasia or carcinoma. Papillary or micropapillary architecture, prominent cytologic atypia, pseudopyloric metaplasia, and disruption of epithelial lining may be seen as part of marked reactive changes and can mimic carcinoma (Fig. 16.34).

2. Peribiliary glands with reactive changes may resemble well-differentiated carcinoma. The presence of a lobular gland pattern favors a benign reactive process, while the presence of nuclear pleomorphism and abnormal mitoses, deeper location in the wall, close proximity to large blood vessels and perineural invasion favor an invasive carcinoma.

Tissue Adjacent to the Superior Mesenteric Artery/ Hepatic Artery

In the setting of post–neoadjuvant therapy resection for PDAC, samples from tissue adjacent to the SMA or hepatic artery may be submitted to determine resectability or to determine the field of intraoperative radiation therapy. The presence of abnormal ducts in this location usually indicates an invasive carcinoma. It is important to note that residual carcinoma with therapy-related changes is often present only in perineural spaces and may be difficult to diagnose with certainty. Deeper sections may be helpful to show more convincing features (Fig. 16.35).

SUGGESTED READINGS

Non-Neoplastic Diseases

1. Banks PA, Bollen TL, Dervenis C, et al. Classification of acute pancreatitis—2012: revision of the Atlanta classification and definitions by international consensus. *Gut*. 2013;62(1):102–111.
2. Basturk O, Coban I, Adsay NV. Pancreatic cysts: pathologic classification, differential diagnosis, and clinical implications. *Arch Pathol Lab Med*. 2009;133(3):423–438.
3. Basturk O, Askan G. Benign tumors and tumorlike lesions of the pancreas. *Surg Pathol Clin*. 2016;9(4):619–641.
4. Bruno MJ, Dutch Pancreatitis Study Group. Improving the outcome of acute pancreatitis. *Dig Dis*. 2016;34(5):540–545.
5. Fléjou JF. Paraduodenal pancreatitis: a new unifying term and its morphological characteristics. *Diagn Histopathol*. 2012;18:31–36.
6. Gregg JA, Monaco AP, McDermott WV. Pancreas divisum. Results of surgical intervention. *Am J Surg*. 1983;145:488–492.
7. Hariri A, Siegelman SS, Hruban RH. Duodenal diverticulum mimicking a cystic pancreatic neoplasm. *Br J Radiol*. 2005;78(930):562–564.
8. Kiernan PD, ReMine SG, Kiernan PC, et al. Annular pancreas. *Arch Surg*. 1980;115:46–50.
9. Klöppel G. Chronic pancreatitis, pseudotumors and other tumor-like lesions. *Mod Pathol*. 2007;20(suppl):113–131.
10. Klöppel G, Adsay NV. Chronic pancreatitis and the differential diagnosis versus pancreatic cancer. *Arch Pathol Lab Med*. 2009;133:382–387.
11. Lankisch PG, Apte M, Banks PA. Acute pancreatitis. *Lancet*. 2015;386(9988):85–96.
12. Majumder S, Chari ST. Chronic pancreatitis. *Lancet*. 2016;387 (10031):1957–1966.
13. Pauser U, Kosmahl M, Kruslin B, et al. Pancreatic solid and cystic hamartoma in adults: characterization of a new tumorous lesion. *Am J Surg Pathol*. 2005;29(6):797–800.
14. Stram M, Liu S, Singhi AD. Chronic pancreatitis. *Surg Pathol Clin*. 2016;9(4):643–659.
15. Yadav D, Lowenfels AB. The epidemiology of pancreatitis and pancreatic cancer. *Gastroenterology*. 2013;144(6):1252–1261.
16. Yamaguchi H1, Aishima S, Oda Y, et al. Distinctive histopathologic findings of pancreatic hamartomas suggesting their "hamartomatous" nature: a study of 9 cases. *Am J Surg Pathol*. 2013; 37(7):1006–1013.

Exocrine Neoplasms

17. Abraham SC, Klimstra DS, Wilentz RE, et al. Solid-pseudopapillary tumors of the pancreas are genetically distinct from pancreatic ductal adenocarcinomas and almost always harbor beta-catenin mutations. *Am J Pathol*. 2002;160:1361–1369.
18. Abraham SC, Wu TT, Hruban RH, et al. Genetic and immunohistochemical analysis of pancreatic acinar cell carcinoma. frequent allelic loss on chromosome 11p and alterations in the APC/ beta-catenin pathway. *Am J Pathol*. 2002;160:953–962.
19. Abraham SC, Wu TT, Klimstra DS, et al. Distinctive molecular genetic alterations in sporadic and familial adenomatous polyposis-associated pancreatoblastomas: frequent alterations in

the APC/b-catenin pathway and chromosome 11. *Am J Pathol.* 2001;159:1619–1627.
20. Adsay NV, Merati K, Andea A, et al. The dichotomy in the preinvasive neoplasia to invasive carcinoma sequence in the pancreas. differential expression of MUC1 and MUC2 supports the existence of two separate pathways of carcinogenesis. *Mod Pathol.* 2002;15:1087–1095.
21. Adsay V, Mino-Kenudson M, Furukawa T, et al. Pathologic evaluation and reporting of intraductal papillary mucinous neoplasms of the pancreas and other tumoral intraepithelial neoplasms of pancreatobiliary tract: recommendations of Verona Consensus Meeting. *Ann Surg.* 2016;263(1):162–177.
22. Basturk O, Coban I, Adsay NV. Pancreatic cysts. pathologic classification, differential diagnosis and clinical implications. *Arch Pathol Lab Med.* 2009;133:423–438.
23. Basturk O, Hong SM, Wood LD, et al. A Revised classification system and recommendations from the Baltimore Consensus Meeting for Neoplastic Precursor Lesions in the Pancreas. *Am J Surg Pathol.* 2015;39(12):1730–1741.
24. Brosens LA, Hackeng WM, Offerhaus GJ, et al. Pancreatic adenocarcinoma pathology: changing "landscape." *J Gastrointest Oncol.* 2015;6(4):358–374.
25. Chari ST, Yadav D, Smyrk TC, et al. Study of recurrence after surgical resection of intraductal papillary mucinous neoplasm of the pancreas. *Gastroenterology.* 2002;123:1500–1507.
26. Furukawa T, Hatori T, Fujita I, et al. Prognostic relevance of morphological types of intraductal papillary mucinous neoplasms of the pancreas. *Gut.* 2011;60(4):509–516.
27. Hruban RH, Adsay NV, Albores-Saavedra J, et al. Pancreatic intraepithelial neoplasia (PanIN). a new nomenclature and classification system for pancreatic duct lesions. *Am J Surg Pathol.* 2001;25:579–586.
28. Iacobuzio-Donahue CA, Klimstra DS, Adsay NV, et al. DPC-4 protein is expressed in virtually all human intraductal papillary mucinous neoplasms of the pancreas. Comparison with conventional ductal carcinomas. *Am J Pathol.* 2000;24:1544–1548.
29. Klimstra DS, Heffess CS, Oertel JE, et al. Acinar cell carcinoma of the pancreas. A clinicopathologic study of 28 cases. *Am J Surg Pathol.* 1992;16:815–837.
30. Klimstra DS, Pitman MB, Hruban RH. An algorithmic approach to the diagnosis of pancreatic neoplasms. *Arch Pathol Lab Med.* 2009;133:454–464.
31. Klimstra DS, Wenig BM, Adair CF, et al. Pancreatoblastoma. A clinicopathologic study and review of the literature. *Am J Surg Pathol.* 1995;19:1371–1389.
32. Lüttges J, Feyerabend B, Buchelt T, et al. The mucin profile of noninvasive and invasive mucinous cystic neoplasms of the pancreas. *Am J Surg Pathol.* 2002;26:466–471.
33. Lüttges J, Zamboni G, Longnecker DS, et al. The immunohistochemical mucin expression pattern distinguishes different types of intraductal papillary mucinous neoplasms of the pancreas and determines their relationship to mucinous noncystic carcinoma and ductal adenocarcinoma. *Am J Surg Pathol.* 2001;25:942–948.
34. Mino-Kenudson M, Fernández-del Castillo C, Baba Y, et al. Prognosis of invasive intraductal papillary mucinous neoplasm depends on histological and precursor epithelial subtypes. *Gut.* 2011;60(12):1712–1720.
35. Molberg KH, Heffess C, Delgado R, et al. Undifferentiated carcinoma with osteoclast-like giant cells of the pancreas and periampullary region. *Cancer.* 1998;82:1279–1287.
36. Muraki T, Reid MD, Basturk O, et al. Undifferentiated carcinoma with osteoclastic giant cells of the pancreas: clinicopathologic analysis of 38 cases highlights a more protracted clinical course than currently appreciated. *Am J Surg Pathol.* 2016;40(9):1203–1216.
37. Reid MD, Choi H, Balci S, et al. Serous cystic neoplasms of the pancreas: clinicopathologic and molecular characteristics. *Semin Diagn Pathol.* 2014;31(6):475–483.
38. Tanaka M. Fernández-del Castillo C, Adsay V, et al. International consensus guidelines 2012 for the management of IPMN and MCN of the pancreas. *Pancreatology.* 2012;12(3):183–197.
39. Teres B, Cavard C. Diagnosis and molecular aspects of solid-pseudopapillary neoplasms of the pancreas. *Semin Diagn Pathol.* 2014;31(6):484–490.
40. Wilentz RE, Albores-Saavedra J, Hruban RH. Mucinous cystic neoplasms of the pancreas. *Semin Diagn Pathol.* 2000;17:31–42.
41. Wilentz RE, Albores-Saavedra J, Zahurak M, et al. Pathologic examination accurately predicts prognosis in mucinous cystic neoplasms of the pancreas. *Am J Surg Pathol.* 1999;23:1320–1327.
42. Wood LD, Klimstra DS. Pathology and genetics of pancreatic neoplasms with acinar differentiation. *Semin Diagn Pathol.* 2014;31(6):491–497.
43. Wu J, Matthaei H, Maitra A, et al. Recurrent GNAS mutations define an unexpected pathway for pancreatic cyst development. *Sci Transl Med.* 2011;3(92):92ra66.
44. Yamaguchi H, Shimizu M, Ban S, et al. Intraductal tubulopapillary neoplasms of the pancreas distinct from pancreatic intraepithelial neoplasia and intraductal papillary mucinous neoplasms. *Am J Surg Pathol.* 2009;33(8):1164–1172.
45. Zamboni G, Scarpa A, Bogina G, et al. Mucinous cystic tumors of the pancreas: clinicopathological features, prognosis, and relationship to other mucinous cystic tumors. *Am J Surg Pathol.* 1999;23:410–422.

Endocrine Neoplasms

46. Basturk O, Yang Z, Tang LH, et al. The high-grade (WHO G3) pancreatic neuroendocrine tumor category is morphologically and biologically heterogenous and includes both well differentiated and poorly differentiated neoplasms. *Am J Surg Pathol.* 2015;39(5):683–690.
47. Capelli P, Martignoni G, Pedica F, et al. Endocrine neoplasms of the pancreas. pathologic and genetic features. *Arch Pathol Lab Med.* 2009;133:350–364.
48. Klöppel G, Heitz PU. Pancreatic endocrine tumors. *Pathol Res Pract.* 1988;183:155–168.
49. Shi C, Klimstra DS. Pancreatic neuroendocrine tumors: pathologic and molecular characteristics. *Semin Diagn Pathol.* 2014;31(6):498–511.

17

Non-Neoplastic Disorders of the Liver

Daniela S. Allende, MD, MBA and Lisa M. Yerian, MD

MAJOR HISTOLOGIC PATTERNS OF INJURY

Because the liver presents with a relatively small repertoire of responses to injury, there is significant histologic overlap among liver diseases, making specific diagnosis challenging. A pattern-based approach enables the pathologist to generate a relatively short list of differential diagnoses, which can then be distinguished based on histologic findings and available clinical data to establish an informative diagnosis that guides clinical management. Some liver diseases (e.g., autoimmune hepatitis [AIH] and Wilson's disease) can present with more than one pattern of injury.

The major histologic patterns of injury are as follows:

- Hepatitic pattern of injury
  - Acute hepatitis (panlobular)
  - Chronic hepatitis (portal predominant)
- Steatotic-steatohepatitic pattern of injury
- Cholestatic pattern of injury
- Vascular pattern of injury
- Miscellaneous patterns
  - "Almost normal biopsy"
  - Granulomatous hepatitis
  - Massive or submassive hepatic necrosis
- Metabolic and storage disorders
  - Iron storage disorder
  - Copper storage disorder (Wilson's disease)
  - α1-Antitrypsin (α1AT) deficiency
  - Glycogen storage disorder
  - Lysosomal storage disorder (LSD)

ACUTE HEPATITIS PATTERN OF INJURY

Whereas clinically, the term *acute hepatitis* denotes a particular pattern of acute-onset liver disease in a patient without preexisting liver disease, this pattern of injury is defined histologically by a lobular-predominant pattern of inflammation and hepatocyte injury. The clinical picture in most patients with acute hepatitis varies from asymptomatic to mild, vague gastrointestinal (GI) or flu-like symptoms, including nausea and malaise. Laboratory testing demonstrates marked serum aspartate aminotransferase (AST) and alanine aminotransferase (ALT) elevations, but serum bilirubin and alkaline phosphatase (ALP) are normal or only mildly elevated. A subset of patients with clinical features of acute hepatitis exhibit histologic features of an acute hepatitis pattern of injury on biopsy. A biopsy is not indicated in most patients but may be performed to confirm acute hepatitis, exclude entities other that are clinically similar but histologically distinct (e.g., Wilson's disease, ischemic hepatitis, or Budd-Chari syndrome [BCS]), assess for features of chronic liver disease, or evaluate for acute exacerbation of AIH.

Histologically, an acute hepatitis pattern of injury is characterized by a *predominantly lobular pattern of injury* that exhibits lobular inflammatory cell infiltrates accompanied by hepatocyte injury manifest as hepatocyte swelling and necrosis of individual hepatocytes ("acidophil bodies") or hepatocyte clusters ("spotty necrosis"). The resulting loss of the normal, orderly hepatocyte cord arrangement ("lobular disarray") (Figs. 17.1A–C). Depending on the severity of injury, marked hepatocellular regenerative changes, including mitoses, multinucleation ("giant cell transformation"), and hepatocellular rosettes (Fig. 17.1D) may also be present. The lobular inflammation is lymphocyte predominant with Kupffer cell hyperplasia. Neutrophils are neither an important finding nor a defining feature of this pattern. There is no fibrosis in uncomplicated acute hepatitis, although patients with chronic liver disease may develop superimposed acute hepatitis or an acute exacerbation of the chronic disease. Biopsies obtained after the acute phase of the illness may be nearly normal, showing only residual Kupffer cell hyperplasia or aggregates of ceroid-laden histiocytes on periodic acid–Schiff (PAS) with diastase stain (PAS-D; Fig. 17.1E). There is no formal grading scheme for the acute hepatitis pattern of injury.

The differential diagnosis for an acute hepatitis pattern of injury includes acute viral hepatitis caused by hepatotropic viruses (hepatitis A or E or the acute

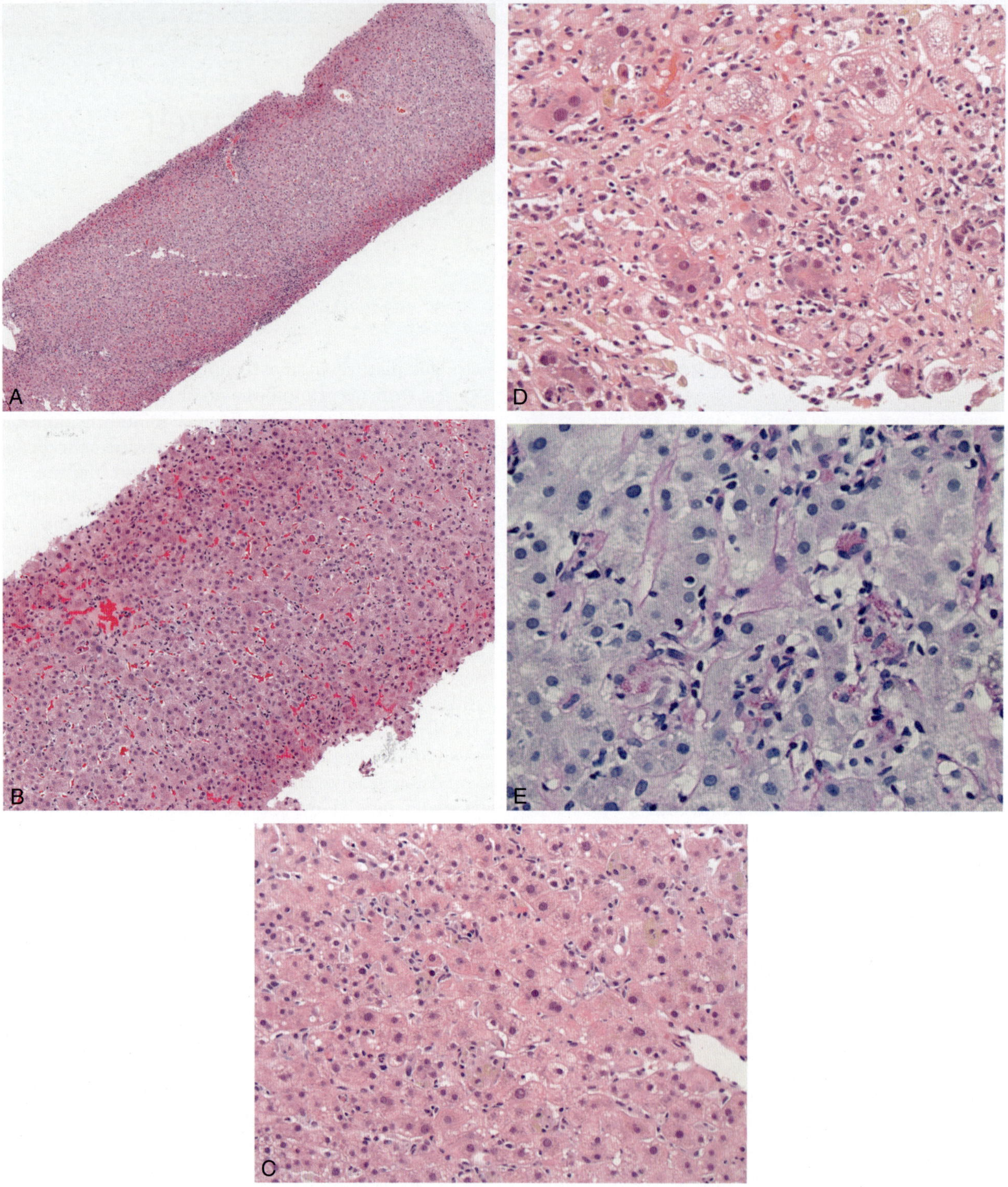

FIGURE 17.1

A, Acute hepatitis pattern of injury on low magnification. **B**, Lobular infiltrates are composed of lymphocytes and Kupffer cells. **C**, Lobular hepatocellular disarray and infiltrating inflammatory cells are typical. **D**, Rosettes and multinucleated hepatocytes are seen in more severe cases. **E**, Periodic acid–Schiff–diastase stain can highlight Kupffer cells in more subtle cases.

phase of hepatitis B, C, or D infection), nonhepatotropic viruses, or drug-induced liver injury (DILI). Acute exacerbation of AIH is also in the clinical and histologic differential diagnosis, although it is considered an a priori chronic disease. DILI and AIH are discussed later in this chapter. A nonspecific form of hepatic inflammation in the absence of clinical illness or hepatocyte injury can be seen in patients undergoing abdominal surgery (so-called "surgical hepatitis"). This entity should not be confused with acute hepatitis.

TABLE 17.1
Viral Hepatitis

Virus	Hepatitis A	Hepatitis B	Hepatitis C	Hepatitis D	Hepatitis E
Type of virus	Single-stranded RNA	Partially double-stranded DNA	Single-stranded RNA	Single-stranded circular defective RNA	Single-stranded RNA
Viral family	Hepatovirus; related to picornavirus	Hepadnavirus	Flaviviridae	Subviral particle in *Deltaviridae* family	Calicivirus
Route of transmission	Fecal–oral (contaminated food or water)	Parenteral (IV drug use), sexual contact, perinatal	Parenteral; intranasal cocaine use is a risk factor	Parenteral	Fecal–oral
Mean incubation period	2–4 weeks	1–4 months	7–8 weeks	Same as for HBV	4–5 weeks
Frequency of chronic liver disease	Never	10%	>85%	Never	5% (coinfection); ≤70% for superinfection
Diagnosis	Detection of serum IgM antibodies	Detection of HBsAg or antibody to HBcAg	PCR for HCV RNA; third-generation ELISA for antibody detection	Detection of IgM and IgG antibodies; HDV RNA in serum; HDAg in liver	PCR for HEV RNA; detection of serum IgM and IgG antibodies
Treatment	Supportive	α-Interferon, lamivudine	Direct-actin antivirals, protease inhibitors, polymerase inhibitors	α-Interferon	Supportive

ELISA, Enzyme-linked immunosorbent assay; *HBcAg*, hepatitis B core antigen; *HBsAg*, hepatitis B surface antigen; *HBV*, hepatitis B virus; *HCV*, hepatitis C virus; *HDAg*, hepatitis D antigen; *HEV*, hepatitis E virus; *IV*, intravenous; *PCR*, polymerase chain reaction.

ACUTE VIRAL (HEPATOTROPIC) HEPATITIS

Acute viral hepatitis represents the prototype acute hepatitis pattern of injury. It is caused by hepatotropic viruses A, B, C, D, and E (Table 17.1). Hepatitis A and E are transmitted through contaminated food and water. Hepatitis A is highly endemic in parts of Africa and Asia, and hepatitis E is highly endemic in Mexico and parts of Africa and Asia. Pregnant women are more susceptible to hepatitis E infection and exhibit a more severe clinical course. Hepatitis B and C are bloodborne pathogens that can also be sexually transmitted. Hepatitis B infection may be further complicated by coinfection or superinfection with hepatitis D, which follows the same route of transmission.

CLINICAL FEATURES

Acute viral hepatitis is often asymptomatic or mildly symptomatic. Patients present with mild symptoms of systemic disease, including malaise, fatigue, low-grade fever, flu-like, or GI symptoms. Adults can develop a more complicated clinical course with prominent cholestasis and even fulminant hepatitis (1%–3% of cases) with massive parenchymal necrosis necessitating liver transplantation.

Physical examination typically reveals jaundice, right upper quadrant tenderness, and hepatomegaly.

LABORATORY VALUES

Most patients show markedly elevated serum AST and ALT levels (often >15-fold normal levels). Bilirubin and ALP may also be elevated. Viral serologies may be negative during the early course of disease. Polymerase chain reaction (PCR)–based testing is frequently used as a confirmatory test.

ACUTE VIRAL (HEPATOTROPIC) HEPATITIS—FACT SHEET

Definition

- Acute hepatitis caused by hepatitis A, B, C, D or E virus infection

Incidence and Location

- The incidence is underestimated because many cases are asymptomatic
- Hepatitis A, B, and C are common worldwide, with hepatitis B more common in Southeast Asia and sub-Saharan Africa
- Hepatitis A is highly endemic in parts of Africa and Asia
- Hepatitis E is highly endemic in Mexico and parts of Africa and Asia

Morbidity and Mortality

- Mortality rate for acute hepatitis A is low, but up to 22% with clinical apparent hepatitis require hospitalization; mortality rate is higher (~1.8%) in patients older than 50 years

- Mortality for hepatitis E is greater in pregnant women; death rate is approximately 5%

Gender, Race, and Age Distribution

- Occurs equally in males and females
- All races and age groups are affected

Clinical Features

- Asymptomatic or mild systemic symptoms, including malaise, low-grade fever, and flulike or gastrointestinal complaints
- Jaundice and pruritus if cholestatic
- Transaminase levels elevated 5- to 10-fold normal

Prognosis and Therapy

- Vaccines are available to prevent hepatitis A and B infection
- Treatment of patients with hepatitis A and E is usually supportive; the infection is self-limited
  Acute hepatitis B virus infection in neonates carries a 90% risk of progression to chronic liver disease, but only 5% to 10% of adults will develop chronic hepatitis B
- Untreated acute hepatitis C carries a 20% to 50% chance of spontaneous resolution of disease

PATHOLOGIC FEATURES

GROSS FINDINGS

The liver may be swollen and congested with a yellow or green discoloration or shrunken with a "loose" capsule in extensive parenchymal injury or collapse. In cases of submassive or massive hepatic necrosis (Fig. 17.2), the liver may be friable and hemorrhagic with obvious areas of necrosis upon sectioning.

MICROSCOPIC FINDINGS

Acute viral hepatitis represents the prototype acute hepatitis pattern of injury, exhibiting the diffuse lobular-predominant inflammation and hepatocyte injury with lobular disarray (see Figs. 17.3A and B). Acidophil bodies are prominent, and in severe cases, portions of lobules or entire contiguous lobules may undergo necrosis (see Fig. 17.3C).

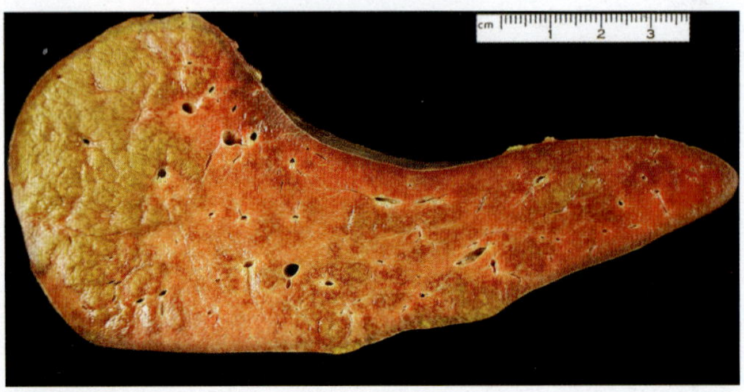

FIGURE 17.2

Massive hepatic necrosis in acute viral hepatitis. The liver is shrunken and soft; islands of regenerating hepatocytes (right) may be localized to one area and mimic a neoplasm.

As part of parenchymal regeneration, there may be pronounced regenerative bile ductular reaction. Cholestasis may be present, including in some cases of hepatitis E (Fig. 17.3D). Portal inflammation may be present but is usually less prominent than the lobular inflammation and injury. Biopsies taken after the initial illness may show only residual Kupffer cell hyperplasia. There is no fibrosis unless the patient has preexisting chronic liver disease.

ACUTE VIRAL (HEPATOTROPIC) HEPATITIS—PATHOLOGIC FEATURES

Gross Findings

- Hepatomegaly
- Congestion; possibly yellow or green discoloration if cholestasis
- In fulminant hepatitis, the liver is friable with hemorrhagic and necrosis areas and the capsule is flaccid

Microscopic Findings

- Lobular disarray caused by hepatocyte injury or necrosis, regeneration, and Kupffer cell hyperplasia
- Predominantly panlobular mononuclear inflammatory infiltrate
  Cholestasis may be present
- Bridging necrosis to submassive or massive necrosis only in severe cases

Differential Diagnosis

- Drug-induced liver injury
- Nonhepatotropic viral hepatitis
- Acute exacerbation of autoimmune hepatitis

ANCILLARY STUDIES

In cases with extensive necrosis, the trichrome stain may be difficult to interpret. In contrast to the bright blue staining collagen in fibrosis, areas of collapsed parenchyma show pale, grayish-blue staining of the collapsed reticulin framework. Reticulin stain highlights the areas of collapse of the normal reticulin framework. Immunohistochemistry (IHC) for viral antigens is not applied in clinical practice because the diagnosis is established through serologic and PCR-based testing.

DIFFERENTIAL DIAGNOSIS

The differential diagnoses include nonhepatotropic viral infections, chronic viral hepatitis, DILI, and AIH. Distinguishing these entities often requires clinical information (e.g., history of travel, new drug or toxins) along with viral serologies and serum autoantibody titers.

Nonhepatotropic viral infections may follow a variable clinical course depending on the specific underlying infection. Classic histologic clues to these diagnoses are discussed in the following section. In chronic viral hepatitis, the inflammatory cell infiltrates are centered within the portal tracts and fibrosis is common.

Prominent lobular inflammation and hepatocyte injury can be seen in AIH; however, AIH is usually associated with brisk interface activity, plasma cells, elevated serum autoantibodies, and polyclonal hypergammaglobulinemia. Exclusion of drug- or toxin-induced injury may be difficult clinically and histologically. Wilson's disease can mimic any clinical or histologic pattern of injury, including acute hepatitis, and a low threshold for performing serum ceruloplasmin and tissue copper quantitation is warranted. The differential diagnosis for submassive or massive necrosis includes infections (e.g., herpes simplex virus [HSV]), vascular injury, and DILI.

Prognosis and Therapy

Viral hepatitis A and E are self-limited diseases that are associated with full recovery within weeks in most patients; treatment is supportive. Most patients with acute hepatitis B virus (HBV) and 20% to 50% of patients with acute hepatitis C experience spontaneous resolution of infection. Newer, highly successful interferon-free antiviral therapies for hepatitis C are available for those who do not clear the virus. Fulminant hepatic failure is rare in patients with hepatitis C but may lead to organ failure and liver transplant.

NONHEPATOTROPIC VIRAL INFECTIONS

Epstein-Barr virus (EBV), cytomegalovirus (CMV), and HSV are the most common nonhepatotropic viruses that cause an acute hepatitis pattern of injury. These infections are typically mild and self-limited except when they occur in infants or immunocompromised patients, in whom they may follow a complicated clinical course with parenchymal necrosis and even hepatic failure and death (especially in HSV infection). The nonhepatotropic viral infections do not progress to chronic hepatitis.

CLINICAL FEATURES

Epstein-Barr virus hepatitis is usually mild and self-limited and may occur in patients of any age as a complication of infectious mononucleosis or in patients without a clinical picture of infectious mononucleosis. Although most patients (≤80%) with infectious mononucleosis exhibit liver enzyme abnormalities, symptomatic hepatitis is uncommon. Symptoms of EBV hepatitis include anorexia, flu-like symptoms, nausea or vomiting, abdominal pain, and weight loss. Jaundice may be seen. Laboratory testing reveals serum lymphocytosis with elevated bilirubin and ALP and ALT elevations that are usually more modest than those seen in patients with hepatotropic viral infections. EBV-associated acute liver failure is rare but described in immunocompetent and immunocompromised patients.

The course of CMV hepatitis varies with the age and immune status of the patient. In immunocompetent hosts, the disease frequently follows a self-limited clinical course and is often asymptomatic. In immunosuppressed hosts, including neonates, older patients, and organ transplant recipients, the infection can manifest with fever, jaundice, and hepatosplenomegaly. Rare fulminant cases have been reported. Patients with CMV hepatitis may show mild hyperbilirubinemia, increased ALP, and increased transaminases (often not exceeding fivefold upper limit of normal).

Herpes simplex virus hepatitis is rare and most often seen in neonates and other immunocompromised patients. The clinical symptoms include fever, mucosal ulcers, hepatomegaly, and systemic constitutional symptoms. AST and ALT are markedly elevated as a reflection of the extensive parenchymal necrosis associated with this infection. HSV hepatitis is rapidly progressive and usually fatal.

NONHEPATOTROPIC VIRAL INFECTIONS—FACT SHEET

Definition

- Nonprogressive forms of hepatitis caused by viruses that do not preferentially affect the liver, including Epstein Barr virus (EBV), cytomegalovirus (CMV), and herpes simplex virus (HSV)

Incidence and Location

- EBV: clinically evident liver disease occurs in minority of patients with infectious mononucleosis and can be seen in the absence of infectious mononucleosis symptoms; worldwide distribution
- CMV: low incidence of clinically evident disease; worldwide distribution
- HSV: low incidence; worldwide distribution

Morbidity and Mortality

- EBV: low
- CMV: low in immunocompetent patients
- HSV: high

Gender, Race, and Age Distribution

- EBV: adolescents and young adults; both genders equally affected
- CMV: clinically apparent hepatitis in immunosuppressed and rarely in immunocompetent patients; both genders equally affected
- HSV: neonates and other immunosuppressed patients; both genders equally affected

Clinical Features

- EBV: often subclinical; anorexia, flulike symptoms, abdominal pain, jaundice, and splenomegaly
- CMV: usually subclinical; fever and hepatosplenomegaly
- HSV: severe acute hepatitis that often evolves into acute liver failure

Prognosis and Therapy

- Variable prognosis, depending on underlying infection and immune status of the host
- Good prognosis in immunocompetent patients with CMV and EBV hepatitis
  Worse prognosis for HSV hepatitis
  Supportive treatment and antivirals (ganciclovir for CMV and acyclovir for HSV infection)
- No propensity to develop chronic hepatitis or progressive fibrosis

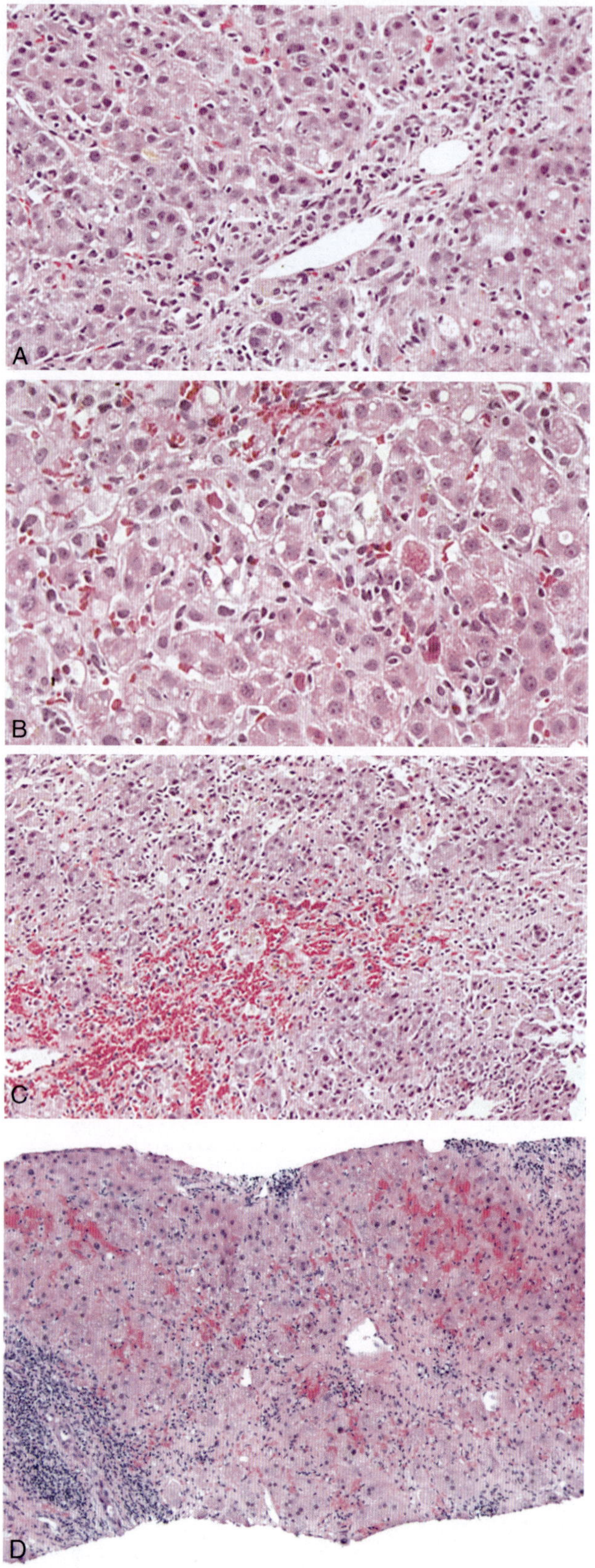

FIGURE 17.3

A, Both portal and lobular inflammation are seen in acute hepatitis; the inflammatory infiltrate is mixed, but mononuclear cells predominate. **B**, Hepatocyte necrosis and regeneration, inflammation, and Kupffer cell hyperplasia contribute to the busy appearance of the lobule (lobular disarray). **C**, Portal-central bridging may be seen in more severe cases and may be an adverse prognostic feature in older patients. **D**, Hepatitis E with classic lobular inflammation and cholestatic changes.

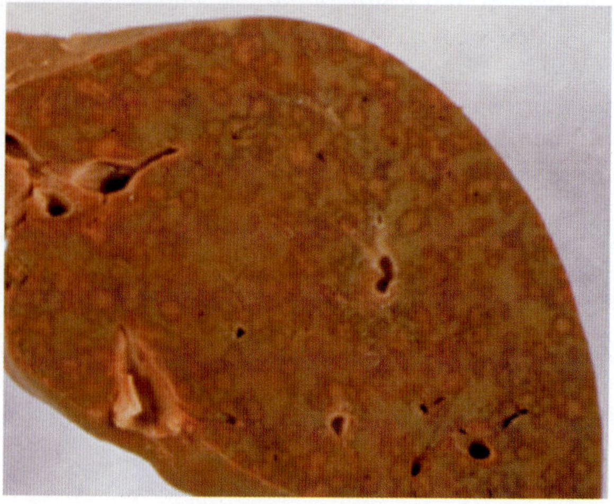

FIGURE 17.4

Areas of geographic necrosis with hyperemic borders are seen in herpes simplex hepatitis.

Pathologic Features

Gross Findings

Mild hepatomegaly and variable congestion are common in all nonhepatotropic viral infections. An HSV-infected liver may show a hyperemic and mottled cut surface with foci of geographic necrosis (Fig. 17.4).

Microscopic Findings

In general, nonhepatotropic viral hepatitis exhibits histologic features similar to those described in hepatotropic virus infections, including lobular-predominant inflammation and hepatocyte injury.

The most characteristic histologic feature of EBV hepatitis is "sinusoidal lymphocytosis" characterized by a diffuse sinusoidal infiltrate typically composed of small lymphocytes arranged in a single-file "string-of-beads" pattern (Fig. 17.5A). Acidophil bodies are rare. Small lobular Kupffer cell aggregates may be present. The portal tracts demonstrate mild lymphocytic infiltrates but significant interface hepatitis. Immunosuppressed patients may show more pronounced necroinflammatory activity and even bile duct injury. Extensive necrosis is only seen in those with fulminant EBV hepatitis (Fig. 17.5B).

Cytomegalovirus hepatitis histologically mimics EBV infection in immunocompetent hosts. The typical intranuclear or intracytoplasmic viral inclusions that are often present in immunocompromised patients may not be seen. As with other causes of acute hepatitis, lobular inflammation and injury predominate. Acidophil bodies and spotty necrosis are common. Neutrophilic microabscesses may be seen but are neither sensitive nor specific for CMV hepatitis. Diagnostic viral inclusions can be detected on hematoxylin and eosin (H&E) stain or IHC in infected endothelial cells, hepatocytes, or biliary epithelial cells (Fig. 17.6).

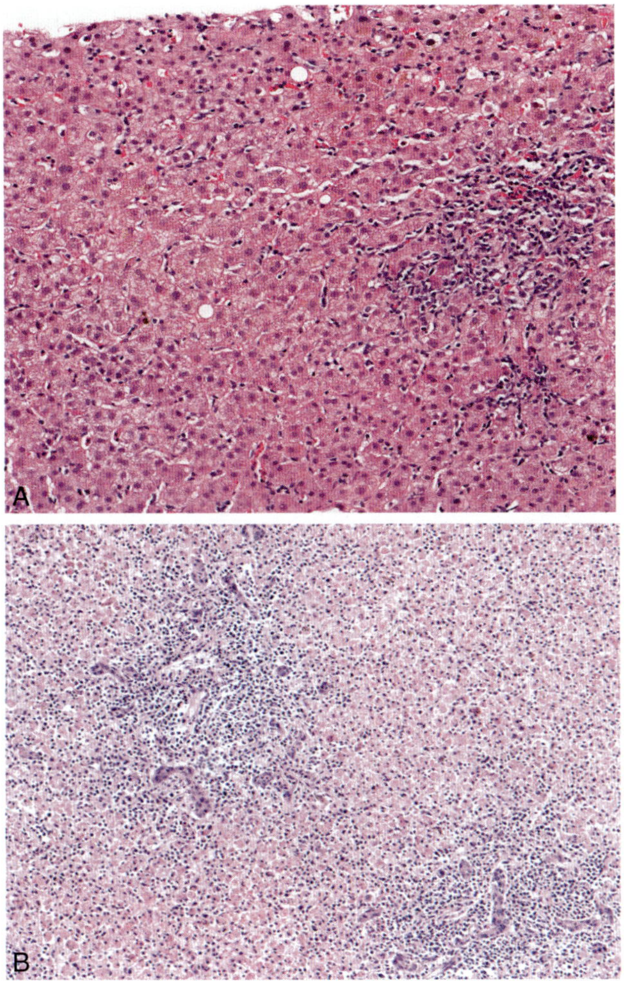

FIGURE 17.5

A, Prominent sinusoidal lymphocytosis with minimal hepatocellular injury is characteristic of Epstein-Barr virus (EBV) hepatitis. **B**, In a small subset of cases, EBV infection can lead to massive hepatic necrosis.

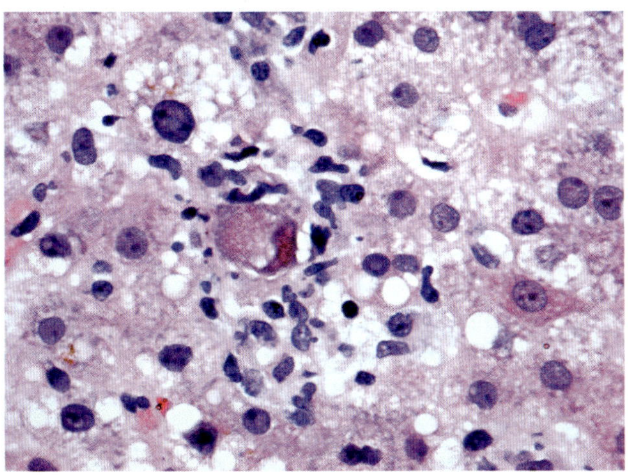

FIGURE 17.6

In immunocompromised hosts, enlarged cells with intranuclear inclusions are found in variable numbers. Associated microabscesses are often seen in liver transplant cases but are not specific for cytomegalovirus infection.

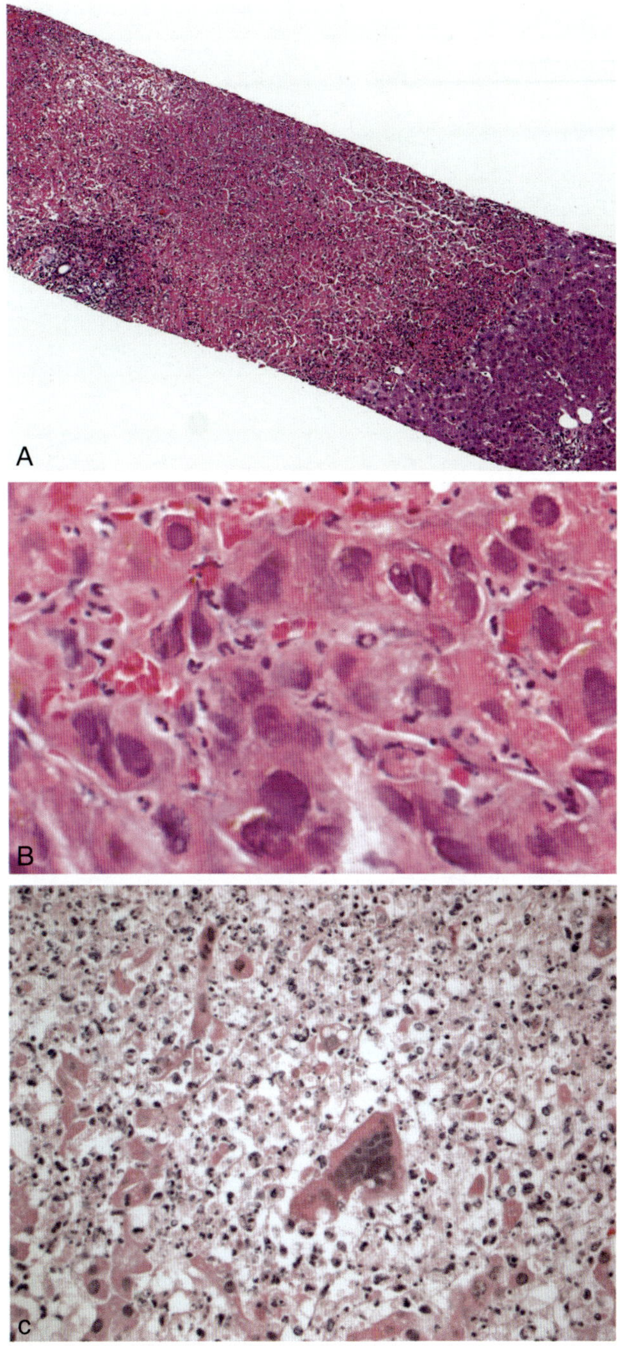

FIGURE 17.7

A, Herpes simplex hepatitis with areas of geographic necrosis. **B**, Infected cells contain ground-glass nuclear inclusions. **C**, Multinucleated cells may be seen in a background of extensive necrosis in this case.

Herpes simplex virus hepatitis has distinct histologic features, which, when present, should promptly suggest this diagnosis. The hepatic parenchyma typically shows irregular foci of nonzonal or "geographic" necrosis (Fig. 17.7A) with relatively mild lobular and portal chronic inflammation. Diagnostic viral inclusions (Cowdry type A) with multinucleation, margination, and molding are usually present within viable hepatocytes adjacent to foci of necrosis (Figs. 17.7B and C). IHC may be needed to confirm the diagnosis.

NONHEPATOTROPIC VIRAL INFECTIONS—PATHOLOGIC FEATURES

Gross Findings

- Hepatomegaly
- Herpes simplex virus (HSV): geographic necrosis with hyperemic borders

Microscopic Findings

- Epstein-Barr virus (EBV): sinusoidal lymphocytic infiltrate ("string of pearls")
- Cytomegalovirus (CMV): neutrophilic microabscesses and intranuclear or cytoplasmic inclusions
- HSV: geographic necrosis and Cowdry A-type inclusions

Ancillary Studies

- EBV: scattered positive lymphocytes on chromogenic in situ hybridization
- CMV: positive viral inclusions on immunohistochemistry
- HSV: positive viral inclusions on immunohistochemistry

Differential Diagnosis

- Other causes of acute hepatitis, including the hepatotropic viruses (hepatitis A, B, C, D, E)
- Drug-induced liver injury
- Other hepatic infections

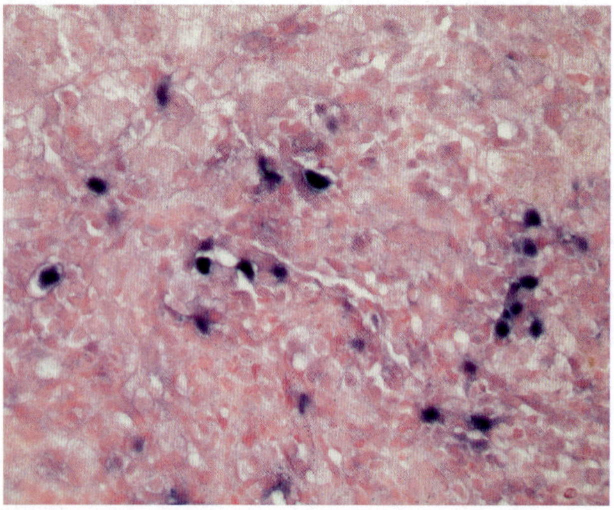

FIGURE 17.8

Epstein-Barr virus (EBV)-encoded small RNA demonstrate occasional positive cells in a case of Epstein-Barr virus hepatitis.

ANCILLARY STUDIES

Serologic testing and PCR-based assay are used clinically to establish the diagnosis and exclude other causes of hepatitis. Immunohistochemical stains (especially for CMV and HSV) and chromogenic in situ hybridization (CISH) for EBV-encoded RNA (EBER) are widely available. EBER-positive lymphocytes are rare in EBV-infected patients; most of the lymphocytes seen in EBV hepatitis do not show positive EBV staining (Fig. 17.8).

DIFFERENTIAL DIAGNOSIS

The differential diagnosis includes other causes of acute hepatitis, including hepatotropic and other nonhepatotropic viral infections (adenovirus, human herpesvirus 6A, parvovirus), other hepatic infections, and DILI. In cases of suspected EBV hepatitis, specimens showing "atypical lymphocytes" should be investigated carefully to exclude the involvement of a lymphoproliferative disorder.

In cases with extensive hepatic necrosis, ischemia and DILI should be considered. The zonal distribution of necrosis (predominantly zone 3), clinical history, and absence of viral inclusions are helpful in distinguishing these entities.

PROGNOSIS AND THERAPY

In immunocompetent patients, the disease course is self-limited, and symptoms usually resolve in 4 to 6 weeks. In immunocompromised individuals, the disease follows a more severe course and may result in acute liver failure.

In most patients, antiviral therapy is not required. Ganciclovir is administered to CMV-infected patients who are at risk of severe or life-threatening illness. HSV is often treated with acyclovir, but the outcome is generally poor.

CHRONIC HEPATITIS PATTERN OF INJURY

Chronic hepatitis is defined histologically as a pattern of ongoing hepatitis with portal-based inflammation and fibrosis in which hepatocytes are the primary site of injury. Symptoms vary and are often vague or nonspecific, consisting of constitutional symptoms, abdominal pain, nausea, and malaise. Many patients are asymptomatic, and some may present with decompensated cirrhosis or acute liver failure. The histologic differential diagnosis for this pattern of injury is broad and includes causes of chronic hepatitis (chronic viral hepatitis [hepatitis B and hepatitis C], AIH, and DILI) in addition to certain inherited diseases (Wilson's disease and α1AT deficiency) and early stages of primary biliary disorders (primary sclerosing cholangitis [PSC], primary biliary cholangitis [PBC]).

A liver biopsy may be performed to confirm the overall pattern of injury, establish the diagnosis, grade and stage the disease, and assess for other superimposed patterns of injury (e.g., steatosis) that may impact management and prognosis. The histologic hallmarks of chronic hepatitis pattern of injury are the dense portal inflammatory cell infiltrates and often fibrosis. The portal infiltrates are predominantly lymphocytic and may be admixed with other inflammatory cells, including plasma cells. Interface activity (piecemeal necrosis) and variable necroinflammatory lobular activity are often also seen. Periods of disease flare typically show more prominent interface activity and lobular necroinflammatory activity, including confluent necrosis in severe cases. Some cases show mild bile duct injury, but destructive bile duct lesions are not a feature. Bile ductular proliferation may be evident in advanced fibrosis or extensive necrosis.

Biopsies from patients with chronic hepatitis (hepatitis B or C; AIH) may be assigned a semiquantitative "grade" and "stage" to indicate the degree of necroinflammatory activity and fibrosis, respectively. There are several semiquantitative systems for grading and staging chronic hepatitis, including the Ishak, Knodell, Scheuer, Metavir, and Batts and Ludwig systems (Table 17.2). All have been clinically validated with good interobserver reproducibility. The choice of system is often made in partnership with the clinical team to ensure clear and consistent communication. Many centers prefer the Batts and Ludwig system, in which necroinflammatory activity (grade) (Fig. 17.9) and fibrosis (stage) (Fig. 17.10) are assessed using a 0 to 4 scale. Specimen adequacy is an important consideration. An adequate liver biopsy is at least 2 cm in length and contains at least 11 portal tracts. Subcapsular biopsy samples (including subcapsular wedge biopsies) cannot be accurately staged because the normal extension of the hepatic capsule a few millimeters into the subcapsular parenchyma may be interpreted as fibrosis and result in over-staging. The limitations of subcapsular or suboptimal (small or fragmented biopsies) should be clearly stated in the pathology report. If bridging necrosis is present, the trichrome

TABLE 17.2
Batts and Ludwig Staging System

Grading	Staging
0: portal inflammation only, no interface activity, no lobular inflammation	0: none
1: portal inflammation, minimal patchy interface activity, spotty lobular necroinflammatory activity	1: fibrous portal expansion
2: mild portal inflammation, mild interface activity involving some or all portal tracts, mild lobular necroinflammatory activity	2: periportal fibrosis (allows rare delicate thin septa)
3: portal inflammation, moderate interface activity involving all portal tracts, moderate lobular necroinflammatory activity with noticeable hepatocellular injury	3: bridging fibrosis
4: portal inflammation, severe interface activity, severe lobular necroinflammatory activity with bridging necrosis	4: cirrhosis

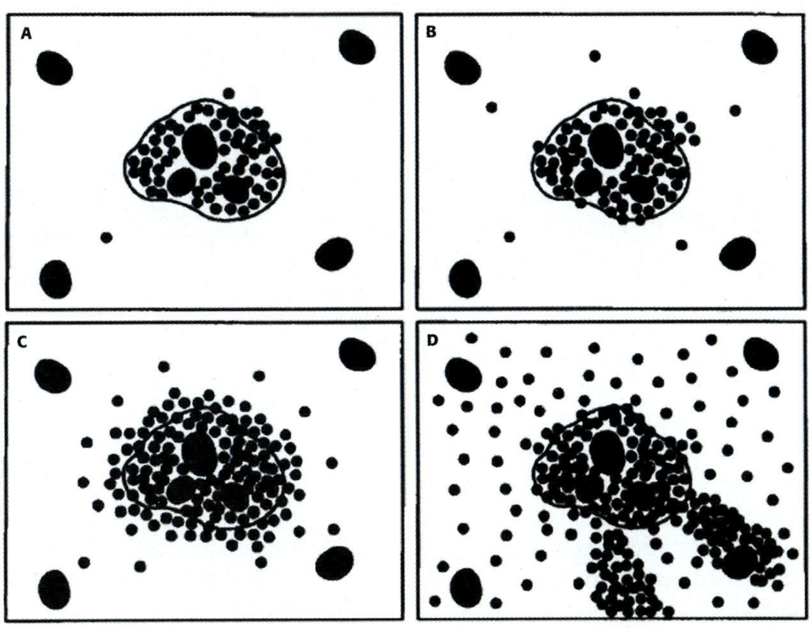

FIGURE 17.9
Grading chronic hepatitis based on Batts and Ludwig classification system. **A**, Minimal activity (grade 1): mild portal inflammation with scant piecemeal necrosis and no lobular necrosis. **B**, Mild activity (grade 2): mild portal inflammation, piecemeal necrosis and scant lobular inflammation. **C**, Moderate activity (grade 3): moderate portal inflammation, piecemeal necrosis and lobular spotty necrosis. **D**, Severe activity (grade 4): marked portal inflammation, brisk piecemeal necrosis, considerable spotty necrosis, and areas of confluent necrosis leading to bridging. (From Batts KP, Ludwig J. Chronic hepatitis. An update on terminology and reporting. *Am J Surg Pathol.* 1995;19:1409–1417.)

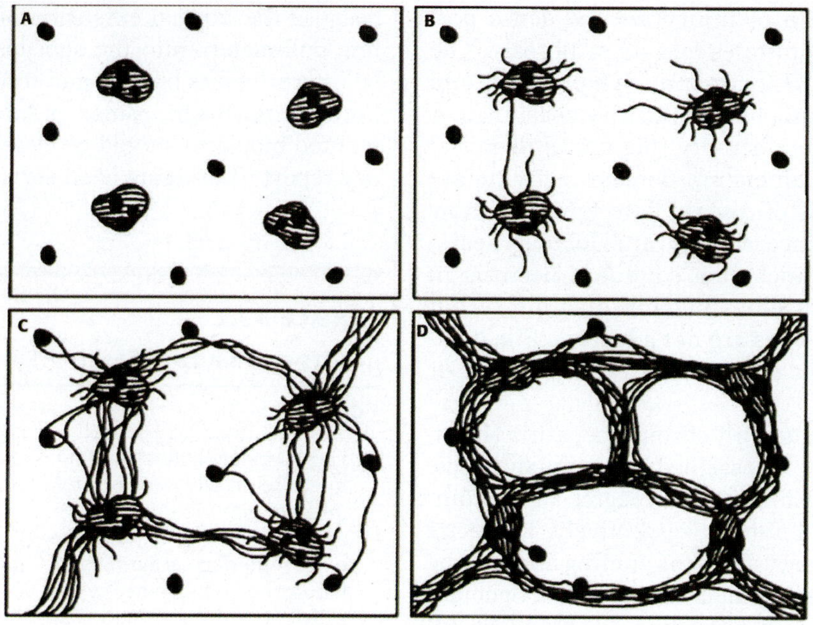

FIGURE 17.10

Staging chronic hepatitis based on Batts and Ludwig classification system. **A**, Portal fibrosis (stage 1): mild fibrous portal expansion of portal tracts. **B**, Periportal fibrosis (stage 2): fine strands of connective tissue in zone 1 with only rare portal–portal septa. **C**, Bridging (septal) fibrosis (stage 3): connective tissue bridges that link portal tracts to other portal tracts and central veins, minimally distorted architecture but no regenerative nodules. **D**, Cirrhosis (stage 4): bridging fibrosis and nodular regeneration. (From Batts KP, Ludwig J. Chronic hepatitis. An update on terminology and reporting. *Am J Surg Pathol*. 1995;19:1409–1417.)

stain may be difficult to interpret, and areas of reticulin collapse may result in overestimation of the degree of fibrosis.

CHRONIC VIRAL HEPATITIS

CLINICAL FEATURES

Chronic viral hepatitis has a wide spectrum of clinical manifestations, ranging from asymptomatic infection to decompensated cirrhosis. Symptomatic patients have mild, nonspecific symptoms such as fatigue, anorexia, and weight loss. Patients with cirrhosis may present with esophageal varices, hepatosplenomegaly, spider angiomata, ascites, peripheral edema, muscle wasting, and abdominal collateral blood vessels.

Serum transaminase levels are usually elevated in the 2- to 10-fold range of normal, although patients with mild chronic viral hepatitis may have normal transaminase levels. ALP and bilirubin levels are usually normal to mildly elevated unless hepatic decompensation occurs. Low-titer nonspecific autoantibodies, especially anti–liver/kidney microsomal 1 antibodies (anti-LKM1) and smooth muscle actin (SMA), have been reported in this setting. Fibrosing cholestatic hepatitis (FCH) is a severe, rapidly progressive form of hepatitis B or C that occurs in immunosuppressed or immunocompromised patients.

CHRONIC VIRAL HEPATITIS—FACT SHEET

Definition

- Chronic viral (hepatitis B, C) infection

Incidence and Location

- Common worldwide
- Approximately 3% of world population (~184 million) has hepatitis C infection
  Approximately 240 million people (3.7%) worldwide are chronically infected with hepatitis B (defined as hepatitis B surface antigen positive for at least 6 months)
- Less than 1% of the population in Western Europe and North America is chronically infected with hepatitis B, but the prevalence in endemic regions is up to 10%

Morbidity and Mortality

- Chronic viral hepatitis accounts for a significant number of deaths per year worldwide (estimated as 786,000 cases caused by hepatitis B and ~500,000 cases caused by hepatitis C in 2010)
- Risk of hepatocellular carcinoma is high in chronic viral hepatitis, particularly hepatitis B

Gender, Race, and Age Distribution

- Both genders and all races are equally affected
- Wide age range for both hepatitis B and hepatitis C; hepatitis B is commonly acquired perinatally in high-incidence areas

Clinical Features

- Commonly asymptomatic at diagnosis or may present with mild nonspecific symptoms
- Patients with late-stage disease exhibit signs of chronic liver disease

Prognosis and Therapy

- Treatment for chronic hepatitis B includes oral antiviral agents, such as tenofovir or entecavir. Interferon injections may be considered in certain cases. A vaccine is available to prevent infection
- Newer, highly effective treatment options for hepatitis C include interferon-free regimens with direct antiviral agents
  The prognosis for hepatitis B is related to severity of liver disease at presentation
- The prognosis for hepatitis C is variable; risk factors for progression of untreated or refractory disease include presence of fibrosis in liver biopsy, immune status, alcohol use, viral genotype, age older than 50 years at infection, and male gender

PATHOLOGIC FEATURES

GROSS FINDINGS

Early-stage chronic viral hepatitis shows no specific macroscopic features of chronic viral hepatitis. The liver becomes firm as fibrosis progresses. Late-stage disease is grossly evident as cirrhosis.

MICROSCOPIC FINDINGS

The microscopic findings include the characteristic features of chronic hepatitis pattern of injury: portal inflammation with or without fibrosis and variable degrees of interface hepatitis and lobular necroinflammatory activity. The portal tracts are expanded by inflammatory infiltrates composed of mostly lymphocytes with variable plasma cells and other inflammatory cells. Lymphoid follicles with prominent germinal centers may be seen (Fig. 17.11A). Mild bile duct injury with intraepithelial lymphocytes may be seen, but there are no destructive bile duct lesions. Interface activity, also known as "interface hepatitis" or "piecemeal necrosis," is a frequent feature (Fig. 17.11B). It is characterized by extension of the portal inflammation beyond the "limiting plate" into the periportal hepatic lobule and accompanying hepatocyte injury or necrosis.

In most cases, lobular inflammation consists of randomly scattered lobular collections of mononuclear cells associated with hepatocyte injury or acidophil bodies (Fig. 17.11C), but confluent and even bridging necrosis can be seen (Fig. 17.11D). Ground-glass hepatocytes (Fig. 17.11E) are a characteristic feature of HBV infection but are only seen in patients with chronic HBV in the setting of active viral replication.

Fibrosis in chronic viral hepatitis is portal-based and evolves to extend into the periportal region (Fig. 17.12). Bridging fibrosis occurs as portal–portal or portal–central fibrous septa. The end result is cirrhosis.

OTHER FINDINGS

Steatosis in hepatitis C can occur in patients with concomitant nonalcoholic fatty liver disease (NAFLD) and as a direct effect of the virus in patients with hepatitis C virus (HCV) genotype 3 infection. HCV infection is also associated with greater insulin resistance and metabolic syndrome, and, when present, both steatosis and insulin resistance predict rapid progression of fibrosis, poor response rate to interferon therapy (even in HCV genotype 3 infection), and an increased risk of hepatocellular carcinoma.

FIBROSING CHOLESTATIC HEPATITIS

The FCH variant of HBV and HCV is an aggressive form of hepatitis that typically occurs in immunosuppressed patients. FCH is characterized by prominent perisinusoidal/pericellular fibrosis occurring in the periportal region, ductular reaction, hepatocellular injury including hepatocyte swelling and ground-glass inclusions (in HBV), and prominent intracellular and canalicular cholestasis (Fig. 17.13). The biopsy usually lacks significant inflammatory infiltrates.

CHRONIC VIRAL HEPATITIS—PATHOLOGIC FEATURES

Gross Findings

- Firm consistency if increased fibrosis
- Cirrhotic livers with brown discoloration and greenish hue, particularly in cases with end-stage cholestasis

Microscopic Findings

- Mononuclear portal-predominant inflammatory infiltrates
- Interface hepatitis is variable
- Lobular activity is manifested by acidophilic bodies and scattered foci of lobular inflammatory infiltrates
- Confluent necrosis may be seen in severe disease or with superimposed acute injury
- Fibrosis is portal based and evolves to involve the periportal areas, with eventual portal–portal and portal–central bridging and cirrhosis

Differential Diagnosis

- Autoimmune hepatitis
- Drug-induced liver injury
- Early chronic cholestatic conditions (primary sclerosing cholangitis, primary biliary cholangitis)
- Lymphoma or leukemic infiltrate
- Wilson's disease
- α1-Antitrypsin

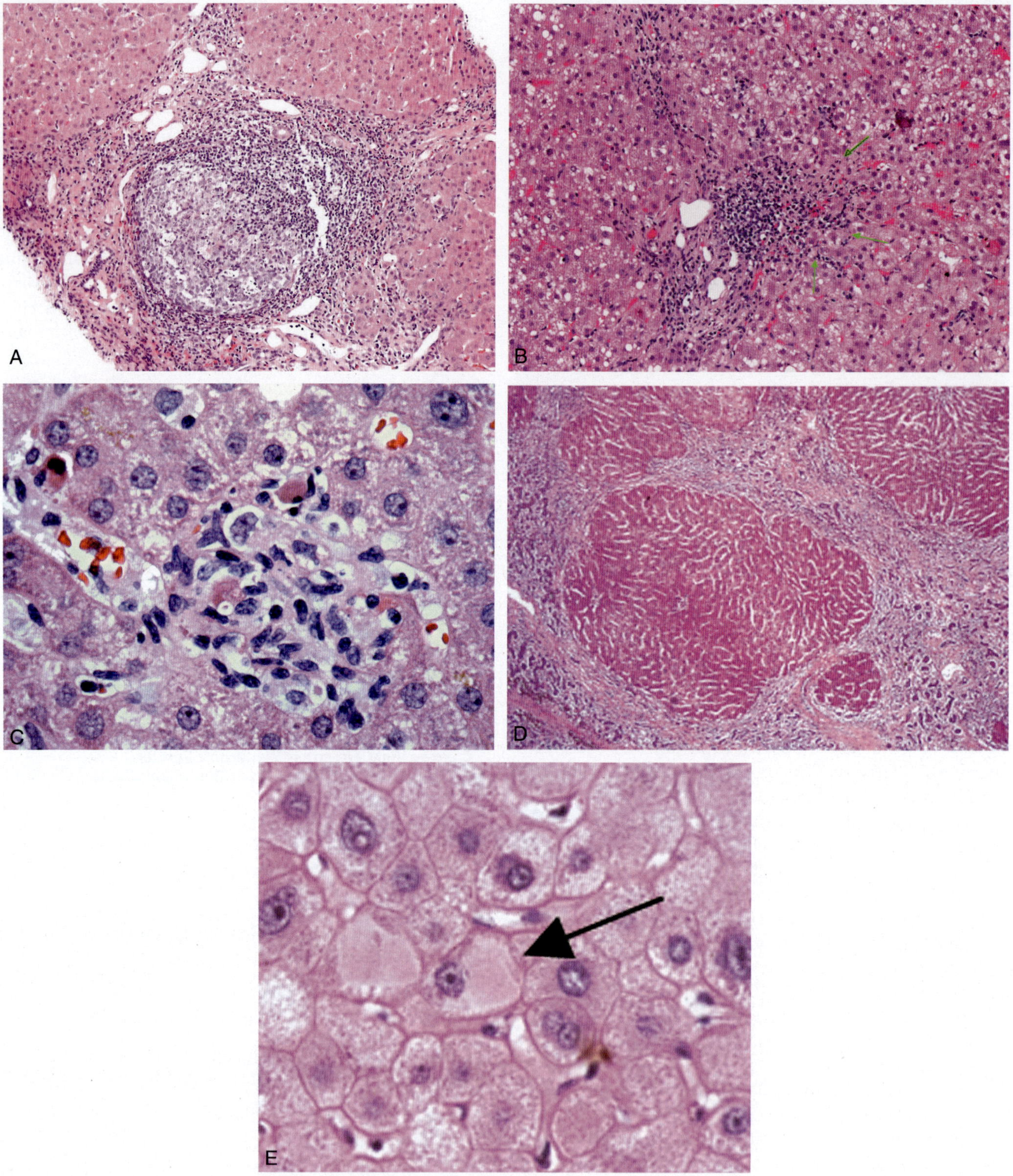

FIGURE 17.11

A, Portal tracts are expanded by an exuberant inflammatory infiltrate with prominent germinal center in this case of chronic viral hepatitis. Interlobular bile ducts show no significant injury. **B**, Lymphocytic inflammation extending into the lobular region (interface hepatitis, *arrows*), causing focal hepatocyte injury. **C**, Lobular activity is variable; small collections of mononuclear inflammatory cells mark sites of lytic necrosis of hepatocytes. **D**, Massive hepatic necrosis in acute viral hepatitis. Collapse of the parenchymal framework may be mistaken for cirrhosis. Bile ductular reaction is common. **E**, Ground glass cytoplasmic inclusions in hepatitis B infection.

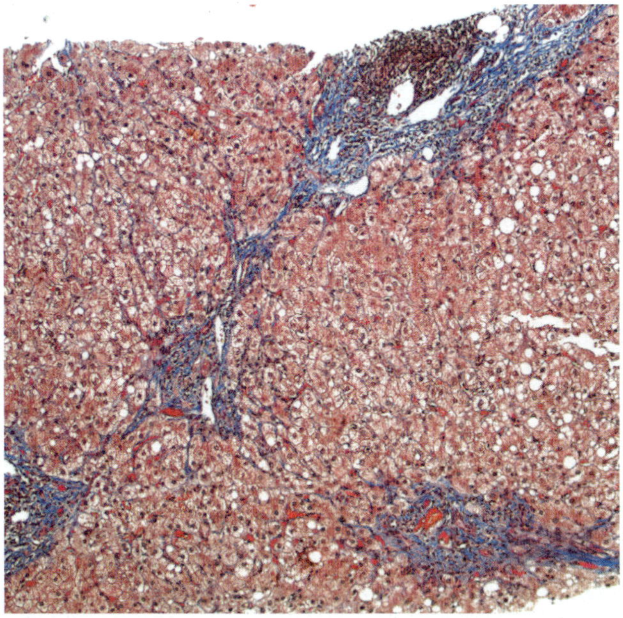

FIGURE 17.12

Portal-based fibrosis is the norm in chronic hepatitis, in this case, periportal to early bridging fibrosis.

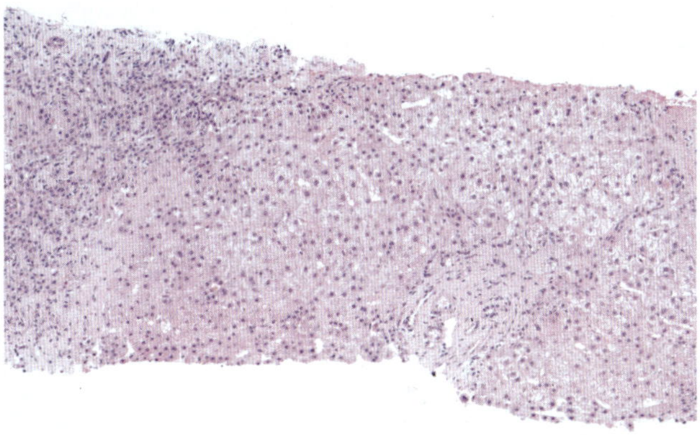

FIGURE 17.13

Diffuse swelling of hepatocytes with pale appearance and bile ductular proliferation, characteristic of early stages of fibrosing cholestatic hepatitis C.

Ancillary Studies

For chronic HBV and HBC infection, the diagnosis is based on serologic testing and confirmatory RNA or DNA by PCR to exclude false-positive serologies (as can occur in the setting of AIH). Cytoplasmic and nuclear accumulation of hepatitis B core antigen (HBcAg) (Fig. 17.14A) may be detected by IHC and correlates with active replication of the virus. However, immunohistochemical stains for surface (Fig. 17.14B) and core antigens (HBV and HCV) are rarely helpful or required in daily practice.

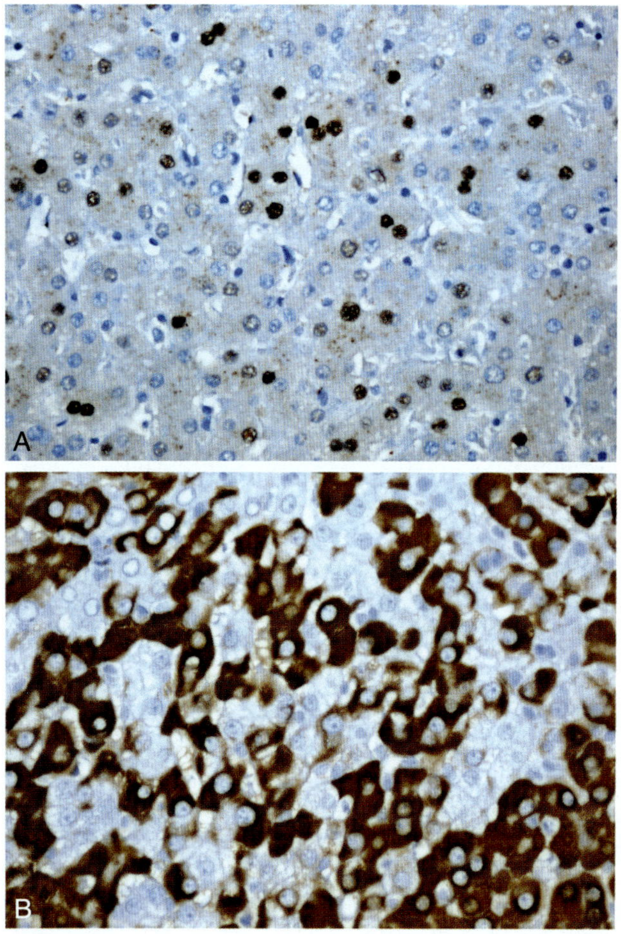

FIGURE 17.14

A, Core antigen (HBcAg) immunohistochemistry showing nuclear positivity in approximately half of the nuclei in this biopsy, with only trace amounts of core antigen seen in the cytoplasm. Cytoplasmic HBcAg staining correlates with high necroinflammatory activity. **B**, Immunohistochemistry for hepatitis B surface antigen shows accumulation of HBsAg in hepatocytes.

Differential Diagnosis

The histologic differential diagnosis of chronic viral hepatitis primarily includes AIH, primary biliary disorders, Wilson's disease, α1AT deficiency, DILI, and low-grade lymphoproliferative disorders. Serologic and PCR-based testing are essential in distinguishing these entities. Ground-glass hepatocytes are associated with chronic HBV infection but are only present in the setting of active viral replication. Similar-appearing cytoplasmic inclusions ("pseudo-ground-glass change") have been described in other conditions, such as cyanamide toxicity, type IV glycogen storage disease (GSD). Lafora disease, uremia, transplant recipients, patients taking numerous medications, and immunosuppressed patients. Extensive plasma cell inflammatory infiltrates and more extensive interface activity with concurrent lobular necroinflammatory activity favor AIH.

Like chronic viral hepatitis, the early stages of PBC and PSC show portal-based inflammation and fibrosis. Elevated serum ALP, positive antimitochondrial antibodies (AMAs) (in PBC), or endoscopic retrograde cholangiopancreatography (ERCP) (in the case of PSC) help distinguish these entities from chronic viral hepatitis.

Wilson's disease usually affects young individuals and can be clinically excluded by the serum ceruloplasmin level, 24-hour urine copper levels, and quantitative copper on liver tissue analysis. A1AT deficiency is characterized by the accumulation of PAS-positive, diastase-resistant cytoplasmic globules in hepatocytes.

Drug-induced liver injury (discussed later in this chapter) must also be considered; medication history is key to diagnosis. Rarely, lymphoproliferative disorders, in particular low-grade B-cell lymphomas, can mimic chronic hepatitis. Monotonous or expansile lymphoid infiltrates should raise suspicion for lymphoma. Immunohistochemical stains and flow cytometry help differentiate lymphoma from chronic hepatitis.

Prognosis and Therapy

Patients with chronic hepatitis B infection can be treated with oral antiviral agents. The treatment suppresses viral replication and thus slows the progression to cirrhosis and improves long-term survival. In general, the regimens include a combination of interferon and nucleos(t)ide analogues, including tenofovir or entecavir. Vaccines are available.

The therapeutic map for hepatitis C is rapidly changing with the introduction of newer interferon-free regimens that are highly effective in achieving sustained serologic response. The newer antiviral drugs are more effective and better tolerated than interferon-based therapies.

Fibrosing cholestatic hepatitis C (hepatitis B or hepatitis C) has been linked to rapid disease progression, liver failure, and poor prognosis, although newer antiviral therapies for hepatitis C in particular may be responsible for better outcomes in this subset of cases.

AUTOIMMUNE HEPATITIS

CLINICAL FEATURES

Autoimmune hepatitis is an immune-mediated hepatitis characterized by a combination of clinical, laboratory, and histologic findings of hepatitis that predominantly affects young to middle-aged women. It is an a priori chronic form of hepatitis with phases of acute exacerbations. The presenting symptoms are highly variable and include anorexia, jaundice, hepatomegaly, and abdominal pain. However, the diagnosis should be considered in any patient with elevated transaminases of any duration. Between 10% and 20% of patients present with acute liver failure, but presentation with clinical features of an acute or chronic hepatitis is far more common.

Transaminase elevation is a consistent feature of AIH, and nearly all patients exhibit elevated serum immunoglobulin (Ig) G levels at the time of diagnosis. Autoantibodies including anti–smooth muscle antibodies (ASMAs) and antinuclear antibodies (ANAs), can be detected in most patients but are not required for the diagnosis. Anti-LKM1 are most often seen in young female patients (including adolescents and children). These autoantibodies are not specific and can be present in other conditions including alcoholic liver disease, NAFLD, PBC, and PSC, among others. Hepatitis C antibodies can also be falsely positive in patients with AIH and remain positive after effective HCV treatment; for this reason, confirmatory RNA testing is used to confirm or exclude HCV infection. Hyperbilirubinemia and ALP elevations may be seen in patients with severe hepatitis and extensive hepatocyte injury and in the setting of AIH–PBC overlap.

Given the multiple elements (clinical, serologic, and histologic) that contribute to the diagnosis, a detailed scoring system for diagnosing AIH was established by the International Autoimmune Hepatitis Group and later simplified by Hennes et al. (Table 17.3). Rapid response to immunosuppression is typical.

TABLE 17.3

Parameters Included in the Simplified Scoring System for the Diagnosis of Autoimmune Hepatitis

Parameters
ANA or SMA titers ≥1:40 → 1 point
ANA or SMA titers ≥1:80 or LKM titer ≥1:40 or SLA positive → 2 points
(The sum of both results was limited to 2 points)
IgG levels >UNL → 1 point
IgG levels >1.10 UNL (>10% above UNL) > 2 points
Liver histology compatible or typical for AIH → 1, or 2 points
Exclusion of viral hepatitis → 2 points
Cumulative score interpretation:
• ≥6: probable AIH
• ≥7: definite AIH

AIH, Autoimmune hepatitis; *ANA*, antinuclear antibodies; *Ig*, immunoglobulin; *LKM*, liver-kidney microsomal antibodies; *SLA*, *SMA*, smooth muscle actin; *UNL, upper normal limit.*

Based on Hennes EM, Zeniya M, Czaja AJ, et al. Simplified criteria for the diagnosis of autoimmune hepatitis. *Hepatology*. 2008;48(1):169–176.

AUTOIMMUNE HEPATITIS—FACT SHEET

Definition

- Ongoing immune-mediated hepatitis

Incidence and Location

- Incidence is approximately 0.1 to 1.9 per 100,000 per year in Northern Europe and North American white populations
- Rare in Asia and Africa

Morbidity and Mortality

- High rate of complications (from cirrhosis to acute liver failure) if left untreated
- 50% 5-year mortality rate if untreated

Gender, Race, and Age Distribution

- Predominantly young to middle-aged women
- More common in patients of European descent

Clinical Features

- Often presents abruptly, similar to acute viral hepatitis
- Anorexia, jaundice, hepatomegaly, abdominal pain
- May present with arthralgia and skin rash
- Marked elevation of transaminases
- Polyclonal hypergammaglobulinemia
- Positive autoantibodies: antinuclear antibodies, SMA, and/or liver-kidney microsomal antibodies

Prognosis and Therapy

- Ongoing and variable clinical course, often with flares
- Corticosteroids and other immunosuppressants significantly improve survival

Pathologic Features

Gross Findings

The gross appearance of the liver in AIH is variable. For patients presenting with an acute fulminant course, massive hepatic necrosis results in a shrunken liver with a flaccid capsule. Islands of regenerating or preserved hepatic parenchyma often show greenish hue caused by cholestasis. The liver is firm in advanced fibrosis and diffusely nodular in cirrhosis.

Microscopic Findings

Autoimmune hepatitis most commonly presents a chronic hepatitis pattern of injury followed by acute hepatitis and cholestatic hepatitis patterns. The classic histologic findings include a chronic hepatitis with well-developed interface hepatitis and lobular necroinflammatory activity. Most cases reveal dense portal lymphoplasmacytic infiltrates, often with plasma cell aggregates. Prominent plasma cells are a frequent but not required feature. Interface hepatitis is often prominent in untreated AIH (Fig. 17.15A). The lobules demonstrate several foci of necroinflammatory activity, including perivenular plasma cell–rich inflammatory cell infiltrates and hepatocyte necrosis. Acidophil bodies may be frequent, and patients experiencing an acute exacerbation may show diffuse hepatocyte swelling with lobular disarray (Fig. 17.15B). Kupffer cell hyperplasia can be seen, but well-formed epithelioid granulomas are not a feature of AIH. A panel of pathology experts recently published a set of criteria to aid in the histologic diagnosis of AIH. In this publication (Lohse et al., 2022), portal or lobular lymphoplasmacytic infiltrates along with more than mild interface activity and portal based fibrosis remain importan features in the diagnosis.

Bile duct injury, if present, tends to be patchy, mild, and most commonly associated with lymphocytic injury. Destructive bile duct lesions or "florid duct lesions" are not a feature of AIH and, if present, should raise concern for an AIH–PBC overlap syndrome, DILI, or other forms of liver disease. Portal-based fibrosis is often present at initial presentation.

In a subset of cases, an acute hepatitis or acute-on-chronic hepatitis pattern of injury predominates. In these biopsies, the lobular inflammation and injury predominates, with prominent hepatocellular swelling, lobular disarray, and regenerative changes, including hepatocellular rosettes (Fig. 17.15C) and bile ductular proliferation. In severe cases, extensive necroinflammatory activity leads to bridging necrosis and even massive hepatic necrosis with parenchymal collapse (Fig. 17.15D). Transformation of hepatocytes into syncytial multinucleated giant cells (acute hepatitis with giant cell transformation) can also be present. Hepatocanalicular cholestasis may be seen in the acute phase of exacerbation and present as an acute cholestatic hepatitis pattern of injury.

AUTOIMMUNE HEPATITIS—PATHOLOGIC FEATURES

Gross Findings

- Cases of acute fulminant disease may show massive hepatic necrosis
- In end-stage disease, the liver shows evidence of cirrhosis

Microscopic Findings

- Chronic hepatitis pattern of injury
- Usually well-established interface hepatitis and lobular necroinflammatory activity in untreated disease
  Plasma cells may be prominent in portal tracts and perivenular locations
- Variable fibrosis, from portal expansion to portal–portal or portal–central bridging and cirrhosis

Genetics

- Genetic predisposition associated with human leukocyte antigen A1-B8-DR haplotype

Differential Diagnosis

- Viral hepatitis (especially hepatitis B and C)
- Primary biliary cholangitis and primary sclerosing cholangitis
- Drug-induced liver injury

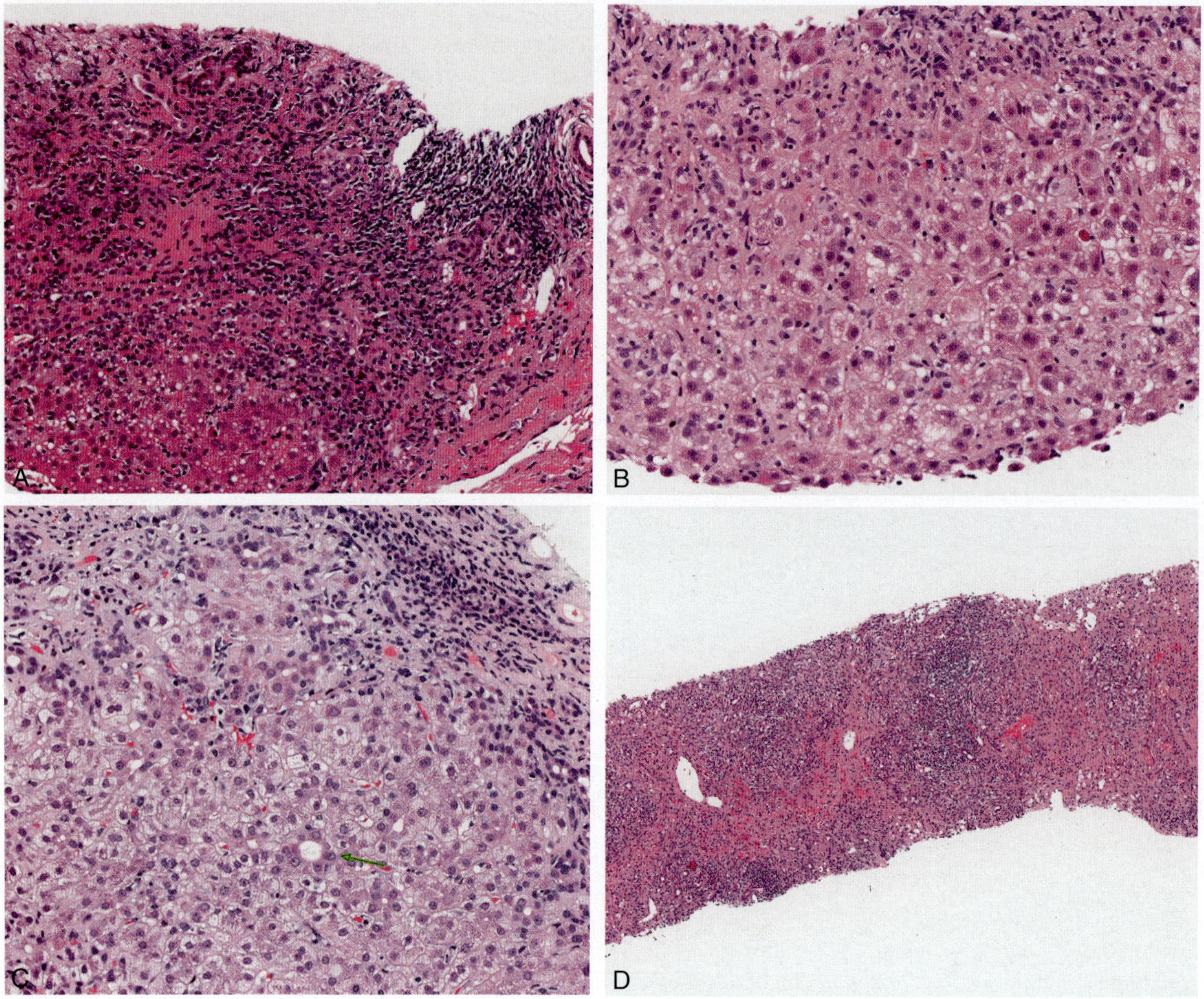

FIGURE 17.15

A, Interface hepatitis and lobular activity are often pronounced in autoimmune hepatitis; plasma cells in clusters in the inflammatory infiltrate are a helpful but relatively nonspecific feature of AIH. **B**, Lobular disarray with scattered acidophil bodies. **C**, Hepatocyte regeneration may lead to formation of hepatocyte rosettes (*arrow*). **D**, Cases with severe acute AIH can demonstrate extensive lobular necrosis and collapse.

These histologic changes may be significantly reduced or even absent after immunosuppressive therapy.

Differential Diagnosis

The differential diagnosis for AIH includes chronic viral hepatitis, DILI, and early stages of primary biliary disorders, among others. Viral serologies and PCR-based testing are used to exclude chronic viral hepatitis, which often shows less extensive interface hepatitis and lobular necroinflammatory activity than AIH. As opposed to PBC, AIH exhibits only minimal bile duct injury without duct destruction and a hepatitic rather than cholestatic pattern of liver enzyme abnormalities.

Drugs can cause an AIH-like clinical and histologic picture with autoantibodies and hypergammaglobulinemia at any time after initiating the medication. Drugs associated with an AIH-like pattern of injury include nitrofurantoin, minocycline, diclofenac, infliximab, atorvastatin, and other statins and hydralazine, methyldopa, and anti–tumor necrosis factor-α (anti–TNF-α) agents, among others. DILI is a diagnosis of exclusion and requires clinical correlation. The LiverTox website is a helpful database to search for medications known to induce liver injury. Wilson's disease can rarely present with features of AIH; however, clinical and laboratory findings are helpful in separating these entities.

Prognosis and Therapy

The goals of treatment are to induce or maintain remission and prevent progression of disease. Most patients experience a rapid response to immunosuppressive therapy, which typically includes steroids with or without azathioprine. Treatment-refractory cases are well recognized. Relapse is common upon withdrawal of immunosuppression, but most patients quickly recover after restarting therapy. Liver transplantation is indicated for cirrhotic patients as well as for patients with massive hepatic necrosis.

FATTY LIVER DISEASE OR STEATOHEPATITIS PATTERN OF INJURY

The term *fatty liver disease* is used to describe a histologic pattern of injury that characteristically includes steatosis at least at some point during the course of disease. Steatosis is associated with a wide spectrum of clinical disorders, such as obesity, hyperinsulinemia, metabolic disorders, malnutrition, medications, and others (Table 17.4). Steatosis and steatohepatitis are distinguished based on their histologic features and prognoses. Steatosis occurs in the absence of features of steatohepatitis and carries the lowest risk of progressive disease. Alcoholic steatohepatitis (ASH) and nonalcoholic steatohepatitis (NASH) are both characterized by progressive fibrosis and common histologic features, including steatosis, lobular inflammation, hepatocellular injury, and pericellular or perisinusoidal fibrosis.

TABLE 17.4
Conditions That Cause Steatosis

Causes of Macrovesicular Steatosis	Causes of Microvesicular Steatosis
Obesity or metabolic	Acute fatty liver of pregnancy
Total parental nutrition	Inherited disorders of fatty acid metabolism
Rapid starvation	Reye's syndrome
Hypothyroidism	Mitochondrial cytopathies
Jejunoileal bypass	Medications
Wilson's disease	• Amiodarone
Abetalipoproteinemia	• Valproate
Weber-Christian disease	• Nucleoside analog reverse transcriptase inhibitors
Infection (hepatitis C)	• Tetracycline
Alcohol	Wolman's disease
Medication	Acute iron toxicity
• Amiodarone	Cholesterol ester storage disease
• Tamoxifen	Jamaican vomiting disease
• Steroids	Labrea fever
• Estrogen	Multiple hornet stings
• Antiretroviral agents	*Bacillus cereus* toxins
• Tetracycline	Alcoholic foamy degeneration
• Minocycline	Navajo neuropathy
	Inherited urea cycle disorders
	Pearson's syndrome

NONALCOHOLIC FATTY LIVER DISEASE

CLINICAL FEATURES

Nonalcoholic fatty liver disease refers to steatosis and steatohepatitis occurring in the absence of significant alcohol use and attributed to metabolic factors that are associated with increased risk of cardiovascular disease and death known as the metabolic syndrome: abdominal obesity, atherogenic dyslipidemia, hypertension, insulin resistance, and prothrombotic or proinflammatory states. NAFLD is common in developed countries and has also been recognized as an emerging health problem in the pediatric population. Patients are usually asymptomatic and often incidentally discovered because of mildly elevated transaminase levels. Many patients who were previously diagnosed with "cryptogenic cirrhosis" likely had cirrhosis secondary to end-stage NAFLD.

NONALCOHOLIC FATTY LIVER DISEASE—FACT SHEET

Definition
- Steatosis, mostly macrovesicular, occurring in patients with features of the metabolic syndrome
- May also exhibit features of steatohepatitis (ballooning hepatocyte degeneration, inflammation) and fibrosis

Incidence and Location
- More common in developed countries; estimated prevalence in the US population is 20% to 40%

Morbidity and Mortality
- May progress to cirrhosis
- Patients with steatohepatitis and fibrosis are at greatest risk of cirrhosis

Gender, Race, and Age Distribution
- Common in both men and women of all races
- Nonalcoholic fatty liver disease increasingly diagnosed in obese children, teenagers, and young adults

Clinical Features
- Mostly asymptomatic, slightly abnormal liver tests (and alanine aminotransferase > aminotransferase) or hepatomegaly
- Associated with obesity, insulin resistance or diabetes, hypertriglyceridemia, and other dyslipidemias (metabolic syndrome)

Radiologic Features
- Fatty liver infiltration on ultrasound on magnetic resonance imaging

Prognosis and Therapy
- Fibrosis on index biopsy is associated with progressive disease and poor outcome
- Treatment includes lifestyle modifications that include weight loss and blood glucose control; antidiabetic drugs and bariatric surgery have shown to have significant benefit

Pathologic Features

Gross Findings

In severe steatosis, the liver is grossly enlarged, yellow, and greasy (Fig. 17.16).

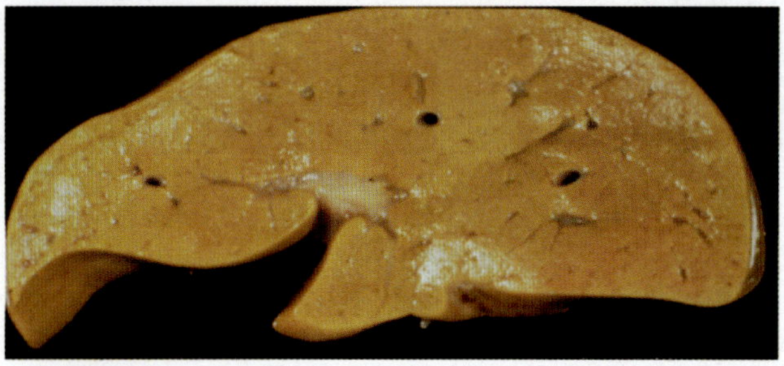

FIGURE 17.16

Accumulation of fat leads to an enlarged yellow liver in nonalcoholic fatty liver disease (NAFLD).

Microscopic Findings

Nonalcoholic fatty liver disease encompasses a range of histologic findings, including mild steatosis to steatohepatitis (NASH) and even end-stage cirrhosis.

Steatosis is a key feature of NAFLD. A minimum of 5% macrovesicular steatosis (large or small droplets) (Fig. 17.17A), often exclusively or predominantly macrovesicular (Fig. 17.17B) or mixed, should be present for the diagnosis. Microvesicular steatosis is less common and is characterized by very small fat vacuoles that impart a granular or "fluffy" appearance to the hepatocyte cytoplasm (Fig. 17.17C). Microvesicular steatosis may be present as scattered cells or in contiguous patches in NAFLD. Steatosis is classified as none (<5%), mild (5%–33%), moderate (34%–66%), or severe (>66%).

Nonalcoholic steatohepatitis can be distinguished from steatosis by the presence of ballooning hepatocyte degeneration (a key diagnostic feature) and inflammation (Fig. 17.17D). Ballooned hepatocytes (Fig. 17.17E) stand out from the background hepatocytes because of

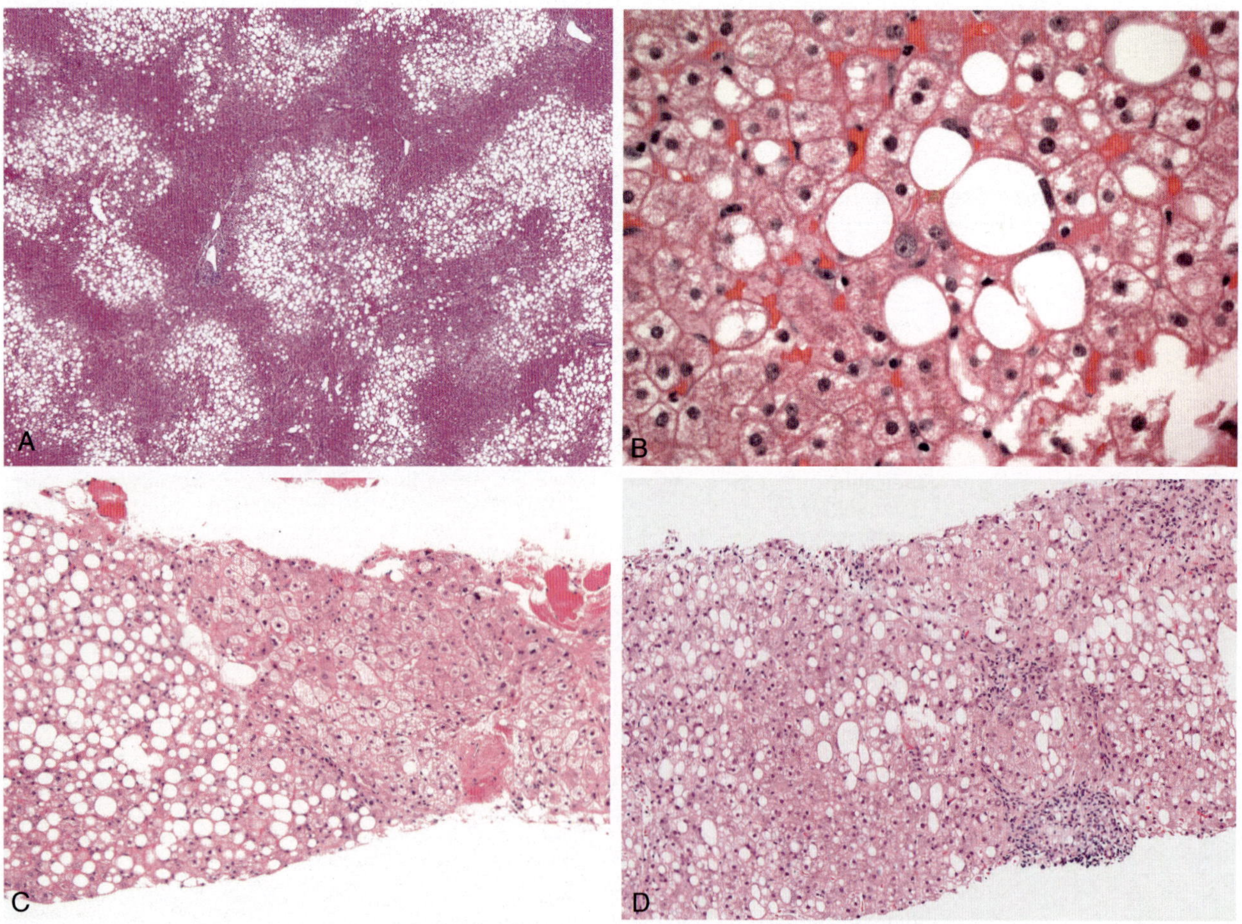

FIGURE 17.17

Steatohepatitis. **A**, Macrovesicular steatosis is readily identified on low power by the large rounded clear vacuoles that represent fat accumulation in hepatocytes. Note the conspicuous zones 2 and 3 distribution of steatosis commonly seen in NAFLD. **B**, Mainly large droplets of macrovesicular steatosis. **C**, A patch of microvesicular steatosis (*right* of the photo) is seen admixed with areas of macrovesicular steatosis (*left*) in this case. **D**, Histologic features of steatohepatitis

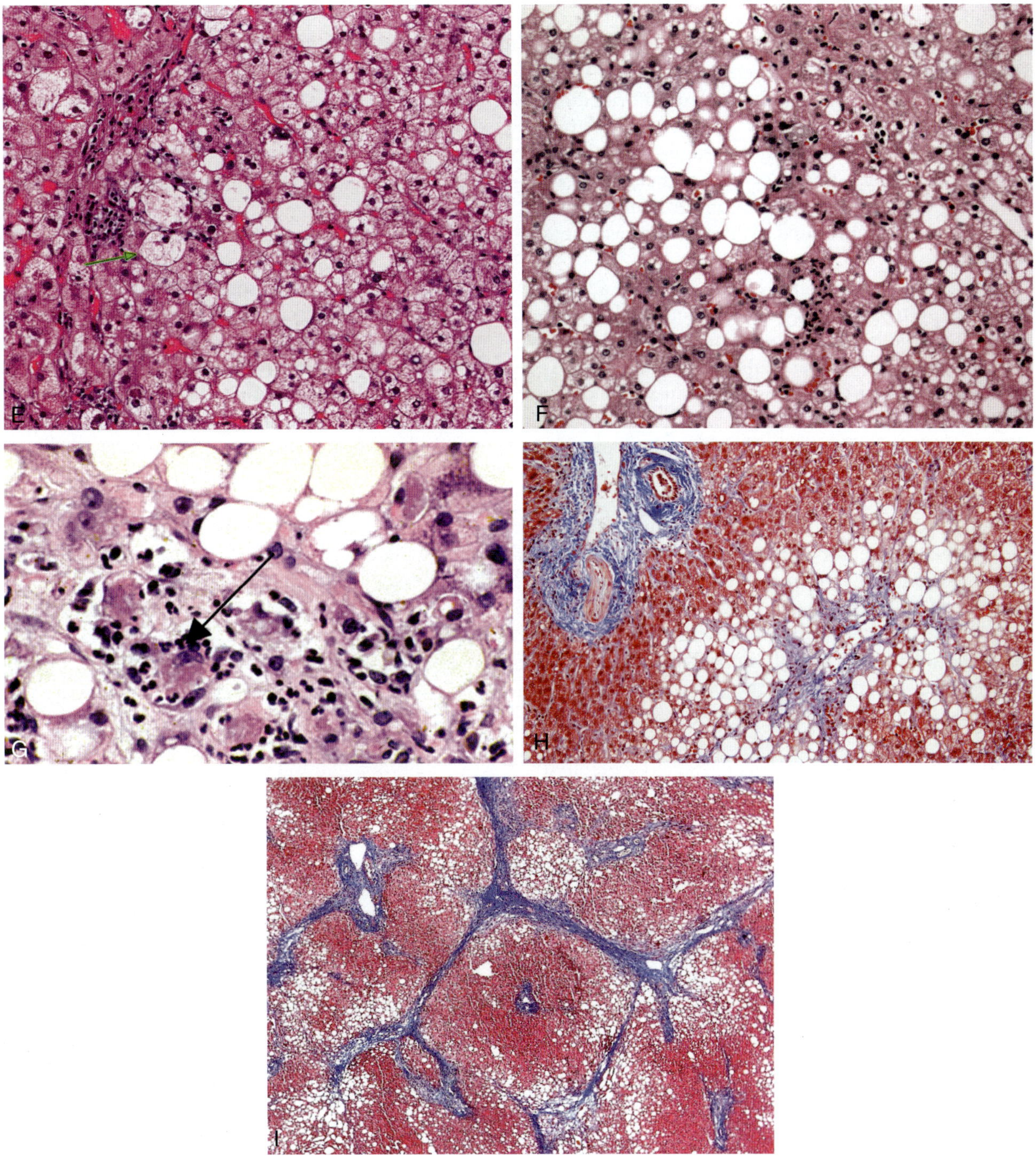

FIGURE 17.17, Cont'd

include steatosis, ballooning, and lobular inflammation. **E**, Ballooning degeneration of hepatocytes with Mallory hyaline (*arrow*) and focal accumulation of mononuclear inflammatory cells in the lobule are features of nonalcoholic steatohepatitis. Mallory's hyaline, ropey eosinophilic cytoplasmic accumulation of intermediate filaments is more common in alcoholic steatohepatitis. **F**, Lobular inflammation may include lymphocytes, Kupffer cells, and neutrophils. **G**, Mallory hyaline is chemotactic for neutrophil and frequently associated with "satellitosis." **H**, Fibrosis in steatohepatitis generally begins in centrilobular areas as delicate pericellular fibrosis in a "chicken wire" pattern. **I**, As advanced fibrosis develops, central-central bridging may be prominent, as in this case.

their large size and pale, irregular wispy or clumpy cytoplasm and disrupted cell membranes. They tend to be most prominent in zone 3, where they are associated with perisinusoidal fibrosis and steatotic hepatocytes. Classic ballooned hepatocytes may contain Mallory-Denk bodies, although this is not a required feature. Mallory-Denk bodies (also termed *Mallory bodies* or *Mallory hyaline*) are abnormally folded intermediate filaments recognized histologically as eosinophilic ropy or globular structures in hepatocyte cytoplasm. Mallory-Denk bodies are not specific to NASH and can be seen in a variety of settings, including alcoholic liver disease, chronic cholestatic conditions, Wilson's disease, and some tumors.

The inflammation seen in NASH includes a mixture of neutrophils, lymphocytes, plasma cells, and macrophages in the hepatic lobules and/or portal tracts (Figs. 17.17F and G). Whereas lobular inflammation is usually more prominent in adults, children may exhibit predominantly or exclusively portal inflammation (see later discussion). Lobular neutrophils are often present but are not required for the diagnosis of steatohepatitis. Portal inflammation is inconspicuous in most cases and is usually composed of mature lymphocytes and rare plasma cells. Greater portal inflammation occurring in the absence of chronic hepatitis (e.g., hepatitis C) has been linked to faster progression of disease, especially in pediatric patients, and with more severe disease in adults. If portal inflammation exceeds the extent of lobular inflammation, the possibility of coexisting chronic hepatitis or other liver disease should be considered, particularly when interface activity is seen. Megamitochondria, patchy glycogenosis, glycogenated nuclei, and lipogranulomas may also be seen in patients with steatohepatitis, although these features are not required for diagnosis.

Fibrosis in adult patients with NASH begins in the centrilobular region (Fig. 17.17H). In the early stages, delicate pericellular fibrosis is best highlighted by the trichrome stain. With progressive disease, portal and periportal fibrosis develops, and fibrous septa form between portal tracts and central veins or between portal tracts with subsequent evolution to cirrhosis. "Burned-out" steatohepatitis presenting in the cirrhotic stage (Fig. 17.17I) often shows only focal residual features of steatohepatitis and may be difficult to recognize histologically. Many cases of "cryptogenic cirrhosis" likely represent end-stage NAFLD.

Pediatric Nonalcoholic Fatty Liver Disease

Nonalcoholic fatty liver disease is the leading cause of liver disease in children. Some children show a similar histologic picture as seen in adults (type 1 pediatric NAFLD), whereas others have a distinct pattern of injury termed *type 2 pediatric NAFLD* and characterized by zone 1–predominant steatosis, portal inflammation, and portal or periportal scarring. Some children may show a combination of these patterns. The minimal diagnostic criteria for recognizing children at greatest risk of progressive disease are unclear, and some pathologists have used the term *borderline, zone 1, steatohepatitis* to indicate potentially progressive disease in biopsies exhibiting zone 1–predominant or panacinar steatosis, portal inflammation (usually mild) (Fig. 17.18A), and portal fibrosis (Fig. 17.18B) but little or no ballooning or Mallory bodies.

In 2005, the semiquantitative "NAFLD Activity Score" (NAS; Table 17.5) was published by the NASH Clinical Research Network (CRN). This score was intended for use in research trials to standardize reporting and assess changes in component features that might be seen in serial biopsies. The NAS represents the unweighted sum of steatosis, lobular inflammation, and hepatocyte ballooning scores. As in chronic hepatitis, grade is reported separately from stage (extent of fibrosis).

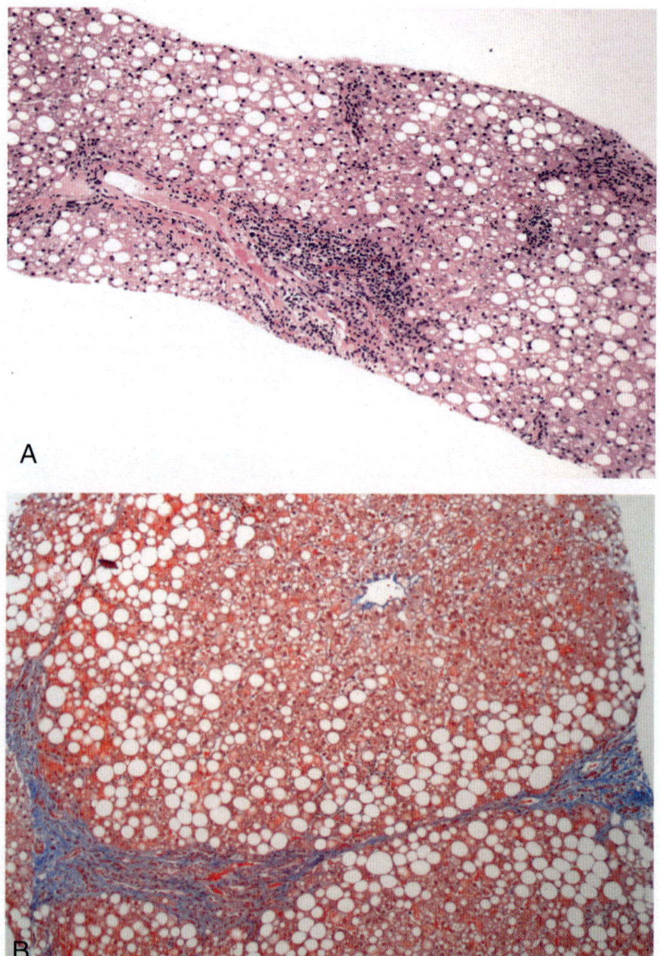

FIGURE 17.18

Pediatric steatohepatitis. **A**, As opposed to adult NASH, these cases may reveal more prominent portal inflammation and **B**, portal-based fibrosis.

TABLE 17.5

Nonalcoholic Steatohepatitis Clinical Research Network Nonalcoholic Fatty Liver Disease Activity Score

Activity Score (0–8)[a]	Fibrosis Score (0–4)[b]
Steatosis (0–3)	1a: zone 3 perisinusoidal fibrosis requiring trichrome
0: <5%	
1: 5%–33%	1b: zone 3 perisinusoidal fibrosis on H&E
2: 34%–66%	
3: >66%	1c: portal fibrosis only
Lobular inflammation (0–3)	2: zone 3 + portal or periportal
1: <2 foci per 20× field	
2: 2–4 foci per 20× field	
3: >4 foci per 20× field	
Ballooning (0–2)	3: bridging fibrosis
0: none	
1: few	
2: many	
	4: Cirrhosis

[a]Overall pattern of nonalcoholic fatty liver disease.
[b]Using Masson's trichrome.
H&E, Hematoxylin and eosin.
Adapted from Kleiner DE, Brunt EM, Van Natta M, et al. Nonalcoholic Steatohepatitis Clinical Research Network. Design and validation of a histologic scoring system for nonalcoholic fatty liver disease. *Hepatology*. 2005;41:1313–1321.

NONALCOHOLIC FATTY LIVER DISEASE—PATHOLOGIC FEATURES

Gross Findings

- Liver is enlarged, yellow, and greasy

Microscopic Findings

- Steatosis, variable amount, predominantly macrovesicular
- Ballooning hepatocyte degeneration in steatohepatitis
  Lobular inflammation
  Mallory's hyaline may be conspicuous
- Early stages of steatohepatitis show centrilobular, pericellular fibrosis that evolves to involve portal tracts and eventually bridging fibrosis and cirrhosis

Differential Diagnosis

- Alcoholic liver disease
- Drug-induced liver injury
  Hepatitis C
- Other metabolic disorders, especially Wilson's disease

DIFFERENTIAL DIAGNOSIS

Because of the histologic similarities, NAFLD cannot be reliably distinguished from alcoholic liver disease on the basis of biopsy findings alone; this distinction is made clinically. That said, there are some differences between these entities. For example, steatosis is an important feature of NASH but is not always seen in alcoholic liver disease. Furthermore, canalicular cholestasis, bile ductular proliferation, veno-occlusive lesions, sclerosing hyaline necrosis, and alcoholic foamy degeneration (pure microvesicular steatosis) are features of alcoholic liver disease and are not commonly seen in NAFLD.

Drug reaction should also be considered in the differential diagnosis. Many medications, including estrogens, tamoxifen, and glucocorticoids, can cause steatosis, and amiodarone toxicity, for example, can cause a pattern of injury similar to ASH with frequent Mallory bodies.

Autoimmune hepatitis is sometimes considered in the clinical differential diagnosis of NAFLD, and nonspecific elevation of autoantibodies (ANA, SMA, AMA) can be identified in up to 20% of individuals with NAFLD. When autoantibodies are detected in the presence of prominent portal inflammation, a careful search for diagnostic features of coexisting chronic liver diseases such as AIH or PBC is warranted. Chronic HBV or HCV can coexist with NAFLD and should also be excluded clinically.

ANCILLARY STUDIES

Some studies have shown the utility of cytokeratin (CK) 8/18, hsp70, p62, and ubiquitin immunohistochemical stains in the identification of ballooned hepatocytes, but these stains are not used in clinical practice.

PROGNOSIS AND THERAPY

Although there are ongoing clinical trials, diet and exercise and, in select patients, bariatric surgery remain the mainstay therapy for NASH. Steatosis appears to follow a relatively stable course, but steatohepatitis shows a greater propensity to progress to significant fibrosis or cirrhosis (~28% of patients progress to bridging fibrosis or cirrhosis over 5–10 years).

ALCOHOLIC LIVER DISEASE

CLINICAL FEATURES

Excess alcohol consumption is a leading cause of liver failure in the United States and worldwide. Significant alcohol use has been variably defined for research purposes. The National Institutes of Health–funded NASH CRN defined a limit of 20 g/day for men and 10 g/day for women for inclusion in their studies on NAFLD. Risk for severe hepatic injury correlates with daily intake, with 80 g/day of alcohol being a risk factor for severe hepatic injury. However, only 10% to 15% of people with alcoholism develop cirrhosis.

Like NAFLD, alcoholic liver disease can present as steatosis, alcoholic hepatitis, or cirrhosis. Hepatic steatosis presents with hepatomegaly and mild elevation of serum liver test results (in particular AST > ALT in a >2:1 ratio). Steatosis resolves with cessation of alcohol intake. Acute alcoholic hepatitis (acute alcoholic intoxication) may be life threatening. Patients often present with malaise, anorexia, weight loss, jaundice, and altered sensorium. In this setting, hyperbilirubinemia may be seen in addition to more pronounced elevation of transaminases. The clinical presentation of alcoholic cirrhosis is similar to other forms of cirrhosis.

ALCOHOLIC LIVER DISEASE—FACT SHEET

Definition

- Spectrum of liver disease caused by alcohol use, including steatosis, alcoholic hepatitis, and cirrhosis

Incidence and Location

- 10% to 15% of people with chronic alcoholism develop cirrhosis; true incidence of milder forms of alcoholic liver disease is unknown
- Worldwide distribution

Morbidity and Mortality

- For hepatic steatosis, full recovery is expected with cessation of alcohol intake
- Severe acute alcoholic hepatitis is associated with up to 50% mortality rate; it may progress to cirrhosis or occur in the setting of cirrhosis
- For alcoholic cirrhosis, the 5-year survival rate is approximately 50% for those who continue to consume alcohol; hepatocellular carcinoma is a common complication

Gender, Race, and Age Distribution

- More common in men
- All races are equally affected
  Alcoholic cirrhosis is more common in older adults
- Hepatic steatosis and alcoholic hepatitis may be seen in younger adults

Clinical Features

- Steatosis presents with hepatomegaly; mild elevation of transaminases (aspartate aminotransferase > alanine aminotransferase in a >2:1 ratio)
- Alcoholic hepatitis usually follows an episode of binge drinking and is associated with systemic symptoms, such as malaise or anorexia, with or without fever; liver enzymes can be markedly elevated with or without hyperbilirubinemia
- Alcoholic cirrhosis presents with typical signs of cirrhosis

Prognosis and Therapy

- Steatosis has an excellent prognosis with cessation of alcohol consumption
- Alcoholic hepatitis may slowly resolve or may progress to cirrhosis; treatment is cessation of ethanol consumption and supportive therapy
- Alcoholic cirrhosis has a poor prognosis in patients who continue to drink, with a 5-year survival rate of 50%; treatment is supportive or liver transplantation

Pathologic Features

Gross Findings

The liver in patients with steatosis and alcoholic hepatitis is often enlarged, yellow, soft, and greasy. In alcoholic cirrhosis, the liver is enlarged initially, with a finely granular capsular surface and firm texture (Fig. 17.19).

Microscopic Findings

Alcoholic steatosis is commonly macrovesicular and zone 3 in distribution. With abstinence, steatosis may rapidly disappear, but residual foci lobular inflammation and lipogranulomas may be observed.

The diagnosis of alcoholic hepatitis (also known as alcoholic steatohepatitis has overlapping histologic features with NASH: steatosis with lobular inflammation and liver cell injury (ballooned hepatocytes and acidophil bodies), often with Mallory-Denk bodies (Fig. 17.20A). The degree of steatosis is variable. The lobular inflammation may be neutrophil rich with neutrophils in clusters around ballooned hepatocytes containing Mallory-Denk bodies ("satellitosis") (Fig. 17.20B). In cases with pronounced hepatocellular injury, there is evidence of hepatocellular dropout, readily highlighted by the reticulin stain. Most cases show only mild or complete absence of mononuclear cell inflammatory infiltrate within the portal tracts.

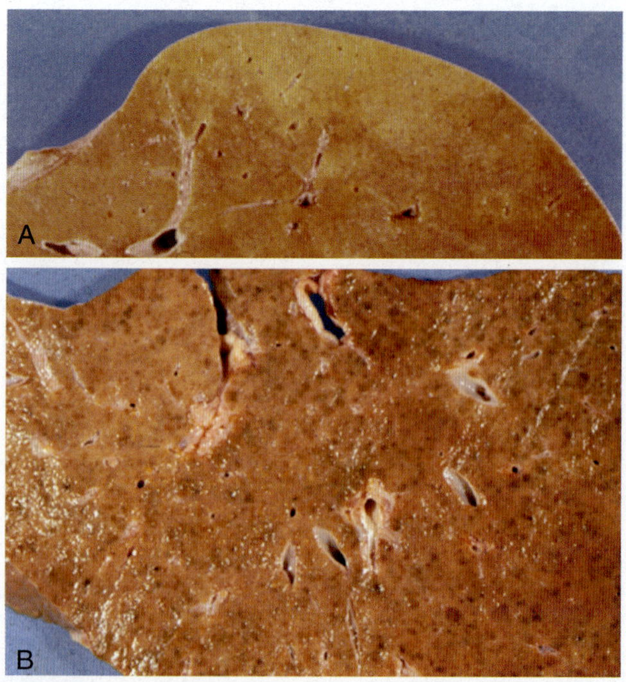

FIGURE 17.19

A, The liver with steatosis is enlarged, soft, and yellow. The fat may be irregularly distributed. **B**, Cirrhosis due to excess alcohol consumption is micronodular, with a uniform cut surface.

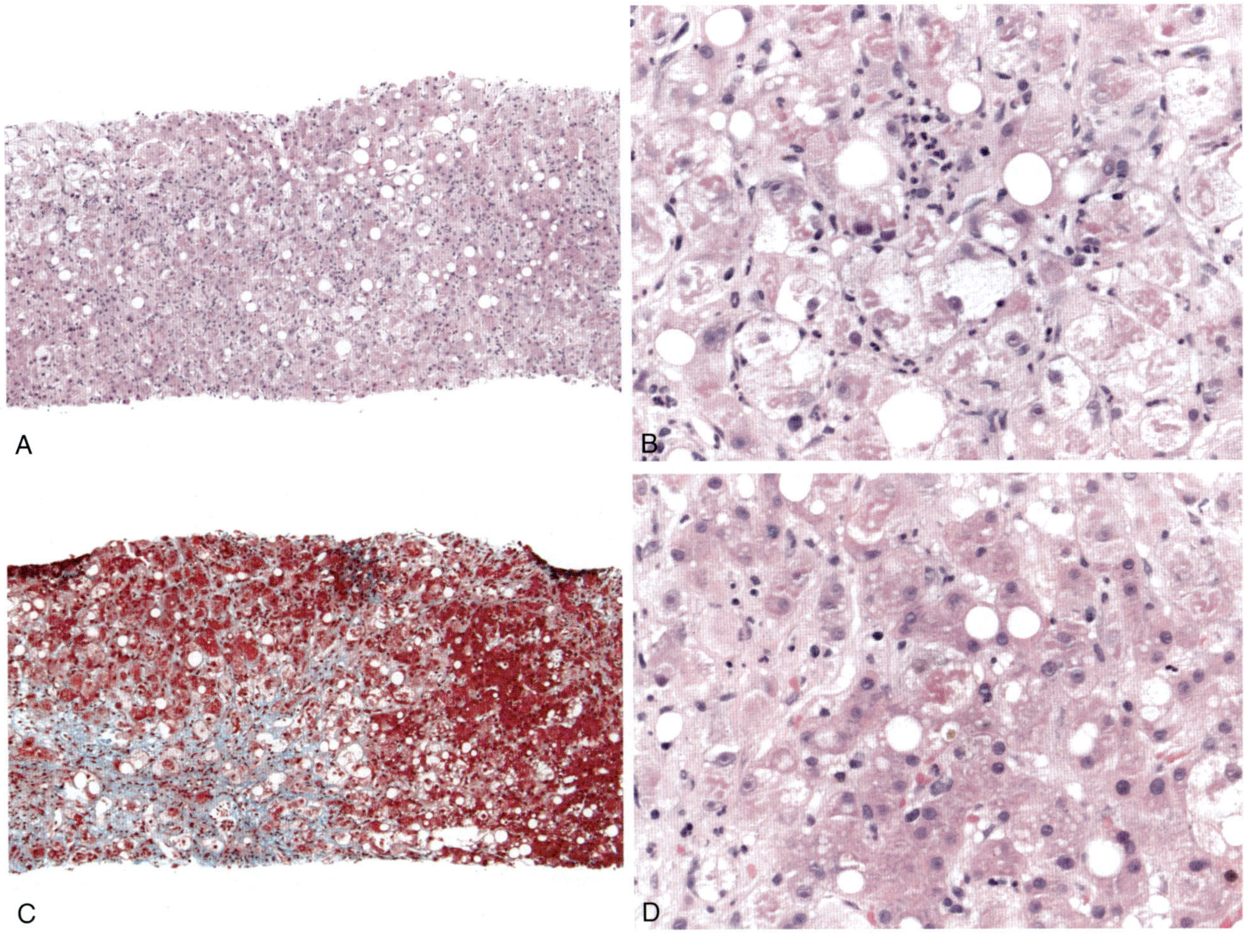

FIGURE 17.20

A, In alcoholic steatohepatitis, the amount of steatosis is variable; hepatocyte injury, Mallory's hyaline accumulation (*arrow*), and a neutrophilic infiltrate are key diagnostic features. **B**, Mallory hyaline is often present and associated with "satellitosis." **C**, Pericellular fibrosis in alcoholic hepatitis has a chicken-wire appearance and is most prominent in the centrilobular region, where ballooned hepatocytes are frequently present. **D**, Cholestatic steatohepatitis is almost always seen in the setting of alcohol-induced injury.

Zone 3 pericellular and perisinusoidal fibrosis is a characteristic feature of alcoholic hepatitis. Collagen surrounds individual hepatocytes in a "chicken wire" pattern (Fig. 17.20C). As fibrosis progresses, central–central and central–portal fibrous bridges form, eventually resulting in micronodular cirrhosis. Scoring systems specifically designed for alcoholic liver disease (e.g., the system by Altamirano et al., 2014) are not widely used in clinical practice.

Although similarity between ASH and NASH exists, some patterns of injury described in alcoholic liver disease do not occur in NASH: (1) cholestatic steatohepatitis (Figs. 17.20D), (2) alcoholic foamy degeneration, and (3) sclerosing hyaline necrosis. Patients with cholestatic disease are often jaundiced with elevated ALP and gamma-glutamyl transferase (GGT). Biopsy shows prominent canalicular and hepatocellular cholestasis with or without bile ductular proliferation, mimicking bile duct obstruction. Alcoholic foamy degeneration is characterized by marked centrilobular microvesicular steatosis, often with prominent megamitochondria and cholestasis. Macrovesicular steatosis and neutrophilic inflammation is usually absent. *Sclerosing hyaline necrosis* is characterized by marked centrilobular hepatocellular necrosis and dropout. These patients later develop confluent fibrosis that obliterates the central veins (veno-occlusive lesions).

Alcoholic Liver Disease—Pathologic Features

Gross Findings

- Steatosis: liver is enlarged, yellow, and greasy because of lipid accumulation
- Alcoholic hepatitis: liver may be enlarged; yellow discoloration and firm consistency with progressive fibrosis

Microscopic Findings

- Steatosis: macrovesicular steatosis, predominantly centrilobular but can be panlobular
- Alcoholic steatohepatitis: hepatocyte ballooning degeneration, Mallory-Denk bodies, variable steatosis, neutrophilic inflammation, zone 3 pericellular and perisinusoidal fibrosis, progressing to central–portal bridging fibrosis

- Alcoholic cirrhosis: delicate central–portal fibrous septa in early stages form micronodules, later mixed macronodular and micronodular cirrhosis pattern

Differential Diagnosis

- Nonalcoholic fatty liver disease
- Drug-induced liver injury
  Chronic cholestatic conditions
- Wilson's disease

Differential Diagnosis

Nonalcoholic fatty liver disease is the major differential diagnosis for alcoholic liver disease, and frequently NASH and ASH cannot be differentiated based on histologic features alone. In general, neutrophilic-rich infiltrates, prominent Mallory's hyaline, cholestasis, and conspicuous pericellular sinusoidal fibrosis should favor the diagnosis of alcohol-induced injury over NASH.

Drug-induced liver injury is an important consideration if a history of alcohol use cannot be established. Amiodarone toxicity causes phospholipidosis and prominent Mallory-Denk bodies, which can mimic alcoholic hepatitis.

Cholestatic ASH, large duct obstruction, and other chronic cholestatic conditions can show overlapping histologic features; however, the clinical history of alcohol use and clinical exclusion of large duct obstruction should be helpful in sorting this differential. In young patients, Wilson's disease should be also considered as a potential cause and should be distinguished using clinical and ancillary laboratory tests.

Prognosis and Therapy

The long-term prognosis depends on the severity of liver injury and alcohol abstinence. Alcoholic steatosis tends to resolve within 1 to 3 months of stopping alcohol consumption. On the other hand, alcoholic hepatitis can progress to cirrhosis. Sclerosing hyaline necrosis carries a poor prognosis and often leads to portal hypertension and ascites. Treatment includes alcohol cessation and nutritional interventions and, for patients with more severe disease, prednisolone or pentoxifylline. Liver transplantation is an option for patients who achieve abstinence.

Cholestatic Pattern of Injury

A cholestatic pattern of injury can be seen in disease processes that affect parts of the biliary tree. The clinical presentation depends on the underlying disease, but in general, patients present with pruritus and fatigue, and laboratory testing reveals elevation of ALPH, bilirubin, and GGT. Clinically, cholestasis is associated with certain signs and symptoms that correspond, at least in part, to elevated serum levels of bilirubin, bile acids, and cholesterol. However, pathologically, it is defined by morphologic consequences of biliary retention and injury to the biliary tree. It is important to note that cholestasis by itself is quite nonspecific and does not necessarily indicate a primary cholestatic disorder. It can be seen in many other conditions, including drug injury, viral hepatitis, Wilson's disease, and alcoholic liver disease.

Cholestasis may be classified by time frame (acute vs chronic cholestasis) or by the pattern and location of cholestasis: bland cholestasis, canalicular cholestasis, ductular cholestasis, ductal cholestasis, or ductular reaction or proliferation.

Acute Versus Chronic Cholestasis

Acute cholestasis often results from acute biliary obstruction but can also occur in sepsis and DILI. Histologic features of acute biliary obstruction include portal stromal edema, bile ductular proliferation with accompanying neutrophils. The lobules show canalicular cholestasis and bile plugs. Portal edema is a more specific histologic feature; however, it is uncommon and lacks sensitivity. Occasionally, bile infarcts and bile lakes are identified, and their presence indicates large bile duct obstruction.

Chronic cholestatic conditions such as chronic biliary obstruction, PBC, PSC, drugs or toxins, total parenteral nutrition (TPN) toxicity, sarcoidosis, graft-versus-host disease, bile transporter mutations, IgG4 cholangitis, and ischemic cholangitis, among others, show histologic features of chronic cholestasis. A key feature is periportal "cholate stasis" caused by accumulation of bile salts in hepatocytes, imparting a rarefied, feathery appearance to the cytoplasm of periportal hepatocytes. Intracytoplasmic copper accumulation within periportal hepatocytes can be highlighted by rhodanine and orcein stains, and periportal Mallory-Denk bodies are often seen. Other features include feathery degeneration of hepatocytes, hepatocyte rosette formation, and ductular proliferation. Over time, scarring progresses to a biliary-type cirrhosis, which exhibits a characteristic low-power appearance of irregular, serpiginous, or "jigsaw-shaped" nodules and periportal cholate stasis.

Patterns and Manifestations of Cholestasis

Bland cholestasis is defined by the presence of lobular canalicular and hepatocellular cholestasis in the absence of inflammation and hepatocyte injury. Bland cholestasis is typically related to DILI (Fig. 17.21A).

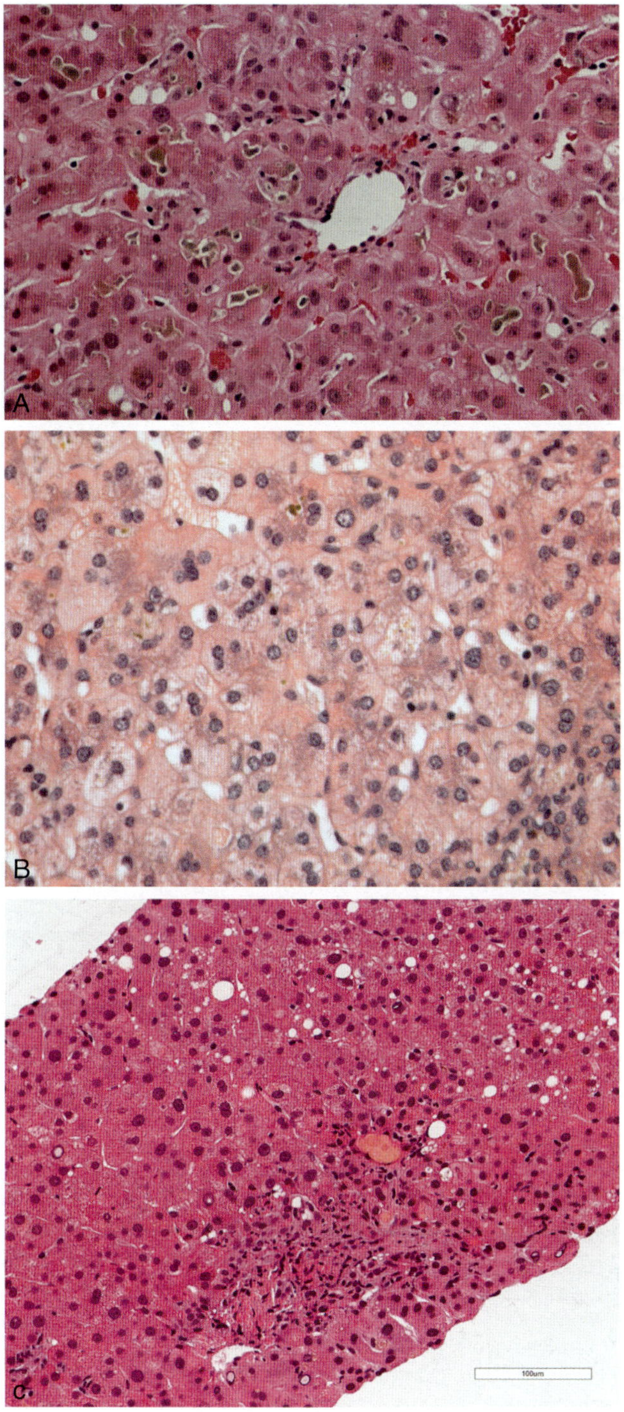

FIGURE 17.21

A, Bland cholestasis associated with drug-induced liver injury. **B**, Most commonly, canalicular and hepatocellular cholestasis as a result of cholestatic liver injury. **C**, Ductular cholestasis involves the interlobular bile ducts, classically described in the setting of "cholangitis lenta."

Medications associated with bland cholestasis include androgenic steroids, estrogen, azathioprine, and others. Less frequently, bland cholestasis occurs in benign recurring intrahepatic cholestasis, thyroid disorders, or intrahepatic cholestasis of pregnancy and as a paraneoplastic syndrome.

Canalicular cholestasis refers to bile within the bile canaliculi, which are not visible on routine H&E in the normal liver. *Hepatocellular cholestasis* indicates bile accumulation within hepatocyte cytoplasm. Hepatocellular and canalicular cholestasis often coexist (*hepatocanalicular cholestasis*) (see Fig. 17.19B).

Ductal cholestasis is uncommon and indicates the presence of bile within the lumen of a native interlobular bile duct. *Ductular cholestasis* indicates the presence of bile plugs within the lumens of proliferating bile ductules (see later). Also termed *cholangitis lenta* (Fig. 17.21C), this finding can be seen in patients with sepsis. *Ductular reaction or proliferation* is a nonspecific finding that can be seen in a broad array of settings, including biliary obstruction, as a regenerative phenomenon in the setting of hepatocyte injury, with drug-induced injury, sepsis, parenteral nutrition, advanced hepatic fibrosis, and others.

DISORDERS OF THE BILE DUCTS

LARGE DUCT OBSTRUCTION

CLINICAL FEATURES

The clinical diagnosis of large duct obstruction is based on imaging studies. Mechanical blockage of extrahepatic (large) intrahepatic ducts in the setting of biliary lithiasis is usually manifested by colicky right upper quadrant abdominal pain and elevated ALP, GGT, and serum bilirubin levels. In cases of malignant obstruction, patients often present with painless jaundice. Fever is only present when there is superimposed ascending bacterial cholangitis.

LARGE DUCT OBSTRUCTION—FACT SHEET

Definition

- Obstruction of large bile ducts by any cause, such as biliary stones, fibrosis, impingement by external structures/lesions (e.g., hematoma, abscess, tumor), or intrinsic biliary lesions

Incidence and Location

- Common worldwide

Morbidity and Mortality

- Histologic changes can be reversible upon resolution of the underlying obstruction
- Long-standing biliary obstruction may progress to cirrhosis
- Severe secondary ascending (bacterial) cholangitis; can lead to abscesses and strictures

Gender, Race, and Age Distribution

- Men and women equally affected; obstruction secondary to gallstones more common in women
- All races affected; gallstones more common in some populations.
- Wide age range, depending on cause of obstruction

Clinical Features

- Cholestatic pattern of liver enzymes
- Colicky abdominal pain suggests biliary obstruction from stones Painless jaundice suggests obstruction from malignancy
- Fever may be seen in the setting of superimposed bacterial cholangitis

Radiologic Features

- Ultrasonography may show dilated intrahepatic or extrahepatic ducts and may identify the cause of obstruction
- Endoscopic ultrasonography and endoscopic retrograde cholangiopancreatography are very helpful in determining the site of obstruction and diagnostic/therapeutic interventions

Prognosis and Therapy

- Treatment is relief of obstruction by surgery, endoscopic or percutaneous drain or stent placement, endoscopic removal of stones, or endoscopic dilation of stricture
- Prognosis depends on the underlying cause but is generally good for nonmalignant causes of obstruction

Radiologic Features

Imaging studies remain the gold standard for diagnosing of large duct obstruction. Ultrasonography may show dilated intrahepatic and extrahepatic bile ducts above the level of obstruction as well as biliary stones. Endoscopic ultrasonography or ERCP is more helpful in the setting of malignant obstruction because this procedure provides information on the exact site of obstruction and allows clinicians to obtain biopsy samples to place stents or dilate strictures. Compared with ERCP, magnetic resonance cholangiopancreatography (MRCP) is noninvasive; superior in visualizing the bile ducts proximal to a site of obstruction; and provides additional information regarding hepatic parenchyma, vascular structures, and lymph nodes.

Pathologic Features

Gross Findings

Biliary sludge or stone material may be seen in the obstructed biliary tree, and areas of extravasated bile may form bile lakes or bile infarcts. Dilated extrahepatic and intrahepatic bile ducts, thickening of the bile duct wall, and ulceration of the bile duct mucosa may be seen with malignant obstruction. Advanced stages of chronic biliary obstruction can result in biliary-type cirrhosis characterized by irregular nodules and greenish discoloration of the liver parenchyma.

Microscopic Findings

Liver biopsy does not play a major role in the work-up and diagnosis of large duct obstruction because the histologic features are largely nonspecific, and the diagnosis of large duct obstruction is generally based on imaging studies. Portal tract abnormalities appear as early as 4 to 5 days after obstruction and include mixed portal inflammation, bile duct proliferation, and portal stromal edema (Fig. 17.22A). The portal inflammation consists of numerous neutrophils (secondary to bile ductular proliferation) and scattered lymphocytes and plasma cells (Fig. 17.22B). Canalicular cholestasis and bile plugs may be present. When present, bile infarcts and bile lakes are very specific for large duct obstruction (Figs. 17.22C and D). Some patients may develop superimposed ascending cholangitis with numerous *intraluminal* neutrophils within bile ducts, portal edema, and bile ductular proliferation.

With prolonged biliary obstruction, periportal hepatocytes show cholate stasis, copper accumulation, and Mallory hyaline inclusions. Mild periductal fibrosis may occur but bile duct loss is unusual in large duct obstruction. Advanced fibrosis with prominent bile ductular proliferation may develop in the setting of chronic biliary obstruction (Fig. 17.22E).

Large Duct Obstruction—Pathologic Features

Gross Findings

- Intrabiliary stones
- Bile lakes and infarcts Strictures or thickening of the bile duct wall
- Biliary-type cirrhosis with green discoloration

Microscopic Findings

Early Findings

- Canalicular and hepatocellular cholestasis
- Portal tract edema, more pronounced around interlobular bile ducts Variable portal mixed inflammatory infiltrates
- Bile ductular reaction accompanied by neutrophils

Late Findings

- Bile infarcts and bile lakes
- Periportal cholate stasis with Mallory bodies and copper accumulation
- Periductal fibrosis and biliary type cirrhosis

Differential Diagnosis

- Primary sclerosing cholangitis
- Primary biliary cholangitis
- Ischemic cholangiopathy and other forms of secondary sclerosing cholangitis
- Immunoglobulin G4–related cholangitis
- Drug-induced liver injury
- Sepsis
- Total parenteral nutrition toxicity

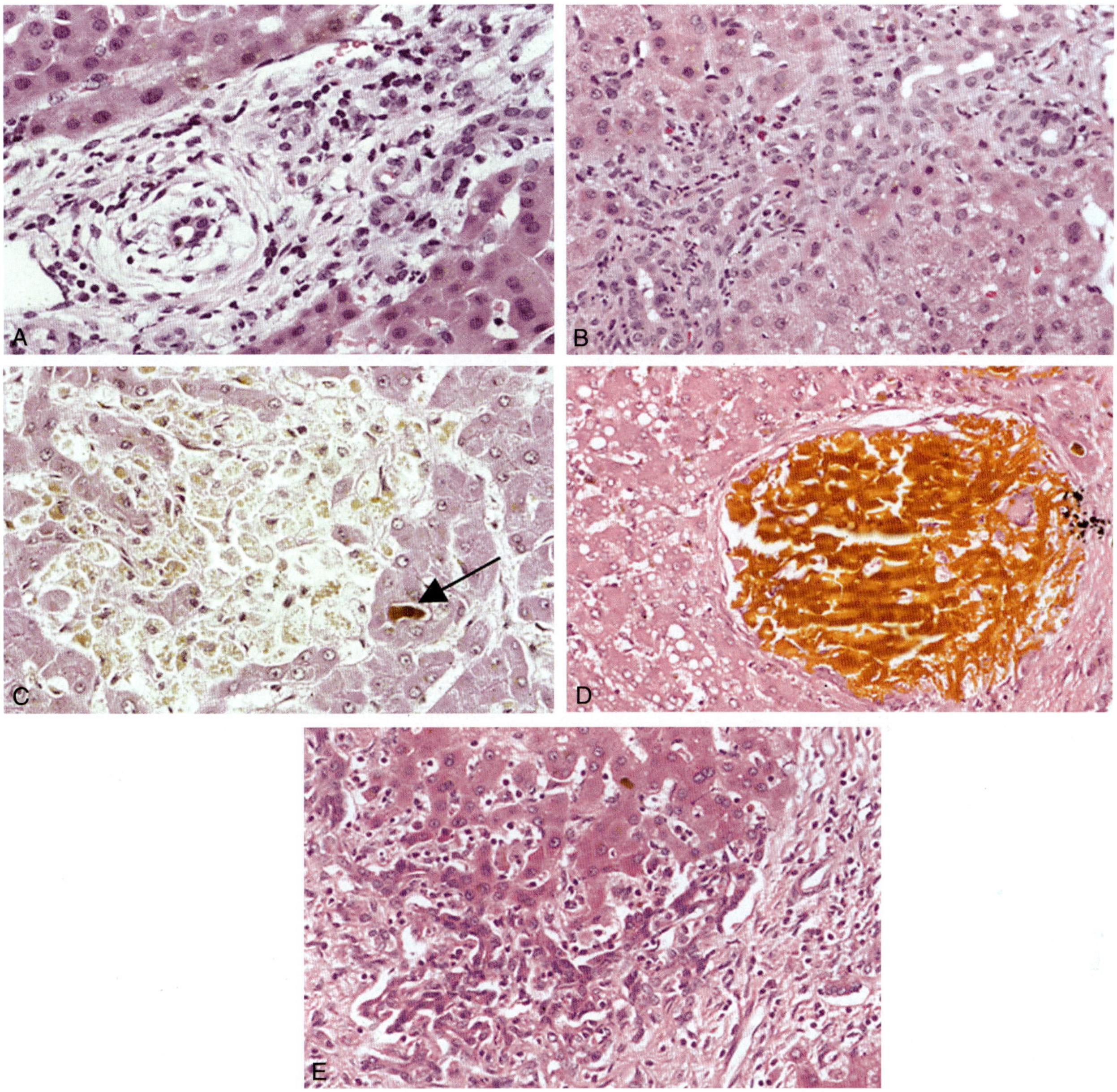

FIGURE 17.22

A, Early in biliary obstruction, the portal tracts are edematous, with only a modest increase in inflammatory cells. The edema is particularly pronounced around interlobular bile ducts. **B**, If obstruction is not relieved, bile ductular reaction at the periphery of the portal tract develops. **C**, In later stages of biliary obstruction, hepatocyte necrosis with release of accumulated bile (bile infarct) may be seen. Note canalicular cholestasis (*arrow*), more prominent in centrilobular regions. **D**, Bile lakes are seen in late-stage large duct obstruction. **E**, In biliary cirrhosis due to large duct obstruction, bile ductular reaction is prominent at the periphery of the regenerative nodules.

Differential Diagnosis

Imaging studies are required to exclude large duct obstruction as a cause of cholestasis. If large duct obstruction has been excluded, other entities, including drug reaction, sepsis, and TPN toxicity, should be excluded clinically.

In later stages, PBC, PSC, ischemic cholangiopathy, and IgG4-related cholangitis enter the differential diagnosis. In addition to the classic clinical findings, patients with PBC and IgG4-related cholangitis usually exhibit more dense portal inflammatory infiltrates and more prominent bile duct injury. In PBC, bile duct injury is recognized as "florid duct lesions" (see later), and in IgG4-related cholangitis, IgG4-positive plasma cells are prominent. PSC is usually detected on imaging studies, although biopsy may be required if the imaging findings are lacking or equivocal. Early ischemic cholangiopathy shows eosinophilia of bile duct epithelial cells and formation of bile duct casts, whereas late disease can lead to scarring and duct loss. All of these entities can lead to bile duct loss, which is not a feature of bile duct obstruction.

Prognosis and Therapy

Identifying and removing the cause of obstruction typically restores normal biliary function. Cirrhosis is uncommon in this setting.

PRIMARY BILIARY CHOLANGITIS

CLINICAL FEATURES

Primary biliary cholangitis (formerly known as primary biliary cirrhosis) is a chronic, progressive autoimmune disorder leading to destruction of the intrahepatic bile ducts. It usually affects middle-aged to older females. Most patients (~95%) show AMAs, although AMA-negative cases are well documented and follow an identical clinical course. ANA positivity can be found in 90% of patients with AMA-negative PBC. Patients often present with fatigue and pruritus in early stages. Jaundice is only seen in later stages. The diagnosis of PBC is based on the presence of any two of the following three criteria: (1) biochemical evidence of cholestasis (mainly ALP elevation), (2) detection of AMAs, and (3) characteristic histology (nonsuppurative destructive cholangitis of the interlobular bile ducts, or "florid duct lesions"). Accordingly, biopsy is typically only required to establish the diagnosis in patients who are AMA negative or in whom another diagnosis is suspected.

PRIMARY BILIARY CHOLANGITIS—FACT SHEET

Definition

- Progressive chronic cholestatic liver disease characterized by destruction of intrahepatic bile ducts and positive antimitochondrial antibodies (AMA)

Incidence and Location

- Variable prevalence reported, from 3.7 to 65 per 100,000
- More common in Western countries

Morbidity and Mortality

- Progressive disease leading to cirrhosis
- Morbidity related to cirrhosis and chronic cholestasis
- Slight increased risk for hepatocellular carcinoma

Gender, Race, and Age Distribution

- 90% are female and white
- Most patients are 40 to 60 years old at diagnosis

Clinical Features

- Strongly associated with AMA
- Asymptomatic in early stages; may be detected by elevated alkaline phosphatase (may be normal in early-stage disease), fatigue, pruritus
- Late symptoms related to chronic cholestasis include jaundice

Prognosis and Therapy

- Ursodeoxycholic acid improves serum biochemical liver tests, delays histologic progression, and improves survival
- Liver transplantation for patients with decompensated cirrhosis

Pathologic Features

Gross Findings

Gross abnormalities are only present in the late stages of PBC when the liver shows features of biliary-type cirrhosis (Fig. 17.23).

Microscopic Findings

Histologic features of chronic nonsuppurative cholangitis are typically seen in the interlobular bile ducts. In early PBC, the portal tracts contain dense inflammatory infiltrates composed of lymphocytes, histiocytes, and plasma cells. There may be patchy spillover of the portal inflammation beyond the limiting plate, but significant hepatocyte injury or necrosis is not a feature of PBC. The portal inflammation is characteristically centered around the interlobular bile duct, which shows evidence of injury in the form of intraepithelial lymphocytosis, nuclear disarray, cytoplasmic eosinophilia, and cytoplasmic vacuolization.

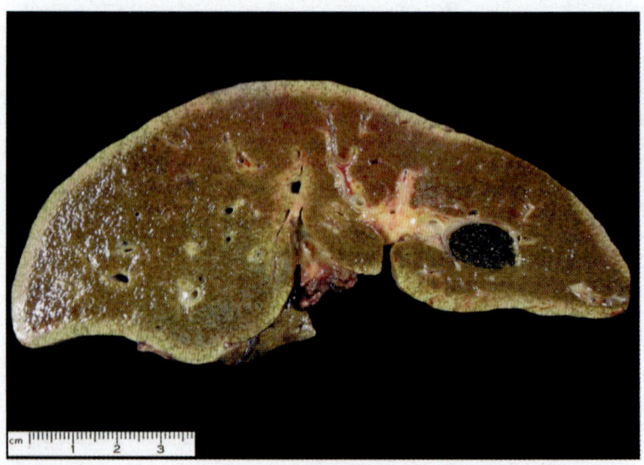

FIGURE 17.23

Biliary cirrhosis with bile discoloration and vague nodularity on the cut surface. Note area of biliary dilatation containing dark-colored calculi.

These changes are often accompanied by loose histiocyte aggregates or granulomas, often poorly formed. This constellation of inflammation and bile duct injury is the characteristic histologic finding of PBC, termed *florid duct lesion* (Fig. 17.24A). Granulomas are not required for the diagnosis of PBC. Lobular inflammation is typically minimal and may include scattered foci of inflammation and/or granulomas.

Late-stage PBC shows features of chronic cholestasis (periportal cholate stasis with periportal Mallory bodies), bile duct loss, and variable degrees of fibrosis (Figs. 17.24B–D).

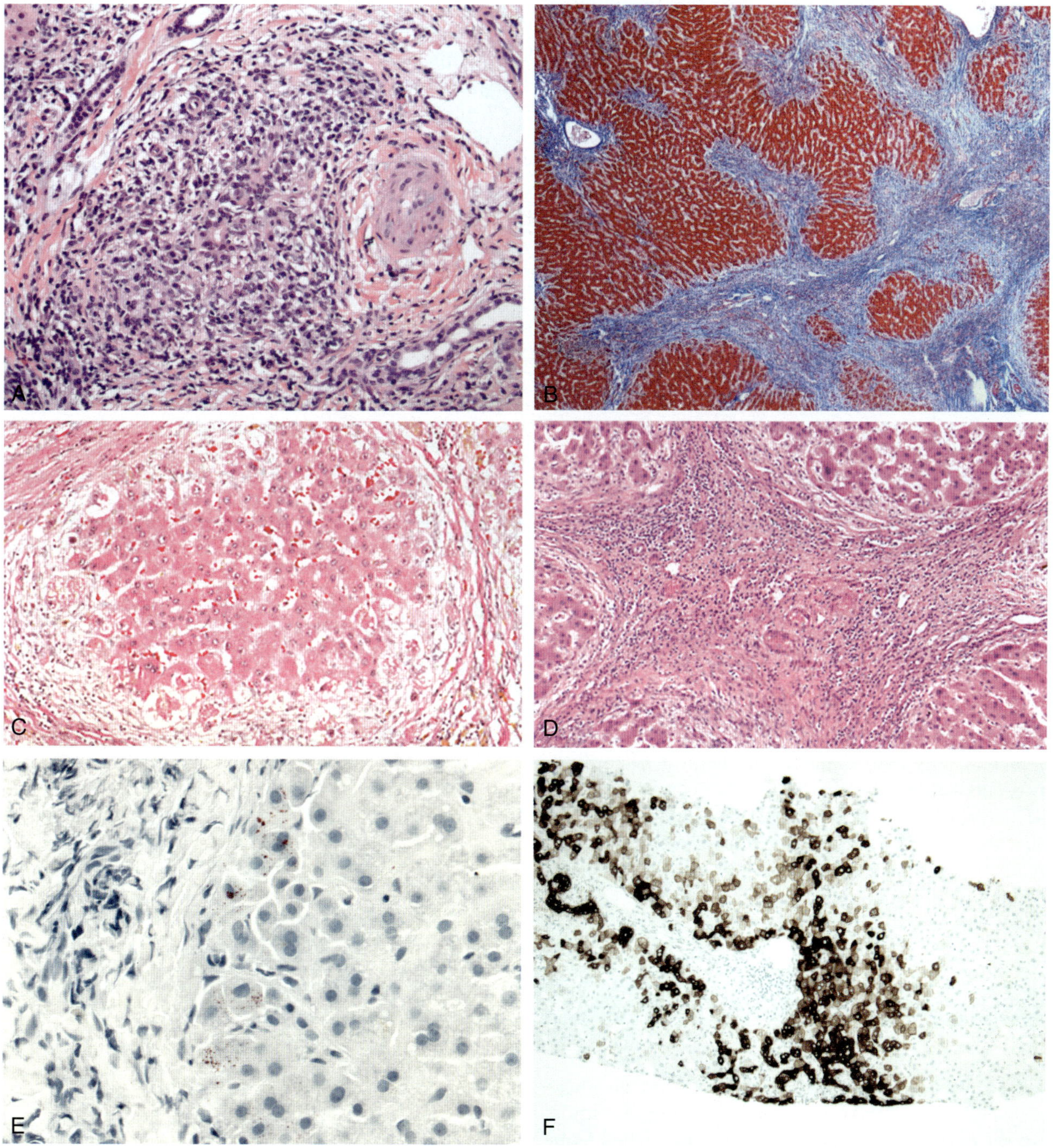

FIGURE 17.24

Primary biliary cirrhosis: **A**, Granulomatous destruction of interlobular bile ducts and intraepithelial lymphocytosis (florid-duct lesion) is present in this case of stage I primary biliary cirrhosis. Larger bile ducts (>80 μm) are typically preserved, as in this example. **B**, In cirrhosis due to PBC, the regenerating nodules have an irregular "jigsaw puzzle piece" outline. **C**, Periseptal hepatocytes appear pale due to accumulation of bile salts (cholate stasis), a common feature in chronic cholestasis. **D**, In late-stage PBC, ductopenia is common, with few or no residual bile ducts and little bile ductular reaction. **B**, Rhodanine stain reveals copper deposition in periportal hepatocytes. **F**, CK7 can be helpful in highlighting the interlobular ducts if present along with staining periportal hepatocytes.

Several staging systems (e.g., Scheuer and Ludwig) have been proposed for staging PBC but are variably used in clinical practice.

Primary Biliary Cholangitis—Pathologic Features

Gross Findings

- Biliary-type cirrhosis in late stages, with green discoloration

Microscopic Findings

- Dense portal inflammatory cell infiltrates, including large numbers of lymphocytes and often plasma cells
- "Florid duct lesions": lymphocyte-mediated bile duct injury with nuclear disarray, cytoplasmic eosinophilia, and vacuolization
  Granulomas or loose collections of histiocytes associated with bile duct injury
  Variable bile ductular proliferation
- Late-stage primary biliary cholangitis (PBC) exhibits features of chronic cholestasis, duct loss and biliary-type cirrhosis

Genetics

- Increased prevalence among first-degree relatives; variety of reported human leukocyte antigen haplotypes

Differential Diagnosis

- Primary sclerosing cholangitis
- Autoimmune hepatitis (AIH)
  AIH–PBC overlap syndrome
  Chronic viral hepatitis, especially hepatitis C
  Granulomatous diseases, including sarcoidosis
- Drug-induced liver injury

Ancillary Studies

Rhodanine or orcein stains highlight copper deposits within periportal hepatocytes in the setting of chronic cholestasis of any cause and can be helpful to confirm the presence of a chronic cholestatic condition (Fig. 17.24E). Cytokeratins (CK7 or CK19) can be used to identify and count interlobular bile ducts, especially when ductopenia is suspected. CK7 often stains periportal hepatocytes (biliary metaplasia of hepatocytes) in chronic biliary disorders (Fig. 17.24F).

Differential Diagnosis

The differential diagnosis for PBC depends on the stage of the disease. Given the prominent portal inflammation seen in the early stages, PBC must be distinguished from chronic viral hepatitis and AIH. Histologic clues, AMA status, and serologic and PCR-based assays for viral hepatitis are helpful in this distinction. Distinguishing AIH from PBC may be difficult because the clinical features overlap, both are often ANA positive, patients with PBC can be AMA negative, and PBC can be patchy in distribution. Whereas PBC is associated with cholestatic liver enzymes (ALP or GGT elevations), AIH is characterized by striking transaminase elevations. Although mild bile duct injury can be seen in AIH, bile duct destruction is not a feature of AIH. Interface hepatitis is a key feature of AIH, but significant lobular hepatocyte injury is not a feature in PBC.

Compared with PBC, peripheral needle biopsy in patients with PSC usually shows nonspecific histologic features with less prominent portal inflammation. Clinical and imaging findings are key in separating these entities (Table 17.6). Sarcoidosis is associated with destruction of bile ducts, granulomas, cholestatic liver serology, and an irregular pattern of fibrosis. However, sarcoidosis is usually associated with well-formed granulomas, includes scarring within and around foci of granulomatous inflammation, lacks AMA positivity, and often shows other systemic manifestations of the disease.

TABLE 17.6

Clinicopathologic Features of Primary Biliary Cholangitis and Primary Sclerosing Cholangitis

	Primary Biliary Cholangitis	Primary Sclerosing Cholangitis
Age	Median age, 50 years (30–70 years)	Median age, 30 years
Gender	Predominantly female (90%)	Predominantly male (70%)
Clinical course	Progressive	Unpredictable but progressive
Associated conditions	Sjögren's syndrome (70%) Scleroderma (5%) Rheumatoid arthritis Thyroid disease (20%)	Inflammatory bowel disease (UC more common than CD) Pancreatitis (≤25%) Idiopathic fibrosing diseases (retroperitoneal fibrosis)
Serology incidence	95% AMA positive 20% ANA positive 60% ANCA positive	0%–5% AMA positive (low titer) 6% ANA positive 82% ANCA positive
Radiology	Normal	Strictures and beading of large bile ducts; "pruning" of smaller ducts
Duct lesion	Florid duct lesion; loss of small ducts	Concentric periductal fibrosis with epithelial injury; loss of small ducts

AMA, Antimitochondrial antibody; *ANA*, antinuclear antibody; *ANCA*, antineutrophil cytoplasmic antibody.

PROGNOSIS AND THERAPY

If untreated, PBC follows a progressive clinical course. Most but not all asymptomatic patients develop significant liver disease. Survival is variable, ranging from 6 to 12 years after presentation for untreated symptomatic patients to several decades for asymptomatic patients. Ursodeoxycholic acid is an effective treatment, especially when started early in the course of the disease, and has been shown to reduce morbidity (delays histologic progression and risk of developing esophageal varices) and improve survival (≤84% at 10 years). Patients with "AMA-negative PBC" are treated like AMA-positive patients and exhibit the same outcomes as those with AMA positivity. Liver transplantation is the only effective therapy for late-stage disease.

PRIMARY SCLEROSING CHOLANGITIS

CLINICAL FEATURES

Primary sclerosing cholangitis is a chronic progressive, fibroinflammatory condition of the bile ducts that results in biliary cirrhosis and hepatic failure. It can only be reliably diagnosed when all other causes of secondary cholangitis, such as postoperative bile duct injury, biliary lithiasis, ischemic cholangiopathy, and IgG4-related cholangitis, among others, can be excluded clinically.

In its classic form, PSC typically affects extrahepatic and large intrahepatic bile ducts. In a minority of patients (5%), only small ducts are affected ("small duct PSC"). Males are more commonly affected (male-to-female ratio, 2–3 to 1), and disease onset usually occurs before 50 years of age. Patients with PSC show an increased prevalence of human leukocyte antigen (HLA) B8 and DR3 antigens. Most, if not all, patients with PSC have inflammatory bowel disease; however, only 2.5% to 7.5% of patients with ulcerative colitis have PSC. Patients with PSC and ulcerative colitis are at increased risk for cholangiocarcinoma and pancreatic adenocarcinoma.

LABORATORY FINDINGS

Serologic studies reveal cholestatic biochemistry (usually ALP elevations), often with normal bilirubin levels. A diagnosis of PSC is established upon identification of multifocal beading, stricturing and irregularity of the extrahepatic biliary system, and dilation of the intrahepatic biliary tree on cholangiography (ERCP or MRCP) (Fig. 17.25). Liver biopsy is only performed in patients lacking imaging findings and in those suspected to have small duct PSC.

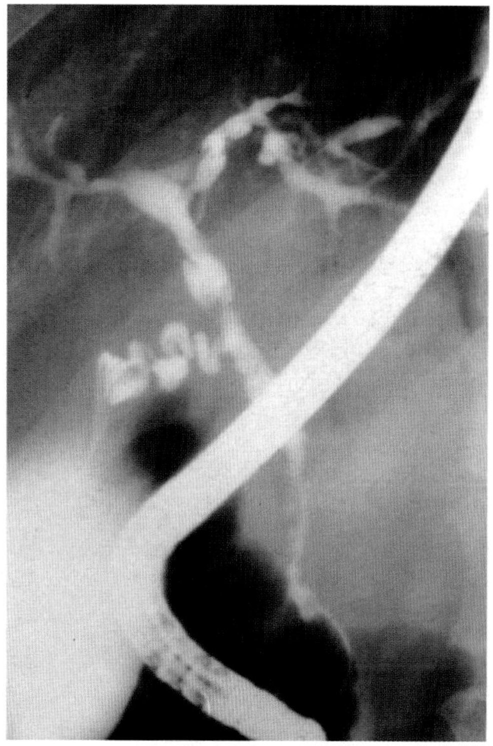

FIGURE 17.25
Primary sclerosing cholangitis. Extrahepatic and large intrahepatic bile ducts show alternating areas of beading and structuring.

PRIMARY SCLEROSING CHOLANGITIS—FACT SHEET

Definition
- Chronic biliary disease characterized by inflammation and fibrosis of biliary tree, involving both intra- and extrahepatic bile ducts

Incidence and Location
- Up to 5% prevalence in patients with ulcerative colitis
- Prevalence in US population ranges from 1 to over 16 per 100,000

Morbidity and Mortality
- Progressive disease, with a median survival period from diagnosis 9 to 18 years if liver transplant is not an option
- Complications include bacterial cholangitis and biliary stones
- Increased risk of neoplasia: adenocarcinoma bile ducts, colon, pancreas

Gender, Race, and Age Distribution
- More common in young men (<70%) of northern European descent; rare in Asia
- Mean age at diagnosis is approximately 40 years
- Also occurs in children

Clinical Features
- Strongly associated with ulcerative colitis and other autoimmune diseases
- Presentation ranges from asymptomatic to cirrhosis
- Fluctuating jaundice, fatigue, and weight loss are common presenting symptoms
- Elevated alkaline phosphatase

Radiologic Features

- Endoscopic retrograde cholangiopancreatography and magnetic resonance cholangiopancreatography can identify multifocal strictures and beading involving the extra- and intrahepatic biliary tree

Prognosis and Therapy

- No effective medical treatment
- Patients with dominant bile duct strictures may be treated with balloon dilation, stent placement, or surgery
- Liver transplantation for end-stage disease results in a greater than 80% 5-year survival rate

Pathologic Features

Gross Findings

In late-stage PSC, the liver is grossly cirrhotic and bile stained. Hilar fibrosis may be prominent, as are extrahepatic biliary strictures. Dense hilar scarring may mimic the appearance of cholangiocarcinoma.

Microscopic Findings

Larger bile ducts are not sampled in peripheral liver biopsies. As a result, liver biopsies from patients with PSC may be completely normal or only show nonspecific features. Thus, the absence of histologic findings on needle core biopsies does not exclude a diagnosis of large duct PSC.

The classic histologic features of PSC include periductal, concentric onion-skinning fibrosis associated with mild portal inflammation and bile duct injury (Fig. 17.26A). The bile duct epithelium is often flattened and may show vacuolization or eosinophilia of the cytoplasm with pyknotic nuclei. As the injury progresses, bile ducts may disappear, leaving an area of scar (tombstone or "fibro-obliterative" lesions) (Fig. 17.26B). The portal inflammatory infiltrates are usually sparse and primarily composed of lymphocytes with scattered plasma cells and eosinophils. The hepatic lobules are usually unremarkable in the early stage of the disease. With progressive disease, the parenchyma shows features of chronic cholestasis as well as changes of large duct obstruction such as bile ductular proliferation, canalicular cholestasis, and portal edema. In liver explant specimens, larger intrahepatic bile ducts are often dilated and contain inspissated bile plugs and sludge (Fig. 17.26C). The walls of large bile ducts are fibrotic and contain chronic inflammatory cells (Fig. 17.26D). Reactive epithelial atypia within injured ducts can be difficult to distinguish from biliary dysplasia.

Primary Sclerosing Cholangitis—Pathologic Features

Gross Findings

- Biliary-type cirrhosis in late stages
- Large intrahepatic and extrahepatic ducts may show dilation and strictures

Microscopic Findings

- Concentric ("onion skinning") periductal fibrosis
- Bile duct injury that leads to ductopenia and "tombstone" lesion (fibro-obliterative scars)
  Mild portal inflammatory infiltrates
- Chronic cholestatic changes and biliary type cirrhosis in late stages

Genetics

- Strong association with human leukocyte antigen haplotypes B8 and DR3

Differential Diagnosis

- Large bile duct obstruction
- Immunoglobulin G4 disease
  Ischemic cholangiopathy (ischemic cholangitis)
  Primary biliary cholangitis
- Idiopathic adulthood ductopenia

Differential Diagnosis

The differential diagnosis for PSC includes large bile duct obstruction, IgG4-related cholangitis, ischemic cholangitis, and PBC.

Chronic large duct obstruction may be difficult to distinguish from PSC because of overlapping clinical and histologic findings. However, chronic large duct obstruction seldom leads to loss of interlobular bile ducts, a feature characteristic of PSC.

In contrast to PSC, IgG4 cholangitis typically affects older men (mean age 60 years or older). Most patients have concomitant autoimmune (type I) pancreatitis. Imaging findings mimic those of PSC and include segmental strictures in the distal extrahepatic biliary tree. However, IgG4 cholangitis may show mass-forming lesions. Whereas ductopenia and fibro-obliterative lesions are more common in PSC, IgG4-positive plasma cell infiltration and perivenulitis are prominent in IgG4 cholangitis and storiform fibrosis can be seen. As a general rule, greater than 10 IgG4 positive plasma cells/hpf in biopsy specimens and greater than 50/hpf in resection specimens support a diagnosis of IgG4 cholangitis, but the sensitivity and specificity of this finding is low. Unlike PSC, the pathologic findings of IgG4 cholangitis, especially strictures, resolve with steroid therapy.

Most causes of ischemic cholangitis are iatrogenic in nature, including vascular injury at cholecystectomy, hepatic artery infusion with chemotherapeutic agents,

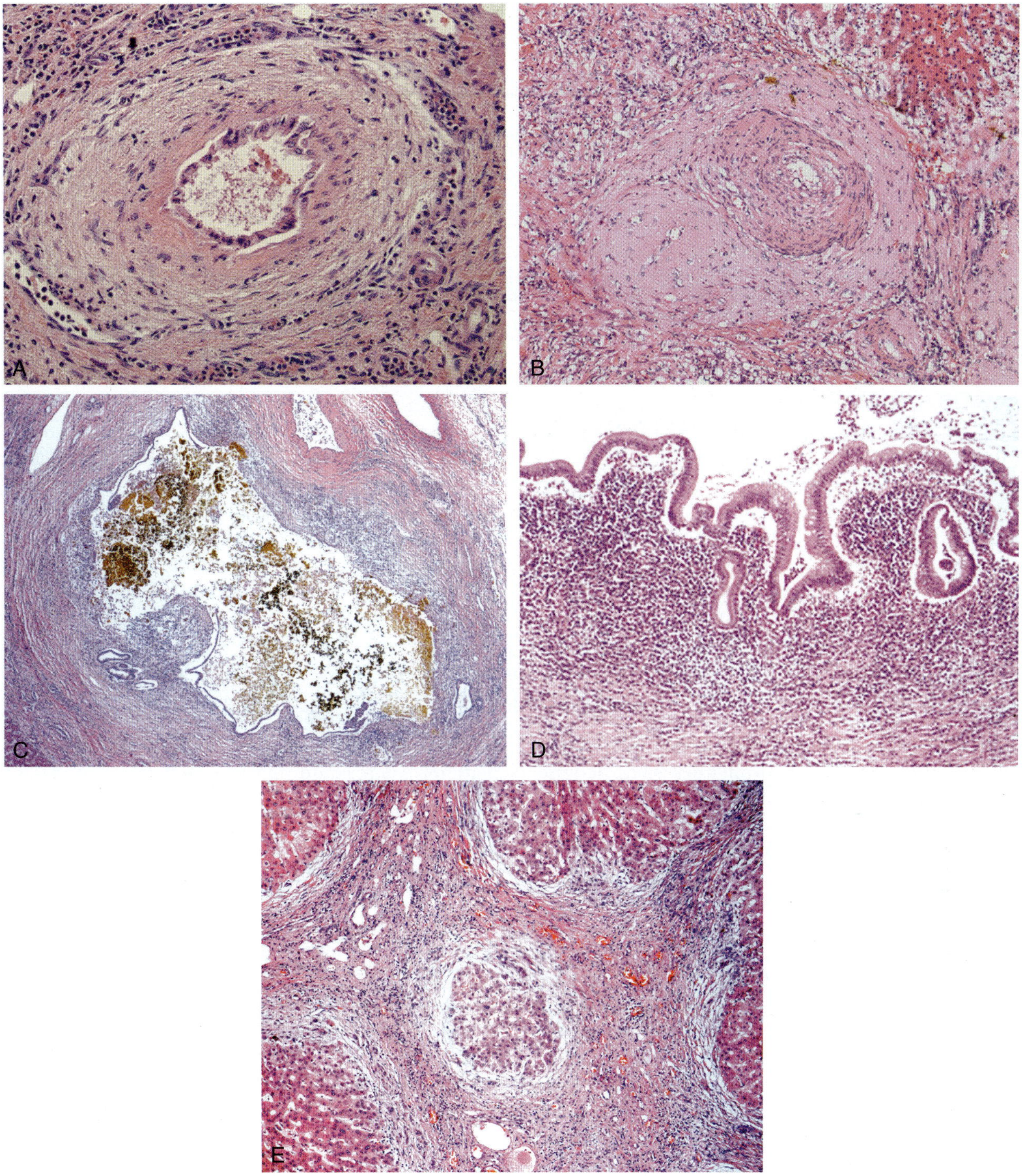

FIGURE 17.26

A, Interlobular bile ducts in PSC show a characteristic periductal pattern of "onion-skin" fibrosis. Also note the biliary epithelial injury. **B**, Fibroobliterative lesion mark the area of destroyed interlobular bile ducts in late-stage PSC. **C**, Large bile ducts in PSC often contain inspissated bile and biliary stones. **D**, The epithelium of large bile ducts is heavily infiltrated by mononuclear inflammatory cells; the underlying wall is fibrotic. **E**, The end result of PSC is biliary cirrhosis with ductopenia.

radiotherapy, and liver transplantation. However, human immunodeficiency virus (HIV), hereditary hemorrhagic telangiectasia, polyarteritis nodosa, and atherosclerosis are also associated with this entity. Unlike PSC, acute ischemic injury results in formation of biliary casts, bile duct necrosis, and bilomas. Fibrosing strictures of the biliary tree dominate the chronic stage.

Last, histologic overlap with PBC is occasionally a problem. However, knowledge of the clinical setting, serologic tests, and radiographic appearance generally helps in this distinction.

Prognosis and Therapy

The natural history of PSC is variable. PSC is commonly complicated by bacterial cholangitis, and cholangiocarcinoma is a major complication seen in up to 13% of patients with PSC. Immunosuppression is ineffective, and liver transplantation is the treatment of choice for late-stage disease. The mean duration of survival (without transplantation) ranges between 9 and 18 years from the time of diagnosis.

OVERLAP SYNDROMES (AUTOIMMUNE HEPATITIS, PRIMARY BILIARY CHOLANGITIS, AND PRIMARY SCLEROSING CHOLANGITIS)

A minority of patients with AIH exhibit clinical, serologic, and histologic features of one or more autoimmune liver diseases, such as PBC or PSC. These "overlap" syndromes may present as two concurrent or sequential diseases. Standardized diagnostic criteria are lacking, so the prevalence of overlap syndromes remains unclear. In general, a diagnosis of overlap syndrome requires clear, objective clinical and histologic features of AIH in combination with those of PBC or PSC.

The AIH–PBC overlap syndrome describes patients with clinical and histologic evidence of both AIH and PBC. Delineation of an overlap syndrome is somewhat challenging and controversial because overlap exists in the clinical and histologic features of otherwise typical AIH and PBC. For example, mild lymphocytic infiltration of bile ducts and cholestatic features can be seen in patients with AIH, but autoantibodies (ANA and ASMA) and plasma cells are detected in most patients with PBC. The presence of any of these features in isolation does not indicate the presence of an overlap syndrome.

Although diagnostic criteria for AIH–PBC overlap syndrome are not standardized, the European Association for the Study of Liver Disease guidelines require the presence of at least two of three specific criteria for AIH and PBC independently along with interface hepatitis. The criteria for AIH include (1) ALT levels at least five times the upper limit of normal, (2) IgG levels at least twice the upper limit of normal or positive ASMA, and (3) liver biopsy with moderate or severe periportal or periseptal lymphocytic piecemeal necrosis. The criteria for PBC are (1) ALP levels at least twice the upper limit of normal or GGT levels at least five times the upper limit of normal, (2) positive AMA, and (3) liver biopsy showing a florid duct lesion.

The AIH–PSC overlap syndrome is less common and usually occurs in children, adolescents, and young adults with autoimmune liver disease. The two diseases may occur concurrently but more commonly present sequentially in adults, with AIH frequently presenting before PSC. Histologic features of AIH–PSC overlap syndrome include those of AIH combined with periductal concentric fibrosis and bile duct injury. However, the diagnosis of PSC is often based on cholangiography rather than biopsy findings.

VASCULAR PATTERN OF INJURY

Vascular pathology of the liver can manifest with a broad spectrum of clinicopathologic findings, including abdominal pain, hepatomegaly, jaundice, portal hypertension, and mass-forming and diffuse nodular appearance of the parenchyma, among others. Vascular compromise can be secondary to reduced inflow (e.g., hepatic artery or portal vein thrombosis, obstruction), outflow obstruction (BCS, congestive heart failure) or systemic hypotension or hypovolemia (Table 17.7). The dual blood supply of liver provides protection against ischemia. However, an acute ischemic event is often uncompensated and results in hepatocyte necrosis. Because of the lower oxygen availability and higher metabolic activity, zone 3 hepatocytes are the first to be affected.

The clinical presentation of arterial flow impairment depends on the nature and timing of injury. Patients with acute, marked ischemic injury ("shock

TABLE 17.7
Common Causes of Vascular Pattern of Injury

Pathogenic Event	Entities
Ischemic injury	Hepatic artery disease (thrombosis or obstruction) discussed in Chapter 20 on liver transplantation) • Ischemic cholangiopathy: affecting bile ducts • Ischemic lobular injury: affecting lobular parenchyma Portal vein thrombosis (discussed later) or shock liver in setting of systemic hypotension • Ischemic injury affecting lobular parenchyma
Congestive injury	Hepatic vein disease • Budd-Chiari syndrome • Congestive (cardiac) hepatopathy Sinusoidal disease • Sinusoidal obstruction syndrome • Peliosis
Portal hypertensive injury	Portal vein disease • Portal vein thrombosis or obstruction • Nodular regenerative hyperplasia • Hepatoportal sclerosis

liver") show marked transaminase elevations (typically >5000 U/L) followed by a rapid decline. Hepatic arterial ischemia compromises blood flow to the peribiliary arterial plexus. Therefore, patients with arterial ischemia may show features of acute biliary injury (like bile duct epithelial cell necrosis and bile leaks) followed by progressive scarring, stricture formation, and loss of bile ducts. These changes are associated with marked elevation of serum ALP and bilirubin levels.

Acute and chronic venous outflow impairment present with distinct clinical and histologic pictures. Patients with acute impairment may present with hepatomegaly with or without splenomegaly, followed by jaundice in cases of severe injury. Progressive scarring can develop in patients with chronic outflow impairment. Laboratory findings are variable and may include elevated ALP elevations or ALT elevations reflecting hepatocellular injury.

BUDD-CHIARI SYNDROME

There is lack of agreement on the definition of BSC. Based on recommendations from the European Group for the Study of Vascular Disorders of the Liver, BCS should be used as an eponym for *hepatic venous outflow tract obstruction* independent of the level or mechanism of obstruction. Obstruction of venous outflow can occur at the level of hepatic veins (small or large branches), inferior vena cava (IVC), or both. By definition, the term excludes venous outflow obstruction from the other major causes of hepatic venous outflow obstruction: sinusoidal obstruction syndrome/veno-occlusive disease (SOS/VOD) and right-sided cardiac decompensation. Several conditions such as hypercoagulable states, membranous obstruction of IVC (especially in Asia and South Africa), and mechanical intrinsic or extrinsic compression of veins have been associated with BCS. Up to 30% of cases are idiopathic.

CLINICAL FEATURES

The prevalence of BCS is low, ranging from 0.2 to 2 cases per 1 million population. It is more common in Asia than in Western countries. Most affected Western patients tend to be young women, but in Asia, patients are middle aged, and there is no specific gender predilection. The clinical presentation ranges from complete absence of symptoms to fulminant hepatic failure. In most cases, the disease progresses through acute, subacute, or chronic stages. Asymptomatic BCS accounts for up to 20% of cases and is thought to be related to formation of large hepatic vein collaterals. Classical symptoms of BCS include fever, abdominal pain, hepatomegaly, ascites, lower extremity edema, GI bleeding, and hepatic encephalopathy. Jaundice and portal hypertension are uncommon. Superimposed features of portal venous obstruction are common in patients with severe BCS. Hepatic venography is considered the gold standard for establishing the diagnosis. Alternatively, less invasive techniques, such as Doppler ultrasonography and magnetic resonance imaging (MRI) or computed tomography (CT) scan with contrast, are also helpful. Imaging studies often reveal caudate lobe hypertrophy in 75% of patients. Regenerative nodules are more common in patients with chronic BCS.

LABORATORY FINDINGS

Liver enzymes, including transaminases and ALP, can be normal or variably increased.

PATHOLOGIC FEATURES

MACROSCOPIC FINDINGS

In the acute setting, the liver may be enlarged with congestion. Later stages may reveal evidence of fibrosis and nodularity. The large hepatic veins may contain organizing thrombi or obstructing membranes or webs.

MICROSCOPIC FINDINGS

Thrombosis of large veins cannot be appreciated on biopsy specimens, but small vein thrombosis with intimal thickening can be evident in some cases. The classic features in the acute phase include zone 3 congestion, sinusoidal dilation, liver plate atrophy, and red blood cells in spaces of Disse (Fig. 17.27). Zone 3 necrosis and parenchymal collapse may be present in rapidly

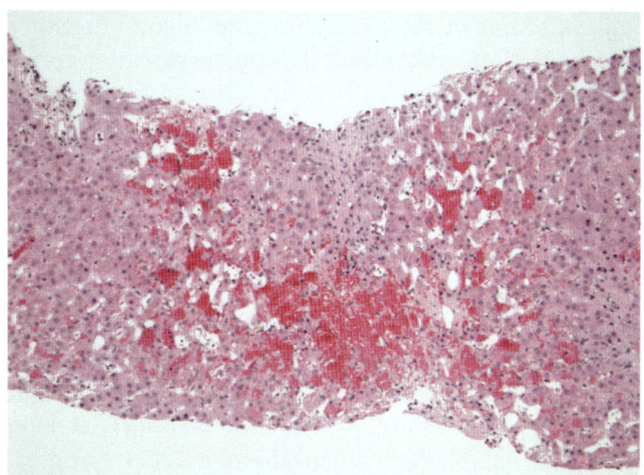

FIGURE 17.27

Budd Chiari reveals congestion and sinusoidal dilation in zone 3, the distinction from congestive hepatopathy is mainly made through correlation with clinical history.

progressive cases. Nodular regenerative hyperplasia (NRH) and macroregenerative nodules are more typical of chronic BCS. These findings are attributed to superimposed obstruction of intrahepatic portal vein branches and increased arterial flow in the affected areas. In cases of pure hepatic vein involvement, the specimen may show central–central fibrous septa, a phenomenon known as reverse nodularity. If the cause of BCS cannot be reversed, patients may ultimately develop advanced irregular fibrosis or even cirrhosis.

Differential Diagnosis

The differential diagnosis for BCS includes congestive hepatopathy, biliary obstruction, and other causes of sinusoidal dilation and congestion. Congestive hepatopathy is distinguished based on the clinical features and is discussed later in this chapter. BCS can mimic chronic biliary disorders because approximately 50% of patients may show mild bile ductular proliferation and ALP elevations. In these cases, the lack of portal or periportal fibrosis and bile duct injury along with the presence of centrilobular injury should favor BCS. Other causes of sinusoidal dilation and congestion in the differential diagnosis include DILI (estrogen, azathioprine, oxaliplatin), collagen vascular diseases, Crohn's disease, HIV infection, sickle cell anemia, and hemophagocytic syndrome, among others.

Prognosis and Therapy

The prognosis depends on the clinical presentation. In acute BCS, the mortality rate is high. In chronic BCS, an overall 80% 5-year survival rate has been reported. Hepatocellular carcinoma remains a rare complication in this population. The treatment depends on the underlying cause but in most cases includes a combination of anticoagulation, thrombolysis, portosystemic venous shunt, or angioplasty with stent. Ultimately, transplantation is required in some cases.

CONGESTIVE (CARDIAC) HEPATOPATHY

Congestive hepatopathy, also known as *cardiac-related venous congestion* or *chronic passive venous congestion*, refers to hepatic parenchymal changes resulting from right ventricular failure. A diagnosis of congestive hepatopathy is established when there are (1) structural heart disease impairing right heart function, (2) signs and symptoms of right heart failure, (3) serology consistent with cholestasis, and (4) exclusion of other possible causes of liver damage.

CLINICAL FEATURES

Patients with congestive hepatopathy present with dull right upper quadrant pain, nausea, vomiting, anorexia, and mild jaundice. A pulsatile liver or positive hepatojugular reflux is often present. Ascites occurs in up to 25% of patients. Most patients often have long-standing history of cardiovascular or pulmonary disease, which, if left untreated, leads to cirrhosis and complications of portal hypertension.

Laboratory findings may vary depending on the clinical presentation. Transaminases can be increased two to three times the normal range in most cases, mainly in patients with low cardiac output. Total bilirubin is often mildly elevated. In addition, abnormalities in GGT and ALP are associated with elevated vascular pressures.

On imaging, classic features include hepatomegaly, cirrhosis, and variably ascites as well as features of portal hypertension and its complications.

Pathologic Features

Macroscopic Findings

The liver is often enlarged, tense, and congested. The cut surface is classically described as "nutmeg liver," presenting a variegated mottled discoloration that results from passive congestion and hypoperfusion. Extensive fibrosis usually develops in the later stages of the disease.

Microscopic Findings

Early findings of congestive hepatopathy include centrilobular sinusoidal dilation with hepatocellular atrophy (Fig. 17.28A). In severe cases, there are necrosis and dropout of centrilobular and accumulation of ceroid-laden macrophages. Inflammation is typically absent or inconspicuous. Cholestasis, when present, is mild and only seen in severe cases. The iron stain may show increased storage iron within Kupffer cells in the centrilobular areas (Fig. 17.28B). Another unique finding is that the centrilobular hepatocytes may show intracytoplasmic eosinophilic hyaline globules (the so-called congestion-associated globules) composed of a combination of serum proteins that are PAS positive and diastase resistant. These should not be confused with cytoplasmic globules found in α1AT deficiency, which are typically located within the periportal hepatocytes.

In long-standing cases, perivenular or perisinusoidal fibrosis develops and eventually progresses to bridging fibrosis between adjacent central veins (Fig. 17.28C). The distribution of fibrosis is quite variable within the sampled hepatic parenchyma. At this stage, there may be evidence of variable compensatory hepatocyte hyperplasia.

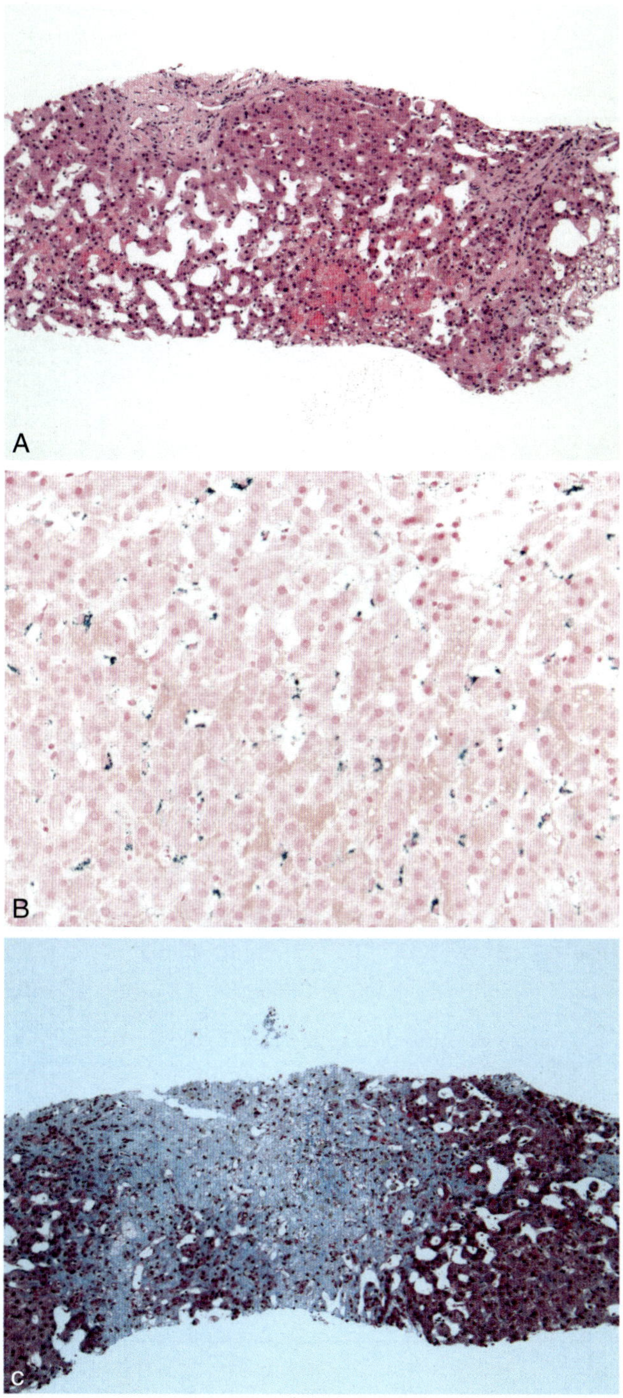

FIGURE 17.28

Congestive hepatopathy. **A**, Marked centrilobular sinusoidal congestion and dilatation is often present with extravasated red blood cells, hepatocellular atrophy and drop out. **B**, Nonspecific iron accumulation can be seen in Kupffer cells within the sinusoids. **C**, Fibrosis is mainly centrilobular with progression to obliteration of central veins.

Differential Diagnosis

The clinical presentation and history are usually sufficient to indicate the correct diagnosis. A liver biopsy is only performed to exclude any concurrent hepatic disorder. In patients with no history of a cardiac or pulmonary disorder, the differential diagnosis for histologic findings includes BCS, peliosis, and other causes of sinusoidal dilation mentioned earlier in this chapter.

Prognosis and Therapy

Therapy is directed towards treating the underlying cause and improving cardiac function through lifestyle modifications and medications. Congestive hepatopathy is reversible during early stages of the disease.

SINUSOIDAL OBSTRUCTION SYNDROME

Hepatic SOS (also known as VOD) is a potentially life-threatening complication that is most commonly observed in patients undergoing hematopoietic stem cell transplantation (HSCT). It was originally described nearly 100 years ago in Jamaican individuals consuming pyrrolizidine alkaloid–containing African bush tea and in those consuming inadequately winnowed wheat or herbal traditional remedies in India and Egypt. Myeloablative high-dose chemoradiation treatment in the context of HSCT is the most common cause of SOS. Other causes include solid organ transplant, systemic inflammatory conditions, and chemotherapeutic agents (oxaliplatin, azathioprine, and others). An autosomal recessive condition of SOS with immunodeficiency has also been described. The term *veno-occlusive disease* was used to denote the fibrous obliteration of small hepatic vein branches, including the terminal hepatic venules. However, recent animal model experiments have shown that the main injury in SOS occurs at the level of hepatic sinusoids, and the centrilobular venous involvement that occurs after this acute phase of sinusoidal injury becomes less apparent. Thus, SOS is currently diagnosed even in the absence of the characteristic hepatic venous lesions.

CLINICAL FEATURES

Sinusoidal obstruction syndrome is not associated with a specific age or gender. Clinical features of SOS include hepatomegaly, weight gain caused by fluid accumulation or ascites, and hyperbilirubinemia. A Doppler ultrasound study demonstrating hepatomegaly, ascites, reversal of portal venous flow, and attenuation of hepatic venous flow, in the absence of other causes, is highly suggestive of SOS.

Laboratory Findings

Liver function tests usually show hyperbilirubinemia and elevated transaminase and serum ALP levels.

Pathologic Features

Macroscopic Findings

The liver may be enlarged and congested with foci of hemorrhage. In severe SOS, the liver shows a bluish-red, marbled appearance. There may be evidence of dilated blood-filled spaces (peliosis hepatis) on cut section.

Microscopic Findings

The liver biopsy findings may be patchy in distribution and vary over the course of the disease. In the acute phase of SOS, there is prominent zone 3 sinusoidal dilation along with sinusoidal congestion, hepatocellular atrophy, and centrilobular necrosis. The endothelial injury initially results in subendothelial edema and later leads to obliteration of central veins (Fig. 17.29A). A Movat stain may be required to identify the "obscured veins." In the chronic phase, congestion is minimal. Instead, there is dense perivenular fibrosis radiating into the parenchyma dominates, with complete obliteration of the central veins and hemosiderin deposition (Fig. 17.29B).

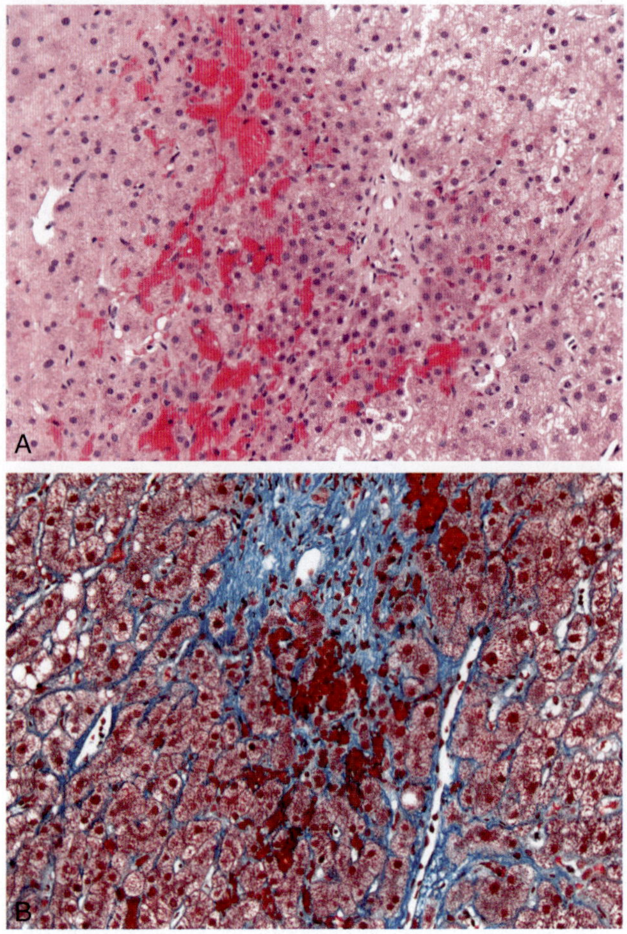

FIGURE 17.29

Sinusoidal obstruction syndrome. **A**, Obliteration of a central vein chemotherapy induced. **B**, Trichrome stain shows fibrosis of the central vein, in other instances, Movat stain can be helpful in highlighting the presence of a vein wall.

Differential Diagnosis

The differential diagnosis for SOS includes other causes of zone 3 congestion and sinusoidal dilation. BCS shows centrilobular parenchymal changes similar to SOS; however, occlusion of the central veins is diagnostic of SOS. Severe SOS may mimic drug-induced liver injury by exhibiting hepatocyte necrosis, cholestasis, and inflammation. However, the occlusive venous changes of SOS help in distinguishing the two causes.

Prognosis and Therapy

Treatment is targeted toward preventing fluid overload and vascular compromise to the liver with anticoagulant therapy and methylprednisolone. Proposed strategies for SOS prevention include reduced conditioning for HSCT, treatment with ursodeoxycholic acid, and using a combination of chemotherapeutic agents to lower drug toxicity. Although significant progress has been made to improve outcomes, SOS remains a serious complication with a mortality rate of up to 30%.

PORTAL VEIN THROMBOSIS OR OBSTRUCTION

CLINICAL FEATURES

The clinical features of portal vein disease depend on whether the process involves the large (extrahepatic) portal vein or smaller intrahepatic branches. Large portal vein thrombosis may present acutely as a catastrophic and potentially lethal event or follow an insidious clinical course, whereas obstruction of the smaller branches is often asymptomatic. Whereas the more acute clinical course occurs in the setting of sepsis, abdominal trauma or surgical interventions, or intravascular tumor spread, a silent clinical course is often associated with various causes, including cirrhosis, systemic inflammatory disease, vasculitis, prothrombotic states, medications, sarcoidosis, or schistosomiasis, among others. Occlusion of smaller portal veins branches is linked to obstruction as well as inflammatory and toxic injury of diverse nature.

Occlusion of the main portal vein or its branches produces abdominal pain, portal hypertension, ascites, and GI bleeding caused by esophageal varices. Severe continuous and colicky abdominal pain with bloody diarrhea often signifies concomitant mesenteric vein thrombosis and intestinal infarction. Imaging studies can confirm obstruction of larger branches and assess possible causes such as extrinsic compression by tumors.

PATHOLOGIC FEATURES

Macroscopic Findings

The portal vein may show a partially obstructed lumen with thickening of the vessel wall. For cases presenting more acutely, fresh intraluminal thrombus may be evident in addition to areas of parenchymal congestion and necrosis. In advanced cases, there may be scarring or nodularity of the vein.

Microscopic Findings

Depending on the phase of the disease, the portal vein and its branches may show organizing or recanalized thrombus (Fig. 17.30). More severe injury is associated with centrilobular hepatocyte swelling, hepatocellular dropout, and hepatocellular necrosis as a result of ischemia. NRH may be seen in cases of chronic episodes of suboptimal portal vein flow.

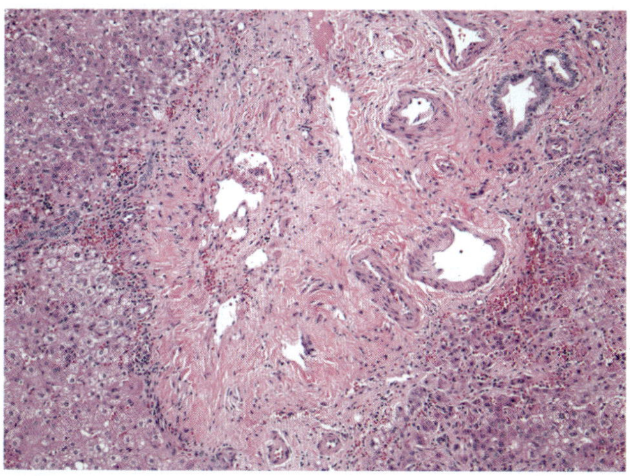

FIGURE 17.30

A portal tract demonstrates thrombosis and recanalization of the portal vein in long standing cirrhosis.

Differential Diagnosis

In most cases, portal vein thrombosis or obstruction occurs as a superimposed phenomenon in patients with cirrhosis and portal hypertension. Other causes of noncirrhotic portal hypertension, including hepatoportal sclerosis (HPS; see section on Hepatoportal Sclerosis), should be considered.

Prognosis and Therapy

Anticoagulation therapy for at least 3 months is the mainstay therapy for acute portal vein thrombosis. In patients with chronic portal vein thrombosis, variceal banding or sclerotherapy is used to control bleeding resulting from portal hypertension.

NODULAR REGENERATIVE HYPERPLASIA

Nodular regenerative hyperplasia develops in the setting of abnormal blood flow to the liver and is characterized by the presence of multiple 1- to 2-mm nodules distributed diffusely throughout the parenchyma. NRH is part of a spectrum of hepatic disorders that cause noncirrhotic portal hypertension and manifest histologically as HPS, SOS, and incomplete septal cirrhosis. NRH has been associated with several conditions, including drug-induced injury (e.g., oxaliplatin, azathioprine), portal vein thrombosis, prothrombotic states, immunologic disorders (e.g., HIV, collagen vascular diseases, liver allograft, celiac disease, common variable immunodeficiency), and multiple tumors in the liver.

CLINICAL FEATURES

The clinical presentation varies depending on the underlying cause, and patients may manifest signs of portal hypertension or may be completely asymptomatic. Imaging may show only focal nodularity (nodular transformation of the hilum) or diffuse nodularity of the liver that raises suspicion for cirrhosis.

Laboratory Findings

Laboratory findings may reveal elevation of ALP and transaminase levels.

Pathologic Features

Macroscopic Findings

Diffuse nodularity mimicking cirrhosis is seen grossly, but palpation of the cut surface confirms the lack of scarring associated with the nodules.

Microscopic Findings

The hepatic parenchyma has a vaguely nodular appearance at low magnification. However, there is no accompanying fibrosis. The parenchymal nodularity is caused by atrophy of zone 3 hepatocytes and compensatory enlargement of hepatocytes in zones 1 and 2 (Fig. 17.31A). Reticulin stain is extremely helpful in highlighting the vague nodularity and collapse of the reticulin framework (within zone 3) in subtle cases (Fig. 17.31B). Sinusoidal dilation is often present. Special attention should be paid to the vasculature and superimposed findings that could serve as a clue to the underlying cause.

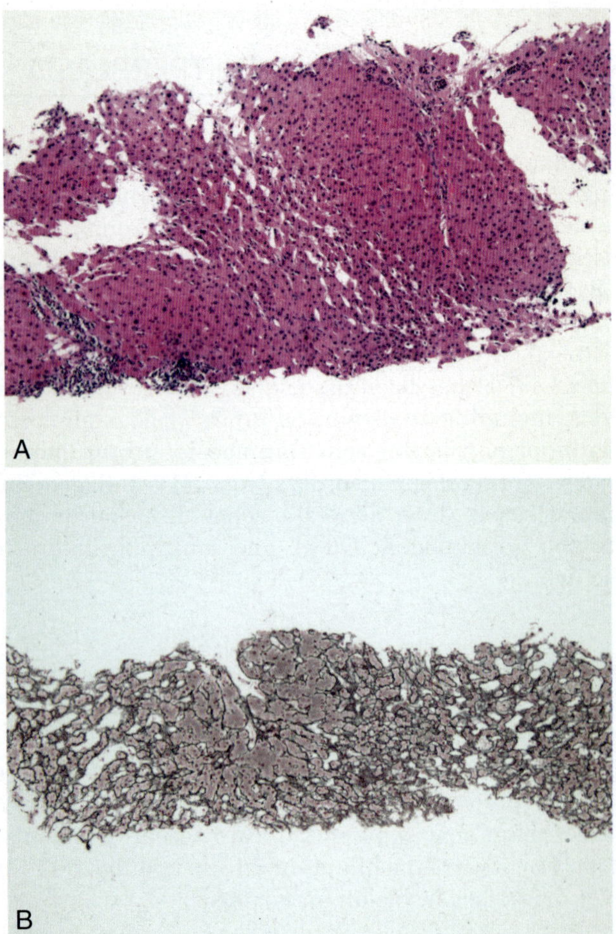

FIGURE 17.31

Nodular regenerative hyperplasia. **A**, A low power magnification reveals a vaguely nodular architecture due to the relative preservation of zone 1 hepatocytes and atrophy of zone 3-2 hepatocytes. **B**, Reticulin stain emphasizes the collapse of the reticulin framework, with accentuation of the nodularity particularly useful in subtle cases.

Differential Diagnosis

The main clinical differential diagnosis is cirrhosis. The lack of fibrosis on trichrome stain as well as typical findings on reticulin stain is helpful in distinguishing NRH from cirrhosis. In patients with portal hypertension and no evidence of cirrhosis, other causes of noncirrhotic portal hypertension (see later) should be excluded both clinically and histologically.

Prognosis and Therapy

The treatment of patients with NRH is directed towards treating the underlying cause. The prognosis largely depends on the severity of underlying disease and management of complications related to portal hypertension.

HEPATOPORTAL SCLEROSIS

The term *noncirrhotic portal hypertension* encompasses a variety of conditions that manifest as portal hypertension but do not show histologic evidence of cirrhosis. The underlying causes can be divided into "primary causes" in which the cause is unknown (idiopathic noncirrhotic portal hypertension) and "secondary causes" caused by a variety of conditions such as SOS, hepatic venous outflow impairment, extrahepatic portal venous thrombosis, schistosomiasis, or congenital hepatic fibrosis, among others. HPS is a presinusoidal cause of noncirrhotic portal hypertension. Other names for this entity include Banti's disease, noncirrhotic portal fibrosis, obliterative portal venopathy, and noncirrhotic intrahepatic portal hypertension. Although the exact cause of HPS remains unclear, hypercoagulability, infection, and immunologic abnormalities have been suggested to play a role.

CLINICAL FEATURES

Most cases have been reported in Asia (mostly young men in India and middle-aged women in Japan); this disease is rare in Western countries. The clinical manifestations include anemia or pancytopenia and features of portal hypertension (splenomegaly, varices with or without hematemesis, and elevated portal pressure) in the absence of cirrhosis with patent large portal and hepatic veins and normal to mildly elevated liver function tests. Encephalopathy is rare.

Pathologic Features

Macroscopic Findings

The liver may appear completely normal or may show a wrinkled capsular surface. Gross nodularity is uncommon.

Microscopic Findings

The main goal of liver biopsy is to evaluate for any potential cause of portal hypertension and confirm or exclude cirrhosis. The histologic findings of HPS may be patchy. Typical cases show portal fibrosis and abnormalities of the intrahepatic portal veins such as phlebosclerosis, portal vein dilation or arterialization, and herniation of the portal veins into the periportal tissue (Fig. 17.32). There may be accompanying sinusoidal dilation and perisinusoidal fibrosis. In addition, portal tract remnants (portal tracts with an overall size smaller than twice the diameter of their bile ducts) have been associated with this entity. NRH and incomplete thin septa are also described and can be highlighted on reticulin and trichrome stains. In most cases, the bile ducts are intact. The lobular parenchyma is generally unremarkable except for patchy foci of hepatocellular atrophy. In long-standing cases, the hepatic veins show obliteration of the lumens and phlebosclerosis with marked parenchymal atrophy.

Differential Diagnosis

Hepatoportal sclerosis is a diagnosis of exclusion. Compared with primary extrahepatic portal vein thrombosis, HPS is more frequently seen in men and often shows more portal tract remnants, phlebosclerosis, portal vein arterialization, and NRH. Portal vein dilation is often more severe in primary extrahepatic portal vein thrombosis. However, these histologic features have a low overall specificity, and other clinical findings, including vascular imaging studies for portal vein thrombosis, are often required to separate these entities.

Prognosis and Therapy

The prognosis in Western countries has been regarded as poor compared with Asian cohorts that demonstrate a 100% 5-year survival rate. Treatment is symptomatic

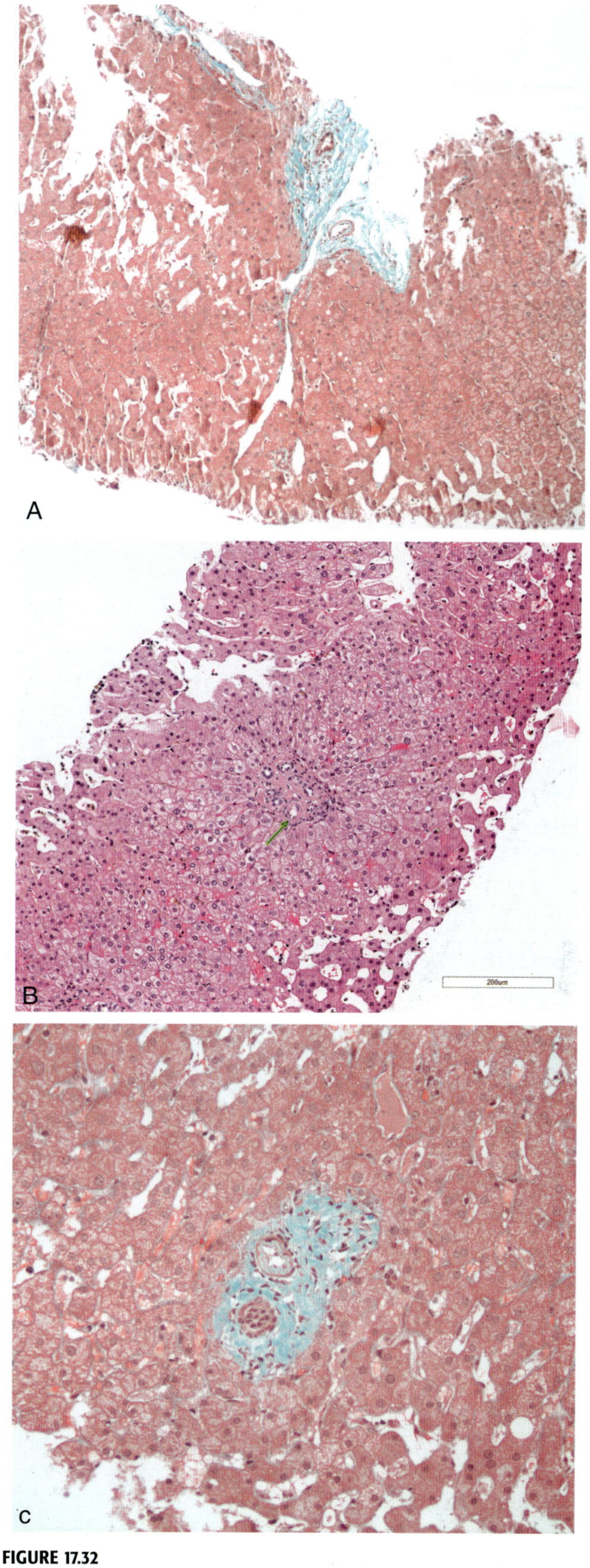

FIGURE 17.32

Hepatoportal sclerosis. **A**, Herniation of portal veins extending into the lobule. **B**, Long-standing cases may show complete obliteration/loss of portal veins. **C**, Trichrome stain can aid identified the lack of portal veins in portal tracts.

and includes beta-blockers, endoscopic sclerotherapy, and endoscopic band ligation of varices. In patients with more severe variceal bleeding or symptomatic hypersplenism, portosystemic shunt surgery or splenectomy may be required.

PELIOSIS HEPATIS

Peliosis hepatis is a rare entity characterized by the presence of multiple blood-filled cysts that are randomly distributed throughout the liver. These cystic lesions are thought to be a consequence of ruptured sinusoids. The disease may involve other organs such as the lungs, spleen, and lymph nodes. Peliosis hepatis has been associated with steroid use (anabolic, oral contraceptives), danazol, tamoxifen, thorotrast, methotrexate, vinyl chloride exposure, azathioprine, leukemia and lymphoma, and *Bartonella henselae* infection.

CLINICAL FEATURES

The diagnosis is often incidental at the time of autopsy. Patients can also present with intraabdominal bleeding as a result of ruptured cysts. *Bartonella* infection can be detected using serologic studies, cultures, and PCR-based assays.

PATHOLOGIC FEATURES

MACROSCOPIC FINDINGS

The hepatic parenchyma shows multiple round, blood-filled spaces ranging from 0.2 to 5 cm in diameter. These spaces may be separated by foci of fibrosis. Long-standing cases of peliosis may show foci of dystrophic calcification.

MICROSCOPIC FINDINGS

The characteristic finding is the presence of blood lakes surrounded by hepatic cords and lacking an endothelial lining (Fig. 17.33). Reticulin stain is useful in demonstrating the absence of reticulin framework in areas of peliosis. Adjacent lobular parenchyma may show sinusoidal dilation, fibrosis, organizing thrombosis, and calcification. In bacillary peliosis, the organisms are usually extracellular or within Kupffer cells and can be easily highlighted by Warthin-Starry stain. Bacillary peliosis may also be associated with vascular proliferation, similar to that observed in bacillary angiomatosis.

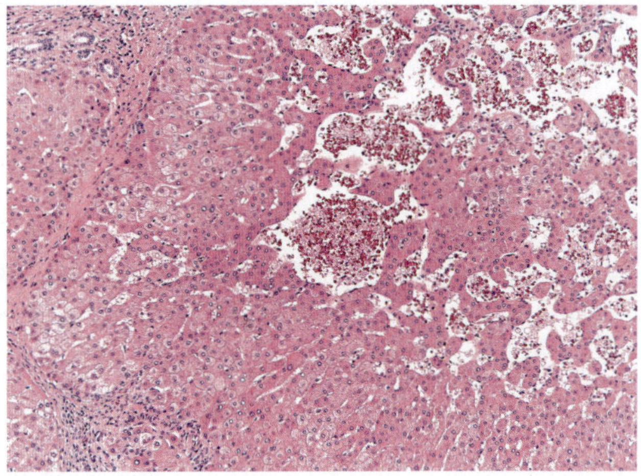

FIGURE 17.33
Peliosis. Dilated blood-filled spaces surrounded by hepatocytes and lacking an endothelial lining.

ANCILLARY STAINS

Warthin-Starry stain highlights the organisms of *B. henselae*.

DIFFERENTIAL DIAGNOSIS

Extensive sinusoidal dilation may mimic peliosis hepatic, but intact sinusoidal walls and well-maintained reticulin framework in areas of sinusoidal dilation help distinguish these entities.

PROGNOSIS AND THERAPY

Most cases are incidentally found and require no specific therapy. Erythromycin or doxycycline therapy is used to treat *B. henselae* infection, but relapses are known to occur.

DRUG-INDUCED LIVER INJURY

Drug-induced liver injury results from deleterious effects of compounds present in medications, toxins, herbal products, and dietary supplements that are primarily metabolized in the liver. Because many cases are asymptomatic and DILI is largely underreported, the true incidence is difficult to estimate. The mechanism of injury is either "intrinsic" (dose dependent) or "idiosyncratic" (non–dose dependent). Acetaminophen toxicity is the prototype of intrinsic injury and one of the leading causes of DILI. Idiosyncratic DILI accounts for approximately 15% of cases of acute liver failure in the United States. Idiosyncratic DILI can be further subdivided into hypersensitivity (immune-mediated processes, one-third of cases) and metabolism-mediated injury (two-thirds of cases).

Several risk factors have been proposed for idiosyncratic reactions, including HLA genotypes (e.g., HLA-DRB1*15 and *6 in amoxicillin–clavulanate toxicity), mitochondrial enzyme (cytochrome P450, N-acetyltransferase 2, UDP-glucuronosyltransferases, and glutathione S-transferases) gene polymorphisms, and as gene variants (mitochondrial DNA polymerase c gene [*POLG*] in sodium valproate toxicity). Age may be a risk factor as well because children are at a greater risk for developing DILI in the setting of valproate therapy and aspirin use, but older individuals may be more susceptible to isoniazid and toxicity induced by amoxicillin–clavulanate.

CLINICAL FEATURES

Although most patients are asymptomatic and show only mild elevation of liver enzymes ("biochemical hepatitis"), some develop symptoms related to cholestatic or hepatic injury. Hypersensitivity reactions are associated with fever, rash, edema, and peripheral eosinophilia. Severe DILI can occasionally result in acute liver failure, a complication more frequently encountered in women than men.

Temporal association between exposure to the agent and onset of symptoms is useful in some cases, although other agents may induce a delayed response after months or years of use.

More recent antiretroviral drugs (etravirine, raltegravir, elvitegravir, dolutegravir) exhibit lower toxicity characterized by hepatocellular injury and hypersensitivity reactions. Tyrosine kinase inhibitors (lapatinib, pazopanib, ponatinib, regorafenib, and sunitinib) more frequently show transient elevation of transaminases caused by hepatocellular injury ($\leq$50% of cases), but severe hepatotoxicity has also been documented. Monoclonal antibodies are widely used in today's practice. Whereas rituximab and bevacizumab have not shown significant hepatotoxicity, other agents such as ipilimumab and trastuzumab have been associated with hepatocellular injury and rarely with more severe hepatocellular injury, especially when used in combination with other chemotherapeutic drugs. Newer therapies with check point inhibitors have shown to induce multiple patterns of injury including hepatitic, cholangitic, mixed, steatotic patterns as well as nonspecific changes.

Among anti–TNF-α agents, infliximab has been reported as the most common implicated agent in DILI, with a hepatocellular pattern of injury in 75% of cases.

Herbal and dietary supplement (HDS) use has increased significantly over the past several years in the United States. Even though the US DILI Network has been reporting anecdotal cases, the incidence of DILI associated with HDS is unknown. Weight loss supplements (e.g., Hydroxy cut and OxyElite) were among the most common type of HDS implicated in DILI and more frequently induced hepatocellular injury.

LABORATORY FINDINGS

Given the heterogeneous clinical manifestation, there is no diagnostic test or histologic finding that can unequivocally confirm the diagnosis. Based on the liver enzyme profile, cholestatic, hepatitis, and mixed patterns can be recognized. Some patients may reveal autoantibodies including ANA and SMA, resulting in an AIH-like picture.

DRUG-INDUCED LIVER INJURY—FACT SHEET

Definition

- Hepatic injury secondary to exposure to a chemical compound

Incidence and Location

- Difficult to estimate with certainty; approximately 10% of cases of all "hepatitis" are suspected to be a drug reaction
- Up to 25% of acute liver failure cases

Morbidity and Mortality

- Depends on severity of injury and offending agent
- Low mortality for mild reactions and prompt withdrawal of injurious agent
- High mortality rate with direct hepatotoxins

Gender, Race, and Age Distribution

- Both genders; women more susceptible to acute liver failure
- All ages affected, although variations are noted among age groups

Clinical Features

- Range from asymptomatic to mild hepatitis, cholestasis, and hepatomegaly
- Severe liver injury can result in symptoms associated with acute liver failure

Prognosis and Therapy

- Primary treatment is withdrawal of the culprit
- Immunosuppressive therapy may be required in patients with an autoimmune hepatitis–like pattern
- Supportive measures and liver transplantation in severe life threatening cases of acute liver failure
- Prognosis depends on severity of injury, but most cases resolve without sequelae

PATHOLOGIC FEATURES

GROSS FINDINGS

In acute severe DILI, the liver shows massive hepatic necrosis and hemorrhage. In cholestatic DILI, the liver is bile stained. Long-standing DILI can induce fibrosis, which may be evident grossly.

Microscopic Findings

The purposes of the liver biopsy are to assess the severity of the injury (necrosis or fibrosis) and exclude other causes and guide therapy. DILI can cause virtually any known pattern of injury (Fig. 17.34). More recently, the DILI Network (United States) has described 18 distinct histologic patterns of DILI (Table 17.8). Among these, acute (including acute resolving hepatitis) and chronic hepatitic, cholestatic, and mixed hepatitis–cholestatic patterns are the most frequently encountered

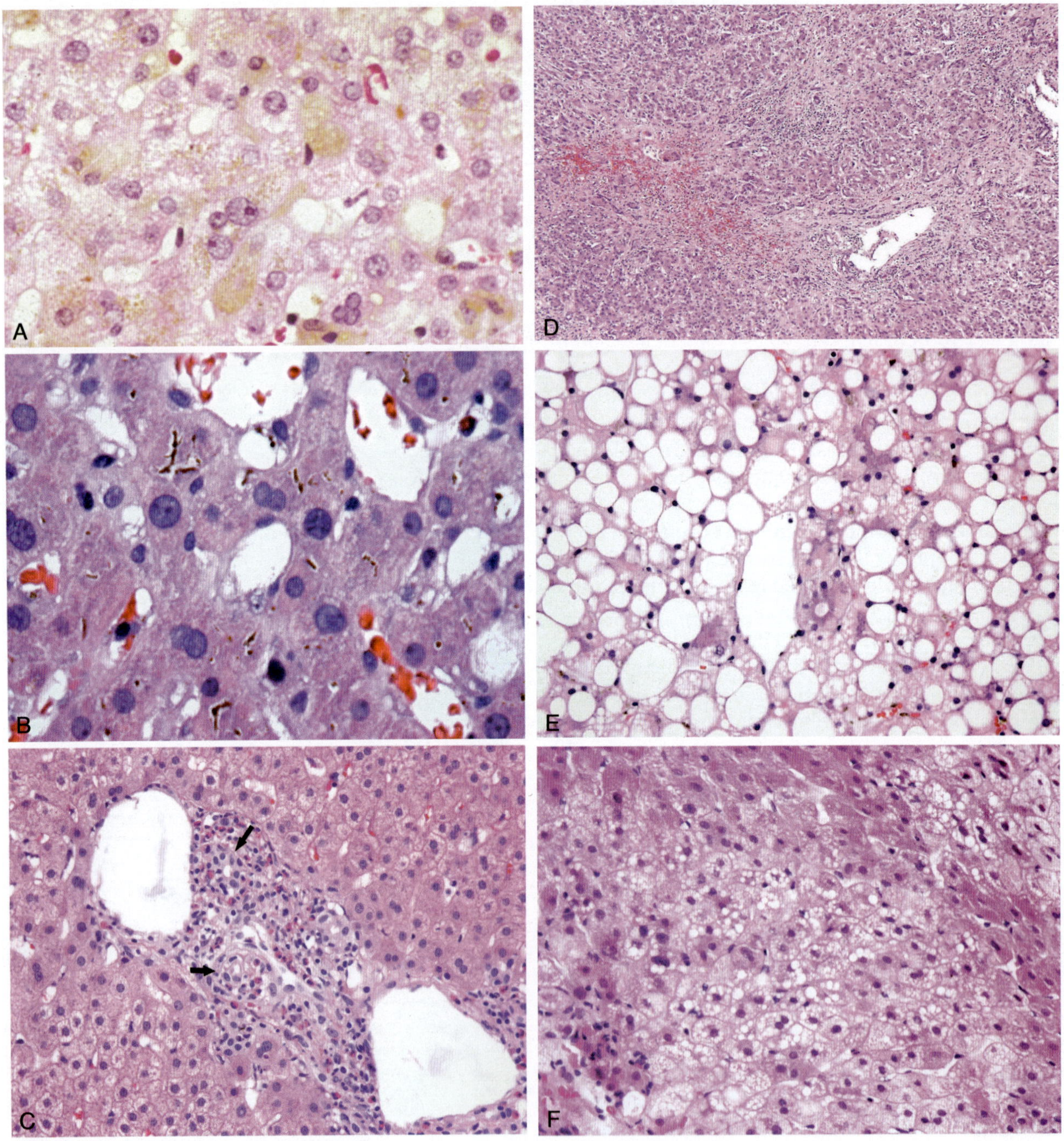

FIGURE 17.34

Toxic injuries. **A**, Bland cholestasis, with accumulation of bile in canaliculi and hepatocytes without significant portal inflammation, is a pattern of injury sometimes associated with estrogen administration. **B**, Canalicular cholestasis is usually more prominent in zone 3 in drug-related hepatic injury. **C**, Bile duct injury and destruction (*arrow*) result in prolonged cholestasis in some cases of drug reaction. Also note the markedly increased number of eosinophils in this example. **D**, Massive hepatic necrosis has led to parenchymal collapse in this case of hepatic injury due to isoniazid; nests of regenerating hepatocytes are separated by collapsed stroma. **E**, Macrovesicular steatosis is a common but nonspecific pattern of toxic injury. **F**, Microvesicular steatosis is less common than

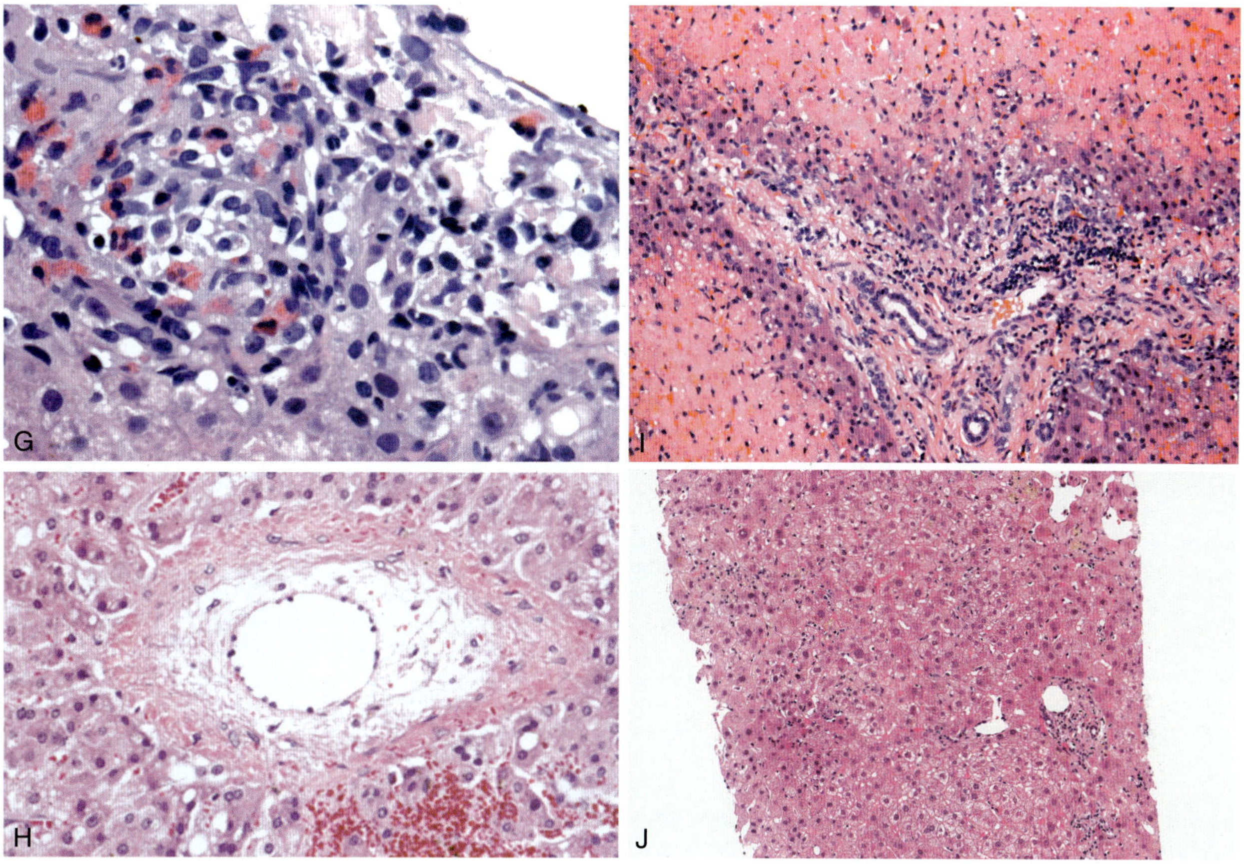

FIGURE 17.34, Cont'd
macrovesicular fatty change. This pattern is classically seen in Reye's syndrome, associated with aspirin use in children, or in valproic acid and tetracycline toxicity. **G**, Granulomas are a common pattern of injury due to drugs and may feature a prominent eosinophilic infiltrate. **H**, Veno-occlusive disease, or sinusoidal obstruction syndrome, affects central veins and is associated with high-dose chemotherapy used in bone marrow transplantation. The lumen of the central vein is narrowed by edematous fibrous tissue. **I**, Some injurious agents, such as halothane, carbon tetrachloride, and acetaminophen, may cause prominent zonal necrosis without significant inflammation. **J**, Resolving acute hepatitis of injury is among the most commonly seen in DILI and characterized by subtle collections of ceroid-laden Kupffer cells and lymphocytes sparse in the lobules that can be highlighted on PAS-D stain.

patterns. In fact, the inability to classify a biopsy into one of these histologic patterns is a strong indicator of DILI. Within the hepatitic pattern, most patients present with portal tract and lobular inflammation. Many patients exhibit features of acute resolving hepatitis at the time of biopsy with rare lymphocytes and PAS-D–positive Kupffer cells in small aggregates around rare acidophil bodies or within portal tracts. Eosinophilic infiltrates may be prominent in cases of hypersensitivity type DILI. Among the cases with cholestatic pattern of injury, bland cholestasis is a frequent observation. Nonspecific hepatocellular changes in DILI are well recognized and include "induced" hepatocytes (abundant homogeneous pale cytoplasm), "two-tone" hepatocytes (areas of pale cytoplasm and others of eosinophilic granular cytoplasm), and PAS-positive pseudo-ground-glass inclusions.

Because of the broad range of offending agents and varying patterns of injury, data on PubMed and the LiverTox website (http://livertox.nlm.nih.gov) are extremely helpful for finding associations with specific substances.

Fibrosis is uncommon because most patients recover from acute DILI. However, it can be seen with long-term amiodarone and methotrexate use. In the case of methotrexate toxicity, Roenigk grade is often reported to assess (Table 17.9).

TABLE 17.8

Drug-Induced Liver Injury Patterns

Pattern of Injury	Associated Drugs and Toxins
Acute hepatitis	Fluoroquinolones; statins, minocycline, isoniazid, interferon, infliximab, nitrofurantoin, diclofenac, cephalexin, and methyldopa
Autoimmune-like hepatitis	Minocycline, nitrofurantoin, hydralazine, methyldopa, statins, fenofibrate, α- and β-interferon, infliximab and etanercept
Chronic hepatitis	Nitrofurantoin, methyldopa
Acute (bland) cholestasis	Estrogens, androgenic steroids
Chronic cholestasis	Floxuridine
Cholestatic hepatitis, ductopenia, vanishing bile duct syndrome (paucity of bile ducts in <50% of portal tracts)	Amoxicillin–clavulanate, fluoroquinolones, azithromycin, trimethoprim–sulfamethoxazole, anabolic steroids, ibuprofen, valproic acid, total parental nutrition
Granulomas	Phenytoin, interferon-α, allopurinol, diphenylhydantoin
Macrovesicular steatosis	Methotrexate, tamoxifen, irinotecan, oxaliplatin, protease inhibitors
Microvesicular steatosis	Valproic acid, tetracycline, nucleoside–nucleotide analogs
Steatohepatitis	Amiodarone, tamoxifen, methotrexate, steroids
Zonal necrosis	Acetaminophen, carbon tetrachloride
Massive or submassive necrosis	Isoniazid, nitrofurantoin, methyldopa
Sinusoidal obstruction syndrome and other vascular injury patterns	Chemotherapeutic agents, steroids, Jamaican bush tea
Mixed or unclassifiable injury	A combination of two or more other patterns or significant change that does not qualify for another pattern No specific drugs associated
Minimal nonspecific changes	Minor changes such as minimal inflammation or steatosis that do not qualify as normal or for another pattern; no specific drug associated

Adapted from Kleiner DE, Chalasani NP, Lee WM, et al. Hepatic histological findings in suspected drug-induced liver injury: systematic evaluation and clinical associations. *Hepatology*. 2014;59(2):661–670

Drug-Induced Liver Injury—Pathologic Features

Gross Findings

- Variable; dependent on severity of injury
- Normal in minimal cases, to steatosis, hepatomegaly, and even necrosis
- In cases of massive hepatic necrosis, liver is shrunken and flaccid with islands of residual viable or regenerating parenchyma

Microscopic Findings

- Variable; 18 different histologic patterns of drug-induced liver injury described
- Acute and chronic hepatitis, cholestasis, and cholestatic hepatitis among the most frequent patterns

Differential Diagnosis

- Viral hepatitis
- Autoimmune hepatitis
- Biliary disorders, such as primary biliary cholangitis or large duct obstruction
- Sarcoidosis
- Fatty liver disease
- Vascular injury

TABLE 17.9

Roenigk Scoring System for Methotrexate

Grade	Histologic Findings	Clinical Implications
1	Normal to mild steatosis, nuclear variability, and/or portal inflammation	Continue therapy
2	Moderate to marked steatosis, nuclear variability, and/or portal inflammation	Continue therapy
3	A: mild fibrosis B: moderate to severe fibrosis	A: can continue therapy but repeat biopsy in 6 months B: should not be given methotrexate therapy unless there are exceptional circumstances
4	Cirrhosis	Should not be given methotrexate therapy unless there are exceptional circumstances

Adapted from Roenigk HH Jr. Auerbach R, Maibach HI, Weinstein GD. Methotrexate in psoriasis: revised guidelines. *J Am Acad Dermatol*. 1988;19 (1 Pt 1):145–156.

Differential Diagnosis

The differential diagnosis for DILI is broad because drug and toxic reactions can mimic other liver diseases. Diagnosis relies on identification of an offending agent, and other causes of hepatic injury must be excluded.

Prognosis and Therapy

Treatment for patients with DILI includes withdrawal of the offending agent followed by supportive therapy. For mild liver injury, the prognosis is excellent. More severe liver injury, such as massive hepatic necrosis, may be life threatening, in which case liver transplantation is indicated. Chronic DILI is often associated with cholestatic pattern of injury and can ultimately lead to cirrhosis.

MISCELLANEOUS PATTERNS OF INJURY

"ALMOST NORMAL" BIOPSY OR NONSPECIFIC FINDINGS

In certain circumstances, marked elevation of liver enzymes does not necessarily correlate with obvious histologic findings or a definitive diagnosis. Table 17.10 includes frequent differential diagnoses under this pattern of injury.

Scattered mononuclear infiltrates within portal tracts (Fig. 17.35A) are commonly seen in this differential diagnosis. Biopsies reveal scant lymphocytes and occasional plasma cells without significant lobular or interface

TABLE 17.10

Causes of "Almost Normal" Pattern of Injury

Histologic Finding	Suspected Diagnosis	Ancillary Stain
Slight nodularity (clinically suspected cirrhosis)	Nodular regenerative hyperplasia	Reticulin stain
Dilated sinusoids	Sickle cell disease	
Sinusoidal infiltration	Tumor infiltrating sinusoids (including lymphoma) Collagen vascular diseases Hemophagocytic syndrome Systemic inflammatory conditions	
Periportal eosinophilic cytoplasmic globules	α1-Antitrypsin deficiency	PAS-D stain
Eosinophilic amorphous deposits in sinusoids and/or vessels	Amyloid	Congo red stain Mass spectrophotometry
Scattered mononuclear infiltrates in lobules or portal tracts with Kupffer cell aggregates	Celiac disease Common variable immunodeficiency Crohn's disease "Resolving acute hepatitis pattern of injury" in DILI and self-limited infections Collagen vascular diseases	PAS-D can highlight scattered Kupffer cells
Large pale hepatocytes (classic diabetic patient in metabolic acidosis)	Glycogenic hepatopathy	
Prominent, herniated portal veins with or without nodular architecture (portal hypertension, suspected cirrhosis of unknown cause)	Causes of noncirrhotic portal hypertension, including hepatoportal sclerosis	Reticulin stain
Reduced number of bile ducts with or without bile ductular proliferation, minimal cholestatic changes	Vanishing bile duct syndrome in drug reaction and others Primary sclerosing cholangitis	Orcein or rhodamine to highlight copper deposition PAS-D, CK7, or CK19 may aid bile duct identification
Minimal cholestasis without inflammation or bile duct changes	"Bland lobular cholestasis" in the setting of sepsis, thyroid disease, or DILI	
Enlarged hepatic stellate cells (Ito cells) with lipid-filled vacuolated cytoplasm and indented nuclei	Hypervitaminosis A	
Amphophilic cytoplasmic change in hepatocytes (ground-glass or pseudo ground-glass inclusions)	Hepatitis B infection Polypharmacy Cyanamide therapy Type IV glycogen storage disease Uremia Lafora's disease	PAS or PAS-D

CK, Cytokeratin; *DILI*, drug-induced liver injury; *PAS*, periodic acid–Schiff; *PAS-D*, periodic acid–Schiff–diastase.

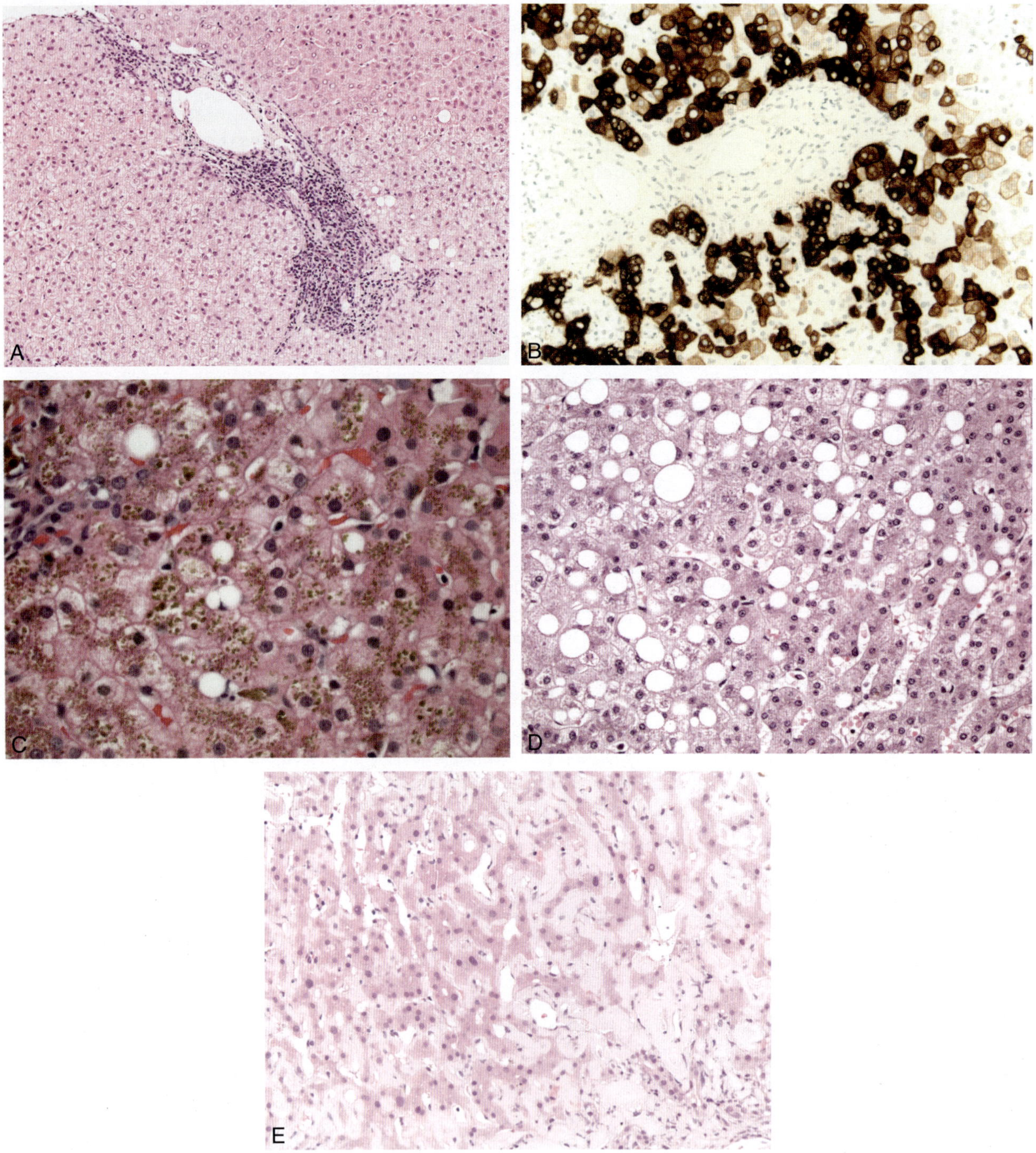

FIGURE 17.35

Almost normal pattern: **A**, Sparse chronic inflammatory infiltrates within portal tracts, in this case associated with minimal bile ductular proliferation. **B**, CK7 stain demonstrates the lack of an interlobular bile duct and highlights periportal hepatocytes in a case of primary sclerosing cholangitis with ductopenia. **C**, Ito cells (hepatic stellate cells) are not visualized under normal conditions but become hyperplastic and hypertrophic in certain diseases such as hypervitaminosis A. The picture demonstrates Ito cell hyperplasia with cells that exhibit vacuolated cytoplasm with septations. **D**, In comparison, a case of macrovesicular steatosis with large vacuoles of fat within hepatocytes without septations. **E**, Globular eosinophilic and amorphous deposits within sinusoids and involving the portal tracts, consistent with amyloidosis.

activity. These findings need to be correlated with the clinical impression but raise the possibility of medication-induced injury, chronic biliary obstruction (in particular if there is bile ductular reaction or cholestatic findings), early primary biliary disorders such as PBC and PSC, and resolving acute hepatitis in the setting of infections or even AIH. This could also represent a nonspecific finding without clinical significance in some cases.

Ductopenia (Fig. 17.35B) is defined as the loss of bile ducts. In general, up to 10% to 20% of portal tracts may lack an interlobular bile duct, particularly those of smaller size. The diagnosis of ductopenia can be rendered when 50% or more of portal tracts do not show a bile duct, and in most cases, at least 20 portal tracts are required for a more accurate diagnosis. In clinical practice, the term *bile duct loss* can be used in cases that do not fulfill the criteria for ductopenia but demonstrate absence of bile ducts in more than 20% of portal tracts. Ductopenia is typically associated with primary biliary disorders (PBC and PSC), but it can also occur in the setting of drug-induced injury (antibiotics, total parental nutrition), can be idiopathic, and can occur as a paraneoplastic syndrome. CK7 stain is helpful in highlighting the native bile ducts. PAS-D stain reveals positive staining of the basement membrane of the interlobular bile ducts, so it should also be useful when assessing this.

Ito cell hyperplasia (Fig. 17.35C and D), also known as hepatic stellate cells, is found in a sinusoidal distribution within the space of Disse but is not visible on routine H&E stain under normal conditions. In pathologic states such as hypervitaminosis A, Ito cells are the main sites for storage, and they become hyperplastic and hypertrophic, compressing sinusoids, which imparts a honeycomb appearance to the liver. Ito cells exhibit cytoplasmic vacuolation and septations with indented dark nuclei, a characteristic that can help in the differential diagnosis from steatosis in hepatocytes.

Amyloidosis (Fig. 17.35E) in the liver is often not a subtle diagnosis but can be an incidental finding. The characteristic eosinophilic amorphous deposits in a sinusoidal distribution, involving the stroma of portal tracts or involving the wall of small arterioles. In doubtful cases, Congo red stain or sulfated Alcian blue can confirm the diagnosis. Mass spectrophotometry is the gold standard for subtyping the variant of amyloid.

HEPATIC GRANULOMAS

Granulomas are reported in 5% to 10% of all liver biopsies. The most common causes of hepatic granulomas are infections (Fig. 17.36A), PBC, sarcoidosis (Fig. 17.36B), DILI, systemic inflammatory conditions, immunologic deficiencies, lymphomas (especially Hodgkin lymphoma), and nonspecific reaction adjacent to a mass lesion. In up to one-third of patients, granulomas are idiopathic in nature. Table 17.11 outlines the different forms of granulomatous injury and corresponding causes. A definitive diagnosis often requires a thorough review of the clinical history or medication list, extensive serologic work-up, culture, and imaging studies. The treatment and prognosis depend on the underlying cause.

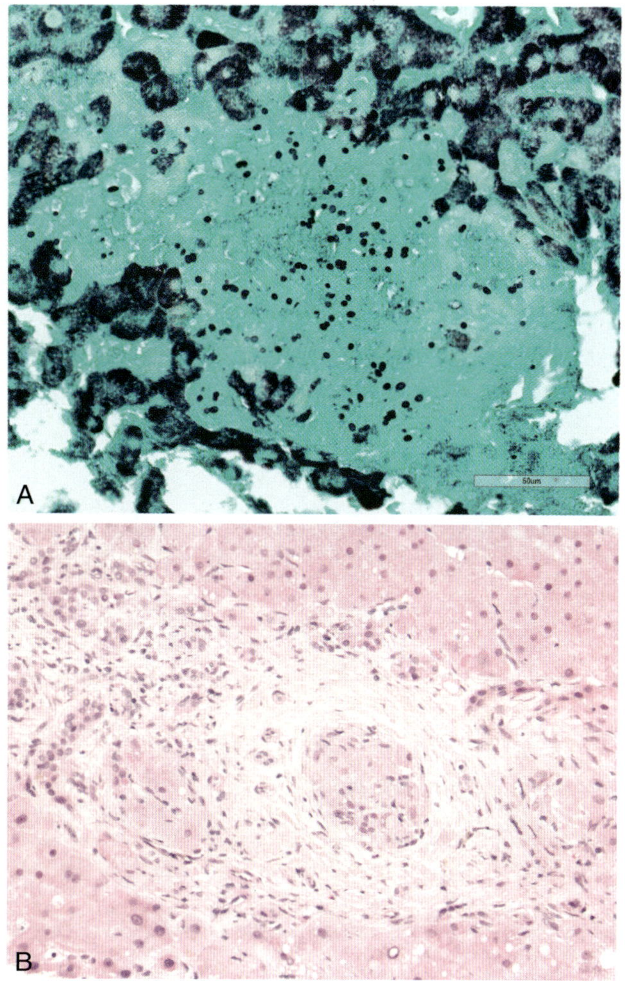

FIGURE 17.36

A, Histoplasma capsulatum found in a case of granulomatous inflammation in the liver on GMS stain. **B**, In cases of sarcoidosis, granulomas are well formed and can be encountered in the portal tracts.

NECROSIS

Liver necrosis can result from several different causes (Table 17.12). The distribution of necrosis and severity are helpful in suggesting the possible etiology. A zonal distribution of necrosis, especially zone 3, is associated with certain drugs or toxins and vascular injury. In contrast, a geographic or "random" pattern of necrosis favors an infectious cause. Interface activity with spotty necrosis and coexistence of a lobular inflammatory infiltrate suggests infection (commonly viral) or immune-mediated injury. Autoimmune hepatitis and DILI should be suspected if there is bridging necrosis and hepatocellular collapse. Most cases of focal necrosis resolve; however, significant necrosis may evolve to fibrosis in a subset of cases.

Submassive or massive hepatic necrosis is a nonspecific pattern of injury in which large areas of the parenchyma or entire hepatic lobule are destroyed (Fig. 17.37). The trichrome stain can be difficult to interpret in these

TABLE 17.11
Types of Granulomas in the Liver and Common Associations

Granulomas Type	Description	Causes
Epithelioid	Well-formed aggregates of macrophages with abundant eosinophilic dense cytoplasm May have necrosis and destroy liver architecture	Infections (fungal, mycobacterial, others) Sarcoidosis DILI CVID
Microgranulomas	Small aggregates (less than 10 cells) of Kupffer cells with admixed lymphocytes usually.	Nonspecific CVID
Fibrin ring granulomas	Epithelioid granuloma with a central lipid vacuole surrounded by a fibrin ring	Q fever Leishmaniasis Rickettsia typhus Toxoplasmosis CMV EBV infection *Mycobacterium avium–intracellulare* Typhoid fever Allopurinol Hodgkin's lymphoma
Lipogranulomas	Histiocytes contain lipid vacuoles	Fatty liver disease Hepatitis C Mineral oil Nonspecific
Granulomatous bile duct injury	Portal-based granulomas with associated bile duct injury; rarely cholestasis	PBC (granulomas often poorly formed) DILI
Foreign body granulomas	Birefringent material upon polarization of H&E-stained slide; occasional multinucleated giant cells	Beryllium Talc Drug abuse

CMV, Cytomegalovirus; *CVID*, common variable immunodeficiency; *DILI*, drug-induced liver disease; *EBV*, Epstein-Barr virus; *H&E*, hematoxylin and eosin; *PBC*, primary biliary cholangitis.
Adapted from Lamps L. Hepatic granulomas: a review with emphasis on infectious causes. *Arch Pathol Lab Med*. 2015;139:867–875.

TABLE 17.12
Common Entities Associated With Liver Necrosis

Pattern of Necrosis	Diagnosis
"Bland necrosis," often zonal	DILI or toxins Ischemia
Spotty necrosis	Viral infections Autoimmune hepatitis
Bridging necrosis	Autoimmune hepatitis DILI or toxins
Confluent necrosis • Random, geographic necrosis • Submassive or massive necrosis	Infection (HSV, others) DILI or toxins Ischemia Autoimmune hepatitis

DILI, Drug-induced liver disease; *HSV*, herpes simplex virus.

cases. Reticulin stain is particularly useful in such cases because they demonstrate areas of parenchymal collapse that may be distinguished from fibrosis. Although this is relatively uncommon, it may be life threating, and liver transplant may be indicated.

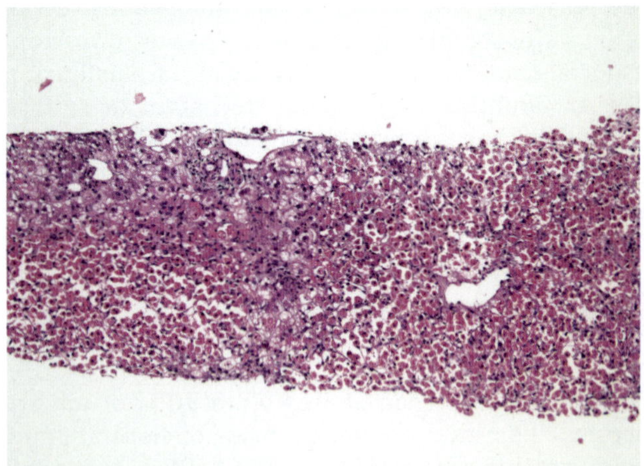

FIGURE 17.37
Submassive hepatic necrosis involving zones 2 and 3 mainly in a patient with drug toxicity.

METABOLIC DISEASES

IRON OVERLOAD

Excessive accumulation of iron in the liver may be a manifestation of mutations of iron-related genes

TABLE 17.13
Most Common Mutations in Iron-Related Genes Involved in Iron Overload

Iron Accumulation Predominantly in Hepatocytes					IRON ACCUMULATION PREDOMINANTLY IN KUPFFER CELLS			
Entity	**Gene Mutated**	**Subtype**	**Transmission**	**Onset (decade)**	**Entity**	**Gene Mutated**	**Transmission**	**Onset (decade)**
Hemochromatosis	*HAMP*	Type 2 A (juvenile)	Recessive	Second to third	A(hypo)transferrinemia	*Tf*	Recessive	First to second
	HJV	Type 2B (juvenile)						
	TFR2	Type 3			A(hypo)ceruloplasminemia	*CP*		Second to third
	HFE	Type 1		Third to fifth	Ferroportin disease (type A)	*1SLC40A1* (hypo-functional)	Dominant	Forth to fifth
Ferroportin disease (type B)	*SLC40A1* (hyper-functional)		Dominant					

Adapted from Torbenson M. Biopsy interpretation of the liver. In: Epstein, ed. Wolters Kluwer; 2015:303.

(primary) or secondary to other acquired or genetic disorders such as anemia of chronic disease, systemic inflammatory conditions, tumors, and even fatty liver disease. Although primary iron overload was thought to be mainly hepatocellular in distribution, rare conditions with primarily Kupffer iron accumulation have been described in recent years (summarized in Table 17.13).

HEREDITARY HEMOCHROMATOSIS

Hereditary hemochromatosis (HH) is an inherited disorder caused by a group of different gene mutations that result in excess iron storage. HH is the most common genetic disorder in whites, with a 1 in 200 prevalence rate of homozygous mutations. That said, heterozygous mutations have been reported in up to 15% of the overall population. All currently known forms of HH are caused by an abnormal production, regulation, or activity of hepcidin. Hepcidin regulates iron metabolism, so a deficiency in hepcidin triggers increased iron absorption from duodenal enterocytes and release of iron from macrophages because of overexpression of ferroportin. High levels of iron in plasma lead to transferrin saturation and increased nontransferrin bound iron that is rapidly accumulated in different tissues (liver, heart, endocrine glands). The most common *HFE* mutation is C282Y missense mutation, which prevents formation of a disulfide bond necessary for binding of HFE protein to β2-microglobulin. Other less common mutations are H63D and S65C. The juvenile variant of hemochromatosis is caused by mutations of the hemojuvelin *(HJV)* and hepcidin *(HAMP)* genes. Other mutations related to the iron metabolism are described in Table 17.13.

CLINICAL FEATURES

Clinical manifestations of HH depend on the specific gene mutation and homozygous versus heterozygous status. More severe forms usually present early in life and are related to genes that play a critical role in hepcidin synthesis, such as *HAMP* and *HJV*. In such cases, there is extensive organ involvement, and cardiac insufficiency and endocrine gland dysfunction are frequent symptoms at diagnosis. Other less severe forms, such as *HFE* mutations, have a more variable clinical presentation and are often influenced by external factors such as alcohol consumption, blood donation, and menstruation, among others. Patients often present between 40 and 60 years of age. Women present later because of the protective effects of menstruation. Some patients are discovered incidentally through abnormal iron studies, but others present with lethargy, hepatomegaly, arthropathy, hypogonadism, abdominal pain, and skin pigmentation. Heart failure, diabetes mellitus, and cirrhosis are late manifestations.

LABORATORY FINDINGS

Patients typically present with increased iron serum concentration, transferrin saturation, and/or serum ferritin as well as total iron-binding capacity. In this setting, molecular genetic testing for HFE and non-HFE mutations is often indicated.

HEREDITARY HEMOCHROMATOSIS—FACT SHEET

Definition

- Inherited disorders of iron overload leading to chronic organ injury (including the liver, heart, and endocrine glands) and cirrhosis

Incidence and Location

- Most common identified genetic disorder in white populations
- Rare in patients of non-European descent

Morbidity and Mortality

- Deposition of iron in the liver, heart, joints, and endocrine tissues leads to organ damage and dysfunction (cirrhosis, diabetes mellitus, congestive heart failure, hypogonadism)
- Increased risk for hepatocellular carcinoma

Gender, Race, and Age Distribution

- Both sexes affected
- White populations
- Earlier onset in juvenile hemochromatosis

Clinical Features

- Common presenting symptoms are arthralgias, skin pigmentation, diabetes mellitus, and hepatomegaly
- Endocrine and cardiac manifestations may be presenting symptoms in younger patients (juvenile hemochromatosis)

Prognosis and Therapy

- Phlebotomy is the treatment of choice; chelating agents are less effective
- 10-year survival rate of cirrhotic patients is 60%
- Hepatocellular carcinoma occurs as a late complication in up to one-third of cases

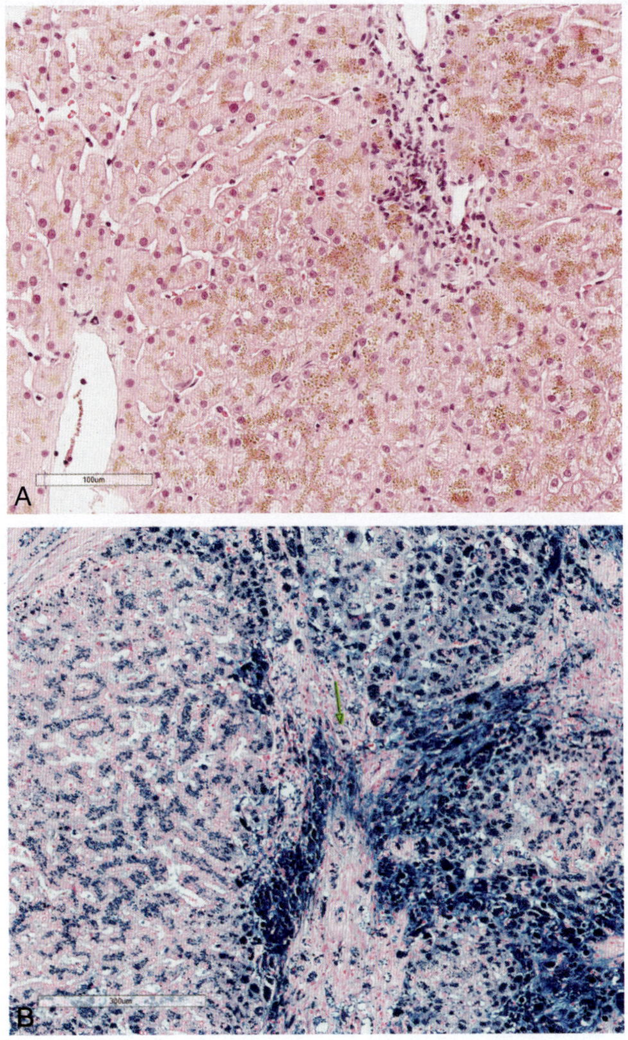

FIGURE 17.38

A, In hereditary hemochromatosis, iron accumulates in hepatocytes before spilling over to Kupffer cells. The iron deposition is in a zonal distribution, with accumulation predominantly in periportal hepatocytes in early stages of the disease. The iron deposition progresses and involves the entire lobule, as seen in this case. **B**, Prussian blue stain for iron is helpful in highlighting the increased iron storage in HH, which is primarily hepatocellular but also noted in stromal cells and biliary epithelium (*arrow*).

Pathologic Features

Gross Findings

Early stages of HH show grossly normal or slightly darkened liver parenchyma. As the disease progresses, patients may develop hepatomegaly, and the liver may show a characteristic rust discoloration. In cases complicated by hepatocellular carcinoma, the tumor may lack iron deposits (iron-free foci) and appear distinct compared with the darker background cirrhosis.

Microscopic Findings

The defining histologic feature is the presence of finely granular yellow-brown iron deposits within the periportal hepatocytes (Fig. 17.38A). These are easily confirmed by an iron stain. As iron continues to accumulate, the deposits extend to involve the rest of the lobule. In late stages, there is a milder degree of iron deposition within Kupffer cells and bile duct epithelial cells. Lobular or portal inflammation is usually absent or inconspicuous. Periportal fibrosis evolves to bridging and cirrhosis.

Iron grading systems are used to provide a semiquantitative assessment of the overall hepatic storage of iron. The four—scale system that is most commonly used in clinical practice is as follows: 1+, zone 1 iron storage only; 2+, zones 1 and 2 involved; 3+, panlobular but not intense iron deposition; and 4+, panzonal and intense iron deposits (Fig. 17.38B). In cases of nonhepatocellular (reticuloendothelial cells) iron deposition, a three-tier scale is used: mild, moderate, and severe trace iron deposition. The modified Scheuer system also represents a popular alternative option for grading iron storage. This is a five-tier system that evaluates hepatocellular and reticuloendothelial cells' iron storage separately as well. Detailed description of the different grades is provided in Table 17.14.

TABLE 17.14

Modified Scheuer System for Grading Iron Storage

Grade	Description
0	Iron granules absent or iron granules barely seen at 400×
1	Iron granules resolved at 250×
2	Iron granules resolved at 100×
3	Iron granules resolved at 25×
4	Iron granules resolved at 10× or iron granules visible without magnification

HEREDITARY HEMOCHROMATOSIS—PATHOLOGIC FEATURES

Gross Findings

- Hepatomegaly
- Early cirrhosis is micronodular, evolving to macronodular cirrhosis Rusty discoloration
- The pancreas, spleen, heart, and other organs may be involved

Microscopic Findings

- Deposition of iron in zone 1 hepatocytes, with subsequent accumulation in zones 2 and 3 hepatocytes
- Lesser degree of iron deposition in Kupffer cells and duct epithelial cells

Genetics

- Most are autosomal recessive inheritance (except juvenile hemochromatosis—dominant)
- Most common *HFE* hereditary hemochromatosis (HH) are related to C282Y (80% of all *HFE* HH) and H63D mutations
- Non-*HFE* HH include juvenile hemochromatosis (*HJV* and *HAMP* gene mutations), transferrin receptor 2 hemochromatosis (*TRF2* gene mutations), and type B ferroportin disease (*SLC40A1* mutation)

Differential Diagnosis

- Secondary iron overload
- Hemolytic anemias and other hematologic disorders Blood transfusions
- Hemosiderosis in alcoholic liver disease, hepatitis C, hemodialysis, and metabolic syndrome

ANCILLARY STUDIES

Special stains for iron such as Prussian blue stain are helpful in confirming accumulation of iron in hepatocytes and differentiating it from other brown pigments such as bile and lipofuscin. The hepatic iron index (HII) can be assessed in paraffin-embedded tissue, and a value greater than 1.9 is consistent with HH. Increased HII correlates with severity of iron deposition observed on histochemical iron stains. However, in isolation, increased HHI is not diagnostic of HH. It also has limited utility in pediatric patients because reference values for the test have been validated for the adult population and not in the younger age group. MRI has an acceptable accuracy for assessing liver iron concentration as well as differentiating hepatocellular from Kupffer cell iron deposition.

DIFFERENTIAL DIAGNOSIS

Besides identifying the specific mutation, HH must be distinguished from secondary pattern of iron overload. Whereas iron accumulation in hepatocytes is more pronounced in HH, secondary iron overload is characterized by a mixed hepatocellular and Kupffer cell iron deposition. Additional studies (HHI and mutational status) are helpful to distinguish these patterns.

PROGNOSIS AND THERAPY

The prognosis is linked to the specific gene involved as it determines severity and onset of disease. The overall 10-year survival rate in patients with cirrhosis who undergo treatment is approximately 70%. Dysplastic nodules and hepatocellular carcinoma are late complications. The goal of treatment is to reduce serum ferritin levels through regular phlebotomy sessions. Iron chelation agents may be indicated in patients in whom phlebotomy is contraindicated.

SECONDARY IRON OVERLOAD

CLINICAL FEATURES

Secondary iron overload is more common than HH and frequently associated with dietary factors (excessive consumption of iron pills), transfusions, chronic liver disease (hepatitis C, alcoholism, fatty liver), chronic anemia (thalassemia, sideroblastic anemia, anemias associated with defective heme synthesis, and sickle cell disease), porphyria, and chronic systemic inflammatory diseases. Clinical features in secondary iron overload are related to the underlying cause rather than liver parenchymal damage caused by iron deposition.

PATHOLOGIC FEATURES

GROSS FINDINGS

Even though macroscopic findings may be similar to those seen in HH, secondary iron overload tends to be less severe; therefore cirrhosis is rare.

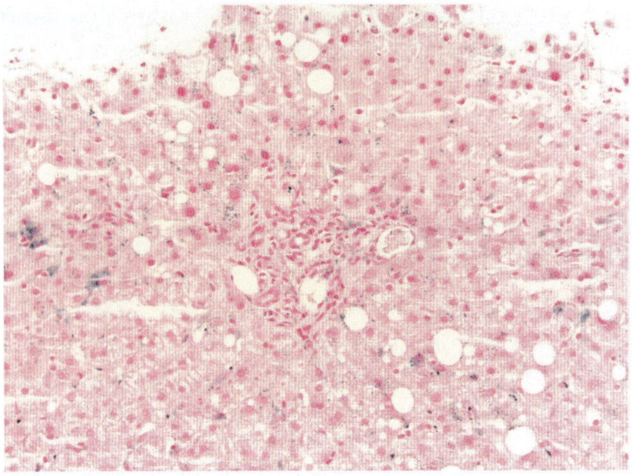

FIGURE 17.39

Secondary iron overload often presents as mild increased iron deposits in Kupffer cells and hepatocytes in Prussian blue stain.

Microscopic Findings

In secondary iron overload, the main site of iron accumulation is the reticuloendothelial cells (Fig. 17.39), with subsequent involvement of hepatocytes and biliary epithelial cells. As in HH, inflammation is not prominent, and the biopsy may reveal other features of an underlying chronic liver disease. Fibrosis is less common than in HH.

Differential Diagnosis

Marked iron deposition in Kupffer cells as opposed to hepatocytes favors secondary iron overload rather than HH. Clinical history, genetic testing for *HFE* mutations, and quantitative iron determination are often necessary for a definitive diagnosis.

Prognosis and Therapy

The prognosis is determined by that of the underlying disease. Therapeutic interventions have two goals: treatment of the underlying disease and iron chelation to reduce tissue injury.

COPPER ACCUMULATION DISORDER

WILSON'S DISEASE

Wilson's disease is an autosomal recessive disorder of copper metabolism. The underlying defect is caused by mutations in the *ATP7B* gene located on chromosome 13. *ATP7B* encodes a protein responsible for transporting copper into hepatocyte secretory pathways. The majority of affected individuals are compound heterozygotes; no consistent correlation between genotype and clinical manifestations has been observed.

CLINICAL FEATURES

Wilson's disease presents with a wide range of clinical features and histologic findings. A high level of suspicion is warranted in young patients (younger than 40 years) with liver disease of unclear cause, especially if neurologic or psychiatric symptoms are also present. Hepatic manifestations dominate in early stage of the disease and can be seen in up to 40% of patients at diagnosis. As a result of the liver injury, transaminases are elevated, and patients can have signs of cirrhosis. Some patients present with acute liver failure in the setting of significant hepatocellular necrosis, usually accompanied by hemolytic anemia caused by abrupt release of massive amounts of copper from the liver. Liver disease is followed by neurologic and psychiatric symptoms in teens and young adults that include dysphagia, dysarthria, tremor, involuntary movements, seizures, dementia, depression, and schizophrenia, among others. The well-known Kayser-Fleischer rings are caused by the deposition of copper in the limbus of the cornea and may be detected on slit-lamp examination but are not pathognomonic because they can also be seen in iatrogenic copper overload. Other organs such as the heart, joints, and endocrine glands can be affected as well.

Laboratory Findings

Low serum ceruloplasmin and elevated 24-hour urinary copper concentrations can be encountered. Quantitative hepatic copper in tissue is elevated (>250 μg/g dry weight).

WILSON'S DISEASE—FACT SHEET

Definition

- Inherited disorder of copper metabolism caused by decreased copper excretion

Incidence and Location

- Prevalence of 1 in 30,000 to 1 in 45,000 individuals

Morbidity and Mortality

- Progressive disorder with variable clinical presentation, leading to cirrhosis if untreated
- Copper deposition in brain, particularly in basal ganglia and cerebral cortex, leads to extrapyramidal motor disorders
- Fulminant hepatitis with nonimmune hemolytic anemia and massive release of copper into the bloodstream

Gender, Race, and Age Distribution

- Occurs equally in males and females
- All races
- Most patients present before 40 years of age

Clinical Features

- Liver disease (acute hepatitis, chronic liver disease, cirrhosis) and neurologic or psychiatric manifestations are the most frequent presenting features
- Kayser-Fleischer rings can be seen in patients with neurologic disease but are not pathognomonic
- Low serum ceruloplasmin; increased serum copper and 24-hour urinary copper
- Increased quantitative hepatic copper in tissue (>250 μg/g)

Prognosis and Therapy

- Copper chelating agents such as D-penicillamine prevent disease progression
- Liver transplantation for patients with end-stage liver disease or fulminant hepatic failure

Pathologic Features

Gross Findings

The macroscopic appearance depends on the stage and clinical presentation. In early stages, the liver may be normal or mildly enlarged with steatosis. In cases of acute liver failure, extensive parenchymal necrosis can be seen with occasional islands of residual viable parenchyma. In late stages, there may be macronodular cirrhosis.

Microscopic Findings

Wilson's disease can present with any of the common patterns of liver injury such as a steatohepatitic, cholestatic, or even chronic hepatitis pattern (Figs. 17.40A and B). In a series of 110 patients, cirrhosis was the most common form of liver disease (38%), followed by acute liver failure (27%) and acute hepatitis (19%). Early Wilson's disease may reveal minimal nonspecific changes, including glycogenated nuclei, minimal

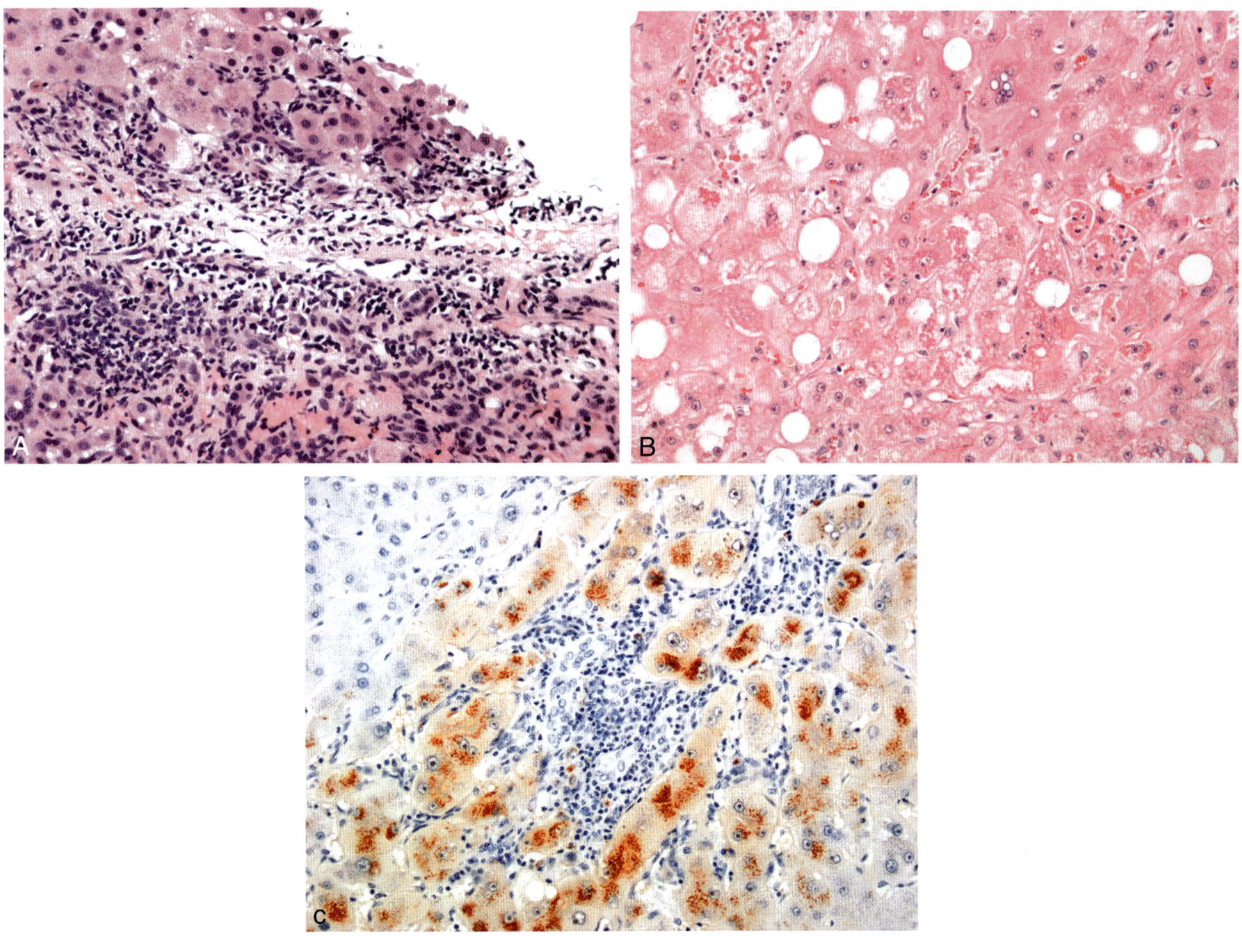

FIGURE 17.40

A, Wilson's disease often shows a nonspecific chronic hepatitis pattern of injury, with portal chronic inflammation and focal interface hepatitis. **B**, Steatohepatitis can be seen as part of the spectrum of Wilson's disease with extensive ballooning degeneration and Mallory hyaline formation. **C**, Rhodanine (copper) stain highlights increased copper binding protein in Wilson's disease with cytoplasmic accumulation of copper.

mononuclear inflammation, and steatosis. Some patients may exhibit ballooned hepatocytes and Mallory hyaline along with previously described features; this pattern can be mistaken for NASH. A chronic hepatitis pattern of injury is relatively common, and in some cases, a mixed hepatitis and cholestatic pattern can be seen. Occasionally, patients may present with acute liver failure, in which case the liver shows submassive or massive hepatic necrosis. With disease progression, fibrosis begins in the periportal region and eventually evolves to cirrhosis. Copper cannot be usually identified on H&E stain but may be visualized with special stains such as rhodanine or orcein as granular cytoplasmic staining in periportal or periseptal hepatocytes and within the lobules (Fig. 17.40C).

Wilson's Disease—Pathologic Features

Gross Findings

- Early: normal or mildly enlarged, steatotic
- Massive hepatic necrosis in acute liver failure
- Late: macronodular cirrhosis

Microscopic Findings

- Early: nonspecific, fatty liver disease, chronic hepatitis pattern of injury, cholestatic liver disease
- Hepatocellular necrosis, fibrosis leading to cirrhosis
- Periportal or periseptal hepatocyte often show copper accumulation (rhodanine stain)

Genetics

- Autosomal recessive disorder
- Multiple known mutations in *ATP7B* gene on chromosome 13

Differential Diagnosis

- Acute or chronic viral hepatitis
- Autoimmune hepatitis
- Nonalcoholic fatty liver disease
- Cryptogenic cirrhosis
- Drug-induced liver injury
- Idiopathic copper toxicosis
- Endemic Tyrolean infantile cirrhosis
- Indian childhood cirrhosis

Differential Diagnosis

The histologic differential diagnosis of Wilson's disease includes a broad differential diagnosis because Wilson's disease can mimic any pattern of injury in the liver. Because most cases are diagnosed in young patients, other entities such as drug toxicity, viral hepatitis, and AIH need to be excluded clinically. Laboratory findings and viral serologies are helpful but may not be available in cases with acute liver failure. Quantitative copper analysis of dry hepatic tissue is useful in supporting a presumptive diagnosis of Wilson's disease.

Less common diseases of increased copper storage (other than Wilson's disease) include idiopathic copper toxicosis, Indian childhood cirrhosis, and endemic Tyrolean infantile cirrhosis. These can be distinguished from Wilson's disease by clinical presentation in childhood and greater level of copper accumulation than Wilson's disease.

Prognosis and Therapy

Copper-chelating agents (e.g., D-penicillamine) in combination with dietary restriction of copper is the treatment of choice in preventing progression of disease. Liver transplantation is needed in cases of acute liver failure or cirrhosis.

Rarely, hepatocellular carcinoma and cholangiocarcinoma have been reported in patients with chronic Wilson's disease.

α1-Antitrypsin Deficiency

α1-Antitrypsin, a plasma serine protease inhibitor, plays a key role in controlling tissue degradation by forming complexes with proteases, such as elastase, trypsin, chymotrypsin, and thrombin. This function is particularly critical in the lungs, where α1AT inhibits leukocyte elastase and prevents degradation of alveolar walls by this enzyme. More than 100 genetic variants of α1AT have been identified; most are associated with normal levels and function of the protein. The deficiency state is most commonly caused by homozygosity for the PI*Z allele, in which alanine is substituted for leucine at amino acid 213, causing self-aggregation of the protein. This abnormal form of the protein is trapped within the endoplasmic reticulum of hepatocytes and appears as intracytoplasmic eosinophilic globules.

CLINICAL FEATURES

The most common clinical disorder associated with α1AT deficiency is pulmonary emphysema. Approximately 10% of patients with α1AT deficiency present with liver disease in infancy, manifested as neonatal cholestasis, and up to 25% of affected individuals develop cirrhosis in childhood. Some of the genetic variants may be mildly symptomatic, and others may not reveal clinical manifestations until adulthood when patients present with signs of cirrhosis.

Laboratory Findings

The diagnosis can be determined based on serum levels of α1AT, which are low (<100 mg/dL) in these patients.

This is followed by genotyping by PCR testing or gene sequencing to assess the specific variant of the disease. In addition, normal or mildly elevated transaminases are often seen.

α1-ANTITRYPSIN DEFICIENCY—FACT SHEET

Definition

- Autosomal recessive disorder leading to accumulation of α1-antitrypsin (α1AT) in hepatocytes, with decreased serum α1AT

Incidence and Location

- Homozygous state occurs in 1 in 6700 to 1 in 2000 births in North America
- Geographic variation, with highest incidence in Northern Europe, particularly Scandinavia

Morbidity and Mortality

- Increased risk for emphysema, hepatocellular carcinoma, and glomerulonephritis
- Increased risk for cirrhosis (roughly 20% older than age 50 years)

Gender, Race, and Age Distribution

- Both genders
- All ages
- More common among people of Northern European ancestry

Clinical Features

- Persistent jaundice in neonates
- Hepatosplenomegaly or ascites in late childhood
- Cryptogenic cirrhosis in adults
- Low serum α1AT levels
- Abnormal protein identified by serum electrophoresis, polymerase chain reaction assay, or gene sequencing

Prognosis and Therapy

- Avoid or stop smoking and liver toxins such as alcohol
- Supportive therapy
- Liver transplantation for end-stage cirrhosis

Pathologic Features

Gross Findings

There are no specific gross manifestations of this disease in the early phase. Cirrhosis caused by α1AT deficiency is typically macronodular in appearance.

Microscopic Findings

The diagnostic histologic feature of α1AT deficiency is the presence of globular eosinophilic PAS-positive, diastase-resistant cytoplasmic inclusions within periportal hepatocytes (Figs. 17.41A and B). The distribution can be uneven throughout the parenchyma. With increasing age, there is an increase in the number as well as the size of inclusions. Importantly, the inclusions are not evident in infants younger than 12 weeks of age; in this setting, the PAS stain is less helpful. When the clinical presentation is that of cholestatic disease (often in infants), other histologic findings include canalicular cholestasis, giant cell transformation of hepatocytes, ductopenia, and ballooning of hepatocytes. There may be granular accumulation of α1AT within the hepatocytes, which is only highlighted by IHC. In adults, the α1AT globules are present often in a background of chronic hepatitis pattern of injury (with or without cirrhosis).

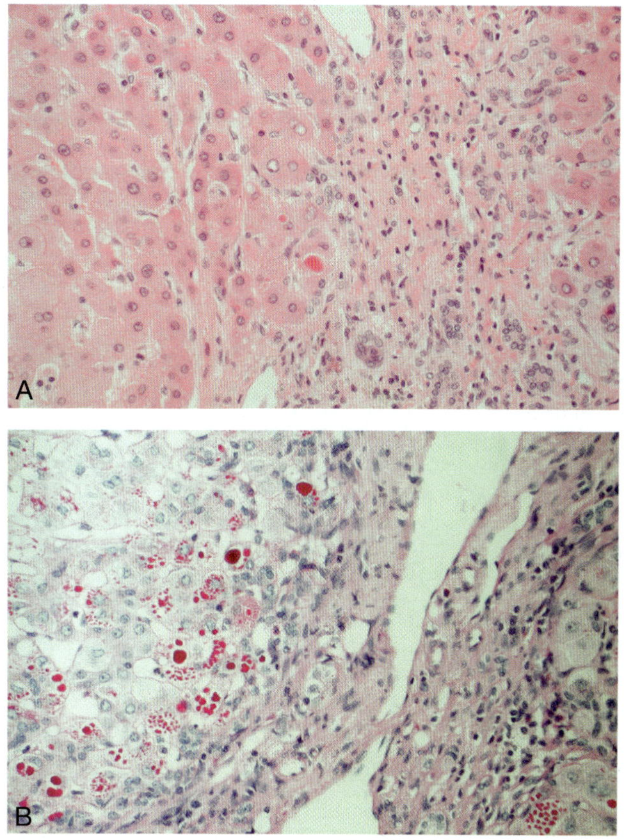

FIGURE 17.41

A, Rounded eosinophilic cytoplasmic inclusions in periportal hepatocytes represent accumulation of α1AT in endoplasmic reticulum in α1AT deficiency. **B**, The inclusions are PAS-positive, diastase resistant.

Ancillary Studies

α1-Antitrypsin cytoplasmic inclusions are strongly positive on PAS and resistant to diastase digestion. Negative stains should not exclude the diagnosis in infants younger than 12 weeks of age. Both granular and globular forms can be highlighted by IHC.

α1-Antitrypsin Deficiency—Pathologic Features

Gross Findings

- Hepatomegaly with bile staining in young children
- Cirrhosis in late stages

Microscopic Findings

- Periodic acid–Schiff–positive, diastase-resistant eosinophilic cytoplasmic globules in hepatocytes in patients older than 12 weeks (not present in young infants or neonates)
- Globules are more prominent in periportal hepatocytes and represent accumulation of α1-antitrypsin (α1AT) in endoplasmic reticulum
  In neonates, bile ducts may be decreased in number
- Chronic hepatitis pattern of injury with cirrhosis in adults

Ultrastructural Findings

- Amorphous proteinaceous material in endoplasmic reticulum

Genetics

- Autosomal recessive disorder
- Gene is located on chromosome 14q
  α1AT is a single-chain protease inhibitor in the Serpin family
- M form is the normal form; Z form is the abnormal form of the protein resulting from a single base substitution

Immunohistochemistry

- α1AT accumulation is more pronounced in periportal hepatocytes
- Granular accumulation in neonates, without globule formation

Differential Diagnosis

- Neonatal hepatitis
- Biliary atresia
- Paucity of intrahepatic bile ducts
- Chronic viral hepatitis
- Cryptogenic cirrhosis
- Nonspecific hyaline globules
- Congestion associated globules

Differential Diagnosis

In children, the main differential diagnosis is with other causes of neonatal cholestasis, and protein electrophoretic testing is needed for a definitive diagnosis.

In general, identification of characteristic cytoplasmic inclusions is highly suggestive of α1AT deficiency. Occasionally, nonspecific cytoplasmic inclusions can be noted in end-stage liver diseases that mimic α1AT globules. However, these globules are usually much smaller in size.

Prognosis and Therapy

Older men are at a greater risk for cirrhosis and rarely hepatocellular carcinomas.

Interventions include smoking cessation and avoidance of drugs or toxins in the liver. Therapy is supportive, and there is no rationale for replacement therapy with α1AT because the liver injury is caused by an inherent defect in metabolism and accumulation of the protein within hepatocytes.

GLYCOGEN STORAGE DISEASES

Glycogen storage diseases are inherited disorders of glycogen metabolism that result in accumulation of excess or structurally abnormal glycogen in the liver and other organs such as the heart, kidney, and skeletal muscle because of specific enzymatic defects in glycogen metabolism pathways. Almost all GSDs are autosomal recessive in nature, with the exception of GSD IX, which shows an X-linked mode of inheritance (Table 17.15).

CLINICAL FEATURES

Even though each entity has specific findings, there is a significant overlap in clinical presentation. Many patients present in early infancy and childhood with hepatomegaly, hypoglycemia, and failure to thrive. Some GSD present in adulthood with muscle weakness and hepatomegaly. Some patients are at risk for developing hepatic adenomas and hepatocellular carcinomas, documented in the literature mostly among those with GSD type Ia but also in types Ib, III, and VI.

GLYCOGEN STORAGE DISEASE—FACT SHEET

Definition

- Inherited disorders of glycogen metabolism leading to abnormal accumulation of glycogen in the liver

Incidence and Location

- Type I: 1 in 100,000
- Type II: fewer than 1 in 100,000 live births
- Other types: very rare

Morbidity and Mortality

- Failure to thrive
- Patients with type I survive into adulthood but may have focal segmental glomerulosclerosis and hepatic adenomas
- Type II is variable in severity
- Patients with type IV often die in the early perinatal period
- Type VI is relatively benign; adults are asymptomatic

Gender, Race, and Age Distribution

- Males and females are equally affected, except for some subtypes of type IX, which are X linked
- Age at presentation is variable and depends on type, although most cases present in infancy

TABLE 17.15
Glycogen Storage Diseases With Hepatic Manifestations

Glycogen Storage Disease	Clinical Presentation	Enzyme Deficiency	Histopathologic Findings
Type 0	Hepatomegaly, hypoglycemia	Glycogen synthetase	Steatosis
Type Ia (von Gierke's disease)	Growth retardation, hepatomegaly, lactic acidemia, hyperlipidemia	Glucose-6-phosphatase	Glycogenosis and macrovesicular steatosis; glycogenated nuclei, possibly fibrosis; hepatic adenomas
Type Ib	As for Ia; neutropenia and impaired PMN function, some with IBD	Glucose-6-phosphatse	As for Ia
Type II (Pompe's disease)	Variable; cardiomegaly, hypotonia (floppy baby syndrome), hepatomegaly; adult presentation with only muscle weakness with breathing complications	Lysosomal acid α-glucosidase	Glycogenosis, intralysosomal glycogen accumulation (PAS-positive cytoplasmic vacuoles); lacks fibrosis
Type III (Cori's disease)	Similar to type I but less severe Type IIIa: liver and muscle involvement Type IIIb: only liver involvement	Amylo-1, 6-glucosidase	Glycogenosis, glycogenated nuclei; fibrosis with progression to cirrhosis, hepatic adenomas
Type IV (Andersen's disease)	Hepatosplenomegaly and failure to thrive; hypoglycemia is uncommon	Amylo-1,4-1,6 transglucosidase	Ground glass inclusions (PAS positive, partially diastase resistant) Two forms: nonprogressive and classic hepatic form with cirrhosis before age 5 years
Type VI (Hers' disease)	Hepatomegaly, failure to thrive; variable hypoglycemia and hyperlipidemia, usually mild	Liver phosphorylase E	Predominantly glycogenosis with variable steatosis, fibrosis, hepatic adenomas
Type IX	As for type VI	Liver phosphorylase kinase	Marked glycogenosis (PAS positive, diastase sensitive), fibrosis leading to cirrhosis
Type XI (Fanconi Bickel syndrome)	Failure to thrive, hypoglycemia, moon face, fat deposition in shoulders and abdomen	GLUT2 transporter	Glycogenosis and macrovesicular steatosis

IBD, Inflammatory bowel disease; *PAS*, periodic acid–Schiff; *PMN*, polymorphonuclear leukocytes.

Clinical Features

- Definitive diagnosis requires biochemical determination of enzyme defect
- Patients present with variable hepatomegaly, hypoglycemia, and failure to thrive

Prognosis and Therapy

- Treatment is dietary supplementation with glucose drip feedings and uncooked cornstarch in type I, high-protein diets in types II and III, and uncooked cornstarch in type VI
- Prognosis depends on type: good for type VI, poor for type IV, and intermediate for other types

Laboratory Findings

Patients can present with hypoglycemia with hyperlactatemia. Increased serum creatine kinase levels are described. Other laboratory abnormalities include hyperuricemia, hyperlipidemia, hypercalciuria, and azotemia. Elevated biotinidase activity has been suggested as a useful biomarker for hepatic GSDs. In addition, determination of liver enzyme activities and molecular genetic analysis by next-generation sequencing are needed for further classification.

Pathologic Features

Gross Findings

The liver in most GSD types is enlarged and pale. Some forms of GSDs reveal advanced fibrosis or cirrhosis. Distinct lesions can be seen in patients who develop hepatocellular adenomas or carcinomas.

Microscopic Findings

Most patients demonstrate diffuse glycogen accumulation in enlarged hepatocytes, which results in a pale appearance on H&E stain with distinct cell membranes (described as mosaic appearance) (Fig. 17.42A). PAS further supports the presence of cytoplasmic glycogen (Fig. 17.42B). In some forms, glycogenated nuclei and macrovesicular steatosis may be prominent (see Fig. 17.42C). Ground-glass cytoplasmic inclusions are classically described in GSD type IV.

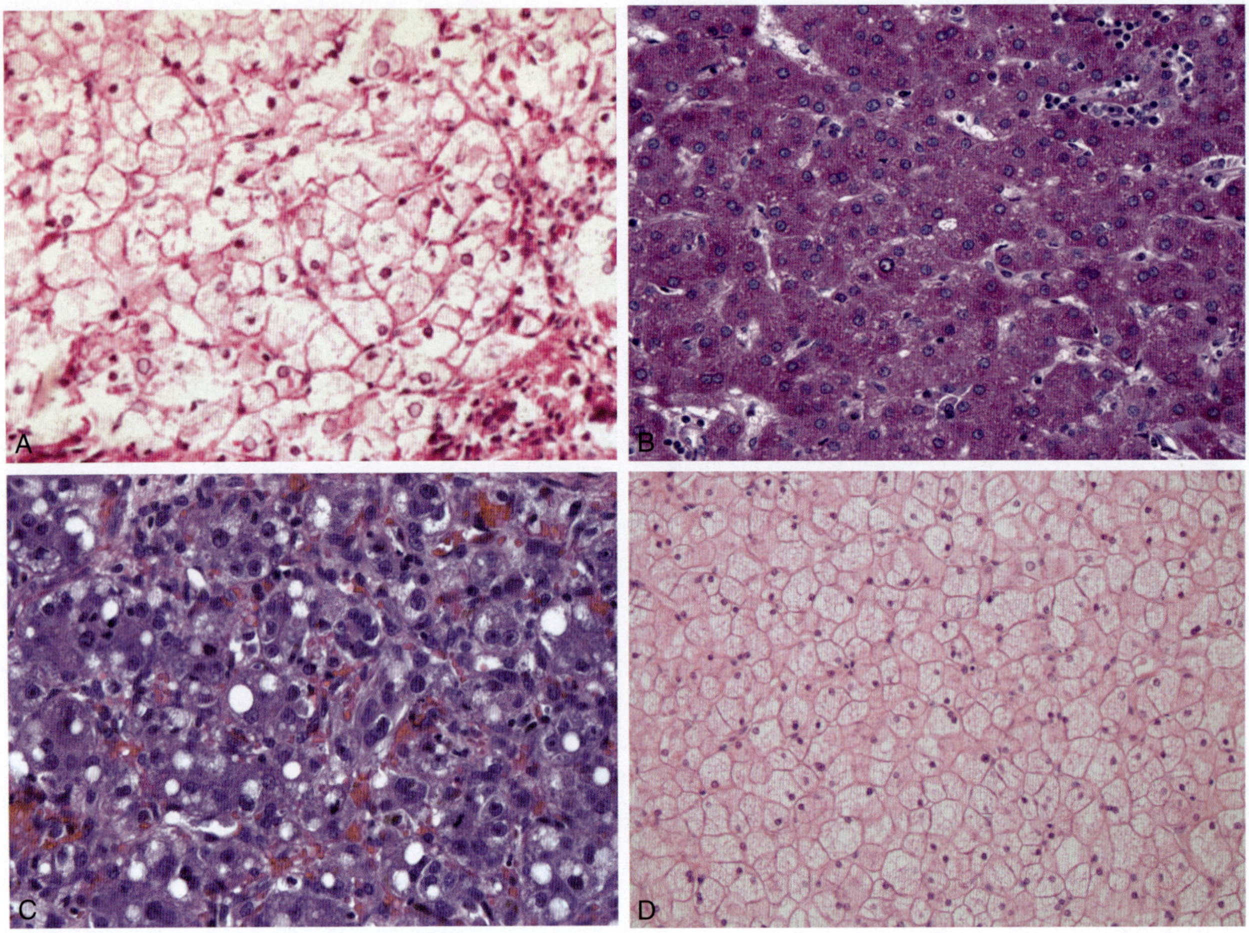

FIGURE 17.42

A, Cytoplasmic accumulation of glycogen in hepatocytes leads to a clear appearance with distinct cell membranes on hematoxylin and eosin stain (mosaic pattern). **B**, PAS stain highlights the glycogen accumulation (shown), with removal of glycogen with diastase digestion. **C**, Type II GSD does not show a mosaic pattern; hepatocytes contain lipid vacuoles. **D**, Histologic findings of GSD type IX.

Fibrosis tends to develop in certain cases (typically in GSD types III, IV, VI, and IX) (see Fig. 17.42D) and can lead to cirrhosis. Although histologic findings may raise suspicion for GSD, a definitive diagnosis often requires further metabolic work-up. The general approach when suspecting a GSD should be to snap freeze a portion of the tissue, submit a sample in glutaraldehyde for electron microscopy, and process the rest of the sample for routine stains.

Glycogen Storage Disease—Pathologic Features

Gross Findings

- Hepatomegaly
- Pale discoloration
  Variable fibrosis, cirrhosis in certain cases
- Liver masses: hepatocellular adenomas or carcinomas

Microscopic Findings

- Hepatocytes are enlarged by glycogen accumulation, with pale cytoplasm
- Mosaic pattern caused by compression of sinusoids and accentuation of hepatocyte cell membranes (type II lacks mosaic pattern)
- In type IV, hepatocytes contain rounded ground glass cytoplasmic inclusions
- Fibrosis leading to cirrhosis may be found in types III, IV, VI, and IX

Ultrastructural Findings

- Large pools of glycogen displace cytoplasmic organelles
- In type I, double-contoured vesicles are seen in the endoplasmic reticulum
- In type II, glycogen accumulates in lysosomes
- In type IV, non–membrane-bound inclusions are seen

Genetics

- Autosomal recessive inheritance, except for some subtypes of type IX, which are X linked

Differential Diagnosis

- Glycogenic hepatopathy
- Type IV: Lafora's disease

Ancillary Studies

Ultrastructural Findings

By electron microscopy, monoparticulate glycogen fills the cytoplasm displacing normal organelles. Intranuclear glycogen may also be identified in some types of GSD. In type IV GSD, fibrillar aggregates characteristic of amylopectin are present.

Differential Diagnosis

One of the main differential diagnoses is glycogenic hepatopathy (GH); however, a history of diabetes mellitus and overall clinical presentation of GH (hepatomegaly, abdominal pain, and elevated transaminases in a patient with poorly controlled diabetes) is helpful. GSDs may show considerable morphologic overlap with each other, and definitive diagnosis relies on biochemical testing of fresh, frozen, or other target liver tissue.

Prognosis and Therapy

The prognosis depends on the specific type because some present in early infancy and carry a high mortality rate, but others present in adulthood and are mildly symptomatic.

For most GSDs, no specific treatment is available. Dietary manipulation can prevent hypoglycemia and promote growth. Liver transplantation is considered in patients with cirrhosis.

Lysosomal Storage Disorders. Lysosomal storage disorders most commonly involve glycolipid, phospholipid, or mucopolysaccharide metabolism and result in accumulation of storage products within cytoplasmic membrane-bound vesicles. The excessive undegraded substrate usually accumulates in reticuloendothelial cells in the liver, nervous system, and muscle. There are more than 50 LSDs described. Most are inherited in an autosomal recessive manner (Table 17.16).

CLINICAL FEATURES

The clinical presentation depends on the disorder. In severe cases, the substrate accumulation starts in utero and often results in hydrops fetalis. Most patients exhibit multiorgan involvement with organomegaly (an enlarged liver and spleen are most common) and neurologic symptoms, including visual abnormalities, seizures, and neurodegenerative signs. In addition, hematologic and psychiatric manifestations can be encountered. The diagnosis is confirmed through specific enzyme assays, lysosomal enzyme activity in tissue cultures, and mutational analysis.

TABLE 17.16

Clinical Features of Selected Lysosomal Storage Diseases

Disorder	Inheritance	Clinical Features	Clinical Outcome
Mucopolysaccharidoses (MPS) (seven distinct types, most common: Hunter, Hurler, and Morquio diseases)	Autosomal recessive (six types); X-linked for MPS II	Multisystem involvement; organomegaly; abnormal facies; mental retardation in some types	Chronic progressive course; survival depends on specific disease type and severity and ranges from early childhood to old age
Gaucher disease types 1, 2, and 3	Autosomal recessive	Hepatosplenomegaly, all types; CNS degeneration, types 2 and 3	Type 1: 6–80 years Type 2: <2 years Type 3: second to fourth decades of life
Niemann-Pick disease types A, B, and C	Autosomal recessive	Type A: failure to thrive; hepatosplenomegaly; neurologic degeneration Type B: variable presentation, no neurologic involvement Type C: progressive neurologic degeneration, hepatosplenomegaly	Type A: fatal by age 3 years Types B and C: survival into adulthood
Acid lipase deficiency (Wolman's disease)	Autosomal recessive	Hepatosplenomegaly; steatorrhea, adrenal calcification	Wolman's disease is fatal by 1 year
Metachromatic leukodystrophy	Autosomal recessive	Gait disturbances, mental regression, dementia, seizures	Variable; may be slowly progressive over decades
Mucolipidoses (I cell disease and pseudo-Hurler polydystrophy)	Autosomal recessive	Severe psychomotor retardation; abnormal facies, hepatomegaly in I-cell disease; joint abnormalities and growth retardation in pseudo-Hurler polydystrophy	Death in first decade for I-cell disease; survival into adulthood for pseudo-Hurler polydystrophy

CNS, Central nervous system.

LYSOSOMAL STORAGE DISORDERS—FACT SHEET

Definition

- Inherited disorder of degradation of substances normally broken down in lysosomes such as sphingolipidoses (e.g., Gaucher disease, Niemann-Pick disease), mucopolysaccharidoses (e.g., Hurler's disease, Hunter's disease), mucolipidoses, oligosaccharidosis, and acid lipase deficiency (Wolman's disease, cholesterol ester storage disease)

Incidence and Location

- Rare disorders but collectively represent 1 in 7000 to 1 in 10,000 births
- Gaucher disease is most common

Morbidity and Mortality

- Depends on biochemical defect

Gender, Race, and Age Distribution

- For most of these disorders, males and females are affected equally
- Certain ethnic groups may be at a greater risk (e.g., Ashkenazi Jews: Gaucher disease; Irish descent: Tay-Sachs)
- Most are diagnosed in infancy or childhood, but some may present in late adulthood (type I Gaucher disease)

Clinical Features

- Variable; hepatomegaly and neurologic symptoms are common

Prognosis and Therapy

- Bone marrow transplantation has been performed for some of the lysosomal storage disorders
- Liver transplantation is rarely indicated and is not curative
- Prognosis depends on the disease

Laboratory Findings

Abnormal liver function ranges from a clinical picture of neonatal hepatitis with marked elevation of transaminases to established cirrhosis. Elevated excretion of oligosaccharides and glycosaminoglycans can be assessed in urine. Enzymatic activity and DNA mutation analysis in blood are useful in classifying the underlying disease.

Pathologic Features

Gross Findings

Similar to GSDs, hepatomegaly is common, but in patients with LSD, the cut surface has a yellow to orange discoloration. In advanced cases, there may be obvious scarring or cirrhosis.

Microscopic Findings

The characteristic finding in most LSDs is accumulation of foamy material ("the substrate") within reticuloendothelial cells and sometimes hepatocytes (Table 17.17 and Fig. 17.43). On a histologic basis, specific findings may be a clue to the diagnosis. For example, enlarged Kupffer cells with a "crinkled paper" appearance of the cytoplasm are present in Gaucher disease. Certain cases evolve to fibrosis and cirrhosis, although the true incidence depends on the underlying disease and medical interventions.

TABLE 17.17

Histopathologic Features in Select Lysosomal Storage Disorders

Disorder	Microscopic Features
Mucopolysaccharidoses (liver involvement in types I, II, III, VI, and VII)	Vacuolization of Kupffer cells and hepatocytes, well demonstrated on colloidal iron stain; liver fibrosis and cirrhosis may develop
Gaucher disease	Accumulation of storage material in Kupffer cells; striated or wrinkled cytoplasm (PAS negative); progressive fibrosis in some cases but rarely cirrhosis; hepatocytes not affected
Niemann-Pick disease	Progressive increase in lipid-laden foamy histiocytes in hepatic sinusoids; hepatocyte vacuolization; cirrhosis in some cases; cholestasis with giant cell transformation in type C; oil red O and Luxol fast blue positive, but PAS is negative
Acid liposomal lipase deficiency (Wolman's disease)	Microvesicular steatosis; vacuolated and enlarged, pale-staining Kupffer cells and hepatocytes; needle-shaped birefringent crystals in hepatocytes; fibrosis and cirrhosis; oil red O stain positive
Metachromatic leukodystrophy	Light brown granules in Kupffer cells, portal macrophages, and biliary epithelium; metachromatic with cresyl violet staining of frozen sections
Mucolipidoses	Vacuolated hepatocytes, Kupffer cells, and portal fibroblasts

PAS, Periodic acid–Schiff.

Ancillary Studies

Trichrome and PAS-D stains can highlight the striations in the cytoplasm of Gaucher cells. In Niemann-Pick disease, the cells storing sphingomyelin reveal a foamy pale cytoplasm that can be easily identified on PAS stain because of the dark staining of hepatocytes. Colloidal iron stain demonstrates mucosubstances in Kupffer cells and hepatocytes in mucopolysaccharidosis.

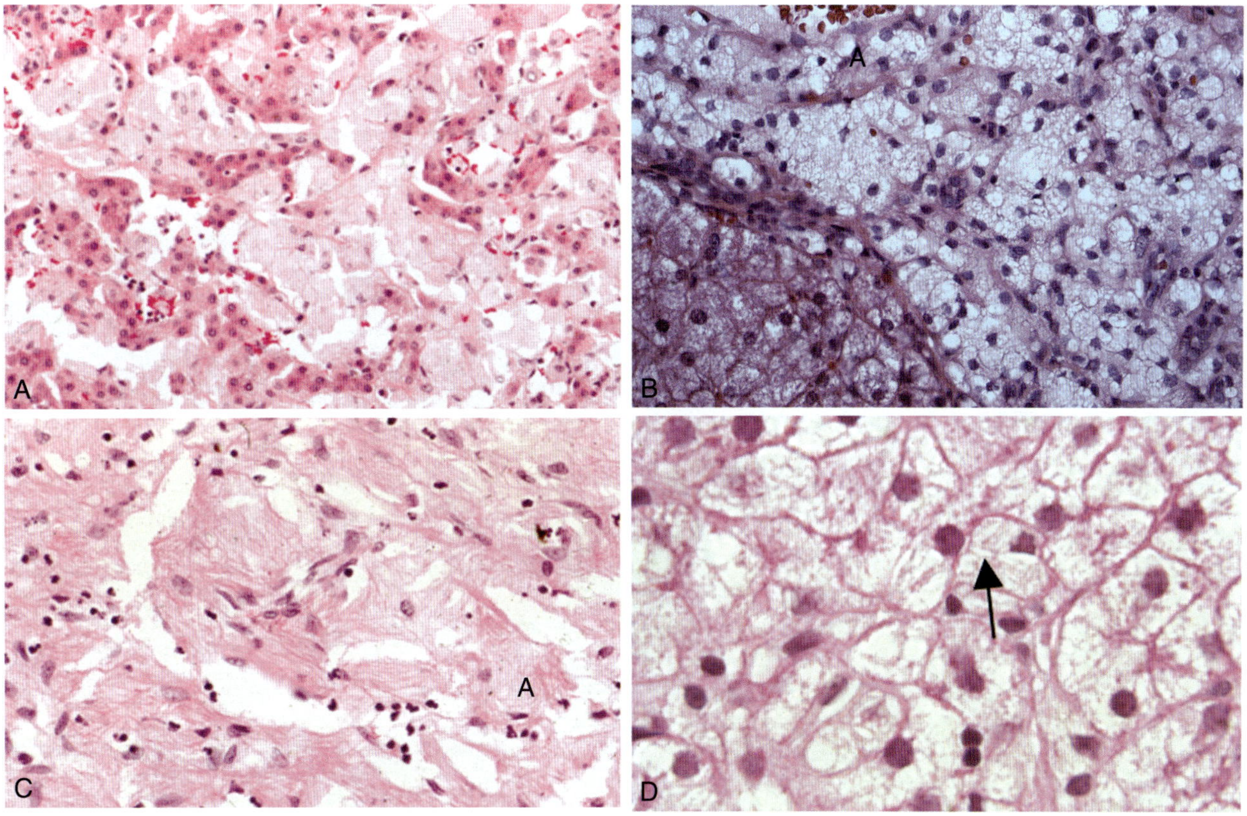

FIGURE 17.43

Lysosomal storage diseases. **A**, In Gaucher's disease, Kupffer cells are markedly distended and accumulate in hepatic sinusoids; hepatocytes do not accumulate glucosylceramide and are thus uninvolved, although they may show atrophic changes. **B**, The Gaucher cells are characterized by striated or wrinkled cytoplasm. **C**, In Niemann-Pick disease, both Kupffer cells (*top*) and hepatocytes develop cytoplasmic vacuoles. Fibrosis is typically not prominent. **D**, In Wolman's disease, both hepatocytes and Kupffer cells are swollen and pale staining. Lipid droplets may be seen in hepatocytes. Needle-shaped birefringent crystals of cholesterol may be inconspicuous (*arrow*).

Lysosomal Storage Disorders—Pathologic Features

Gross Findings
- Hepatomegaly with yellow-orange discoloration

Microscopic Findings
- Reticuloendothelial cells are enlarged and may appear vacuolated, foamy, or exhibit striated cytoplasm
- Steatosis is present in cholesteryl ester storage disease

Ultrastructural Findings
- Lysosomal or lamellar inclusions
- Membrane-bound vacuoles containing granular or fibrillar material in some disorders

Genetics
- Most are autosomal recessive
- Some exhibit an X-linked pattern of inheritance

Differential Diagnosis
- The specific diagnosis is established by biochemical or genetic testing

Ultrastructural Findings

Electron microscopy shows lysosomal inclusions, usually granular or fibrillar. In Niemann-Pick disease, the inclusions resemble myelin. Lipid droplets and cholesterol clefts are seen in Wolman's disease and cholesterol ester storage disease.

Differential Diagnosis

Although some of the LSDs have characteristic liver findings, definitive diagnosis is based on demonstration of decreased enzyme activity in appropriate tissues or with diagnostic molecular assays.

Prognosis and Therapy

Most cases are diagnosed in infancy. The reported survival is 5 to 10 years after diagnosis (see Table 17.16). Whereas some LSDs are fatal in early childhood, milder forms are compatible with a normal lifespan. There is no cure for LSDs, and the treatment is symptomatic. Enzyme replacement therapy can be beneficial, if available. HSCT is performed as therapy for some of the LSDs, including mucopolysaccharidosis types I and VI and attenuated forms of metachromatic leukodystrophy.

GLYCOGENIC HEPATOPATHY

CLINICAL FEATURES

Glycogenic hepatopathy is typically seen in adult and pediatric patients with type I diabetes mellitus who have poorly controlled blood glucose levels. Patients with GH classically have a history of poorly controlled blood glucose and present with hepatomegaly, abdominal pain, and markedly elevated transaminases after an episode of marked or prolonged hyperglycemia that required intense insulin therapy. Mauriac's syndrome, originally described in children with type 1 diabetes, consists of hepatic glycogenosis with associated growth retardation, dwarfism, delayed puberty, and cushingoid features.

PATHOLOGIC FEATURES

MICROSCOPIC FINDINGS

The most striking feature is the prominent hepatocyte swelling with cytoplasmic rarefaction and accentuation of cell membranes. Diffuse glycogenated nuclei are common, as are giant megamitochondria. The overall liver architecture remains intact, and there are absent to minimal steatosis, inflammation, acidophil bodies, and fibrosis. PAS stain is not needed for the diagnosis, but if performed, it highlights the abundant cytoplasmic glycogen (Fig. 17.44).

DIFFERENTIAL DIAGNOSIS

The differential diagnosis of GH includes GSDs, as well as other genetic disorders. The clinical setting in which these occur is helpful in making this distinction. Cases with diffuse microvesicular steatosis can mimic GH. Microvesicular steatosis occurs in a very limited number of clinical situations (e.g., acute fatty liver of pregnancy, Reye syndrome) and the hepatocytes reveal a pale, foamy appearance that differs from the rarefied cytoplasm with distinct nuclear membranes seen in GH. Patchy or diffuse glycogenosis in the setting of NAFLD is common. That said, those patients have a different clinical presentation, and the biopsy often shows steatosis or features of NASH.

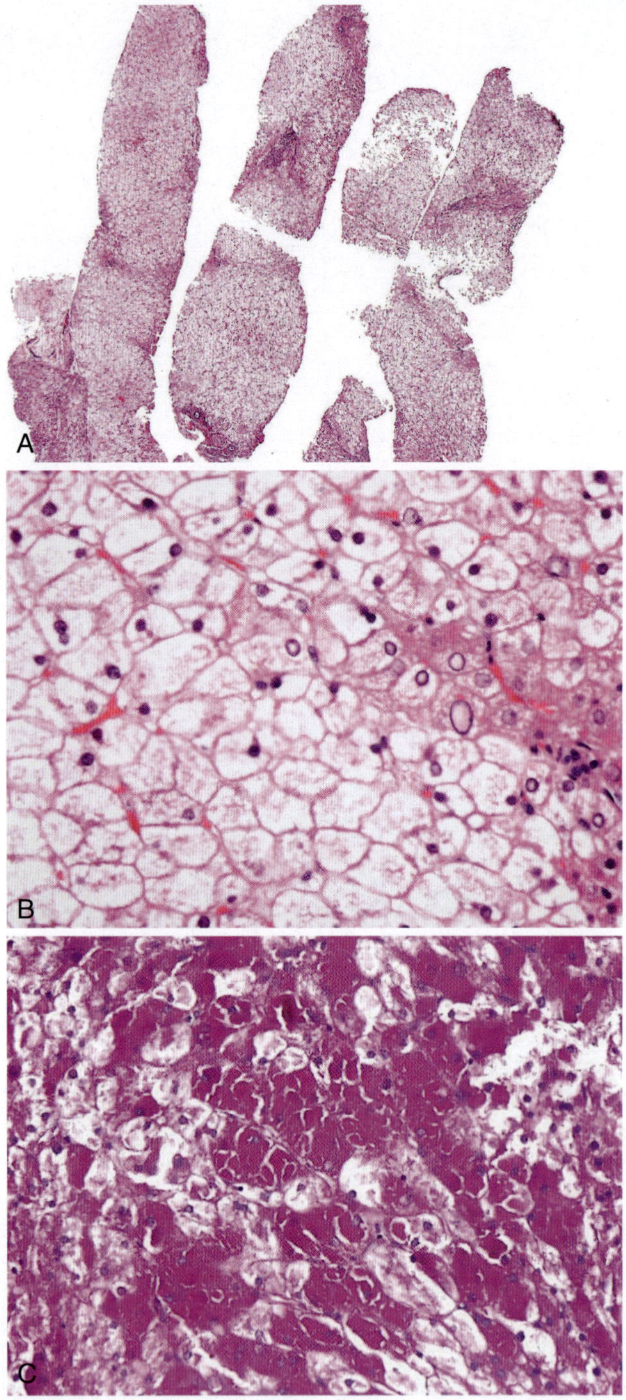

FIGURE 17.44

Glycogenic hepatopathy. **A**, Prominent cytoplasmic clearing is present throughout this biopsy sample from a 14-year-old patient with poorly controlled type 1 diabetes and elevated transaminases. **B**, Hepatocytes show uniform cytoplasmic distention and glycogenated nuclei. **C**, PAS stain demonstrating abundant intracytoplasmic glycogen.

Prognosis and Therapy

Clinical findings and histologic features gradually resolve with adequate blood glucose control.

PORPHYRIAS

CLINICAL FEATURES

The porphyrias are a group of eight inherited metabolic disorders associated with abnormalities in the heme biosynthetic pathway. Acute intermittent porphyria (AIP), porphyria cutanea tarda (PCT), and erythropoietic protoporphyria (EPP) are inherited in an autosomal dominant fashion and can be associated with significant liver disease. Based on the clinical presentation, porphyrias are divided into acute and cutaneous forms. The acute attacks often follow a prodrome and are timated because many case triggered by several events such as hormonal changes, drugs, smoking, or fasting, among others. AIP usually presents after puberty with episodes of severe abdominal pain, sympathetic symptoms, and motor neuropathy. Life-threatening neurologic and adrenergic symptoms can develop. Patients with PCT present with erosive photodermatosis and chronic blisters in sun-exposed skin. Most cases coexist with hemochromatosis, alcoholic liver disease, hepatitis C or HIV infection, ethanol use, and estrogen administration. The most common clinical manifestation of EPP is lifelong acute photosensitivity in sun-exposed skin that starts in childhood and includes burning, stinging, and pruritus. Cholelithiasis is common, and a minor subset of patients develop cholestatic liver failure.

PORPHYRIAS—FACT SHEET

Definition
- Disorders of biosynthesis of porphyrins and heme
- Acute intermittent porphyria (AIP), porphyria cutanea tarda (PCT), and erythropoietic protoporphyria (EPP) often affect the liver

Prevalence and Location
- AIP prevalence is 1 to 2 in 100,000; it is more common in European countries
- PCT is most common porphyria in the United States
- EPP prevalence is 1 in 75,000 to 1 in 200,000 worldwide

Morbidity and Mortality
- Most patients with AIP recover fully; it can be life threatening during acute attacks
- PCT is associated with collagen vascular diseases, acquired immunodeficiency syndrome (AIDS), and hepatitis C, among others
- Patients with EPP can develop cirrhosis

Gender, Race, and Age Distribution
- AIP: more common in women; peak in third decade
- PCT: sporadic PCT (80%) occurs in male patients in fourth decade of life; familial PCT is equally common in males and females
- EPP: males affected twice as often as females; peak in third decade

Clinical Features
- AIP: abdominal pain, sympathetic and neurologic symptoms
- PCT presents with blisters on sun-exposed skin
- EPP: acute photosensitivity on sun-exposed skin

Prognosis and Therapy
- Treatment in general is supportive and symptomatic
- Patients with AIP are treated with intravenous lyophilized alkaline heme; good prognosis
- PCT: approximately 65% develop cirrhosis; increased risk for hepatocellular carcinoma
- Treatment for PCT is avoidance of sun exposure and alcohol; phlebotomy to decrease iron stores if increased; chloroquine is effective in some cases
- EPP: hematin is effective treatment; liver transplantation for patients with cirrhosis

Pathologic Features

Gross Findings

Gross findings are nonspecific, except in end-stage liver disease when micro- or macronodular cirrhosis can be evident. The liver may show a dark brown to black discoloration in some cases.

Microscopic Findings

Microscopic changes in the liver in AIP are nonspecific and include cholestatic changes, steatosis, and accumulation of iron in Kupffer cells and hepatocytes.

In PCT, distinctive cytoplasmic uroporphyrins may be identified. These inclusions are autofluorescent needle-shaped structures in the cytoplasm of hepatocytes and can be seen on light microscopy or fluorescent microscope. They can be difficult to identify in routinely processed sections and are best appreciated in unstained sections. Nonspecific histologic findings in PCT include variable hemosiderosis, mild chronic portal inflammation, steatosis, and fibrosis (Figs. 17.45A and B).

Erythropoietic protoporphyria is characterized by the presence of dense dark brown pigment in Kupffer cells, canaliculi, and bile ducts. This pigment is birefringent and shows characteristic central, dark Maltese cross configuration under polarized light (Fig. 17.45C). Cholestasis is common.

Cirrhosis occurs in a small subset of cases and may be complicated by the development of hepatocellular carcinoma.

PORPHYRIAS—PATHOLOGIC FEATURES

Gross Findings

- Explanted livers show cirrhosis or marked green discoloration if cholestatic liver failure
- Black discoloration in particular in erythropoietic protoporphyria (EPP)

Microscopic Findings

- Acute intermittent porphyria (AIP): nonspecific steatosis; increased iron deposition in Kupffer cells and hepatocytes
- Porphyria cutanea tarda (PCT): needle-shaped cytoplasmic inclusions of uroporphyrin are birefringent, best seen in unstained paraffin sections
- Other findings in PCT are hepatic steatosis, iron deposition, and fibrosis
- EPP: cholestasis, dark autofluorescent-dense pigment in canaliculi, bile ducts, and Kupffer cells that display central Maltese cross upon polarization
- Cirrhosis and hepatocellular carcinoma in a small subset

Ultrastructural Findings

- PCT: crystalline inclusions
- EPP: protoporphyrin crystals have a "starburst" pattern

Differential Diagnosis

- AIP: drug reaction, chronic viral hepatitis
- PCT: chronic viral hepatitis, iron overload
- EPP: cholestatic disorders, including extrahepatic biliary obstruction

ANCILLARY STUDIES

Deposits of uroporphyrin in PCT and protoporphyrin in EPP exhibit red autofluorescence in sections examined under ultraviolet light.

DIFFERENTIAL DIAGNOSIS

Microscopic findings of porphyrias are largely nonspecific. However, with an appropriate clinical history, the finding of characteristic inclusions in PCT and in EPP may be helpful. A definitive diagnosis requires correlation with porphyrin precursors in urine, feces, and plasma fluorescence emission spectroscopy in plasma. DNA mutational analysis remains the gold standard for diagnosing this group of disorders.

PROGNOSIS AND THERAPY

The treatment is mainly supportive and symptomatic. Infusion of intravenous lyophilized alkaline heme is used to treat acute crises in patients with AIP. Patients with PCT may be treated with phlebotomy to reduce hepatic iron stores and chloroquine. Patients with EPP are treated with β-carotene and avoidance of sun exposure.

Liver transplant may be needed in some cases, but EPP can recur in the allograft.

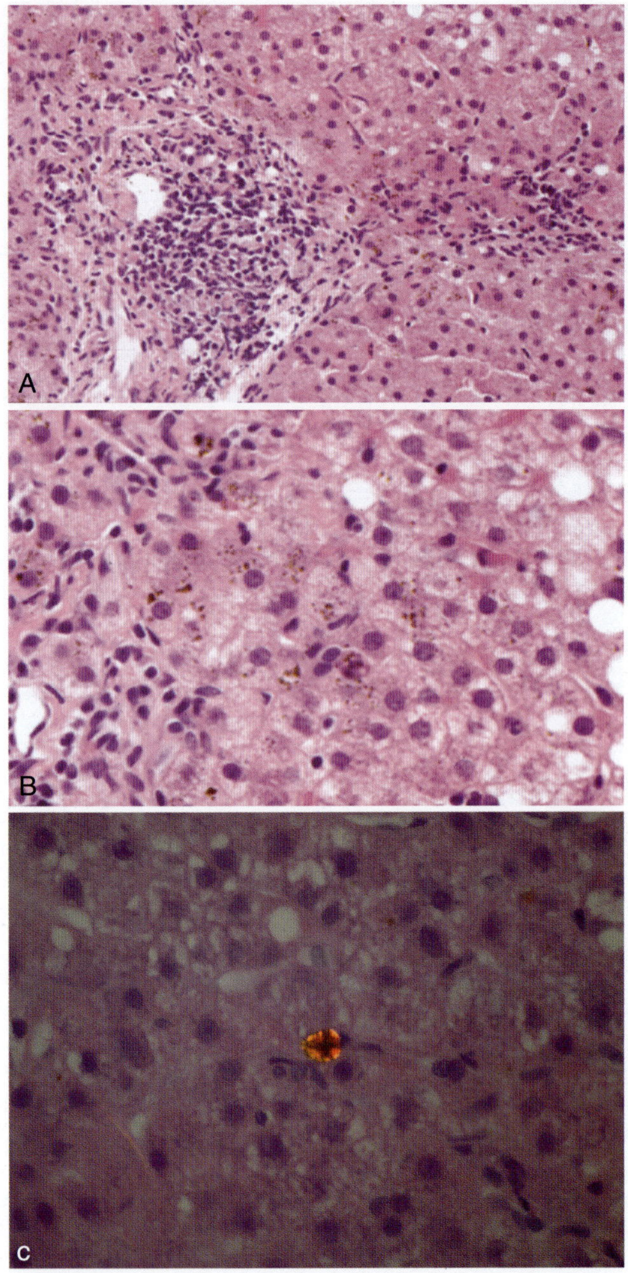

FIGURE 17.45

A, The liver in porphyria cutanea tarda (PCT) may exhibit nonspecific changes such as portal chronic inflammation and mild interface hepatitis. **B**, Iron accumulation in periportal hepatocytes is a common feature. **C**, In cases of EPP, a dark autofluorescent dense pigment within canaliculi, bile ducts and/or Kupffer cells will display a central Maltese cross upon polarization.

SUGGESTED READINGS

Acute and Chronic Hepatitis Pattern of Injury

1. Batts KP, Ludwig J. Chronic hepatitis. An update on terminology and reporting. *Am J Surg Pathol*. 1995;19:1409–1417.
2. Ennes EM, Zeniya M, Czaja AJ, et al. International Autoimmune Hepatitis Group. Simplified criteria for the diagnosis of autoimmune hepatitis. *Hepatology*. 2008;48(1):169–176.
3. Theise ND. Liver biopsy assessment in chronic viral hepatitis: a personal, practical approach. *Mod Pathol*. 2007;20(suppl 1): S3–S14.
4. De Torres M, Poynard T. Risk factors for liver fibrosis progression in patients with chronic hepatitis C. *Ann Hepatol*. 2003;2: 5–11.
5. Czaja AJ. Diagnosis and management of autoimmune hepatitis. *Clin Liver Dis*. 2015;19:57–79.
6. Manns MP, Czaja AJ, Gorham JD, et al. Diagnosis and management of autoimmune hepatitis. *Hepatology*. 2010;51:1–31.
7. Lohse AW, Sebode M, Bhathal PS, et al. Consensus recommendations for histological criteria of autoimmune hepatitis from the International AIH Pathology Group: results of a workshop on AIH histology hosted by the European Reference Network on Hepatological Diseases and the European Society of Pathology: results of a workshop on AIH histology hosted by the European Reference Network on Hepatological Diseases and the European Society of Pathology. *Liver Int*. 2022;42(5):1058–1069.
8. Hennes EM, Zeniya M, Czaja AJ, et al. Simplified criteria for the diagnosis of autoimmune hepatitis. *Hepatology*. 2008; 48(1):169–176.

Steatosis–Steatohepatitis Pattern of Injury

9. Ratziu V, Bellentani S, Cortez-Pinto H, et al. A position statement on NAFLD/NASH based on the EASL 2009 special conference. *J Hepatol*. 2010;53(2):372–384.
10. Ford ES. Prevalence of the metabolic syndrome defined by the International Diabetes Federation among adults in the U.S. *Diabetes Care*. 2005;28:2745–2749.
11. Cornier MA, Dabelea D, Hernandez TL, et al. The metabolic syndrome. *Endocr Rev*. 2008;29:777–822.
12. Flegal KM, Carroll MD, Ogden CL, et al. Prevalence and trends in obesity among US adults, 1999–2008. *JAMA*. 2010;303: 235–241.
13. Matteoni CA, Younossi ZM, Gramlich T, et al. Nonalcoholic fatty liver disease: a spectrum of clinical and pathological severity. *Gastroenterology*. 1999;116:1413–1419.
14. Harrison SA, Torgerson S, Hayashi PH. The natural history of nonalcoholic fatty liver disease: a clinical histopathological study. *Am J Gastroenterol*. 2003;98(9):2042–2047.
15. Powell EE, Cooksley WG, Hanson R, et al. The natural history of nonalcoholic steatohepatitis: a follow-up study of forty-two patients for up to 21 years. *Hepatology*. 1990;11(1):74–80.
16. Younossi ZM, Stepanova M, Rafiq N, et al. Pathologic criteria for nonalcoholic steatohepatitis: interprotocol agreement and ability to predict liver-related mortality. *Hepatology*. 2011;53:1874–1882.
17. Brunt EM, Janney CG, Di Bisceglie AM, et al. Nonalcoholic steatohepatitis: a proposal for grading and staging the histological lesions. *Am J Gastroenterol*. 1999;94:2467–2474.
18. Tiniakos DG, Vos MB, Brunt EM. Nonalcoholic fatty liver disease: pathology and pathogenesis. *Annu Rev Pathol*. 2010; 5:145–171.
19. Yeh MM, Brunt EM. Pathology of nonalcoholic fatty liver disease. *Am J Clin Pathol*. 2007;128:837–847.
20. Tiniakos DG. Liver biopsy in alcoholic and non-alcoholic steatohepatitis patients. *Gastroenterol Clin Biol*. 2009;33:930–939.
21. Kleiner DE, Brunt EM. Nonalcoholic fatty liver disease: pathologic patterns and biopsy evaluation in clinical research. *Semin Liver Dis*. 2012;32:3–13.
22. Schwimmer JB, Behling C, Newbury R, et al. Histopathology of pediatric nonalcoholic fatty liver disease. *Hepatology*. 2005;42: 641–649.
23. Carter-Kent CA, Yerian LM, Brunt EM, et al. Nonalcoholic steatohepatitis in children: a multicenter clinicopathological study. *Hepatology*. 2009;50:1113–1120.
24. Schwimmer JB. Definitive diagnosis and assessment of risk for nonalcoholic fatty liver disease in children and adolescents. *Semin Liver Dis*. 2007;27:312–318.
25. Brunt EM, Kleiner DE, Wilson LN, et al. Portal chronic inflammation in nonalcoholic fatty liver disease (NAFLD): a histologic marker of advanced NAFLD-Clinicopathologic correlations from the nonalcoholic steatohepatitis clinical research network. *Hepatology*. 2009;49:809–820.
26. Ayak NC, Vasdev N, Saigal S, et al. End-stage nonalcoholic fatty liver disease: evaluation of pathomorphologic features and relationship to cryptogenic cirrhosis from study of explant livers in a living donor liver transplant program. *Hum Pathol*. 2010;41(3): 425–430.
27. Ayata G, Gordon FD, Lewis WD, et al. Cryptogenic cirrhosis: clinicopathologic findings at and after liver transplantation. *Hum Pathol*. 2002;33:1098–1104.
28. Vuppalanchi R, Gould RJ, Wilson LA, et al. Clinical significance of serum autoantibodies in patients with NAFLD: results from the nonalcoholic steatohepatitis clinical research network (NASH CRN). *Hepatol Int*. 2012;6:379–385.
29. Lackner C, Gogg-Kamerer M, Zatloukal K, et al. Ballooned hepatocytes in steatohepatitis: the value of keratin immunohistochemistry for diagnosis. *J Hepatol*. 2008:821–828.
30. Kleiner DE, Brunt EM. Nonalcoholic fatty liver disease: pathologic patterns and biopsy evaluation in clinical research. *Semin Liver Dis*. 2012;32:2–13.
31. Kleiner DE, Brunt EM, Van Natta M, et al. Nonalcoholic Steatohepatitis Clinical Research Network. Design and validation of a histologic scoring system for nonalcoholic fatty liver disease. *Hepatology*. 2005;41:1313–1321.
32. Lucey MR, Mathurin P, Morgan TR. Alcoholic hepatitis. *N Engl J Med*. 2009;360:2758–2769.
33. Adinolfi LE, Restivo L, Marrone A. The predictive value of steatosis in hepatitis C virus infection. *Expert Rev Gastroenterol Hepatol*. 2013;7:205–213.
34. Machado MV, Cortez-Pinto H. Insulin resistance and steatosis in chronic hepatitis C. *Ann Hepatol*. 2009;8(suppl 1):S67–S75.
35. Lok AS, Everhart JE, Chung RT, et al. Evolution of hepatic steatosis in patients with advanced hepatitis C: results from the hepatitis C antiviral long-term treatment against cirrhosis (HALT-C) trial. *Hepatology*. 2009;49:1828–1837.
36. Bedossa P, Moucari R, Chelbi E, et al. Evidence for a role of nonalcoholic steatohepatitis in hepatitis C: a prospective study. *Hepatology*. 2007;46:380–387.
37. Yeh MM, Brunt E. Pathological features of fatty liver disease. *Gastroenterology*. 2014;147:754–764.
38. Alpert L, Hart J. The pathology of alcoholic liver disease. *Clin Liver Dis*. 2016;20:473–489.
39. Altamirano J, Miquel R, Katoonizadeh A, et al. A histologic scoring system for prognosis of patients with alcoholic steatohepatitis. *Gastroenterology*. 2014;146(5):1231–1239. e1–e6.

Cholestatic Pattern of Injury

40. European Association for the Study of the Liver. EASL Clinical Practice Guidelines: management of cholestatic liver diseases. *J Hepatol*. 2009;51(2):237–267.
41. Lindor KD, Gershwin ME, Poupon R, et al. Primary biliary cirrhosis (AASLD Practice Guidelines). *Hepatology*. 2009;50: 291–308.
42. Chan AW, Chan RC, Wong GL, et al. Evaluation of histological staging systems for primary biliary cirrhosis: correlation with clinical and biochemical factors and significance of pathological parameters in prognostication. *Histopathology*. 2014;65(2): 174–186.
43. Wendum D, Boëlle PY, Bedossa P, et al. Primary biliary cirrhosis: proposal for a new simple histological scoring system. *Liver Int*. 2015;35(2):652–659.
44. Lindor KD, Kowdley KV, Harrison ME. ACG clinical guideline: primary sclerosing cholangitis. *Am J Gastroenterol*. 2015;110: 646–659.
45. Chapman R, Fevery J, Kalloo A. Diagnosis and management of primary sclerosing cholangitis. *Hepatology*. 2010;51:660–678.
46. Boberg KM, Chapman RW, Hirschfield GM. Overlap syndromes: the International Autoimmune Hepatitis Group (IAIHG)

position statement on a controversial issue. *J Hepatol*. 2011;54: 374–385.
47. Washington MK. Autoimmune liver disease: overlap and outliers. *Mod Pathol*. 2007;20(suppl):S15–S30.
48. Sarcognato S. Sacchi D. Grillo F, et al. Autoimmune biliary diseases: primary biliary cholangitis and primary sclerosing cholangitis. *Pathologica*. 2021;113(3):170–184.

Vascular Pattern of Injury

49. Fan CQ, Crawford JM. Sinusoidal obstruction syndrome (hepatic veno-occlusive disease). *J Clin Exp Hepatol*. 2014;4(4):332–346.
50. Ibarrola C, Castellano VM, Colina F. Focal hyperplastic hepatocellular nodules in hepatic venous outflow obstruction: a clinicopathological study of four patients and 24 nodules. *Histopathology*. 2004;44:172–179.
51. Tanaka M, Wanless IR. Pathology of the liver in Budd-Chiari syndrome: portal vein thrombosis and the histogenesis of veno-centric cirrhosis, veno-portal cirrhosis, and large regenerative nodules. *Hepatology*. 1998;27:488–496.
52. Plessier A, Valla DC. Budd-Chiari syndrome. *Semin Liver Dis*. 2008;28:259–269.
53. Cazals-Hatem D, Vilgrain V, Genin P, et al. Arterial and portal circulation and parenchymal changes in Budd-Chiari syndrome: a study in 17 explanted livers. *Hepatology*. 2003;37:510–519.
54. Kakar S, Batts K, Poterucha JJ, et al. Histologic changes mimicking biliary disease in liver biopsies with venous outflow impairment. *Mod Pathol*. 2004;17(7):874–878.
55. Weisberg IS, Jacobson IM. Cardiovascular diseases and the liver. *Clin Liver Dis*. 2011;15(1):1–20.
56. Fiel MI, Schiano TD, Klion FM, et al. Recurring fibro-obliterative venopathy in liver allografts. *Am J Surg Pathol*. 1999;23:734–737.
57. DeLeve LD, Valla DC, Garcia-Tsao G, American Association for the Study Liver Diseases. Vascular disorders of the liver. *Hepatology*. 2009;49(5):1729–1764.
58. Hartleb M, Gutkowski K, Milkiewicz P. Nodular regenerative hyperplasia: evolving concepts on underdiagnosed cause of portal hypertension. *World J Gastroenterol*. 2011;17(11):1400–1409.
59. Ghabril M, Vuppalanchi R. Drug-induced nodular regenerative hyperplasia. *Semin Liver Dis*. 2014;34(2):240–245.
60. Verheij J, Schouten J, Komuta M, et al. Histological features in western patients with idiopathic non-cirrhotic portal hypertension. *Histopathology*. 2013;62:1083–1091.
61. Bioulac-Sage P, Le Bail B, Bernard PH, et al. Hepatoportal sclerosis. *Semin Liv Dis*. 1995;15(4):329–339.
62. Schouten JN, Garcia-Pagan JC, Valla DC, et al. Idiopathic noncirrhotic portal hypertension. *Hepatology*. 2011;54:1071–1081.
63. Okudaira M, Ohbu M, Okuda K. Idiopathic portal hypertension and its pathology. *Semin Liver Dis*. 2002;22:59–72.
64. Corpa MV, Bacchi MM, Bacchi CE, et al. Peliosis hepatis associated with lymphoplasmacytic lymphoma: an autopsy case report. *Arch Pathol Lab Med*. 2004;128:1283–1285.
65. Czapar CA, Weldon-Linne CM, Moore DM, et al. Peliosis hepatis in the acquired immunodeficiency syndrome. *Arch Pathol Lab Med*. 1986;110:611–613.
66. Alet PF, Moonka D. Peliosis hepatis: old disease, new cause. *Gastroenterology*. 1991;101(3):864–866.

Drug-Induced Liver Injury

67. Kleiner DE, Chalasani NP, Lee WM, et al. Hepatic histological findings in suspected drug-induced liver injury: systematic evaluation and clinical associations. *Hepatology*. 2014;59(2):661–670.
68. Fisher K, Vuppalanchi K, Saxena R. Drug induced liver injury. *Arch Pathol Lab Med*. 2015;139:876–887.
69. Ramachandran R, Kakar S. Histologic patterns in drug induced liver disease. *J Clin Pathol*. 2009;62:481–492.
70. Leiner DE. The pathology of drug-induced liver injury. *Semin Liver Dis*. 2009;29(4):364–372.
71. Bunchorntavakul C, Reddy KR. Drug hepatotoxicity. Newer agents. *Clin Liver Dis*. 2017;21:115–134.
72. Zheng EX, Navarro VJ. Liver injury from herbal, dietary, and weight loss supplements: a review. *J Clin Transl Hepatol*. 2015; 3:93–98.
73. Leise MD, Poterucha JJ, Talwalkar JA. Drug induced liver injury. *Mayo Clin Proc*. 2014;89(1):95–106.
74. Cohen JV, Dougan M, Zubiri L, et al. Liver biopsy findings in patients on immune checkpoint inhibitors. *Mod Pathol*. 2021;34:426–437.

Miscellaneous Patterns of Injury: Granulomas

75. Lamps L. Hepatic granulomas: a review with emphasis on infectious causes. *Arch Pathol Lab Med*. 2015;139:867–875.
76. Torbenson M. *Biopsy interpretation of the liver*. In: Epstein, ed: Wolters Kluwer; 2015:99–119.

Metabolic Diseases

Iron Metabolism

77. Pietrangelo A. Hemochromatosis: an endocrine liver disease. *Hepatology*. 2007;46(4):1291–1301.
78. Pietrangelo A, Caleffi A, Corradini E. Non-HFE hepatic iron overload. *Semin Liver Dis*. 2011;31(3):302–318.
79. Pietrangelo A. Genetics, genetic testing, and management of hemochromatosis: 15 years since hepcidin. *Gastroenterology*. 2015;149(5):1240–1251.

Copper Metabolism

80. Johncilla M, Mitchell K. Pathology of liver in copper overload. *Semin Liver Dis*. 2011;31(3):239–244.
81. El-Youssef M. Wilson disease. *Mayo Clin Proc*. 2003;78: 1126–1136.
82. Roberts EA, Schilsky ML. American Association for Study of Liver Diseases (AASLD). Diagnosis and treatment of Wilson disease: an update. *Hepatology*. 2008;47(6):2089–2111.
83. Stromeyer FW, Ishak K. Histology of the liver in Wilson's disease. *Am J Clin Pathol*. 1980;73(1):12–24.
84. Guindi M. Wilson disease. *Semin Diagn Pathol*. 2019;36(6):415–422.

α1 Antitrypsin

85. Fairbanks KD, Tavill AS. Liver disease in alpha 1-antitrypsin deficiency: a review. *Am J Gastroenterol*. 2008;103(8):2136–2141.
86. Talbot IC, Mowat AP. Liver disease in infancy. Histological features and relationship to alpha 1 antitrypsin phenotype. *J Clin Pathol*. 1975;28:559–563.
87. Schneider CV, Hamesch K.Gross A, et al. Liver Phenotypes of European Adults Heterozygous or Homozygous for Pi⊠Z Variant of AAT (Pi*MZ vs Pi*ZZ genotype) and Noncarriers. *Gastroenterology*. 2020;159(2):534–548. e11.

Glycogen and Lysosomal Storage Diseases

88. Ozen H. Glycogen storage diseases: new perspectives. *World J Gastroenterol*. 2007;13(18):2541–2553.
89. Wolsdorf JI, Holm IA, Weinstein DA. Glycogen storage disease: phenotypic, genetic, and biochemical characteristics, and therapy. *Endocrinol Metab Clin*. 1999;28(4):802–824.
90. Roy A, Finegold MJ. Biopsy diagnosis of inherited liver disease. *Surg Pathol Clin*. 2010;3:743–768.
91. Chen M, Wang J. Gaucher disease: review of the literature. *Arch Pathol Lab Med*. 2008;132(5):851–853.
92. Wang R, Bodamer O, Watson M, et al. Lysosomal storage diseases: diagnostic confirmation and management of presymptomatic individuals. *Genet Med*. 2011;13:457–484.

Glycogenic Hepatopathy

93. Torbenson M, Chen YY, Brunt E, et al. Glycogenic hepatopathy: an underrecognized hepatic complication of diabetes mellitus. *Am J Surg Pathol*. 2006;30(4):508–513.

Porphyrias

94. Foran SE, Abel G. Guide to porphyrias. A historical and clinical perspective. *Am J Clin Pathol*. 2003;119(supp l):S86–S93.
95. Chemmanur AT, Bonkovsky HL. Hepatic porphyrias: diagnosis and management. *Clin Liver Dis*. 2004;8(4):807–838.
96. Puy H, Gouya L, Deybach JC. Porphyrias. *Lancet*. 2010;375(9718) :924–937.
97. Arim Z, Lyoumi S, Nicolas G, et al. Porphyrias: a 2015 update. *Clin Res Hepatol Gastroenterol*. 2015;39(4):412–425.

18

Liver Neoplasms

■ **Safia N. Salaria, MD, Amitabh Srivastava, MD, and Daniela S. Allende, MD, MBA**

Primary hepatocellular neoplasms are much less common than metastatic tumors to the liver. The former may arise from either the epithelial or mesenchymal component of the hepatic parenchyma and rarely may also show both lines of differentiation. Hepatocellular neoplasms may be benign or malignant (Table 18.1). The differential diagnosis of a well-differentiated hepatocellular proliferation is typically between focal nodular hyperplasia (FNH), hepatic adenoma (HA), and a well-differentiated hepatocellular carcinoma (HCC). These can usually be distinguished based on morphologic features and a small panel of ancillary stains. HAs are now known to be composed of distinct subsets of tumors with well-characterized genetic alterations that must be subclassified accurately because of varying risks of malignant transformation in these distinct categories. Rarely, the distinction between benign and malignant hepatocellular neoplasms may be challenging, particularly in a biopsy specimen, and the terms *atypical hepatic adenoma* and *well-differentiated hepatocellular neoplasm of uncertain malignant potential* have been used in such cases. Poorly differentiated tumors pose a greater challenge because they may represent a HCC or intrahepatic cholangiocarcinoma (CC) or a metastatic carcinoma, sarcoma, or malignant melanoma. Distinguishing primary versus metastatic tumor in this scenario often requires a larger panel of ancillary stains, and often correlation with imaging findings may be the only way to render a definite diagnosis.

EPITHELIAL TUMORS HEPATOCELLULAR TUMORS FOCAL NODULAR HYPERPLASIA

Focal nodular hyperplasia is a localized disorganized non-neoplastic proliferation of hepatocytes that is believed to be centered around a vascular anomaly, usually an arterial malformation, and may coexist with hepatic cavernous hemangiomas (CHs) in about 20% of cases. Current theories propose outflow obstruction and hepatic congestion as etiologic factors. It accounts for approximately 10% of hepatocellular mass lesions with an overall prevalence of 0.9%. The majority (80%) of cases are solitary, but patients with multiple FNHs who also have one or more concurrent hepatic hemangioma, berry aneurysms, and brain tumors (astrocytoma and meningioma) have also been described and are considered to have the multiple FNH syndrome.

■ CLINICAL FEATURES

Focal nodular hyperplasia is found mainly in women of reproductive age (80%–95%), but these tumors are not hormone dependent and unaffected by oral contraceptive use and pregnancy. Up to 15% of cases occur in children and may be associated with glycogen storage disease type Ia. FNH is usually an incidental finding and nonspecific abdominal pain is the most common complaint in symptomatic patients. FNH may increase in size over time. The background liver and the serum α-fetoprotein (AFP) level is normal in almost all cases. Some lesions may occur in association with portal vein thrombosis, Budd-Chiari syndrome, or hereditary hemorrhagic telangiectasia. The pathogenesis is thought be outflow tract obstruction that leads to collapse, fibrosis, and nodular regeneration. Expression of angiopoietin 1 and 2 is altered compared with normal liver with an increase in *ANGPT1*-to-*ANGPT2* ratio.

FOCAL NODULAR HYPERPLASIA—FACT SHEET

Definition

- Non-neoplastic mass lesion caused by nodular overgrowth of hepatocytes in region of altered hepatic blood flow

Incidence and Location

- Up to 0.9%
- 2% of hepatic tumors in children
- No geographic predilection

Morbidity and Mortality

- Low morbidity
- Rupture is rare
- No increase in mortality

Gender, Race, and Age Distribution
- More common in women than men (male-to-female ratio, 9 to 1)
- Occurs in all age groups
- No race predilection

Clinical Features
- Usually incidental finding
- Rarely associated with abdominal pain, hepatomegaly, or tenderness
- Associated with extrahepatic vascular lesions

Radiologic Features
- Central scar by ultrasonography, computed tomography (CT), or magnetic resonance imaging
- Doppler imaging may detect feeding artery
- Hypodense lesion on CT with enhancement during arterial phase

Prognosis and Therapy
- Prognosis is excellent
- Observation is adequate for asymptomatic lesions
- Surgical resection for symptomatic or enlarging lesions or lesions that cannot be diagnosed with certainty on imaging

TABLE 18.1
Hepatic Mass Lesions

Epithelial Mass Lesions	Nonepithelial Mass Lesions
BENIGN	Benign
Hepatocellular	Hemangioma
Focal fatty change	Angiomyolipoma
Focal nodular hyperplasia	Infantile hemangioendothelioma
Hepatic adenoma	Mesenchymal hamartoma
Macroregenerative nodule	Inflammatory "pseudotumor"
Dysplastic nodules	
• Low grade	
• High grade	
Biliary	
Biliary cyst	
Bile duct adenoma	
Bile duct hamartoma	
flat precursor (biliary intraepithelial neoplasia)	
Mucinous cystic neoplasm	
Intraductal papillary neoplasm of the bile duct	
MALIGNANT	Malignant
Hepatocellular Carcinoma	Epithelioid hemangioendothelioma
Hepatoblastoma	Angiosarcoma
Intrahepatic	Undifferentiated (embryonal) sarcoma
Intrahepatic Cholangiocarcinoma	Lymphoma
• Mucinous cystic neoplasm with associated invasive carcinoma	
• Intraductal papillary neoplasm with associated carcinoma	
• Metastasis	Other rare sarcomas

Radiologic Features

Typical features of FNH on computed tomography (CT) or magnetic resonance imaging (MRI) include a central scar, and angiography or Doppler ultrasonography can show a centrifugal hypervascularity with numerous enlarged peripheral vessels imparting a "wheel-spoke" appearance. A technetium-99 sulfur colloid scan shows normal or increased uptake. Imaging studies are about 70% sensitive for a preoperative diagnosis of FNH, and false-positive results are rare.

Pathologic Features

Gross Findings

Focal nodular hyperplasia is usually a subcapsular, well-circumscribed, bulging, tan, nodular mass. Size can vary widely, but most lesions measure less than 5 cm in diameter. The most characteristic finding is the presence of a central stellate scar with radiating fibrous septa that subdivide the mass into multiple smaller nodules (Fig. 18.1). The central scar may be inconspicuous in smaller lesions. Hemorrhage, necrosis, and bile staining are rare. The background liver is normal in most cases.

Microscopic Findings

Focal nodular hyperplasia is composed of nodules of hepatocytes surrounded by fibrous septa that contain thick hepatic artery branches along with a variable degree of bile ductular proliferation. Interlobular bile ducts and portal vein branches are markedly decreased or absent. The central scar is composed of dense collagen (Fig. 18.2A) and contains numerous thick-walled dystrophic arteries and bile ductules (Fig. 18.2B). The histologic features of the lesion overall resemble biliary type of cirrhosis with marked ductular proliferation, but the background liver is completely normal. The hepatocytes in FNH lesions are similar to those in the surrounding liver, although they may be somewhat larger and paler and may incorporate variable quantities of fat

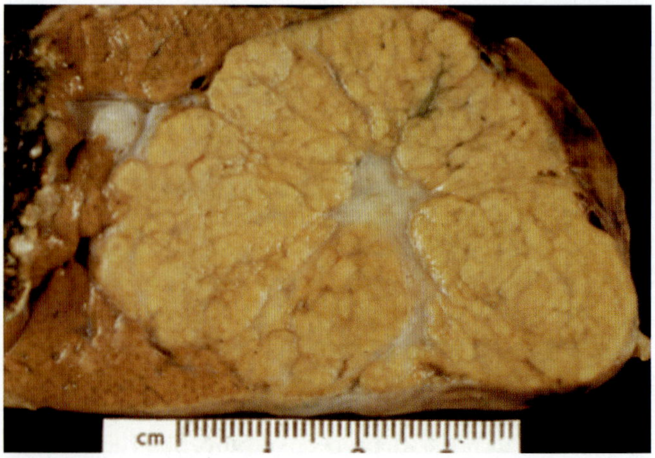

FIGURE 18.1
Focal nodular hyperplasia is a sharply circumscribed mass in a background of normal liver and shows a multinodular cut surface with a characteristic central scar.

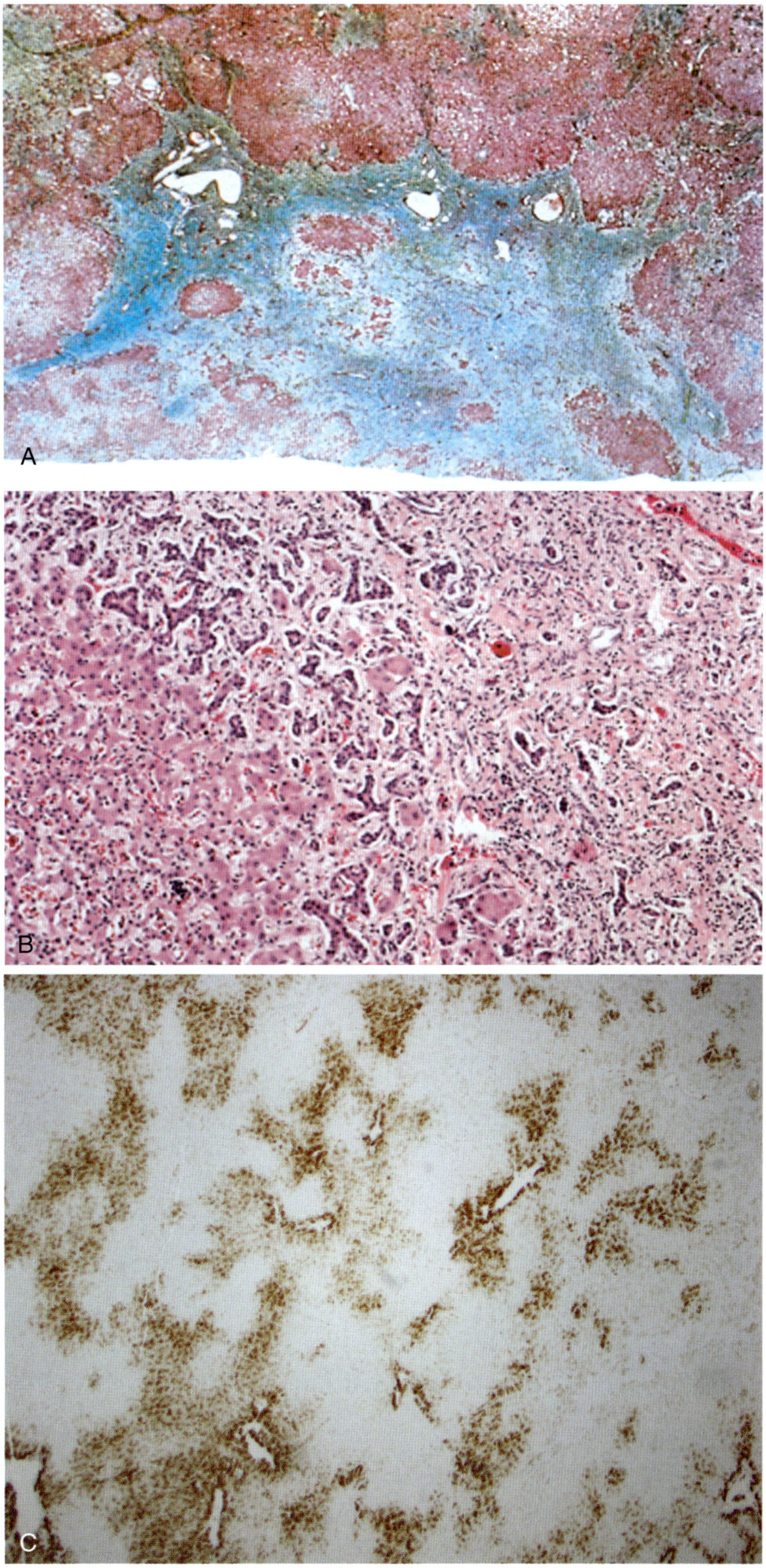

FIGURE 18.2

The central stellate scar is composed of dense hyalinized collagen and thick arteries (**A**), and a variable degree of bile ductular proliferation is typically present at the interface of the scar and hepatic parenchyma (**B**). A map-like staining pattern on glutamine synthetase immunostain (**C**) is diagnostic of focal nodular hyperplasia but may be challenging to interpret in a small biopsy specimen.

or glycogen. Nuclear pleomorphism, prominent nucleoli, and mitotic figures are not found in FNH. Mild chronic inflammation may be present within the lesion. The variant formerly referred to as "telangiectatic FNH" has been shown to be a form of HA by molecular analysis. Other variations on the typical appearance described earlier include prominent steatosis, steatohepatitis, and even large cell change.

Focal Nodular Hyperplasia—Pathologic Features

Gross Findings

- Single subcapsular lesion
- Variable size; average size is smaller than 5 cm
- Central stellate scar with radiating septa

Microscopic Findings

- Nodular overgrowth of normal-appearing hepatocytes
- Large-caliber vessels in central stellate scar
- Bile ductular proliferation in scar
- Appears like "localized cirrhosis"

Genetics

- Polyclonal proliferation
- Increased angiopoietin (1:2 ratio)
- β-Catenin pathway activated without mutations in *CTNNB1* or *AXIN1*

Differential Diagnosis

- Cirrhosis
- Hepatic adenoma

Ancillary Studies

Immunohistochemistry

A characteristic "map-like" staining pattern is seen in these lesions on a glutamine synthetase (GS) immunostain as a result of activation of the β-catenin pathway (Fig. 18.2C) and can be very helpful in establishing the diagnosis in lesions without the characteristic central scar. The positive areas of staining are markedly expanded anastomosing zones around hepatic veins, but this may not be easily identified in small biopsy samples.

Differential Diagnosis

Focal nodular hyperplasia may be confused on biopsy with cirrhosis; with HA, especially the telangiectatic variant; and less likely with well-differentiated HCC. The localized nature of the lesion and its origin in normal liver excludes cirrhosis. The presence of bile ductular proliferation, a central scar, and nodular architecture distinguishes FNH from all subtypes of HA with the exception of inflammatory HA, which still represents a difficult differential diagnosis because of the significant histologic overlap. Sinusoidal dilation, steatosis, and isolated arteries favor a diagnosis of inflammatory HA. Whereas FNH shows a map-like pattern of staining on GS, inflammatory HA can be negative, patchy positive, or diffusely positive if β-catenin mutations occurred. Inflammatory HAs are also diffusely positive for serum amyloid A (SAA) or C-reactive protein (CRP). Well-differentiated HCC are typically not a challenge in this differential because they show more pronounced cellular atypia, thickened hepatic cords with loss of reticulin, and positivity for glypican-3 in a subset of cases.

Prognosis and Therapy

The majority of FNH is stable, nonprogressive lesions that do not undergo malignant transformation and can therefore be followed safely by imaging without the need for surgical resection. Unlike HAs, FNHs rarely rupture or cause intraperitoneal bleeding. Surgical management is reserved for enlarging tumors, those that cause symptoms, or cases in which the diagnosis cannot be established with certainty on imaging findings alone.

HEPATIC ADENOMA

CLINICAL FEATURES

Hepatic adenoma is a benign hepatocellular neoplasm arising in normal livers. The overwhelming majority of cases (90%) develop in women in their childbearing years, and long-term oral contraceptive steroid (OCS) use is a common risk factor. In men, use of anabolic or androgenic steroids is a risk factor for HA. HAs are rarely found in children and are usually associated with metabolic disorders such as glycogen storage disease (especially types I and III), diabetes mellitus, and Hurler's disease. Obesity and metabolic syndrome are also risk factors for the development of HAs.

A majority of HAs are found incidentally and are asymptomatic; however, patients with larger tumors can present with a palpable mass or with acute abdominal pain secondary to hemorrhage within the tumor. Intraperitoneal rupture produces hemoperitoneum and may lead to shock. Serum AFP levels are normal. The lesions are usually solitary but may be multiple, and when more than 10, the condition is described as *hepatic adenomatosis*. There are distinctive subtypes of HA

(*HNF1A*-inactivated, inflammatory, β-catenin activated, GLI family zinc finger 1 [*GLI-1*] rearranged, unclassified). The overall risk of malignant transformation is 4% to 8% and linked to high-risk features such as male gender, androgen use, and β-catenin mutations. Risk of bleeding has been recently described as associated with HA with *GLI-1* rearrangements.

HEPATIC ADENOMA–FACT SHEET

Definition

- Benign hepatocellular neoplasm with low risk of malignant transformation

Incidence and Location

- 3.4 per 100,000 in long-term users of oral contraceptives (OCPs)
- Approximately 1.3 per million in women who have never used OCPs
- Higher incidence in Western countries than in Asia

Morbidity and Mortality

- Hemorrhage in approximately 25% of patients; usually in tumors larger than 5 cm
- Mortality rate of 6% to 20% in patients with hemorrhage

Gender, Race, and Age Distribution

- More common in young to middle-aged women (average age, 30 years)
- Rare in men; increased in those with anabolic steroid use
- In children, seen mainly in setting of glycogen storage disease types I and III, in whom they occur before age 20 years (male-to-female ratio, 2 to 1)
- No race predilection

Clinical Features

- More than 90% of patients have history of oral contraceptive use for more than 5 years
- Most common complaint is right upper quadrant abdominal pain
- Occasionally seen in patients taking anabolic steroids

Radiologic Features

- Vascular lesion on computed tomography, with irregular enhancement
- Magnetic resonance imaging shows well-defined mass, low signal to slightly hyperintense on T1-weighted images

Prognosis and Therapy

- Surgical resection (if >5 cm or high-risk factors)
- Withdrawal of estrogens to reduce tumor size
- Liver transplantation is considered for adenomatosis
- Malignant transformation to hepatocellular carcinoma is uncommon (4%–8%)

RADIOLOGIC FEATURES

Hepatic adenoma is visualized as a vascular lesion on CT scan, with irregular enhancement. MRI shows a well-defined mass with low to slightly hyperintense signal on T1-weighted images.

PATHOLOGIC FEATURES

GROSS FINDINGS

Hepatic adenoma is a well-circumscribed, often subcapsular mass in the right lobe of an otherwise noncirrhotic liver. Ruptured HAs may be obscured by blood clot and difficult to recognize, but the tumor is usually pale or more yellow compared with the adjacent liver (Fig. 18.3). Fibrous septa may be present as a result of a previous infarct.

MICROSCOPIC FINDINGS

On first glance, most HAs represent a nodular proliferation of bland-appearing hepatocytes arranged in cords that are one to two cells thick and separated by sinusoids lined by inconspicuous Kupffer cells. However, no normal portal tracts are present, and there is a notable lack of any biliary epithelium. Another key feature of HA is the presence of haphazardly distributed arteries and thin-walled veins (Fig. 18.4). Hepatocellular rosettes (pseudoglands) are rare in HA and should not be confused with bile ducts. Extensive pseudoglandular proliferation raises concern for a diagnosis of well-differentiated HCC.

The hepatocytes of HA frequently display clear or vacuolated cytoplasm because of accumulation of glycogen or fat. Cytoplasmic inclusions representing α1-antitrypsin (α1AT), megamitochondria, and Mallory's hyaline are occasionally found. Focal cellular pleomorphism and prominent nucleoli may be seen, especially in tumors associated with androgenic steroid use. Mitoses, vascular invasion, and stromal invasion are not seen in HA and are suggestive of malignancy. Various degenerative changes occur in HA and include dilated sinusoids and larger blood-filled (peliosis-like) spaces, myxoid stroma, and areas of necrosis, infarct, and hematoma.

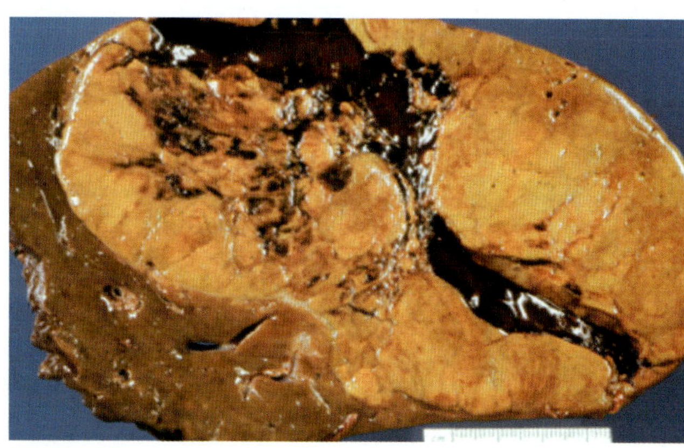

FIGURE 18.3

Hepatic adenomas are sharply circumscribed lesions of variable size that also occur in a background of normal liver. Intralesional hemorrhage is common, as in this example, in adenomas that activate sonic hedgehog signaling because of fusion of inhibin subunit beta E (INHBE) promoter with GLI family zinc finger 1 (Gli-1).

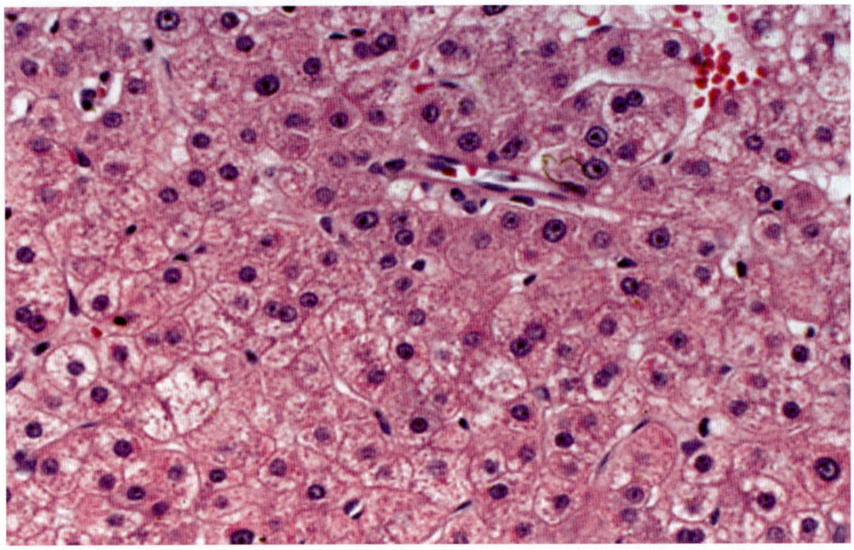

FIGURE 18.4

Hepatic adenomas show isolated arteries, and with the exception of the inflammatory variant, these tumors lack portal tracts and bile ductules. The hepatocytes are monomorphic with cords of normal thickness, preserved reticulin, and minimal atypia. Nuclear abnormalities are more common in the β-catenin–mutated adenomas.

TABLE 18.2

Classification of Hepatic Adenomas

Hepatic Adenoma Type	HNF1α (30%)	β-Catenin Mutated (20%–25%)	Inflammatory (35%–40%)	Sonic Hedgehog (<5%)	Unclassified
Clinical features	Females	Males	Females and males, alcohol, obesity	Significant risk of intralesional hemorrhage	None
Pathologic features	Steatosis, ≥ 10 adenomas (adenomatosis)	Cytologic atypia, pseudogland formation	Inflammatory infiltrate in portal tract–like structures; dilated sinusoids; bile ductular component	Bleeding even in small lesions	No distinctive associations
Genetics	*HNF1A, MODY3, CYP1B1* mutations	*CTNNB1* mutations	*IL6* signal transducer, *FRK, STAT3, GNAS, JAK1* mutations	*INHBE-Gli-1* fusion	None
Progression to HCC	Rare	Increased	Rare; almost always in β-catenin–mutated subset	None	None
Diagnostic IHC findings	Loss of LFABP	Aberrant nuclear β-catenin	Positive SAA and/or CRP	Positive PTGDS or ASS1	None

ASS1, Argininosuccinate synthase 1; *CRP*, C-reactive protein; *HCC*, hepatocellular carcinoma; *LFABP*, liver fatty acid binding protein; *PTGDS*, prostaglandin D2 synthase; *SAA*, serum amyloid A.
Includes inflammatory hepatic adenoma (HA) c̄ β-catenin mutation.

The current World Health Organization (WHO) classification of HAs is based on genotype-phenotype correlation. Based on presence of HNF1α or β-catenin mutation and expression of SAA or CRP in tumors that show a conspicuous inflammatory infiltrate, HAs can be subclassified into four categories: (1) HAs with mutations of the *HNF1α* gene; (2) HAs with β-catenin gene mutation; (3) inflammatory HA positive for serum amyloid A (SAA) or CRP; (4) sonic hedgehog HA harboring somatic deletions of inhibin subunit beta E (*INHBE*) leading to *INHBE* and *GLI-1* fusions; and (5) unclassified HA, tumors that do not fit any of these categories (Table 18.2). *HNF1α*-inactivated tumors are the second most common (30%–35% of HAs) and show prominent steatosis without cellular atypia or inflammation (Figs. 18.5A and B). β-catenin–activated HA (10%–15%) is more common in male patients and tend to show cytologic and architectural atypia, overlapping features between HA and HCC. Inflammatory HAs are the most frequent (35%–40%) and show pseudoportal tracts, bile ductular proliferation, inflammatory infiltrates, and prominent sinusoidal dilation (telangiectatic areas) (Figs. 18.5 C and D). Lesions previously classified as "telangiectatic FNHs" are now classified as inflammatory HA based on clonality studies and expression of SAA and CRP. A new subtype has been described recently that shows activation of the sonic

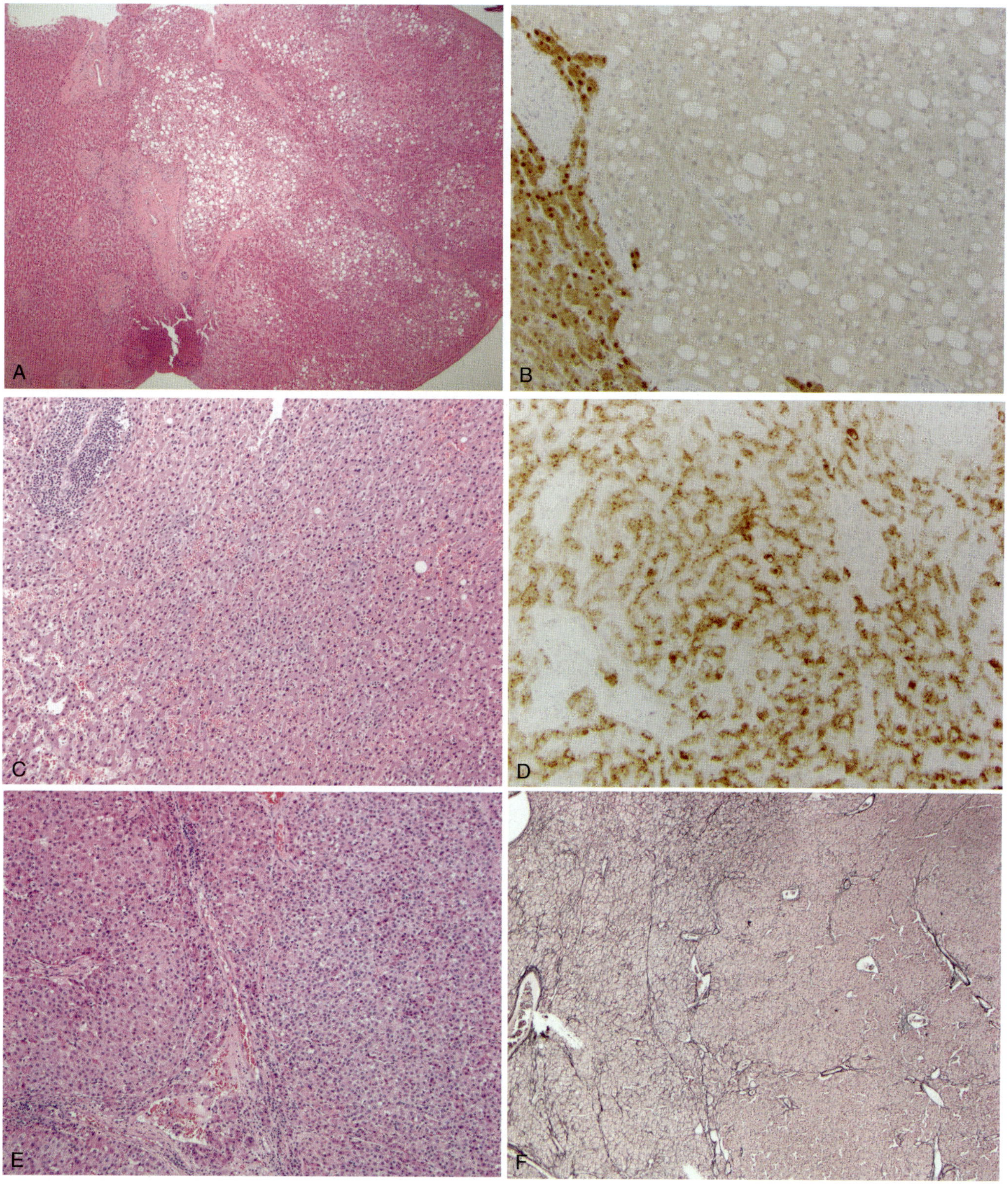

FIGURE 18.5

HNF1A-mutated adenomas (HAs) show prominent steatosis in the majority of cases (**A**). Loss of staining for liver fatty acid binding protein on immunohistochemistry is diagnostic (**B**). Portal tract–like structures with lymphoid aggregates and dilated (telangiectatic) sinusoids are characteristic of inflammatory HAs (**C**) that stain positively with serum amyloid A (**D**) or C-reactive protein. Malignant transformation to carcinoma occurs rarely in HAs and manifests as increased cell density (**E**), cellular atypia, and loss of reticulin (**F**) in the malignant foci.

hedgehog pathway caused by *INHBE* deletion and consequent *INHBE-GLI-1* fusion. This subtype confers an increased high risk of hemorrhage, even in small tumors.

The term *adenomatosis* is sometimes used for cases with multiple (>10) adenomas. Because the etiologic associations appear to be similar for multiple and solitary adenomas, distinction between these two groups is probably not warranted on clinicopathologic grounds. HNF1A and inflammatory HA are the most common subtypes that may present with adenomatosis. It is also important to remember that different HA subtypes may occur in the same liver.

Hepatic Adenoma—Pathologic Features

Gross Findings

- Yellow, tan, or red-brown solitary nodule in noncirrhotic liver
- Most measure 5 to 15 cm
- May be hemorrhagic or multiple (>10 is labeled adenomatosis)

Microscopic Findings

- Benign hepatocytes without acinar architecture or portal tracts
- Thin-walled vascular channels and isolated arteries scattered throughout tumor
- Tumor cells may show prominent steatosis (usually in the *HNF1α*-inactivated subtype); loss of liver fatty acid–binding protein is diagnostic
- Bile ductular reaction is not present within the lesion (except in inflammatory hepatic adenoma [HA])
- Prominent sinusoidal dilation (telangiectasia) and lymphoid infiltrates in portal tract–like structures are seen in inflammatory HA; serum amyloid A and C-reactive protein positive
- Nuclear atypia may be prominent in β-catenin–activated HA; nuclear β-catenin and/or diffuse glutamine synthetase positivity
- Intralesional hemorrhage in sonic hedgehog subtype of HA

Differential Diagnosis

- Focal nodular hyperplasia
- Well-differentiated hepatocellular carcinoma

Ancillary Studies

The most useful immunohistochemical stain in the differential diagnosis from FNH is GS, map-like pattern of staining is diagnostic of FNH but can be challenging to determine in small biopsy samples. A panel of immunostains has been proposed to further classify HAs including β-catenin, liver fatty acid–binding protein (LFABP), SAA, or CRP. Loss of LFABP is diagnostic of HNF1α-mutated HA, positivity for SAA or CRP supports the diagnosis of inflammatory HA, and nuclear β-catenin expression is indicative of a β-catenin–activated HA. Diffuse homogenous GS positivity is considered a surrogate for β-catenin mutations, leading to strong activation of this pathway such as exon 3 mutations. Diffuse heterogenous GS expression is observed in other β-catenin mutations (exon 3 S45). Some authors have reported overexpression of ASS1 in sonic hedgehog HAs, but this finding remains under investigation.

Differential Diagnosis

Focal nodular hyperplasia shows a central scar, prominent bile ductular proliferation at the interface of hepatocellular nodules and stroma and a map-like staining pattern on GS. HA is characterized by isolated arteries, lack of normal portal tracts, absence of bile duct proliferation (with the exception of the inflammatory subtype), and hepatic cord architecture that is uniformly one to two cells thick. Diffuse presence of pseudoglandular architecture should raise suspicion for well-differentiated HCC. A diagnosis of HCC is based on classic radiologic features, thickened hepatic cords with loss of reticulin staining, prominent nuclear, and architectural atypia (Figs. 18.5E and F) and in some cases, positivity for glypican-3 or heat shock protein 70. Foci worrisome for HCC in an otherwise typical HA can sometimes be seen. In small biopsy samples, these lesions are classified as either hepatocellular neoplasm with uncertain malignant potential or as atypical hepatocellular neoplasm. In resection specimens, these tumors can be classified as HA as long as the atypical foci constitute less than 5% of the tumor and do not fulfill the criteria for HCC.

Prognosis and Therapy

Rupture with subsequent massive bleeding into the peritoneal cavity is the most common cause of death related to HA. Because of this risk, HAs increasing in size on surveillance are often resected. In many institutions, patients with lesions larger than 5 cm are treated surgically. This management algorithm is likely to change with the recognition of the specific sonic hedgehog subtype of HA associated with hemorrhage. Liver transplantation is occasionally performed for very large lesions or adenomatosis. There is a low risk for transformation to HCC and is typically seen in the β-catenin activated HAs.

MACROREGENERATIVE AND DYSPLASTIC NODULES

Numerous terms have been applied to grossly distinct large hepatocellular nodules arising in the setting of cirrhosis. Macroregenerative nodules (MRNs) are larger than surrounding nodules but do not display any atypical features. Dysplastic nodules (DNs) exhibit atypical architectural or cytologic features but do not meet histologic criteria for HCC.

MACROREGENERATIVE NODULES AND DYSPLASTIC NODULES—FACT SHEET

Definition

- Macroregenerative nodule (MRN): large dominant nodule in cirrhotic liver
- Dysplastic nodule (DN): putative precursor lesion to hepatocellular carcinoma; does not meet definite histologic criteria of malignancy

Incidence and Location

- Reflect the etiology of the underlying cirrhosis

Morbidity and Mortality

- Related to the risk for development of hepatocellular carcinoma

Gender, Race, and Age Distribution

- Similar to etiology of underlying cirrhosis

Clinical Features

- Arise in setting of cirrhosis
- Usually seen in explant specimens

Radiologic Features

- Indistinguishable from cirrhotic nodules
- Do not fulfill radiologic criteria for hepatocellular carcinoma (HCC)

Prognosis and Therapy

- Excision for DNs, when possible, facilitates definite pathologic classification, but more commonly, these lesions are ablated, given the risk of surgical intervention in cirrhotic patients

Prognosis depends on status of underlying cirrhosis

- High risk for development of HCC

Pathologic Features

Gross Findings

Macroregenerative nodules and DNs are usually similar to other cirrhotic nodules, although they may be paler, slightly larger in size, or more bile stained. A thick fibrous capsule or a variegated cut surface is more suggestive of a small HCC. MRNs are larger than other cirrhotic nodules and are larger than 1 cm and may measure up to 5 cm or more in diameter (Fig. 18.6). High-grade DNs resemble MRNs grossly but may appear less well circumscribed.

Microscopic Findings

Most of the MRNs in cirrhosis are multiple and contain portal tracts scattered throughout the nodule. The hepatocytes within these nodules are identical to those in the surrounding liver. The hepatocellular plates are one or two cells thick. Prominent bile ductular reaction may be seen in the adjacent fibrous tissue. The reticulin framework is intact and similar to a typical cirrhotic nodule.

Dysplastic nodules are regarded as precursors to HCC. They demonstrate increased nuclear density (twice that of normal) and are graded as low or high grade. Portal tracts are preserved in low- and high-grade DNs, and the hepatocytes show a monomorphic appearance with increased cell density or cytologic atypia (Fig. 18.7). Cytologic and architectural abnormalities are minimal in low-grade DNs. There is often slight increase in nuclear density (<1.3 times compared with the adjacent parenchyma), large cell change (nuclear enlargement but preserved N/C ratio, pleomorphism, hyperchromasia) and possibly multinucleation. In contrast, high-grade DNs show small cell change characterized by smaller size and a greater nuclear-to-cytoplasmic ratio than the surrounding hepatocytes (approximately two times), nuclear hyperchromasia, cytoplasmic basophilia, and mild nuclear pleomorphism. Architectural and cytologic atypia, including pseudoglandular formations, are common in high-grade DNs, but reticulin architecture is well preserved in both low- and high-grade DNs. Loss of iron deposition when compared with the background cirrhotic liver is a useful feature of high-grade dysplasia arising in a DN. It is common to see an HCC in close proximity to a high-grade DN. The progression from MRN to DN and ultimately HCC is noted by decreased ductular reaction as demonstrated by loss of cytokeratin (CK) 19 immunohistochemical labeling, but this is not necessary for the diagnosis.

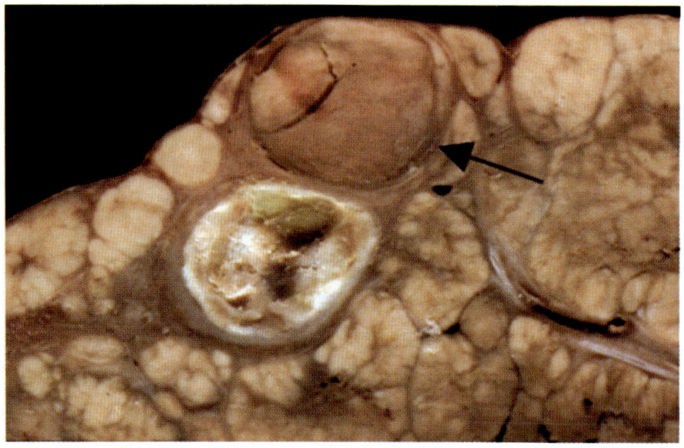

FIGURE 18.6

The macroregenerative nodule in this cirrhotic liver *(arrow)* is distinguishable from the background cirrhosis by its larger size. The variegated nodule of similar size in the same specimen is a small hepatocellular carcinoma.

Prognosis and Therapy

Dysplastic nodules are considered an important precursor to HCC. Ablation or resection of the lesion is recommended because of the potential to develop into HCC. MRNs cannot always be reliably distinguished from low-grade DNs on imaging grounds, and patients with apparent MRNs on imaging studies are kept under surveillance by periodic imaging. Between 10% and 30% of high-grade DNs are reported to progress to HCC within 3 years, but a substantial proportion do not progress and can even

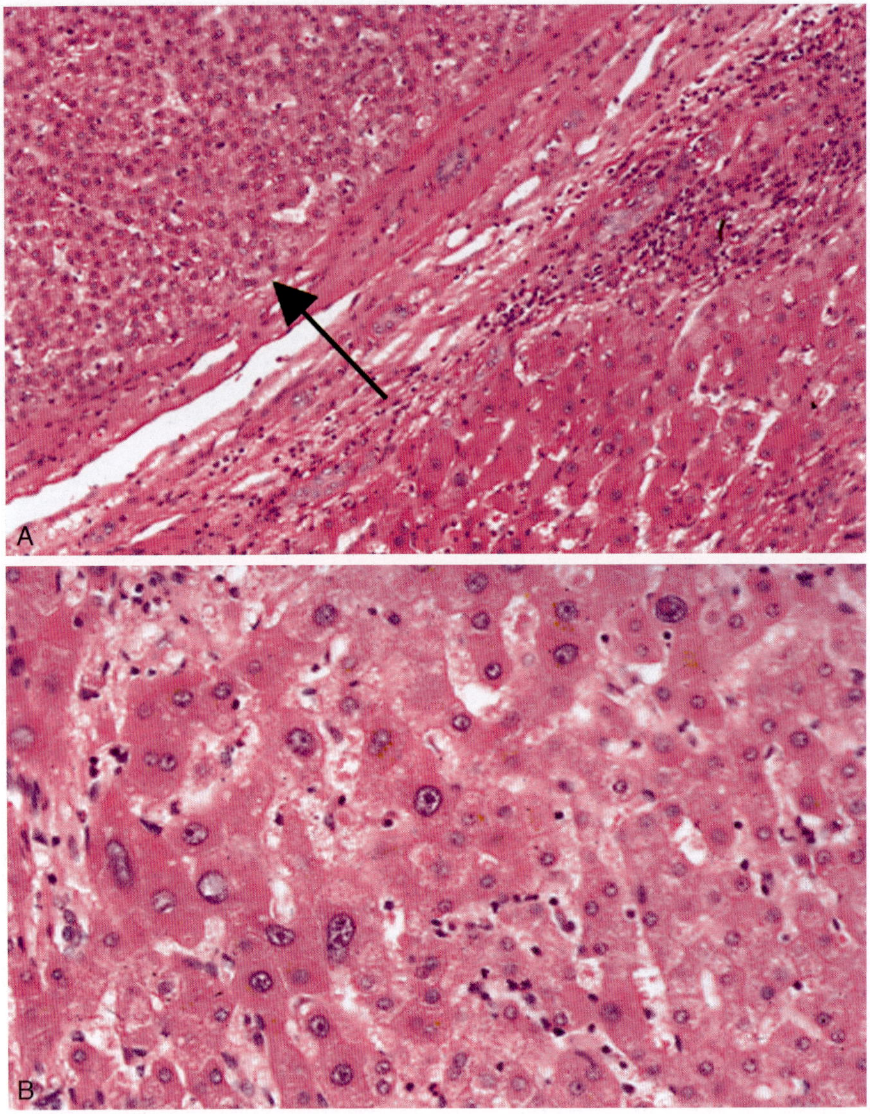

FIGURE 18.7

Dysplastic nodules (DNs) retain portal tracts and may exhibit small cell change *(arrow)* that is recognized by the presence of densely packed hepatocytes smaller than those of the surrounding liver (**A**). Large cell change shows enlarged hepatocytes with atypical, irregular nuclei and large nucleoli (**B**). Abnormal architectural features of hepatocellular carcinoma are not seen in DNs.

Macroregenerative Nodules and Dysplastic Nodules—Pathologic Features

Gross Findings

- Macroregenerative nodule (MRNs) are larger than other nodules in cirrhotic liver; there is no difference in color or texture
- Dysplastic nodules (DNs) may be of any size; may be paler than other cirrhotic nodules and bile stained

Microscopic Findings

- MRNs are similar to other nodules in the cirrhotic liver
- Low-grade DNs show minimal nuclear atypia and only slight architectural abnormalities; large cell change may be seen; portal tracts could be present within nodule
- High-grade DNs can show small cell change and focal pseudoglandular formation
- Trabeculae are two cells thick, and reticulin framework is preserved in dysplastic nodules
- Increased mitotic activity may be seen in high-grade DNs, but it is more commonly associated with the diagnosis of hepatocellular carcinoma (HCC)

Genetics

- MRNs are polyclonal
- Low- and high-grade DNs may be monoclonal or polyclonal, but high-grade DNs tend to have a molecular profile more reminiscent of HCC

Differential Diagnosis

- Hepatocellular adenoma
- HCC

regress spontaneously. Imaging surveillance and biopsy are key to guiding management in these patients.

Differential Diagnosis

Separation of low-grade DNs from MRNs, as well as high-grade DNs from HCC, may be difficult on hematoxylin and eosin (H&E) examination alone. Features more often seen in HCC are diffuse architectural atypia (more than three cell thick cords, pseudoglandular formation, reticulin loss), marked cellular atypia with increased mitoses, and increased number of unpaired arteries or vascular invasion, which is helpful but rarely seen in early lesions.

HEPATOCELLULAR CARCINOMA

CLINICAL FEATURES

Hepatocellular carcinoma is the most common type of primary epithelial tumor in the liver. Although relatively uncommon in Western countries, HCC is one of the most prevalent malignant tumors worldwide, responsible for 20% to 40% of cancer deaths in regions of high incidence, such as sub-Saharan Africa and Southeast Asia. In low-incidence areas, HCC is a tumor of older men. In areas of higher incidence, HCC occurs in the third or fourth decade of life because of the high prevalence of perinatally acquired hepatitis B.

Virtually any chronic liver disease may predispose toward HCC. The most common predisposing condition is cirrhosis from any cause, with hepatitis B, hepatitis C, and alcoholic liver disease being the most common causes. Obesity-related liver disease is increasingly recognized as a risk factor for HCC, and genetic hemochromatosis carries a particularly high risk. The annual risk for HCC developing in a cirrhotic liver is estimated at 1% to 6%.

Patients may present with abdominal pain or fullness, a mass, or clinical signs and symptoms of cirrhosis. HCC rarely presents with metastases. The most useful serum marker is elevation of AFP, which may be highly elevated in patients with large tumors. Of note, serum AFP levels may also be elevated viral hepatitis and cirrhosis. High AFP levels are also seen in hepatoid variants of gastric adenocarcinomas and germ cell tumors containing a yolk sac component.

HEPATOCELLULAR CARCINOMA—FACT SHEET

Definition

- Malignant neoplasm of hepatocytes

Incidence and Location

- Most common primary liver malignancy in adults
- In United States, incidence is 4 per 100,000
- Wide geographic variation in incidence, with high incidence in Southeast Asia and sub-Saharan Africa and low incidence in Western countries

Morbidity and Mortality

- High mortality rate; 5-year survival rate is less than 5%
- Median survival for resectable tumors is up to 45 months; for unresectable tumors, less than 6 months
- Patients with cirrhosis are at risk for development of new tumors

Gender, Race, and Age Distribution

- Male predominance (male-to-female ratio, 2:1 to 5:1)
- Predilection for Asian and African population probably because of chronic viral hepatitis and aflatoxin exposure
- Incidence increases with age in Western countries (peak incidence, seventh decade), but mean age in South Africa is 35 years

Clinical Features

- Associated with chronic hepatitis C and hepatitis B infections and exposure to aflatoxins
- Commonly arises with a background of cirrhosis; obesity is increasingly associated with hepatocellular carcinoma
- Presentation is variable, ranging from decompensated liver disease to malaise, weight loss, and hepatomegaly
- Serum α-fetoprotein is elevated in approximately 50% of cases

Radiologic Features

- Computed tomography or magnetic resonance imaging used for noninvasive diagnosis: based on arterial phase hyperenhancement and portal venous or delayed phase washout
- Ultrasonography used for surveillance in patients with cirrhosis

Prognosis and Therapy

- Prognosis is heavily dependent on status of liver disease
- Treatment is surgical excision when feasible
- Liver transplantation may be indicated when tumors are small and low stage in the setting of cirrhosis
- Palliative treatments include ethanol injection, cryoablation, and chemoembolization
- Chemotherapy has limited benefit

Radiologic Features

Advanced HCC is generally easily detected by ultrasonography, CT, or MRI. HCC on CT is usually low attenuation and may have daughter nodules. Ultrasonography is useful in screening for HCC in cirrhotic livers; a mosaic pattern with peripheral sonolucent region is typical.

Pathologic Features

Gross Findings

Hepatocellular carcinoma arising in a noncirrhotic liver usually grows as a single large mass with or without satellite nodules (Fig. 18.8A) and may also exhibit this pattern in the

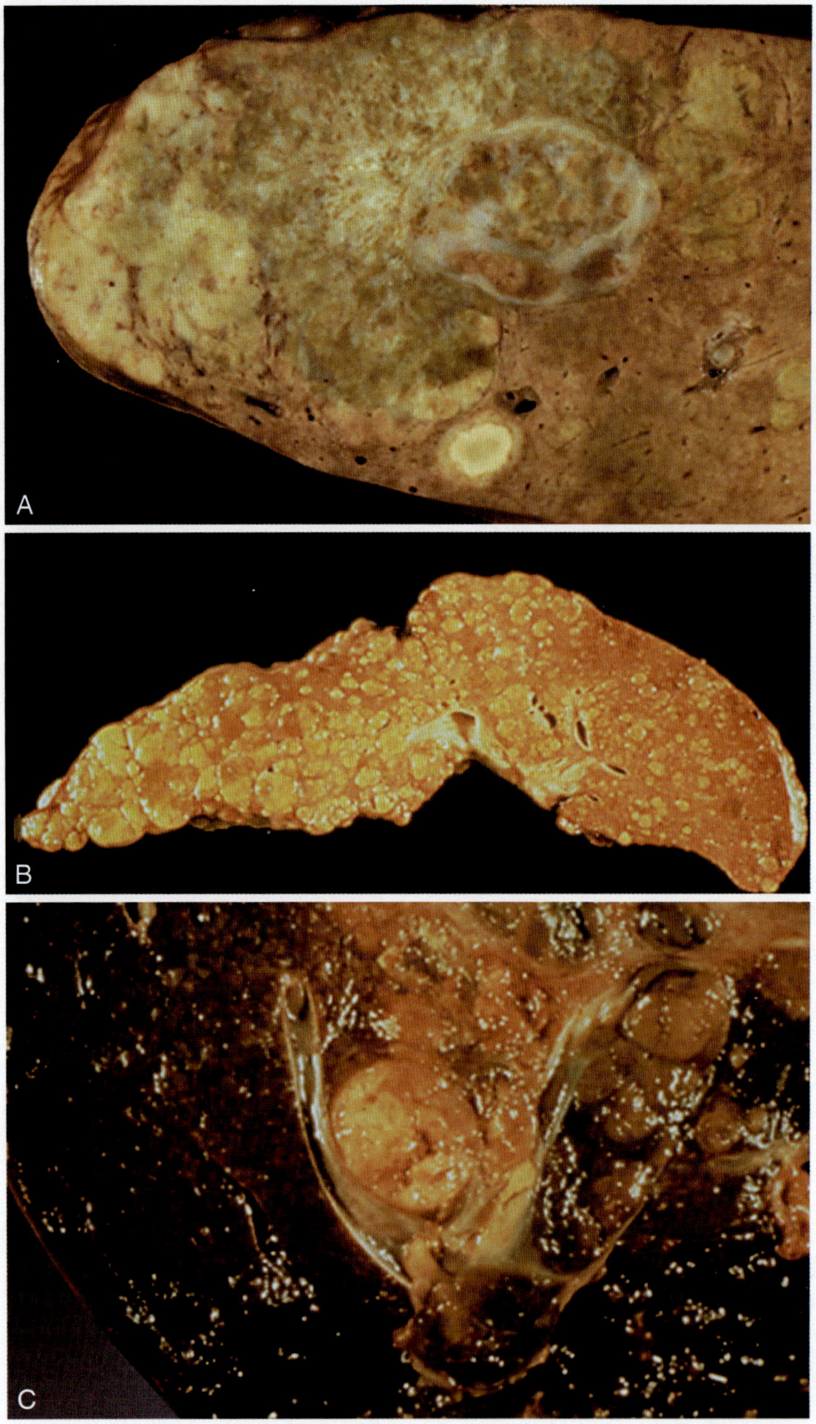

FIGURE 18.8

Variegated appearance and a bile-stained cut surface are characteristic of hepatocellular carcinoma (**A**). Satellite nodules are often present around large lesions. Nodules of carcinoma may be small and diffusely scattered throughout the liver and difficult to distinguish from cirrhosis (**B**). Invasion of large veins is an important prognostic feature to assess on gross examination (**C**).

setting of cirrhosis. However, tumors arising in cirrhosis may grow as numerous small nodules (diffuse type) that may be difficult to distinguish from the background liver (Fig. 18.8B). Tumor nodules are soft, bile stained, or yellow to tan and often variegated because of foci of hemorrhage and necrosis. Separate tumor nodules may represent multicentric growth or may represent tumor spread via intrahepatic vascular routes. Macroscopic portal vein, hepatic vein, or bile duct invasion are present in some cases (Fig. 18.8C). Involvement of the inferior vena cava, sometimes with extension into the right atrium, may be found.

Microscopic Findings

Hepatocellular carcinomas show a wide range of differentiation, and several grades may be present within the same tumor. Well-differentiated HCC shows obvious hepatocellular differentiation with tumor cells arranged in a trabecular pattern lined by endothelial cells. Stroma is typically scant, and bile production by neoplastic cells is pathognomonic of HCC but should not be confused with bile production by trapped non-neoplastic hepatocytes. Cytoplasmic inclusions such as Mallory's hyaline, α1AT inclusions, and fat accumulation are frequently present, often in focal areas of the tumor or in individual tumor nodules. Vascular lakes may simulate peliosis hepatis. The WHO classification divides HCC into well-, moderately, and poorly differentiated grades. Whereas well-differentiated tumors show minimal atypia and resemble normal hepatocytes, poorly differentiated tumors resemble a variety of carcinomas and are not clearly recognizable as hepatocellular on H&E stain. The moderately differentiated spectrum of tumors falls between the two extremes. In the compact or solid areas, compression of broad trabeculae forms sheets with inconspicuous sinusoids (Fig. 18.9A). Pseudoglandular (acinar) formation with dilated rounded spaces rounded by cytologically malignant hepatocytes may be mistaken for adenocarcinoma (Fig. 18.9B). The lumen of these acini may contain bile.

Among the major histologic subtypes are steatohepatitic, clear cell, macrotrabecular massive, scirrhous, chromophobe, neutrophil-rich, lymphocyte-rich, and fibrolamellar hepatocellular carcinoma (FL-HCC). The steatohepatitic subtype (5%–20%) reveals steatosis and ballooning as seen in steatohepatitis (Fig. 18.9D). Because of the fragmentation of the reticulin framework in areas of fat, the differential diagnosis can be challenging. Clear cell HCC (3%–7%) demonstrates clear cell morphology in more than 80% of the tumor (Fig. 18.9E) and carries better prognosis than conventional HCC. Macrotrabecular massive HCC (5%) consists of thickened trabeculae larger than 10 cells thick and has worse prognosis than conventional HCC (Fig. 18.9F). The rare scirrhous HCC (4%) displays prominent fibrous stroma accounting for more than 50% of the tumor (Fig. 18.9G). Neutrophil-rich (<1%), chromophobe (3%), lymphocyte-rich (<1%) (Fig. 18.9H), sarcomatoid (Fig. 18.9I), lipid-rich, HCC with syncytial giant cells (Fig. 18.9J), GCSFP producing HCC, and cirrhotomimetic are rare subtypes.

Hepatocellular Carcinoma—Pathologic Features

Gross Findings

- Single large mass, with or without satellite nodules or multiple nodules diffusely involving the liver
- The tumor is soft, often variegated, and can be bile stained
- Vascular invasion is common, with involvement of portal or hepatic veins

Microscopic Findings

- Wide range of differentiation
- Most tumors have trabecular growth pattern; a pseudoglandular pattern is also common
- Stroma is sparse in most tumors
- Bile production, fat droplets, Mallory's hyaline, and other cytoplasmic inclusions may be seen

Ultrastructural Findings

- Bile canaliculi may be demonstrated

Genetics

- TP53 mutations associated with progression from early to advanced stage
- Frequent allelic losses on multiple chromosomes
- TERT promoter mutations in transformed hepatic adenoma (HA)

Immunohistochemistry

- Tumor cells are positive for HepPar-1 (granular cytoplasmic pattern), glypican 3, and nuclear/cytoplasmic expression of arginase 1
- Fewer than 50% of tumors are positive for α-fetoprotein (AFP)
- Polyclonal carcinoembryonic antigen (CEA) or CD10 demonstrate a canalicular staining pattern; monoclonal CEA is negative
- CAM 5.2 is positive; CK7 and CK20 can be focally expressed

Differential Diagnosis

- HA
- Dysplastic nodule in cirrhosis
- Metastatic tumors, especially neuroendocrine tumors
- Cholangiocarcinoma

Ancillary Studies

Immunohistochemistry

Hepatocellular carcinoma demonstrates canalicular staining pattern with antibodies to CD-10 and polyclonal carcinoembryonic antigen (CEA) (Fig. 18.10), as well as positivity for hepatocyte (HepPar-1), glypican 3, and Arginase-1. Granular cytoplasmic staining pattern with HepPar-1 and nuclear/cytoplasmic staining for Arginase is present in HCC and normal hepatocytes. Glypican 3 is expressed in HCC (with lower sensitivity in well-differentiated HCC) and negative in nonmalignant liver. Arginase-1 has been proposed as the hepatocellular marker with greater sensitivity in poorly differentiated HCC. In situ hybridization for albumin messenger RNA appears to be highly sensitive but not specific because it has been demonstrated in CCs and adenocarcinomas of other sites.

Even though CAM 5.2 is positive in HCC, other keratins (CK7, CK20, CK19, AE1/AE3, Ker 903) area variable expressed and more commonly negative. CK19 expression has been associated with a poor prognosis.

MOC-31 and Ber-Ep4 are negative and can be useful in the differential diagnosis with CC or other adenocarcinomas.

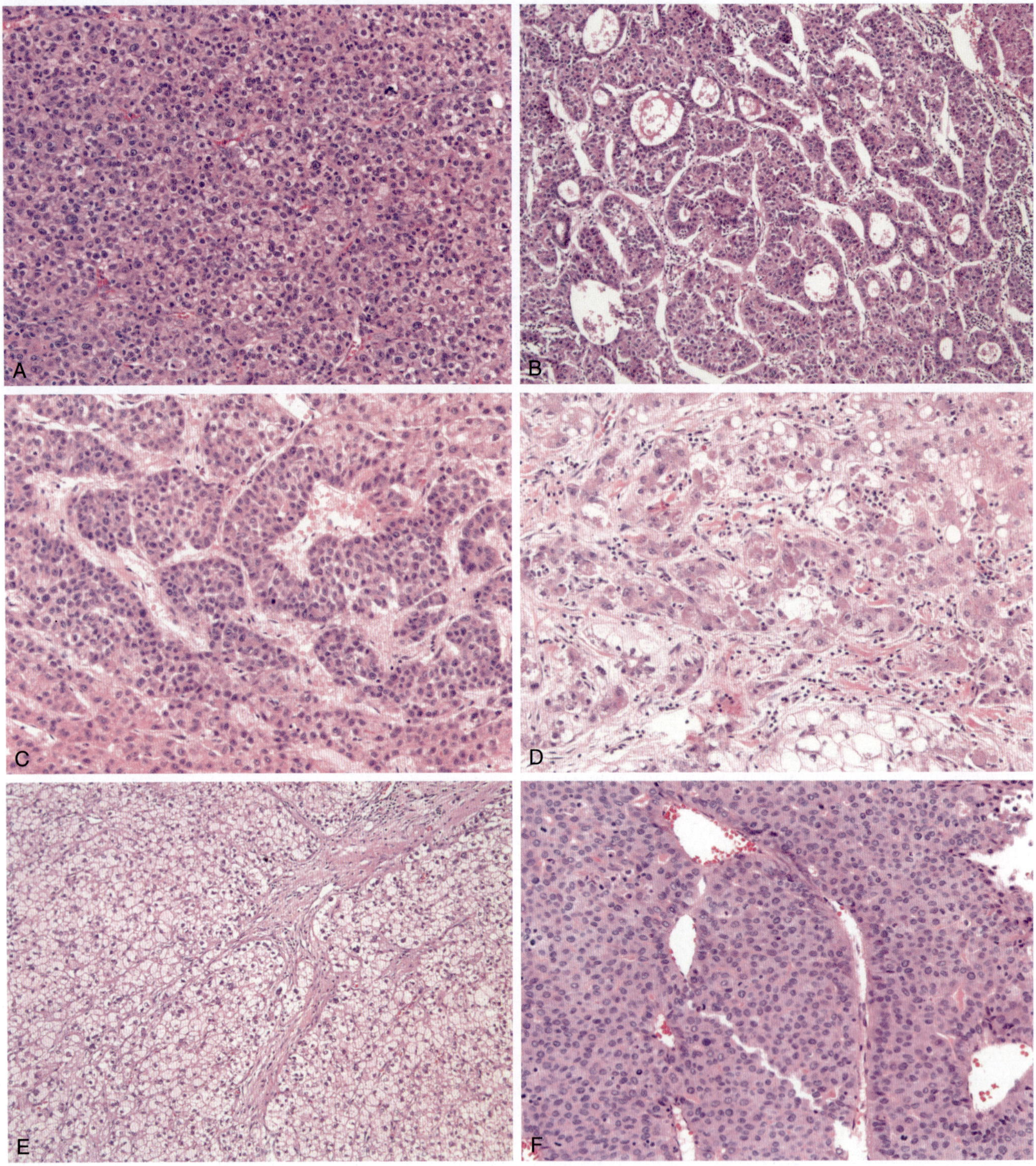

FIGURE 18.9

Hepatocellular carcinomas (HCCs) show a variety of architectural and cytologic patterns. Certain areas of the tumor may reveal a more solid architecture (**A**) or pseudoglandular pattern (**B**) that can mimic an adenocarcinoma. Typical areas of trabecular growth pattern are seen in most cases (**C**). The steatohepatitic subtype of HCC (**D**) can be challenging to diagnosed because it is often cytologically bland and shares morphologic features with fatty liver disease. Ancillary stains such as loss of reticulin in fat-poor areas or positive glypican-3 stain can be helpful. HCC clear cell can mimic other clear cell tumors such as metastatic renal cell carcinoma, so immunostains are needed to sort out the differential diagnoses (**E**). Some HCCs demonstrate a macrotrabecular growth pattern with trabecula of more than 10 cells thick (**F**). The rare scirrhous HCC (**G**) shows prominent collagen bands, but the cytologic features of fibrolamellar HCC are not present. Uncommon subtypes also include lymphocytic-rich HCC (**H**), which shows an immune-rich stroma with greater than 100 tumor-infiltrating lymphocytes in 10 hfp. Sarcomatoid HCC (**I**) mimics an undifferentiated sarcoma and can only be diagnosed by demonstration of a conventional HCC component or positivity for markers of hepatocellular differentiation and HCC with syncytial giant cells (**J**).

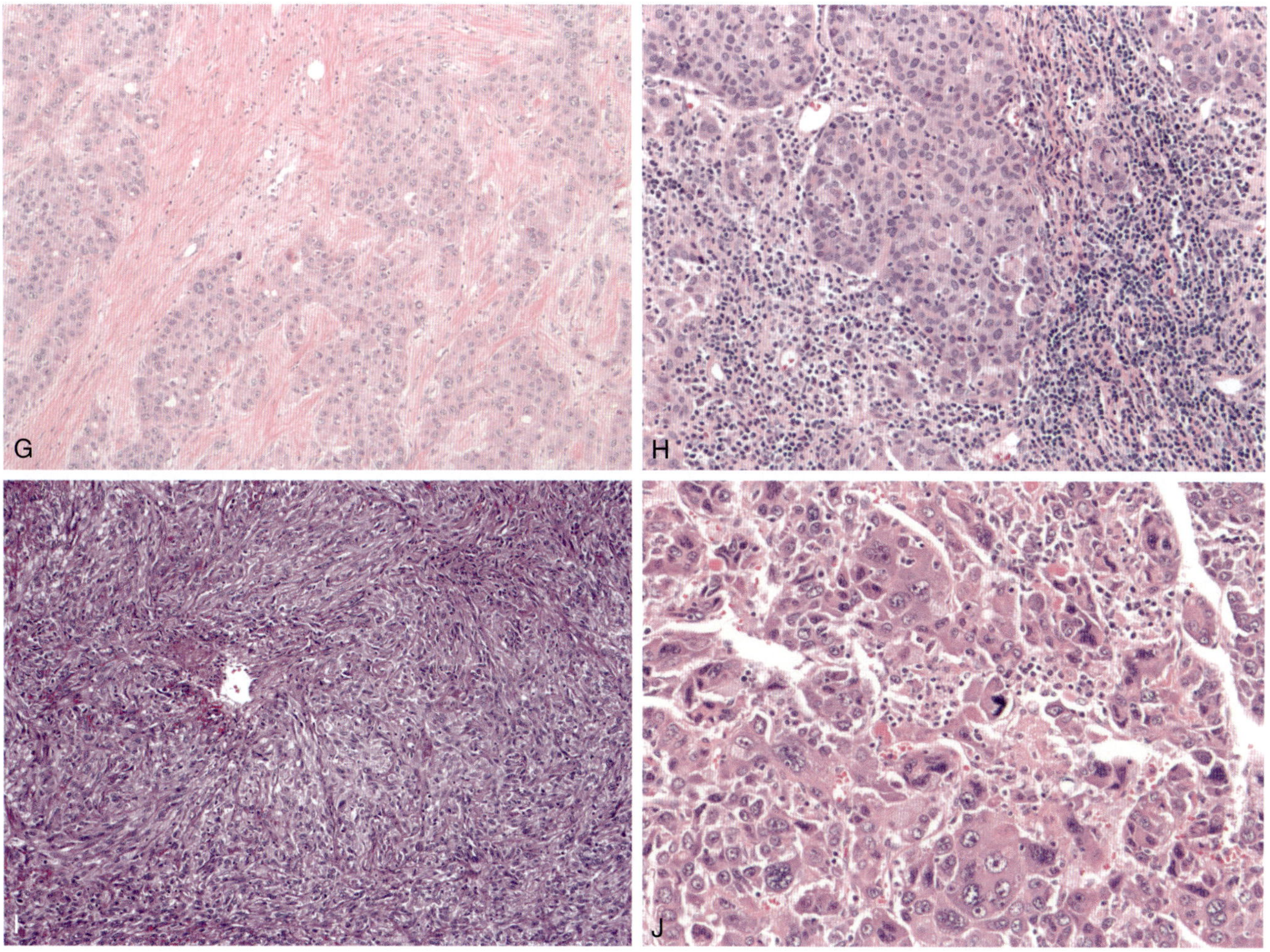

FIGURE 18.9
Continued

Differential Diagnosis

Dysplastic nodule and HA are in the differential diagnosis of well-differentiated HCC (discussed earlier). Neuroendocrine tumors metastatic to the liver, particularly those with oncocytic features (Fig. 18.11A), may be mistaken from HCC because of their trabecular architecture. Diffuse positivity for neuroendocrine markers such as synaptophysin and chromogranin is helpful in making this distinction. Similarly, metastatic breast carcinoma (Fig. 18.11B), adrenocortical carcinoma, oncocytic renal tumors, hepatoid adenocarcinomas, and melanoma may also mimic HCC but can be easily ruled out with a panel of immunostains. Distinction of poorly differentiated and undifferentiated HCC from poorly differentiated CC (Figs. 18.11C and D), high-grade neuroendocrine carcinoma, and certain sarcomas can be challenging and often requires a battery of ancillary stains and correlation with clinical and imaging findings to arrive at the correct diagnosis.

Prognosis and Therapy

The prognosis is determined primarily by HCC stage and the functional status of the liver. Nonoperative palliative therapies include percutaneous ethanol injection, cryoablation, and transcatheter arterial chemoembolization; chemotherapy has largely proven ineffective. At autopsy, metastases, most commonly to the lung and porta hepatis lymph nodes, are found in up to 75% of patients. Bone, adrenal gland, and virtually any site in the body can be involved by metastatic disease. Tumor size, number and location (one or both lobes) of tumor nodules, presence of gross or microscopic vascular invasion, and disease status of the uninvolved liver are the most important prognostic variables. In carefully selected patients, hepatic resection and/or liver transplantation may be performed with success. Small, low-stage, incidentally discovered HCCs in a cirrhotic liver at transplantation do not adversely affect outcome.

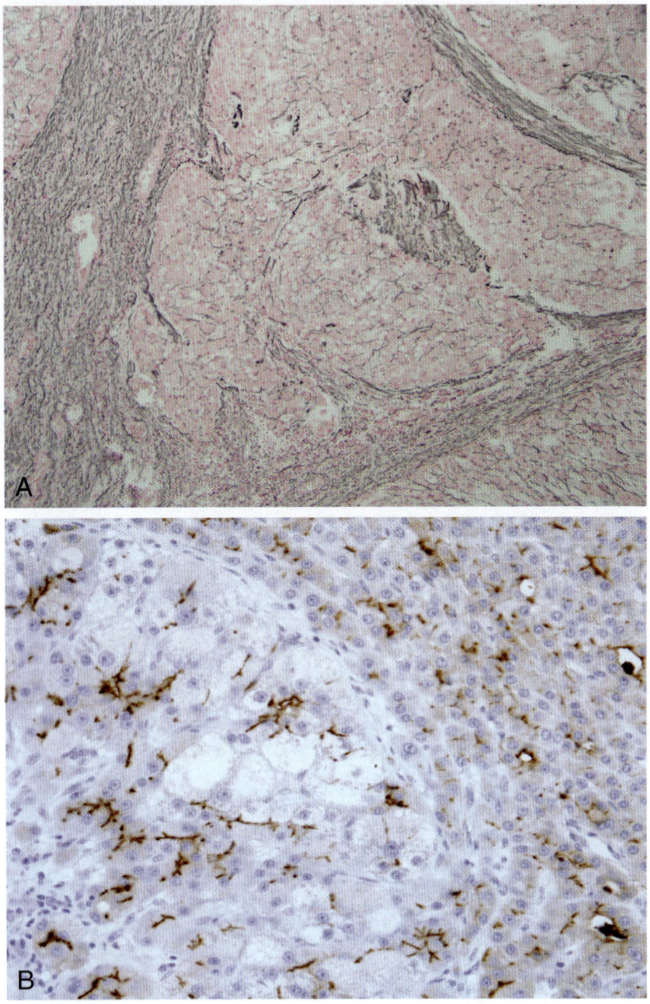

FIGURE 18.10

Ancillary stains are often helpful in diagnosis of hepatocellular carcinoma. Thickened hepatic cord architecture or loss of reticulin on a reticulin stain is diagnostic of malignant transformation (**A**). The presence of a canalicular pattern of staining on a polyclonal carcinoembryonic antigen immunostain is helpful in confirming hepatocellular differentiation (**B**). Arginase-1, HepPar-1, and glypican-3 are other commonly used markers of hepatocellular differentiation.

FIBROLAMELLAR CARCINOMA—FACT SHEET

Definition

- Rare variant of hepatocellular carcinoma (HCC) with characteristic morphology occurring in a noncirrhotic liver

Incidence and Location

- Rare in Asian and African countries
- Age-adjusted incidence rate is approximately 0.02 per 100,000

Morbidity and Mortality

- Overall, more indolent course than typical HCC but stage-matched outcomes similar

Gender, Race, and Age Distribution

- Male to female ratio, 3:4
- No race predilection in US population
- Mean age, 23 years

Clinical Features

- Nausea, weight loss, abdominal pain, malaise
- Not associated with chronic liver disease or cirrhosis
- Normal or mild serum α-fetoprotein elevation

Radiologic Features

- Well-demarcated hypodense tumor on computed tomography scan
- Central scar may mimic focal nodular hyperplasia

Prognosis and Therapy

- Approximately 60% are surgically resectable
- Chemotherapy is reserved for patients with unresectable disease and is not curative
- The most significant determinant of survival is tumor stage
- 5-year survival rate is approximately 60%

FIBROLAMELLAR CARCINOMA

CLINICAL FEATURES

Fibrolamellar HCC (is a rare HCC variant arising in noncirrhotic liver in young patients, 80% between ages of 10–35 years). It is associated with a better prognosis than typical HCC, likely because of the younger age of the patients and their lack of significant underlying liver disease. The outcome in stage-matched fibrolamellar and conventional HCC appears to be similar. Clinical presentation is similar to typical HCC. In most cases, serum AFP levels are normal or only modestly elevated.

PATHOLOGIC FEATURES

GROSS FINDINGS

Most FL-HCCs arise in the left lobe, but large tumors may affect both lobes. The tumors are usually solitary, firm, and well circumscribed and may be bile stained, necrotic, or hemorrhagic. They are typically large, measuring up to 25 cm. A central stellate scar similar to that seen in FNH may be present (Fig. 18.12). The adjacent non-neoplastic liver is unremarkable.

MICROSCOPIC FINDINGS

The tumor cells of FL-HCC are very large, display abundant granular eosinophilic cytoplasm because of large numbers of mitochondria and distinct cell borders, and have a distinctive oncocytic appearance (Fig. 18.13A). A defining feature of FL-HCC is the presence of parallel bands of hyalinized fibrous tissue separating the tumor cells into nests (Fig. 18.13B). Other patterns of fibrosis include haphazard collagen deposition and tumors

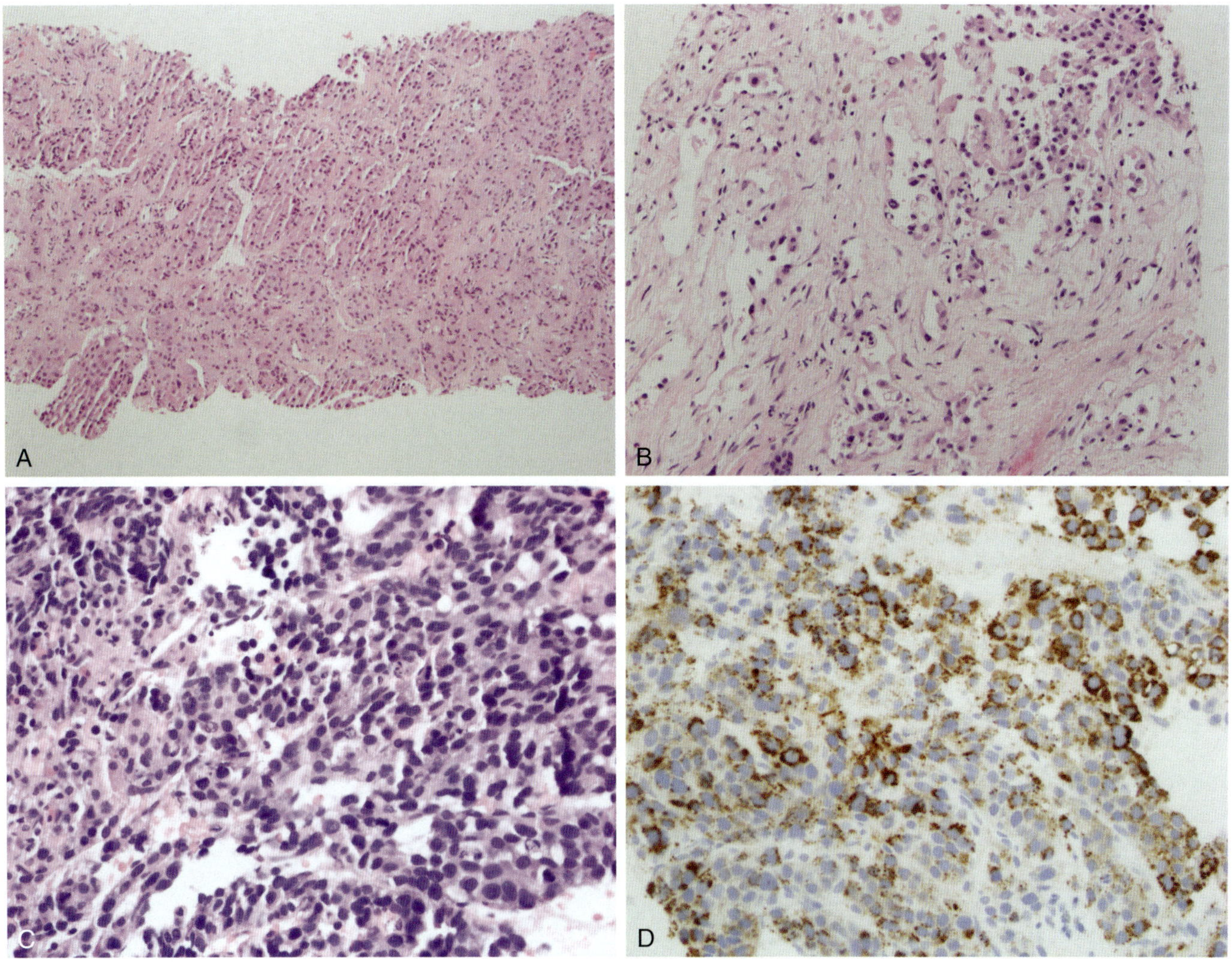

FIGURE 18.11

The differential diagnosis of hepatocellular carcinoma (HCC) is broad and includes primary intrahepatic and metastatic tumors. Tumors with oncocytic change, such as metastatic pancreatic endocrine tumors (**A**) and breast carcinoma (**B**), can mimic HCC but are easily distinguished by appropriate immunostains. Poorly differentiated HCC with small cell undifferentiated morphology (**C**) can be challenging to separate from metastatic melanoma, carcinoma, or lymphoma. Positive staining for HepPar-1 (**D**), glypican-3, or arginase-1 is essential for definitive diagnosis.

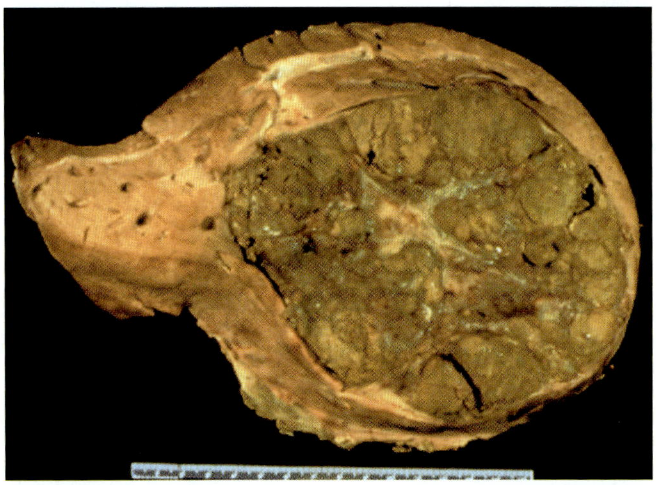

FIGURE 18.12

Fibrolamellar hepatocellular carcinoma is usually a solitary mass arising in a noncirrhotic liver and may also show a central stellate scar.

showing areas with little or no intratumoral fibrosis (least common pattern). Cytoplasmic eosinophilic hyaline globules, which may be Periodic Acid–Schiff (PAS) positive and diastase resistant, may represent α1AT. Cytoplasmic pale bodies contain fibrinogen and are present in about 50% of cases (Fig. 18.13C). In a subset of cases, pseudoglandular formation and mucin production can be seen, but these findings do not constitute a component of adenocarcinoma. Most FL-HCC are moderately differentiated, but they can contain foci of carcinoma that are poorly differentiated. In addition to staining with HepPar-1, albumin in situ hybridization (ISH), and arginase-1, FL-HCC is positive for CK7 (Fig. 18.13D) and CD68 (Fig. 18.13E). Polyclonal CEA demonstrates a canalicular staining pattern.

Recent molecular data have shown that FL-HCC show activation of protein kinase A, most commonly through a *DNAJB1-PRKACA* fusion transcript, secondary to somatic intrachromosomal deletion on chromosome 19.

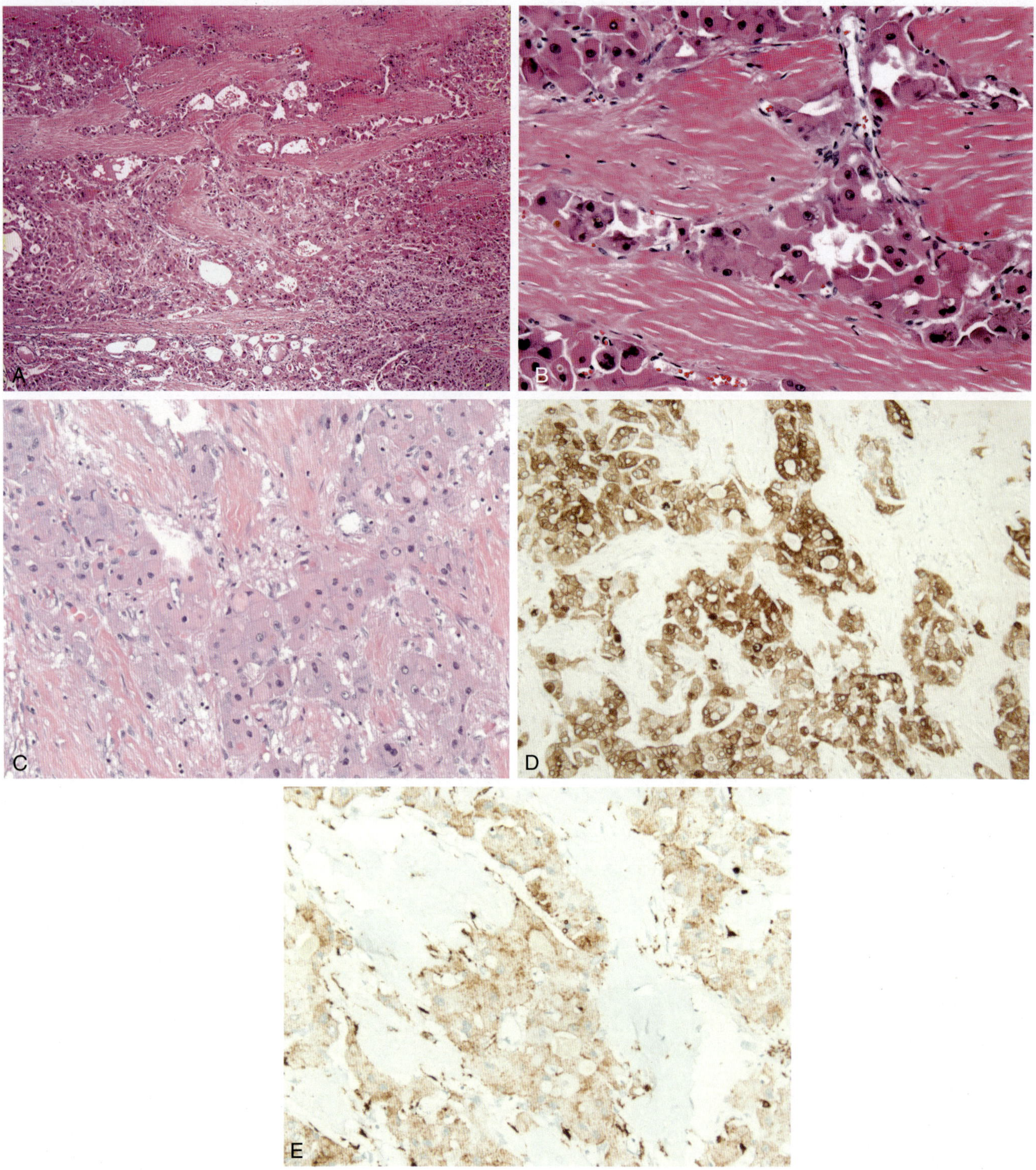

FIGURE 18.13

Fibrolamellar hepatocellular carcinoma is characterized by large and polygonal tumor cells with abundant granular pink cytoplasm and prominent nucleoli (**A**) arranged in cords and nests separated by dense collagen bundles are arranged in parallel layers (**B**). The glassy pink cytoplasmic inclusions (**C**) are also a characteristic feature. Coexpression of cytokeratin 7 (**D**) and CD68 (**E**) in the tumor cells helps support the diagnosis.

This genetic abnormality is diagnostic of FL-HCC in the differential of hepatocellular malignancies. Interestingly, the *DNAJB1-PRKACA* fusion transcript has been also demonstrated in other oncocytic pancreatic and biliary neoplasms, but these are typically not in the differential of FL-HCC so do not constitute a diagnostic challenge.

Ancillary Studies

Ultrastructural Findings

The cytoplasm contains numerous mitochondria, as expected from the oncocytic appearance of the tumor cells. Dense core neuroendocrine-like granules may also be rarely found.

FIBROLAMELLAR CARCINOMA—PATHOLOGIC FEATURES

Gross Findings

- Two-thirds are located in left lobe
- Single mass in 56% of cases
- Firm tan or green circumscribed mass
- Central scar in many cases
- Surrounding liver is noncirrhotic

Microscopic Findings

- Large polygonal, granular oncocytic tumor cells in nests separated by lamellar fibrous stroma
- Cytoplasmic inclusions contain pale bodies (accumulated fibrinogen), Mallory's hyaline, α_1-antitrypsin

Ultrastructural Findings

- Numerous densely packed mitochondria

Genetics

- *DNAJB1-PRKACA* translocation is diagnostic of fibrolamellar hepatocellular carcinoma (HCC)

Immunohistochemistry

- Positive for HepPar-1, albumin in situ hybridization (ISH), arginase 1, CK7 and CD68
- Polyclonal carcinoembryonic antigen positive with a canalicular distribution
- α-Fetoprotein negative

Differential Diagnosis

- Focal nodular hyperplasia
- Conventional hepatocellular carcinoma (HCC)
- Sclerosing or scirrhous variant of HCC
- Cholangiocarcinoma

DIFFERENTIAL DIAGNOSIS

The most common lesions in the differential diagnosis for FL-HCC are FNH, typical HCC, scirrhous HCC, and metastatic tumors with extensive fibrosis. Although FNH and FL-HCC may have central stellate scars, microscopically, the lack of hepatocellular atypia, isolated arteries, bile ductular proliferation, and lamellar collagen distinguishes FNH from FL-HCC. Diffuse lamellar fibrosis combined with oncocytic cellular features is not found in typical HCC. In metastatic carcinomas, the collagen is more haphazardly arranged and lacks the lamellar features characteristic of FL-HCC. The tumor cells in scirrhous HCC are smaller, do not display oncocytic features, and form glandular patterns. Scirrhous HCC arises in liver with chronic liver disease, and Hepar-1 expression is often weak or absent; the opposite is true for FL-CC. Both FL-HCC and scirrhous HCC can be CK7 positive, leading to confusion with CC, which can be easily excluded based on typical morphologic characteristics and presence of markers of hepatocellular differentiation. The presence of *DNAJB1-PRKACA* translocation supports the diagnosis of fibrolamellar HCC.

PROGNOSIS AND THERAPY

Fibrolamellar HCC is often resectable and is thus associated with an overall better outcome than usual HCC, but stage-matched outcomes are similar in both groups. Hepatic transplantation may be considered for nonresectable tumors confined to the liver. The most common metastatic sites are the abdominal lymph nodes, peritoneum, and lung.

HEPATOBLASTOMA

CLINICAL FEATURES

Hepatoblastoma is the most common primary hepatic tumor in children, accounting for about 50% of all primary pediatric hepatic malignancies. The majority occur by 2 years of age, and there is a male predominance (male-to-female ratio, 2 to 1). Patients generally present with an abdominal mass noticed by the parent, but some patients present with precocious puberty related to human chorionic gonadotropin production by the tumor. Approximately 5% of patients have an associated congenital abnormality. Familial adenomatous polyposis is associated with higher risk for hepatoblastoma, as are Beckwith-Wiedemann syndrome and trisomy 18. Although the etiologic factors of hepatoblastoma are unknown, an association with parental smoking and low birth weight is recognized, although it is not clear if an environmental cause is responsible. The serum AFP level is elevated in 90% of cases.

RADIOLOGIC FEATURES

Hepatoblastoma is visualized as a solid or multifocal mass on CT, with calcification in more than half of cases. MRI shows decreased signal relative to the normal liver on T1-weighted images and increased signal on T2-weighted images.

PATHOLOGIC FEATURES

GROSS FINDINGS

Hepatoblastoma is typically a solitary mass that may be quite large, measuring up to 20 cm. Purely epithelial hepatoblastoma is a soft, fleshy mass (Fig. 18.14);

HEPATOBLASTOMA–FACT SHEET

Definition

- Malignant liver tumor occurring in children, mimicking fetal or embryonal liver and often containing heterologous cell types

Incidence and Location

- Rare; annual incidence in the United States is 0.2 per 100,000 children
- 47% of pediatric malignant liver tumors

Morbidity and Mortality

- Overall survival is 65% to 70%

Gender, Race, and Age Distribution

- Male predominance (male-to-female ratio, 2:1)
- No racial predilection
- 90% occur within first 5 years of life

Clinical Features

- More common in low-birth-weight infants
- Presenting symptom is enlarging abdomen noted by parent
- Weight loss and anorexia are less common
- 5% of children with hepatoblastoma have congenital anomalies; known association with familial adenomatous polyposis, Beckwith-Wiedemann syndrome, and trisomy 18
- Human chorionic gonadotropin production may lead to presentation with precocious puberty

Radiologic Features

- Solid or multifocal mass on computed tomography
- Calcification in more than 50% of cases
- Magnetic resonance imaging shows decreased signal relative to normal liver on T1-weighted images and increased signal on T2-weighted images

Prognosis and Therapy

- Tumor stage is the key prognostic factor
- The pure fetal type may have a better prognosis; the small cell undifferentiated pattern has a worse prognosis
- Treatment is surgical excision when possible
- Preoperative chemotherapy allows many previously unresectable cases to be completely resected

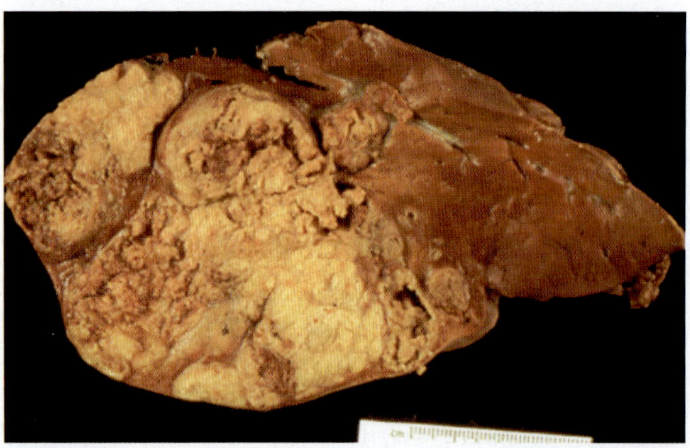

FIGURE 18.14

Hepatoblastoma typically presents as a single, large, soft, fleshy tumor mass.

whereas the fetal type grossly appears similar to normal liver, other patterns show a variegated appearance. Tumors with a prominent mesenchymal component are often firm and may be calcified. Cystic degeneration, necrosis, and hemorrhage may be seen.

MICROSCOPIC FINDINGS

Hepatoblastomas may be classified as either epithelial or mixed epithelial–mesenchymal and are subclassified into a variety of patterns that are usually present in variable combinations (Figs. 18.15A-D).

1. Fetal pattern (30%): Hepatocytes are uniform and similar to normal hepatocytes, although they have a slightly higher nuclear-to-cytoplasmic ratio. An alternating light and dark pattern is characteristic on low power. Mitoses are rare and less than 2 per 10 hpf. The tumor cells form cords two to three cells thick, separated by sinusoids, in a pattern reminiscent of normal liver. However, normal structures such as portal tracts, bile ducts, and ductules are absent. A mitotically active aggressive variant of the fetal type is also recognized.
2. Embryonal pattern (20%): The tumor cells in the embryonal pattern are less differentiated and cohesive than the fetal pattern and have a high nuclear-to-cytoplasmic ratio and coarser chromatin. The trabecular pattern is not well developed, and the tumor cells may form sheets. Mitoses and necrosis are more common than in the fetal pattern.
3. Macrotrabecular pattern (3%): This pattern is characterized by broad trabeculae 10 or more cells thick. Trabeculae may be composed of embryonal or fetal cells.
4. Small cell undifferentiated pattern (3%): This pattern is the least differentiated pattern and resembles other small blue cell tumors of childhood. The tumor is composed of loosely cohesive sheets of uniform small cells with scanty cytoplasm. The tumor cells are positive for keratins.
5. Cholangioblastic pattern (rare): Small ducts are dispersed around or within a hepatocellular component.
6. Mixed epithelial and mesenchymal pattern (44%). Both epithelial and mesenchymal differentiation are present. The primitive mesenchymal component may be primitive, with spindle or stellate cells with little cytoplasm, or display differentiation along chondroid and rhabdomyoblastic lines. Osteoid is the most frequent heterologous element and may be more prominent after chemotherapy. The mesenchymal elements may also be keratin positive, suggesting sarcomatoid differentiation of the epithelial component.
7. A subtype of mixed pattern tumors displays teratoid features and may contain elements of mature teratoma such as keratinized squamous epithelium, intestinal epithelium, and neuroectodermal structures.

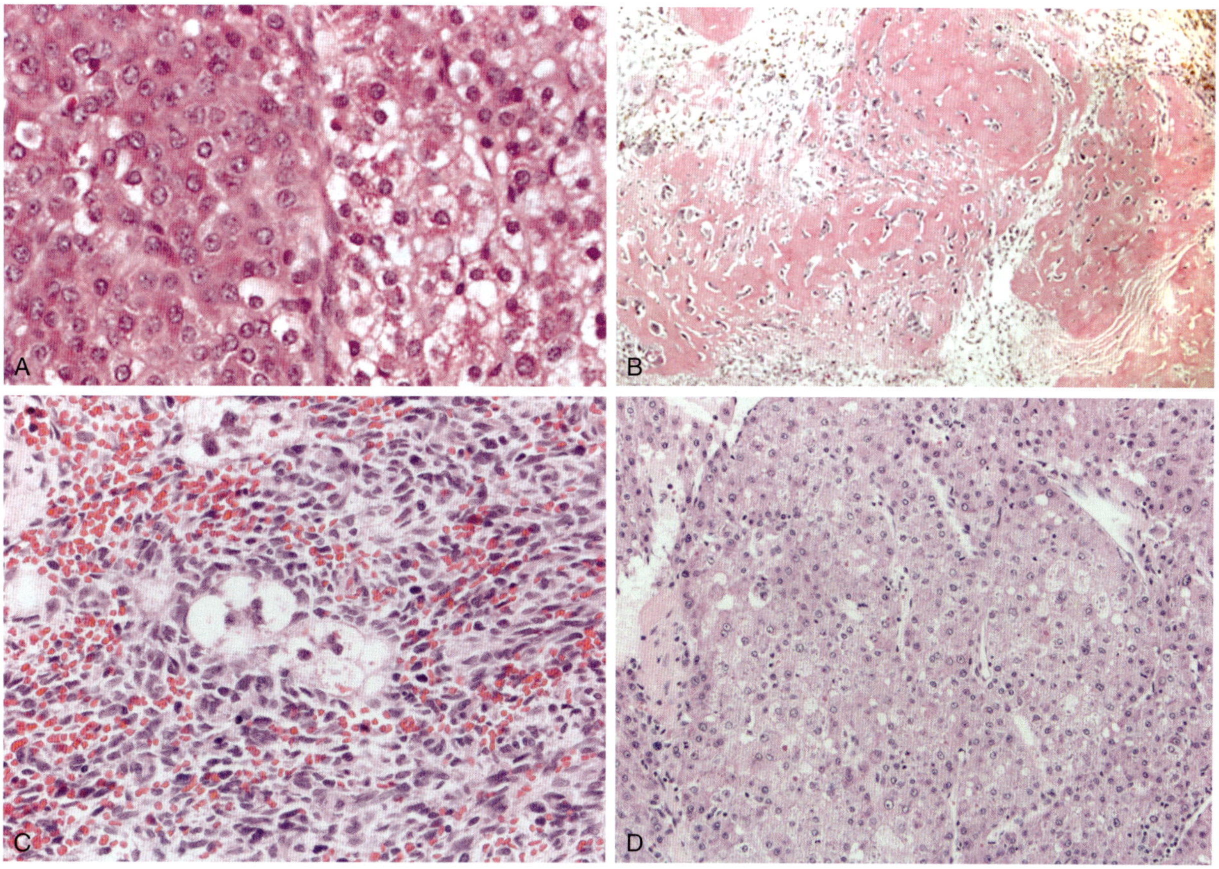

FIGURE 18.15

The fetal pattern of hepatoblastoma exhibits alternating areas of light- and dark-staining tumor cells showing hepatocellular differentiation (**A**). Osteoid is the most common mesenchymal element and may be abundant after chemotherapy (**B**). Some tumors may show rare clusters of differentiated hepatocytes embedded in primitive mesenchymal cells (**C**), and others may show marked differentiation and resemble hepatocellular carcinomas (**D**).

Hepatoblastoma—Pathologic Features

Gross Findings

- Single well-circumscribed mass in 80% of cases
- Pure fetal tumors are soft, tan to brown, and coarsely lobulated
- Mixed epithelial and mesenchymal tumors have a variegated, heterogeneous cut surface

Microscopic Findings

- Pure fetal epithelial pattern (~30%) is composed of sheets of uniform cells resembling fetal hepatocytes
- Embryonal pattern consists of a mixture of fetal-type cells and smaller, less differentiated cells with higher nuclear-to-cytoplasmic ratio
- Macrotrabecular pattern: epithelial hepatoblastoma with trabeculae more than 10 cells thick
- Small cell undifferentiated pattern is composed of discohesive sheets of small cells indistinguishable from other small blue cell tumors of childhood
- Cholangioblastic pattern also shows small duct-like structures
- Mixed epithelial and mesenchymal pattern contains fetal and embryonal epithelial cells and primitive mesenchyme with various mesenchymal tissues such as fibrous tissue, osteoid, and cartilage
- Teratoid pattern contains a variety of tissue types in addition to those found in the mixed pattern, such as skeletal muscle, bone, or squamous epithelium

Ultrastructural Findings

- Small cell tumors have relatively dense cytoplasm with tonofilaments, intercellular junctions, and microvilli
- Glycogen accumulation and bile canaliculi may be seen in epithelial components

Genetics

- WNT/β-catenin abnormalities present in 80%
- Deletions or mutations in *CTNNB1*, *AXIN*, or *APC*
- Two subtypes on gene expression studies:
  1. Genomic instability with overexpression of α-fetoprotein (AFP), CK19, EpCAM, and Myc; these tumors are usually of an immature embryonal phenotype
  2. Genomically stable with lack of above findings that is usually of fetal type

Immunohistochemistry

- Epithelial components are Hepar-1, AFP, and epithelial membrane antigenpositive; immature components may be Hepar-1 negative and glypican-3 positive
- Glutamine synthetase positive in the fetal component
- Pankeratin are variably expressed
- Cytokeratin (CK) 7 and CK19 are positive in the cholangioblastic component
- SWI/SNF related, matrix associated, actin dependent regulator of chromatin, subfamily b, member 1 (SMARCB1) (INI-1) is usually positive; exception is a subset that shows INI-1 loss in small cell undifferentiated component and carries a worse prognosis

Differential Diagnosis

- Hepatocellular carcinoma
- Other small blue cell tumors of childhood

Ancillary Studies

Immunohistochemistry

Positivity for keratins helpful in confirming epithelial differentiation. Markers of hepatocellular differentiation are useful in fetal, embryonal, and small cell undifferentiated subtypes; the latter may be negative for HepPar-1 but may be positive for arginase 1 and glypican 3. INI-1 loss is seen in a subset of small cell undifferentiated subtype of tumors that are associated with a worse prognosis.

Differential Diagnosis

Hepatoblastoma with a predominantly or exclusively small cell component may be difficult to distinguish from the small, round cell tumors such as neuroblastoma, lymphoma, and rhabdomyosarcoma. The presence of more differentiated areas of hepatoblastoma and the tumor cell immunophenotype (CK positive; leukocyte common antigen, neurofilament, and desmin negative) can distinguish small cell hepatoblastoma from other neoplasms. The absence of a renal mass generally excludes Wilms' tumor. The macrotrabecular variant of hepatoblastoma closely resembles HCC; however, HCC is exceedingly rare in the age group affected by hepatoblastoma. Other diagnostic considerations include sarcomas, such as embryonal sarcoma, which can be distinguished by the lack of an epithelial component. Germ cell tumor must be considered in the differential diagnosis but is generally excluded by the focal nature of the teratoid areas in hepatoblastoma.

Prognosis and Therapy

The outcome is dependent on tumor resectability. Most patients are treated with neoadjuvant multiagent chemotherapy, and the rate of resection is greater than 90%. More than 70% of patients have long-term survival. The most frequent metastatic sites are regional lymph nodes and the lung. Liver transplantation may be considered in some cases in which tumor is limited to the liver but is unresectable.

Histologic pattern is generally not an independent predictor of prognosis, although the small cell undifferentiated pattern with INI-1 loss does appear to correlate with a poorer prognosis, and completely resected pure fetal tumors may have a more favorable outcome. Other unfavorable prognostic features are increased mitotic activity, vascular invasion, incomplete tumor resection, and AFP levels of less than 100 ng/mL at diagnosis.

BILIARY TUMORS

BILE DUCT HAMARTOMA

CLINICAL FEATURES

Bile duct hamartomas (BDHs), also known as von Meyenburg complexes, are small, incidental, clinically asymptomatic lesions, reported in up to 27% of all autopsies. BDH is considered part of the spectrum of ductal plate malformation and may be sporadic or related to autosomal dominant polycystic kidney disease, congenital hepatic fibrosis, or other genetic disorders

BILE DUCT HAMARTOMA (VON MEYENBURG COMPLEX)—FACT SHEET

Definition

- Bile duct malformation at the level of the interlobular bile duct caused by failure of involution of the embryonic ductal plate

Incidence and Location

- Common incidental finding at autopsy or surgery
- No geographic predilection

Morbidity and Mortality

- Sporadic lesions are innocuous; not associated with increased morbidity or mortality
- Increased risk for cholangiocarcinoma when present as part of the spectrum of ductal plate malformations

Gender, Race, and Age Distribution

- Equal gender distribution
- No race predilection
- All ages but more common in adults

Clinical Features

- Most commonly sporadic asymptomatic incidental finding
- When multiple and numerous may be part of the spectrum of ductal plate malformation and adult polycystic disease

Prognosis and Therapy

- Treatment is not indicated; lesion is excised for diagnostic purposes when identified during surgery
- Prognosis is excellent—innocuous finding

Pathologic Features

Gross Findings

Bile duct hamartomas appear as single or multiple subcapsular, gray-white, or occasionally green nodules smaller than 0.5 cm in diameter.

Microscopic Findings

Bile duct hamartomas are found directly adjacent to portal tracts and consist of ectatic, branched bile ducts lined by a single layer of bland, low columnar to cuboidal biliary

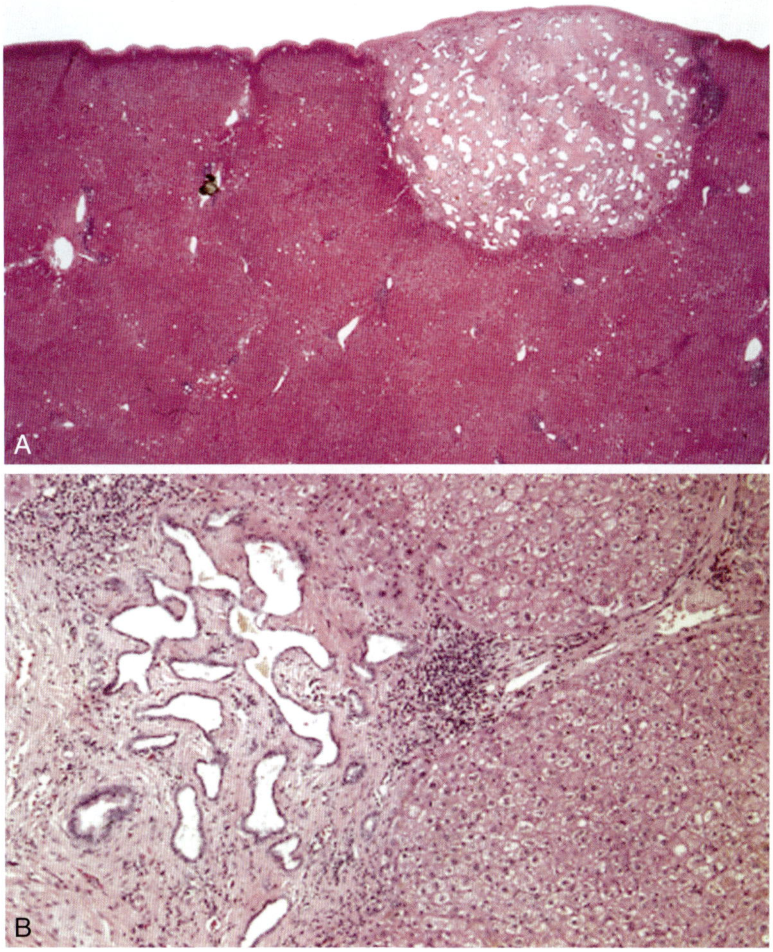

FIGURE 18.16

Bile duct hamartomas are well-circumscribed and frequently subcapsular lesions (**A**) characterized by dilated biliary channels (**B**) that may be filled with inspissated bile.

epithelium (Fig. 18.16). The lumen frequently contains bile. The stroma is dense and hyalinized, with minimal inflammation.

BILE DUCT HAMARTOMA (VON MEYENBURG COMPLEX)—PATHOLOGIC FEATURES

Gross Findings

- Small gray-white nodule, often subcapsular

Microscopic Findings

- Dilated biliary channels embedded in fibrous stroma
- Located at periphery of portal tract
- Channels may contain bile

Differential Diagnosis

- Bile duct adenoma
- Metastatic adenocarcinoma or cholangiocarcinoma

DIFFERENTIAL DIAGNOSIS

A BDH is distinguished from a bile duct adenoma (BDA) by its dilated, rather than compact, biliary channels and the presence of intraluminal bile. It is distinguished from CC by its circumscribed lobular configuration and the lack of cellular atypia.

PROGNOSIS AND THERAPY

Bile duct hamartomas are innocuous incidental findings. Rarely, CC has been reported in association with multiple BDHs, as with other ductal plate malformation disorders.

BILE DUCT ADENOMA

CLINICAL FEATURES

A BDA is an innocuous lesion, usually an incidental finding at autopsy or in the resected liver. It is not clear that a BDA is a true neoplasm, and it is regarded by some investigators as a hamartoma of peribiliary glands.

BILE DUCT ADENOMA—FACT SHEET

Definition

- Small benign lesion composed of acini and tubules, regarded by some as a peribiliary gland hamartoma

Incidence and Location

- No geographic variation in incidence reported
- Considered rare but found in approximately 25% of livers at autopsy when livers were closely examined

Morbidity and Mortality

- No increase in morbidity or mortality

Gender, Race, and Age Distribution

- Male predominance (male-to-female ratio, 3 to 2)
- No race predilection
- Older adults (mean age, 55 years) but all age ranges

Clinical Features

- Incidental finding at surgery or autopsy

Prognosis and Therapy

- Excellent prognosis
- Excised for diagnosis; no treatment indicated

Pathologic Features

Gross Findings

Bile duct hamartomas are solitary, well-circumscribed, firm, gray-white or tan, subcapsular nodules. Most measure 5 mm or less.

Microscopic Findings

Bile duct hamartomas consist of a compact proliferation of simple tubular ducts embedded in a variable amount of fibrous stroma. The tubules have small lumen unlike the dilated channels of a BDH and do not contain intraluminal secretions or bile. The cuboidal or low columnar lining epithelium resembles that of interlobular bile ducts (Figs. 18.17A and B). The cells of a BDA are uniform and usually lack nuclear pleomorphism and hyperchromasia. Mitoses and vascular or lymphatic invasion are not seen. The stromal inflammation is variable. Some variants may be larger in size and show a prominent stromal component ("biliary adenofibroma").

Differential Diagnosis

A BDA is distinguished from a BDH by its lack of intraluminal bile and the compact nature of the proliferation

Bile Duct Adenoma—Pathologic Features

Gross Findings

- Usually solitary, subcapsular lesion
- ≤1 cm, well-demarcated gray-white mass

Microscopic Findings

- Densely packed tubules and acini lined by single layer of cuboidal to columnar cells
- Fibrous stroma with variable inflammatory infiltrate

Immunohistochemistry

- Immunophenotype is that of peribiliary glands: cytokeratin 19, carcinoembryonic antigen, and epithelial membrane antigen positive

Differential Diagnosis

- Bile duct hamartoma (von Meyenburg complex)
- Cholangiocarcinoma
- Metastatic adenocarcinoma, especially pancreatic adenocarcinoma

with small lumina. It is distinguished from CC and metastatic adenocarcinoma, especially pancreatic ductal adenocarcinoma, by its circumscribed nature (lack of infiltrative growth pattern), no mitoses, no intraluminal debris, and the lack of cytologic atypia. Having said that, some BDAs can reveal clear cell and oncocytic change and even harbor cytologic atypia that can lead to diagnostic challenges, especially during intraoperative consultations for subcapsular liver lesion in a patient undergoing Whipple's procedure for a pancreatic mass. On permanent sections, Ki67 stain can help in the differential diagnosis because most BDA demonstrate a low proliferative index (<10%) (Fig. 18.17C).

Prognosis and Therapy

A BDA is an innocuous incidental finding. However, some lesions, particularly larger BDAs, may carry a low risk for malignant transformation.

SOLITARY BILIARY CYST

Clinical Features

Solitary biliary cysts are found in up to 14% of autopsies but rarely come to clinical attention. They occur predominantly in women and are usually asymptomatic. Their origin is obscure, but many may develop from BDHs that become isolated from the biliary tree.

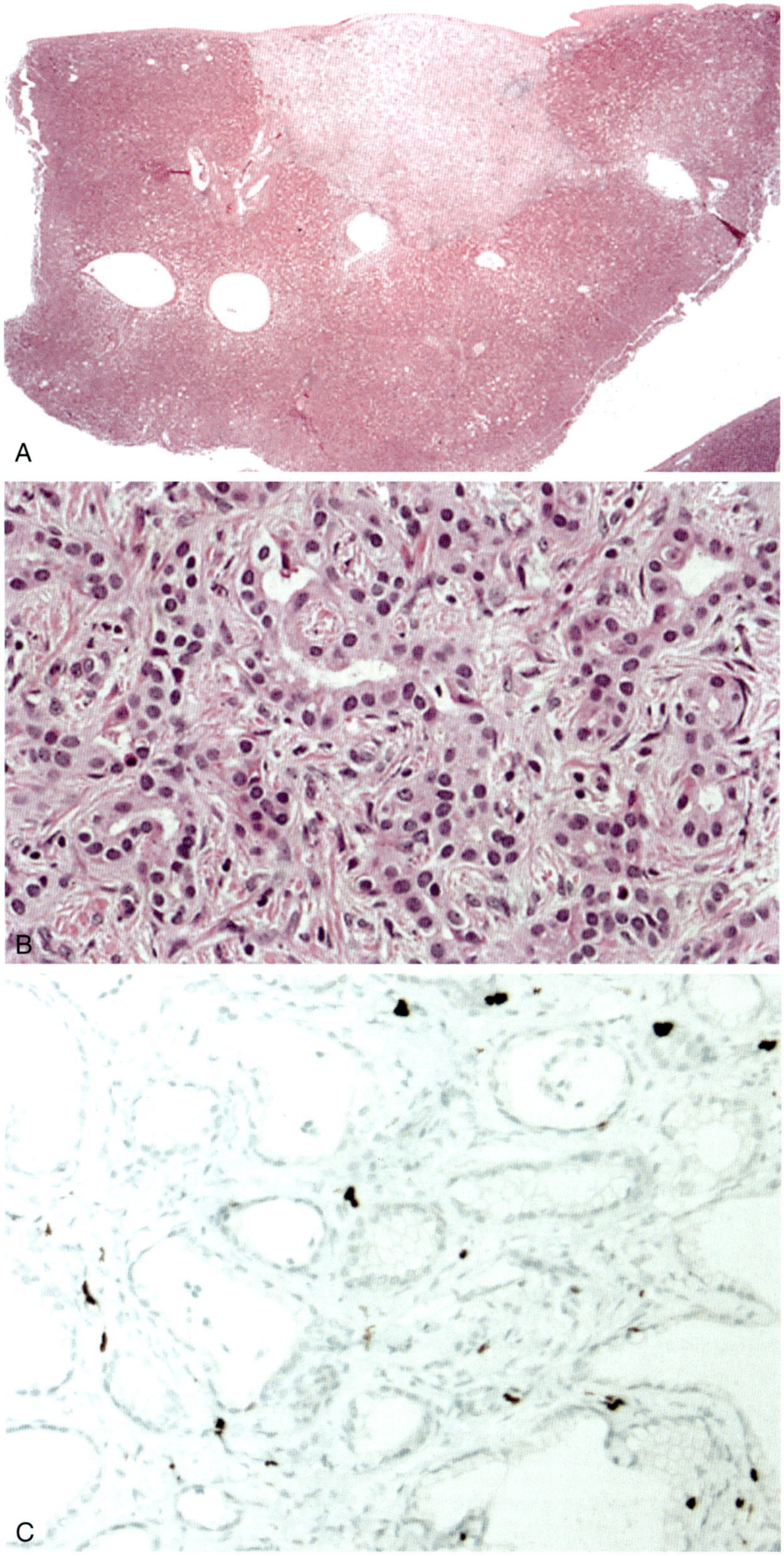

FIGURE 18.17

Bile duct adenomas (BDAs) are small, well-circumscribed lesions, similar to hamartomas (**A**) and composed of a tightly packed proliferation of bland biliary glands with angulated profiles and a narrow lumen (**B**). Ki67 proliferative index is low, often less than 10% in BDAs (**C**).

SOLITARY BILIARY CYST—FACT SHEET

Definition

- Non-neoplastic unilocular cyst lined by single layer of cuboidal to columnar epithelium

Incidence and Location

- Often incidental finding
- Up to 14% of autopsies
- No geographic variation in incidence reported

Morbidity and Mortality

- Clinically insignificant unless large in size and causing symptoms
- Favorable outcome in most cases

Gender, Race, and Age Distribution

- Female predominance (male-to-female ratio, 4 to 1)
- No race predilection
- Rare in children; more common in 30- to 50-year-old age range

Clinical Features

- Smaller cysts are usually asymptomatic
- Abdominal fullness, mass, nausea, rarely jaundice in larger cysts

Radiologic Features

- Circumscribed lesion with water density on computed tomography

Prognosis and Therapy

- Surgical excision, laparoscopic fenestration, or aspiration with sclerotherapy are treatment options

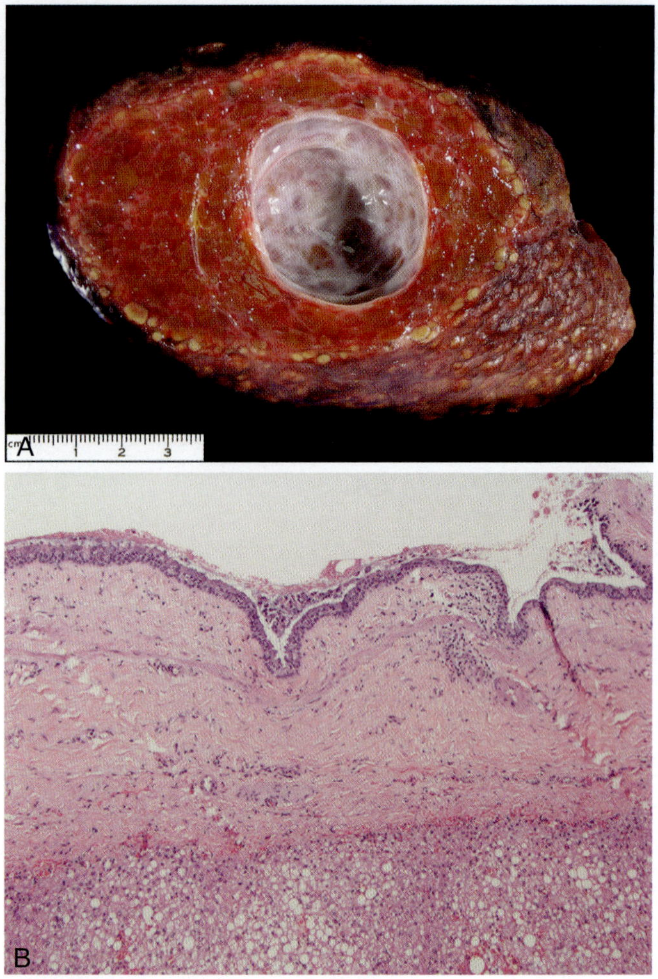

FIGURE 18.18

Biliary cyst is a unilocular, smooth-walled cyst, usually found just under the hepatic capsule (**A**) lined by low cuboidal or markedly attenuated biliary epithelium. In contrast, ciliated foregut type cysts (**B**) are lined by a columnar respiratory-type epithelium with cilia and surrounded by a variable cuff of smooth muscle.

PATHOLOGIC FEATURES

GROSS FINDINGS

Most cysts are subcapsular (Fig. 18.18A) and of variable size that ranges from a few centimeters in incidental lesions to up to 40 cm. Biliary cysts usually contain thin clear yellow fluid, and the cyst lining is flat and glistening. Connection to the biliary tree is not demonstrated.

MICROSCOPIC FINDINGS

Biliary cysts are frequently lined by a single layer of cuboidal, flattened, or columnar biliary-type epithelium. The cyst wall is thin and fibrous and lacks the mesenchymal ovarian-type stroma of biliary cystadenoma, better known as hepatic mucinous cystic neoplasm (MCN). A ciliated lining and smooth muscle in the cyst wall are characteristic of ciliated hepatic foregut cyst (Fig. 18.18B).

PROGNOSIS AND THERAPY

Asymptomatic biliary cysts do not require treatment. Partial or complete surgical excision or cyst fenestration may be performed in symptomatic cases.

SOLITARY BILIARY CYST—PATHOLOGIC FEATURES

Gross Findings

- More common in right lobe
- Round, with smooth lining
- Fluid is usually clear but may be bile stained; fluid may be purulent if secondarily infected

Microscopic Findings

- Single layer of biliary-type epithelium
- Cyst wall is fibrous tissue and lacks ovarian-type mesenchymal stroma
- Ciliated foregut cyst lined ciliated cuboidal epithelium and surrounded by smooth muscle and fibrous tissue

Differential Diagnosis

- Mucinous cystic neoplasm (formerly known as biliary cystadenoma shows ovarian-type stroma)
- Polycystic liver disease (distinguished on gross examination by presence of numerous cysts)

POLYCYSTIC LIVER DISEASE

CLINICAL FEATURES

Polycystic liver disease belongs to the family of fibrocystic disorders of the liver and represents one of the ductal plate malformation disorders, with the malformation occurring at the level of the interlobular bile duct. Patients with polycystic liver disease usually have autosomal dominant polycystic kidney disease. The liver cysts are not present at birth but develop over time as fluid accumulates in the dilated biliary spaces of BDHs (von Meyenburg complexes). Up to 30% of young adults have liver cysts; this prevalence increases to 90% in older patients.

POLYCYSTIC LIVER DISEASE—FACT SHEET

Definition

- Multiple hepatic cysts associated with autosomal dominant polycystic kidney disease

Incidence and Location

- Incidence of autosomal dominant polycystic kidney disease is 1 in 1000
- Numerous hepatic cysts are found in approximately 20% of patients with polycystic kidney disease
- More common in patients of Northern European descent

Morbidity and Mortality

- Morbidity is associated with infection of cysts and development of cholangiocarcinoma
- Death is usually caused by renal disease, not hepatic involvement

Gender, Race, and Age Distribution

- Symptomatic hepatic cysts are more common in women, related to number of pregnancies
- More common in whites
- Average age for manifestation of liver cysts is approximately 53 years; number and size of cysts increase with age

Clinical Features

- Hepatomegaly and upper abdominal pain
- Jaundice and portal hypertension are rare
- Hepatic outflow obstruction may be seen
- Manifestations in other organs include colonic diverticula, cardiac valve abnormalities, and intracranial aneurysms

Radiologic Features

- Multiple circumscribed lesions with water density on computed tomography

Prognosis and Therapy

- Excision or fenestration of cysts is rarely indicated
- Liver transplantation has been performed in selected patients
- Prognosis is related to underlying renal disease

PATHOLOGIC FEATURES

GROSS FINDINGS

Multiple unilocular cysts resembling simple biliary cysts and ranging in size from a few millimeters to over 10 cm in diameter are scattered diffusely throughout the liver or, more rarely, are limited to one lobe (Fig. 18.19).

MICROSCOPIC FINDINGS

Cysts in polycystic liver disease resembled solitary biliary cysts microscopically. Origin from BDHs may be seen (Fig. 18.20).

POLYCYSTIC LIVER DISEASE—PATHOLOGIC FEATURES

Gross Findings

- Numerous cysts of various sizes, sometimes involving one lobe more than the other
- Cysts contain clear colorless or yellow fluid

Microscopic Findings

- Cysts are lined by columnar to flat biliary epithelium
- Origin in von Meyenburg complex may be demonstrated in smaller cysts

Genetics

- Associated with autosomal dominant polycystic kidney disease.
- Mutations in *PKD1* and *PKD2* have been implicated

Differential Diagnosis

- Solitary biliary cyst
- Mucinous cystic neoplasm (formerly known as biliary cystadenoma) shows ovarian-type stroma

PROGNOSIS AND THERAPY

The cysts usually do not compromise hepatic function but may produce hepatomegaly (sometimes massive) and abdominal discomfort. Women are more likely to be symptomatic

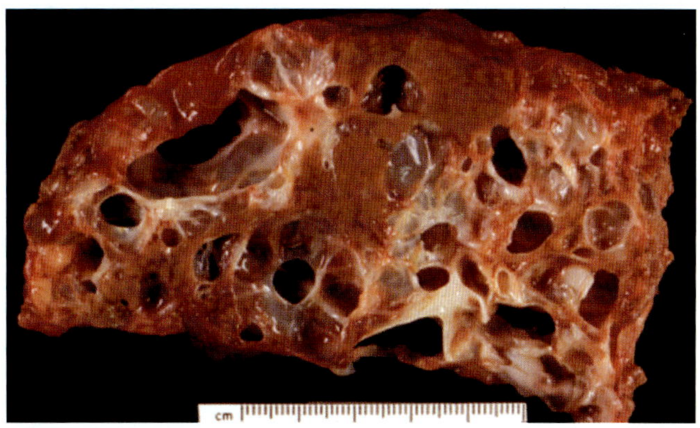

FIGURE 18.19

Polycystic liver disease shows numerous cysts of varying sizes that completely distort the hepatic parenchyma.

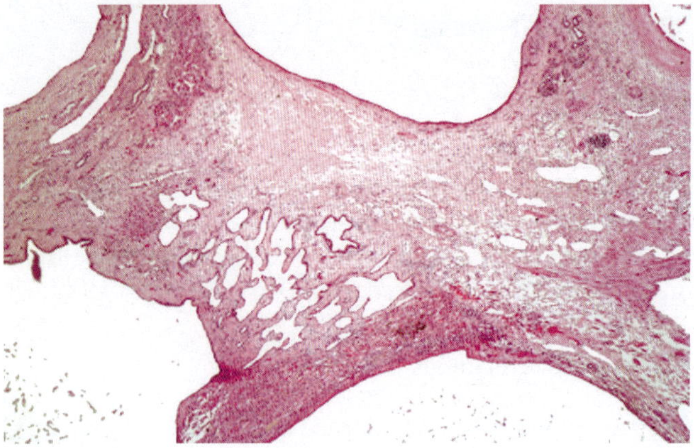

FIGURE 18.20

The cysts are lined by flattened or cuboidal biliary epithelium, and some cysts can be seen in association with small bile duct hamartomas.

from the cysts, and morbidity is related to number of pregnancies, use of oral contraceptives, and severity of renal involvement. Hepatic complications include secondary infection of cysts and development of cholangiocarcinoma (CC). Treatments include resection of more severely affected areas of liver, and in some cases, liver transplantation.

MUCINOUS CYSTIC NEOPLASM

CLINICAL FEATURES

The previous terms *hepatobiliary cystadenoma* and *cystadenocarcinoma* are no longer recommended. These lesions are similar to their pancreatic counterparts and are now designated mucinous cystic neoplasms that are characterized by an ovarian-type stroma. The tumor occurs almost exclusively in women, with the mean age at diagnosis 45 years. It is likely that lesions reported in the past as hepatobiliary cystadenoma or cystadenocarcinoma in men were examples of intraductal papillary neoplasms (IPNs) of the bile duct that lack an ovarian-type stroma. Patients may present with abdominal pain or an abdominal mass. Although most mucinous cystadenomas are intrahepatic, these tumors may also be found in the common bile duct, hepatic duct, cystic duct, and gallbladder. Carcinomas arising in hepatic MCNs are rare and usually arise in older patients.

MUCINOUS CYSTIC NEOPLASM—FACT SHEET

Definition

- Multilocular cystic neoplasm lined by biliary-type or mucinous epithelium surrounded by an ovarian-type stroma

Incidence and Location

- Rare tumors
- Geographic variation in incidence not reported

Morbidity and Mortality

- Survival is excellent for completely resected lesions
- Recurrence rate of approximately 13% for completely resected carcinomas arising in mucinous cystic neoplasms

Gender, Race, and Age Distribution

- Almost exclusively in women
- Mean age is 51 years
- More common in whites
- Carcinomas occur in older patients (mean age, 59 years)

Clinical Features

- Present with upper abdominal discomfort or pain

Radiologic Features

- Solitary, multilocular cystic lesions
- Papillary areas, thickened internal septa, and enhancing mural nodules suggest malignant transformation

Prognosis and Therapy

- Complete surgical excision is the treatment of choice
- Prognosis is excellent for completely resected lesions

PATHOLOGIC FEATURES

GROSS FINDINGS

Intrahepatic MCNs are encapsulated and solitary multicystic lesions ranging from 2.5 to 28 cm in diameter. The cyst fluid is usually clear and mucinous. The cyst lining is flat, with a few coarse trabeculations (Fig. 18.21A). Solid areas suggest an invasive adenocarcinoma arising in mucinous cystic neoplasm (MCN) (Fig. 18.21B). MCNs show no communication to the biliary tree.

MICROSCOPIC FEATURES

The cyst epithelial lining of MCNs is composed of cuboidal to columnar or flattened mucinous epithelium (Fig. 18.22A). Tall columnar mucinous epithelium similar to pancreatic MCNs and intestinal metaplasia can be seen in a subset of tumors (Fig. 18.22B). Neuroendocrine cells, gastric-type epithelium, and squamous metaplasia can also be identified occasionally. A characteristic dense subepithelial mesenchymal spindle cell stroma resembling ovarian stroma is found in almost all cases from women and is not found in lesions occurring in men. The characteristic stroma is usually diffusely noted in the majority (75%) of patients but can be focal and is immunoreactive for estrogen receptor, progesterone receptor, and inhibin.

Mucinous cystic neoplasms typically show a flat lining or papillary intraluminal growth with low- or

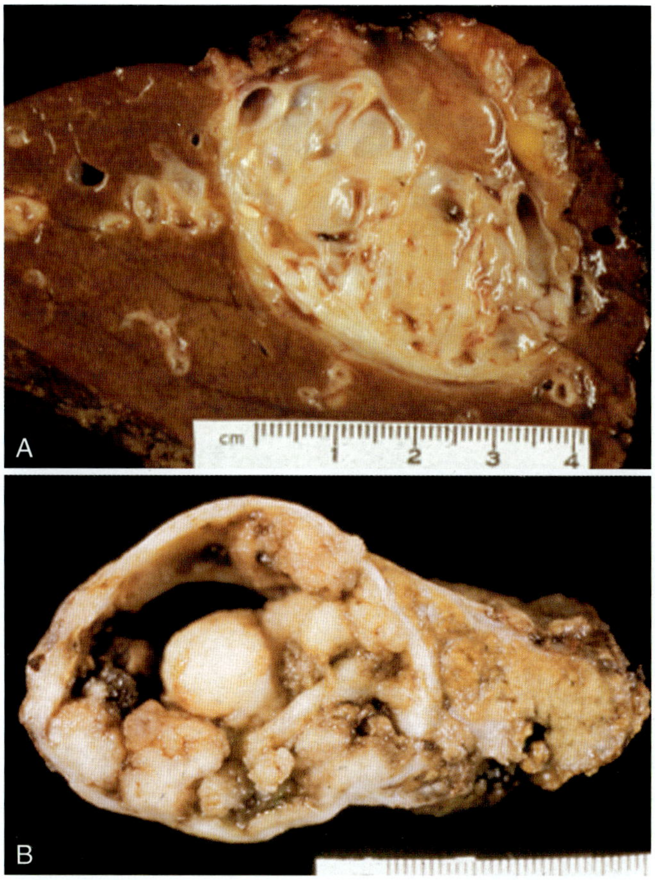

FIGURE 18.21

Mucinous cystic neoplasms (formerly known as biliary cystadenomas) are multilocular lesions arising in a normal liver (**A**). The cyst walls are smooth, without exophytic projections, and the presence of mural nodules is an indication of malignant transformation into a biliary cystadenocarcinoma (**B**).

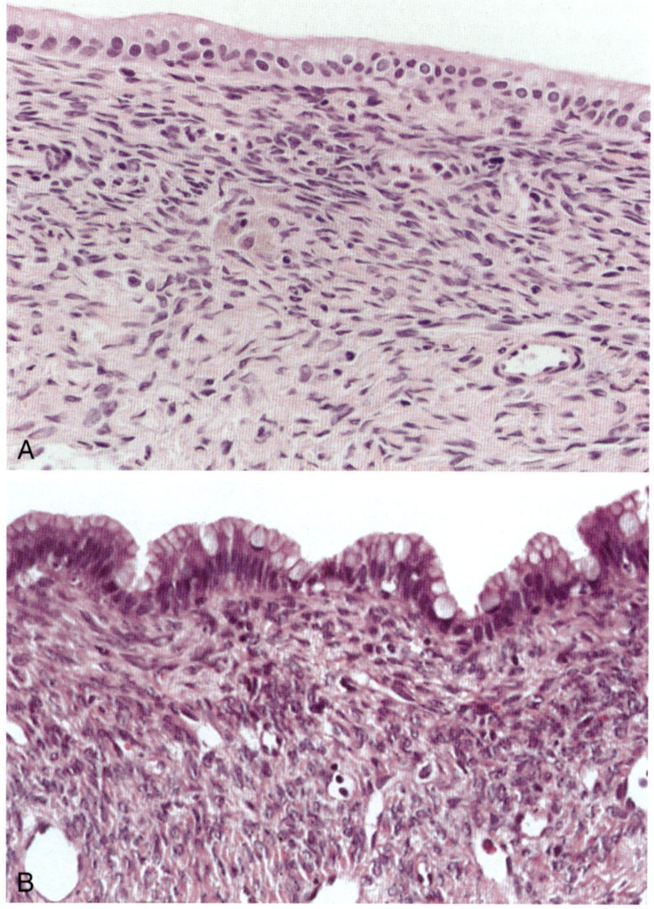

FIGURE 18.22

Mucinous cystic neoplasms are lined by a cuboidal pancreaticobiliary-type epithelium in more than half of all cases that is surrounded by an ovarian-type stroma (**A**). An intestinal type lining epithelium, similar to their pancreatic counterparts, can also be seen in some cases (**B**).

high-grade dysplasia (or both) (Fig. 18.23A). High-grade dysplasia characterized by marked architectural and cytologic atypia is rare in these tumors. An associated invasive adenocarcinoma is present in about 6% of tumors and is characterized by invasion into the adjacent stroma accompanied by a desmoplastic stromal reaction (Fig. 18.23B).

Mucinous Cystic Neoplasm—Pathologic Features

Gross Findings

- Multilocular cystic mass, 2.5 to 28 cm
- Cyst fluid is usually clear but may be blood tinged in tumors associated with carcinoma
- Papillary or solid areas suggest cystadenocarcinoma
- Extensive sampling is necessary to rule out associated carcinoma

Microscopic Findings

- Lined by cuboidal, flat, or columnar mucinous epithelium
- Others show nonmucinous epithelium; intestinal or squamous metaplasia may be present in a subset
- Ovarian-type stroma underlying the epithelium is characteristic
- Most cases show low-grade dysplasia; high-grade dysplasia is rare
- Invasive adenocarcinoma is present in fewer than 10% of cases

Immunohistochemistry

- Epithelium is positive for cytokeratin (CK) 7, CK 8/18, CK 19, epithelial membrane antigen, carcinoembryonic antigen, mucin 1 (MUC1), and/or mucin 5A (MUC5A)
- Ovarian-type stroma is positive for estrogen receptor, progesterone receptor, and inhibin

Differential Diagnosis

- Simple biliary cyst
- Metastatic mucinous adenocarcinoma

Ancillary Studies

Molecular Studies

KRAS mutations are present in about 20% of MCNs, but these lesions lack mutations in *GNAS*, *RNF43*, and *PIK3CA*.

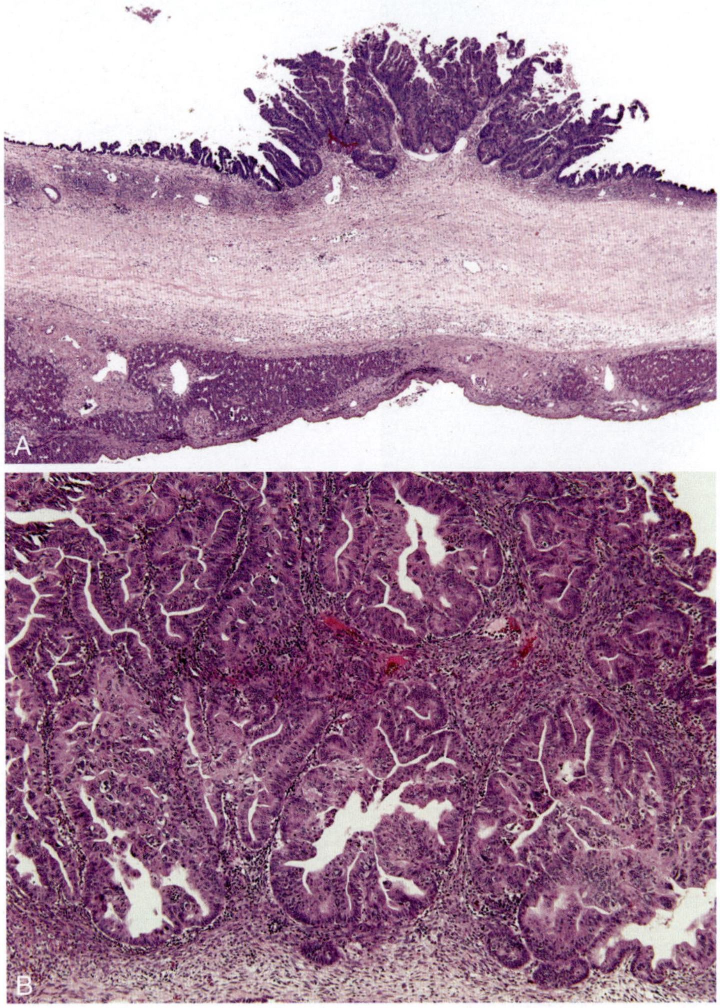

FIGURE 18.23

A majority of mucinous cystic neoplasms (MCNs) show low-grade dysplasia. However, cases with high-grade dysplasia also occur and show a complex papillary proliferation (**A**) correspond to exophytic areas noted on gross examination. Demonstration of invasion into the surrounding stroma is necessary for a diagnosis of invasive adenocarcinoma arising in an MCN (**B**).

Differential Diagnosis

Mucinous cystic neoplasms are distinguished from simple biliary cysts by their multilocular nature, nature of lining epithelium, and ovarian-type stroma.

Prognosis and Therapy

Complete excision of a cystadenoma is the treatment of choice and is curative. Incomplete resection or cyst fenestration usually results in persistent disease. The prognosis for patients with invasive adenocarcinoma arising in an MCN carries a better prognosis than conventional intrahepatic CC.

CHOLANGIOCARCINOMA

CLINICAL FEATURES

Cholangiocarcinomas are generally subdivided into peripheral (small duct) or hilar (large duct) types. Peripheral small duct CC is defined as cholangiocarcinoma arising in a segmental duct or a more peripheral duct. Intrahepatic CC is the second most common primary hepatic malignancy and accounts for nearly 15% of all primary hepatic carcinomas. The cause of CC is usually unknown. However, large duct–type CC may be associated with chronic inflammatory lesions of the bile ducts and conditions associated with bile stasis, including primary sclerosing cholangitis (PSC), parasitic infections with liver flukes such as Clonorchis and Opisthorchis, and recurrent bacterial cholangitis with hepatolithiasis. Large duct–type CCs have also been reported to occur in forms of fibropolycystic liver disease, including the presence of multiple BDHs. Small duct–type CC tends to be associated with nonbiliary type cirrhosis (viral, hemochromatosis, alcohol, obesity or diabetes), Thorotrast, and asbestos.

Cholangiocarcinoma generally occurs in older adults, with most patients between 50 and 70 years of age. Intrahepatic CC is often clinically silent until late in the course; patients typically complain of fever, weight loss, anorexia, and vague abdominal pain. Patients with intrahepatic CC rarely present with jaundice, in contrast to those with hilar CC.

Elevated serum CA19-9 levels, if greatly elevated, may be of utility, although considerable overlap with PSC without cancer is seen. Serum CEA is elevated in about 40 % of PSC patients with CC but is less sensitive and specific than CA19-9. The serum AFP level is not typically elevated.

CHOLANGIOCARCINOMA–FACT SHEET

Definition

- Malignant hepatic neoplasm demonstrating biliary differentiation

Incidence and Location

- Approximately 46,000 cases worldwide per year; 19% of primary liver malignancies
- Incidence is rising
- Geographic variation, with higher incidence in Japan and East Asia compared with the United States

Morbidity and Mortality

- Most patients have unresectable tumors
- Patients undergoing resection have longer survival times (23 months median survival vs 6 months with unresectable tumors)

Gender, Race, and Age Distribution

- Male predominance (male-to-female ratio, 3:2)
- More common in Asian population
- Affects older adults; mean age is 62 years

Clinical Features

- Large duct–type cholangiocarcinoma (CC): associated with inflammatory conditions involving the biliary tree (primary sclerosing cholangitis, recurrent pyogenic cholangitis, parasitic liver diseases, hepatolithiasis)
- Small duct–type CC: associated with risk factors of hepatocellular carcinoma (nonbiliary-type cirrhosis)
- Patients with intrahepatic CC present with nonspecific symptoms (upper abdominal pain, ascites, weight loss, anorexia)
- Patients with hilar CC present with obstructive jaundice

Radiologic Features

- The usual finding on computed tomography is homogeneous low-attenuation mass
- Calcification is present in some cases
- On magnetic resonance imaging, tumors are usually hypointense relative to liver on T1-weighted images and hyperintense on T2-weighted images

Prognosis and Therapy

- Poor prognosis, with median survival period of approximately 6 months in patients with unresectable tumors
- Chemotherapy and radiation therapy are of little benefit
- Survival depends on tumor stage; tumor grade is less important

Radiologic Features

CCs are visualized on CT as a homogeneous low-attenuation mass, with calcification in some cases. On MRI, the tumors are usually hypointense relative to liver on T1-weighted images and hyperintense on T2-weighted images. Cholangiography is useful in visualizing biliary strictures in hilar CC, but distinction from benign lesions may be difficult.

Pathologic Features

Gross Findings

On gross examination, intrahepatic CCs are generally gray-white to tan masses arising in a noncirrhotic liver (Fig. 18.24A). Whereas hilar lesions grow as periductal

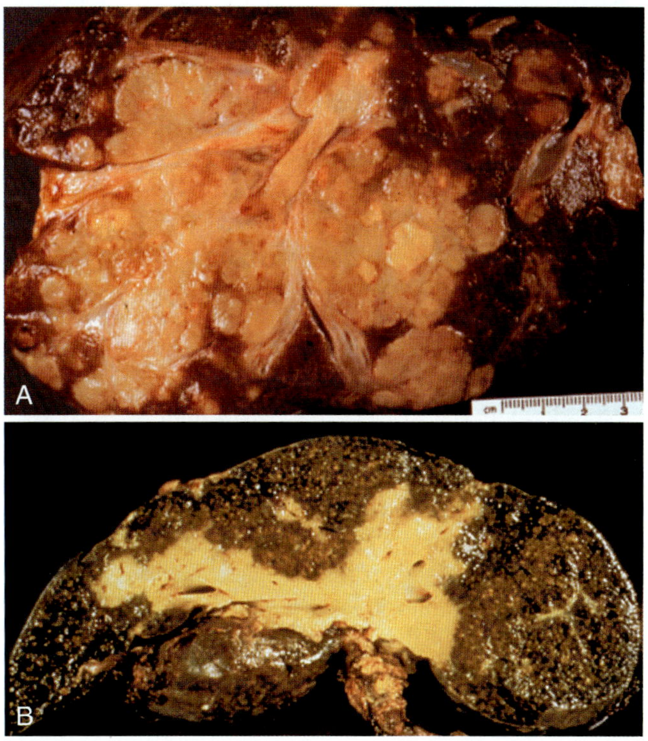

FIGURE 18.24

Peripheral or intrahepatic cholangiocarcinoma arises as a single firm mass, usually in a noncirrhotic liver (**A**). Hilar cholangiocarcinoma leads to biliary obstruction, resulting in severe bile staining, and may be indistinguishable from hilar scarring in primary sclerosing cholangitis (**B**).

and sclerosing mass lesions along the large ducts (Fig. 18.24B), peripheral lesions appear as irregular gray-white mass-forming lesions in the hepatic parenchyma. Large tumors may contain areas of central necrosis or hemorrhage. Central umbilication may be seen in subcapsular tumors. Intrahepatic CCs are grossly classifiable into mass-forming (the most common pattern), periductal infiltrating, and intraductal growth pattern (least common) types. The mass-forming type is often seen in a background of chronic nonbiliary liver disease. The periductal infiltration type shows spreading along portal tracts, resulting in bile duct strictures, but can also infiltrate into the hepatic parenchyma. The intraductal growth type is the least common type, often presenting as a papillary tumor within the dilated bile duct, and are considered part of the spectrum of IPNs of the bile duct.

Most CCs are firm because of the prominent desmoplastic stroma, which may be gritty because of dystrophic calcifications. Satellite lesions resulting from intravascular or intraductal spread may be present. The margins may be infiltrative or deceptively well circumscribed on gross examination. Rarely, involvement of portal or hepatic veins may be seen.

Microscopic Findings

Most CCs are adenocarcinomas with variable grades of differentiation. The most common microscopic pattern is a well- to moderately differentiated adenocarcinoma forming small tubular glands and duct-like structures (Fig. 18.25A) in a background of abundant desmoplastic or hyalinized fibrous stroma. The tumor cells are low cuboidal to columnar, with clear to eosinophilic cytoplasm and round to oval nuclei. Intracellular mucin production may be scant but is usually demonstrable with special stains for mucin. Perineural and lymphovascular invasion is common (Fig. 18.25B). CCs often involve portal tracts, either by spread within portal vein radicals or by spread within the intrahepatic biliary tree. In cases of large duct CC, adjacent bile ducts may demonstrate varying degrees of epithelial dysplasia which is graded as low- and high-grade biliary intraepithelial neoplasia.

Small duct type CC is comprised of malignant tubules that area bland appearing and mimic reactive bile ducts. The growth pattern is in the form of nodules encroaching the hepatic parenchyma.

The bile ductular or cholangiolocarcinoma type resembles a proliferation of primitive biliary ductules with cells that are smaller in size than conventional intrahepatic CC and embedded in a hyalinized stroma. More than 80% of the tumor is composed of ductular structures. They can resemble small caliber tubular structures with slit-like cords, spindled cell morphology with no discernible lumen-like structures. Ductal plate malformation type of CC (Fig. 18.25C) is a deceptively bland-appearing variant that mimics congenital hepatic malformation and is accompanied by a fibrous stroma. The presence of a larger size (lesions >2 cm), infiltrative growth pattern, mitotic figures, intraluminal necrosis, and vascular and perineural invasion are clues toward the diagnosis of carcinoma. Other variants of CCs include signet ring cell, squamous, adenosquamous, sarcomatoid (spindle cell), mucinous or signet ring cell, clear cell, neuroendocrine, and lymphoepithelioma-like variants.

Cholangiocarcinoma—Pathologic Features

Gross Findings

- Intrahepatic cholangiocarcinomas (CCs) may form large single tumor masses or infiltrate diffusely
- Tumors are firm and white to tan
- Satellite nodules are common
- Hilar CCs grow as periductal growth and strictures along large ducts
- Peripheral CC appear as gray white mass-forming lesions in liver parenchyma

Microscopic Findings

- The most common pattern is adenocarcinoma
- Most are composed of small glands lined by cuboidal to columnar mucin-producing epithelium in a dense fibrous stroma
- Perineural invasion is common
- Other adenocarcinoma variants include a bland bile ductular (CC) or ductal malformation-like pattern of CC
- Squamous, signet ring or mucinous, clear cell, neuroendocrine, or sarcomatoid differentiation may also occur

Genetic

- Mutations in *KRAS, TP53, IDH1/2, ARID1A, BAP1, BRAF, and EGFR* are the most common genetic abnormalities
- *GNAS* mutations are reported in minor subset of fluke-associated CC
- IDH1/2, BRAF, and FGFR2 fusions are seen in small duct CC

Immunohistochemistry

- Most are cytokeratin (CK) 7 and CK19 positive
- Variable expression of CK20 (more common in hilar type)
- HepPar-1 and arginase 1 are negative
- Albumin ISH is positive in intrahepatic CC
- MOC31 and Ber-EP4 positive
- polyclonal CEA (pCEA) shows cytoplasmic expression
- Hepatoid variants of CC can show glypican 3 expression
- CDX-2 is usually negative but may show focal weak positivity in some cases
- CD56 and epithelial membrane antigen in small duct–type CC

Differential Diagnosis

- Metastatic adenocarcinoma
- Hepatocellular carcinoma
- Benign lesions such as florid bile ductular proliferation or bile duct adenoma

Ancillary Studies

Immunohistochemistry

Cholangiocarcinomas are positive for CK7 and CK19. Peripheral CCs are usually negative for CK-20, whereas

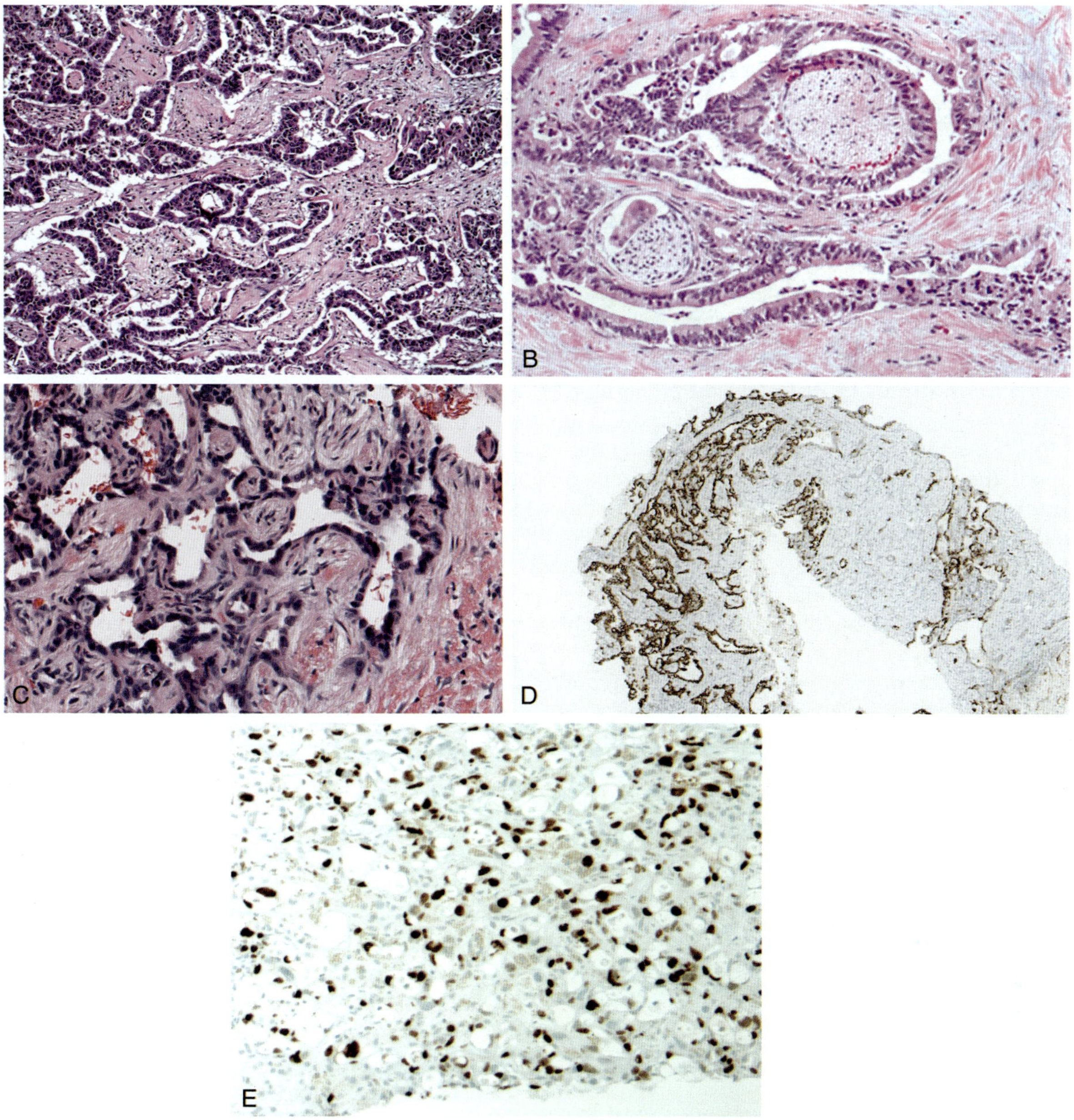

FIGURE 18.25

Cholangiocarcinomas are adenocarcinomas of varying grades that incite a striking desmoplastic response, which can be helpful in distinguishing it from pseudoglandular hepatocellular carcinoma (**A**). Perineural invasion is an almost universal finding in cholangiocarcinomas (CCs) (**B**) but is hardly ever seen in needle biopsies. Within the group of small duct cholangiocarcinomas, a subset can show a ductal plate malformation type of growth pattern (**C**). The small duct cholangiocarcinomas are known to express CD56 (**D**), which can cause diagnostic confusion on some cases. Ki67 stain reveals a proliferation rate of approximately 50% supportive of the diagnosis of malignancy (**E**).

hilar CCs are commonly positive for this marker, particularly carcinomas arising in IPNs. CDX-2 is usually negative in peripheral and hilar CC but may show focal weak reactivity in some tumors. CCs show cytoplasmic reactivity for CEA and usually are negative for AFP, arginase 1, and HepPar-1 but may be positive for albumin in situ hybridization. Glypican 3 can be positive in intrahepatic CC with hepatoid features. MOC 31 and Ber-Ep4 can be helpful in the differential diagnosis with HCC.

CD56 (Fig. 18.25D) and luminal expression of epithelial membrane antigen is described in small duct–type CC.

Differential Diagnosis

The primary challenge in diagnosing most CCs is distinction from metastatic adenocarcinoma, particularly of the pancreas, gastrointestinal tract, breast, and occasionally lung. Immunohistochemical stains are of limited use in distinguishing CC from other primary tumors and correlation with imaging findings to exclude a primary site elsewhere is usually needed for definite diagnosis. Colorectal and lung primary cancers can usually be excluded using a panel of CK7, CK20, CDX2, and thyroid transcription factor 1 (TTF-1). Albumin in situ hybridization has been reported as positive in intrahepatic CC and HCC as well as in adenocarcinomas metastatic to the liver with the exception of pancreatic adenocarcinoma.

Among the most difficult differential are benign BDAs because small duct–type CC can be extremely bland appearing. Histologic findings that support a diagnosis of CC are large size (>2 cm), infiltrative growth pattern, cytologic atypia, mitoses, intraluminal necrosis, and increased Ki67 (often >30%) (Fig. 18.25E).

The distinction between HCC and CC is usually more straightforward. HCCs display a trabecular architecture with scant fibrous stroma, a distinctly different morphology from the usual CC. Polyclonal CEA and CD10 staining in CC usually show a cytoplasmic staining pattern without the canalicular pattern typically seen in HCC. Arginase-1 immunohistochemistry may also be useful in this setting, especially in cases of poorly differentiated lesions. Glypican-3 can be problematic because it is expressed in CC with hepatoid features and in germ cell tumors such as yolk sac within can be in the differential diagnosis.

Ultrastructural examination is seldom indicated, but electron microscopy of CC cells shows typical features of adenocarcinoma, such as microvilli and true lumen formation. Epithelioid hemangioendothelioma (EHE) is easily distinguished from CC by its immunophenotype (ERG, CD31, and calmodulin binding transcription activator 1 [CAMTA 1] positivity) and morphologic features (discussed later).

Molecular Findings

Recent advances in the understanding of molecular pathways leading to CC have described two main subtypes of intrahepatic CC: The first is inflammatory (38% of cases), which is associated with alterations in *PTGS2 (COX-2)*, *GNAS*, and *STAT3*. *Kras* mutations have been described also as early events in CCs arising in PSC). The second subtype is proliferative (62% of cases), which is linked to activation of oncogene pathways, including *Ras, MAPK, c-Met, Braf, Kras, TP53, IDH* mutations, and chromosomal instability. *IDH1/2, Braf* and *FGFR2* fusions are found only in small duct–type CC.

Prognosis and Therapy

Complete resection of the tumor appears to be an important factor in prognosis in CC. The median survival period for patients with resectable intrahepatic CC is around 30 months, and the 5-year survival rate ranges between 35% and 45%. The median survival period for patients with unresectable intrahepatic tumors is only 6 to 7 months, even with adjuvant therapy. Patients with carcinomas arising in IPNs and small duct CC have a better prognosis. At autopsy, 75% of patients have metastases, usually to porta hepatis lymph nodes, peritoneal surfaces, lung, bone, and adrenal gland. Vascular invasion and high tumor stage are important poor prognostic indicators.

Adjuvant (or more recently neoadjuvant) therapy used in this setting includes chemotherapy, radiation, chemoradiation, and transarterial chemoembolization. 5-Fluoracil–based regimens, as well as gemcitabine and cisplatin are agents commonly used for the treatment of intrahepatic CC. Newer therapeutic approaches encompass targeting molecular pathways activated in intrahepatic CC (erlotinib is an epidermal growth factor receptor–inhibiting drug and more recently pemigatinib, which is a fibroblast growth factor receptor inhibitor).

COMBINED HEPATOCELLULAR–CHOLANGIOCARCINOMA

CLINICAL FEATURES

Hepatic neoplasms demonstrating morphologic features of both CC and HCC within the same tumor are classified as combined HCC–CCs. They are rare and share many epidemiologic characteristics with conventional HCC and intrahepatic CC. Imaging features also overlap and are not specific.

COMBINED HEPATOCELLULAR-CHOLANGIOCARCINOMA–FACT SHEET

Definition

- A tumor containing unequivocal morphologic evidence of both hepatocellular carcinoma (HCC) and cholangiocarcinoma (CC)

Incidence and Location

- Rare tumors
- Fewer than 5% of all liver carcinomas
- Geographic variation similar to that of HCC

Morbidity and Mortality

- Survival appears to be better than that of CC but worse than that of HCC
- Overall 3- and 5-year survival rates of 30% and 18%, respectively

Gender, Race, and Age Distribution

- Reported frequently in Asian populations
- Older adults (older than 60 years)
- Male
- Association with underling chronic liver disease is not clear

Clinical Features

- Abdominal pain
- Elevation of α-fetoprotein, CA19-9, and carcinoembryonic antigen levels

Radiologic Features

- No specific radiologic features

Prognosis and Therapy

- Resectability is a good prognostic factor
- Prognosis is worse than pure HCC
- Locoregional therapy is preferred over transplantation

Pathologic Features

Gross Findings

The gross findings are similar to those of HCC. Tumors are usually solitary; however, multiple nodules can be present. The size ranges from 3 to 15 cm. If there is a prominent CC component, the cut surface is often firm and fibrotic. Hemorrhagic and necrotic cut surfaces have also been noted.

Microscopic Findings

There are no data to support a minimum cut-off threshold for the two components. Therefore, any extent of each component is acceptable as long as the evidence is unequivocal. The classical type of combined HCC–CC is composed of conventional-appearing HCC and CC (Fig. 18.26A). Both components range in their differentiation, and immunohistochemical stains can aid in highlighting both components. Intraluminal mucin can be present in the CC component. In clinical practice, hepatocellular markers such as arginase-1 can be used to demonstrate hepatocellular differentiation (Fig. 18.26B), and CK19 is helpful in highlighting CC (Fig. 18.26C). A transitional morphology with stem cell–like features is often present at the interface of the HCC and CC. Positivity for CK19, epithelial cellular adhesion molecule (EpCAM), CD56,

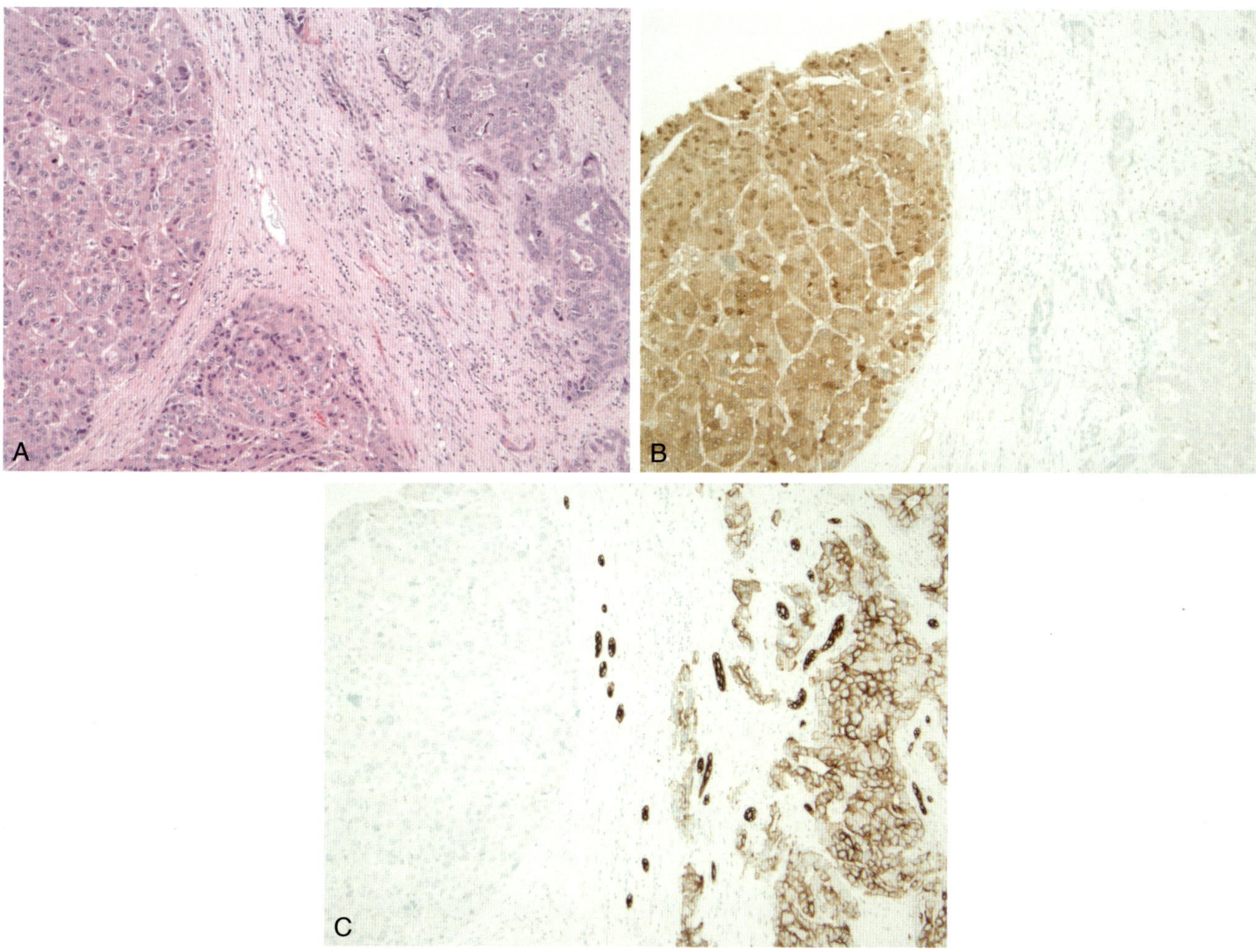

FIGURE 18.26

Combined hepatocellular–cholangiocarcinomas (HCC–CCs) are rare tumors and require demonstration of two histologically distinct components, HCC and CC (**A**). Tumor cells on the left reveal morphologic features of HCC and are positive for markers of arginase-1 (**B**), whereas the foci on the right clearly show a gland forming adenocarcinoma component consistent with CC and expressing cytokeratin 19 supportive of the diagnosis (**C**).

CD117/c-kit stain, and CD133 has been used in the past as evidence of stem cell–like features, but none of these markers are specific for hepatic or cancer stem cells and can be expressed in both components (HCC and CC). The use of the term *combined hepatocellular and cholangiocarcinoma with stem cell features* is no longer recommended in the latest WHO classification. Similarly, mere CK19 positivity in an otherwise typical HCC should not be classified as a combined HCC–CC.

Primary liver carcinomas that show a uniform, monomorphic appearance that is intermediate between hepatocytes and cholangiocytes have been classified as intermediate cell carcinoma of the liver. Immunohistochemical expression of both markers of hepatocellular and cholangiolar differentiation are present within the same cells uniformly throughout the tumor. It is unclear whether these represent a unique tumor type or a variant of combined HCC–CC. A CC component with antler-like anastomosing cords of bile ductular profiles with a high nuclear-to-cytoplasmic ratio may be present as a component of combined HCC–CC. However, when this component is present alone or admixed with other adenocarcinoma variants, it is now classified as an intrahepatic CC.

Combined Hepatocellular-Cholangiocarcinoma—Pathologic Features

Gross Findings

- Solitary or multiple nodules
- 3 to 15 cm in size
- Firm cut surface with areas of necrosis and hemorrhage

Microscopic Findings

- Variable; depends on proportion of hepatocellular carcinoma (HCC) and cholangiocarcinoma (CC) components
- Either component can be well, moderately, or poorly differentiated
- Typically, more fibrosis and desmoplasia compared with pure HCC
- Classic type demonstrates two distinct components morphologically; an intermediate zone of transition may be present
- Pure intermediate-cell tumors are classified as intermediate cell carcinoma rather than mixed tumors
- CC may be present as the CC component in a mixed HCC–CC but if present in pure form, it should be classified as an intrahepatic CC

Differential Diagnosis

- HCC with extensive pseudoglandular formation
- Metastatic carcinoma

Immunohistochemistry

- HepPar-1, Arginase-1, and/or glypican-3 in HCC areas
- Cytokeratin (CK) 19, CK7, or mucicarmine positivity in CC areas
- No marker is specific for liver stem cell phenotype other than keratin expression

Differential Diagnosis

Metastatic carcinomas can be challenging to distinguish combined HCC–CC if the HCC component is minimal. Immunohistochemical studies along with clinical and radiologic correlation can help in making this distinction. Undifferentiated carcinomas, by definition, do not show any evidence of hepatocellular or glandular differentiation but can be identified as epithelial based on keratin positivity. These can also be primary or metastatic tumors, and hence correlation with clinical and imaging findings is necessary.

Prognosis and Therapy

Long-term follow-up for these tumors is currently limited and partly reflects changing diagnostic criteria for various subtypes within the group. Patients with combined tumors who underwent resection or liver transplantation have shown worse survival compared with patients with HCC alone. At present, locoregional therapy (i.e., transarterial chemoembolization, radiofrequency ablation) is preferred.

MESENCHYMAL TUMORS BENIGN HEMANGIOMA

CLINICAL FEATURES

Cavernous hemangioma, the most common primary hepatic tumor, is usually an incidental finding at autopsy. It is more frequent in adults. Symptomatic CH is more common in women, and abdominal pain is the most common symptom. Most CHs are static over time, but the lesions can rapidly increase in size in pregnancy or with estrogen therapy. CHs may occur in conjunction with FNH.

HEMANGIOMA—FACT SHEET

Definition

- Benign vascular tumor of the liver

Incidence and Location

- Common; found in approximately 7% of autopsies
- No geographic variation

Morbidity and Mortality

- Usually incidental, innocuous finding
- Rarely, hemangiomas increase rapidly in size and rupture

Gender, Race, and Age Distribution
- More frequent in women
- More common in adults (mean age, 46 years)
- No race predilection

Clinical Features
- Most patients (>85%) are asymptomatic
- Upper abdominal mass or pain is seen in approximately 50%
- Rupture may be spontaneous or related to trauma

Radiologic Features
- Mass isodense to large blood vessels on computed tomography, with cloud-like peripheral enhancement

Prognosis and Therapy
- Excellent prognosis for incidental lesions
- Rarely, surgical excision is performed for symptomatic lesions

Pathologic Features

Gross Findings

Most CHs are small (<4 cm) solitary lesions, and background liver is normal. They are soft, spongy, and well circumscribed and may be subcapsular or deep within the parenchyma. On sectioning, CH has an empty mesh-like appearance because of escape of blood from the dilated vascular channels (Fig. 18.27).

Microscopic Findings

Cavernous hemangiomas consist of large variably sized vascular spaces lined by bland, flattened endothelial cells (Fig. 18.28). The intervening stroma consists of fibrocollagenous or myxoid tissue. Thrombi in various stages of organization are commonly found within the channels. As these thrombi undergo organization, the CH may undergo sclerosis that begins centrally but may sometimes spread to obscure the entire lesion, resulting in a fibrous nodule.

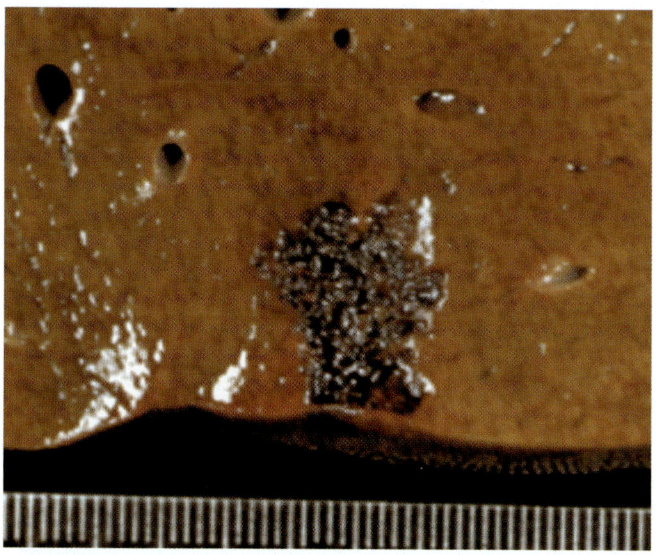

FIGURE 18.27
Cavernous hemangiomas are spongy red-brown lesions, usually incidentally discovered at imaging examinations or at autopsy.

Hemangioma—Pathologic Features

Gross Findings
- Single or multiple
- Vary from smaller than 1 cm to larger than 30 cm
- Spongy honeycombed surface on sectioning

Microscopic Findings
- Well-formed, blood-filled spaces lined by single layer of bland endothelium
- Extensive fibrosis may be seen
- Some vascular spaces may contain recent or organized thrombi

Differential Diagnosis
- Hepatic lymphangioma
- Peliosis hepatis

Differential Diagnosis

Major differential diagnostic considerations include hereditary hemorrhagic telangiectasia, lymphangioma (extremely rare), and peliosis hepatis. In hereditary hemorrhagic telangiectasia (Rendu-Osler-Weber disease), hepatic involvement is rarely symptomatic. Telangiectatic lesions, composed of dilated veins and small capillaries, arise in portal tracts and are frequently found in fibrous septa. In peliosis hepatis, the blood-filled cavities are not lined by endothelium. CH with sclerosis may be confused with other hepatic lesions that may have prominent fibrosis; the relatively acellular nature of the fibrosis should prevent confusion with malignancy. CHs with superimposed thrombosis can reveal areas of cytologic atypia and florid endothelial cell proliferation mimicking angiosarcoma.

Prognosis and Therapy

Most CHs are not associated with any morbidity or increased mortality rate. Asymptomatic CH is not treated and can be followed up with imaging. Symptomatic lesions larger than 10 cm are often treated by resection or enucleation.

INFANTILE HEMANGIOMA

Clinical Features

Infantile hemangioma (IH, previously known as infantile hemangioendothelioma) is the most common

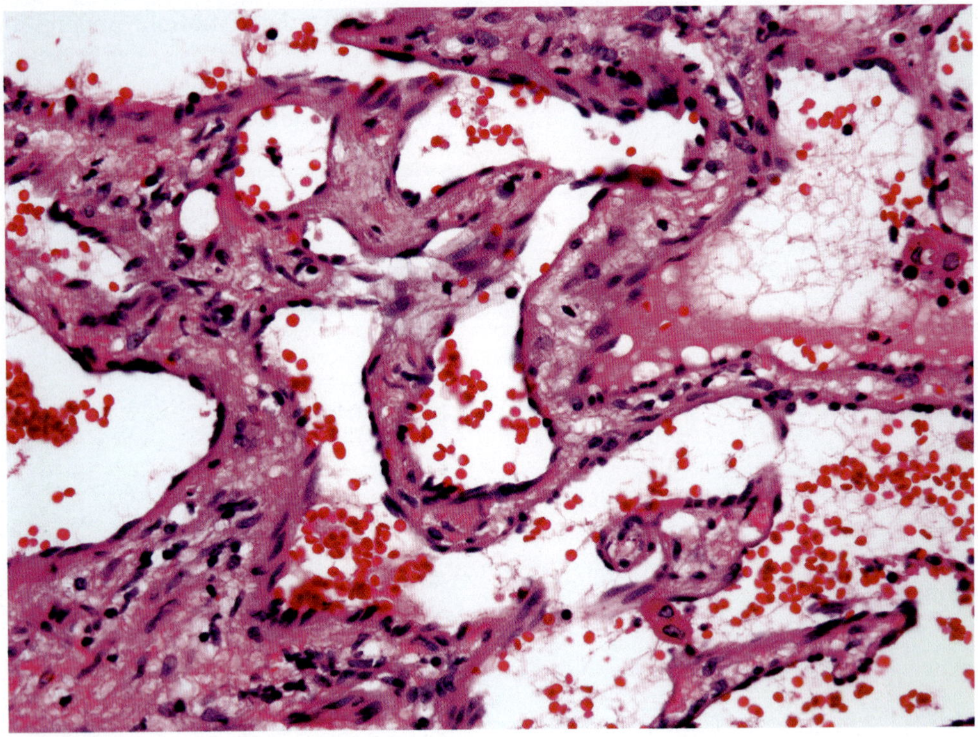

FIGURE 18.28
Large, ectatic blood-filled spaces lined by a single layer of bland endothelial cells are characteristic of cavernous hemangioma.

mesenchymal tumor of the liver in childhood, accounting for about 20% of all primary pediatric hepatic tumors. The vast majority (90%) of patients are younger than 6 months of age at the time of diagnosis. Girls are affected slightly more often than boys. Typical presenting signs include an abdominal mass and high-output cardiac failure, although a significant number of cases are asymptomatic and are discovered incidentally at autopsy after rupture. Platelet sequestration within the lesion may lead to severe thrombocytopenia and bleeding (Kasabach-Merritt syndrome). IH is associated with hemangiomas of the skin and other organs in up to 40% of cases. The serum AFP level is usually normal.

INFANTILE HEMANGIOMA—FACT SHEET

Definition
- Low-grade vascular neoplasm occurring in the first year of life

Incidence and Location
- Approximately 17% of all pediatric liver tumors
- 40% of benign liver tumors in first 21 years of life

Morbidity and Mortality
- Spontaneous regression in up to 10% of cases
- Overall survival rate is 70%
- Most deaths are associated with operative complications or congestive heart failure

Gender, Race, and Age Distribution
- Female predominance (63%)
- No racial predilection
- 90% are seen in first 6 months of life
- Almost all cases present by 2 years of age

Clinical Features
- Many patients are asymptomatic; symptoms are usually nonspecific (nausea, gastrointestinal bleeding, lethargy, liver failure)
- Most present with hepatomegaly and diffuse enlarged abdomen
- 15% present with congestive heart failure
- Associated with extrahepatic hemangiomas in approximately 10% of cases

Radiologic Features
- Hypoechoic or complex mass on ultrasonography
- Low-attenuation mass on nonenhanced computed tomography
- Fine calcifications in 50% of cases
- Magnetic resonance imaging is helpful in determining multifocality
- Enlarged tortuous feeding arteries on arteriography

Prognosis and Therapy
- Surgical resection is often curative for unifocal lesions
- Transplantation is used for large or multifocal lesions
- Hepatic artery embolization is also used for large lesions
- Jaundice and multiple tumor nodules are poor prognostic features

Pathologic Features

Gross Findings

Infantile hemangiomas may be solitary or multiple. The tumor nodules are variable in size and are well circumscribed. Smaller lesions have a vascular appearance and are red to tan, soft, and spongy; larger nodules are variegated and have a gray-white, scarred central area with calcification.

Microscopic Findings

Infantile hemangioma is composed of a proliferation of small, capillary-like, or dilated vascular spaces lined by plump endothelial cells (Figs. 18.29A and B). Occlusion of the lumen by the endothelial cells may be seen, but mitoses are rare except for proliferative areas. Areas of pseudopapillary architecture should not be interpreted as malignant. The vascular channels of IH are separated by loose connective tissue. Extramedullary hematopoiesis is present in most cases. Portal tracts may be identified embedded within the lesion (Fig. 18.29C). Areas indistinguishable from CH are often present in the center of the lesion. Degenerative changes such as thrombi, fibrosis, and stroma calcification are common in larger lesions.

Infantile Hemangioma—Pathologic Features

Gross Findings
- Single tumor in 55%
- Spongy red-brown lesions; may have areas of hemorrhage, necrosis, calcification

Microscopic Findings
- Thin vascular channels lined by single layer of plump endothelial cells
- Myxoid to dense fibrous stroma
- Margins may be well demarcated or infiltrative
- Solid areas with atypical endothelial cells should be diagnosed as angiosarcoma

Genetics
- Most tumors are diploid; aneuploidy may be associated with a poor outcome
- Balanced translocations reported

Immunohistochemistry
- Endothelial cells are positive for vascular markers: ERG, CD31, CD34, glucose transporter 1 (GLUT-1)
- Pericytes surrounding vessels are positive for α-smooth muscle actin
- Low Ki67 proliferation index

Differential Diagnosis
- Hemangioma
- Mesenchymal hamartoma

Ancillary Studies

Immunohistochemistry

The endothelial nature of the lining cells is easily demonstrated by immunohistochemical stains for ERG, glucose transporter 1 (GLUT-1), CD31, and CD34.

Differential Diagnosis

Infantile hemangioma should be differentiated from angiosarcoma. An infiltrative margin can be found in IH and is not a discriminating feature. Mitotic activity is more pronounced in angiosarcoma, there is higher KI67 proliferative index, and hypercellularity caused by densely packed tumor cells and marked cytologic atypia also favors angiosarcoma. Of note, pediatric patients with angiosarcoma are typically older than 1.5 years. The presence of extrahepatic tumors in patients with IH is not indicative of metastatic spread.

When considering benign vascular lesions and vascular malformations in the differential diagnosis, GLUT-1 stain can be helpful because it is only positive in IH. CH lacks the proliferation of numerous small blood vessels found in IH.

Myxoid stroma in IH may be confused with mesenchymal hamartoma (MH), but the presence of calcification suggests the possibility of IH.

Prognosis and Therapy

Roughly 70 % of patients survive at least 7 years; most deaths occur within 1 month of diagnosis. Congestive heart failure and jaundice are the factors most often associated with death, but multiple nodules and the absence of cavernous differentiation are also adverse prognostic features. Solitary lesions may be resected. Ablative therapies may be considered, and in some cases, liver transplantation has been performed. Spontaneous regression may occur in some cases.

MESENCHYMAL HAMARTOMA

Clinical Features

Mesenchymal hamartoma is the second most common benign pediatric tumor. Most patients are male, and 75 % show symptoms by 1 year of age. Serum AFP levels are usually normal but can be slightly elevated for age. The neoplastic nature of MH has not been conclusively established; alternative theories include aberrant development of primitive mesenchyme in portal tracts associated with ductal plate malformation and localized ischemia during development.

Pathologic Features

Gross Findings

Mesenchymal hamartoma is solitary and well circumscribed, is usually large (≤23 cm), and is more common

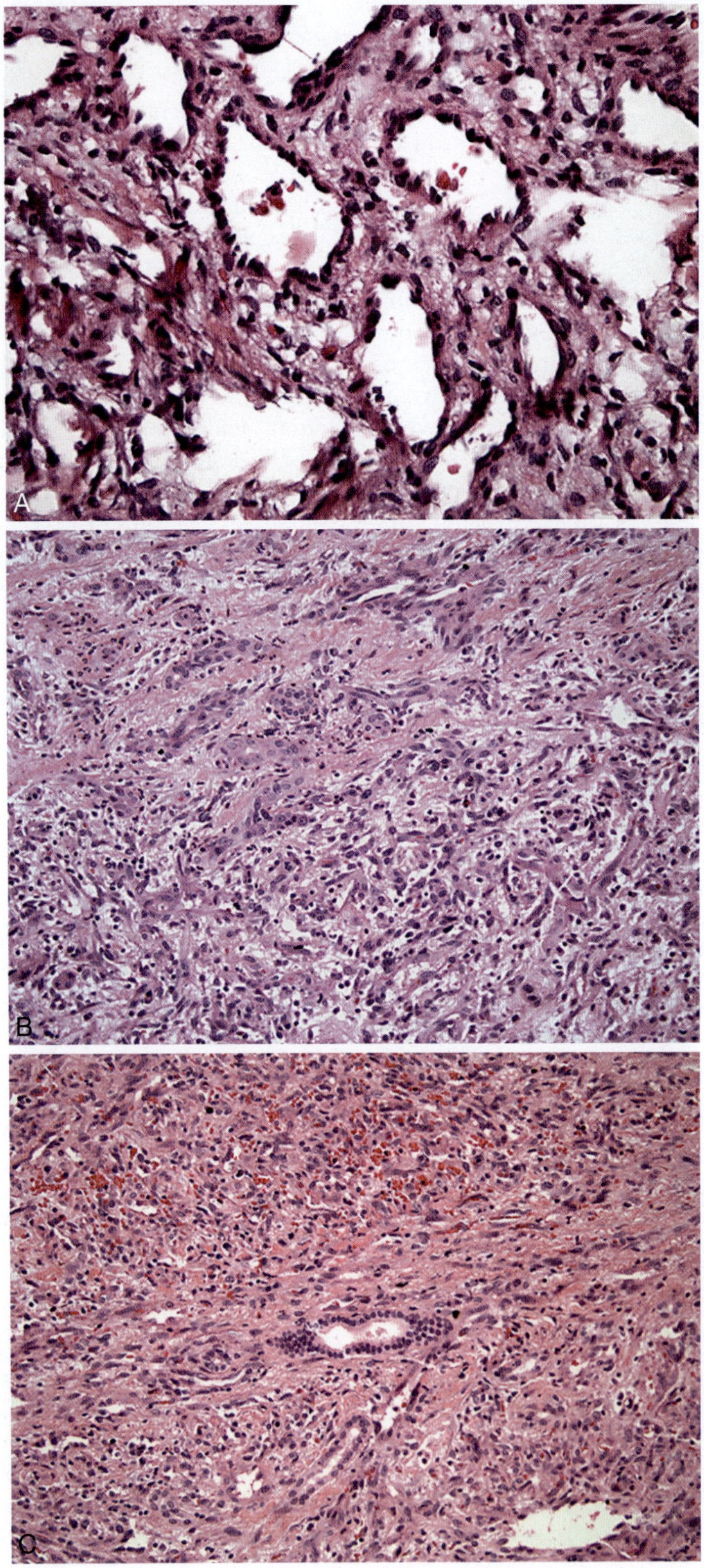

FIGURE 18.29

Infantile hemangioma shows irregular vascular channels separated by loose edematous stroma (**A**) or densely cellular granulation tissue–like areas (**B**) that may harbor entrapped portal tracts (**C**).

MESENCHYMAL HAMARTOMA—FACT SHEET

Definition

- Benign lesion occurring in young children; composed of large fluid-filled cysts surrounded by mesenchymal stroma

Incidence and Location

- 8% of all pediatric liver tumors
- No geographic variation

Morbidity and Mortality

- 90% survival rate
- Mortality and morbidity are primarily related to surgical complications

Gender, Race, and Age Distribution

- Male predominance (male-to-female ratio, 2:1)
- No race predilection
- Median age, 10 months

Clinical Features

- Most common presentation is enlarging abdomen
- Physical examination reveals a nontender mass

Radiologic Features

- Ultrasonography shows complex multicystic mass
- May be detected in utero
- Computed tomography shows variation in cyst size and septal thickness

Prognosis and Therapy

- Surgical excision is the preferred therapy
- Rare examples of embryonal sarcoma arising in conjunction with mesenchymal hamartoma have been reported

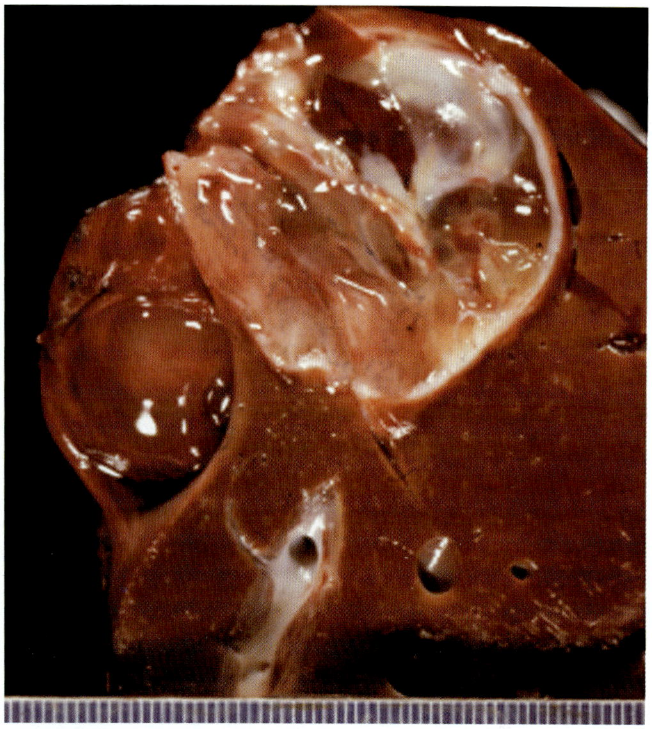

FIGURE 18.30

Mesenchymal hamartomas are large, well-circumscribed lesions with variable sized degenerative cystic spaces with smooth surfaces.

in the right lobe. In most cases, multiple cysts are present, imparting a multilocular appearance (Fig. 18.30). The cysts contain clear or mucoid fluid, do not communicate with the bile duct, and are separated by solid areas that become fibrotic with age.

Microscopic Findings

Mesenchymal hamartoma is characterized by a mixture of different cell types, including mesenchymal elements, bile ducts, nests of hepatocytes, and vessels. The cysts occur secondary to degenerative changes in the mesenchymal component but rarely represent dilated bile ducts lined by attenuated biliary epithelium (Fig. 18.31A). This stroma consists of bland stellate and spindle cells embedded in a myxoid matrix that may show variable fibrosis (Fig. 18.31B). Extramedullary hematopoiesis is an almost universal finding. The bile ducts may show progressive dilation and an aberrant architecture reminiscent of ductal plate malformation. The biliary epithelium is often flattened, with atrophic or degenerative changes, and a periductal neutrophilic infiltrate may be present.

Mesenchymal Hamartoma—Pathologic Features

Gross Findings

- Involves right lobe in 75% of cases
- Pedunculated in up to 30% of cases
- Vary from a few centimeters to more than 30 cm
- Cysts in more than 85% of cases; cysts are filled with clear amber fluid
- Hemorrhage and necrosis are rare and suggest undifferentiated sarcoma

Microscopic Findings

- Mixture of bile ducts, hepatocytes, loose mesenchyme, and vessels
- Degenerative cystic changes lacking epithelial lining are common
- Loose edematous stroma with scattered bland stellate cells
- Dilated bile ducts at periphery of lesion may be surrounded by dense collar of fibrosis
- Extramedullary hematopoiesis is common

Genetics

- Chromosome 19q13.4 alterations (MHLB1), translocations between chromosomes 15 and 19, 11 and 19 are consistently reported and cases with germline DICER1 mutations have also been described. Some authors have reported chromosome 19 inversions in a subset of cases

Differential Diagnosis

- Myxoid change in infantile hemangioma
- Embryonal sarcoma

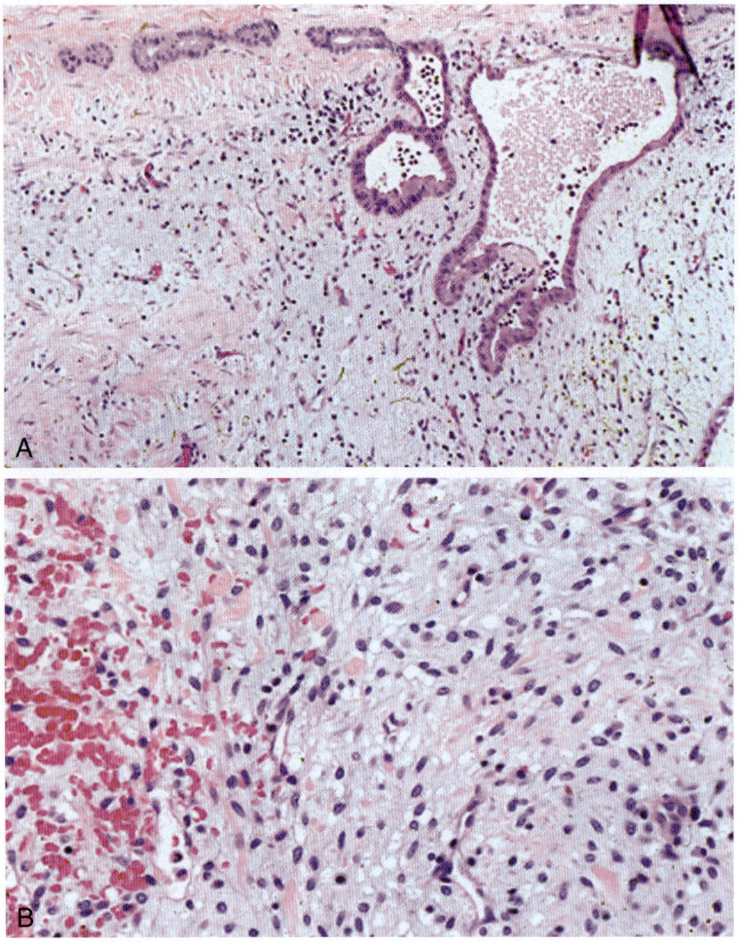

FIGURE 18.31

The bile ducts in mesenchymal hamartoma may undergo progressive cystic dilation (**A**), and the stroma is abundant, loose, edematous, and myxoid with bland stellate stromal cells (**B**).

ANCILLARY STUDIES

Ancillary work-up is not helpful except in ruling out a metastatic tumor or undifferentiated sarcoma.

PROGNOSIS AND THERAPY

The treatment of choice is total excision, which is curative. The perioperative mortality rate is relatively high (≤17%) and is related to technical difficulties with surgical resection. Recurrence of incompletely resected lesions has not been reported. MH has rarely been associated with embryonal sarcoma, raising the possibility of malignant transformation of MH.

ANGIOMYOLIPOMA

CLINICAL FEATURES

Hepatic angiomyolipomas (AMLs) are rare benign tumors that predominantly affect women and belong to the perivascular epithelioid cell tumor family. Although usually detected incidentally, large tumors may cause abdominal discomfort. Tumor rupture with intraabdominal bleeding is an uncommon complication. Association of hepatic AML with tuberous sclerosis occurs in only 6% to 10% of cases compared with 20% to 40% of cases of renal AML. Tumors with a low-fat content are often mistaken for other benign or malignant lesions on imaging studies.

PATHOLOGIC FEATURES

GROSS FINDINGS

Hepatic AMLs are usually solitary, well-circumscribed, nonencapsulated lesions. Tumor size varies from a few millimeters to larger than 36 cm. The gross appearance is highly dependent on the tumor composition. Whereas the fatty component may be evident as soft, yellow regions, the vascular component may appear as hemorrhagic foci (Fig. 18.32). Myomatous areas are soft, white-tan, and homogeneous. Necrosis is not commonly present.

ANGIOMYOLIPOMA—FACT SHEET

Definition

- Rare benign lesion composed of a combination of abnormal blood vessels, myoid cells, and adipocytes

Incidence and Location

- Rare
- No known geographic variation

Morbidity and Mortality

- Generally benign
- Rare malignant examples reported

Gender, Race, and Age Distribution

- Female predominance (1.4:1 to 9:1)
- No known race predilection
- Adult patients; no specific age group

Clinical Features

- Most lesions are asymptomatic and detected incidentally
- Large lesions may present with abdominal pain

Radiologic Features

- Heterogeneous, circumscribed, hyperechoic lesion on ultrasound
- Computed tomography shows a hypodense mass with marked early contrast enhancement, as well as delayed enhancement in the portal venous phase
- Magnetic resonance imaging is very sensitive for the detection of the fatty component on T1-weighted images (high signal intensity)

Prognosis and Therapy

- Surgical excision usually indicated; nonsurgical management may be an option for selected patients
- Excellent prognosis

MICROSCOPIC FINDINGS

Hepatic AMLs are composed of three basic histologic elements: blood vessels, myoid cells, and adipocytes (Fig. 18.33A). Tumors have been classified as angiomatous, myomatous, lipomatous, or mixed, depending on the proportion of each element present in an individual lesion. Although a lipomatous component is usually present in hepatic AMLs, the fatty areas may be inconspicuous and may not be represented in core biopsies. Myoid cells may show different histologic appearances, including spindled,

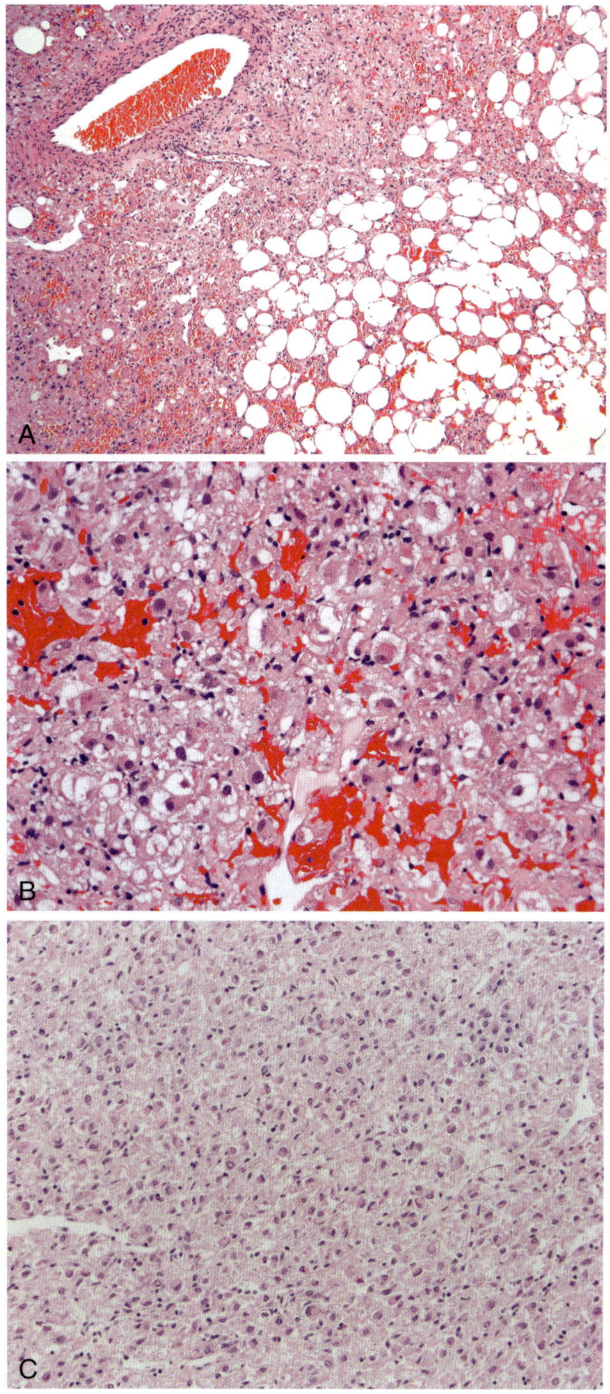

FIGURE 18.33

Angiomyolipomas contain variable amounts of thick-walled vessels, spindle or epithelioid myoid cells, and adipose tissue (**A**). Myoid cells with epithelioid morphology can mimic a variety of epithelial and mesenchymal tumors (**B**). Tumors with minimal or no adipose tissue also occur (**C**). The eccentric nuclei with abundant eosinophilic cytoplasm, reminiscent of rhabdomyoblasts, should raise suspicion for a myomelanocytic tumor involving the liver.

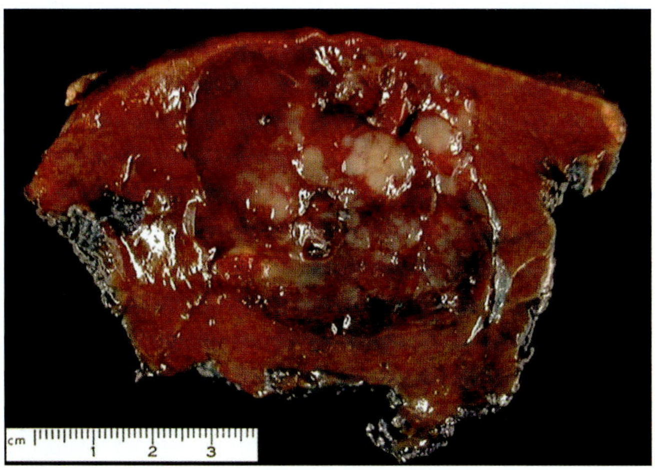

FIGURE 18.32

Hepatic angiomyolipoma is usually a well-circumscribed soft lesion with areas of hemorrhage and adipose tissue in a background of normal liver parenchyma.

epithelioid, and intermediate morphology. Epithelioid myoid cells are commonly present in hepatic AMLs and may cause significant diagnostic difficulties. They are large, polygonal cells with abundant clear to eosinophilic cytoplasm and a round nucleus with a single, often prominent nucleolus (Figs. 18.33B and C). Although mitoses are not numerous, the epithelioid myoid component may show considerable cytologic atypia. Hemosiderin and melanin pigment may be present. The vascular component is comprised of tortuous, thick-walled blood vessels. In addition, extramedullary hematopoiesis may also be present in hepatic AMLs, a feature not typically seen in renal AMLs. An infiltrating growth pattern with tumor invasion of portal tracts and liver parenchyma has been reported in AMLs that had a benign clinical course upon follow-up; these features, therefore, should not be regarded as an indication of malignant behavior. Malignant AMLs resulting in metastatic disease or death are very rare.

Angiomyolipoma—Pathologic Features

Gross Findings

- Well-circumscribed lesion, variable size (0.1–36 cm)
- Gross appearance varies according to tumor composition—combination of hemorrhagic foci (vascular component), white-tan, solid, homogeneous areas (myomatous component), and soft, yellow areas (lipomatous component)
- Normal background liver

Microscopic Findings

- Angiomatous: abnormal, thick-walled vessels
- Myomatous: myoid cells, which may have a spindle cell, epithelioid, or intermediate morphology
- Myoid cells with epithelioid morphology are common in hepatic angiomyolipomas (AMLs) and may be misinterpreted as neoplastic hepatocytes, or another epithelial malignancy
- A lipomatous component usually present but may be inconspicuous
- A subset of tumors may show significant atypia; the presence of diffuse atypia, increased mitoses, or atypical mitoses is associated with aggressive behavior

Genetics

- Most hepatic AMLs are monoclonal lesions, although no characteristic molecular abnormalities have been described
- Similar gene expression profile as activated stellate cells by cDNA microarray

Differential Diagnosis

- Benign and malignant hepatocellular tumors (myomatous variant)
- Metastatic carcinomas and melanoma (myomatous variant)
- Focal fatty change, steatotic hepatocellular tumors (lipomatous variant)
- Hemangioma, vascular malformations (angiomatous variant)

Ancillary Studies

Immunohistochemistry

Hepatic AMLs are myomelanocytic tumors (Fig. 18.34) that are positive for melanocytic (human melanoma black [HMB-45], Melan-A, microphthalmia transcription factor [MiTF], tyrosinase) and smooth muscle markers (desmin, SMA). Pancytokeratin, S100, SOX-10, Hep-Par 1, and arginase-1 are negative and may be used to differentiate AMLs from metastatic carcinomas and hepatocellular lesions.

Differential Diagnosis

Hepatic AMLs with one predominant component may pose diagnostic dilemmas. Angiomatous AMLs must be distinguished from hepatic hemangiomas and vascular malformations, whereas lipomatous AMLs may be confused with focal fatty change and hepatocellular lesions with prominent steatosis. The differential diagnosis of myomatous AML is broader and includes hepatocellular lesions (liver cell adenoma and HCC), metastatic carcinomas from various sites, and metastatic melanomas. Recognition of the additional components of the lesions is the key for a correct diagnosis, which may be confirmed by demonstrating myomelanocytic differentiation on immunohistochemistry. Metastatic carcinomas and hepatocellular lesions can be excluded with CKs and hepatocytic immunohistochemical markers. The nonfatty component of hepatic AML is S-100 negative, which is helpful in excluding metastatic melanomas.

Prognosis and Therapy

Most patients with hepatic AMLs are managed surgically, although observation may be appropriate in selected cases. Hepatic AMLs are generally benign lesions and have an excellent prognosis. Only rare, anecdotal cases of malignant AMLs have been reported.

MALIGNANT ANGIOSARCOMA

CLINICAL FEATURES

Although hepatic angiosarcoma (HAS) is the most common primary malignant mesenchymal tumor of the liver in adults, overall it is quite rare, with only about 200 cases of HAS diagnosed annually worldwide, for an estimated annual occurrence of 10 to 20 cases in the United States. HAS usually occurs in older men and has been associated with vinyl chloride exposure and Thorotrast administration. HAS caused by environmental exposure is associated with a prolonged latency period. Patients present with abdominal pain, fatigue, weight loss, or an abdominal mass.

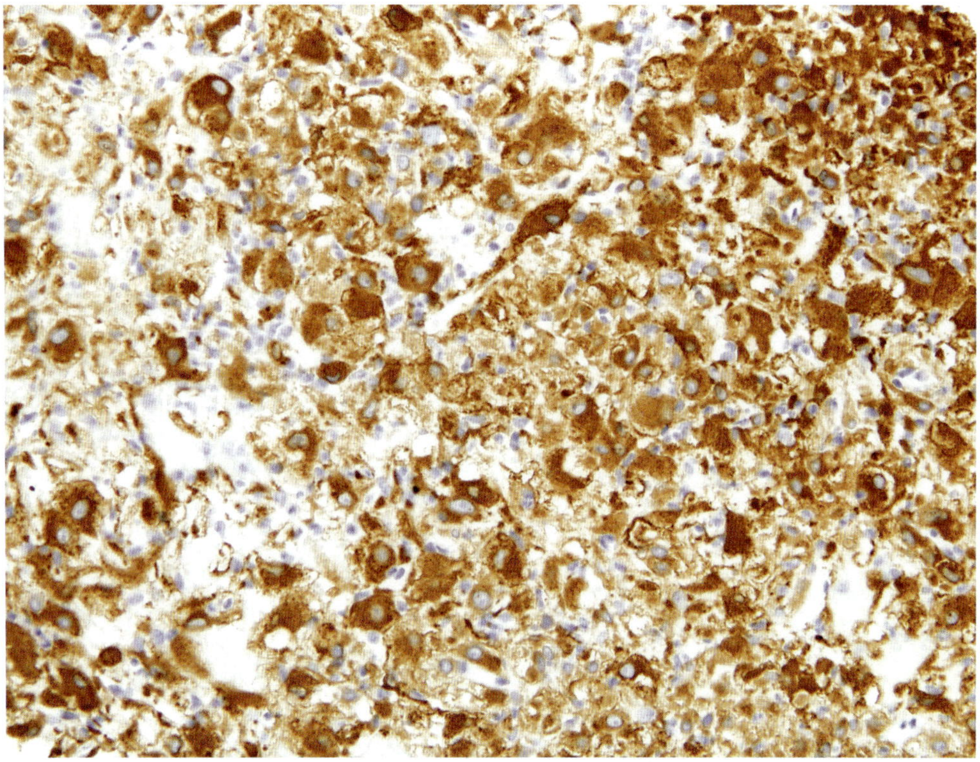

FIGURE 18.34

Positive staining for myoid markers, desmin, or smooth muscle actin, along with strong human melanoma black reactivity (illustrated in this figure), is characteristic of angiomyolipomas. Other markers of melanocytic differentiation (S100, MART1, Sox10) can also be variably positive.

ANGIOSARCOMA—FACT SHEET

Definition

- High-grade malignant neoplasm of endothelial cells

Incidence and Location

- Most common primary hepatic sarcoma
- 200 cases diagnosed worldwide annually

Morbidity and Mortality

- Rapidly fatal tumor, with most patients dead within 6 months of liver failure or hemorrhage

Gender, Race, and Age Distribution

- Male predominance (male-to-female ratio, 3:1)
- No race predilection
- Peak age incidence is in the seventh decade of life

Clinical Features

- Patients may present with symptoms of liver disease, hemoperitoneum caused by tumor ruptures, splenomegaly, or symptoms related to metastasis
- The most important known etiologic factors are exposure to vinyl chloride, Thorotrast, or androgenic steroids

Radiologic Features

- Nonenhanced computed tomography shows hypodense masses that are isodense on delayed postcontrast scans
- Abnormal vascular pattern on angiography

Prognosis and Therapy

- The prognosis is dismal
- Chemotherapy is ineffective
- Surgery and radiation have been used in rare cases

Pathologic Features

Gross Findings

Hepatic angiosarcoma is usually multicentric and involves both lobes. The spleen is often involved at the time of diagnosis. Individual tumor foci are infiltrative, variable in size, and heterogeneous, with solid areas alternating with large blood-filled spaces.

Microscopic Findings

Hepatic angiosarcoma is composed of highly atypical, large, plump, pleomorphic endothelial cells with hyperchromatic nuclei (Fig. 18.35). Solid areas resembling fibrosarcoma and bizarre tumor giant cells may be seen. Mitotic figures are easily identified. At the periphery of the lesion, tumor cells of HAS display a characteristic growth pattern of spread along preexisting sinusoids. Obliteration of sinusoids by tumor cells leads to hepatocyte atrophy. Tumor invasion of portal or hepatic vein branches is common.

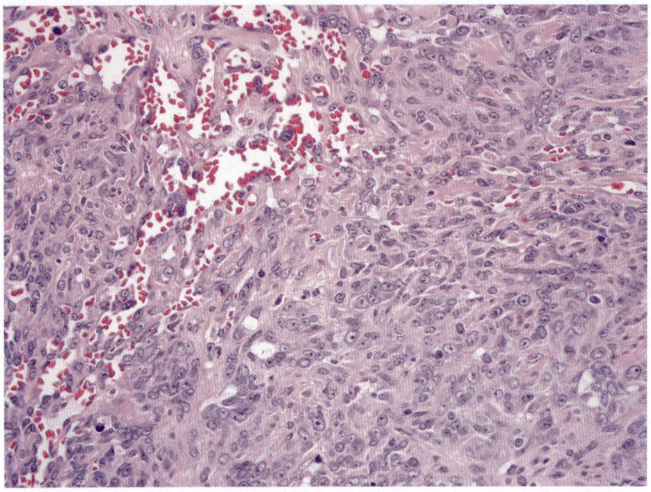

FIGURE 18.35

Angiosarcomas show a cellular proliferation of highly atypical cells that are spindle or epithelioid in shape and may form narrow vascular channels.

ANGIOSARCOMA—PATHOLOGIC FEATURES

Gross Findings

- Gray-white tumor tissue alternates with hemorrhagic areas
- Entire liver is usually involved

Microscopic Findings

- Tumor cells grow along sinusoids and other preformed vascular channels and replace normal endothelial cells
- Tumor cells are highly pleomorphic spindle cells and may grow as solid nodules
- Areas of infarct, atrophy, and fibrosis are frequent

Molecular alterations

- *TP53* mutations mTOR (mammalian target of rapamycin) pathway alterations; PTEN deletions rare

Immunohistochemistry

- Tumor cells are positive for endothelial markers: ERG, CD31, and CD34 (only in 50% of cases)
- Keratin expression can be seen in epithelioid angiosarcoma

Differential Diagnosis

- Other primary or metastatic sarcomas
- Hepatic metastases of angiosarcoma arising in other organs

ANCILLARY STUDIES

ELECTRON MICROSCOPY

Demonstration of Weibel-Palade bodies by electron microscopy may confirm the diagnosis, but ultrastructural examination is rarely necessary.

IMMUNOHISTOCHEMISTRY

Immunoreactivity for vascular markers (ERG, CD31, CD34, FLI-1) confirms the vascular nature of the tumor. Epithelioid angiosarcomas, a minor subset (10%), may be keratin positive, leading to confusion with a carcinoma.

DIFFERENTIAL DIAGNOSIS

Subtle foci, especially at the infiltrate edge of the lesion, may be mistaken for inflammatory or benign vascular disorders. The atypia of the sinusoidal lining cells distinguishes HAS from benign mimics. The pattern of infiltration along sinusoids seen in HAS should not be confused with HCC, in which the hepatocytes, not the endothelial cells, are malignant. Kaposi's sarcoma may be confused with HAS; however, clinical history of acquired immunodeficiency syndrome (AIDS) and positive staining in endothelial cells for human herpesvirus 8 facilitates the diagnosis.

PROGNOSIS AND THERAPY

The prognosis for patients with HAS is dismal, with most patients dying within months of diagnosis. Available therapies are ineffective. Hepatic failure and intraabdominal bleeding are the most common causes of death. At autopsy, most patients have metastases, most frequently to the lung.

EPITHELIOID HEMANGIOENDOTHELIOMA

CLINICAL FEATURES

Epithelioid hemangioendothelioma is a malignant vascular neoplasm most commonly developing in middle-aged women. Common presenting symptoms are abdominal pain and weight loss and, rarely, hepatic rupture or liver failure. Involvement of major hepatic vein branches or terminal hepatic venules may produce hepatic venous outflow obstruction. In about 40% of cases, EHE may be an incidental finding. The cause of EHE is unknown, although OCS use has been suggested as an etiologic factor. Multicentricity is not uncommon in these tumors.

PATHOLOGIC FEATURES

GROSS FINDINGS

Grossly, EHE lesions are usually multiple ill-defined tumor nodules of variable size, with involvement of both

EPITHELIOID HEMANGIOENDOTHELIOMA–FACT SHEET

Definition

- Low-intermediate grade malignant neoplasm of endothelial cells

Incidence and Location

- Rare tumor
- No reported geographic variation

Morbidity and Mortality

- Approximately 75% 5-year survival rate, independent of therapy
- Metastases in 25%, primarily to lung, abdominal lymph node, omentum, and peritoneum; does not preclude long-term survival

Gender, Race, and Age Distribution

- Female predominance (62%)
- No race predilection
- Wide age range (12–86 years)

Clinical Features

- Incidental finding in many cases
- Weakness, anorexia, nausea, jaundice, hepatomegaly
- Two-thirds have elevated alkaline phosphatase levels at presentation

Radiologic Features

- On computed tomography, low-attenuation, peripheral tumor nodules
- Signal halo around nodules on magnetic resonance imaging

Prognosis and Therapy

- Outcome is unpredictable
- Approximately 30% metastasize or involve other organ systems
- Treatment ranges from observation only to chemotherapy and radiation to liver transplantation

lobes. Tumor nodules are typically gray to white, firm, and sometimes gritty. Vascular channels are not appreciated on gross examination.

Microscopic Features

Epithelioid hemangioendothelioma often demonstrates a zonal pattern. At the periphery, portal tracts are spared and are surrounded by a sinusoidal proliferation of tumor cells, with residual intact hepatocytes and scanty myxoid stroma. Progressive obliteration of the sinusoids results in atrophic hepatocyte plates in the midzonal portion of the hepatic acinus. In zone 3, the tumor stroma becomes progressively sclerotic, and central veins may be partially or totally obliterated by tumor cells. However, this feature cannot be evaluated in biopsies, and the diagnosis rests on demonstration of epithelioid tumor cells in cords, small nests, or single cells embedded in a myxohyaline or dense collagenous matrix (Fig. 18.36). Dendritic cells are spindle shaped or stellate. Epithelioid cells are rounded and display a greater amount of eosinophilic cytoplasm. A notable feature is the presence of one or more well-defined intracytoplasmic vacuoles of variable size that represent vascular lumen formation may contain erythrocytes.

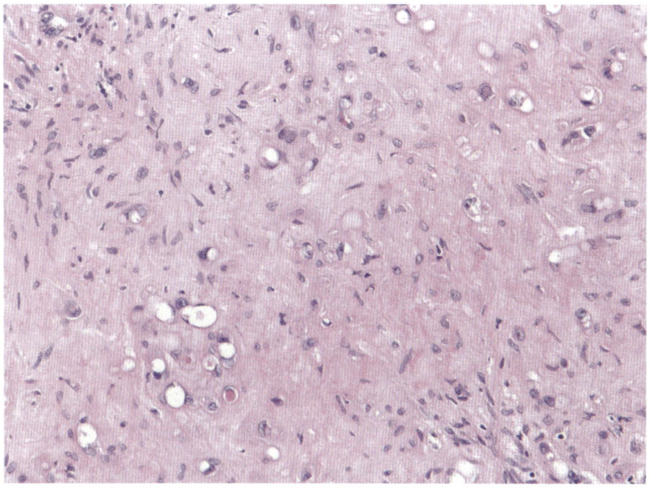

FIGURE 18.36

Neoplastic cells in epithelioid hemangioendothelioma are embedded in collagenous or myxoid stroma and show foci of intracytoplasmic lumen that mimic carcinoma. A subset is also keratin positive and may lead to misdiagnosis (not shown).

EPITHELIOID HEMANGIOENDOTHELIOMA–PATHOLOGIC FEATURES

Gross Findings

- Multiple white to tan firm nodules involving the entire liver
- Margins of lesions appear hyperemic
- Nodules vary from a few millimeters to several centimeters

Microscopic Findings

- Ill-defined lesions
- In early stages, tumor spares portal areas
- Tumor cells grow along sinusoids and cause atrophy of liver cell plates
- Myxoid or collagenous stroma with epithelioid or spindle cells in clusters, nests or single cells
- Cytoplasmic vacuoles represent intracellular vascular lumina and may contain erythrocytes

Immunohistochemistry

- Tumor cells are positive for vascular endothelial markers ERG, CD31, CD34
- Keratin 8/18 expression in a subset of cases
- Positivity for calmodulin binding transcription activator 1 (CAMTA1) (85%–90%) on immunohistochemistry is diagnostic

Differential Diagnosis

- Angiosarcoma
- Cholangiocarcinoma
- Non-neoplastic diseases

Ancillary Studies

Electron Microscopy

Ultrastructural examination reveals Weibel-Palade bodies, characteristic of endothelial cells, and numerous intermediate filaments, which are responsible for the epithelioid histologic appearance.

Immunohistochemistry

The tumor cells demonstrate immunoreactivity for ERG, CD31, and CD34 but are negative for CEA. Nearly 15% of EHEs are positive for keratins. Positivity for CAMTA1 is diagnostic (Fig. 18.37).

Genetics. *WWTR1-CAMTA1* fusion present in approximately 90% of cases and involves chromosomal regions 1p36.3 and 3q25. A minor subset has been shown to harbor a *YAP1-TFE3* gene fusion.

Differential Diagnosis

The differential diagnosis includes other neoplasms such as metastatic adenocarcinoma (particularly the signet ring cell carcinoma), CC, and neuroendocrine neoplasms. These tumors can be distinguished from EHE by their lack of zonal growth pattern, cytologic features, and negative staining for endothelial markers. Although neuroendocrine tumors may contain dense sclerotic stroma, their trabecular growth pattern and other characteristic features make the diagnosis straightforward.

Non-neoplastic lesions such as sclerosed hemangioma, fibrous scarring, granulation tissue, and cirrhosis may also be confused with EHE. Sclerosed hemangiomas are paucicellular and well circumscribed and do not invade veins. The distinction between primary hepatic EHE and metastatic EHE, usually from the lung, is not possible on morphologic grounds.

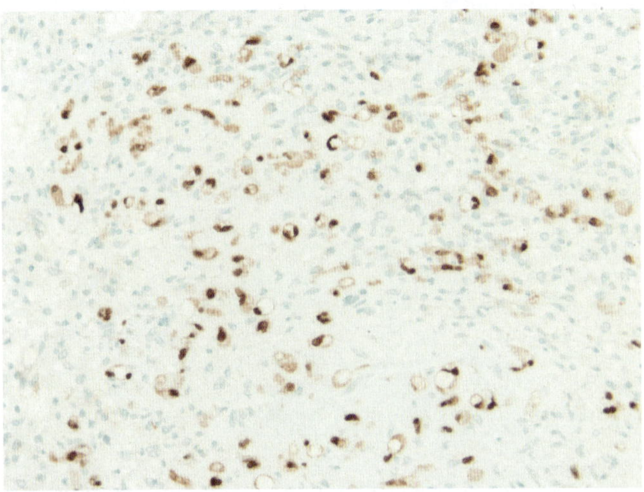

FIGURE 18.37

The neoplastic cells of epithelioid hemangioendothelioma mark strongly with vascular markers, such as ERG, CD31, CD34, but positivity for CAMTA1 (as shown in the figure) is diagnostic for these tumors.

Prognosis and Therapy

The clinical course of EHE is variable and unpredictable. Some patients die within months of initial diagnosis, but roughly 20% survive for at least 5 years. Resection is usually performed if possible, and hepatic transplantation has led to improved survival even in selected unresectable cases showing signs of extrahepatic disease. Prolonged survival with metastatic disease has been reported. Extrahepatic involvement (lung, omentum or mesentery, lymph nodes) is noted in 50% of patients and may reflect multicentricity rather than metastatic spread.

EMBRYONAL SARCOMA OF THE LIVER

CLINICAL FEATURES

Embryonal sarcoma of the liver (ESL) (also previously described as undifferentiated sarcoma, mesenchymal sarcoma, and malignant mesenchymoma) is a rare malignancy occurring almost exclusively in the pediatric population. Most patients with ESL are between 6 and 10 years of age, and more than 90% are 21 years of age or younger. There is no gender predilection. Patients lack a history of chronic liver disease. An abdominal mass or abdominal pain is the most common presentation.

EMBRYONAL SARCOMA OF THE LIVER—FACT SHEET

Definition

- Primitive primary sarcoma of liver; more common in children

Incidence and Location

- Approximately 6% of primary liver neoplasms in childhood

Morbidity and Mortality

- Prolonged survival and cure possible with multiagent chemotherapy followed by surgical resection
- Morbidity related to massive local tumor growth

Gender, Race, and Age Distribution

- Equal distribution between sexes
- No race predilection
- Most common between 6 and 10 years of age; rare in those older than 20 years of age

Clinical Features

- Most patients present with abdominal swelling, with or without a palpable mass

Radiologic Features

- Computed tomography reveals a hypodense mass with solid and cystic areas
- Tumor is usually hypovascular

Prognosis and Therapy

- Multiagent chemotherapy followed by surgical resection
- Combined modality treatment has improved survival; previously reported as 15% 5-year survival rate

Radiologic Features

Embryonal sarcoma of the liver is usually hypodense on CT scan, with solid and cystic areas. The tumor is generally hypovascular.

Pathologic Features

Gross Findings

Embryonal sarcoma of the liver is usually a large, bulky solitary mass measuring up to 30 cm in diameter. On macroscopic examination, the tumor is a well-circumscribed, soft, gray mass; degenerative changes are common and include necrosis, hemorrhage, and cystic degeneration.

Microscopic Findings

Embryonal sarcomas of the liver are composed predominantly of large, highly atypical spindle to stellate cells with ill-defined cell borders embedded in abundant fibromyxoid stroma (Fig. 18.38A). Cell density may be quite variable. Multinucleation, cellular anaplasia, and numerous mitotic figures are usually found. Cytoplasmic hyaline globules that are PAS positive and diastase resistant are a characteristic finding and may represent α1AT uptake by tumor cells (Fig. 18.38B).

Ancillary Studies

Electron Microscopy

Ultrastructural features are consistent with mesenchymal differentiation.

Embryonal Sarcoma of the Liver—Pathologic Features

Gross Findings

- Most occur in the right lobe and measure up to 20 cm in diameter
- Cut surface is gray-white, variegated, and glistening with cystic areas

Microscopic Findings

- Tumor cells are stellate or spindle shaped and loosely arranged in myxoid stroma
- Tumor cells are often bizarre, with numerous mitotic figures
- Multiple eosinophilic periodic acid–Schiff–positive cytoplasmic globules are a characteristic feature

Ultrastructural Findings

- Fibroblastic, smooth muscle, and skeletal muscle differentiation may be demonstrated

Genetics

- No single characteristic abnormalities
- Multiple cytogenetic alterations reported

Immunohistochemistry

- Tumor cells may express cytokeratins, are usually positive for vimentin, and may express α1-antitrypsin and α_1-chymotrypsin

Differential Diagnosis

- Mesenchymal hamartoma
- Mixed epithelial and mesenchymal hepatoblastoma
- Other hepatic sarcomas

Immunohistochemistry

Immunohistochemical studies have indicated variable immunoreactivity with antibodies to desmin, muscle-specific actin, calponin, CD10, CD68, and cytokeratin. HepPar-1, myogenin, MyoD1, CD34, CD117, ALK-1, S100, and β-catenin are usually negative. Areas of specific sarcomatous differentiation are positive for markers of their respective lineage.

Differential Diagnosis

The sarcomatoid (spindle cell) variant of HCC is distinguished by identification of typical foci of HCC. Hepatoblastoma should also demonstrate epithelial areas with fetal or embryonal hepatocellular features; despite the dissimilar immunohistochemical profile and morphologic findings, glypican 3 can be expressed in 50% of ESL cases, creating confusion. MH is cytologically bland and paucicellular relative to ESL.

Prognosis and Therapy

Survival in patients with ESL has improved with modern therapy. Multiagent chemotherapy followed by complete

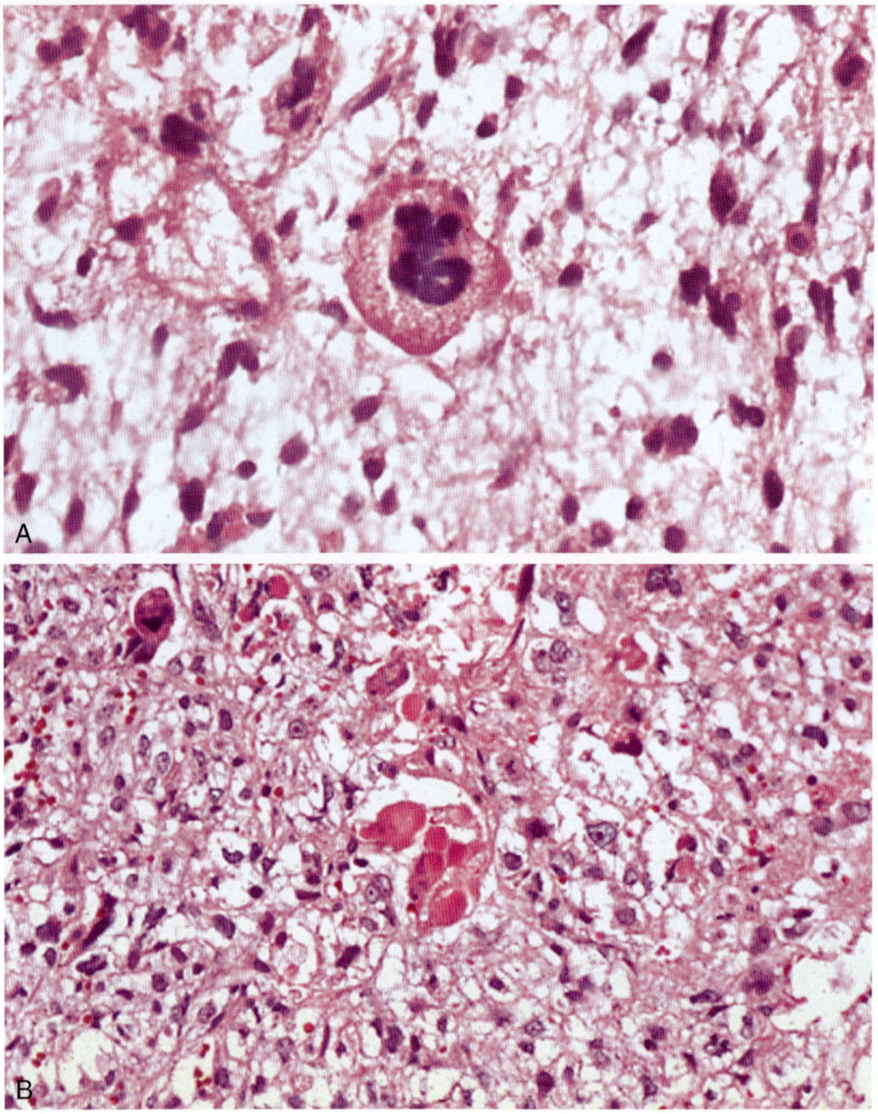

FIGURE 18.38

Embryonal sarcoma of the liver shows large, bizarre tumor cells in a cellular background of neoplastic spindle to stellate cells (**A**). Cytoplasmic globular inclusions are common (**B**) and may be positive for α1-antitrypsin.

resection has resulted in long-term disease-free survival (>10 years) in some cases. The lung, pleura, and peritoneum are the most common sites of metastasis.

PRIMARY HEPATIC LYMPHOMA

CLINICAL FEATURES

Primary hepatic lymphoma is rare and represents fewer than 0.5 % of all extranodal non-Hodgkin's lymphomas. However, reported cases vary in lymph node, bone marrow, and splenic involvement, resulting in difficulties in comparing clinicopathologic features. In particular, the spleen is often involved at the time of detection.

A male predominance is seen among reported cases, which includes a wide age range. Patients may present with abdominal pain with hepatomegaly; liver test results are variably abnormal. Human immunodeficiency virus (HIV), hepatitis B virus, hepatitis C virus, and autoimmune diseases have been implicated in some cases. Please see Chapter 19 for additional details on hepatic lymphomas.

PATHOLOGIC FEATURES

GROSS FINDINGS

In most cases, a single large mass or multiple bulky deposits are present in the liver (Fig. 18.39). A diffusely infiltrative pattern may also be seen, depending on the type of lymphoma.

PRIMARY HEPATIC LYMPHOMA—FACT SHEET

Definition

- Malignant lymphoid neoplasm confined to the liver

Incidence and Location

- Rare; only approximately 0.4% of extranodal non-Hodgkin's lymphomas
- No geographic predilection

Gender, Race, and Age Distribution

- Male predominance (male-to-female ratio, 2:1)
- No racial predilection
- Usually occurs in adults (median age, 53 years)

Clinical Features

- Reported in setting of chronic viral hepatitis (hepatitis B and hepatitis C) and AIDS
- Patients present with abdominal pain, distension, and hepatomegaly

Radiologic Features

- Lesions are hypoechoic on ultrasonography
- Low-attenuation lesions with variable enhancement on computed tomography

Prognosis and Therapy

- Prognosis is poor for HIV-positive and cirrhotic patients
- Approximately 60% 2-year survival rate
- Combination chemotherapy is generally used

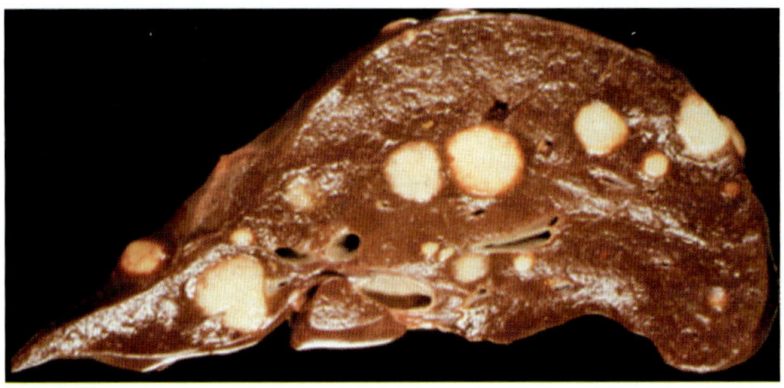

FIGURE 18.39

Hepatic lymphomas can present as multiple nodular masses mimicking a metastatic carcinoma.

Microscopic Findings

Most cases are of B-cell lineage, with the diffuse large cell type accounting for more than 75% of cases. However, reported cases include many of the lymphoma histologic subtypes, including primary extranodal marginal zone lymphoma and hepatosplenic T-cell lymphoma. Some B-cell lymphomas are manifested primarily by the presence of a relatively monomorphic portal infiltrate (Fig. 18.40). T-cell lymphomas tend to demonstrate a sinusoidal infiltrative pattern.

PRIMARY HEPATIC LYMPHOMA—PATHOLOGIC FEATURES

Gross Findings

- Large cell lymphomas produce bulky white to yellow masses
- A discrete mass may not be evident

Microscopic Findings

- Most are diffuse large cell B-cell lymphomas
- T-cell lymphomas are more likely to infiltrate sinusoids diffusely

Immunohistochemistry

- Depends on type of lymphoma; most hepatic lymphomas are CD20+ (see Chapter 19 for additional information)
- Sinusoidal T-cell lymphomas are CD3+, CD45RO+ (see Chapter 19 for additional information)

Differential Diagnosis

- Chronic hepatitis is distinguished by the mixed nature of the infiltrate and characteristic pattern of tissue damage and inflammation
- Epstein-Barr virus hepatitis is best distinguished by clinical findings

Differential Diagnosis

The presence of a lymphoid infiltrate that does not fit a recognized pattern of inflammatory disease in the liver should prompt consideration of hepatic lymphoma. Although immunohistochemical markers for various lymphoid markers may be helpful, gene rearrangement studies may be necessary. Lymphoma is not usually mistaken for carcinoma in the liver; immunostains for CK and leukocyte common antigen are useful in making this distinction.

Prognosis and Therapy

In general, the prognosis depends on the specific type of lymphoma and the presence or absence of underlying liver disease. Treatment has included surgery, chemotherapy, and radiation therapy. Patients with HIV infection or cirrhosis have a poor prognosis.

METASTASES

CLINICAL FEATURES

Metastatic tumors account for the overwhelming majority of all hepatic malignancies in noncirrhotic livers in Western countries. In cirrhotic livers, however, primary

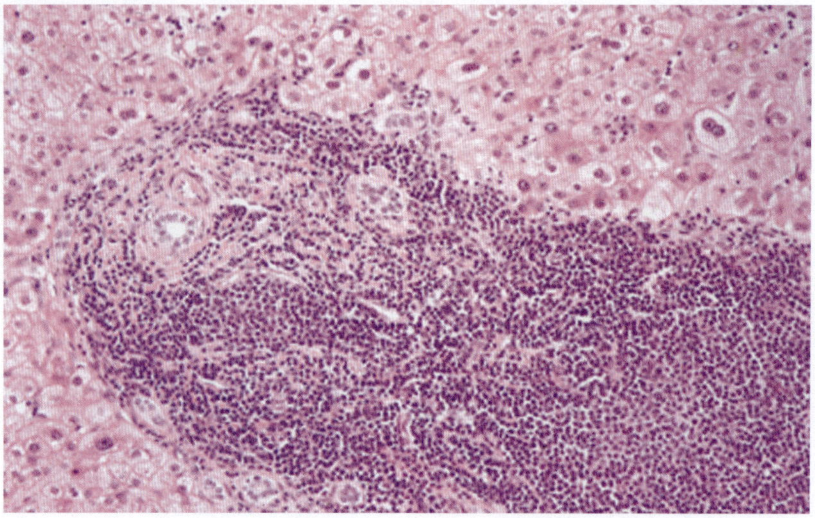

FIGURE 18.40

Low-grade B-cell lymphomas involving the liver often present as a monomorphic portal infiltrates of small lymphocytes, a pattern that can mimic chronic hepatitis. The neoplastic infiltrate is typically dense and monomorphic and shows marked expansion of the portal tracts.

hepatic malignancies are more common than metastatic tumors. Carcinomas of the lung, breast, colon, and pancreas are the most common primary sites in adults; neuroblastoma, Wilms' tumor, and rhabdomyosarcoma are the most common primary sites in children.

Clinical features range from asymptomatic to fulminant hepatic failure because of the diffuse replacement of the liver. Obstructive jaundice may occur secondary to tumor growth within large bile ducts or compression of the extrahepatic biliary tree by involved perihilar lymph nodes.

HEPATIC METASTASES–FACT SHEET

Definition

- Malignant tumor that secondarily involves the liver

Incidence and Location

- Most common malignant neoplasm involving liver
- 40% of patients dying from cancer have liver metastases
- No geographic variation

Morbidity and Mortality

- High morbidity, with many patients having signs of liver failure
- High mortality rate, with most patients dying within 2 years of diagnosis

Gender, Race, and Age Distribution

- Depends on primary site of cancer

Clinical Features

- The most common primary sites are lung, breast, colon, and pancreas
- Hepatomegaly, anorexia, and weight loss are common
- Jaundice may be seen when tumors near the hilum cause large duct obstruction
- Patients may present with acute liver failure from massive diffuse hepatic involvement

Radiologic Features

- Imaging studies show multiple hepatic lesions
- Solid, hypoechoic masses on ultrasonography
- Computed tomography appearance is variable, usually decreased attenuation
- Magnetic resonance imaging shows high lesion-to-liver contrast

Prognosis and Therapy

- Treatment is usually palliative (systemic or intrahepatic artery chemotherapy; chemoembolization, or cryotherapy)
- Resection of isolated hepatic metastases from colorectal cancer produces an approximately 30% 5-year survival rate for carefully selected patients
- Prognosis is related to growth characteristics of tumor, extent of hepatic involvement, and comorbid conditions

PATHOLOGIC FEATURES

GROSS FINDINGS

In most cases, multiple tumor deposits of varying sizes are present (Fig. 18.41A), although in some cases, the liver parenchyma is diffusely replaced, and nodules are not apparent on gross examination (Fig. 18.41B). Large subcapsular nodules may demonstrate central necrosis and fibrosis, producing umbilication. Highly vascular tumors such as choriocarcinoma, angiosarcoma, and thyroid carcinoma appear hemorrhagic.

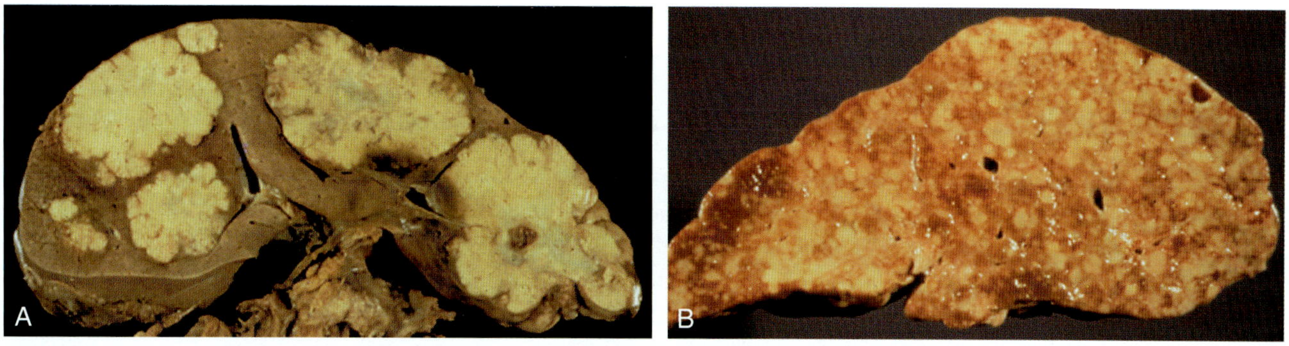

FIGURE 18.41

Metastatic carcinoma is the most common malignancy involving the liver. Whereas metastatic colon cancer may be solitary or multicentric and typically shows abundant necrosis (**A**), metastatic breast cancer may produce diffuse involvement without discrete mass formation (**B**).

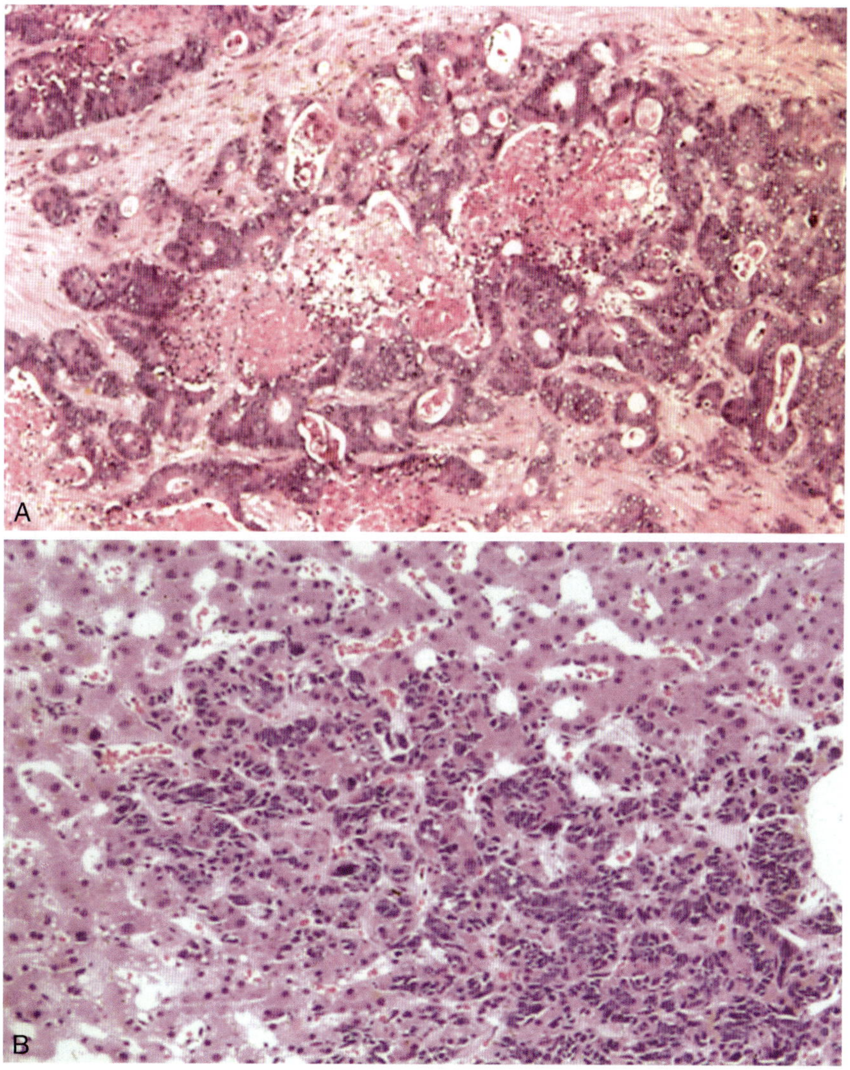

FIGURE 18.42

Metastatic colon cancer resembles the primary tumor, and abundant central necrosis is characteristic (**A**). Small cell neuroendocrine carcinoma metastatic to the liver may infiltrate the liver diffusely in a sinusoidal pattern (**B**) and result in fulminant hepatic failure.

Microscopic Findings

Metastases usually retain the histologic features of the primary tumor (Fig. 18.42). Intrasinusoidal growth should not be mistaken for a trabecular architecture or origin from hepatocytes. Vascular invasion of portal vein radicals may be noted. Colon carcinoma may involve large bile ducts, with an intrabiliary growth pattern that mimics CC.

Hepatic Metastases—Pathologic Features

Gross Findings

- Usually multiple irregular nodules of varying sizes
- Central necrosis with retraction produces an umbilicated appearance
- Tumors are firm because of desmoplastic stromal response

Microscopic Findings

- Features are similar to primary tumors
- Metastatic adenocarcinoma may grow within bile ducts and simulate cholangiocarcinoma (CC)

Fine-Needle Aspiration Biopsy Findings

- Features are similar to those of primary tumors

Differential Diagnosis

- Hepatocellular carcinoma
- CC
- Primary hepatic sarcomas
- Benign bile duct lesions

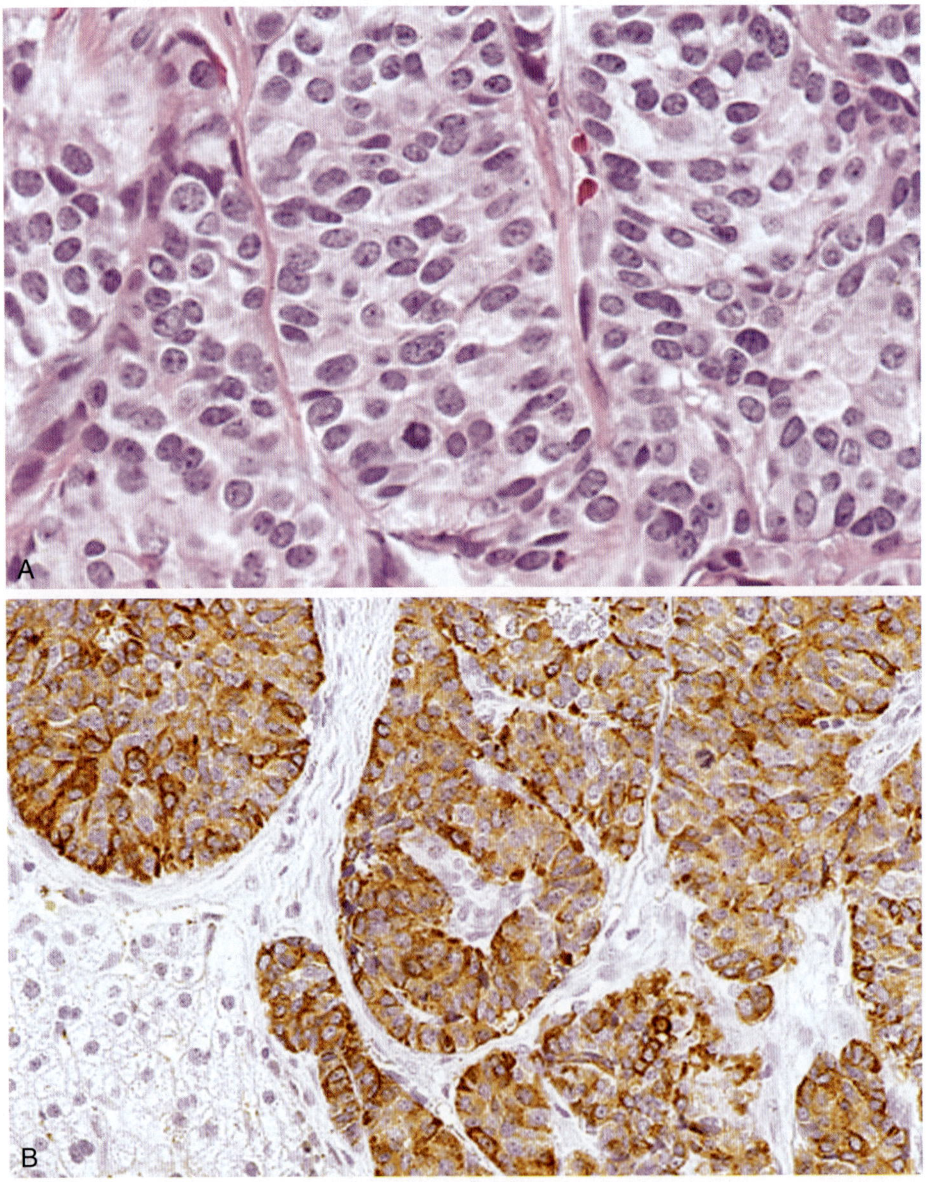

FIGURE 18.43

Metastatic well-differentiated neuroendocrine tumors from a pancreatic or gastrointestinal primary cancer also commonly spread to the liver. A trabecular or nested growth pattern with monomorphic tumor cells that show fine nuclear chromatin is characteristic (**A**), and the diagnosis is easily established by positivity for markers of neuroendocrine differentiation such as chromogranin (**B**) or synaptophysin.

Differential Diagnosis

Hepatocellular carcinoma displays a trabecular growth pattern and obvious hepatocellular differentiation, including bile production, in many cases. A panel of immunohistochemical markers including Hepar-1, CD10 or polyclonal CEA, arginase-1, and glypican-3 distinguishes most HCCs from metastases. If metastatic neuroendocrine carcinoma is a consideration, positivity for chromogranin, INSM1, and/or synaptophysin is generally diagnostic (Fig. 18.43). For carcinomas or adenocarcinomas, a panel that includes CK7 and CK20 to suggest the site of origin is recommended. CDX2 and TTF-1 immunohistochemistry may help distinguish metastatic gastrointestinal (especially midgut) carcinoids from metastatic pulmonary carcinoids, whereas polyclonal PAX8 and Islet1 positivity favors a pancreatic primary. PAX8 serves also as a Mullerian marker. GATA-3 is positive in breast and bladder primary tumors but can be weakly expressed in pancreatobiliary tumors. SF-1 can be useful when adrenal lesions are noted. NKX3.1 and PSA or PSAP can be positive in prostatic adenocarcinomas. In general, metastatic adenocarcinoma from the pancreas, extrahepatic biliary tree, and gastrointestinal tract may be difficult to distinguish from primary intrahepatic cholangiocarcinoma (ICC) and correlation with clinical history and imaging findings is key to making this distinction.

Prognosis and Therapy

Most patients with hepatic metastases die within 1 year, and treatment is largely aimed at palliation. Exceptions include patients with metastatic neuroendocrine tumors; these patients may enjoy prolonged survival. Carefully selected patients with colorectal metastases with single or few tumor deposits and no extrahepatic spread are candidates for surgical resection.

SUGGESTED READINGS

1. Nault JC, Cauchy G, Balabaud C, et al. Molecular classification of hepatocellular adenoma associates with risk factors, bleeding, and malignant transformation. *Gastroenterology*. 2017;152(4): 880–894.e6.
2. Beaufrère A, Paradis V. Hepatocellular adenomas: review of pathological and molecular features. *Hum Pathol*. 2021 Jun;112:128-137.
3. Joseph NM, Ferrell LD, Jain D, et al. Diagnostic utility and limitations of glutamine synthetase and serum amyloid-associated protein immunohistochemistry in the distinction of focal nodular hyperplasia and inflammatory hepatocellular adenoma. *Mod Pathol*. 2014 Jan;27(1):62-72.
4. Aishima S, Iguchi T, Fujita N, et al. Histological and immunohistological findings in biliary intraepithelial neoplasia arising from a background of chronic biliary disease compared with liver cirrhosis of non-biliary aetiology. *Histopathology*. 2011;59(5):867–875.
5. Aishima S, Oda Y. Pathogenesis and classification of intrahepatic cholangiocarcinoma: different characters of perihilar large duct type versus peripheral small duct type. *J Hepatobiliary Pancreat Sci*. 2015;22(2):94–100.
6. Akita M, Fujikura K, Ajiki T, et al. Dichotomy in intrahepatic cholangiocarcinomas based on histologic similarities to hilar cholangiocarcinomas. *Mod Pathol*. 2017;30(7):986–997.
7. Albores-Saavedra J, Córdova-Ramón JC, Chablé-Montero F, et al. Cystadenomas of the liver and extrahepatic bile ducts: morphologic and immunohistochemical characterization of the biliary and intestinal variants. *Ann Diagn Pathol*. 2015;19(3):124–129.
8. Amason T, Borger DR, Corless C, et al. Biliary adenofibroma of liver: morphology, tumor genetics, and outcomes in 6 cases. *Am J Surg Pathol*. 2017;41(4):499–505.
9. Ariizumi S, Kotera Y, Katagiri S, et al. Combined hepatocellular-cholangiocarcinoma had poor outcomes after hepatectomy regardless of Allen and Lisa class or the pre-dominance of intrahepatic cholangiocarcinoma cells within the tumor. *Ann Surg Oncol*. 2012;19(5):1628–1636.
10. Bioulac-Sage P, Cube G, Taouji S, et al. Immunohistochemical markers on needle biopsies are helpful for the diagnosis of focal nodular hyperplasia and hepatocellular adenoma subtypes. *Am J Surg Pathol*. 2012;36(11):1691–1699.
11. Bioulac-Sage P, Laumonier H, Laurent C, et al. Benign and malignant vascular tumors of the liver in adults. *Semin Liver Dis*. 2008;28(3):302–314.
12. Borzio M, Fargion S, Borzio F, et al. Impact of large regenerative, low grade and high grade dysplastic nodules in hepatocellular carcinoma development. *J Hepatol*. 2003;39(2):208–214.
13. Brunt E, Aishima S, Clavien PA, et al. cHCC-CCA: consensus terminology for primary liver carcinomas with both hepatocytic and cholangiocytic differentation. *Hepatology*. 2018;68(1):113–126.
14. Burt AD, Alves V, Bedossa P, et al. Data set for the reporting of intrahepatic cholangiocarcinoma, perihilar cholangiocarcinoma and hepatocellular carcinoma: recommendations from the International Collaboration on Cancer Reporting (ICCR). *Histopathology*. 2018;73(3):369–385.
15. Calderaro J, Cauchy G, Imbeaud S, et al. Histological subtypes of hepatocellular carcinoma are related to gene mutations and molecular tumour classification. *J Hepatol*. 2017;67(4):727–738.
16. Nguyen CT, Caruso S, Maille P, et al. Immune Profiling of Combined Hepatocellular- Cholangiocarcinoma Reveals Distinct Subtypes and Activation of Gene Signatures Predictive of Response to Immunotherapy. *Clin Cancer Res*. 2022 Feb 1; 28(3):540-551.
17. Cancer Genome Atlas Research Network. Comprehensive and integrative genomic characterization of hepatocellular carcinoma. *Cell*. 2017;169(7):1327–1341.e23.
18. Cazals-Hatem D, Rebouissou S, Bioulac-Sage P, et al. Clinical and molecular analysis of combined hepatocellular-cholangiocarcinomas. *J Hepatol*. 2004;41(2):292–298.
19. Devaney K, Goodman ZD, Ishak KG. Hepatobiliary cystadenoma and cystadenocarcinoma. A light microscopic and immunohistochemical study of 70 patients. *Am J Surg Pathol*. 1994;18(11):1078–1091.
20. Ding GH, Liu Y, Wu MC, et al. Diagnosis and treatment of hepatic angiomyolipoma. *J Surg Oncol*. 2011;103(8):807–812.
21. Evason KJ, Grenert JP, Ferrell LD, et al. Atypical hepatocellular adenoma-like neoplasms with β-catenin activation show cytogenetic alterations similar to well-differentiated hepatocellular carcinomas. *Hum Pathol*. 2013;44(5):750–758.
22. Fujikura K, Akita M, Abe-Suzuki S, et al. Mucinous cystic neoplasms of the liver and pancreas: relationship between KRAS driver mutations and disease progression. *Histopathology*. 2017;71(4):591–600.
23. Goodman ZD, Ishak KG. Angiomyolipomas of the liver. *Am J Surg Pathol*. 1984;8(10):745–750.
24. Ishak KG, Sesterhenn IA, Goodman ZD, et al. Epithelioid hemangioendothelioma of the liver: a clinicopathologic and follow-up study of 32 cases. *Hum Pathol*. 1984;15(9):839–852.
25. Ismail H, Dembowska-Bagiriska B, Broniszczak D, et al. Treatment of undifferentiated embryonal sarcoma of the liver in children-single center experience. *J Pediatr Surg*. 2013; 48(11):2202–2206.

26. Jiao Y, Pawlik TM, Anders RA, et al. Exome sequencing identifies frequent inactivating mutations in BAP1, ARID1A and PBRM1 in intrahepatic cholangiocarcinomas. *Nat Genet.* 2013; 45(12):1470–1473.
27. Kiani B, Ferrell LD, Qualman S, et al. Immunohistochemical analysis of embryonal sarcoma of the liver. *Appl Immunohistochem Mol Morphol.* 2006;14(2):193–197.
28. Kim WJ, Hwang S, Lee YJ, et al. Clinicopathological features and long-term outcomes of intraductal papillary neoplasms of the intra-hepatic bile duct. *J Gastrointest Surg.* 2016;20(7): 1368–1375.
29. Komuta M, Spee B, Vander Borght S, et al. Clinicopathological study on cholangiolocellular carcinoma suggesting hepatic progenitor cell origin. *Hepatology.* 2008;47(5):1544–1556.
30. Kozaka K, Sasaki M, Fujii T, et al. A sub-group of intrahepatic cholangiocarcinoma with an infiltrating replacement growth pattern and a resemblance to reactive proliferating bile ductules: 'bile ductular carcinoma'. *Histopathology.* 2007;51(3):390–400.
31. Lack EE, Schloo BL, Azumi N, et al. Undifferentiated (embryonal) sarcoma of the liver. Clinical and pathologic study of 16 cases with emphasis on immunohistochemical features. *Am J Surg Pathol.* 1991;15(1):1–16.
32. Lauwers GY, Grant LD, Donnelly WH, et al. Hepatic undifferentiated (embryonal) sarcoma arising in a mesenchymal hamartoma. *Am J Surg Pathol.* 1997;21(10):1248–1254.
33. Lauwers GY, Terris B, Balis UJ, et al. Prognostic histologic indicators of curatively resected hepatocellular carcinomas: a multi-institutional analysis of 425 patients with definition of a histologic prognostic index. *Am J Surg Pathol.* 2002;26(1):25–34.
34. Liau JY, Tsai JH, Yuan RH, et al. Morphological subclassification of intrahepatic cholangiocarcinoma: etiological, clinicopathological, and molecular features. *Mod Pathol.* 2014;27(8):1163–1173.
35. Makhlouf HR, Ishak KG, Goodman ZD. Epithelioid hemangioendothelioma of the liver: a clinicopathologic study of 137 cases. *Cancer.* 1999;85(3):562–582.
36. Matsuura S, Aishima S, Taguchi K, et al. 'Scirrhous' type hepatocellular carcinomas: a special reference to expression of cytokeratin 7 and hepatocyte paraffin 1. *Histopathology.* 2005;47(4): 382–390.
37. Moeini A, Sia D, Zhang Z, et al. Mixed hepatocellular cholangiocarcinoma tumors: cholangiolocellular carcinoma is a distinct molecular entity. *J Hepatol.* 2017;66(5):952–961.
38. Oikawa T, Ojima H, Yamasaki S, et al. Multistep and multicentric development of hepatocellular carcinoma: histological analysis of 980 resected nodules. *J Hepatol.* 2005;42(2):225–229.
39. Park YN, Kojiro M, DiTommaso L, et al. Ductular reaction is helpful in defining early stromal invasion, small hepatocellular carcinomas, and dysplastic nodules. *Cancer.* 2007;109(5): 915–923.
40. Sasaki M, Sato Y, Nakanuma Y. Mutational landscape of combined hepatocellular carcinoma and cholangiocarcinoma, and its clinicopathological significance. *Histopathology.* 2017;70(3): 423–434.
41. Selby DM, Stocker JT, Waclawiw MA, et al. Infantile hemangioendothelioma of the liver. *Hepatology.* 1994;20(1 Pt 1):39–45.
42. Selves J, Meggetto F, Brousset P, et al. Inflammatory pseudotumor of the liver. Evidence for follicular dendritic reticulum cell proliferation associated with clonal Epstein-Barr virus. *Am J Surg Pathol.* 1996;20(6):747–753.
43. Shehata BM, Gupta NA, Katzenstein HM, et al. Undifferentiated embryonal sarcoma of the liver is associated with mesenchymal hamartoma and multiple chromosomal abnormalities: a review of eleven cases. *Pediatr Dev Pathol.* 2011;14(2):111–116.
44. Sia D, Hoshida Y, Villanueva A, et al. Integrative molecular analysis of intrahepatic cholangiocarcinoma reveals 2 classes that have different outcomes. *Gastroenterology.* 2013;144(4):829–840.
45. Tsui WM, Colombari R, Portmann BC, et al. Hepatic angiomyolipoma: a clinicopathologic study of 30 cases and delineation of unusual morphologic variants. *Am J Surg Pathol.* 1999;23(1):34–48.
46. Tsui WM, Loo KT, Chow LT, et al. Biliary adenofibroma. A heretofore unrecognized benign biliary tumor of the liver. *Am J Surg Pathol.* 1993;17(2):186–192.
47. Ward SC, Huang J, Tickoo SK, et al. Fibrolamellar carcinoma of the liver exhibits immunohistochemical evidence of both hepatocyte and bile duct differentiation. *Mod Pathol.* 2010;23(9): 1180–1190.
48. Zatkova A, Rouillard JM, Hartmann W, et al. Amplification and overexpression of the IGF2 regulator PLAG1 in hepatoblastoma. *Genes Chromosomes Cancer.* 2004;39(2):126–137.
49. Zen Y, Jang KT, Ahn S, et al. Intraductal papillary neoplasms and mucinous cystic neoplasms of the hepatobiliary system: demographic differences between Asian and Western populations, and comparison with pancreatic counterparts. *Histopathology.* 2014;65(2):164–173.

19

Gastrointestinal Lymphoma

Michael Cruise, MD, PhD

The gastrointestinal (GI) tract is the most common site of extranodal lymphoma, which should not be a surprise as the GI system contains approximately 70% of the lymphoid tissue and 80% of the plasma cells (most of those being immunoglobulin [Ig] A expressing). Anywhere from 20% to 48% of primary extranodal lymphomas have been reported to occur in the GI tract. Additionally, recent reports provide evidence of increasing incidence rates of primary GI lymphoma in North American population with 0.13 per 100,000 in 1999 up to 2.7 per 100,000 in 2007. A 2018 report from Japan also places the current incidence at around 2.97 per 100,000. Furthermore, there appear to be specific populations such as those from northern Italy, Asia, Native Americans, the Netherlands, and Mexico with an increased incidence of GI lymphoma of up to 13.2 cases per 100,000.

The primary sites of involvement of the GI tract are the stomach and the small bowel. In developed countries, most occur in the stomach; however, in developing countries and the Middle East, the small bowel is the most common site of involvement. In general, approximately 50% to 75% of primary GI lymphomas occur in the stomach but only make up 1% to 7% of gastric malignancies. In the stomach, lymphomas are evenly divided between marginal zone lymphoma and diffuse large B-cell lymphoma (DLBCL). The small bowel is the primary site in 15% to 35% of GI lymphomas, and 25% of small bowel neoplasms are GI lymphomas. DLBCL represents the majority of cases (30%–50%) followed by follicular lymphoma (FL), marginal zone lymphoma, Burkitt lymphoma (BL), and primary intestinal T-cell lymphomas. Approximately 10% to 20% of GI lymphomas arise in the colon, but these account for only between 0.2% and 1% of colorectal malignancies.

Overall, in the GI tract, the number of B-cell lymphomas greatly outnumber T-cell lymphomas, and in the GI tract, aggressive lymphomas outnumber the mature (low-grade) B-cell lymphomas. However, given the increased endoscopic evaluations and improved resolutions, an increased number of smaller lesions, of mature B-cell lymphoma, are being identified.

Although almost any lymphoma or leukemia can involve the GI tract, this chapter focuses on primary GI lymphomas (including hepatic lymphomas) and updates the proposed terminology from the 2017 update to the fourth edition of the World Health Organization (WHO) Classification of Hematological malignancies Table 19.1. Several updates are pertinent to the GI lymphomas, including the new category of indolent T-cell lymphoproliferative disorder of the GI tract and duodenal-type FL. There is also the reclassification of B-cell lymphoma unclassifiable with features intermediate between DLBCL and BL to high-grade lymphoma with or without *MYC* and *BCL2* or *BCL6* translocation. Additionally, the accumulation of clinical and molecular data has shown that the two subtypes of enteropathy-associated T-cell lymphoma (EATL) are two distinct disease processes, and their names have been changed to reflect this realization. Specifically, the entity formerly known as type I EATL is now only designated as enteropathy-associated T-cell lymphoma, and the entity known as type II EATL will be designated as monomorphic epitheliotropic intestinal T-cell lymphoma (MEITL). Additionally, other entities that can affect the GI tract, Epstein-Barr virus (EBV)–positive DLBCL, EBV-positive mucocutaneous ulcer, and indolent T- and natural killer (NK) cell proliferation, have been added to the WHO classification.

MATURE B-CELL NEOPLASMS

EXTRANODAL MARGINAL ZONE B-CELL LYMPHOMA OF MUCOSA ASSOCIATED LYMPHOID TISSUE (MALT LYMPHOMA)

Clinical Features

The most common primary low-grade B-cell lymphoma of the GI tract is extranodal marginal zone B-cell lymphoma of mucosa-associated lymphoid tissue (MALT lymphoma). This lymphoma can develop in either primary or secondary MALT. Extranodal marginal zone lymphomas primarily occur in the stomach with decreasing incidences in the small bowel and colon.

TABLE 19.1

2017 World Health Organization Updated Classification of Mature Lymphoid, Histiocytic, and Dendritic Neoplasms

MATURE B-CELL NEOPLASMS
Chronic lymphocytic leukemia/small lymphocytic lymphoma
Monoclonal B-cell lymphocytosis[a]
B-cell prolymphocytic leukemia
Splenic marginal zone lymphoma
Hairy cell leukemia
Splenic B-cell lymphoma/leukemia, unclassifiable
Splenic diffuse red pulp small B-cell lymphoma
Hairy cell leukemia-variant
Lymphoplasmacytic lymphoma
Waldenstrom macroglobulinemia
Monoclonal gammopathy of undetermined significance (MGUS), IgM[a]
Monoclonal gammopathy of undetermined significance (MGUS), IgG/A[a]
Plasma cell myeloma
Solitary plasmacytoma of bone
Extraosseous plasmacytoma
Monoclonal immunoglobulin deposition diseases[a]
Extranodal marginal zone lymphoma of mucosa-associated lymphoid tissue (MALT lymphoma)
Nodal marginal zone lymphoma
Pediatric nodal marginal zone lymphoma
Follicular lymphoma
In situ follicular neoplasiaa
Duodenal-type follicular lymphoma[a]
Pediatric-type follicular lymphoma[a]
Large B-cell lymphoma with IRF4 rearrangement[a]
Primary cutaneous follicle center lymphoma
Mantle cell lymphoma
In situ mantle cell neoplasia[a]
Diffuse large B-cell lymphoma (DLBCL), not otherwise specified (NOS)
Germinal center B-cell typea
Activated B-cell type[a]
T-cell/histiocyte-rich large B-cell lymphoma
Primary DLBCL of the central nervous system
Primary cutaneous DLBCL, leg type
EBV-positive DLBCL, NOS[a]
EBV-positive mucocutaneous ulcer[a]
DLBCL associated with chronic inflammation
Lymphomatoid granulomatosis
Primary mediastinal (thymic) large B-cell lymphoma
Intravascular large B-cell lymphoma
ALK1 large B-cell lymphoma
Plasmablastic lymphoma
Primary effusion lymphoma
Human herpesvirus 8–positive DLBCL, NOS[a]
Burkitt lymphoma
Burkitt-like lymphoma with 11q aberration[a]
High-grade B-cell lymphoma, with MYC and BCL2 and/or BCL6 rearrangements[a]
High-grade B-cell lymphoma, NOS[a]
B-cell lymphoma, unclassifiable, with features intermediate between DLBCL and classical Hodgkin lymphoma

Approximately 75% to 85% of MALT lymphomas of the GI tract involve the gastric mucosa with the remaining involving the small bowel and colon.

Compared with the distal GI tract, the stomach is normally devoid of primary lymphoid tissue, and any lymphoid tissue present is secondary to inflammatory, infections, or autoimmune causes. So, it should not be surprising that the majority of gastric MALT lymphomas are associated with *Helicobacter pylori* infection. The inflammatory response to the infection leads to the formation of secondary lymphoid tissue in which the lymphoma develops.

In other sites in the GI tract, the extranodal marginal zone lymphoma can develop in the normal primary lymphoid tissue, especially in the distal small bowel and the colon. Although extranodal marginal zone lymphoma of

TABLE 19.1

2017 World Health Organization Updated Classification of Mature Lymphoid, Histiocytic, and Dendritic Neoplasms

MATURE T AND NATURAL KILLER NEOPLASMS
T-cell prolymphocytic leukemia
T-cell large granular lymphocytic leukemia
Chronic lymphoproliferative disorder of natural killer (NK) cells
Aggressive NK cell leukemia
Systemic EBV-positive T-cell lymphoma of childhood[a]
Hydroa vacciniforme–like lymphoproliferative disorder[a]
Adult T-cell leukemia/lymphoma
Extranodal NK-/T-cell lymphoma, nasal type
Enteropathy-associated T-cell lymphoma
Monomorphic epitheliotropic intestinal T-cell lymphoma[a]
Indolent T-cell lymphoproliferative disorder of the gastrointestinal tract[a]
Hepatosplenic T-cell lymphoma
Subcutaneous panniculitis-like T-cell lymphoma
Mycosis fungoides
Sezary syndrome
Primary cutaneous CD30-positive T-cell lymphoproliferative disorders
Lymphomatoid papulosis
Primary cutaneous anaplastic large cell lymphoma
Primary cutaneous gamma delta T-cell lymphoma
Primary cutaneous CD8-positive aggressive epidermotropic cytotoxic T-cell lymphoma
Primary cutaneous acral CD8-positive T-cell lymphoma[a]
Primary cutaneous CD4-positive small/medium T-cell lymphoproliferative disorder[a]
Peripheral T-cell lymphoma, NOS
Angioimmunoblastic T-cell lymphoma
Follicular T-cell lymphoma[a]
Nodal peripheral T-cell lymphoma with TFH phenotype[a]
Anaplastic large-cell lymphoma, ALK1
Anaplastic large-cell lymphoma, ALK2[a]
Breast implant–associated anaplastic large-cell lymphoma[a]
HODGKIN LYMPHOMA
Nodular lymphocyte–predominant Hodgkin lymphoma (HL)
Classical Hodgkin lymphoma
Nodular sclerosis classical HL
Lymphocyte-rich classical HL
Mixed cellularity classical HL
Lymphocyte-depleted classical HL
POSTTRANSPLANT LYMPHOPROLIFERATIVE DISORDERS
Plasmacytic hyperplasia posttransplant lymphoproliferative disorder (PTLD)
Infectious mononucleosis PTLD
Florid follicular hyperplasia PTLD[a]
Polymorphic PTLD
Monomorphic PTLD (B- and T-/NK cell types)
Classical Hodgkin lymphoma PTLD
HISTIOCYTIC AND DENDRITIC CELL NEOPLASMS
Histiocytic sarcoma
Langerhans cell histiocytosis
Langerhans cell sarcoma
Indeterminate dendritic cell tumor
Interdigitating dendritic cell sarcoma
Follicular dendritic cell sarcoma
Fibroblastic reticular cell tumor
Disseminated juvenile xanthogranuloma
Erdheim-Chester disease+a

Modified from Swerdlow SH, Campo E, Harris NL, et al, eds. *WHO Classification of Tumours: Pathology and Genetics. Tumours of Haematopoietic and Lymphoid Tissues*. Revised 4t. Lyon, France: IARC; 2017. http://publications.iarc.fr/Book-And-Report-Series/Who-Iarc-Classification-Of-Tumours/Who-Classification-Of-Tumours-Of-Haematopoietic-And-Lymphoid-Tissues-2017.

[a]Changes from the 2008 classification.

MALT occurs less often in the small bowel, there is a unique form of MALT lymphoma that is primarily seen in patients from the Mediterranean and Middle Eastern areas that is referred to as *immunoproliferative small intestinal disease* (IPSID), which is discussed separately in this chapter.

Pathologic Features

Gross Findings

Endoscopically, lymphomas generally have a nonspecific appearance. MALT lymphomas of the stomach generally have a benign appearance often mimicking multifocal gastritis with ulceration. However, the findings can vary significantly and include multiple ulcerations, polypoid masses (mucosal or submucosal), mucosa erythema or edema, granular or nodular mucosal changes, thickened or hypertrophic gastric folds, or a combination of features. Endoscopic ultrasonography can be useful and tends to yield a more details view of the lesion and pattern of involvement.

Our ability to detect small bowel lesions has increased with the advent of capsule endoscopy and double-balloon push enteroscopy. Typically, the appearance in the small bowel is of an ulcerated or fibrotic area or polypoid mass, or it may have a stricture appearance. In the colon, MALT lymphomas are more likely to have a whitish or whitish-red polypoid lesion. Given the endoscopic overlap with other common nonhematopoietic entities, cases are only rarely submitted with a high suspicion for lymphoma or are submitted fresh for ancillary testing such as flow cytometry.

Microscopic Findings

As the name implies, the neoplastic cells are derived from the marginal zone of the germinal centers and have a centrocyte to "monocytoid" appearance. They demonstrate abundant pale to clear cytoplasm with slightly irregular nuclei and inconspicuous nucleoli. Although the neoplastic cells are B cells, the lesions can contain a prominent T cells, or plasma cell infiltrate. Typically in GI MALT lymphomas, the lamina propria is expanded by the neoplastic lymphocytes that infiltrate through the muscularis mucosa as well as into the glandular epithelium with destructive lymphoepithelial lesions (Fig. 19.1A and B). Lymphoepithelial lesions consist of at least three neoplastic B cells infiltrating the glands with distortion or destruction of the glands (see Fig. 19.1B). Actual lymphoepithelial lesions are typically thought to be pathognomonic for marginal zone lymphoma. However, lymphoepithelial-like lesions can be seen in multiple etiologies and in these cases, they consist of the epithelium infiltrated by T cells.

The lymphoepithelial lesions are more prominent in the stomach than the small bowel and colon, where they can be quite rare. Unfortunately, MALT lymphoma of the small bowel and colon can resemble expanded reactive MALT and Peyer's patches. The marginal zone lymphoma cells expand from the marginal zone but can also infiltrate and colonize the reactive germinal centers (Fig. 19.1F and G). Reportedly, up to one-third of gastric cases demonstrates a component of plasma cell differentiation. These can also lead to amyloid deposition and light chain accumulation. There can be scattered larger atypical cells, which are admixed with the smaller neoplastic cells; however, if there are diffuse sheets of the larger neoplastic cells, the diagnosis would be DLBCL. In the evaluation of cases for MALT lymphoma, one can use the Wotherspoon criteria (Table 19.2) as a useful framework to separate reactive gastritis (Wotherspoon 1 and 2) from suspicious lesions (Wotherspoon 3 and 4) from MALT lymphoma (Wotherspoon 5).

Ancillary Studies

Immunohistochemical stains are often an essential part of rendering the diagnosis of MALT lymphoma. However, unfortunately, unlike most other low-grade B-cell lymphomas, only a proportion of cases will have an aberrant immunophenotype. The neoplastic cells are B cells and express B-cell lineage markers, CD20, PAX5, and CD79a. Additionally, because they are derived from marginal zone B cells, they also express BCL-2 but are negative for germinal center markers CD10, BCL6, and LMO2. The germinal center markers can highlight the residual germinal centers and helps accentuate follicular colonization by the lymphoma cells. There is no aberrant coexpression of CD5, cyclin D1, LEF1, SOX11, or CD23 on the neoplastic cells. Marginal zone lymphomas can demonstrate aberrant coexpression of CD43 (Fig. 19.1C, D, and E) but generally only in a minority of cases (up to 25% of gastric cases and 30%–40% of the colon or small bowel cases). In cases with prominent plasma cell differentiation, immunohistochemistry (IHC) or in situ hybridization for κ and λ light chains can be used to differentiate the clonal plasma cells from reactive plasma cells that are present as part of the inflammatory background. Additionally, the presence or absence of *Helicobacter* organisms should be documented in all gastric lymphoma or carcinoma cases either by hematoxylin and eosin (H&E), Giemsa, or immunohistochemical stains (Fig. 19.1H).

In borderline cases (e.g., Wotherspoon 3 and 4), when CD43 coexpression cannot be demonstrated, B-cell gene rearrangement studies by polymerase chain reaction (PCR) may be helpful. In the distal small intestine

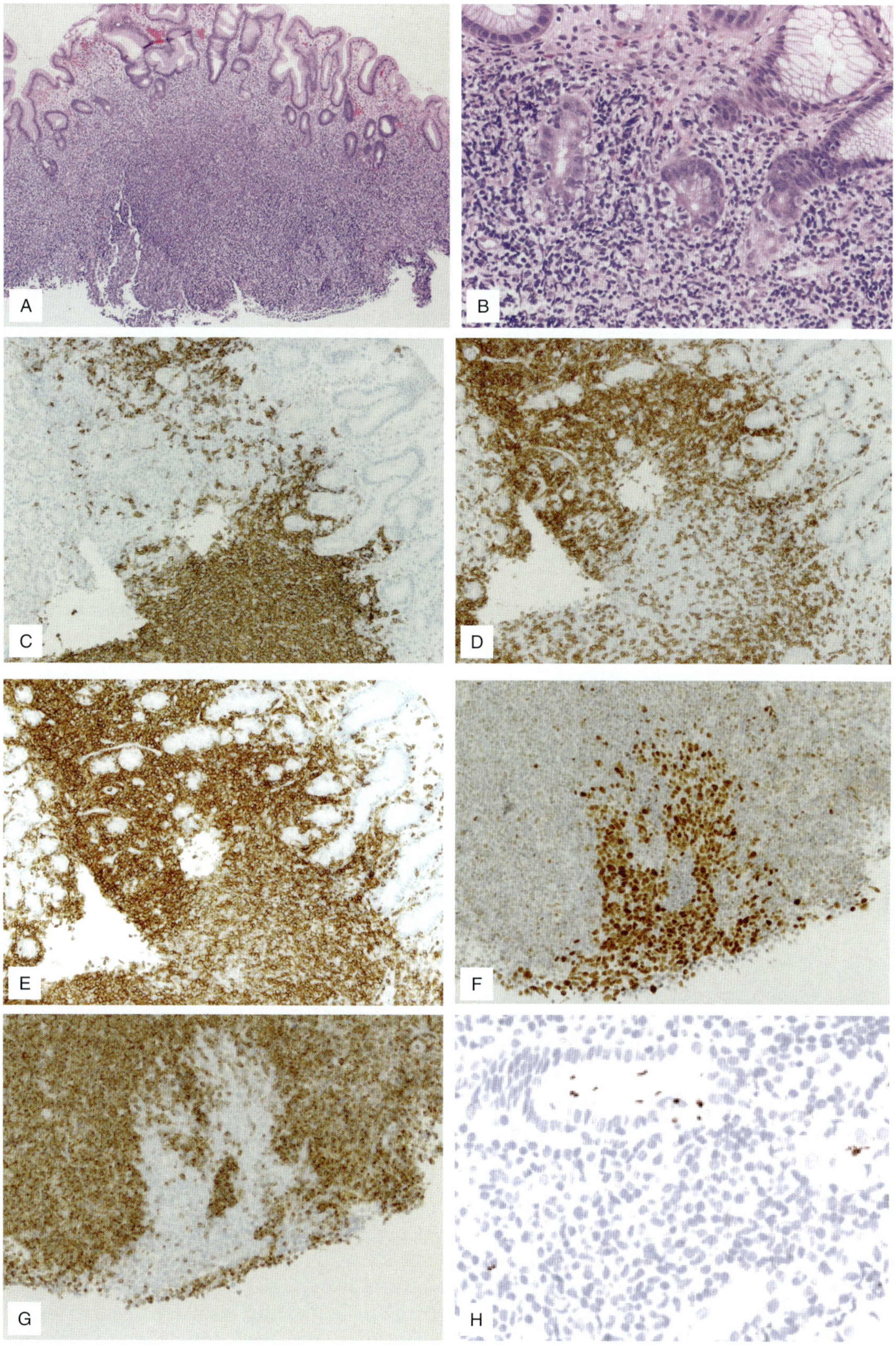

FIGURE 19.1

Mucosa-associated lymphoid tissue (MALT) lymphoma. **A**, At low magnification, the lamina propria is markedly expanded by small lymphocytes. Residual oxyntic glands are present within the neoplastic infiltrate. **B**, The infiltrate is composed of monomorphic, monocytoid lymphocytes with abundant clear cytoplasm, well-defined cell borders, and eccentric small nuclei. The lymphocytes invade the gastric glandular epithelium to form lymphoepithelial lesions. The lymphocytes are primarily CD20+ B cells (**C**) admixed with a background of CD3 positive T cells (**D**). The B cells demonstrates aberrant CD43 expression (**E**). MALT lymphomas can demonstrate colonized germinal centers. The lymphoma cells expressing BCL2 (**G**) can be seen infiltrating the BCL6-expressing germinal center (**F**). As in all cases of possible lymphomas and gastric carcinoma, the presence or absence *Helicobacter pylori* (**H**) should be determined.

TABLE 19.2

Histological Differential Scoring of Lymphoid Infiltrations in the Stomach According to Wotherspoon et al. (1993)

Score	Diagnosis	Histologic Features
0	Normal	Scattered plasma cells in lamina propria; no lymphoid follicles
1	Chronic active gastritis	Small clusters of lymphocytes in lamina propria; no lymphoid follicles; no lymphoepithelial lesions
2	Chronic active gastritis with florid lymphoid follicle formation	Prominent lymphoid follicles with surrounding mantle zone and plasma cells; no lymphoepithelial lesions
3	Suspicious lymphoid infiltrate, probably reactive	Lymphoid follicles surrounded by small lymphocytes that infiltrate diffusely in lamina propria and occasionally into epithelium
4	Suspicious lymphoid infiltrate, probably lymphoma	Lymphoid follicles surrounded by marginal zone cells that infiltrate diffusely in lamina propria and into epithelium in small groups
5	MALT lymphoma	Presence of dense infiltrate of marginal zone cells in lamina propria with prominent lymphoepithelial lesions

Adapted from Wotherspoon A, Doglioni C, Diss T, et al. Regression of primary low-grade B-cell gastric lymphoma of mucosa-associated lymphoid tissue type after eradication of Helicobacter pylori. *Lancet*. 342:575-577, 1993.
MALT, Mucosa-associated lymphoid tissue.

TABLE 19.3

Groupe d' Etude des Lymphomes de l'Adulte Histologic Grading System for Posttreatment Evaluation of Gastric Mucosa-Associated Lymphoid Tissue

Interpretation	Lymphoid Infiltrate	Lymphoepithelial Lesions	Stromal Changes
Complete histological remission	Absent or scattered plasma cells and small lymphoid cells in the LP	Absent	Normal or empty LP and/or fibrosis
Probable minimal residual disease	Aggregates of lymphoid cells Or lymphoid nodules in the LP/MM and/or SM	Absent	Empty LP and/or fibrosis
Responding residual disease	Dense, diffuse or nodular, extending around glands in the LP	Focal LEL or absent	Focal empty LP and/or fibrosis
No change	Dense diffuse or nodular	Present but may be absent	No changes

Adapted from Copie-Bergman C, Wotherspoon AC, Capella C, et al. Gela histological scoring system for post-treatment biopsies of patients with gastric MALT lymphoma is feasible and reliable in routine practice. *Br J Haematol*. 2013;160:47-52.
LEL, Lymphoepithelial lesions; *LP*, lamina propria; *MM*, muscularis mucosa; *SM*, submucosa.

where normal B cells can coexpress CD43, B-cell gene rearrangement studies are often necessary to establish or confirm the diagnosis. Of note, B-cell clonality studies have a use in the initial diagnosis but should not be used as a means to determine therapy response. Specifically, B-cell clones may persist for an extended time after morphologic resolution, and their presence does not affect outcomes. We typically utilize the Groupe d' Etude des Lymphomes de l'Adulte (GELA) histologic scoring system by Copie-Bergman et al. (2013) (Table 19.3) as a way of reporting treatment effect. One should note that even in the absence of lymphoma that treated *Helicobacter* gastritis takes months to more than 1 year for histology to become "normal."

Several cytogenetic abnormalities have been associated with MALT lymphoma. There are four recurrent chromosomal translocations associated with MALT lymphoma, and they vary in their prominence at various anatomic sites. These include t(11;18)(q21;q21)/API2-MALT1, t(1;14)(p22;q32)/IgH-BCL10, t(14;18)(q34;q21)/IgH-MALT1, and t(3;14)(p14.1;q32)/FOXP1-IGH. Only two are associated with GI MALT lymphoma, t(11;18) and t(1;14). The t(11;18) translocation has been reportedly seen in 6% to 16% of gastric and 12% to 56% of intestinal MALT lymphomas. Only rare gastric (0%–5%) or intestinal (0%–13%) MALT lymphoma cases have the t(1;14). The most common genetic abnormalities in MALT lymphoma are trisomies involving chromosomes 3 and 18. Interestingly, although t(11;18) (API2/MALT1) lymphomas tend to be less responsive to *Helicobacter* eradication therapy, they also have little to no potential to progress to DLBCL.

CD43 Pitfall

The diagnosis of marginal zone lymphoma can be challenging because most cases lack an aberrant immunophenotype. A minority of cases aberrantly expressed is CD43. CD43 is normally expressed by T cells and plasma cells but can be aberrantly expressed by B-cell lymphomas. It is essential to remember that it is not specific for marginal zone lymphoma. Typically, CD43 on the B cells in MALT lymphomas demonstrates a dimmer expression than T cells, and if the CD43 expression on the B cells is as strong as or stronger than the background T cells, other possible mature B cells must be considered. Specifically, aberrant CD43 expression can be seen in mantle lymphoma, small lymphocytic lymphoma (SLL) and chronic lymphocytic leukemia (CLL), as well as BL. Additionally, there are populations of normal B cells in the terminal ileum and proximal right colon that generally express CD43. In certain situations, the lymphomas have a prominent population of T cells and plasma cells, and one must be cautious not to misinterpret these cells as aberrant B cells.

Differential Diagnosis

Often the most challenging differential diagnosis is between chronic active *Helicobacter* gastritis versus MALT lymphoma. The infection leads to a reactive lymphoid infiltrate, creating acquired MALT with reactive germinal centers and surrounding mantle and marginal zones. During the transition from gastritis to lymphoma, both the number of *Helicobacter* organisms and the amount of acute inflammation typically decreases. Of note, although the neoplastic B cells are not *Helicobacter* antigen dependent, the reactive T cells appear to be *Helicobacter* antigen driven. These activated T cells active or stimulate B cells (both neoplastic and non-neoplastic) via CD40-CD40L interaction.

This differential between gastritis and lymphoma can at times be extremely challenging. Although strict adherence and application of the Wotherspoon criteria are not typically required, it does provide a useful framework for classifying reactive gastritis from cases that are suspicious for or diagnostic for MALT lymphoma. A differentiating point is the presence of epithelial invasion and glandular destruction by a B-cell process. As outlined earlier, aberrant CD43 expression and detection of a clonal B cell process are useful in the differentiation between a reactive inflammatory process and lymphoma.

The other primary differential includes the other mature B-cell lymphomas. Both mantle cell lymphoma (MCL) and FL are discussed in further detail later. Briefly, MCL demonstrates an abnormal phenotype with aberrant expression of CD5, CD43, cyclin D1, and SOX11 by the neoplastic B cells. MALT lymphomas can have a nodular appearance overlapping with that of low-grade FL. However, FL has a distinctive immunophenotype with an expression of germinal center markers CD10, BCL6, LMO2 with aberrance coexpression for BCL2. FL is negative for CD43. Another mature B-cell lymphoma that can mimic MALT lymphoma is SLL or CLL. These can also have similar cytomorphologic appearance (although typically with less cytoplasm). SLL and CLL lymphoma cells are typically B cell markers CD19, CD20, PAX5, and CD79a as well as aberrant expression of CD43, CD5, CD23, and CD200. SLL and CLL also demonstrate aberrant coexpression of LEF1 in the neoplastic B cells. The expression of LEF1 is typically seen in T cells and can be seen in aggressive B-cell lymphomas.

Prognosis and Therapy

Long-term remission is generally the rule, not the exception, in low-grade MALT lymphomas, especially the gastric subtype. The continued proliferation of gastric MALT lymphoma cells in patients with *H. pylori* is dependent on the presence of *H. pylori*–specific T cells and not caused by antigen and direct B-cell receptor interactions. The majority of patients respond to *Helicobacter* eradication antibiotic therapy with long-term remissions seen in up to 70% to 80% of cases. Certain features are associated with failure of *Helicobacter* eradiation therapy. Specifically, the presence of either the t(11;18) and t(1;14) translocation is associated with BCL10 expression, and these patients are more likely to fail *Helicobacter* eradication therapy. Approximately, 6 weeks after *Helicobacter* eradication therapy, patients should be tested for the continued presence of the organisms (either by biopsy or another method, such *H. pylori* fecal antigen test). Specifically, with the rise in clarithromycin as well as metronidazole and levofloxacin antibiotic-resistant strains, more than 20% of patients need a second round of antibiotic therapy to eliminate the infection.

Additionally, when the lymphoma has extended beyond the submucosa, the lesion tends to be more resistant to conservative therapy. Generally, MALT lymphomas are sensitive to radiation therapy with an excellent response rate. Additionally, some patients may be managed with single-agent rituximab or rituximab with additional chemotherapy. Transformation to DLBCL may occur but typically in fewer than 10% of cases. Interestingly, DLBCL cases that are associated with *Helicobacter* may also respond to *Helicobacter* eradication therapy only.

MALT LYMPHOMA—FACT SHEET

Definition

- Low-grade extranodal marginal zone B-cell lymphoma that arises from mucosa-associated lymphoid tissue (MALT)

Incidence and Location

- Most common location is stomach (75%–85%), followed by the small bowel and colon/rectum
- Account for fewer than 1% to 4% of primary gastric neoplasms and up to 50% of gastric lymphomas
- Associated with *Helicobacter pylori* gastritis in the stomach

Morbidity and Mortality

- Indolent behavior in most low-grade lesions with excellent prognosis
- Minority of lesions (<10%) show transformation to high-grade B-cell lymphoma

Gender, Age, and Race Distribution

- Slight female predominance in gastric MALT lymphoma and male predominance in small intestinal MALT lymphoma
- Presents in the fifth and sixth decades of life

Clinical Features

- Physical examination is normal in 55% to 60%
- Abdominal pain
- Bleeding
- Intestinal obstruction or perforation
- Weakness, night sweats, or fever
- Palpable abdominal mass
- Hematemesis and melena are rare

Prognosis and Treatment

- Good prognosis associated with age younger than65 years, low-grade histology, and/or initial complete remission
- 5-year survival rates for gastric MALT lymphoma: 50% to 90%
- 5-year survival rate for small intestinal MALT lymphoma: 50% to 80%
- Progression to diffuse large B-cell lymphoma (DLBCL) may occur in 8% of MALT lymphomas
- Adverse prognostic factors include extension beyond the bowel wall, nodal involvement, and transformation to DLBCL

MALT LYMPHOMA—PATHOLOGIC FEATURES

Gross, Endoscopic, and Radiology Findings

- Ulcerated, polypoid, granular, nodular, or edematous and hyperplastic mucosal folds
- Single or multiple mucosal or submucosal masses
- Stricture (in small bowel or colon cases)
- Most commonly found in the gastric body or the prepyloric area

Microscopic Findings

- Infiltrate of small monocytoid lymphocytes often mixed with immunoblasts and plasmacytoid cells
- Lymphoepithelial lesions
- Infiltrate expands interfollicular space and effaces normal architecture
- Prominent plasma cell differentiation in up to a third of gastric cases
- Reactive follicles occasionally present with the colonization of the follicles
- Presence of moderate nuclear atypia, Dutcher bodies, and prominent lymphoepithelial lesions are features highly suggestive of lymphoma

Immunohistochemistry

- Positive B-cell markers (CD19, CD20, PAX5, CD79), BCL2+, CD3-, CD5-, LEF1-, Cyclin D1-, SOX11- BCL6-, LMO2-, CD10-, and low Ki-67 proliferation index
- Minority of cases (20%–40%) are CD43+

Genetic Abnormalities

- t(11;18)(q21;q21) , API2/MALT1
- t(1;14) results in *BCL1* and *IGH* fusion leading to overexpression of BCL10
- Trisomy of chromosomes 3 and 18

Differential Diagnosis

- Reactive lymphoid hyperplasia such as chronic *Helicobacter* gastritis or autoimmune gastritis
- Mantle cell lymphoma (Cyclin D1+, SOX11+, CD5+, BCL2+, CD43+, LEF1-, CD23-, CD10-, BCL6-, LMO2-)
- Follicular lymphoma (CD10+, BCL6+, LMO2+, BCL2+, CD43-, CD5-, cyclin D1-, SOX11-, LEF1-, CD23-)
- Small cell lymphoma/Chronic lymphocytic leukemia (CD5+, LEF1+, CD43+, CD23+, CD43+, BCL2+, SOX11-, CD10-, BCL6-, LMO2-, cyclin D1-)
- DLBCL

IMMUNOPROLIFERATIVE SMALL INTESTINAL DISEASE (α HEAVY CHAIN DISEASE)

Immunoproliferative small intestinal disease (also known as α heavy chain disease, Mediterranean lymphoma, and diffuse small intestinal lymphoma) is a subtype of extranodal marginal lymphoma of mucosa associated lymphoid tissue. The production of α heavy chains without associated light chains characterizes this disease. IPSID occurs almost exclusively the Mediterranean, Middle Eastern, and North African countries. However, the disease has also been reported in places with a prominent population of migrants, including Asia, Europe, and the United States. This lymphoma accounts for up to 75% of the GI lymphomas that occur in adolescents and adults in the Middle East.

CLINICAL FEATURES

Immunoproliferative small intestinal disease typically affects adolescent and younger adults with a median age of 25 years. Patients typically present with abdominal pain with chronic diarrhea and malabsorption (often severe), resulting in malnutrition and weight loss. In these patients, the malnutrition can lead to peripheral edema, muscle spasms, and digital clubbing. GI tract obstruction, bleeding, and perforation is uncommon. However, these patients can also present with enteroenteric fistula as well as lactose intolerance, hypocalcemia, and organomegaly. Common risk factors for IPSID include low socioeconomic status, poor sanitation, endemic parasitic infestation, and history of infantile infectious enteritis. Importantly, in areas with improving sanitary conditions, the frequency of the disease is decreasing. Similar to the association of *H. pylori* infection and gastric marginal zone lymphoma, IPSID is thought to be associated with an infectious etiology. Specifically, *Campylobacter jejuni* has been shown to be associated with IPSID, although other possible infectious agents have also been suggested. As mentioned earlier, patients with IPSID produce an altered α heavy chain that can be secreted and then detected in body fluids. Up to 70% of patients can have an α heavy chain paraprotein, which typically is at its highest levels early in the disease course and may diminish as the disease progresses.

Pathologic Features

Gross and Endoscopic Findings

Immunoproliferative small intestinal disease can be divided into three stages based on gross and microscopic features and the extent of involvement. The lymphoma typically involves the proximal portion of the small bowel but can involve any other part of the small bowel. Additionally, gastric and colonic lesions have been reported. Stage A is confined to the small bowel and mesenteric lymph node. There are typically no gross lesions. Stage B disease typically demonstrates a mildly modular or cobblestone appearance. In stage C disease, patients have can have single or multiple larger masses.

Microscopic Findings

Immunoproliferative small intestinal disease demonstrates a histologic spectrum ranging from low-grade histologic changes seen in stage A and B to high-grade histology seen in stage C. Because this is considered a specialized subtype of MALT lymphoma, most patients demonstrate features typical of MALT lymphomas. Specifically, IPSID tends to demonstrate marked plasmacytic differentiation. In stage A, there is a lymphoplasmacytic infiltrate with lymphoepithelial lesions. Similar to typical MALT lymphomas, there are often reactive follicles surrounded by marginal zone with an expansion of the lamina propria. The changes are limited to the mucosa and often demonstrate widened or blunted villi. In stage B disease, the neoplastic cells demonstrate similar morphologic features as those of stage A. However, the infiltrate becomes nodular, imparting an endoscopic appearance of thickened mucosal folds, nodularity, flatting, or cobblestoning of the small bowel mucosa. The infiltrate also extends beyond the mucosa through the muscularis propria to involve the submucosa or muscularis propria. Stage C disease represents large cell transformation in which large masses are seen in the small bowel. The neoplastic cells often retain a plasmacytoid appearance but are often quite pleomorphic and bizarre appearing. Additionally, the mesenteric lymph nodes can be involved in any stage. Typically, in early-stage disease, the lymph node sinuses are expanded by plasma cells with progressive involvement of the marginal zone and colonization of the follicular centers.

Ancillary Studies

The neoplastic cells are positive for B-cell markers CD20, PAX5, and CD79a as well as BCL2. They can also aberrantly express CD43 but are negative for germinal center markers CD10, BCL6, and LMO2. Additionally, the neoplastic cells are negative for aberrant coexpression of CD5, cyclin D1, LEF1, and CD23. The plasmacytic component can be highlighted by plasma cell marker CD138.

One of the distinctive features of IPSID is the presence of an aberrant α heavy-chain protein in which the Ig lacks the variable heavy chain domain as well as the first constant domain producing a truncated Ig that cannot bind to the light chain. This protein can be detected in the plasma or serum. Additionally, the α Ig heavy chains can be demonstrated in the cytoplasm of the infiltrating B cells, plasma cells, and transformed large cells. The Ig heavy chain is clonally arranged. However, other recurrent genetic abnormalities have not been described. Specifically, the t(11;18) translocation described in other MALT lymphomas has not been demonstrated in IPSID.

Differential Diagnosis

The differential diagnosis for IPSID depends on the stage of the disease. As described earlier, one of the most challenging differentials is between lymphoma and reactive lymphoid process. In stage A, the initial consideration is often that of gluten-sensitive enteropathy (GSE) or celiac disease. However, in GSE, the intraepithelial lymphocytes are significantly increased with associated villous atrophy. Typically, patients with GSE are from northern European ancestry and respond to a gluten-free diet. Also, the infiltrate in GSE is CD3+ T cells, whereas IPSID is populated by CD20+ B cells. Additionally, other intestinal T-cell lymphomas often present with a similar diffuse infiltrate like IPSID; however, these are easily differentiated by CD3 and CD20 immunostains.

The nodular lymphoid aggregates of stage B disease can mimic reactive lymphoid hyperplasia as well as FL and MCL. Reactive follicular hyperplasia is common in the distal small bowel, but lymphoid aggregates in the proximal small bowel necessitate additional work up. The reactive processes also lack prominent lymphoepithelial lesions that are typical of MALT-lymphoma or IPSID. Compared with other low-grade lymphomas, IPSID demonstrates a prominent plasma cell or plasmacytoid differentiation with lymphoepithelial lesions. The neoplastic cells are not as monotonous as is typical of MCL and do not demonstrate aberrant expression of cyclin D1 or SOX11. FL consists of centrocytes with germinal center differentiation and aberrant BCL2 expression.

The differential diagnosis of stage C disease is that of high-grade malignancies, including EATL, DLBCL malignancies, plasmablastic lymphoma (PBL), and even poorly differentiated carcinoma or melanoma. Often among and between the pleomorphic neoplastic cells are residual low-grade neoplastic cells that can help with these differentials

Prognosis and Therapy

There are no treatment guidelines for patients with IPSID; however, in patients with early-stage disease, the use of broad-spectrum antibiotic therapy has led to remission, similar to *Helicobacter* eradication for gastric MALT lymphoma. In more advanced cases with visible tumor masses, chemotherapy with rituximab (e.g., R-CHOP [rituximab, cyclophosphamide, doxorubicin, vincristine, and prednisone]) is typically used, with reported remission and long-term survival rate of up to 70%. Ultimately, in situations with obstructing tumors, treatment with radiation, surgery, or both may be required.

Immunoproliferative Small Intestinal Disease—Pathologic Features

Gross, Endoscopic, and Radiology Findings

- May have normal macroscopic appearance
- Thickened mucosal folds and nodularity or cobblestoning
- Advanced disease presents with large masses
- Typically involves the proximal small intestine but may also involve any part of the small intestine, and involvement of stomach and colon have been reported
- Mesenteric lymph node involvement is a common finding in all stages of the disease
- Direct extension into adjacent structures is a feature of advanced disease

Microscopic Findings

- Stage A: dense lymphoplasmacytic infiltrate with features of a typical mucosa-associated lymphoid tissue (MALT lymphoma), including lymphoepithelial lesions, but is restricted to the mucosa
- Stage B: similar features to stage A with prominent nodular infiltrate and germinal center colonization, infiltrate extends through the muscularis mucosa into the submucosa, and no evidence of large cell transformation
- Stage C: large masses with a transformation to large cell lymphoma, plasmacytoid differentiation often evident along with centroblasts, immunoblasts, and pleomorphic cells

Immunohistochemistry

- CD20+, CD19+ PAX5+, CD79a+, BCL2+, CD5-, CD10-, BCL6- and CD23-; may be positive for CD43. The plasmacytic component is positive for CD138
- α-Immunoglobulin heavy chains in the cytoplasm (typically without light chain expression) of the infiltrating plasma cells, centrocytes, and transformed blast cells

Differential Diagnosis

- Low-stage disease: reactive lymphoid hyperplasia, mantle cell lymphoma, celiac disease, indolent T-cell lymphoma, and follicular lymphoma
- High-stage disease: large B-cell lymphoma, enteropathy-associated T-cell lymphoma, melanoma, and other poorly differentiated malignancies

Immunoproliferative Small Intestinal Disease—Fact Sheet

Definition

- IPSID and α heavy-chain disease are considered subtypes of MALT lymphoma that produces α heavy chain that can be either secreted or nonsecreted by the neoplastic cells

Incidence and Location

- Primarily in Mediterranean, Middle East, and North Africa
- In these areas, immunoproliferative small intestinal disease accounts for up to 20% of non-Hodgkin lymphomas and 75% of all small bowel neoplasms

Gender, Race, and Age Distribution

- Young adults with a median age of 25 to 30 years; no gender to only a slight male predominance

Clinical Features

- Severe chronic intermittent diarrhea, abdominal pain, weight loss ultimately leading to severe carbohydrate and lipid malnutrition
- Protein-losing enteropathy can be seen
- Nearly half of patients have peripheral edema, tetany, and clubbing of digits

Prognosis and Treatment

- Patients with early-stage disease respond to antibiotics
- Established disease: radiation therapy and/or combination chemotherapy combined with nutritional support
- Because intestinal involvement is generally diffuse, surgery is rarely indicated
- Prognosis is variable; it was previously poor, but the chance of 5-year survival might be as high as 70%

FOLLICULAR LYMPHOMA (INCLUDING PRIMARY DUODENAL-TYPE FOLLICULAR LYMPHOMA)

Although outside of the GI tract, the two most common lymphomas are FL and DLBCL; FL is far less common in the GI tract. Specifically, systemic FL makes up to 40 % of all non-Hodgkin lymphomas (NHLs) and up to 70 % of mature B-cell lymphoma. However, FL only accounts for 1 % to 6 % of primary GI lymphomas. FL is a neoplasm of follicle (germinal) center cells and consists of smaller centrocytes admixed with larger centroblasts. There is a unique variant of FL that occurs in the GI tract and was initially referred to as primary intestinal FL in the 2008 edition of the WHO Classification of Tumours of the Haematopoietic and Lymphoid Tissues. In the 2017 update to the WHO classification, the lesion is referred to as duodenal-type follicular lymphoma (DTFL). These are unique and have a different course than systemic FL's involvement of other locations in the GI tract. DTFL primarily occurs in the second portion of the duodenum or periampullary. DTFL is a localized polypoid variant of this disease typically limited to a stage IE disease and tends to have an indolent course. DTFL is rare with current estimates of occurring once in 3000 to 7000 endoscopic evaluations. In one recent review of 1109 GI FL cases, 63.6 % of cases involved the small bowel with 18.2 % involving the stomach and 18.2 % in the colon.

Pathologic Features

Gross and Endoscopic Findings

Follicular lymphomas can have a variety of appearances. DTFL presents as small polyps in the duodenum (often distal). Typical FLs can form obstructive lesions, especially when they involve the terminal ileum, as well as ulcerated lesions. Similar to MCL, they can have a multiple "lymphomatous polyposis"–like appearance. Increasing numbers of FLs are diagnosed incidentally on screening colonoscopy or esophagogastroduodenoscopy. Capsule endoscopy, as well as barium studies and computed tomography scans, can assist in identifying multiple small polyps or intussusception. Imaging may also highlight involved mesenteric lymph nodes.

Microscopic Findings

The neoplastic cells are composed of two B-cell types that are found in follicle or germinal centers, centrocytes, and centroblasts. The centrocytes are small and have angulated and cleaved nuclei with inconspicuous nucleoli. The centroblasts are larger cells that have round to oval nuclei that can occasionally appear indented or cleaved. Centroblasts have one to three nucleoli, and the cells are typically greater than three times the size of normal lymphocytes. The number of these large centroblasts in a high-power field (hpf) determines the grade of the tumor with up to 5 centroblasts being grade 1, 6 to 15 being grade 2, and greater than 15 being grade 3. The current WHO combines grade 1 and 2 into a low-grade category. There are two growth patterns, a nodular and a diffuse growth pattern. The diffuse pattern can have a prominent sclerotic component and on biopsies can lack any nodular architecture.

Typically, FL presents as nodules composed primarily of centrocytes. Compared with normal germinal centers, the neoplastic nodules lack tangible body macrophages and significant mitotic figures (Fig. 19.2A and B). Occasionally, only the diffuse portion is biopsied, which can mimic the other low-grade B-cell lymphomas. DTFL almost exclusively consists of centrocytes in a predominantly follicular pattern (Fig. 19.2A) and is limited to the mucosa or submucosa. If the lymphoma demonstrates high-grade features, has extensive diffuse growth pattern, extends into or beyond the muscularis propria, or demonstrates extensive lymph node involvement, it be consistent with systemic FL involvement of the GI lymphoma and should not be considered a DTFL.

Ancillary Studies

The neoplastic cells are positive for B-cell markers CD19, CD20, PAX5, and CD79a (Fig. 19.2C). The neoplastic cells are derived from the germinal center and as such are typically positive for CD10, BCL6, and LMO2 (Fig. 19.2E and F). However, in some cases, CD10 can be weak or lost. The neoplastic cells demonstrate aberrant coexpression of BCL2 (Fig. 19.2G). Most FLs will be positive for the standard BCL2 (clone 124); however, because mutations can occur in the *BCL2* gene, the use of an alternative BCL2 clone (clone EP36/E17) is sometimes necessary to confirm the diagnosis. The neoplastic cells are negative of CD3, CD43 (Fig. 19.2D), CD5, Cyclin D1, Sox-11, and Lef1. Typically, whereas neoplastic follicles in low-grade lymphomas have a Ki-67 labeling index of less than 10 %, normal reactive germinal centers have an elevated Ki-67 (>90 %) labeling index. The dendritic cell networks are highlighted by immunostains for CD21, CD23, and CD35. Compared with the nodal and extranodal types, the DTFLs tend to have to a diminished follicular dendritic cell network, often resulting in a "hollowed-out" appearance with the stain restricted to the periphery (Fig. 19.2H). Additionally, unlike the systemic forms, the duodenal-type variant often express IgA as well as the mucosal homing receptor α-β7.

Follicular lymphomas demonstrate clonal rearrangements of the Ig heavy chain and light chains. Additionally, almost all FLs have cytogenetic abnormalities with the most common involving translocation of the *BCL2* gene,

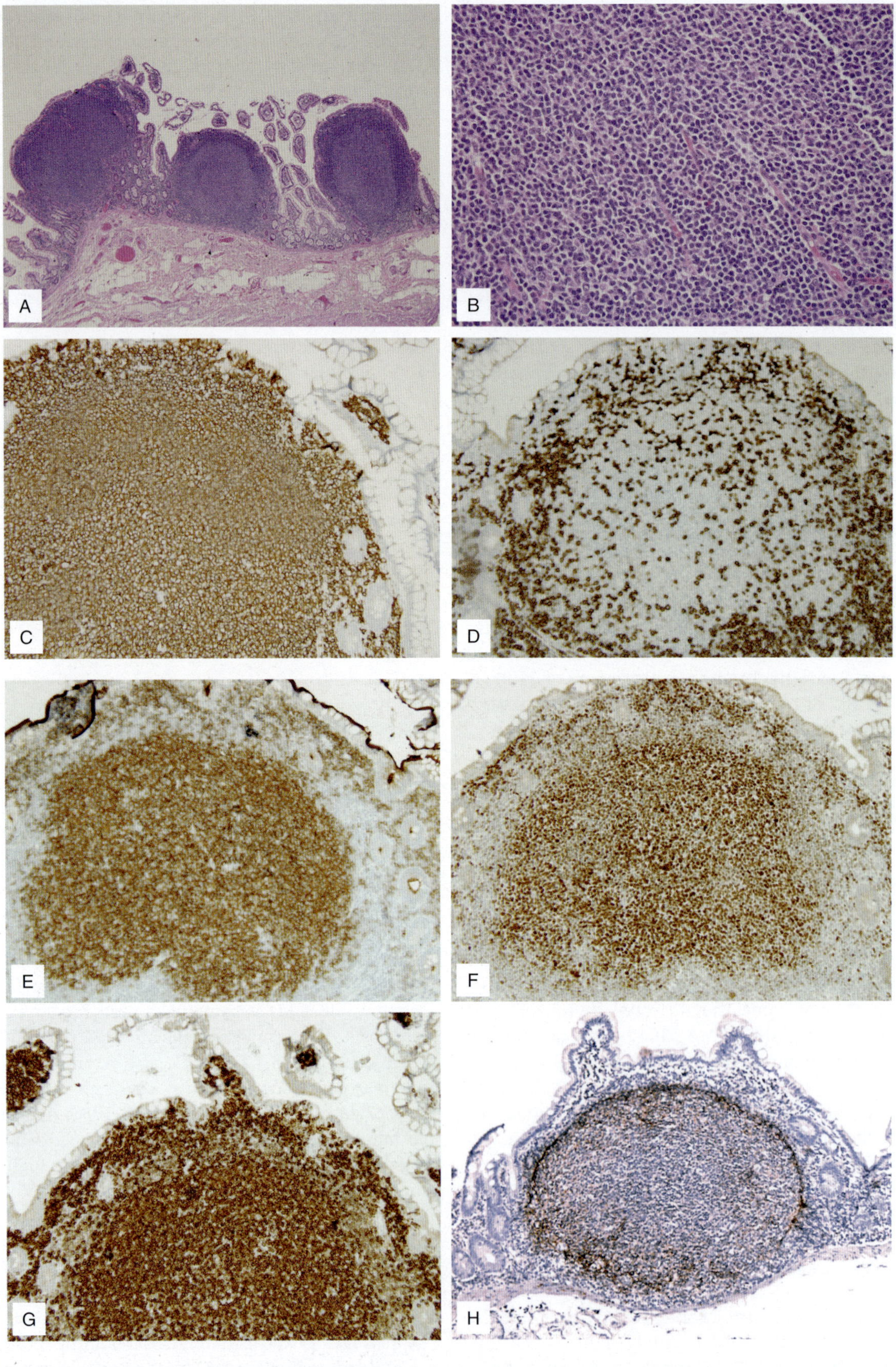

FIGURE 19.2

Follicular lymphoma. **A**, At low magnification, the neoplastic infiltrate is composed of mixture of small centrocytes with nuclear irregularities and no nucleoli and larger centroblasts with vesicular chromatin and prominent nucleoli (**B**). The lymphoid nodules are CD20+ B cells (**C**) that are negative for aberrant coexpression for CD43 (**D**). These germinal center–derived cells expression CD10 (E) and BCL6 (**F**) with aberrant expression of BCL2 (**G**). In cases of duodenal follicular lymphoma, the CD21 highlights diminished follicular dendritic cell network often resulting in a "hollowed-out" appearance with the stain restricted to the periphery (**H**).

which can be identified in up to 90% of low-grade FLs. The most common is the translocation involving the *BCL2* and *IGH* genes, t(14;18)(q32;q21), with rare cases involving the *BCL2* and light chain gene t(2;18)(p12;q21). The majority of DTFLs tested to date only have a *BCL2/IGH* translocation. Outside of this variant, only 10% of cases have only the t(14;18) with most demonstrating additional abnormalities. Other frequent abnormalities, which can be seen in non-DTFL forms, include *BCL6* rearrangements or *BCL6* 5' mutations, as well as +7, +12, +18, 17p deletion, and 6q23-36 abnormalities. A translocation involving *IRF4* can rarely be seen in cases of grade 3 FLs. Interestingly, DTFL (compared with systemic) demonstrates elevated expression of CCL20 and MADCAM1 similar to marginal zone lymphoma.

Differential Diagnosis

The differential diagnosis includes benign reactive lymphoid proliferation, such as follicular hyperplasia and rectal tonsil, as well as other low-grade B-cell lymphomas. Specifically, many conditions in the GI tract can lead to nodular lymphoid hyperplasia, and the distal small bowel usually demonstrates prominent lymphoid aggregates with well-defined germinal centers. Most reactive nodular FL hyperplasia can be differentiated from FL on histology evaluation. Reactive lymphoid hyperplasia demonstrates expanded polarized germinal centers with intact marginal and mantle zones. The germinal centers also demonstrate prominent mitotic activity with high Ki-67 labeling index and multiple tingible body macrophages. These reactive germinal centers express germinal center markers BCL6, CD10, and LMO2 but are negative for aberrant BCL2 expression. The reactive process typically demonstrates increased mitotic index with Ki-67 of greater than 90%; however, neoplastic follicles typically demonstrate less than 10% Ki-67 staining. Most of the other mature B cells lymphomas (marginal zone, mantle, and SLL) can have a nodular growth pattern, and immunohistochemical features are often vital in the differential. BCL2 expression helps differentiate FL from benign germinal centers, but most other mature B-cell lymphomas also expression the antiapoptotic protein BCL2.

Prognosis and Therapy

The prognosis of patients with FL can be variable depending on the grade and stage of the lesion. There is a specific prognostic system for FL (Follicular Lymphoma International Prognostic Index score), which includes age older than 60 years, serum lactate dehydrogenase, hemoglobin level, Ann Arbor stage, and number of involved nodal areas. Compared with a systemic variant of lymphoma, DTFL has a particular indolent course. Specifically, DTFL is a localized disease to the mucosa and submucosa with only rare cases demonstrating evidence of nodal disease, and none of these cases demonstrated high-grade transformation. Patients with asymptomatic DTFL can be treated with a watch-and-wait approach. In general, therapy for patients with low-grade FL is directed at symptom relief and includes resection or excision, single-agent chemotherapy (rituximab only), or radiation therapy. Low-grade FLs are typically considered noncurative and are a chronic disease with a median survival time of greater than 12 years. Follow-up is aimed at evaluation for high-grade transformation or progression to DLBCL or high-grade B-cell lymphoma (HGBL; double-hit lymphomas). Grade 3a lesions tend to have a more aggressive course than grade 1 and 2 lesions requiring therapy. However, those treated with doxorubicin-containing regiments demonstrate similar overall survival to grade 1 and 2 lesions.

Patients with FL grade 3B are treated like those with DLBCL.

FOLLICULAR LYMPHOMA–FACT SHEET

Definition

- Lymphoma that is derived from follicular or germinal center B cells and consists of centrocytes and centroblasts often with a nodular or follicular growth pattern

Incidence and Location

- Accounts for 1% to 6% of primary non-Hodgkin gastrointestinal lymphomas
- Accounts for 30-% to 40% of nodal non-Hodgkin lymphomas

Morbidity and Mortality

- Duodenal-type follicular lymphoma (DTFL) demonstrates indolent behavior with an excellent prognosis
- Low-grade (World Health Organization [WHO] grade 1 or 2) lesions with an excellent prognosis
- Grade 3 lesions have a more aggressive course

Gender, Age, and Race Distribution

- Equal male and female distribution
- Median age is 55 to 59 years
- Two to three times as prevalent in whites than blacks

Clinical Features

- Often is asymptomatic and found incidentally
- May present with abdominal pain or obstructive type symptoms

Prognosis and Treatment

- Patients with DTFL have an excellent prognosis and are often treated with a watch-and-wait approach
- Low grade (WHO grade 1–2) lesions are incurable but may be treated with a watch-and-wait approach, chemotherapy (including rituximab alone), or radiation
- Grade 3 lesions are more aggressive, requiring therapy. With aggressive therapy, these patients have similar outcomes to grade 1 or 2 lesions and in some cases can become disease free

Follicular Lymphoma—Pathologic Features

Gross, Endoscopic, and Radiology Findings
- Nodularity or granularity of the mucosa
- Can present as diffuse lesions with transmural involvement occasionally with changes of obstruction or rarely perforation

Microscopic Findings
- Follicular, diffuse, or combination of follicular and diffuse growth patterns
- Mixture of small-cleaved B cells (centrocytes) admixed with large B cells (centroblasts)

Immunohistochemistry
- Positive B cell markers (CD19, CD20, PAX5, CD79), germinal cell differentiation (CD10, BCL6, LMO2)
- Positive for aberrant coexpression of BCL2 (standard BCL2 clone124 but might need an alternative clone, e.g., EP36/E17)
- CD21, CD23, and CD35 highlight follicular dendritic cell networks, which can appear "hollowed out" in the duodenal-type variant
- Negative for CD3, CD5, Lef1, Cyclin D1, CD43, and MUM1
- Low Ki-67 proliferation index compared with reactive follicular hyperplasia

Genetic Abnormalities
- t(14;18) chromosomal rearrangement (IGH/BCL2)
- Rearranged immunoglobulin H and light chains

Differential Diagnosis
- Benign follicular lymphoid hyperplasia
- Low-grade follicular lymphoma: other low-grade B-cell lymphomas such as marginal zone lymphoma, small lymphocytic lymphoma, mantle cell lymphoma
- High-grade follicular lymphoma: diffuse large B-cell lymphoma, high-grade lymphoma, and poorly differentiated carcinoma

MANTLE CELL LYMPHOMA

Clinical Features

Mantle cell lymphoma is a small cell lymphoma that morphologically resembles a mature or low-grade B-lymphoma but typically has an aggressive clinical course. MCL is typically a disease of older adults (mean age, 60 years) with a male predominance (at least 2:1). Unfortunately, almost 70% to 80% of patients have advanced disease (stage IV) at the time of diagnosis. In some series, greater than 80% of these patients have GI tract involvement. Although any part of the GI tract can be involved, the small bowel, specifically the ileum, is the most common site. MCL was the first to be associated with lymphomatous polyposis. At the time of initial diagnosis of MCL in the GI tract, patients can be asymptomatic but may also present with abdominal pain, diarrhea, hematochezia, weight loss, and fatigue.

Pathologic Features

Gross, Endoscopic, and Radiologic features

When MCL involves the GI tract, it typically involves multiple sites with a predilection for involvement of the distal small bowel and colon. However, involvement of the stomach and duodenum can also be seen. MCL tends to present as either isolated polyps or masses or multiple small nodules or polyps and can vary in size from submillimeter to several centimeters. The numerous small polyps of lymphoma are referred to as lymphomatous polyposis. MCL can also present as ulcerated lesions (more common in the stomach), increased bowel wall thickness, or obstructive masses. Additionally, capsule endoscopy and barium radiography can demonstrate multiple small polyps in the small bowel or colon. Alternatively, imaging may demonstrate bowel wall thickening or obstructive masses as well as mesenteric and retroperitoneal lymphadenopathy or hepatic or splenic enlargement.

Microscopic Findings

Mantle cell lymphoma can grow in three architectural patterns, including mantle, nodular, and diffuse. In the GI tract, the lesions tend to be nodular or diffuse; however, mantle zone pattern and in situ disease can be seen. Typically, the lymphoma is centered in the mucosa and submucosa with a diffuse or nodular pattern. The infiltrate often displaces the glands, and although there can be glandular destruction, lymphoepithelial lesions are not typically seen.

The lymphomatous infiltrate is composed of small lymphocytes with scant cytoplasm and irregular nuclei. The classical variant cells are typically very monomorphic or monotonous compared with other mature or low-grade lymphomas or reactive conditions (Fig. 19.3A and B). In the background, there are often scattered epithelioid macrophages, which can give the section a "starry-sky" appearance. There are only rare larger cells, which tend to be follicular dendritic cells and not large neoplastic cells. Another classic finding is the presence of hyalinized small vessels throughout the lesion. Mitotic figures are easy to identify but are usually less than 1 to 2/hpf. There are two aggressive variants of MCL, the blastoid and the pleomorphic variants. The blastoid variant is typically monomorphic medium to large cells resembling lymphoblasts and can resemble cells of acute leukemia or lymphoma. This variant typically also contains tingible body macrophages and increased mitotic index of greater than 3 mitoses/hpf. As the name suggests, pleomorphic MCL demonstrates variable size from large anaplastic-looking cells to small lymphocytes seen in the classic variant. The proliferation index is between that of the blastoid variant and the classic variant. Often the morphologic features overlap and are challenging to differentiate from DLBCL.

Ancillary Studies

The neoplastic cells are positive for B-cell markers CD20, CD19, CD79a, and PAX5 (Fig. 19.3C). Additionally, the neoplastic B cells aberrantly expression CD5 and CD43 and are negative for CD3 (Fig. 19.3D and E). There is normal expression for BCL-2; however, the cells typically lack expression of germinal center markers CD10, BCL6, and LMO2. The B cells are also typically negative for aberrant coexpression for LEF1 and CD23 (Fig. 19.3H). By flow cytometry, MCL is typically positive for the FMC7 (an epitope of CD20). MCL demonstrates nuclear expression of cyclin D1 (BCL1) in the vast majority of cases (Fig. 19.3F). Fortunately, SOX11 is expressed in most cases of cyclin D1 positive and negative cases as well as the blastoid and pleomorphic variants (Fig. 19.3G). There can be expression of MUM1/IRF4 in a minority of the lymphoma cells. Mantle cells typically express surface IgM or IgD heavy chain with a restricted surface light chain expression, typically lambda restricted.

Fluorescent in situ hybridization (FISH) and cytogenetic studies typically demonstrate the classic translocation associated with MCL, which is t(11;14)(q13;q32), involving the *cyclin D1* gene and the *IGH* gene. The t(11;14) is seen in the vast majority of cases; however, there is a minor population of MCL that does not have the cyclin D1 translocation. In these cases, t(2;12) (p12;p13) translocation, fusing cyclin D2 to the κ light-chain gene locus, or a t(6;14)(p21;q32) translocation, fusing IGH and cyclin D3, have been identified. Additionally, several other cytogenetic alterations have been reported, including gains in 3q, 7p, 8q, 12q, and 18q and loss of 1p, 6q, 8p, 9p, 10p, 11q, 13, and 17p. Additionally, tetraploidy and complex karyotypes are more often associated with pleomorphic or blastoid variants. MYC (8q24) translocations can also be seen in blastoid MCL and tend to predict an aggressive clinical course.

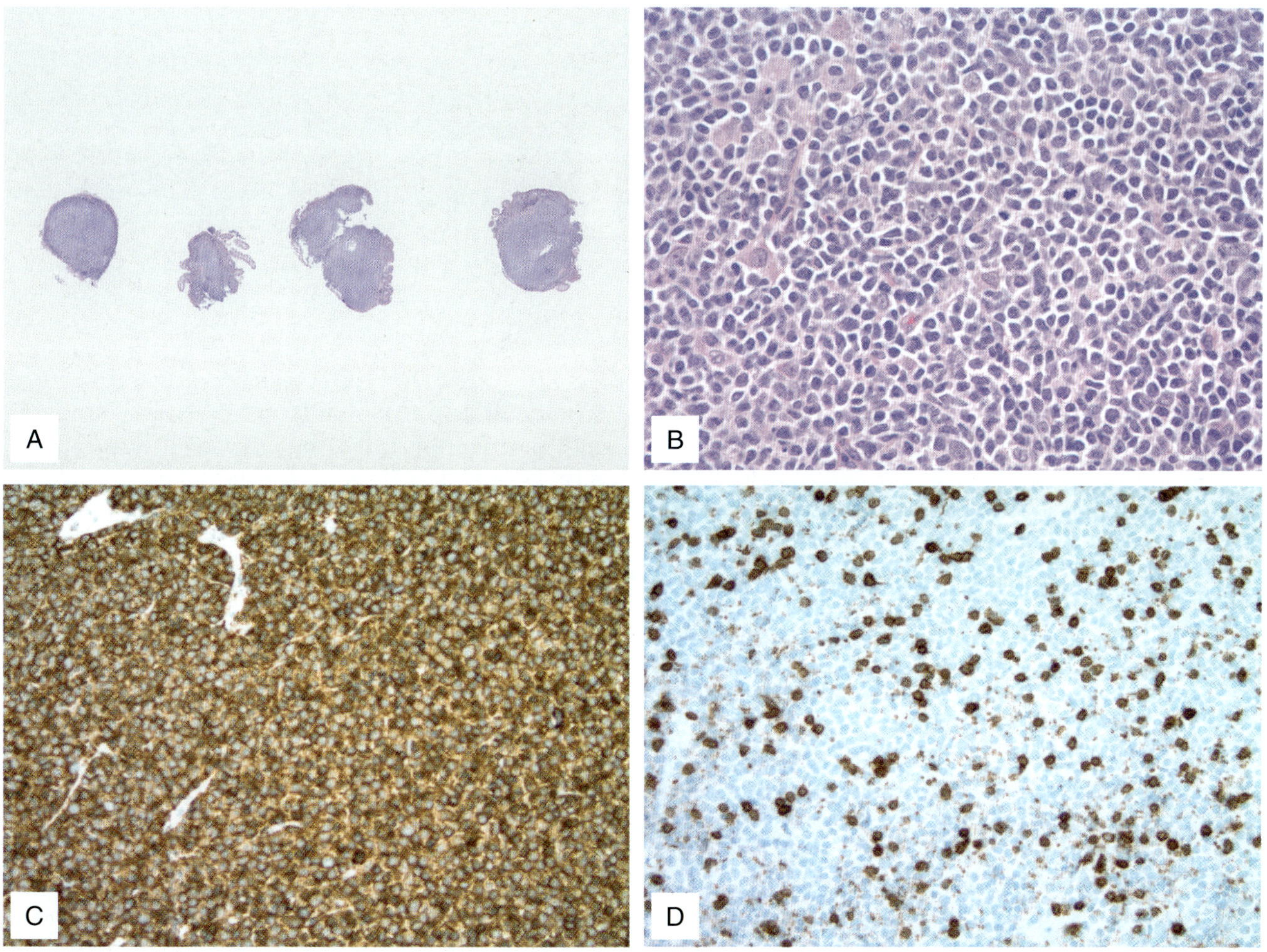

FIGURE 19.3

Mantle cell lymphoma. **A**, Mantle cell lymphoma often forms polypoid masses in the gastrointestinal tract (lymphomatous polyposis) and can be seen in the biopsy of multiple polyps (low magnification). **B**, At high magnification, the infiltrate is composed of a monomorphic population of small lymphocytes with minimally irregular nuclei and scattered epithelioid histocytes. These lymphocytes are B cells with expression of CD20 (C) and aberrant expression of CD5

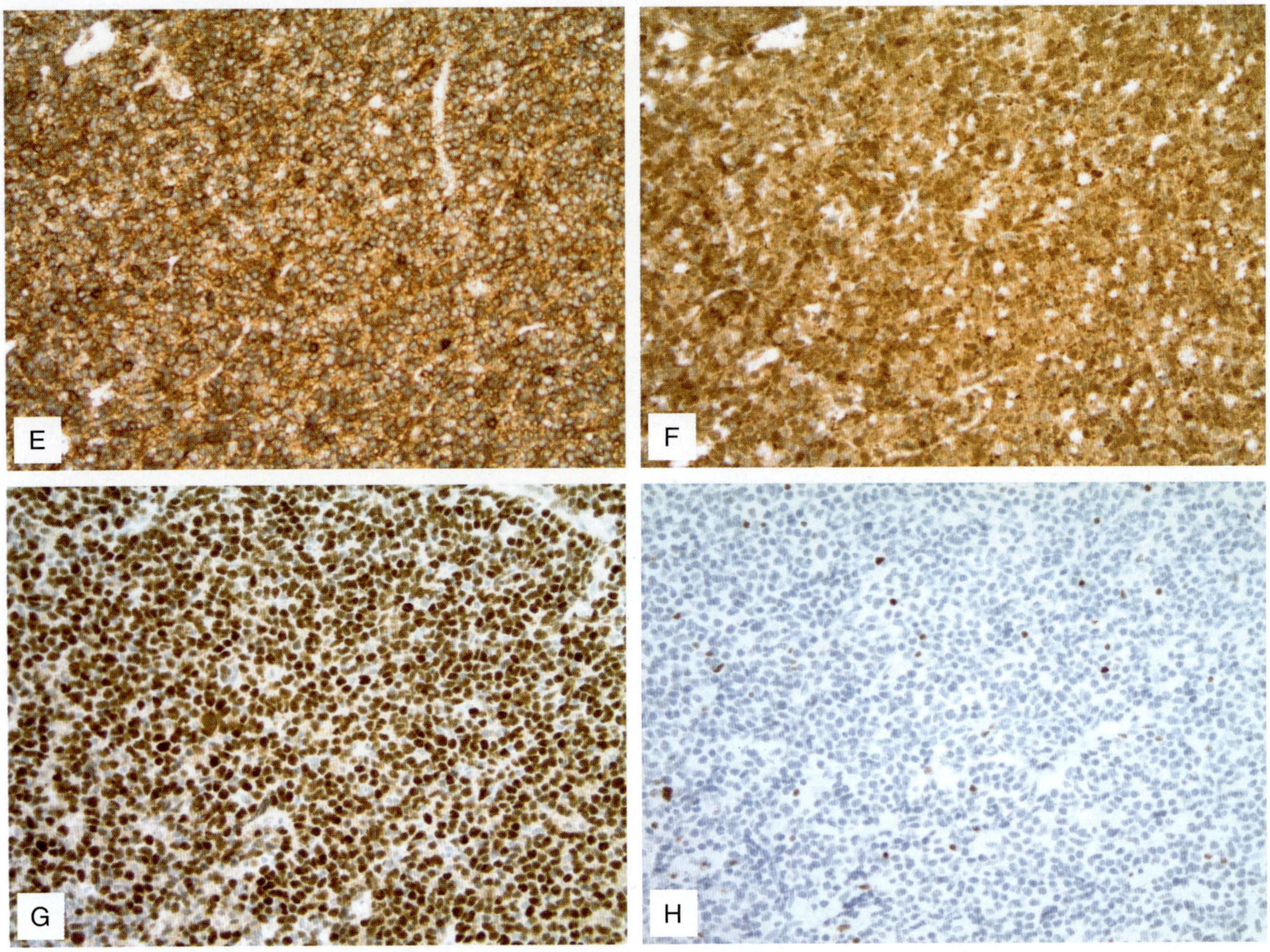

(**E**). The background T cells is highlighted by CD3 (**D**). These neoplastic cells are positive for cyclin D1 (**F**) and SOX11 (**G**) expression. These neoplastic B cells are negative for LEF1 (H) expression that is typically seen in small lymphocytic lymphoma and chronic lymphocytic leukemia.

Differential Diagnosis

The primary diagnostic considerations are other low-grade lymphomas such as marginal zone lymphoma, FL, and SLL. Specifically, lymphomatous polyposis can be caused by MCL, FL, or marginal zone lymphoma. From a cytomorphologic perspective, MCL cells are very monotonous appearing with slight nuclear irregularities, but they lack the typical cleaved morphology of FL cells and the monocytoid appearance of marginal zone lymphoma cells. Given that many of the biopsies suffer from extensive crush artifacts, increased importance is placed on immunohistochemical and cytogenetic findings. Specifically, although both FL and MCL are positive for pan-B-cell markers and BCL2, FL cell also expresses germinal center markers CD10, BCL6, and LMO2, which are negative in MCL. Conversely, MCL expresses CD5, cyclin D1, SOX11, and CD43, and patients typically have systemic disease as well. SLL or CLL can also be a systemic disease, and like MCL, expresses pan-B-cell markers, BCL-2, CD5 and CD43. However, SLL is typically positive for LEF1, but the MCL is positive for cyclin D1 and SOX11. A notable pitfall is that the proliferation centers of SLL or CLL can be cyclin D1 positive by immunohistochemical stains.

Prognosis and Therapy

Typically, at the time of diagnosis, the patient already has systemic disease. Surgery generally has limited utility unless there are obstructive type symptoms or if there was persistent hemorrhage. Survival is poor and worse in patients with blastoid or pleomorphic variants or classic type with a Ki-67 index of greater than 40% to 50%. The overall median survival period is 3 to 5 years from the time of diagnosis. Unfortunately, the majority of patients are not curable even with aggressive chemotherapy and newer therapeutic modalities.

MANTLE CELL LYMPHOMA—FACT SHEET

Definition

- Mature appearing B-cell lymphoma with often aggressive clinical course
- Typically systemic disease with secondary involvement of the gastrointestinal (GI) tract
- Can present as lymphomatous polyposis

Incidence

- Represents 3% to 10% of non-Hodgkin lymphomas
- More than 80% of patient with systemic disease can also have GI involvement

Gender, Race, and Age Distribution

- Mean age at presentation is 60 years
- Male predominance (greater than 2:1, males to females)

Clinical Features

- Abdominal pain
- Diarrhea
- Hematochezia
- Weight loss
- Fatigue
- Widespread disease (hepatosplenomegaly and lymphadenopathy)
- Asymptomatic

Prognosis and Treatment

- Generally considered an incurable disease
- Median survival of 3 to 5 years; patients with blastoid and pleomorphic types have a worse prognosis
- Mitotic index correlates with prognosis with greater than 50 mitoses per mm2 corresponding to a worse prognosis
- Systemic chemotherapy is the treatment of choice
- Aggressive chemotherapy followed by autologous stem cell transplantation may benefit younger patients
- Surgery has a role in cases with bowel obstruction or continuous bleeding

MANTLE CELL LYMPHOMA—PATHOLOGIC FEATURES

Gross, Endoscopic, and Radiology Findings

- Predilection for the colon and small intestine in nearly all cases, but gastric and duodenal involvement are also common
- An isolated mass or multiple polyps throughout the GI tract
- Multiple polyps referred to as *lymphomatous polyposis*
- Polyps range from 0.5 cm to 2 cm; larger polyps common in the ileocecal region
- Nodules or polypoid tumors may be ulcerated with or without normal intervening mucosa
- Involvement by and extension into regional fibroadipose mesentery is common
- Barium radiographs can show numerous luminal round filling defects or tumor mass
- Abdominal computed tomography reveals intestinal wall thickening, mass lesion, retroperitoneal lymphadenopathy, and hepatic or splenic enlargement

Microscopic Findings

- Small to medium sized with scant cytoplasm
- Irregular nuclear outlines (but no deep clefts) and indistinct nucleoli
- Mitotic figures can be easily identified
- Most common architectural pattern is diffuse, but a nodular pattern and true mantle zone pattern can be seen
- Reactive follicles may be intermixed and compressed by the lymphoma
- Some epithelial involvement, but no actual lymphoepithelial lesions

Immunohistochemistry

- Positive for B-cell markers (CD20, CD19, PAX5, CD79a) and BCL2
- Aberrant positive expression of CD5, CD43, FMC7, Cyclin D1, and SOX11
- Negative for germinal center markers (CD10, BCL6, LMO2), markers associated with small lymphocytic lymphoma and chronic lymphocytic leukemia (CD23 and LEF1), and TdT
- Surface immunoglobulin expression (usually immunoglobulin [Ig] M or IgD) with light chain restriction, typically lambda restricted is present
- Ki-67 important prognostic marker; greater than 40% to 50% associated with an adverse prognosis

Genetic Abnormalities

- Typical genetic alteration - t(11;14)(q13;q32) chromosomal rearrangement cyclin D1 with Ig heavy chain (CCND1/IGH)
- Cyclin D1 negative variant typically has rearrangements involving CCND2 or CCND3
- t(2;12) (p12;p13) translocation, fusing cyclin D2 to the κ light-chain gene locus or a t(6;14)(p21;q32) translocation, fusing IGH and CCND3
- MYC (8q24) alterations, including the t(8;14)(q24;q32) translocation, have been seen in blastoid variant cases and tend to correlate with aggressive clinical course
- Clonally rearranged IgH and/or light chain

Differential Diagnosis

- Reactive follicular hyperplasia (polarized germinal centers, without aberrant expression of CD5, CD43, cyclin D1, SOX11, or LEF1 on B cells)
- Follicular lymphoma (CD10+, BCL6+, LMO2+, CD5-, Cyclin D1-, SOX11-, CD43-)
- Mucosa-associated lymphoid tissue (CD10-, CD5-, Cyclin D1-, SOX11-, CD43+/-)
- Small lymphocytic lymphoma (CD10-, CD5+, LEF1+, SOX11-, Cyclin D1 typically negative but can be positive in proliferation centers, CD43+, CD23+, FMC7-)

LARGE CELL AND AGGRESSIVE B-CELL LYMPHOMAS

In addition to mature B-cell lymphomas, the GI tract is commonly involved by diffuse and aggressive large B-cell lymphoma. The entities that can commonly involve the GI tract and are discussed later include DLBCL, not otherwise specified (DLBCL, NOS); Epstein-Barr virus–positive DLBCL, NOS; high-grade B-cell lymphoma; PBL; and BL. At the end of this section, EBV-positive mucocutaneous ulcer is also discussed

DIFFUSE LARGE B-CELL LYMPHOMA

Clinical Features

This is the most common nodal and extranodal NHL. DLBCL is one of the most common lymphomas involving the GI tract and can involve any portion of the GI tract. Unlike those with mature low-grade B-cell lymphomas, patients with DLBCL are more likely to be symptomatic from ulcerations, GI bleed, obstruction, or perforation. However, some patients may be asymptomatic. DLBCL can either arise de novo or may occur as progression or transformation of low-grade lesions. It is essential to make a note of any possible existing or concurrent low-grade lymphoma. For example, DLBCL of the GI tract is most frequently encountered in the stomach. Some patients show histologic evidence of concurrent low-grade B-cell lymphoma (marginal zone lymphoma). For gastric DLBCLs, *Helicobacter* infections have shown to be involved both in MALT lymphoma associated DLBCL and de novo DLBCL. The presence of *Helicobacter* organisms should be noted in any gastric carcinoma or lymphoma. In the revised 2017 WHO classification, EBV-infected lymphoma and double-hit lymphoma are classified separately as EBV-positive DLBCL, NOS, and HGBL, respectively

Pathologic Features

Gross Findings

Grossly, DLBCL can have a variety of appearances. DLBCL of the stomach typically presents as solitary or multifocal ulceration and most commonly involves the gastric body or fundus. Additionally, in the minority of cases, DLBCL can present as polypoid lesions or diffusely infiltrative lesion, leading to a "linitis plastica" appearance. In the small bowel, DLBCL also typically presents as an ulcerated lesion but can also occur as a single polypoid lesion or multiple polyps or polyposis. DLBCL can also have an infiltrative pattern that presents as a stricture or perforation. In the colon, DLBCL typically presents as a bulky annular lesion that is most often suspected to be a carcinoma. Typically, regional lymph nodes are involved, especially in nongastric cases.

Microscopic Findings

The histologic features of DLBCL are the same in the GI tract as in other locations. The lesions are composed of a proliferation of large to intermediate-sized lymphoid cells that typically have a diffuse growth pattern. The large neoplastic cells form sheets of neoplastic cells but may be intermixed with a low-grade (mature) B-cell lymphoma or with the prominent T-cell background. The neoplastic cells can be morphologically heterogeneous and can be divided into three variants: centroblasts, immunoblasts, and anaplastic. Occasionally in these lesions, cell size can be challenging to determine. A helpful way to determine the cell size is to compare it with the nucleus of endothelial cells or benign histiocytes. The most common variant and appearance of the neoplastic cells are the centroblasts. Centroblasts are large B cells with round to oval nuclei with multiple (two to four) small nuclei that are typically attached to the nuclear membrane. The cells show minimal amount of cytoplasm. The immunoblasts are large cells typically with a single large nucleolus. These have more cytoplasm than centroblasts, and in some cases, acquire a more plasmablastic type appearance with ample basophilic cytoplasm. The anaplastic variant has large to extremely large neoplastic cells with pleomorphic to bizarre nuclei.

In the GI tract, DLBCLs can often also demonstrate lymphoepithelial lesions with the neoplastic cells invading and destroying the glandular epithelium.

Ancillary Studies

The large neoplastic cells typically express B-cell markers, CD20, CD22, CD79a, PAX5, and CD19. In cases of lymphoma treated with rituximab, the neoplastic cells lack expression of CD20; therefore, alternative B-cell markers are needed to confirm the diagnosis. Additionally, in cases that are more plasmablastic, the neoplastic cells can express CD138. Importantly, as part of the workup, the DLBCL should be classified by cell of origin into either germinal center B-cell type or activated B-cell type (also known as nongerminal center type). Most practices prefer to use the Hans criteria and use CD10, BCL6, and MUM1 immunostains in which expression by greater than or equal to 30% of neoplastic cells is considered positive. For the Hans criteria, the germinal center subtype is either positive for CD10, or the cells are CD10-/BCL6+/MUM1-; the nongerminal center type is CD10-/BCL6- or CD10-/BCL6+/MUM1+. Additionally, immunohistochemical stains for MYC and BCL2 are typically performed with MYC considered positive if greater than 40% of the neoplastic cells are positive and BCL2 is considered positive if 50% of the neoplastic cells are positive. Importantly, immunohistochemical stains cannot be used as a surrogate for double hit rearrangement status, which requires FISH testing. Ki-67 proliferation rate typically ranges between 40% to greater than 95%. There is a small number of CD5 + DLBCLs, which represent de novo DLBCL, but cyclin D1 and SOX11 are needed to exclude the pleomorphic or blastoid variants.

Generally, Biomed B-cell clonality studies are not necessary. Typically, when the DLBCL occurs with a low-grade B-cell lymphoma, these two entities are clonally related, both by light chain restriction and at the DNA sequence level. FISH for BCL2, BCL6, and MYC are typically performed and will be discussed more in the section on HGBL.

Differential Diagnosis

The differential diagnosis includes other aggressive lymphomas, including HGBL, BL, anaplastic large cell lymphoma, EBV-positive DLBCL, PBL, and acute leukemia/lymphoma as well as poorly differentiated carcinomas.

It is most important to distinguish primary DLBCL from secondary lymphoma and other aggressive B-cell lymphomas as the treatments are quite different. The differentiation between DLBCL and HGBL is further discussed in a later section on HGBL. DLBCL can be differentiated from BL by the prototypical morphologic features of BL (as discussed later). One should keep in mind that not all cases of aggressive lymphoma with a high Ki-67 index are BLs because DLBCL and HGBL can both have Ki-67 indices that approach 100%.

Immunohistochemical stains for markers of immaturity such as CD34 and CD117 may also be useful in the differentiation of GI involvement by acute leukemia/lymphoma. Occasionally, large cell lymphoma can have a particularly cohesive appearance or an infiltrative pattern that may raise the possibility of carcinoma. In these instances, immunohistochemical stains for keratins are helpful in excluding this possibility.

Prognosis and Therapy

Standard therapy for patients with GI tract DLBCL mirrors the approach to nodal DLBCL: chemotherapy with rituximab and CHOP. This may be followed by radiation therapy. Surgery is typically reserved for cases with complications from obstruction, extensive hemorrhage, or perforation. Additionally, after surgery, these patients require adjuvant chemotherapy. The role of antibiotic therapy in DLBCL of the stomach has not been extensively studied; however, several groups report lasting regression of de novo DLBCL and DLBCL with MALT lymphoma after antibiotic therapy alone.

DIFFUSE LARGE B-CELL LYMPHOMA—FACT SHEET

Definition

- High-grade B-cell neoplasm composed of large, pleomorphic B cells with a diffuse growth pattern

Incidence and Location

- Most commonly involves the stomach but can involve any portion of the gastrointestinal tract

Morbidity and Mortality

- Aggressive clinical behavior
- Mortality varies with the extent of disease and other clinical parameters

Gender, Race, and Age Distribution

- Median age is in the sixth to seventh decade of life
- Slightly more common in males than in females

Clinical Features

- Presents with pain, dyspepsia, sometimes asymptomatic
- Rapidly enlarging mass may cause site-specific symptoms

Prognosis and Treatment

- Preliminary data suggest that gastric diffuse large B-cell lymphoma with *Helicobacter* infection may be effectively treated with antibiotics
- Aggressive but potentially curable with multiagent chemotherapy (R-CHOP [rituximab, cyclophosphamide, doxorubicin, vincristine, and prednisone])
- Overall 5-year disease-free survival rate ranges from 50% to 80%

DIFFUSE LARGE B-CELL LYMPHOMA—PATHOLOGIC FEATURES

Gross, Endoscopic, and Radiology Findings

- Ulcerative or mass-forming lesion

Microscopic Findings

- Diffuse infiltration by large lymphoid cells
- Most commonly have oval to round vesicular nuclei with multiple nucleoli and scant to moderate cytoplasm
- Effacement of normal structures

Immunohistochemical

- Positive for pan-B markers CD19, CD20, PAX5, CD79a
- Occasional CD138 or CD30 expression
- Hans criteria (considered positive if ≥30% of lymphoma cells) CD10, BCL6, MUM1
- Variable coexpression: CD10 (30%–50%), BCL6 (60%–90%), MUM1 (35%–65%), CD5 (5%–10%)
- BCL2 considered positive if 50% or greater of tumor cells are positive
- MYC considered positive if 40% or greater of tumor cells are positive
- Ki-67 proliferation index 40% to greater than 90%

Genetic Abnormalities

- Up to 30% have a BCL6 translocation

- 20% to 30% have a BCL2 translocation
- Up to 10% have an MYC translocation (single hit)

Differential Diagnosis

- Aggressive B-cell lymphomas, including high-grade B-cell lymphoma, Burkitt lymphoma, plasmablastic lymphoma, Epstein-Barr virus–positive large B-cell lymphoma
- Blastic or pleomorphic mantle cell lymphoma
- Acute leukemia/lymphoma
- Poorly differentiated carcinoma

HIGH-GRADE B-CELL LYMPHOMA

CLINICAL FEATURES

This is a new entity in the 2017 update to the fourth edition of the WHO classification. There are two categories of HGBL. The first replaces the prior entity known as B-cell lymphoma unclassifiable with features intermediate between DLBCL and BL or those HGBLs with a blastoid morphology that does not fit into another entity. The second category includes large B-cell lymphomas with MYC and BCL2 and/or BCL6 translocation (double- or triple-hit lymphomas.). This category should be used for de novo cases and should not be used for the progression of previously known lymphoma. These lymphomas can present similarly to DLBCL of the GI tract but are thought to have a more aggressive course.

PATHOLOGIC FEATURES

GROSS FINDINGS

The gross appearance is similar to that of other aggressive lymphomas. The lesions can be polypoid or show a masslike growth. These typically have a high proliferation rate that leads to bulky masses. Additionally, the lymphoma tends to demonstrate transmural involvement with extension into the surrounding mesenteric tissue. This can lead to ulceration as well as stricture formation, bowel obstruction, or perforation. On cut sections, these lesions have a characteristic fish flesh appearance, often accompanied by areas of hemorrhage and tumor necrosis.

MICROSCOPIC FINDINGS

The entity covers two categories that can have various morphologic and immunohistochemical profiles. The high-grade B-cell lymphoma with MYC and BCL2 and/or BCL6 rearrangements typically have the morphologic appearance similar to DLBCL, NOS. Although the lesions have a diffuse growth pattern, these can have a variable proliferation index ranging from low (<60%) to as high as BL (>95%). As such, the entities cannot be distinguished on morphologic grounds alone and require cytogenetic or FISH studies for classification. High-grade B-cell lymphoma, NOS, is a somewhat of wastebasket term in that it is used for lesions that do not fit into another mature aggressive large B-cell lymphoma category. These can resemble DLBCL or BL or may have a blastoid morphology.

ANCILLARY STUDIES

These mature large B cells express B-cell markers CD20, CD19, PAX5, and CD79a and lack TdT expression. The Ki-67 index can be quite variable and cannot be used to predict if the lymphoma has MYC, BCL2, or BCL6 translocations. The majority of cases demonstrate a germinal center phenotype with expression of CD10 and BCL6, with a minority of these lymphomas expressing MUM1. Those with a BCL2 translocation are diffusely positive for BCL2. cMYC protein expression can also be variable, and although 40% positivity in the lymphoma is interpreted as positive, this cannot be used as a surrogate for MYC translocation. FISH is an essential part of the workup for these cases. The translocations can be complex, and break-apart probes are helpful in demonstrating these abnormalities. Specially, FISH for MYC, BCL2, and BCL6 is recommended when working up cases of aggressive B-cell lymphoma.

DIFFERENTIAL DIAGNOSIS

The differential diagnosis includes other aggressive B-cell lymphomas. Specifically, the morphologic features have extensive overlap with DLBCL, NOS, and molecular studies for MYC, BCL2, and BCL6 are required. Additionally, the lymphoma can mimic BL; however, the lesion fails to meet the current definition of BL. Specifically, cytologically, HGBL can be more pleomorphic with various cell sizes. Additionally, Burritt lymphoma usually does not express BCL2. Pleomorphic or blastic variants of MCL can demonstrate overlapping morphologic features, but MCL can be excluded with cyclin D1 and SOX11 expression. Additionally, HGBL can have a blastic morphology and cytologically resemble acute lymphoblastic leukemia/lymphomas. The acute lymphoblastic leukemias typically express markers of immaturity such as TdT with variable expression of CD34. The B-lymphoblastic leukemia/lymphomas express PAX5 and cytoplasmic CD22 and CD79a and are typically CD10 positive while CD20 is variable to absent. T-lymphoblastic leukemia/lymphomas are positive for CD3 (may be cytoplasmic only) and often positive for CD1a and/or CD99.

PROGNOSIS AND THERAPY

Overall, the prognosis is poor with reported median survival time between 4.5 and 18.5 months. Unfortunately, these patients do not respond to standard R-CHOP therapy that is the standard of care for patients with DLBCL, NOS. Although this not standardized therapy for these patients, they are often treated more aggressively with some variation of an EPOCH-R (rituximab, etoposide phosphate, prednisone, vincristine sulfate [Oncovin], cyclophosphamide, and doxorubicin hydrochloride hydroxydaunorubicin]) therapy and require central nervous system (CNS) prophylaxis. Unfortunately, a significant proportion of cases are refractory to even aggressive therapy, and relapses are common.

HIGH-GRADE B-CELL LYMPHOMA–FACT SHEET

Definition

- Highly aggressive B-cell neoplasm, new 2016 World Health Organization category replaces lymphomas previous known as B-cell lymphoma unclassifiable with features between diffuse large B-cell lymphoma and Burkitt lymphoma as well as the double- and triple-hit lymphomas
  - Two subtypes: high-grade B-cell lymphoma (HGBL) with MYC and BCL2 and/or BCL6 rearrangements and HGBL, not otherwise specified

Incidence and Location

- Specific data are not available for HGBL involving the gastrointestinal tract
- Typically involves older patients sixth or seventh decade of life; can involve younger patients
- Male predominance
- Typically present with widespread disease involving more than one extranodal site, and more than half have bone marrow or central nervous system involvement

Prognosis and Treatment

- Typically, poor prognosis with median survivals time of 4.5 to 18.5 months
- The mainstay of treatment is intensive combination chemotherapy regimens, often resistant to R-CHOP (rituximab, cyclophosphamide, doxorubicin, vincristine, and prednisone) therapy
- Surgical therapy has a role in the treatment of obstruction or intussusception, debulking, and perforation

HIGH-GRADE B-CELL LYMPHOMA–PATHOLOGIC FEATURES

Gross Findings

- Solid tan-white cut surface (fish flesh appearing) often associated with hemorrhage and necrosis
- In the gastrointestinal tract, the lesions are often ulcerated, and mass forming, or transmural and in some cases can present as obstructive mass or perforation

Microscopic Findings

- High-grade B-cell lymphoma (HGBL) with MYC and BCL2 and/or BCL6 rearrangements
  - Variable morphology:50% to 85% have morphology of DLBCL, not otherwise specified (NOS)
  - Can have morphology similar to Burkett lymphoma, although more pleomorphic nuclei
  - Solid growth pattern with minimal small lymphocytes
  - Variable mitotic figures and apoptotic cells (occasional starry-sky pattern)
- HGBL, NOS
  - More closely resembles Burkitt lymphoma than diffuse large B-cell lymphoma (DLBCL); some have a blastic appearance
  - Solid growth pattern of medium- to large-sized cells
  - Often no stromal reaction
  - Prominent mitotic figures and prominent apoptosis

Immunohistochemistry

- Positive for pan-B markers CD19, CD20, PAX5, and CD79a
- Typically, positive for BCL6 with variable expression of CD10
- Minority of cases are MUM1 positive (20%)
- Negative for CD5, cyclin D1, and TdT
- Ki-67 is variable (between 30% and 100%)
- Those with MYC and *BCL2* translocations typically demonstrates MYC and BCL2 protein expression

Genetic Abnormalities

- "Double hit" demonstrates translocations involving *MYC*, including t(8;14) and *BCL2*
- "Triple hit" demonstrates translocations involving *MYC, BCL2,* and *BCL6*
- Complex cytogenetic abnormalities

Differential Diagnosis

- Diffuse large cell lymphoma
- Burkitt lymphoma
- Epstein-Barr virus–positive DLBCL
- Acute lymphoblastic leukemia/lymphoma

EPSTEIN-BARR VIRUS–POSITIVE DIFFUSE LARGE B-CELL LYMPHOMA, NOT OTHERWISE SPECIFIED

CLINICAL FEATURES

In the previous edition of the WHO classification, EBV-positive DLBCL, NOS, was known as EBV-positive DLBCL of the elderly. This entity had an age cut-off of 50 years; however, subsequent work demonstrated that this lesion was not limited to this older patient population. Although most commonly seen in patients older than 50 years of age, it can occur at any age. In some cases, this lesion is thought to be secondary to immunosenescence secondary to aging.

This entity has a predilection for extranodal sites, especially the GI tract. Up to 10% of patients may have both nodal and extranodal disease. The percent of DLBCL case that falls under this category increases with age with a peak of 20% to 30% of DLBCL cases in patients older than 90 years old. Clinically, they can present similar to other aggressive or large B-cell lymphoma as outlined previously.

Pathologic Features

Gross Findings

Grossly, EBV-positive DLBCL, NOS has similar features as DLBCL (see the DLBCL section earlier).

Microscopic Findings

Morphologically, EBV-positive DLBCL, NOS, resembles other EBV-positive lesions. Specifically, this lymphoma can have a polymorphic appearance with numerous scattered large neoplastic cells. These large neoplastic cells typically have a Reed-Sternberg or Hodgkin-like appearance or transformed immunoblasts (Fig. 19.4E). The number of neoplastic cells can be quite variable, occasionally have a more monomorphic appearance forming solid sheets of neoplastic cells (challenging to distinguish from conventional DLBCL) to those with only rare scattered neoplastic B cells admixed with mature-appearing T cells and histiocytes. The background inflammatory cells may out-number the neoplastic cells and be reminiscent of a T-cell/histiocytic rich large B-cell lymphoma or classical mixed cellularity Hodgkin lymphoma. This lymphoma may have extensive tumor necrosis as well as angioinvasion.

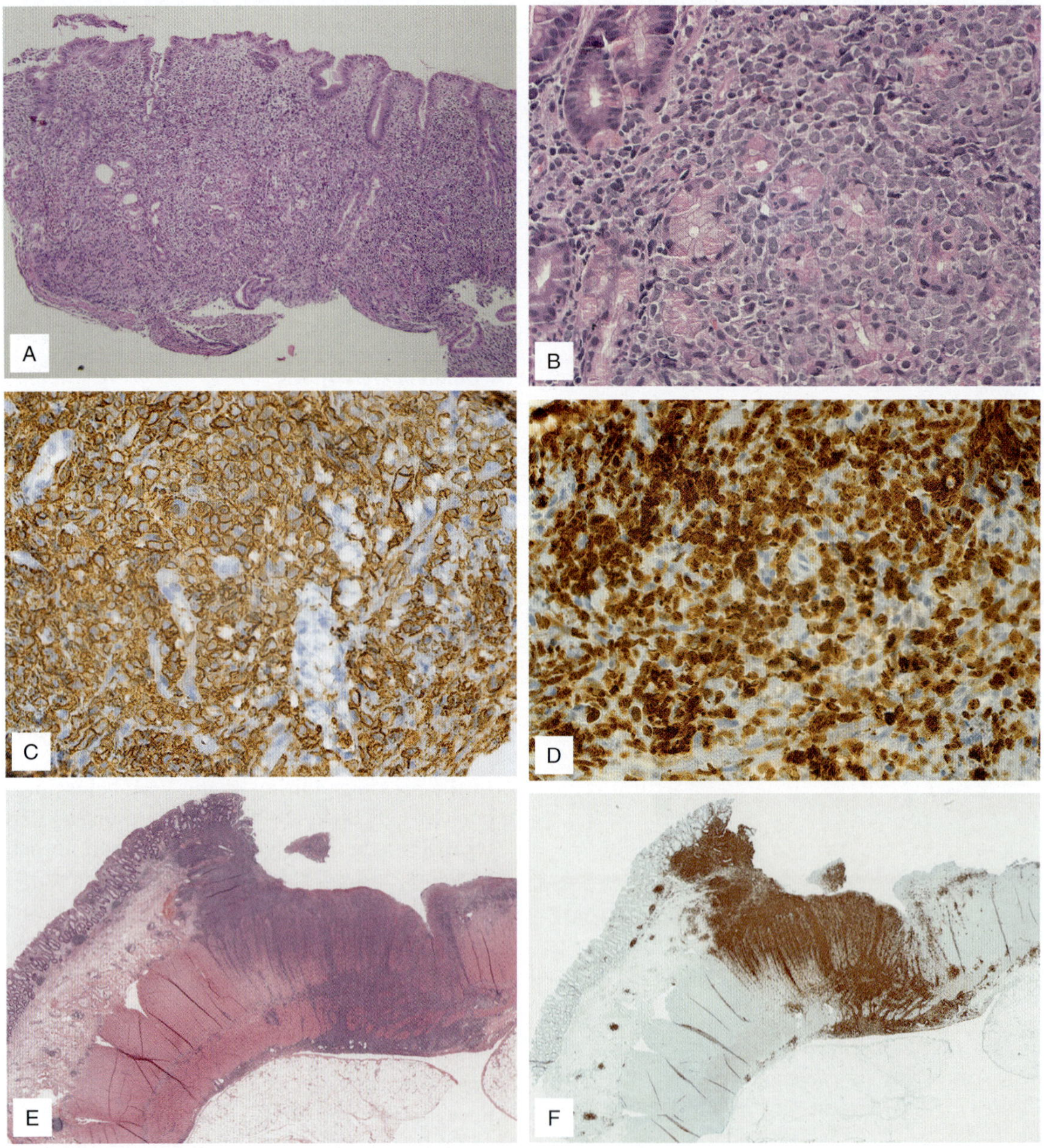

FIGURE 19.4

Aggressive B-cell lymphoma. **A**, At low magnification, this diffuse large B-cell lymphoma (DLBCL) can involve the gastric mucosa. A dense lymphoid infiltrate with a pushing border is noted. **B**, The infiltrate is composed of sheets of pleomorphic large cells with prominent nucleoli and moderate amounts of cytoplasm infiltrating into and destroying the overlying glandular epithelium. **C**, Immunohistochemical stain for CD20 shows a membranous staining pattern of the B cells and emphasizes the pleomorphic nature of these cells. **D**, This lesion can have various Ki-67 labeling, including near 100% of cells as in this example. **E**, This

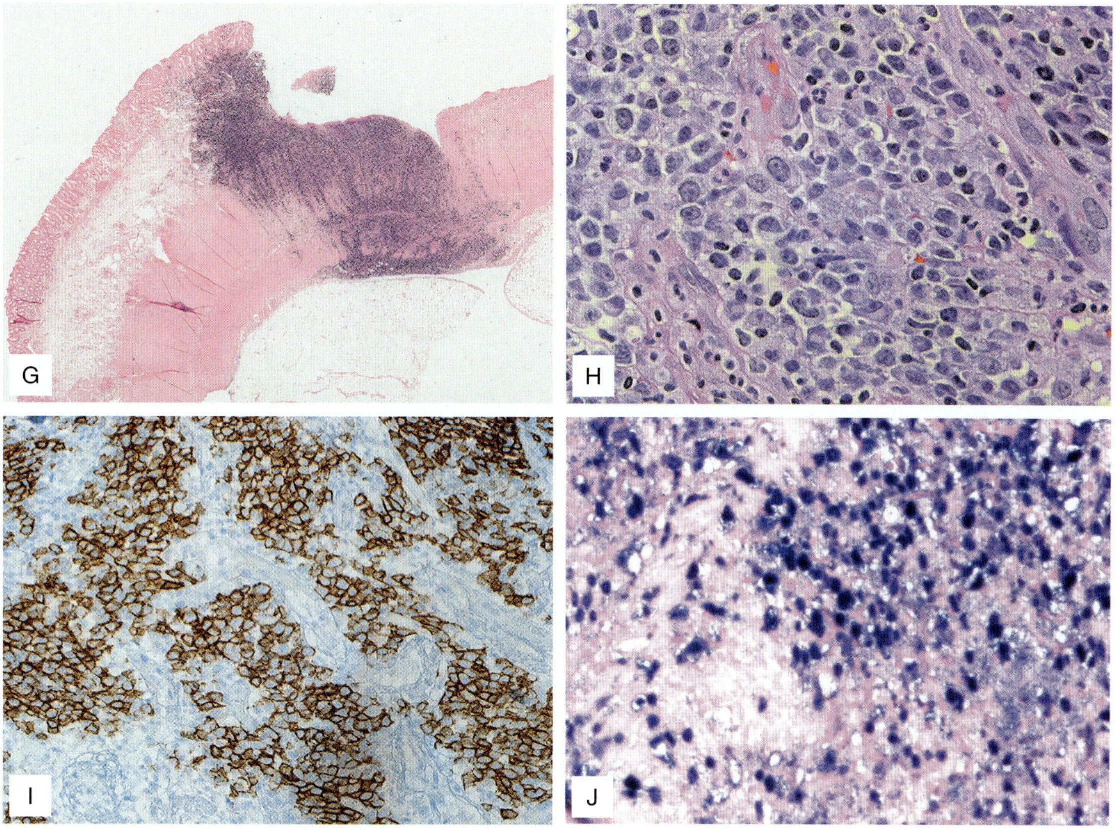

example of Epstein-Barr virus (EBV)–positive DLBCL demonstrates transmural infiltration with associated ulceration. This lesion demonstrates extensive expression of the B-cell marker CD20 (**F**). The in situ hybridization for Epstein-Barr encoding region (EBER) highlights the extensive number of EBV-infected cells (**G**). This example of plasmablastic lymphoma (hematoxylin and eosin) demonstrates large neoplastic cells with eccentric nuclei with prominent. The neoplastic cells have amble basophilic cytoplasm and often has paranuclear clearing (**H**). The neoplastic cells are positive for CD138 (I) as well as positive for EBV by in situ hybridization (**J**).

Ancillary Studies

The large neoplastic cells are positive for pan-B-cell markers CD20, PAX5, and CD79a (Fig. 19.4F). These neoplastic B cells typically demonstrate a nongerminal center phenotype with expression of MUM1 and absence of staining for LMO2, CD10, and BCL6. Additionally, the neoplastic cells also express CD30, but only a small number of cases (15%) coexpress CD15. By definition, the majority of the neoplastic cells should be positive for EBV by in situ hybridization for Epstein-Barr encoding region (ISH-EBER) (Fig. 19.4G). The neoplastic cells are also positive for PDL1.

Differential Diagnosis

The differential diagnosis for EBV-positive DLBCL includes DLBCL, NOS; PBL; posttransplant lymphoproliferative disorder; human herpesvirus 8 (HHV8)–positive DLBCL; EBV-positive mucocutaneous ulcer as well as classical Hodgkin lymphoma and granulation tissue. The monomorphic variant of EBV-positive DLBCL can appear identical to EBV-negative DLBCL but can be differentiated by ISH-EBER. Additionally, EBV-positive DLBCL lymphoma can be differentiated from HHV8-positive DLBCL by the presence of HHV8 infected cells. After an organ transplant, patients can develop a lymphoma that is morphologically similar to EBV-positive DLBCL; however, the clinical history of transplantation drives the diagnosis. PBLs lack expression of B-cell differentiation markers CD20 and PAX5. EBV-positive mucocutaneous ulcers usually have a band of CD30+ EBV-positive lymphocytes at the deepest leading edge, a finding that is absent in EBV-positive DLBCL. The cases with a prominent background of T cells and histiocytes can resemble T-cell/histiocyte-rich large B-cell lymphoma. However, T-cell/histiocyte-rich large B-cell lymphomas are negative for EBV-infected cells. In cases in which there is associated necrosis and ulceration, the diagnosis can be partially obscured by the mixed inflammation and necrosis and resemble granulation tissue of ulcer exudate. Sometimes the neoplastic cells are b difficult to identify on H&E along, and often a PAX5 (and or CD20) along with ISH-EBER can be extremely useful.

Prognosis and Therapy

The prognosis in these cases tends to be worse with age. Specifically, the presence of symptoms and age older than 70 years are poor prognostic features. In older adult patients, a median survival period of 2 years is reported, and if there are B symptoms, the median survival period decreases to 9 months. In younger patients, the prognosis is excellent with long-term remission seen in more than 80 % of cases.

EPSTEIN-BARR VIRUS–POSITIVE DIFFUSE LARGE B-CELL LYMPHOMA, NOT OTHERWISE SPECIFIED–FACT SHEET

Definition

- Epstein-Barr virus (EBV)–positive clonal B-cell proliferation, a new 2017 World Health Organization category, replaces lymphoma previous known as EBV-positive diffuse large B cell lymphoma of the elderly. The current diagnostic criteria removed the age requirement. It excludes other EBV-positive lymphomas

Incidence and Location

- Most cases occur in patients after the age of 50 but can occur at any age
- Typically involves older patients sixth or seventh decade of life; can involve younger patients
- Male predominance (male-to-female ratio, 1.2–3.6:1)
- Typically involves extranodal sites in older adults and nodal disease in patients younger than 40 years of age

Prognosis and Treatment

- Prognosis is worse with older age
- The presence of B symptoms and age older than 70 years are poor prognostic indicators
- Patients younger than 40 years of age have a better prognosis with most achieving long-term remission
- Combined chemotherapy with rituximab

Epstein-Barr Virus–Positive Diffuse Large B-Cell Lymphoma, Not Otherwise Specifiedpathologic Features

Gross Findings

- In younger patients, primary enlarged lymph nodes
- Older patients with extranodal disease and in the gastrointestinal tract present with ulceration or mass-forming lesion

Microscopic Findings

- Large neoplastic cells with a Reed-Sternberg or Hodgkin-like appearance or transformed immunoblasts
    - Polymorphic variant with a background of mixed inflammatory cells, neoplastic cells often the minority cell population
    - Monomorphic variant with increased under of neoplastic cells forming sheet; similar to Epstein-Barr virus (EBV)–negative diffuse large B-cell lymphoma (DLBCL)
- Often with ulceration and large areas of necrosis or granulation-type tissue

Immunohistochemistry

- Positive for pan-B markers CD19, CD20, PAX5, and CD79a
- Positive for MUM1 and negative for germinal center markers CD10 and BCL6
- Negative for CD5, cyclin D1, and TdT
- Positive for CD30 with infrequent CD15 coexpression
- Neoplastic cells are positive for EBV (in situ hybridization for Epstein-Barr encoding region)

Differential Diagnosis

- EBV negative diffuse large cell lymphoma
- Plasmablastic lymphoma
- human herpesvirus 8–positive DLBCL, not otherwise specified
- EBV-positive mucocutaneous ulcer
- Classical Hodgkin lymphoma
- T-cell/histiocyte-rich large B-cell lymphomas
- Granulation tissue

PLASMABLASTIC LYMPHOMA

Clinical Features

Plasmablastic lymphomas is a clinically aggressive lymphoma. The disease typically affects patients who are immunosuppressed through immunosenescence, infectious causes, after transplant, or medications. The typical presentation is the oral cavity, but the GI tract is the second most common site, and these two represent the primary site in the vast majority of cases. In human immunodeficiency virus (HIV)–positive patients, the lesions tend to occur in the anus or distal rectum. Patients with HIV tend to present with disseminated disease more often than patients in the posttransplant setting or those that are immunocompetent. Those with disseminated disease tend to have bone marrow involvement. Typically, lymph nodes involvement is rare and affects fewer than 10 % of patients (slightly higher percentage of nodal involvement in the posttransplant setting).

Similar to patients with other types of GI lymphomas or malignancies, these patients typically present with abdominal pain, weight loss, anorexia, melena, or painless rectal bleeding. Additionally, many patients have diarrhea, and only rarely have patients presented with obstruction.

Pathologic Features

Gross Findings

Plasmablastic lymphoma presents most commonly with an ulcerated mass lesion. Otherwise, the gross appearance is similar to other aggressive lymphomas, appearing as a bulky polypoid masslike lesion. This can lead to strictures, obstructions, or perforation. On cut sections, these lesions have a typical fish flesh appearance with areas of hemorrhage and necrosis.

Microscopic Findings

Plasmablastic lymphoma demonstrates a spectrum of cytologic features ranging from cells with an immunoblastic appearance to those with plasmacytic/plasmacytoid features and plasmablasts. The neoplastic cells have a more solid or cohesive growth pattern. The nuclei are enlarged and typically round and eccentric with prominent single or multiple nucleoli. They have ample amount of basophilic cytoplasm that often shows paranuclear clearing. The lymphoma typically has a high proliferation rate with scattered apoptosis giving it a starry-sky pattern (Fig. 19.4H). The tumors also have areas of geographic necrosis. Typically, there is only a minor component of infiltrating T cells.

Ancillary Studies

The neoplastic cells are positive for markers of plasma cell differentiation, including CD138, CD38, VS38, and MUM1 (Fig. 19.4I). Additionally, expression of CD79a can be seen in up to 40% of cases. Importantly, the lymphoma lacks expression of other B-cell markers CD20 and PAX5 and has variable expression of cytoplasmic light chains. Although the tumor is negative for pan-keratins, the lesion can express epithelial membrane antigen (EMA; often weakly). This lymphoma lacks expression of BCL6 and BCL2 with up to 20% expressing CD10. Expression for CD56 can be seen in up to 25% of cases, which can make it challenging to differentiate from a plasmablastic progression of myeloma. The neoplastic cells are negative for CD3 and CD5 with only rare cases expressing CD43. EBV (ISH-EBER) is positive in around 70% of cases (Fig. 19.4J). By definition, this lesion is negative for HHV-8 expression. This lymphoma is typically positive for MYC by IHC with 50% to 75% of patients demonstrating an *MYC* translocation.

Differential Diagnosis

Often with the cohesively appearing neoplastic cells, this lesion can resemble nonhematopoietic malignancies such as carcinoma or melanoma. Immunohistochemical stains for keratin (i.e., CAM5.2, AE1/3, OSCAR) can assist in excluding carcinoma, and melanoma can be excluded with immunostains for S100 or SOX10. A possible pitfall is the use of EMA, which is expressed in carcinomas but can often be expressed in plasmablastic or plasmacytic lesions. Also remember that in addition to plasmablasts and plasma cells that CD138 is also a good epithelial and carcinoma marker. The differential also includes anaplastic large cell lymphoma and ALK-positive B-cell lymphomas; however, PBL is negative for ALK expression. Also, some DLBCLs can have a plasmablastic appearance, but DLBCL is positive for CD20 and PAX5, unlike PBL. HHV8-positive DLBCL often has a plasmacytic/plasmablastic morphology, but the presence of HHV8-positive cells assists in the exclusion of this entity.

The starry-sky pattern can resemble BL as well as acute leukemia/lymphoma; however, PBL is negative for CD20 (and other B0cell markers) and TdT. Often the more challenging differential is with plasma cell neoplasm with plasmablastic differentiation. Unfortunately, CD56 can also be expressed on PBL, limiting its usefulness. Cyclin D1 is expressed in a proportion of plasma cell neoplasms and can be useful. However, often the differential can be solved with a patient's history of plasma cell myeloma. Also, plasma cell myelomas (or plasmacytomas) occur in immunocompetent people and typically lack EBV-infected tumor cells. Additionally, the presence of an M protein on serum electrophoresis or symptoms of hypercalcemia, renal insufficiency anemia, or bone lesions would support a plasma cell myeloma.

Prognosis and Therapy

The prognosis of this lymphoma is dismal. The majority of patients will succumb to this lymphoma with a median survival time of 6 to 11 months. The presence of a *MYC* translocation is associated with worse outcomes. Unfortunately, there is no true standard of care therapy for these patients.

PLASMABLASTIC LYMPHOMA—FACT SHEET

Definition

- Highly aggressive neoplasm composed of immunoblasts and plasmablasts
  - Excludes human herpesvirus and ALK-positive lymphomas

Incidence and Location

- Predominantly involves adults with immunodeficiency (human immunodeficiency virus, posttransplant, immunosenescence)
- Primarily involved oral cavity and luminal gut

Clinical Features

- Typically presents as an ulcerative mass
- Presents with abdominal pain, weight loss, anorexia, melena, or painless rectal bleeding
- Disseminated disease is found at presentation in 75% of patients

Prognosis and Treatment

- Poor prognosis with median survivals of period of 6 to 11 months
- No standard therapy
- Rarely, surgical therapy has a role in treatment for obstruction or intussusception, debulking, and perforation

Plasmablastic Lymphoma—Pathologic Features

Gross Findings

- Ulcerated (often circumscribed) mass
- Solid tan-white cut surface (fish flesh appearing) often associated with hemorrhage and necrosis
- Lymph nodes involved in fewer than 10% of cases

Microscopic Findings

- Solid or cohesive growth pattern of immunoblasts or large neoplastic cells with plasmablastic differentiation
- Cells with eccentric nuclei with abundant typically with abundant basophilic cytoplasm with prominent single or multiple nucleoli
- Some demonstrate a paranuclear hof (clearing)
- High proliferation rate, often with a starry-sky pattern and associated tumor necrosis

Immunohistochemistry

- Positive for plasma cell markers CD138, MUM1, CD38, VS38c, and EMA
- Negative for B-cell markers CD20 and PAX5 as well as CD45
- Can be positive for CD79a; 40% of cases
- Positive for cMYC IHC expression
- Epstein-Barr virus (EBV) (in situ hybridization for Epstein-Barr encoding region) in 70% of cases
- Minority of cases positive for CD10 (20%) or CD56 (25%)
- Negative for BCL6, BCL2, CD5, cyclin D1, TdT, CD30, human herpesvirus (HHV) 8, and ALK
- Ki-67 index greater than 95%

Genetic Abnormalities

- 50% of cases demonstrate an *MYC* rearrangement
- Complex karyotypes

Differential Diagnosis

- DLBCL and Burkitt lymphoma
- HHV8- or EBV-positive diffuse large B-cell lymphoma
- Acute lymphoblastic leukemia/lymphoma
- Poorly differentiated carcinoma or melanoma

BURKITT LYMPHOMA

Clinical Features

Burkitt lymphoma is a highly aggressive B-cell neoplasm; however, it is often a curable lymphoma. The disease typically presents in extranodal sites or as acute leukemia. There are three recognized epidemiologic variants of BL, and they differ in their geographic distribution, clinical presentation, and molecular and morphologic aspects. These include endemic, sporadic, and immunodeficiency-associated BL, and all these variants are seen in the GI tract. Regardless of the variant, they present with bulky abdominal disease with a high tumor burden.

The endemic form of BL is found primarily in equatorial Africa, where it is the most common childhood malignancy in children 4 to 7 years of age. This form typically presents in the head and neck region with jaw, orbit, or paraspinal lesions in 50% to 70% of cases. In some cases, it can present as an ileal or ileocecal mass that serves as a leading point for intussusception or intestinal obstruction. This form is strongly associated with EBV infection with the EBV genome seen in more than 95% of the neoplastic cells.

Sporadic BL is seen throughout the world, where it mainly occurs in children or younger adults. In nonendemic areas, BL accounts for 1% to 2% of lymphomas but 30% to 50% of childhood lymphomas. Significantly fewer cases are associated with EBV (20%–30% of cases). The majority of sporadic BL cases present as an abdominal mass with the ileocecal area being the primary site of involvement. However, any part of the GI tract may be involved because cases of gastric or rectal BL are common. Patients can present with complaints of abdominal pain or obstructive-type symptoms.

Immunodeficiency-associated BL is primarily seen with HIV infection. Although BL can be the first manifestation of AIDS, BL often occurs when the patients still have relatively high CD4 counts. The risk of development of BL in patients with HIV also appears to be similar in the pre and post–highly active antiretroviral therapy era. Additionally, only 25% to 40% of immunodeficiency-associated BL are also associated with EBV infection. In addition to GI involvement, nodal localization and bone marrow involvement are frequent.

Pathologic Features

Gross Findings

In GI BL cases, there exists a predilection for the involvement of the ileocecal region and less often the rectum and stomach. Given the high proliferation rate, they typically present as large bulky masses that completely replace the bowel wall. The lesions often infiltrate transmurally into the surrounding mesenteric tissue with areas of necrosis and hemorrhage. Similar to other higher grade lymphomas, the lesion has a typical fish flesh appearance. Interesting, the lymph nodes are not involved by BL, but the tissue around the lymph may be involved.

Microscopic Findings

The tumor is characterized by the infiltration of monomorphic medium-sized lymphocytes that often has a cohesive appearance. The nuclei have clumped chromatin with multiple small nucleoli. The cytoplasm is densely basophilic with classic lipid vacuoles, which are seen best on touch preps or cytology specimens. The most recognized feature is the starry-sky background, which is composed of multiple tingible body macrophages with apoptotic debris (Fig. 19.5A and B). Given the high proliferation rate, mitotic figures and apoptosis are readily identified in all cases. Rarely, cases may show a florid granulomatous reaction. In older adults and patients with the immunodeficiency-associated variant, the cells can show a greater degree of nuclear pleomorphism or harbor a plasmablastic morphology.

Ancillary Studies

The neoplastic cells express pan-B-cell markers CD19, CD20, PAX5, and CD79a (Fig. 19.5C). Additionally, they express germinal center markers BCL6 and CD10 (Fig. 19.5D) and show aberrant expression of CD43. Importantly, BCL2 is either negative or there may be weak patchy staining (Fig19.5D). TdT is usually negative. In addition, the cells are negative for cyclin D1, CD23, and CD5. They also show aberrant coexpression of LEF1, and a subset are positive for SOX11. The neoplastic cells are strongly positive for surface IgM with light chain restriction. Given the high mitotic rate, the Ki-67 index is nearly 100% of cells (Fig19.5 F). (ISH-EBER) highlights the EBV infected cells.

The tumor cells demonstrate Ig gene rearrangement. The prototypic cytogenetic abnormality BL is translocations involving the *MYC* (8q24) loci. The

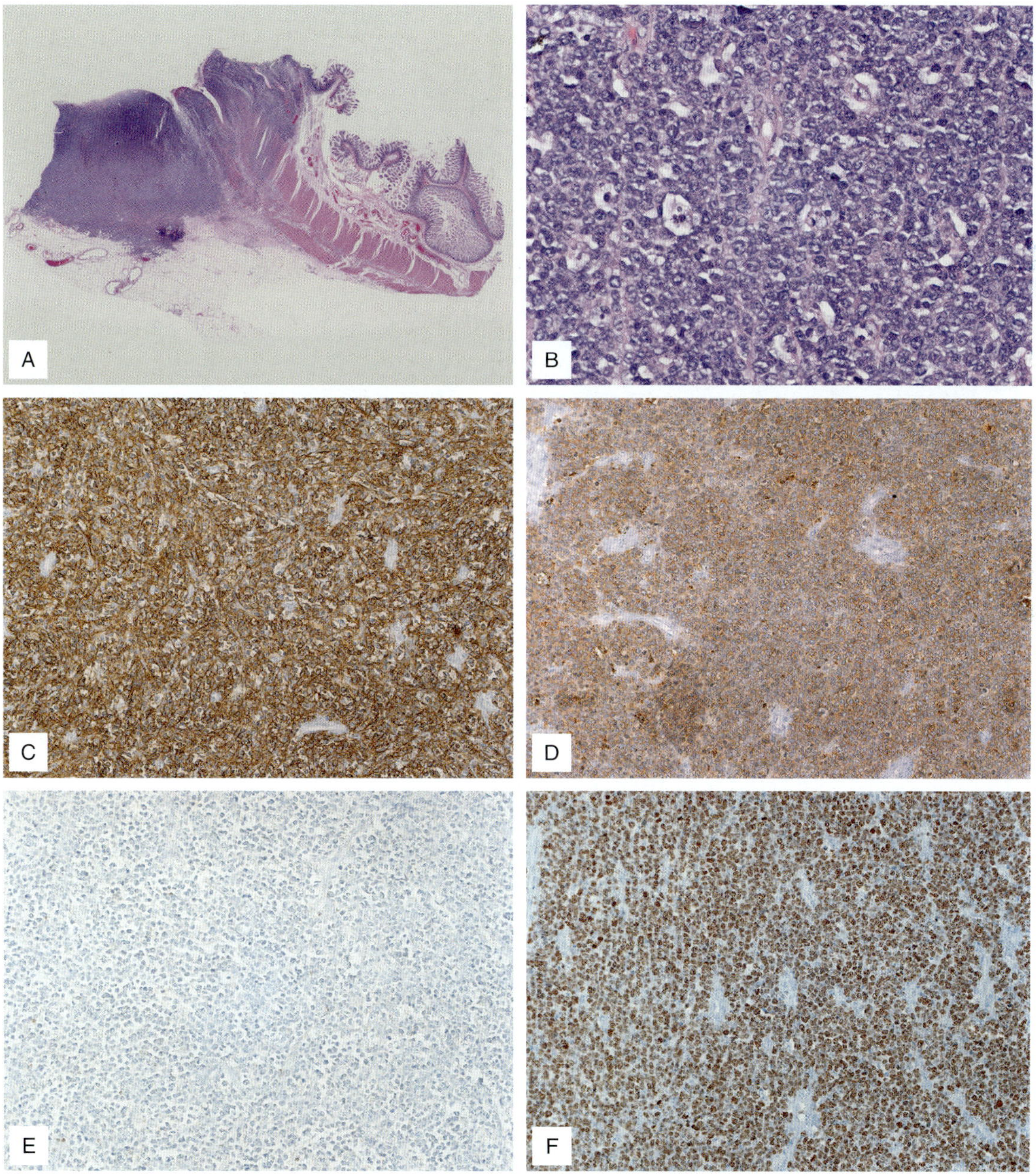

FIGURE 19.5

Burkitt lymphoma. **A**, At low power, this lymphoma commonly involves the small bowel with transmural inflammation and obstruction or perforation **B**, At high power, the neoplastic infiltrate is composed of a highly monotonous, monomorphic population of medium-sized lymphocytes with round nuclei, finely clumped chromatin; several small nucleoli; and scant cytoplasm admixed with tangible-body macrophages containing apoptotic debris lead to a "starry-sky" appearance within the dense infiltrate. **C**, The neoplastic cells are B cells as highlighted by CD20. The neoplastic cells are typically strongly positive for CD10 (**D**) but should

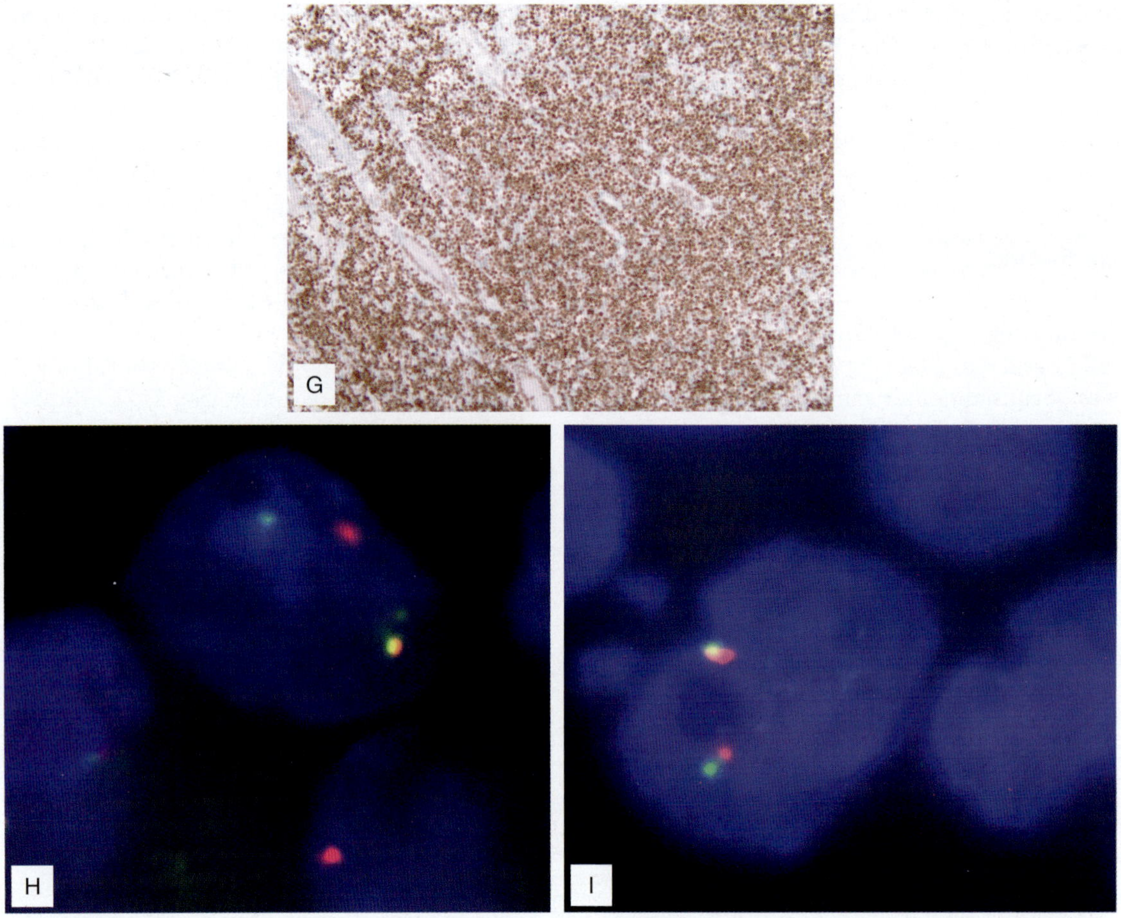

be negative for BCL2 (**E**). An immunohistochemical stain for Ki-67 (**F**) shows nuclear positivity in virtually all neoplastic cells, corresponding to a high proliferative index. Burkitt lymphoma has MYC protein overexpression (**G**). Florescent in situ hybridization using break apart probes demonstrates rearrangement of the *MYC* gene (**H**) and normal intact *BCL2* gene (**I**).

most common *MYC* translocation is with the heavy chain gene t(8;14)(q24q32). However, less commonly, the *MYC* translocations can involve one of the light chain genes IGK (2q11) or IGL (22q11), resulting in t(2;8) or t(8;22). The translocations involving *MYC* result in increased MYC protein expression. Immunohistochemical stains for MYC label the majority of cells in BL cases (Fig. 19.5G). Up to 10% of classic BLs can lack detectable *MYC* rearrangements. The presence of *BCL2* and *BCL6* rearrangements suggest an alternative diagnosis such as high-grade B-cell lymphoma (Fig. 19.5H and I).

Differential Diagnosis

The differential diagnosis includes other high-grade lymphomas and acute leukemia. Typically, DLBCL is more pleomorphic than BL. Although other aggressive lymphomas can have increased proliferation index, few have 100% Ki-67 index that is so typical of BL. Additionally, many of the aggressive lymphomas can have BCL2 expression, which is absent in BL. There can also be morphologic overlap between BL and lymphoblastic lymphoma. Lymphoblastic lymphoma lacks expression of mature B-cell markers (e.g., CD20) and is positive for TdT.

Prognosis and Therapy

Burkitt lymphoma is a highly aggressive tumor; however, with aggressive therapy, it can be potentially curable in the majority of patients. Specifically, intense chemotherapy leads to long-term survival in 70% to 90% of cases. The prognosis depends on clinical stage and is generally is better in children than in adults. Poor prognostic factors include involvement of bone marrow and/or CNS by BL as well as high serum LDH or large (>10 cm) unresectable masses. In immunodeficiency-associated BL, BL remains curable, and the overall prognosis is related more to the underlying HIV or immunodeficiency pathology than to the lymphoma itself. Surgical resection or debulking is indicated in patients with present with symptoms of obstruction or perforation.

BURKITT LYMPHOMA—FACT SHEET

Definition

- Highly aggressive B-cell neoplasm
- Occurs in three clinical forms: endemic, sporadic, and immunodeficiency associated
- All three forms may present in the gastrointestinal (GI) tract

Incidence and Location

- Endemic, primarily in equatorial Africa and Papua New Guinea
  - Associated with Epstein-Barr virus (EBV) infection more than 95% of cases
  - Most common childhood malignancy in endemic areas, with peak incident between 4 and 7 years of age
- Sporadic: sen throughout the industrialized world affecting primary children and young adults
  - Only 20% to 30% are associated with EBV infection
  - Accounts for 1% to 2% of all lymphomas and 30% to 50% childhood lymphomas
- Immunodeficiency associated: Seen throughout the world and associated with human immunodeficiency (HIV) infection
  - Up to 25% to 40% are associated with EBV infection

Clinical Features

- All subtypes: bulky disease and frequently widespread with bone marrow involvement and acute leukemia common
- Endemic: mass in the jaw, orbit, or paraspinal lesion; GI tract involvement less common, usually ileocecal
- Sporadic: children present with abdominal mass, typically in the ileocecal region; causes abdominal pain and obstructive symptoms. Adults can have tumors in any part of the GI tract, most commonly in the ileocecal region and the rectum

Prognosis and Treatment

- Highly aggressive tumor but potentially curable in the majority of patients
- Prognosis depends on the stage and is generally better in children
- The mainstay of treatment is intensive combination chemotherapy regimens
- Surgical therapy has a role in the treatment of obstruction or intussusception, debulking, and perforation

BURKITT LYMPHOMA—PATHOLOGIC FEATURES

Gross Findings

- Typically large bulky mass that in the GI tract has a predilection for the ileocecal region and less often rectum and stomach
- Solid tan-white cut surface (fish flesh appearing) often associated with hemorrhage and necrosis
- Lymph nodes typically not involved by tumor but instead are surrounded by tumor
- In the GI tract, the lesions tend to be transmural and in some cases can present as an obstructive mass or perforation

Microscopic Findings

- Intermediate-sized cells with scant cytoplasm with cytoplasmic vacuoles seen on touch and smear preparations that are positive for Oil red O (usually frozen section preparation)
- Round nuclei with finely clumped chromatin containing three to four centrally located small basophilic nucleoli
- Extremely high proliferation rate
- Associated tingle-body macrophages creating a "starry-sky" appearance

Immunohistochemistry

- Positive for pan-B-cell markers CD19, CD20, PAX5, CD79a
- Positive for CD10, BCL6, CD43, and LEF1
- Negative for BCL2, CD5, and cyclin D1
- Ki-67 index is nearly 100%
- Positive for protein expression for MYC
- Positive for surface immunoglobulin M expression with light chain restriction

Genetic Abnormalities

- Translocation involving *MYC*, including t(8;14) *MYC/IGH*, t(2;8) *IGK/MYC*, or t(8;22) *MYC/IGL*
- Negative for *BCL2* and *BCL6* rearrangements

Differential Diagnosis

- Diffuse large cell lymphoma
- High-grade B-cell lymphoma
- Acute lymphoblastic leukemia/lymphoma

EPSTEIN-BARR VIRUS–POSITIVE MUCOCUTANEOUS ULCER

Another recently described entity is termed EBV-positive mucocutaneous ulcer and is an EBV-associated lymphoproliferative process. These lesions are reported to occur in the GI tract, oropharynx, and skin. The cases are reported in immunosuppressed individuals secondary to iatrogenic, primary immunodeficiency, or age-related immunosenescence.

The lesions are typically ulcerated with a shallow punctate or well-demarcated lesion (Fig. 19.6A). There are no associated systemic symptoms or involvement. Histologically, the lesion demonstrates a polymorphic infiltrate with a mixture of small mature-appearing lymphocytes and plasma cells with scattered immunoblasts and large atypical lymphocytes (Fig. 19.6B). These large atypical cells can have Reed-Sternberg–like morphology. In some cases, there may be evidence of angioinvasion. These large atypical lymphocytes are positive for B cell marker PAX5 with variable expression of other B-cell markers (CD20 and CD79a) (Fig. 19.6E). The neoplastic cells are positive for CD30 (Fig. 19.6C), and about 50 % of reported cases are CD15 positive. These large cells are also highlighted by ISH-EBER (Fig. 19.6D). The lesional cells demonstrate an activated or postgerminal center phenotype and typically express MUM1 but are negative for BCL6 and CD10. ISH-EBER highlights the large atypical cells. Most cases are associated with an extensive background of CD3+ and CD8+ T cells, typically with a dense perilesional infiltrate (Fig. 19.6F).

Even though the morphology is highly concerning, these lesions have been reported to have an indolent natural history. Local progression and tissue destruction can occur. Although a few of the lesions have been reported to be self-limited and spontaneously resolve, reduction of immunosuppression is the primary goal of treatment. In cases when this is not an option, chemotherapy with rituximab or local radiation has proven useful.

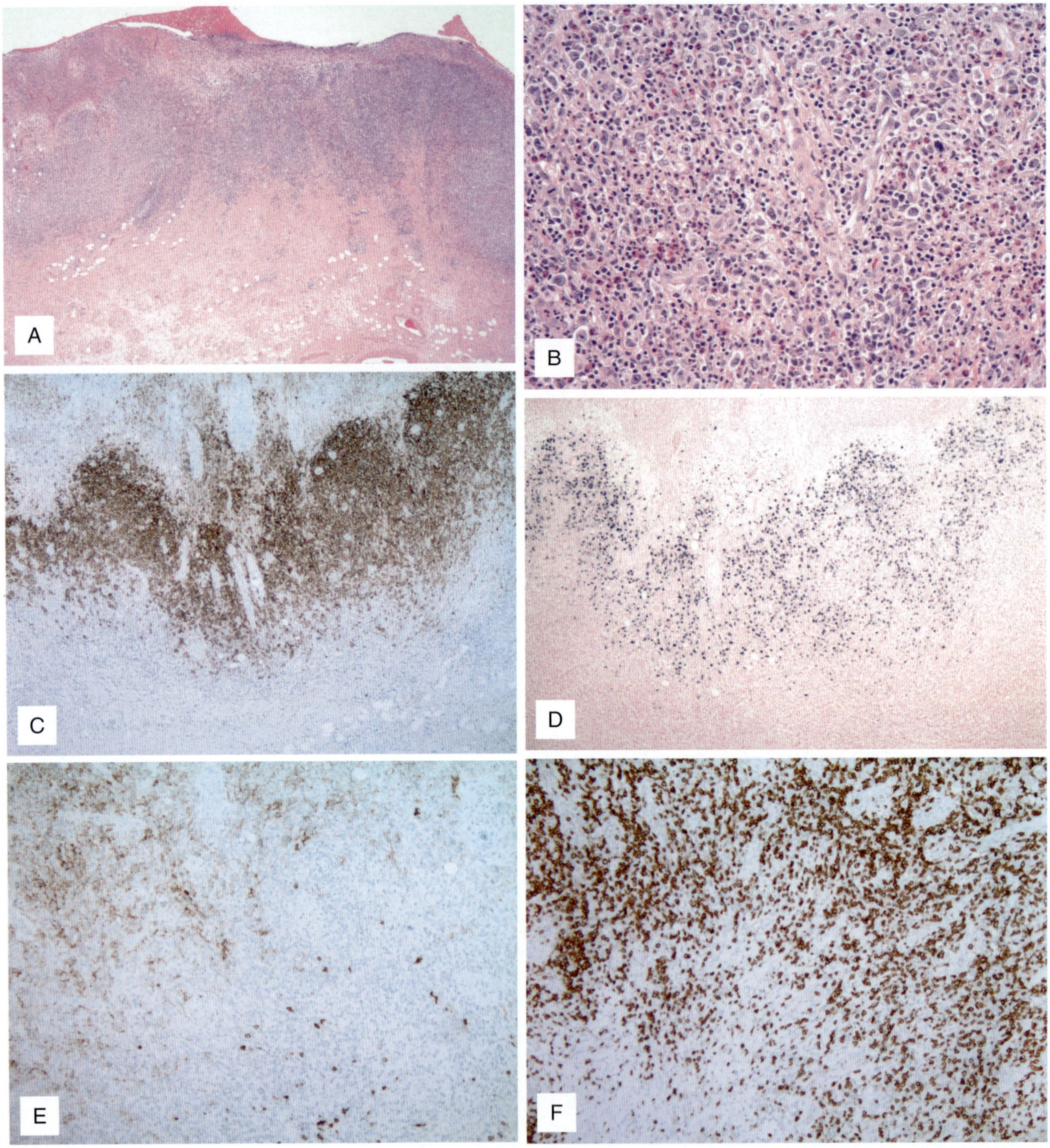

FIGURE 19.6

Epstein-Barr virus (EBV)–positive mucocutaneous ulcer. **A**, At low power, the lesion is ulcerated with a dense inflammatory infiltrate underlying the ulcer. **B**, At high power, the lesion is composed of a polymorphic population of cells, including atypical Reed-Sternberg-like cells. The large atypical cells are typically most prominent at the base of the lesion and strongly expression CD30 (**C**). Additionally, these large atypical cells and a background of small lymphocytes are EBV infected, as highlighted by in situ hybridization for Epstein-Barr encoding region (**D**). There is only focal patchy expression of CD20 (**E**), and the extensive T-cell infiltrate can be seen on CD3 immunostains (**F**).

MATURE T- AND NATURAL KILLER CELL NEOPLASMS

Intestinal T-cell lymphomas are far less common than those of B-cell origin. Although these have a lower incidence, there are subtypes of T-cell lymphomas that are specific to the GI tract. Additionally, the most recent edition of the WHO has reclassified these lesions and added a few preliminary entities.

The most common type of intestinal T-cell lymphoma occurs in the setting of GSE and is referred to as EATL. The lymphoma previously referred to as type II EATL has now been reclassified as MEITL and is not associated with GSE. An additional rare classification is the indolent T-cell lymphoproliferative disorder of the GI tract. Although other T-cell lymphomas only infrequently involve the GI tract, the liver is more commonly affected. Hepatosplenic T-cell lymphoma (HTCL), in particular, frequently involves the liver and well as the spleen. Other T- and NK cell entities that can involve the GI tract include peripheral T-cell lymphoma (PTCL, NOS), and extranodal NK/T-cell lymphoma, nasal type (which is not discussed in this text).

ENTEROPATHY-ASSOCIATED T-CELL LYMPHOMA

CLINICAL FEATURES

Enteropathy-associated T-cell lymphoma is a rare lymphoma representing fewer than 1% of all lymphomas and approximately 5% of all GI tract lymphomas. However, EATL represents up to 60% to 80% of the GI T-cell lymphomas. The vast majority of cases are associated with GSE or celiac disease. Interestingly, it is common for the diagnosis of GSE to occur at the same time as the lymphoma. Although lymphoma can arise in patients with a long-standing history of GSE, it is most commonly seen in adult-onset or presentation of celiac disease or patients who develop dermatitis herpetiformis.

The most common presentation of EATL is a history of abdominal pain and weight loss. Additionally, many patients have symptoms of celiac disease include malabsorption or diarrhea. Patients can also present with hemorrhage and symptoms of obstruction, and up to 50% of patients present with intestinal perforation. In patients with a history of GSE, refractory changes and clinical deterioration, especially in the setting of compliance with a gluten-free diet, should raise a concern for refractory type II celiac disease and the possibility of evolution to EATL. Unfortunately, many patients presenting with EATL appear to have unknown or subclinical GSE, and as such, all patients with T-cell lymphoma of the intestinal tract should also be evaluated for unknown underlying celiac disease. Although most cases are localized disease, when the disease disseminates, it has a predilection to involve the liver, spleen, lung, testes, and skin but only rarely the bone marrow.

PATHOLOGIC FEATURES

GROSS AND ENDOSCOPIC FINDINGS

Enteropathy-associated T-cell lymphoma typically involves the jejunum (90% of cases) occurring as isolated or multifocal lesions, but it can also involve the stomach and large bowel. Typically, the segment of the GI tract involved by the lymphoma has an edematous appearance with large circumferential ulcers and occasional plaques. The lesions can also look similar to celiac disease with loss of mucosal folds. Less commonly, EATL can present as bulky, exophytic, or infiltrating masses. It is common for the lymphoma to infiltrate the mesentery and involve mesenteric lymph nodes.

MICROSCOPIC FINDINGS

The histologic appearance of EATL is variable between individual cases and between different sites in the same patient. The tumor cells are relatively pleomorphic medium to large cells with round or angulated vesicular nuclei, prominent nucleoli, and moderate to abundant pale-staining cytoplasm (Fig. 19.7A and B). Occasionally, the tumor exhibits marked pleomorphism with multinucleated cells bearing a resemblance to anaplastic large cell lymphoma. An associated inflammatory infiltrate of histiocytes, eosinophils, and plasma cells is often present. This inflammatory infiltrate can be so extensive that it may obscure the neoplastic process.

ANCILLARY STUDIES

The neoplastic cells are double-negative T cells, expressing CD3 without expressing CD4 or CD8. The neoplastic cell typically loses expression of CD5 but retains expression of T-cell associated antigens, CD7, CD2, and CD43. Additionally, the neoplastic cells demonstrate a cytotoxic phenotype with expression of TIA1, granzyme B, and perforin. The neoplastic cells also express CD103, typically seen on mucosal homing or intraepithelial lymphocytes. The neoplastic cells are α-β T cells that lack expression of surface T-cell receptor (TCR) as well as CD56. The immunoprofile of the lymphocytes in EATL is the same as that seen in the refractory celiac disease type II. The large cells in EATL usually express CD30 but are negative for ALK. ISH-EBER is usually negative.

Even though the neoplastic cells do not express surface TCR, clonal TCR-β or -γ rearrangements are

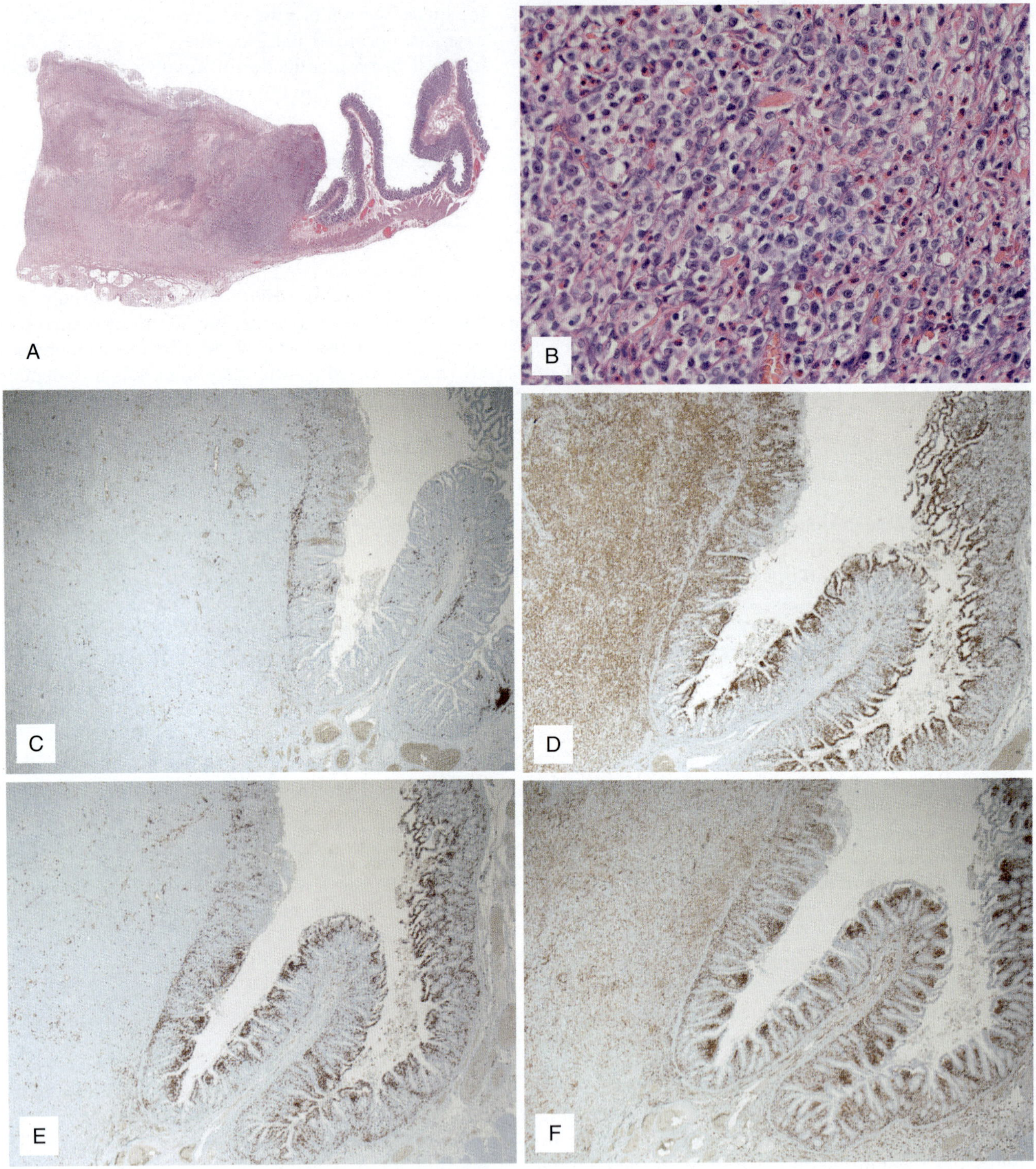

FIGURE 19.7

Enteropathy-associated T-cell lymphoma (EATL). As seen from low power (**A**), EATL in the small bowel shows transmural involvement with marked architectural effacement by a diffuse proliferation of neoplastic T cells. At higher magnification (**B**), the infiltrate is pleomorphic, including scattered anaplastic-appearing cells admixed with small and larger lymphocytes with plasma cells and eosinophils. The infiltrate is negative for CD20 (**C**) but expresses CD3 (**D**). In addition to the neoplastic cells an intraepithelial lymphocytosis can be seen in the small bowel villi. **E**, The neoplastic cells demonstrate loss of CD5 with patchy intact expression of CD5 in the intraepithelial lymphocytes. **F**, The background histocytes are positive for CD4 as are the non-neoplastic T cells in the lamina propria;

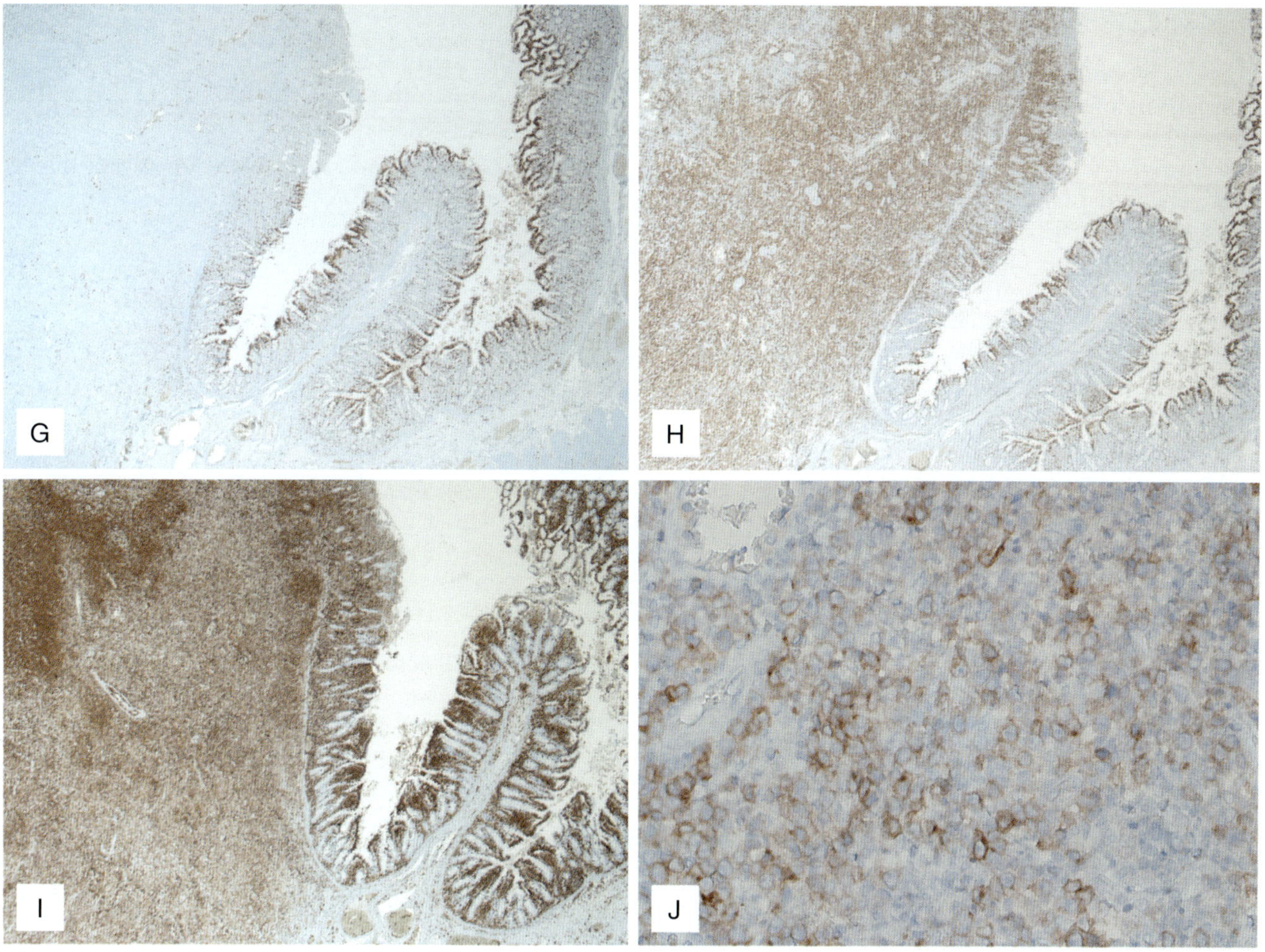

however, the neoplastic cells are negative for CD4. **G**, The intraepithelial lymphocytes are positive for CD8; however, the neoplastic cells are negative for CD8 expression. There is retained expression of CD7 (**H**) and CD43 (**I**) in the neoplastic cells and the intraepithelial lymphocytes. The large pleomorphic neoplastic cells express CD30 (**J**).

found in virtually all cases. Given the correlation with celiac disease, it is not surprising that greater than 90% of patients have HLA-DQA1*0501 or DQB1*0201. Additionally, up to 90% of patients have amplifications of chromosome 9q31 or deletions of 16q12 are prevalent. The lesions also tend to have gains of 1q and 5q.

Differential Diagnosis

In superficial biopsies, the histologic changes overlap with celiac disease and refractory celiac disease. Specifically, they all demonstrate a dense intraepithelial infiltrate of CD3+ T cells with associated villous blunting. The infiltrate in celiac disease is composed of CD3+ CD8+ T cells with intact expression of T cell–associated antigens CD2, CD5, and CD7. Both refractory type II celiac disease and EATL have T cells that have an aberrant phenotype, with double negative T cells (CD3+, CD4-, CD8-) along with loss of CD5 and TCR surface expression with clonal TCR rearrangements. Grossly or endoscopically nonrefractory celiac disease is limited to the mucosa and tends to show loss of folds or fissures and scalloped folds. Refectory celiac disease can have these same features but also can demonstrate erosions and ulcerations. However, when there are obstructing masses, ulcerated nodular mucosa, or stricture, these features suggest the likelihood of an EATL.

Enteropathy-associated T-cell lymphoma typically presents as an infiltrative mass that can resemble an aggressive B-cell lymphoma, which can be distinguished by IHC. Additionally, given the atypical or anaplastic morphology and strong CD30 expression within the large cells, the differential diagnosis includes an anaplastic large cell lymphoma. EATL and anaplastic large cell lymphoma can have similar immunohistochemical features including features of cytotoxic T cells. However, EATL is negative for ALK and CD25. Other mature T and NK cells such as extranodal NK cell lymphoma and PTCL, NOS, also remain in the differential diagnosis. At times, these can be more difficult to distinguish, especially in the absence of a history or clinical features of GSE. Poorly differentiated malignancies (melanoma, carcinoma) can be sorted out by morphologic features and immunohistochemical stains.

Prognosis and Therapy

The prognosis of EATL is unfavorable with a median survival time of only 7 months with reported 1- and 5-year survival rates of 31% to 39% and 0% to 59%, respectively. Most patients succumb to malnutrition and disease progression with complications related to perforation, infection, and peritonitis. Unfortunately, the malnutrition makes most patients intolerant of chemotherapy, and given the diffuse bowel involvement, surgery is typically not useful except in cases of perforation or obstruction. Factors associated with long-term survival include the absence of a previous diagnosis of GSE and completion of an entire course of chemotherapy. Aggressive chemotherapy along with autologous stem cell transplant has shown an overall survival of 60% and progression-free survival of 52%.

ENTEROPATHY-ASSOCIATED T-CELL LYMPHOMA—FACT SHEET

Definition

- An intestinal T-cell lymphoma associated with gluten-sensitive enteropathy

Incidence and Location

- Rare; approximately 5% of all gastrointestinal (GI) tract lymphomas but 60% to 80% of GI T-cell lymphomas
- Geographic distribution is similar to that of celiac disease with the highest incidence in people of Northern European ancestry

Gender, Race, and Age Distribution

- Typically occurs in the seventh decade of life
- Slight male predominance with a male-to-female ratio of 1 to 2.8:1

Clinical Features

- Typical presentation: several months to year history of abdominal pain and weight loss
- May present acutely with acute bleeding, obstruction, or perforation
- Deterioration of celiac disease may herald the presence of lymphoma
- Gluten-sensitive enteropathy (GSE) history, typically of recent onset
- Subclinical GSE may be present
- Most have localized intestinal disease with or without contiguous lymph node involvement
- Disseminated disease has a predilection for the liver, spleen, lung, testes, and skin
- Malnutrition may result in finger clubbing and ichthyosis rash

Prognosis and Treatment

- Prognosis is poor (median survival time, 7 months)
- Patients have complications of peritonitis and malnutrition and later from progressive disease

Enteropathy-Associated T-Cell Lymphoma—Pathologic Features

Gross and Endoscopic Findings

- Most common in the jejunum, either alone or in combination with other sites in the gastrointestinal tract
- Affected bowel segment is often dilated and edematous, with loss of normal mucosal folds
- Large circumferential ulcers, ulcerated plaques, and strictures with intervening areas of normal mucosa
- Bulky exophytic or infiltrating masses are not typical but can be seen in some cases
- Mesenteric lymph node involvement is common

Microscopic Findings

- Variable cytologic appearance between cases and between different sites in the same patient
- Pleomorphic medium-sized to large cells with round or angulated vesicular nuclei, prominent nucleoli, and moderate to abundant pale-staining cytoplasm
- Up to half have marked pleomorphic or anaplastic appearance with multinucleated cells
- Dense inflammatory infiltrate of histiocytes, eosinophils, and plasma cells
- Destruction of the overlying epithelium by the lymphoma cells
- Background mucosa shows changes of gluten-sensitive enteropathy (intraepithelial lymphocytosis, increased lamina propria lymphocytes and plasma cells, villous blunting, and crypt hyperplasia)

Immunohistochemistry

- Most cases are CD3+, CD4-, CD8-, CD7+, CD5- and express cytotoxic granule-associated protein TIA-1, often with granzyme B
- Large pleomorphic cells are typically CD30+ but negative ALK expression
- Negative for surface TCR expression (only up to 25% have cytoplasmic T-cell receptor [TCR] expression)
- Negative for CD56 and CD57 expression
- Neoplastic cells are Epstein-Barr virus (in situ hybridization for Epstein-Barr encoding region) negative

Genetic Abnormalities

- Clonally rearranged TCR genes
- Segmental amplification of chromosome 9p31.3 or deletion at 16q12.1 are seen in up to 80% of cases
- Other common cytogenetic findings are grains in 1q, 5q, and 7q or loss in 8p, 9p, or 13q
- Up to 69% demonstrate evidence of microsatellite instability.
- Patients enriched for HLA-DQ2/DQ8

Differential Diagnosis

- Celiac disease
- Diffuse large B-cell lymphoma
- Extranodal natural killer cell lymphoma
- Peripheral T-cell lymphoma, not otherwise specified
- Poorly differentiated malignancies (melanoma, carcinoma)

MONOMORPHIC EPITHELIOTROPIC INTESTINAL T-CELL LYMPHOMA

Clinical Features

The lymphoma previously referred to as type II EATL is now referred to as MEITL. The name change more closely represents the morphologic appearance of the lymphoma and more clearly delineates this form of lymphoma from EATL. Specifically, MEITL is not associated with GSE. This entity constitutes 34% of the primary intestinal T-cell lymphomas and has a slight male prominence with a reported male-to-female ratio of 1.9 to 2.6:1. Additionally, there is no association with specific human leukocyte antigens. Although MEITL has a worldwide distribution, increased incidence has been documented in patients from an Asian or Hispanic or indigenous origin.

Patients present with symptoms similar to those of other intestinal lymphomas, such as abdominal pain, weight loss, diarrhea, and GI bleeding. However, patients usually do not have a history of malabsorption seen in patients with GSE.

Pathologic Features

Gross and Endoscopic Findings

Grossly, MIETL resembles other lymphomas involving the small bowel. The jejunum is preferentially involved, but the colon can also be involved. Additionally, it is common for the lymphomatous process to infiltrate the mesentery and involve mesenteric lymph nodes. Endoscopically, diffuse mucosal thickening and edema with multiple shallow ulcerations and a nodular or mosaic mucosal pattern are characteristic of the disease. These changes can grossly resemble celiac disease with loss of normal mucosal folds. Occasionally, the lesion can be polypoid or masslike with or without ulceration. Unfortunately, up to 69% of these patients present with perforation or obstruction. Typically, loss of mucosal folds is only present at the site of the lesion. However, in some cases, there is patchy involvement of the mucosa, which can result in a plaque-like appearance. The lymphoma commonly involves the abdominal, inguinal, or mesenteric lymph nodes.

Microscopic Findings

Cytomorphologically, the neoplastic cells are intermediate or medium in size. As the name implies, the cells are monomorphic with a uniformly round noncleaved appearance. These cells also demonstrate clear cytoplasm (Fig. 19.8B) with inconspicuous nucleoli. The neoplastic infiltrate expands the lamina propria and involves the epithelium resulting in widening and blunting of the villi (Fig. 19.8A). Unlike EATL, MEITL does not have significant background inflammation.

Ancillary Studies

The lesion is composed of T cells that express CD3, CD8, and CD56 (Fig. 19.8C, E, and F). The cells retain expression of CD7, CD43, and CD2 expression but are often negative for CD5 (Fig. 19.8D) and CD4. Interestingly, the majority of CD8 are CD8 α homodimers. The lymphoma cells are typically γ-δ T cells but may also be TCR silent. This lymphoma has a cytotoxic phenotype with most expressing TIA-1 and fewer cases expressing granzyme B. More recently, a novel marker, megakaryocyte-associated tyrosine kinase (MATK), has been reported as being positive in up to 90% of cases. Importantly, up to 65% of cases have different immunoprofiles between the mucosal lymphoma cells and the intraepithelial lymphocytes.

The lymphoma has clonal TCR gene rearrangements and has some of the similar genomic changes as EATL. MEITL also demonstrates amplification of 9q and deletion of 16q. Additionally, MEITL can often demonstrate gains in the *CMYC* gene with associated MYC expression seen by IHC. Similar to other γ-δ T cells, MEITL also typically demonstrates *STAT5B* mutation.

Differential Diagnosis

The monomorphic appearance of the mantle cells can be reminiscent of MEITL; however, MCL usually does not show intraepithelial lymphocytosis. Although celiac disease can demonstrate a prominent intraepithelial lymphocytosis and therefore can mimic MEITL, the abnormal T cells in celiac disease are restricted to the epithelium and do not expand the lamina propria. The morphologic and immunohistochemical features of MEITL can overlap with other γ-δ T-cell lymphomas as well as NK or T-cell lymphomas. Specifically, there can be overlap with extranodal NK or T-cell lymphoma nasal type, and PTCL, NOS. Extranodal NK or T-cell lymphoma, nasal type, can frequently involve the GI tract and typically demonstrates villous atrophy. EBV is typically positive in the neoplastic cells, which are positive for CD56 and negative for surface CD3. Additionally, NK or T-cell lymphoma does not typically have an intraepithelial lymphocytosis or an adjacent associated enteropathy. The diagnosis of PTCL, NOS, requires that the T-cell lymphoma does not meet diagnostic features of another defined T-cell lymphoma.

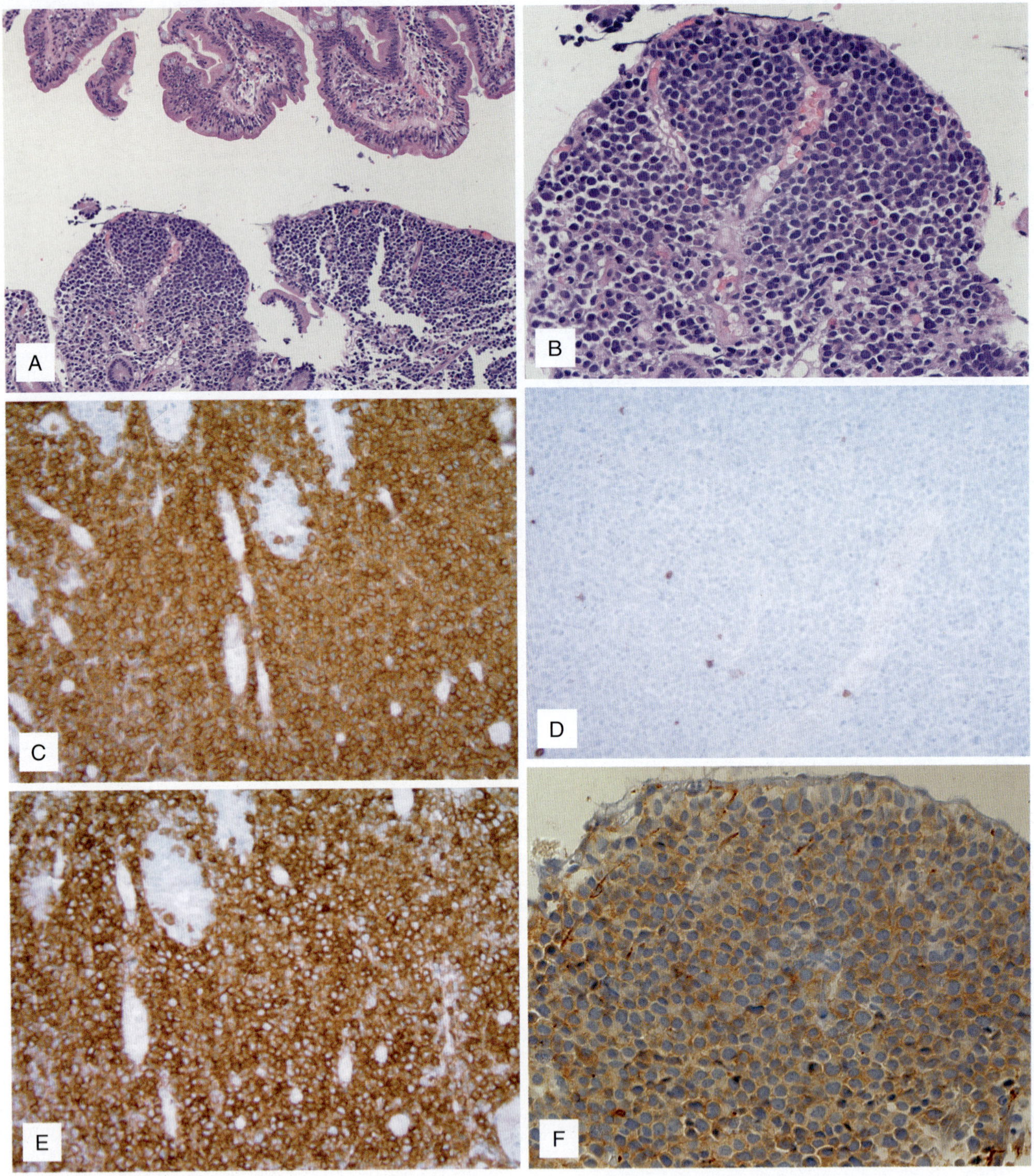

FIGURES 19.8

Monomorphic epitheliotropic intestinal T-cell lymphoma (MEITL), formally known as enteropathy-associated T-cell lymphoma, type II. At low power (**A**), there are a dense intraepithelial lymphocytosis and expansion of the lamina propria. At high power (**B**), the tumor has a very monomorphic population of intermediate-sized lymphocytes with inconspicuous nucleoli. The lymphoma cells are strongly positive for CD3 (**C**), CD8 (**E**), and CD56 (**F**) with loss of expression of CD5 (**D**).

Prognosis and Therapy

The prognosis is poor and similar to EATL with a median survival time of only 7 months, and 1- and 5-year survival rates of 35% and 32%, respectively. There is limited information in regards to prognostic factors and useful treatment regimens. As is typical of lymphoproliferative disorders, an initial response to therapy predicts a better outcome.

Monomorphic Epitheliotropic Intestinal T-Cell Lymphoma—Pathologic Features

Gross, Endoscopic, and Radiologic Findings

- Most common in the jejunum, either alone or in combination with other sites in the gastrointestinal tract
- Affected bowel segment is often dilated and edematous with loss of normal mucosal folds
- Large circumferential ulcers, ulcerated plaques, and strictures with intervening areas of normal mucosa
- Bulky exophytic or infiltrating masses are rarely seen
- Mesenteric and distal lymph node involvement is common

Microscopic Findings

- Uniform (monomorphic) medium-sized round nuclei with a rim of pale cytoplasm
- Florid infiltration of intestinal crypt epithelium with associated with expansion of lamina propria and villous blunting
- Mixed inflammatory background is usually absent
- Intraepithelial lymphocytosis is limited to the area of lymphoma involvement

Immunohistochemistry

- Most cases are CD3+, CD56+, CD8+, CD4-, CD7+, CD5-, and express cytotoxic granule-associated protein TIA-1, often with granzyme B
- Aberrant CD20 expression in up to 20% of cases
- Megakaryocyte-associated tyrosine kinase reported as a novel marker
- Negative for CD30, ALK, and Epstein-Barr virus

Genetic Abnormalities

- Clonal T-cell receptor rearrangement
- Amplified *MYC*
- Activating mutations in *STAT5B*
- Gains in 9q34.3

Differential Diagnosis

- Celiac disease
- MCL
- Extranodal natural killer cell lymphoma
- Peripheral T-cell lymphoma, not otherwise specified

HEPATOSPLENIC T-CELL LYMPHOMA

Clinical Features

Hepatosplenic T-cell lymphoma is a rare neoplasm of gamma δ T cells. This T-cell lymphoma involves and expands the sinusoids of the liver, spleen, and bone marrow. The involvement leads to hepatosplenomegaly without lymphadenopathy. Patients tend to present with B symptoms and pronounced thrombocytopenia. Additionally, patients can present with anemia and often leukopenia along with fever, abdominal pain, and weakness. There can also be variable elevation in liver function tests (aspartate transaminase, alanine transaminase, and alkaline phosphatase).

Hepatosplenic T-cell lymphoma occurs mainly in adolescents and young adults with a male predilection and median age of 35 years. Additionally, up to 20% of patients with HSTL have chronic immunosuppression, including those with a history of solid organ transplantation, Hodgkin lymphoma, acute myelogenous leukemia, malaria infection, pregnancy, and inflammatory bowel disease treated with azathioprine or infliximab or biological agents.

Pathologic Features

Gross and Microscopic Findings

Diffuse hepatic and splenic enlargement is noted with no discrete nodules or masses. The lymphoma predominantly involves the red pulp of the spleen. The liver shows sinusoidal infiltration by tumor cells with relative sparing of portal triads (Fig. 19.9A). The infiltrate consists of a monotonous population of cells with medium-sized nuclei, small inconspicuous nucleoli, and a rim of pale cytoplasm (Fig. 19.9B). Occasional mitotic figures and single-cell necrosis may be noted. Cytologic atypia with large cell changes may be seen, especially with disease progression.

Ancillary Studies

The commonly reported T-cell phenotype is CD2+, CD3+, CD4-, CD5-, CD7+/-, CD8-, with γ-δ TCR expression (Fig. 19.9C&D). CD7 expression may be lost during treatment. NK cell markers CD56 (Fig. 19.9E) and CD16 are often expressed, but CD57 is usually negative. The cells also express the cytotoxic granule-associated proteins, TIA1 (Fig. 19.9F) but are negative for granzyme B and perforin. Although most cases are derived from gamma-delta T-cells, a minority of cases of αβ T cells have also been reported. ISH-EBER is negative. Most cases of HSTL have a specific recurrent chromosomal abnormality, isochromosome 7q, and frequently have *STAT5* mutations. Additionally, trisomy 8 and loss of the Y chromosome have also been reported.

Differential Diagnosis

The differential diagnosis of HTCL includes aggressive NK leukemia/lymphoma, EBV hepatitis, and T-cell large granular lymphocyte leukemia. These other disease entities can also present with hepatomegaly or hepatosplenomegaly. NK leukemia/lymphoma has an aggressive clinical course. The tumor cells in NK cell lymphoproliferative disorders are immunophenotypically similar to HSTL, but they lack expression of a TCR and CD3. The tumor cells share many functional and phenotypic similarities with NK cells and NK-like cytotoxic T cells, resulting in clinical overlap among these malignancies. Morphologic overlap is also seen, although the localization of the HSTL tumor cells within sinusoids in spleen and bone marrow is a feature not seen in other large granular lymphocyte disorders.

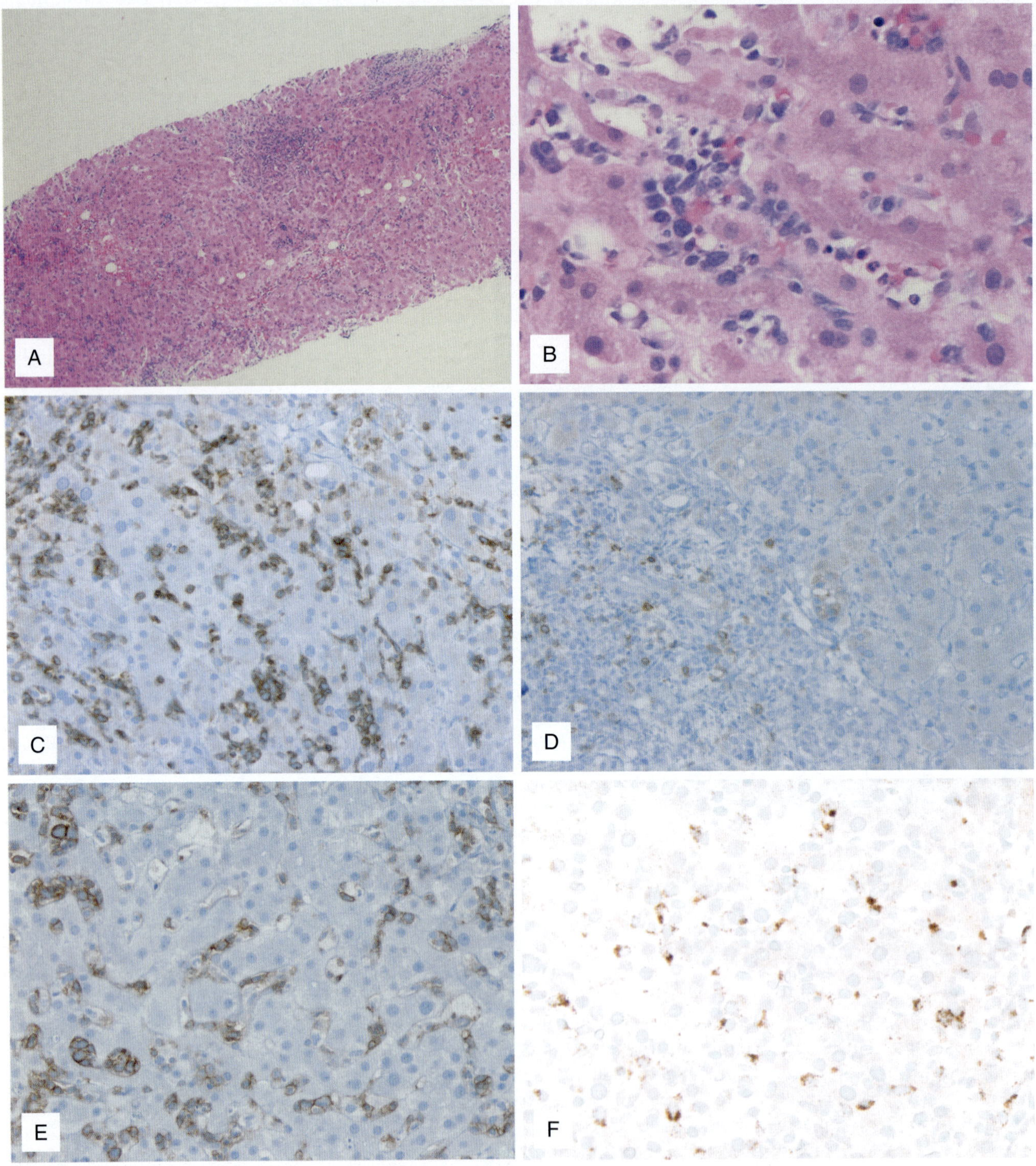

FIGURE 19.9

Hepatosplenic T-cell lymphoma. **A**, A core biopsy of the liver shows a lymphocytic infiltrate involving the sinusoids with relative sparing of the portal triads. **B**, At higher power, the infiltrate is composed of a monotonous population of cells with medium-sized nuclei, small inconspicuous nucleoli, and a rim of pale cytoplasm expanding the sinusoidal spaces. **C**, An immunohistochemical stain for CD3 highlights the predominantly sinusoidal pattern of infiltration by the neoplastic T-lymphocytes. These neoplastic cells demonstrate loss of CD5 expression (**D**) and aberrant expression of CD56 (**E**). These neoplastic cells are cytotoxic and demonstrates expression of TIA1 (**F**).

Prognosis and Therapy

The clinical course is aggressive with a dismal prognosis. Patients may initially respond to chemotherapy, but there is a high relapse rate and short median survival time of 8 months.

HEPATOSPLENIC T-CELL LYMPHOMA—FACT SHEET

Definition

- Extranodal and systemic neoplasm of cytotoxic T cells

Incidence and Location

- Up to 20% arise in the setting of chronic immune suppression
- Involves the spleen, liver, and bone marrow

Gender, Race, and Age Distribution

- Peak incidence in adolescents and young adults
- Male predominance
- Median age of 35 years

Clinical Features

- Marked splenomegaly usually with hepatomegaly
- No lymphadenopathy
- Thrombocytopenia often with anemia and leukopenia
- Systemic symptoms

Prognosis and Treatment

- Aggressive course
- Initial response to chemotherapy
- Median survival less than 2 years

HEPATOSPLENIC T-CELL LYMPHOMA—PATHOLOGIC FEATURES

Gross Findings

- Diffuse enlargement of spleen and liver
- Generally, no specific mass-forming lesion

Microscopic Findings

- Monotonous lymphocytes with medium-sized nuclei and a rim of pale cytoplasm
- Diffuse involvement of the cords and sinuses of the splenic red pulp
- Splenic white pulp atrophy
- Hepatic sinusoid involvement
- Cytologic atypia with large cell or blastic changes seen in disease progression

Immunohistochemistry

- Usually γ-δ T-cell receptor type, but a minority are α-β type
- CD3+, CD56+/-, CD4-, CD8-/+, and CD5-
- Express cytotoxic granule-associated proteins, TIA1
- Negative for granzyme B and perforin
- Epstein-Barr virus is usually negative

Genetic Abnormalities

- Isochromosome 7q present in most cases
- *STAT5B* mutations

Differential Diagnosis

- Extranodal natural killer cell lymphoma
- Peripheral T-cell lymphoma, not otherwise specified

INDOLENT T- AND NATURAL KILLER CELL LYMPHOPROLIFERATIVE DISORDERS

As outlined earlier, T-cell lymphomas are generally considered aggressive neoplasms. However, over the past 2 decades, T and NK lymphomas and lymphoproliferative disorders with an indolent behavior have also been reported. In the 2017 update to the WHO classification system, the provisional entity of indolent T-cell lymphoproliferative disorder of the GI tract was added. Based on a published series and case reports, these T- and NK cell lymphoproliferative disorders can be subdivided into CD4+, CD8+, CD4-/CD8-, and NK lymphoproliferative disorders.

Indolent CD4+ lymphoproliferative disorder of the GI tract was first described in 1994, and since then, a little more than 20 have been reported. Patients tend to present clinically with diarrhea and often with associated weight loss. Rarely, patients present with symptoms of bowel obstruction. Endoscopically, the mucosa may either appear completely normal or may show erosions or ulceration, nodularity, polyps, or a masslike lesion. Generally, at the time of diagnosis, the disease is limited to the GI tract with the majority of the patients demonstrating small bowel involvement. However, in some cases, these proliferations may involve the liver, bone marrow, and lymph node. Morphologically, the lamina propria is expanded by a population of mature-appearing small lymphocytes. The cells tend to have clear cytoplasm with inconspicuous nuclei. Typically, there is no significant intraepithelial lymphocytosis, but the infiltrate can often be seen involving the muscularis mucosa and submucosa. As the name suggests, all cases are positive for CD3 and CD4. These cells are α-βT cells, often with aberrant loss of CD5 and CD7. They are also negative for CD56, CD30, cytotoxic markers, CD103, HHV8, and EBV and demonstrate a low Ki-67 index (<10%). The cases show clonal TCR rearrangements and often other genetic abnormalities; however, there are no common or recurrent genetic abnormalities in these patients. Many of these cases were found on retrospective review, and because clonal T-cell processes have generally be considered to be aggressive malignant processes, most of the patients had undergone aggressive chemotherapy. Interestingly, even with aggressive therapy, 83% of patients demonstrated continued persistent disease at 5 years, with 22% showing continued involvement for longer than 10 years. Only 13% died of disease or treatment-related complications.

Indolent CD8+ T-cell lymphoproliferative disorder was first reported in 2000. The median age at the time of diagnosis is 45 years, and patients typically present with diarrhea along with abdominal pain and bloating. Morphologically, the lamina propria is expanded, and the glands may be displaced; however, destructive lymphoepithelial lesions and changes of celiac disease (including intraepithelial lymphocytosis) are not seen. The lymphocytes are positive for CD3 and CD8 with only a small proportion demonstrating aberrant loss of CD5 and CD7. The lymphocytes are α-β T cells and typically demonstrate expression of cytotoxic marker TIA1. They are positive for intraepithelial T-cell marker CD103 and are negative for CD30 and CD56. All reported patients are negative for EBV. The lymphocytes demonstrate clonal TCR rearrangements, but other recurrent genetic rearrangements have not been documented. Although in the reported cases the median follow-up period was only 2 years (range, 1–19.8), all patients have persistent disease, and no cases of transformation have been reported.

Indolent NK cell lymphoproliferative disorders were first described in 2006 and have been reported as NK cell enteropathy as well as lymphomatoid gastropathy. The disease was either found during asymptomatic gastric screening in the Japanese cohort or in the US and Korea cohorts that presented with abdominal pain. This disease process is often localized to the gastric mucosa but can involve multiple GI sites. The endoscopic appearance is variable, presenting as mucosal nodularity, hyperemic or erythematous lesions, or focal superficial bleeding ulcers. Histologically, the lamina propria is expanded by intermediate- to large-sized lymphocytes that can have a clear to pale eosinophilic cytoplasm, giving the cells a so-called histiocytoid appearance. Occasionally, there is glandular destruction, but changes of more aggressive NK or T-cell lymphoma such as necrosis or angiocentric lesions are not seen.

Immunohistochemically, the lymphocytes demonstrate an NK phenotype with expression of CD56, cytoplasmic (not surface) CD3, CD2, and CD7 and cytotoxic markers TIA1, perforin, and granzyme B. The lymphocytes are negative for CD4 and CD5, and results of ISH-EBER are negative. Because this is an NK process, no TCR rearrangements were identified. Additionally, no recurrent genetic abnormalities were identified.

SUMMARY

Although lymphoproliferative processes in the GI tract are still rare, they appear to be increasing in frequency. An awareness of the various entities is essential. To assist in this, Table 19.4 summarizes the immunohistochemical profiles of lymphoma common to the GI tract.

TABLE 19.4

Immunohistochemical Profiles of Gastrointestinal Lymphoma

	Mature Low-Grade B-Cell Lymphoma				Aggressive B-Cell Lymphoma					T-Cell Lymphoma				Other
	MALT	**Mantle**	**CLL/SLL**	**FL**	**DLBCL, NOS**	**EBV+ DLBCL**	**BL**	**HGBL**	**PBL**	**EATL**	**MEITL**	**HSTL**	**EBVMCU**	**Indolent T-Cell Lymphoma**
CD20	+	+	+	+	+	+	+	+	-	-	- (+ in 20%)	-	+	-
PAX5	+	+	+	+	+	+	+	+	-	-	-	-	+	-
CD79a	+	+	+	+	+	+	+	+	+ in 40% of cases	-	-	-	+	-
CD138	+ in PC	-	-	-	+/- (rarely)	+	-	ND	+	-	-	-	+	-
CD10	-	-	-	+	+ (in 30%–50%)	-	+	Variable	- (+ in 20%)	-	-	-	-	-
BCL2	+	+	+	+	+ (in 47%–84%)	ND	-	+/-[a]	-	-	-	-	ND	-
BCL6	-	+	-	+	+ (in 60%–90%)	-	+	+	-	-	-	-	-	-
LMO2	-	-	-	+	+ (in 45%)	-	-	+/-	ND	-	-	-	ND	-
MUM1	-	+	-	-	+ (in 35%–65%)	+	-	-	+	-	-	-	+	-
Cyclin D1	-	+	-	-	-	-	-	-	-	-	-	-	-	-
SOX11	-	+	-	-	-	-	-	-	-	-	-	-	-	-
LEF1	-	-/+ (in ≤%)	+	-	+ (≤30%–40%)	ND	+	ND	-	ND	ND	-	-	-
CD30	-	-	-	-	+ (in 10%–20%)	+ (in 40%)	-	+/-	-	+	-	-	+	-
CD2	-	-	-	-	-	-	-	-	-	+	+	+	+	+
CD3	-	-	-	-	-	-	-	-	-	+ cytoplasmic	+	+	-	+
CD4	-	-	-	-	-	-	-	-	-	-	-	-	-	+/-
CD5	-	+	+	-	+ (≤10%)	-	-	-	-	-	-	-	-	+
CD7	-	-	-	-	-	-	-	-	-	+	+	+/-	-	+
CD8	-	-	-	-	-	-	-	-	-	+ (20%–30%)	+	-/+	-	+/-
CD43	+ in 40%	+	+	-	+ (≤25%)	-/+	+	ND	-	+	+	+	-	+
CD56	-	-	-	-	-	-	-	-	+	-	+	+	-	-
Tia-1	-	-	-	-	-	-	-	-	-	+	+	+	-	+ (in CD8 +)
MYC	-	-	-	-	+ (≤40%)	-	+	+/-[a]	+	-	-	-	ND	-
EBER	-	-	-	-	-	+ (required)	+ (25%–50%)	-	-	-	-	-	+	-
HHV8	-	-	-	-	-	-	-	-	-	-	-	-	-	-

+, expressed; –, negative for expression, *BL*, Burkitt lymphoma; *CLL*, chronic lymphocytic leukemia; *DLBCL*, diffuse large B-cell lymphoma; *EATL*, enteropathy-associated T-cell lymphoma; *EBER*, Epstein-Barr encoding region; *EBV*, Epstein-Barr virus; *EBVMCU*, Epstein-Barr virus–positive mucocutaneous ulcer; *FL*, follicular lymphoma; *HHV8*, human herpesvirus 8; *HSTL*, hepatosplenic T-cell lymphoma; *MALT*, extranodal marginal zone lymphoma of mucosa-associated lymphoid tissue; *MEITL*, monomorphic epitheliotropic intestinal T-cell lymphoma; *ND*, no or insufficient data; *NOS*, not otherwise specified; *PBL*, plasmablastic lymphoma *PC*, plasma cell; *SLL*, small lymphocytic lymphoma.

[a]In the high-grade B-cell lymphoma (HGBL) with MYC and BCL2 and/or BCL6 rearrangements variant, these cases strongly express BCL2 and MYC.

SUGGESTED READINGS

1. Agbay RLMC, Loghavi S, Medeiros LJ, Khoury JD. High-grade transformation of low-grade B-cell lymphoma. *Am J Surg Pathol.* 2016;40(1):e1–e16.
2. Al-Saleem T, Al-Mondhiry H. Immunoproliferative small intestinal disease (IPSID): a model for mature B-cell neoplasms. *Blood.* 2005;105(6):2274–2280.
3. Bautista-Quach MA, Ake CD, Chen M, Wang J. Gastrointestinal lymphomas: morphology, immunophenotype and molecular features. *J Gastrointest Oncol.* 2012;3(3):209–225.
4. Behdad A, Bailey NG. Comprehensive assessment and classification of high-grade B-cell lymphomas. *Surg Pathol Clin.* 2016; 9(1):41–54.
5. Campo E, Rule S. Mantle cell lymphoma: evolving management strategies. *Blood.* 2015;125(1):48–55.
6. Castillo JJ, Beltran BE, Miranda RN, et al. EBV-positive diffuse large B-cell lymphoma, not otherwise specified: 2018 update on diagnosis, risk-stratification and management. *Am J Hematol.* 2018;93(7):953–962.
7. Chen Y, Chen Y, Chen S, et al. Primary gastrointestinal lymphoma a retrospective multicenter clinical study of 415 cases in Chinese province of Guangdong and a systematic review containing 5075 Chinese patients. *Med (United States).* 2015;94(47):e2119.
8. Choi WT, Gill RM. Hepatic lymphoma diagnosis. *Surg Pathol Clin.* 2018;11(2):389–402.
9. Chouhan J, Batra S, Gupta R, Guha S. Gastrointestinal follicular lymphoma: using primary site as a predictor of survival. *Cancer Med.* 2016;5(10):2669–2677.
10. Cirocchi R, Farinella E, Trastulli S, et al. Surgical treatment of primitive gastro-intestinal lymphomas: a systematic review. *World J Surg Oncol.* 2011;9:145.
11. Copie-Bergman C, Wotherspoon AC, Capella C, et al. Gela histological scoring system for post-treatment biopsies of patients with gastric MALT lymphoma is feasible and reliable in routine practice. *Br J Haematol.* 2013;160(1):47–52.
12. de Leval L, Copie-Bergman C, Rosenwald A, et al. B-cell lymphomas with discordance between pathological features and clinical behavior. *Virchows Arch.* 2017;471(4):439–451.
13. Dojcinov SD, Venkataraman G, Raffeld M, et al. EBV positive mucocutaneous ulcer-A study of 26 cases associated with various sources of immunosuppression. *Am J Surg Pathol.* 2010;34(3): 405–417.
14. Ferreri AJM, Govi S, Ponzoni M. The role of Helicobacter pylori eradication in the treatment of diffuse large B-cell and marginal zone lymphomas of the stomach. *Curr Opin Oncol.* 2013; 25(5):470–479.
15. Foukas PG, de Leval L. Recent advances in intestinal lymphomas. *Histopathology.* 2015;66(1):112–136.
16. Grimm KE, O'Malley DP. Aggressive B cell lymphomas in the 2017 revised WHO classification of tumors of hematopoietic and lymphoid tissues. *Ann Diagn Pathol.* 2019;38:6–10.
17. Haramura T, Haraguchi M, Irie J, et al. Case of plasmablastic lymphoma of the sigmoid colon and literature review. *World J Gastroenterol.* 2015;21(24):7598.
18. Hawkes EA, Wotherspoon A, Cunningham D. Diagnosis and management of rare gastrointestinal lymphomas. *Leuk Lymphoma.* 2012;53(12):2341–2350.
19. Howell JM, Auer-Grzesiak I, Zhang J, et al. Increasing incidence rates, distribution and histological characteristics of primary gastrointestinal non-Hodgkin lymphoma in a North American population. *Can J Gastroenterol.* 2012;26(7):452–456.
20. Huang W, Medeiros LJ, Lin P, et al. MYC/BCL2/BCL6 triple hit lymphoma: a study of 40 patients with a comparison to MYC/BCL2 and MYC/BCL6 double hit lymphomas. *Mod Pathol.* 2018;31(9):1470–1478.
21. Lee P-S, Beneck D, Weisberger J, Gorczyca W. Coexpression of CD43 by benign B cells in the terminal ileum. *Appl Immunohistochem Mol Morphol.* 2005;13(2):138–141.
22. Lightner AL, Shannon E, Gibbons MM, Russell MM. Primary gastrointestinal non-Hodgkin's lymphoma of the small and large intestines: a systematic review. *J Gastrointest Surg.* 2016; 20(4):827–839.
23. Manning MA, Somwaru AS, Mehrotra AK, Levine MS. Gastrointestinal lymphoma. Radiologic-pathologic correlation. *Radiol Clin North Am.* 2016;54(4):765–784.
24. O'Malley DP, Auerbach A, Weiss LM. Practical applications in immunohistochemistry evaluation of diffuse large B-cell lymphoma and related large B-cell lymphomas. *Arch Pathol Lab Med.* 2015;139:1094–1107.
25. O'Malley DP, Goldstein NS, Banks PM. The recognition and classification of lymphoproliferative disorders of the gut. *Hum Pathol.* 2014;45(5):899–916.
26. Perry AM, Warnke RA, Hu Q, et al. Indolent T-cell lymphoproliferative disease of the gastrointestinal tract. *Blood.* 2013;122(22): 3599–3606.
27. Rosenthal A, Younes A. High grade B-cell lymphoma with rearrangements of MYC and BCL2 and/or BCL6: Double hit and triple hit lymphomas and double expressing lymphoma. *Blood Rev.* 2017;31(2):37–42.
28. Smith LB, Owens SR. Gastrointestinal lymphomas: entities and mimics. *Arch Pathol Lab Med.* 2012;136(8):865–870.
29. Smith LB, Hsi ED. Lymphomas of the gastrointestinal tract: an update. *Surg Pathol Clin.* 2013;6(3):405–424.
30. Starr AG, Caimi PF, Fu PF, et al. Dual institution experience of nodal marginal zone lymphoma reveals excellent long-term outcomes in the rituximab era. *Br J Haematol.* 2016;175(2):275–280.
31. Revised 4tSwerdlow SH, Campo E, Harris NL, eds. *WHO Classification of Tumours: Pathology and Genetics. Tumours of Haematopoietic and Lymphoid Tissues.* Lyon: France: IARC; 2017. http://publications.iarc.fr/Book-And-Report-Series/Who-Iarc-Classification-Of-Tumours/Who-Classification-Of-Tumours-Of-Haematopoietic-And-Lymphoid-Tissues-2017.
32. Swerdlow SH, Campo E, Pileri SA, et al. The 2016 revision of the World Health Organization classification of lymphoid neoplasms. *Blood.* 2016;127(20):2375–2390.
33. Swerdlow SH, Jaffe ES, Brousset P, et al. Cytotoxic T-cell and NK-cell lymphomas: current questions and controversies. *Am J Surg Pathol.* 2014;38(10):e60–e71.
34. Takata K, Miyata-Takata T, Sato Y, et al. Gastrointestinal follicular lymphoma: current knowledge and future challenges. *Pathol Int.* 2018;68(1):1–6.
35. Tanaka T, Yamamoto H, Elsayed AA, et al. Clinicopathologic spectrum of gastrointestinal T-cell lymphoma reappraisal based on T-cell receptor immunophenotypes. *Am J Surg Pathol.* 2016; 40(6):777–785.
36. Vaidya R, Habermann TM, Donohue JH, et al. Bowel perforation in intestinal lymphoma: incidence and clinical features. *Ann Oncol.* 2013;24(9):2439–2443.
37. Vetro C, Bonanno G, Giulietti G, et al. Rare gastrointestinal lymphomas: the endoscopic investigation. *World J Gastrointest Endosc.* 2017;7(10):928.
38. Vetro C, Romano A, Amico I, et al. Endoscopic features of gastro-intestinal lymphomas: from diagnosis to follow-up. *World J Gastroenterol.* 2014;20(36):12993–13005.
39. Wang HY, Zu Y. Diagnostic algorithm of common mature B-cell lymphomas by immunohistochemistry. *Arch Pathol Lab Med.* 2017;141(9):1236–1246.
40. Weindorf SC, Smith LB, Owens SR. Update on Gastrointestinal Lymphomas. *Arch Pathol Lab Med.* 2018;142:1347–1351.
41. Wotherspoon AC, Doglioni C, Diss TC, et al. Regression of primary low-grade B-cell gastric lymphoma of mucosa-associated lymphoid tissue type after eradication of Helicobacter pylori. *Lancet (London, England).* 1993;342(8871):575–577.
42. Yabe M., Miranda R.N., Medeiros L.J. Hepatosplenic T-cell Lymphoma: a review of clinicopathologic features, pathogenesis, and prognostic factors. 2018;74:5-16.
43. Yang L, Tang X, Peng X, et al. Clinical characteristics of primary intestinal NK/T cell lymphoma, nasal type: case series and review of the literature. *Pathol Res Pract.* 2018;214(8):1081–1086.
44. Zucca E, Bertoni F. The spectrum of MALT lymphoma at different sites: biological and therapeutic relevance. *Blood.* 2016; 127(17):2082–2092.
45. Ondrejka S, Jagadeesh D. Enteropathy-associated T-cell lymphoma. *Curr Hematol Malig Rep.* 2016;11:504–513.
46. Skinnider BF. Lymphoproliferative disorders of the gastrointestinal tract. *Arch Pathol Lab Med.* 2018;142(1):44–52.

47. Matysiak-Budnik T, Fabiani B, Hennequin C, et al. Gastrointestinal lymphomas: French Intergroup clinical practice recommendations for diagnosis, treatment and follow-up (SNFGE, FFCD, GERCOR, UNICANCER, SFCD, SFED, SFRO, SFH). *Dig Liver Dis*. 2018;50(2):124–131.
48. Matnani R, Ganapathi KA, Lewis SK, et al. Indolent T- and NK-cell lymphoproliferative disorders of the gastrointestinal tract: a review and update. *Hematol Oncol*. 2017;35(1):3–16.
49. Leventaki V, Manning JT, Luthra R, et al. Indolent peripheral T-cell lymphoma involving the gastrointestinal tract. *Hum Pathol*. 2014;45(2):421–426.
50. Xia D, Morgan EA, Berger D, et al. NK-cell enteropathy and similar indolent lymphoproliferative disorders. *Am J Clin Pathol*. 2019;151(1):75–85.

20

Pathology of Liver, Small Bowel, and Pancreas Transplantation

Daniela S. Allende, MD, MBA, Lisa M. Yerian, MD, and Deepa T. Patil, MD

LIVER TRANSPLANTATION

Liver transplantation is performed in patients with liver failure caused by acute or chronic liver disease, selected hepatic tumors, and some metabolic diseases. Approximately 7000 liver transplants (LT) are performed annually in the United States. The graft survival rate at 5 years is greater than 70%, and the patient survival rate is even higher. The most common types of LT are cadaveric and living donor LT. Cadaveric LTs are by far the most common type performed in the United States, accounting for 95% of all LTs. Most cadaveric donor organs derive from brain-dead donors with stable cardiopulmonary function. However, a small percentage of cadaveric donor organs (4%) are procured after cessation of cardiopulmonary function. These donation after cardiac death (DCD) organs are subject to complications related to warm ischemia–induced injury and show reduced graft survival. Cadaveric LT may be performed using a whole donor liver or using a split or reduced size graft. Split grafts enable a donor organ of sufficient size be transplanted into two recipients (often an adult and a child), whereas a reduced size graft is reduced in size to match a single recipient. Living donor LTs currently account for about 5% of LT performed in the United States. Far less common are domino LTs. In this case, an explanted liver from an LT recipient who has a metabolic disease of the liver that can potentially cause severe systemic disease but does not structurally damage the liver (e.g., familial amyloidotic polyneuropathy) is transplanted into another recipient whose condition precludes a long time on the waiting list.

The term *extended criteria* denotes donor organs carrying risk factors associated with a greater risk of poor graft function than standard criteria donor organs. These organs traditionally would not have been used for transplant but are now used in selected recipients in an effort to increase the number of organs available for transplantation. There is no consensus definition of extended criteria organs, but examples include organs with severe steatosis or prolonged warm or cold ischemia times and organs from donors of advanced age, elevated liver enzymes, hepatitis C virus infection, and other factors.

Liver biopsy is a critical diagnostic tool in the care of transplant recipients. It is used in the diagnosis or exclusion of several forms of graft pathology ranging from rejection to technical (biliary, vascular) and infectious complications and is the "gold standard" test for diagnosis of rejection. Biopsy practice varies by center and with recipient factors. Liver biopsies are performed when patients exhibit laboratory abnormalities or other signs or symptoms of graft dysfunction such as fever or abdominal pain. Some centers also perform "protocol" biopsies at set time intervals in the absence of evidence of graft dysfunction.

PRETRANSPLANT DONOR EVALUATION

Protocols for evaluating potential donor organs vary across transplant centers. Frozen sections are commonly used to assess deceased donor organs, although in many instances, no histologic evaluation of the donor organ is performed before transplantation and other factors, such as gross impression of the organ, are used to determine suitability of the graft. Frozen sections are not routinely performed on DCD organs because doing so would prolong the cold ischemia time and increase risk of intrahepatic bile duct strictures. In some centers, preperfusion or "time-zero" biopsies are used to assess for preexisting donor organ pathology at the time of transplantation.

The histologic confirmation of greater than 30% macrovesicular steatosis has long been associated with poor early graft function. However, some studies have shown that grafts with moderate to severe steatosis can be safely in select situations (Fig. 20.1). These apparently conflicting findings are likely caused at least in part by the complex nature of donor selection and differing

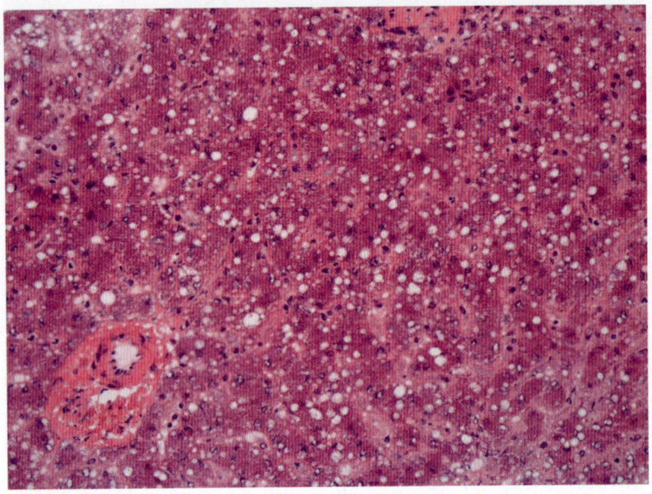

FIGURE 20.1
Frozen sections of a donor liver biopsy with steatosis.

definitions and methods of assessing steatosis. In 2022, The Banf Working Group published recommendation to standardize this assessment. Two forms of macrovesicular steatosis have since been delineated as "large droplet" (a single fat vacuole occupying greater than half of the cell and displacing the nucleus to the periphery) or "small droplet" (one or several discrete vacuoles, each occupying less than half of the cell and not displacing the nucleus). Both forms are distinguished from true microvesicular steatosis (innumerable tiny lipid vacuoles diffusely distributed in the cytoplasm and imparting a foamy appearance to the cell), which may coexist with macrovesicular steatosis but in its pure, diffuse form is uncommon in potential liver donors. There is no universal cutoff for an acceptable amount of steatosis. In most practices, the total amount of macrovesicular steatosis is assessed as the percentage of the hepatocellular component (area) of the biopsy that is involved. Care should be taken not to interpret freeze artifact in frozen liver specimens as fat vacuoles.

In addition to steatosis, pretransplant donor biopsies are used to assess other factors that may affect graft function, including necrosis, inflammation, and fibrosis. These findings are particularly relevant in the assessment of extended criteria donors, who may exhibit features of hepatitis C or other forms of pathology. Mild portal inflammation or bile ductular proliferation may be seen in deceased donor organs and in isolation are not contraindications for transplantation.

PRESERVATION OR ISCHEMIA-REPERFUSION INJURY

Donor organs are subject to injury related to the process of organ procurement, preservation, and reimplantation that is referred to as *preservation injury* or *ischemia-reperfusion injury* (IRI). The mechanism of injury is complex, multifactorial, and attributed to warm and cold ischemic injury followed by reperfusion. Warm ischemic injury occurs in situ and causes hepatocyte damage, whereas cold ischemia occurs after the harvested organ is flushed with cold preservation solution and results in damage of sinusoidal endothelial cells and biliary epithelium. Ischemia results in anaerobic metabolism, cell swelling, and cell death. Microcirculatory damage ensues, and Kupffer cell activation drives a local inflammatory response that is magnified by tissue reperfusion and involves the formation of reactive oxygen species, production of cytokines and chemokines, and activation of the complement systems. These mechanisms further microvascular dysfunction and cellular injury. The injury is exacerbated by preexisting donor pathology (e.g., donor steatosis) and by extended warm or cold ischemia times, whereas the injury is minimal organs with short ischemia times (as in living donors). Some degree of IRI is expected in biopsies obtained in the first 1 to 2 weeks after liver transplantation, and histologic evidence of IRI can persist beyond 2 weeks in more severely injured grafts. When assessing a biopsy in the early posttransplant period, it is helpful to know if the biopsy was performed for clinical concern for rejection or other form of graft dysfunction because biopsies may be obtained during this interval in the absence of clinical concern for graft dysfunction if the patient is taken back to operating room to address bleeding, intraabdominal infection, or fluid collections.

LABORATORY FINDINGS

Ischemia-reperfusion injury is common and typically mild; laboratory findings indicative of this form of graft injury are minor or absent in most patients. Elevated serum lactate levels and persistent serum transaminases elevations in the early posttransplant period are common.

Pathologic Features

Microscopic Features

The histologic findings include predominantly zone 3 hepatocellular injury, which is manifested as perivenular hepatocyte swelling, necrosis, or dropout (Fig. 20.2A). This is usually accompanied by Kupffer cell hyperplasia and regenerative hepatocellular changes such as increased mitotic activity (Fig. 20.2B). Centrilobular perivenular cholestasis is common. Rarely, the degree of preservation or IRI is extensive with areas of confluent or even bridging hepatocyte necrosis and marked

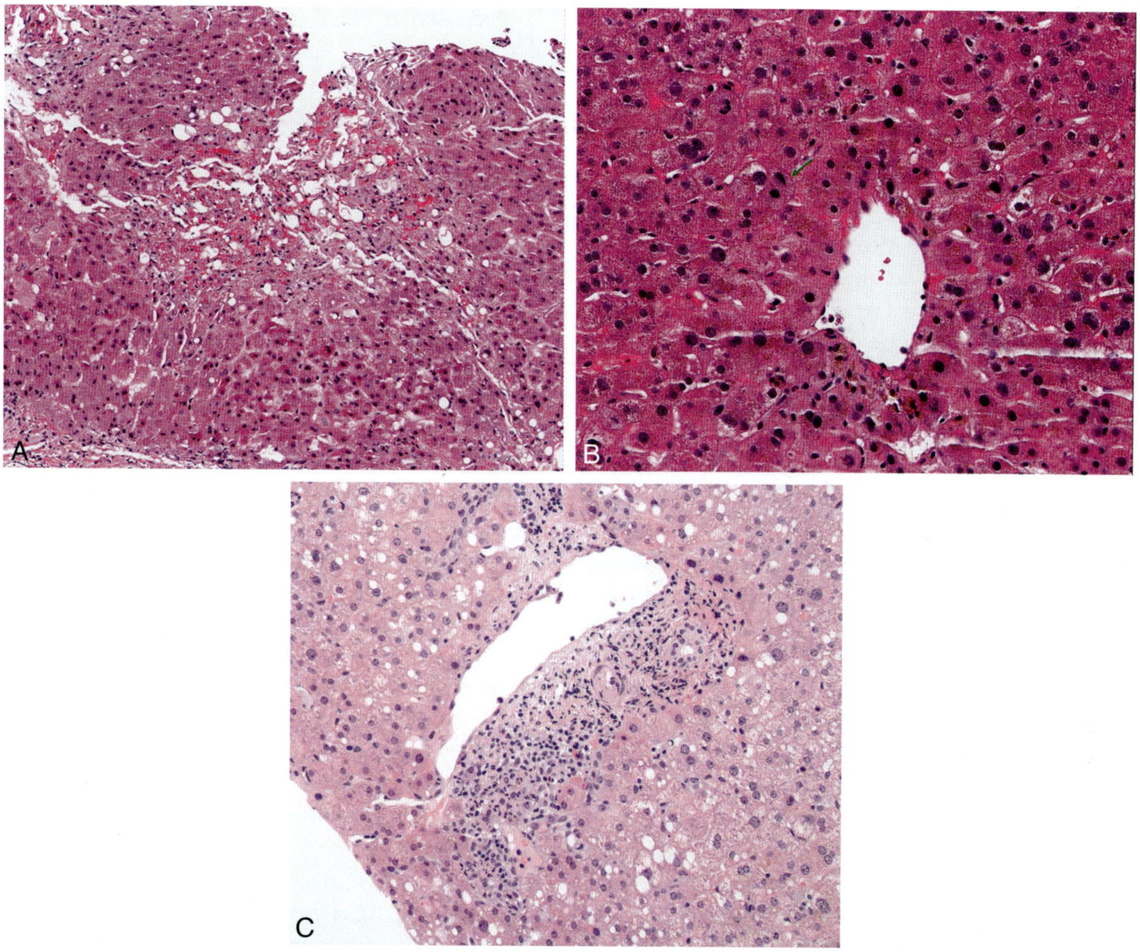

FIGURE 20.2

A, An example of marked preservation or reperfusion injury with hepatocellular dropout in centrizonal regions as well as congestion. **B**, In some cases, regenerative hepatocellular changes, including mitoses and hepatocyte multinucleation, can be seen. **C**, Bile ductular proliferation can be prominent in a subset of cases, raising the differential diagnosis of biliary obstruction.

bile ductular reaction in response to parenchymal collapse. Portal areas may exhibit mild bile ductular proliferation (Fig. 20.2C) and portal neutrophils, and scattered clusters of neutrophils may be seen in the hepatic lobules.

Differential Diagnosis

The major differential diagnosis for IRI includes biliary obstruction, antibody-mediated rejection (AMR), acute T cell–mediated rejection (ACR), and infection. In the early posttransplant period, mild neutrophilic infiltration and ductular proliferation can be seen, but these changes should not be overinterpreted as acute cholangitis. If there is concern for biliary obstruction, this possibility should be excluded clinically with imaging studies. Neutrophil collections within duct lumens and portal edema are required to diagnose acute ascending cholangitis. Neutrophils, cholestasis, ductular reaction, and hepatocyte necrosis are also features of AMR, but AMR shows microvascular changes that are not seen in IRI, and a diagnosis of AMR requires demonstration of C4d positivity and detection of serum donor-specific antibodies. IRI demonstrates less perivenular and portal inflammation than ACR, and the portal infiltrates of early ACR are distinct from those seen in preservation injury, including enlarged, activated-appearing lymphocytes along with other inflammatory cells such as eosinophils. If lobular collections of neutrophils are seen in association with hepatocyte necrosis, a careful search for viral inclusions is warranted.

Prognosis and Therapy

Most patients with mild preservation or IRI show an initial delay in normalization of liver enzymes but eventually recover without significant complications. Severe IRI often reflect preexisting donor disease or graft injury that may lead to long-term complications, including scarring and ischemic cholangiopathy.

ANTIBODY-MEDIATED REJECTION

CLINICAL FEATURES

Antibody-mediated rejection (formerly termed "humoral" rejection) is a pattern of allograft injury mediated by preformed or de novo antidonor antibodies ("donor-specific antibodies" [DSAs]) that bind to antigens on endothelial cells, resulting in antibody-mediated endothelial cell injury and activation of the complement cascade. AMR occurs in recipients of ABO-incompatible grafts or in recipients with preformed or de novo lymphocytotoxic antibodies. Preformed antibodies are encountered in 10% to 15% of LT recipients and are most commonly found in women and patients with autoimmune diseases. De novo DSAs develop after LT in 8% to 15% of liver allograft recipients. Risk factors for de novo DSA include low immunosuppression, young age, cyclosporine use, low Model For End-Stage Liver Disease (MELD) score, and previous transplants. DSAs represent a key diagnostic feature of AMR, and because DSA can occur de novo in LT recipients and may not persist, serum DSA testing should be performed during the posttransplant interval and at the time of biopsy to confirm or exclude a diagnosis of AMR.

Severe, early acute AMR, or "hyperacute rejection," is exceedingly rare, occurs within hours to a few days after transplantation, and is largely limited to recipients of ABO-incompatible grafts. Affected patients develop signs of rapid, acute graft failure within the first 2 weeks after transplantation, including a rapid rise in serum aminotransferases and severe coagulopathy with increased prothrombin times. A more common and less severe form of acute AMR (late-onset acute AMR) develops 1 to 4 weeks after transplant in patients with detectable DSA. Patients present with hyperbilirubinemia, posttransplant transaminasemia, thrombocytopenia, and low serum complement levels. Most patients also have superimposed ACR.

Some patients develop a less well-defined, smoldering, and, in some cases, subclinical form of "chronic AMR" that persists over months or even years and may be linked to persistent or de novo DSAs, late-onset ACR, chronic rejection (CR), and decreased survival. Specific clinical or biochemical features have not been identified. As with acute AMR, patients can develop mixed chronic AMR and T cell–mediated rejection.

PATHOLOGIC FEATURES

GROSS FEATURES

In hyperacute AMR, the liver becomes enlarged with congestion, hemorrhage, and variable degrees of necrosis. Vascular thrombi may be identified.

MICROSCOPIC FEATURES

Severe, early ("hyperacute") acute AMR is rarely biopsied because of the severe coagulopathy that develops in affected patients. Explanted, failed allografts show widespread parenchymal necrosis with congestion and hemorrhage (Fig. 20.3A). Neutrophilic infiltrates may be prominent, and vascular changes, including endothelial cell hypertrophy and inflammation, fibrinoid necrosis, and thrombus formation, can be seen. Bile ducts may also show ischemic injury caused by arterial thrombus.

Early histologic evidence of acute AMR includes centrilobular hepatocyte ballooning and cholestasis, sometimes accompanied by spotty or confluent hepatocyte necrosis (Fig. 20.3B). Portal edema, ductular reaction, and neutrophil-rich portal infiltrates are common yet nonspecific findings (Fig. 20.3C). Microvascular pathology is characteristic and includes endothelial cell hypertrophy or enlargement, capillary dilation, leukocyte sludging or margination, and edema. Sinusoidal infiltration by neutrophils and neutrophil-rich endothelial inflammation or "microvasculitis" affecting portal veins, portal capillaries, and central veins may be seen. More severe cases may show disruption of the microvasculature with portal and periportal hemorrhage, lobular inflammation, and hepatocyte necrosis. Necrotizing arteritis and lymphocytic intimal inflammation can be seen but are rare findings. Focal bile duct necrosis may also be seen because of thrombosis of the peribiliary plexus. Many patients exhibit mixed features of acute AMR and ACR. Tables 20.1 to 20.3 highlight scoring system for AMR.

The histologic features of chronic AMR are less well characterized. The vascular changes of acute AMR are less evident in chronic AMR. Portal, periportal, and perivenular lymphoplasmacytic inflammation with interface activity, perivenular necroinflammatory activity, and scarring are often present (Table 20.4). Portal vein collagenization, biliary strictures, nodular regenerative hyperplasia, and obliterative arteriopathy may also be seen.

ANCILLARY STUDIES

Complement C4d deposition is an indicator of tissue-based complement activation and can be detected by immunohistochemistry (IHC) or immunofluorescence. Diffuse linear or granular microvascular endothelial cell complement C4d deposition involving greater than 50% of portal tracts in greater than 50% of the circumference of portal microvascular endothelia (portal veins and capillaries) is required to establish a diagnosis of definite acute AMR (Fig. 20.3D; see Tables 20.1 and 20.3). C4d positivity may also extend into inlet venules or periportal sinusoids. However, C4d staining is not specific

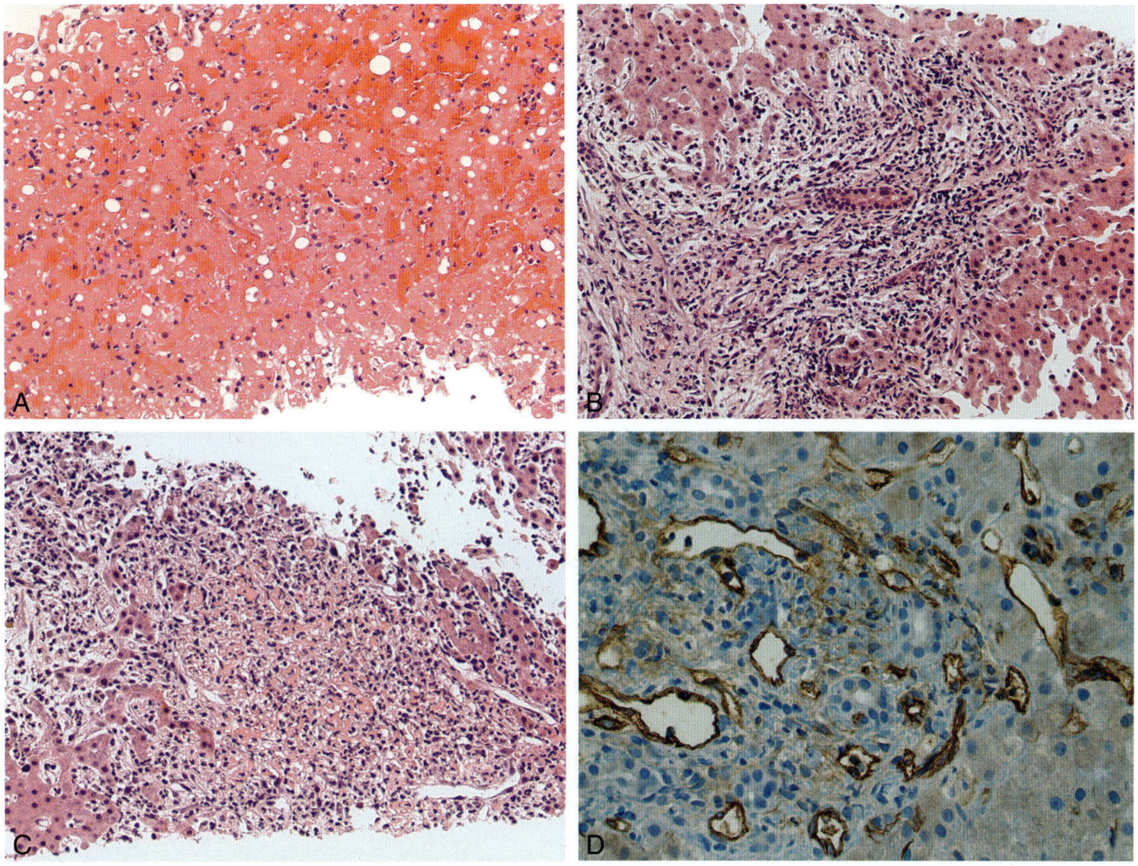

FIGURE 20.3

A, "Hyperacute" antibody-mediated rejection (AMR) demonstrating hepatocellular necrosis and hemorrhage. **B**, Bile duct changes in the setting of acute AMR, including bile ductular proliferation with a neutrophilic-rich infiltrate. **C**, Occasional AMR can show lobular involvement with hepatocellular dropout or necrosis and neutrophilic-rich infiltrates.

TABLE 20.1
Scoring of C4d Deposition

Score	Description
1	No C4d deposition in portal microvasculature
2	Minimal (<10% of portal tracts) C4d deposition in >50% of the circumference of portal microvascular endothelia (portal veins and capillaries)
3	Diffuse (>50% portal tracts) C4d deposition in >50% of the circumference of portal microvascular endothelia (portal veins and capillaries), often with extension into inlet venules or periportal sinusoids

C4d-(immune)-score, formalin-fixed, paraffin-embedded tissue. (Adapted from Banff Working group, Am J Transplant. 2016;16:2816–2835).

for AMR. C4d staining has been described in a variety settings, including in native livers and in other forms of allograft pathology, although usually less widespread and less intense than in acute AMR. Hence, C4d staining in isolation is insufficient to establish a diagnosis of AMR. C4d staining is a feature of chronic AMR but tends to be less diffuse and intense than in acute AMR. Diagnostic criteria for chronic AMR require only focal C4d-positivity (>10% portal tract microvascular endothelia).

Differential Diagnosis

Conditions that mimic hyperacute rejection include severe ischemia or reperfusion injury and allograft ischemia. Clinical data, including risk factors for severe IRI (e.g., prolonged ischemia times or preexisting donor disease) and ABO compatibility, are helpful in distinguishing hyperacute rejection from severe IRI. In the appropriate clinical setting, the clinical history of an ABO-incompatible graft, documentation of preformed

TABLE 20.2

Scoring of Histopathologic Features for Diagnosis of Acute Antibody-Mediated Rejection

Score	Description
1	Portal microvascular endothelial cell enlargement (portal veins, capillaries, and inlet venules) involving a majority of portal tracts with sparse microvasculitis defined as three or four marginated and/or intraluminal monocytes, neutrophils, or eosinophils in the maximally involved capillary with generally mild dilation
2	Monocytic, eosinophilic, or neutrophilic microvasculitis or capillaritis, defined as at least 5 to 10 leukocytes marginated and/or intraluminal in the maximally involved capillary, prominent portal, and/or sinusoidal microvascular endothelial cell enlargement involving a majority of portal tracts or sinusoids, with variable but noticeable portal capillary and inlet venule dilation and variable portal edema
3	As above, with marked capillary dilation, marked microvascular inflammation (≥10 marginated and/or intraluminal leukocytes in the most severely affected vessels), at least focal microvascular disruption with fibrin deposition, and extravasation of red blood cells into the portal stroma and/or space of Disse (subsinusoidal space)

h-score (Adapted from Banff Working group, Am J Transplant. 2016;16:2816–2835).

TABLE 20.3

Criteria for Diagnosis of Acute Antibody-Mediated Rejection

Definite for Acute AMR (All Four Criteria Required)	
1	Histologic pattern of injury consistent with acute AMR, usually including portal microvascular endothelial cell hypertrophy; portal capillary and inlet venule dilation; monocytic, eosinophilic, and neutrophilic portal microvasculitis; portal edema; ductular reaction; cholestasis is usually present but variable; edema and periportal hepatocyte necrosis are more common or prominent in ABO-incompatible allografts; variable active lymphocytic and/or necrotizing arteritis
2	Positive serum DSA
3	Diffuse (C4d score = 3) microvascular C4d deposition on frozen or formalin-fixed, paraffin-embedded tissue in ABO compatible tissues or portal stromal C4d deposition in ABO-incompatible allografts
4	Reasonable exclusion of other insults that might cause a similar pattern of injury; most patients have C4d scores: 3+ h-score = 5 or 6
SUSPICIOUS FOR AMR (BOTH CRITERIA REQUIRED)	
1	Positive serum DSA
2	Nonzero h-score with C4d-score + h-score of 3 or 4
INDETERMINATE FOR AMR (REQUIRES 1 + 2 AND 3 OR 4)	
1	C4d score + h-score is ≥2
2	DSA not available, equivocal, or negative
3	C4d staining not available, equivocal, or negative
4	Coexisting insult might be contributing to the injury

Adapted from Banff Working group, Am J Transplant. 2016;16:2816–2835.
AMR, Antibody-mediated rejection; *DSA*, donor-specific antibodies.

TABLE 20.4

Criteria for Diagnosis of Chronic Active Liver Allograft Antibody-Mediated Rejection

Probable Chronic Active AMR (All Four Criteria Required)	
1	Histologic pattern of injury consistent with chronic AMR
	a.Otherwise unexplained at least mild mononuclear portal and/or perivenular inflammation with interface and/or perivenular necroinflammatory activity
	b.At least moderate portal or periportal, sinusoidal, and/or perivenular fibrosis
2	Recent (within 3 months of biopsy) circulating HLA DSA in serum samples
3	At least focal C4d-positive (>10% portal tract microvascular endothelia)
4	Reasonable exclusion of other insults that might cause a similar pattern of injury
POSSIBLE CHRONIC ACTIVE AMR	
1	As above, but C4d staining minimal or absent

Adapted from Banff Working group, Am J Transplant. 2016;16:2816–2835.
AMR, Antibody-mediated rejection; *DSA*, donor-specific antibodies; *HLA*, human leukocyte antigen.

DSAs, and the vascular changes described earlier all support a diagnosis of hyperacute rejection.

Acute AMR can mimic a variety of conditions, including IRI, ACR, biliary obstruction, ischemia, and sepsis. The vascular features of acute AMR are more helpful in establishing the correct diagnosis than the cholestatic or hepatocellular changes. Clinical information (including imaging studies) is often needed to distinguish these entities, and evaluation of the biopsy for C4d deposition and patient serum for DSAs is warranted in any patient with compatible histology and no clear alternative explanation for their biopsy findings or graft dysfunction. In particular, acute AMR should be considered in patients with histologic features of biliary obstruction in whom there is no clinical evidence of biliary obstruction. In contrast to ACR in which the inflammation is lymphocyte-rich, the portal venous endothelial inflammation seen in acute AMR is more neutrophilic. That said, acute AMR frequently occurs in association with ACR; these diagnoses are not mutually exclusive.

Prognosis and Therapy

The prognosis for AMR is highly variable. Patients with DSAs are at increased risk of CR, chronic inflammation, and progressive fibrosis compared with those without. Most patients with severe, early AMR develop progressive hemorrhagic infarction and graft failure requiring retransplantation, even if the patient survives the acute episode. Late biliary or vascular complications, including ischemic cholangiopathy with biliary strictures, nodular regenerative hyperplasia, or progressive fibrosis, may develop with acute AMR.

Antibody-mediated rejection prevention is preferable to treatment, and AMR can be prevented in most patients by maintaining immunosuppression levels with tacrolimus and in recipients of ABO-incompatible grafts, total plasma exchange, rituximab, and other therapies. Other prevention strategies including avoiding sensitization by reducing blood product usage and administration of antibody-based induction therapy. Therapy for mild acute AMR typically includes immunosuppressive therapy in the form of steroids and tacrolimus, and thymoglobulin. Plasmapheresis, intravenous immunoglobulin (IVIg), rituximab, and other agents may be required in patients with moderate to severe acute AMR.

(ACUTE) T CELL–MEDIATED REJECTION

Clinical Features

T cell–mediated rejection (Banff 2016), previously referred to as acute cellular rejection (ACR), affects around 20% to 40% of all LT recipients. The classical features of ACR described in the 1997 Banff classification are those of "early" ACR, and most often occur within the first 6 months after transplantation. Late ACR is often clinically, biologically, and histologically distinct and is most often seen after 6 months after transplantation, although there is no strict timeline delineating early versus late ACR. Patients with late ACR often have a history of inadequate immunosuppression or prior autoimmune disease.

The clinical features of ACR range from completely asymptomatic patients to those with fever or abdominal pain caused by graft swelling or tenderness. Liver enzyme abnormalities, including elevations of total bilirubin, alkaline phosphatase (ALP), γ-glutamyl transpeptidase (GGT), and serum transaminases, are common in most patients. There may be leukocytosis and eosinophilia.

Pathologic Features

Microscopic Features

The classic histologic triad characteristic of ACR consists of (1) mixed but predominantly mononuclear portal inflammatory cell infiltrates, (2) bile duct inflammation or damage, and (3) subendothelial inflammation of portal veins or terminal hepatic venules ("endotheliitis") (Fig. 20.4A). At least two of these features should be present to establish a diagnosis of ACR. This classic histologic picture most closely reflects the findings seen in patients with ACR occurring within the first 6 months after transplantation and is now often referred to as *early ACR*. The portal inflammatory infiltrates of early ACR include an admixture of enlarged (usually medium or large lymphocytes), "activated-appearing" lymphocytes, neutrophils and often eosinophils (Fig. 20.4B). The bile duct inflammation and damage seen in ACR include intraepithelial lymphocytes and cytologic changes that include cytoplasmic vacuolization, eosinophilia, and uneven spacing of nuclei. Subendothelial inflammation with associated endothelial cell injury and lifting of endothelial cells ("endotheliitis") affects portal veins or terminal hepatic veins (Fig. 20.4C). Hepatic arterial involvement is rare. Recently, isolated "v" lesions (inflammatory, necrotizing, and/or obliterative arteriopathy) have been recognized and associated with impending ACR and/or chronic antibody-mediated rejection.

Late ACR most commonly shows similar features to early ACR, including predominantly mononuclear portal inflammation, inflammatory bile duct damage, and subendothelial inflammation. However, compared with early ACR, the inflammatory infiltrates are more homogenous and mononuclear, and there is less prominent endotheliitis and bile duct damage (Fig. 20.4D). Parenchymal injury in the form of low-grade interface

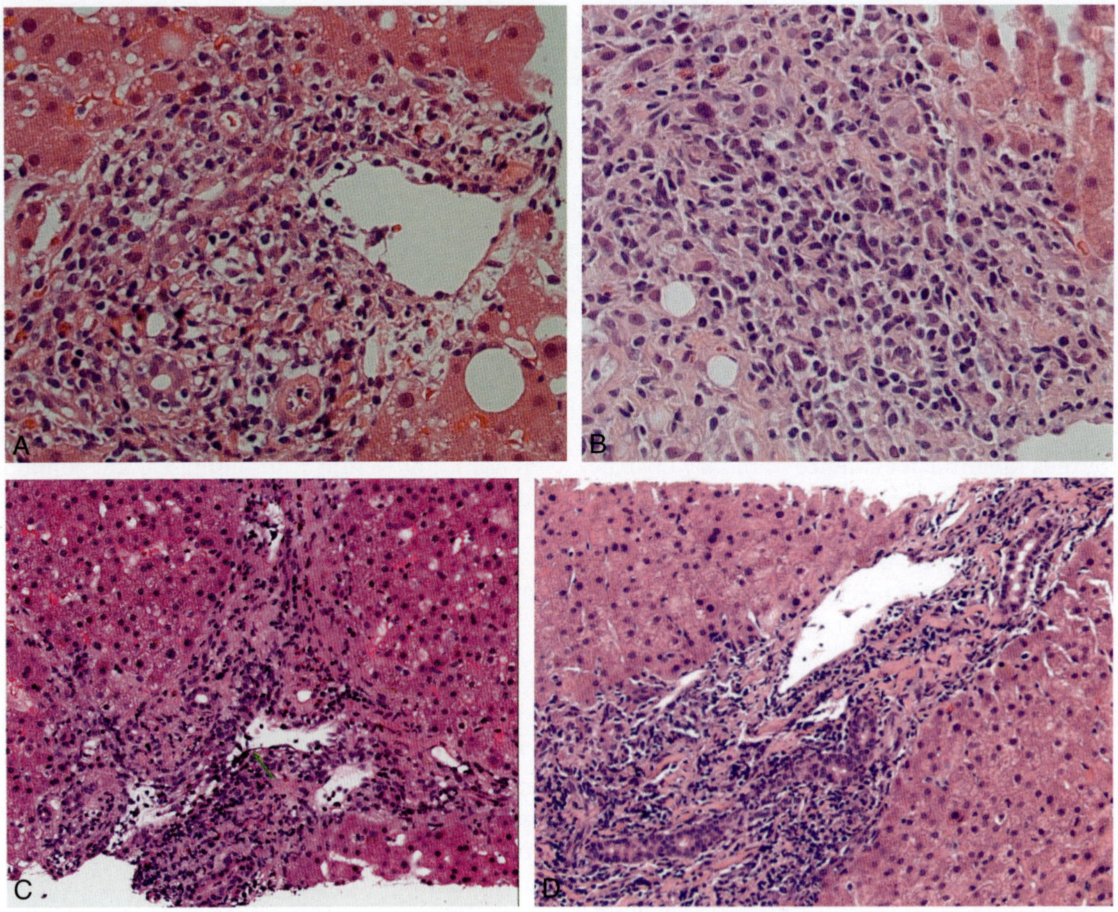

FIGURE 20.4

A, Acute cellular rejection (ACR, T-cell mediated rejection) is characterized by bile duct injury, endotheliitis, and the classic "rejection" type infiltrate. **B**, The typical infiltrate seen in ACR includes enlarged "activated" lymphocytes, numerous eosinophils, and scattered plasma cells. **C**, Endotheliitis is often seen, defined by rejection-type infiltrates involving a vein with associated endothelial injury such as swelling of endothelial cells and possibly lifting of the endothelial lining. **D**, The inflammatory infiltrate seen in late ACR is slightly different and commonly comprises smaller lymphocytes and more prominent plasma cells.

activity, perivenular necroinflammatory activity, or patchy lobular activity is usually present.

Additional patterns of late ACR have been described under a variety of terms, including *central perivenulitis, posttransplant chronic hepatitis, and plasma cell–rich rejection* (also known as *plasma cell hepatitis* or *de novo autoimmune hepatitis [AIH]*). Central perivenulitis is characterized by centrilobular perivenular inflammation with or without hepatocyte dropout, which may occur in combination with portal inflammatory infiltrates or in isolation ("isolated central perivenulitis") (Fig. 20.5). It may or may not be accompanied by portal vein or central vein endotheliitis, and this feature is not required for a diagnosis of ACR in this setting.

Posttransplant chronic hepatitis (also known as idiopathic posttransplant chronic hepatitis) shows histologic features that mimic chronic hepatitis, including mild chronic portal inflammatory infiltrates accompanied by minimal or focal interface activity. The portal infiltrates are more monotonous and the lymphocytes are less activated than those seen in typical ACR. Most cases do not show significant bile duct injury or endotheliitis. Lobular necroinflammatory activity is common and most prominent in the perivenular regions.

Plasma cell–rich rejection encompasses a histologic pattern of immune-mediated graft injury previously described as de novo AIH and posttransplant plasma cell hepatitis. It occurs in patients who lack a history of AIH. The histologic features include dense, plasma cell–rich portal and perivenular infiltrates, often with prominent interface activity and confluent necrosis, and C4d deposits can be demonstrated in the portal microvasculature. The diagnostic criteria for plasma cell–rich rejection are outlined in Table 20.5.

Recently, a pattern of rejection with "hepatitis-like features" was described in patients who completely stop taking immunosuppressive agents. In this pattern, the lobular parenchyma shows activated lymphocytes within the sinusoids ("sinusoidal pattern") or prominent necroinflammatory activity that is randomly

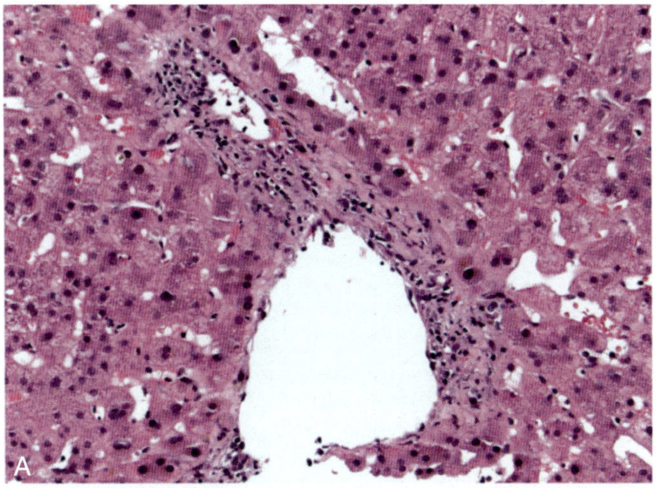

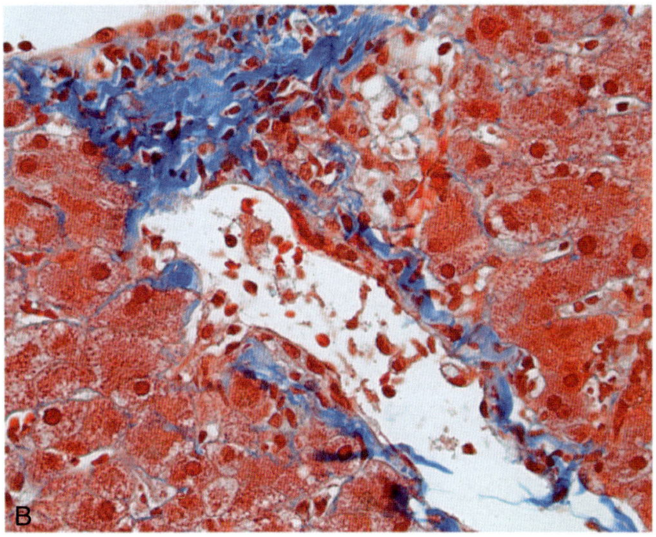

FIGURE 20.5

A, Central perivenulitis, defined as rejection type infiltrates damaging the central veins with associated endothelial injury, can be seen in isolation or associated with more typical portal-based findings. **B**, Delicate perivenular fibrosis highlighted on trichrome stain after recurrent episodes of acute central perivenulitis.

TABLE 20.5

Diagnostic Criteria for Plasma Cell–Rich Rejection

CRITERIA 1 AND 3 ARE REQUIRED FOR DIAGNOSIS. CRITERION 2 IS DESIRABLE BUT NOT STRICTLY REQUIRED FOR DIAGNOSIS.

1.	Portal and/or perivenular plasma cell–rich (estimated >30%) infiltrates with easily recognizable periportal/interface and/or perivenular necroinflammatory activity usually involving a majority of portal tracts and/or central veins
2.	Lymphocytic cholangitis
3.	Original disease other than autoimmune hepatitis

Adapted from Banff Working group, Am J Transplant. 2016;16:2816–2835.

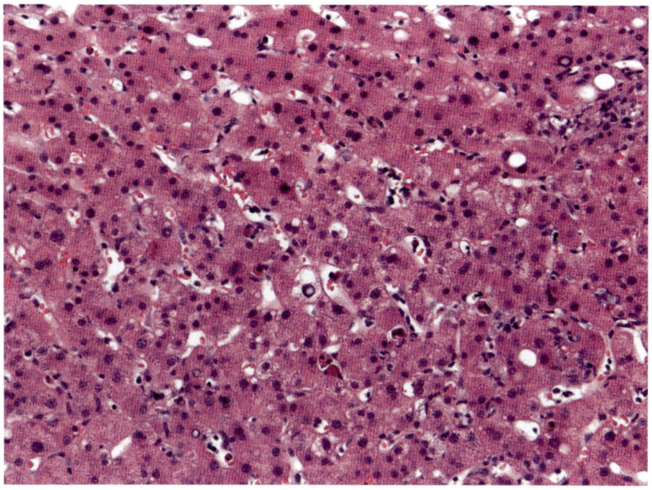

FIGURE 20.6

Hepatitic variant of acute T cell–mediated rejection revealing lobular necroinflammatory activity, mimicking a "hepatitis pattern of injury." In such cases, exclusion of viral infections and medication-induced injury is critical.

distributed throughout the parenchyma (Fig. 20.6). All of these findings may be seen in conjunction with portal-based ACR findings. In early stages, a lesser component of typical ACR involving the portal tracts is noted in close to 50% of cases but later in the posttransplant course that is less often seen.

Grading Acute T Cell–Mediated Rejection

After a diagnosis of ACR is established, the extent of injury is graded using the Banff global assessment as mild, moderate, or severe rejection. According to the 2016 Banff schema, the term *indeterminate for rejection* is used for cases that have portal or perivenular inflammatory infiltrates that could represent rejection but show insufficient tissue damage to meet criteria for a diagnosis of rejection. Mild ACR denotes cases in which rejection-type infiltrates are generally mild, seen in a minority of portal triads or perivenular areas. In portal-based rejection, the infiltrates remain confined within the portal spaces. In patients with isolated perivenular infiltrates, there is no confluent necrosis or hepatocyte dropout in mild ACR. In moderate rejection, the infiltrate expands most or all of the portal triads or perivenular areas with confluent necrosis or hepatocyte dropout limited to a minority of perivenular areas (Fig. 20.7A). Severe ACR shows the features described for moderate ACR and exhibits spillover of the inflammatory infiltrate into periportal areas or moderate to severe perivenular inflammation that extends into the hepatic parenchyma and is associated with perivenular hepatocyte necrosis involving a majority of perivenular areas (Fig. 20.7B). The findings may also be semiquantitatively scored to yield a "Rejection Activity Index" (Table 20.6). The Rejection Activity Index is a

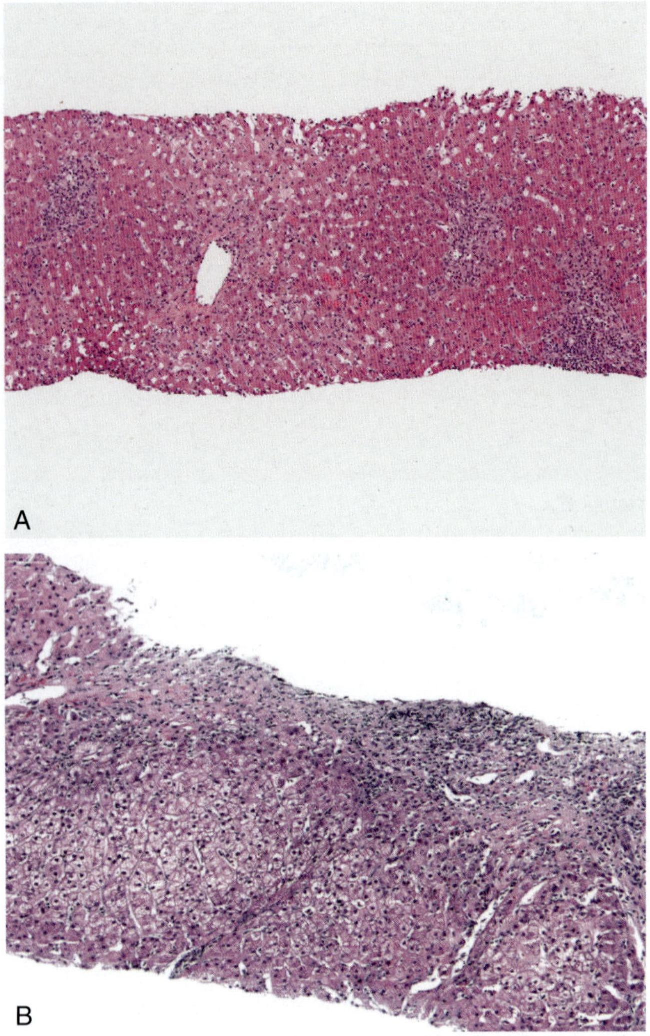

FIGURE 20.7

A, A case of moderate acute T cell–mediated rejection (ACR). By definition, the majority of portal tracts need to be affected by classic features of rejection. **B**, Severe ACR demonstrates not only involvement of the majority of portal tracts but also areas of parenchymal necrosis and often central perivenulitis.

TABLE 20.6

Rejection Activity Index for Grading Acute T Cell–Mediated Rejection

Portal inflammation	1. Mostly lymphocytic inflammation involving, but not noticeably expanding, a minority of the triads
	2. Expansion of most or all portal triads by a mixed infiltrate containing lymphocytes with occasional blasts, neutrophils, and eosinophils
	3. Marked expansion of most or all of the portal triads by a mixed infiltrate containing blasts and eosinophils with inflammatory spillover into the periportal parenchyma
Venous endotheliitis	1. Subendothelial lymphocytic infiltration involving some but not a majority of the portal and/or hepatic venules
	2. Subendothelial infiltration involving most or all of the portal and/or hepatic venules with or without confluent hepatocyte necrosis or dropout involving a minority of perivenular regions
	3. As for 2 above, with moderate or severe perivenular inflammation that extends into the perivenular parenchyma and is associated with perivenular hepatocyte necrosis involving a majority of perivenular regions
Bile duct damage	1. A minority of the ducts are cuffed and infiltrated by inflammatory cells and show only mild reactive changes such as increased epithelial cell nuclear-to-cytoplasmic ratios
	2. Most or all ducts infiltrated by inflammatory cells; more than an occasional duct shows degenerative changes such as nuclear pleomorphism, disordered polarity, and cytoplasmic vacuolization of the epithelium
	3. Inflammation affecting the majority of the bile ducts with most ducts showing marked bile duct injury or duct necrosis
Total	Of possible score of 9:
	RAI 3–4: mild ACR RAI 5–6: moderate ACR RAI 7–9: severe ACR

Adapted from Banff Working group, Am J Transplant. 2016;16:2816–2835.
ACR, acute T cell–mediated rejection; *RAI*, rejection activity index.

numerical score intended to indicate severity of ACR based on the severity of the three features of ACR: portal inflammation, bile duct inflammation or damage, and venous endotheliitis. These grading schemas should only be applied after a diagnosis of ACR is established and should not be used to establish or refute a diagnosis of ACR.

Differential Diagnosis

Depending on the clinical and histologic picture, ACR may need to be differentiated from IRI, AMR, infections, drug-induced liver injury (DILI), biliary and vascular complications, and recurrent disease. In many cases, the clinical history of reduced immunosuppression (through patient history or drug levels) is helpful in establishing the correct diagnosis. IRI is only a diagnostic consideration in the first few weeks after transplantation and usually lacks the prominent portal and perivenular lymphocyte-rich infiltrates seen in ACR.

Biliary obstruction can coexist with ACR and can also mimic the portal inflammatory infiltrates and bile duct injury of ACR, although biliary obstruction may exhibit more neutrophil-rich infiltrates and can be excluded with imaging studies. Neutrophil-rich infiltrates and cholestasis also raise the possibility of AMR; patients with these findings who are not found to have biliary obstruction should be investigated for AMR with serum DSA testing and C4d immunostaining. Prominent eosinophilic or neutrophilic infiltrates and the vascular features of AMR described earlier also warrant further evaluation with C4d staining and serum testing for DSAs. Of note, AMR may coexist with ACR, so establishing a diagnosis of AMR does not exclude additional T cell–mediated rejection.

Both recurrent and de novo hepatotropic viral infections and nonhepatotropic infections can mimic ACR. In early ACR, the mixed "rejection-type" portal infiltrate helps distinguish ACR from other causes of portal inflammation (e.g., chronic viral hepatitis). However, this distinction can be more difficult in late ACR in which the portal infiltrates may be more monotonous and both interface activity and lobular hepatocyte injury can be seen, and the overall histologic picture may be that of a posttransplant chronic hepatitis. Depending on the histologic picture, the findings may mimic chronic hepatitis (hepatitis C, hepatitis B, and AIH), other infections (e.g., cytomegalovirus [CMV] or Epstein-Barr virus [EBV]), or DILI. These other causes should be carefully excluded based on clinical history, laboratory testing, and special stains (CMV and EBV) before initiating heightened immunosuppression. The distinction between ACR and recurrent viral hepatitis C can be challenging but is now a less frequent diagnostic problem with the use of direct-acting antiviral therapies (see later). In the setting of chronic viral hepatitis C, at least 50% of bile ducts or central veins should demonstrate features of ACR to establish a diagnosis of ACR in a patient with chronic hepatitis C to avoid overdiagnosis of ACR and steroid therapy.

The centrilobular hepatocyte dropout and inflammation of central perivenulitis raise a differential diagnosis that includes ischemia, viral hepatitis, AIH, and drug toxicities. Ischemic tends to be less inflamed, and clinical risk factor for ischemia and Doppler studies can be helpful in evaluating the hepatic vasculature. Viral hepatitis and drug toxicities should be excluded as noted earlier. Plasma cell–rich rejection closely mimics AIH. If the patient has no history of AIH before transplantation, a diagnosis of plasma cell–rich rejection should be considered. There is no clear diagnostic distinction between plasma cell–rich rejection and recurrent AIH.

Many recurrent diseases can mimic ACR, and features of recurrent disease and ACR can coexist in the same biopsy. Knowledge of the patient's native liver disease is critical to accurate posttransplant biopsy interpretation. Recurrent viral hepatitis and AIH have already been addressed; both are most likely to mimic late ACR because the features of early ACR are somewhat distinctive with its characteristic mixed and activated portal infiltrates. Primary biliary cholangitis (PBC) can cause bile duct injury and portal inflammation, but the bile duct injury of PBC is often more histiocytic, forming vague granulomas and florid-duct lesions.

Prognosis and Therapy

All patterns of ACR respond to increased immunosuppression, but if left untreated, they may result in progressive graft injury and, in some cases, graft failure. About 10% of patients with ACR develop CR, and patients with moderate or severe ACR and repeated or untreated episodes of ACR are more likely to develop CR, which can lead to graft failure. Patients with late ACR may respond to immunosuppression less well than those with early ACR and may have a higher risk of CR, fibrosis, and graft loss. Up to 27% of adults with posttransplant chronic hepatitis develop progressive fibrosis with bridging fibrosis or cirrhosis.

In most cases of ACR, patients are first treated with adjustment to their baseline immunosuppression regimen, corticosteroids, or both. In patients who do not respond to heightened immunosuppression and initial steroid therapy, antithymocyte globulin with or without rituximab may be used.

Liver Acute Cellular Rejection—Fact Sheet

Incidence

- 20% to 40% of all liver transplant recipients, most during the first 6 months

Demographics

- No gender or race predilection

Clinical Features

- Variable, from asymptomatic to abdominal pain or tenderness, fever
- Elevated transaminases and/or alkaline phosphatase

Therapy and Prognosis

- Respond to immunosuppression
- If untreated, progressive injury leading to graft failure
- 10% evolve to chronic rejection

Liver Acute Cellular Rejection—Pathologic Features

Gross Findings

- Congestion to hemorrhagic changes and necrosis

Microscopic Features

- Classic portal based acute T cell–mediated rejection: rejection-type infiltrates, endotheliitis, and bile duct injury (at least two of the three features required) (grading based on Table 20.6)
- Plasma cell–rich rejection (see Table 20.5)
- Lobular ("hepatitis-like") rejection: lobular rejection–type infiltrates ("sinusoidal pattern") and necroinflammatory injury

Differential Diagnosis

- Opportunistic infections
- Recurrent disease (e.g., hepatitis C)
- Ischemia or reperfusion injury
- Antibody-mediated rejection
- Drug-induced injury
- Biliary and/or vascular complications

CHRONIC (DUCTOPENIC) REJECTION

CLINICAL FEATURES

Unlike ACR, CR (or ductopenic rejection) is uncommon; fewer than 1% to 2% of allografts fail because of CR. Most cases occur more than 12 months after transplant, although cases have been reported as early 3 months after transplant. CR is often related to inadequate immunosuppression and recurrent, untreated, refractory, severe, or persistent ACR. Other risk factors include active CMV infection in the recipient, long cold ischemia time, and older donors. Patients often present with persistent jaundice or persistently elevated bilirubin, elevated ALP, and elevated transaminase. Evidence of arteriopathy and ischemic bile duct injury may be evident on imaging studies as irregular narrowing of the hepatic arterial and biliary trees.

PATHOLOGIC FEATURES

MICROSCOPIC FEATURES

Chronic rejection is characterized by obliterative arteriopathy and bile duct injury with progressive loss of small interlobular bile ducts. The histologic features can be divided into those of "early" and "late" stages, although there is no consistent time frame over which patients progress from early to late CR. A diagnosis of early CR suggests the changes are potentially reversible and can be applied when the majority of ducts exhibit degenerative, atrophic, or senescent changes characterized by cytoplasmic eosinophilia, irregular nuclear spacing, nuclear enlargement, nuclear hyperchromasia, and epithelial attenuation (Fig. 20.8A). Bile duct loss affects fewer than 50% of portal tracts in early CR. Mild portal inflammation and features of ACR, including central perivenulitis and perivenular hepatocyte dropout, are often seen in early CR. These diagnoses are not mutually exclusive, and evidence of both may be present simultaneously. Other changes, including spotty hepatocyte necrosis, centrilobular cholestasis, and perivenular fibrosis, may be seen. Hepatic arteriole loss (portal tracts lacking an arteriole) may be found in occasional (<25%) portal tracts.

In "late" CR, bile duct loss affects a least 50% of the portal tracts in a biopsy containing at least 10 portal tracts. Bile duct counting can be facilitated by cytokeratin (CK) 7 or CK19 staining. In late CR, there are also more extensive degenerative bile duct changes, marked centrilobular hepatocellular swelling and hepatocanalicular cholestasis, and prominent perivenular hepatocyte dropout with more severe perivenular (bridging) fibrosis. Central veins may show luminal obliteration. Late CR may eventually show cirrhosis as well as parenchymal extinction.

Although only rarely identified in needle biopsies, obliterative "foam cell" arteriopathy denotes the accumulation of foamy macrophages within arterial walls, resulting in luminal narrowing and impeding arterial blood flow (Fig. 20.8B). Although this is a very specific feature of CR, it primarily affects medium-sized and large-caliber perihilar arteries not sampled in needle biopsies. In the appropriate clinical context, a diagnosis of CR can be rendered on a needle biopsy if any one of the following features is present: (1) biliary epithelial atrophic changes affecting a majority of the bile ducts with or without bile duct loss, (2) foam cell obliterative arteriopathy, or (3) bile duct loss affecting 50% of the portal tracts.

DIFFERENTIAL DIAGNOSIS

Biliary complications usually show histologic features of cholestasis and a ductular reaction; however, a ductular reaction is less common in CR and its presence favor another cause. Hepatic artery stricture and thrombosis can also cause bile duct injury and duct loss but can be excluded via imaging and vascular studies. Ischemic cholangiopathy caused by microvascular injury is difficult to exclude based on biopsy findings alone; the clinical history is helpful in identifying risk factors of ischemic injury (DCD donor, long ischemia time) versus risk factors for CR.

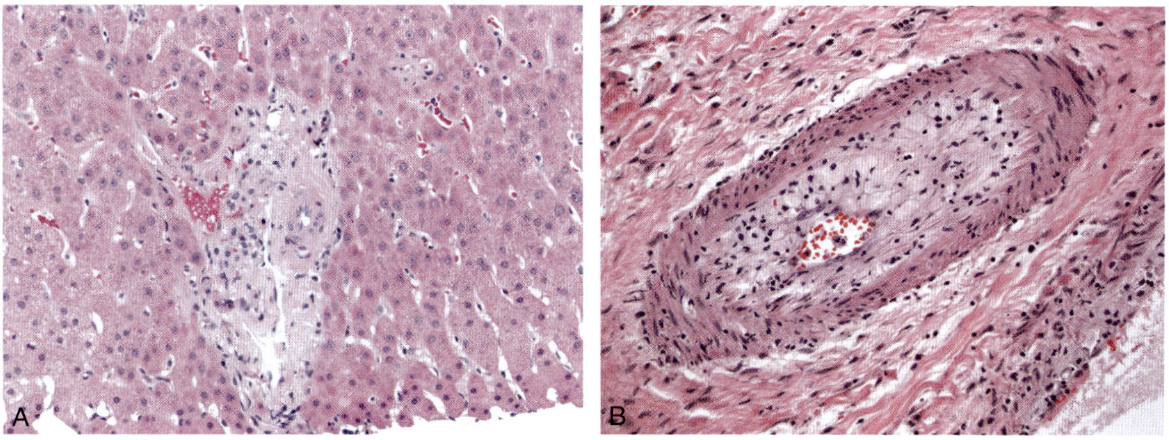

FIGURE 20.8

Chronic rejection (CR). **A**, Bile duct injury is an early feature of CR showing cytoplasmic vacuolization, nuclear disarray and hyperchromasia, attenuated cytoplasm and cytoplasmic eosinophilia. **B**, Foam cell arteriopathy is a well know feature of CR but uncommonly seen, in particular in biopsy specimens.

Given the cholestatic features, recurrent sclerosing cholangitis (primary sclerosing cholangitis [PSC]) and PBC are a common differential. The presence of arterial changes (arterial "pruning") on imaging studies favors CR over PSC. Perivenular fibrosis is a feature of CR not seen in PSC. As seen in PBC in the native liver, recurrent PBC usually shows patchy but, in some portal areas, dense mononuclear inflammatory cell infiltrates with lymphocytic or granulomatous cholangitis that is histologically distinct from the bile duct injury seen in CR.

Prognosis and Therapy

Increased immunosuppression is the mainstay therapy. A lack of response to immunosuppression ultimately leads to retransplantation or death.

Liver Chronic Ductopenic Rejection—Fact Sheet

Incidence

- 1% to 2% allografts fail because of chronic rejection (CR)

Demographics

- No race predilection

Clinical Features

- History of prior episodes of acute T cell–mediated rejection
- Inadequate immunosuppression
- Persistent jaundice
- Elevated bilirubin, alkaline phosphatase, and transaminases

Therapy and Prognosis

- Increase immunosuppression
- Ductopenia can be reversible in some cases
- CR may lead to graft loss, need for retransplantation, or death

Chronic Ductopenic Rejection—Pathologic Features

Gross Features

- Parenchymal scarring, sometimes with biliary type pattern, leading to cirrhosis

Microscopic Features

- Bile duct injury or loss (≥50% portal tracts)
- Obliterative "foam cell" arteriopathy or arteriole loss
- Inflammatory infiltrates (typical less pronounced than in acute T cell–mediated rejection)

Differential Diagnosis

- Recurrent disease (e.g., primary sclerosing cholangitis)
- Vascular complications
- Biliary complications

COMPLICATIONS OF TRANSPLANTATION

Hepatic Artery Thrombosis or Stenosis

Hepatic artery thrombosis (HAT) and hepatic artery stenosis (HAS) are the major arterial complications occurring after liver transplantation. HAT occurs in up to 9% of adult LT recipients, and reported rates of HAS range from 3.5% to 11% among LT recipients. Whereas HAT can present at any time after transplantation, HAS tends to be a later complication, occurring several months to several years after transplantation. Because the bile ducts are perfused by hepatic arterial blood flow, patients with HAT and HAS often present with complications of biliary ischemia, leading to biliary leaks and abscess formation, ischemic biliary strictures, or cholangitis. Patients with early HAT (within

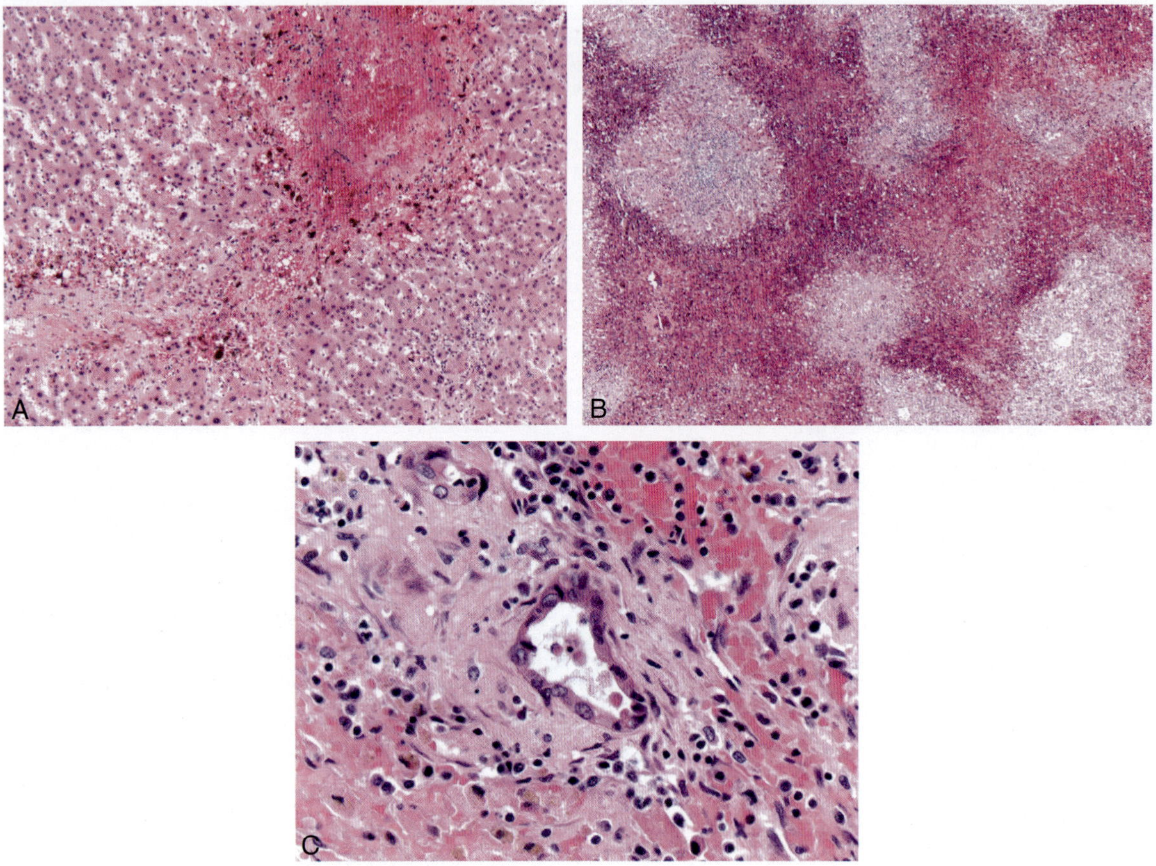

FIGURE 20.9

Hepatic artery thrombosis. **A**, In the acute setting, hemorrhagic changes with focal hepatocellular necrosis accompanied by regenerative hepatocellular changes and increased mitotic activity are seen. **B**, In severe cases, necrosis may be more prominent. **C**, Bile ducts can be injured, leading to bile extravasation and bilomas.

21 days of transplantation) commonly present with fever, abdominal pain, and signs of graft dysfunction or fulminant hepatic failure. Late HAT (at >21 days posttransplantation) exhibits a more insidious onset characterized by more ischemic biliary lesions. Elevated serum transaminases, bilirubin, ALP, and GGT is seen in most patients. Vascular imaging studies are used to assess arterial patency.

Early findings of hepatic arterial compromise include nonspecific centrilobular hemorrhage and hepatocyte dropout or spotty hepatocyte necrosis with increased mitoses and cholestasis (Fig. 20.9A). In severe cases, extensive necrosis of hepatocytes and portal connective tissue is evident (Fig. 20.9B). Ischemic bile ducts with intraluminal biliary casts composed of sloughed necrotic biliary epithelial cells may be seen, with or without bile leaks. These changes are usually more evident in larger segmental bile ducts (Fig. 20.9C). Late changes include those of ischemic cholangiopathy with progressive scarring and biliary strictures.

Hepatic artery thrombosis and HAS are serious complications associated with significant morbidity and mortality. Retransplantation represents the main therapy for HAT. Other therapeutic options include revascularization through arterial reconstruction, surgical thrombectomy, and radiologically guided thrombolysis. Patients with HAS are treated with surgical reanastomosis or interventional vascular procedures such as dilation and vascular stenting. Restenosis is common, occurring after stent placement in about 25% of patients.

PORTAL HYPERPERFUSION INJURY OR SMALL-for-SIZE GRAFT SYNDROME

Portal hyperperfusion (PHP) or small-for-size graft syndrome (SFSS) is a graft complication that primarily occurs in recipients of reduced size grafts (including living donor LT recipients) and in those with adequately sized grafts but with severe portal hypertension. A graft is considered "small for size" if the graft-to-recipient-weight ratio is less than 0.8 or when the ratio of graft volume to standard liver volume is less than 40%. The spectrum of graft injury seen in PHP or SFSS is the result of high portal flows subjected to the reduced vascular bed of a smaller graft liver, a reciprocal decrease in arterial flow, and downstream effects, including bile duct ischemia. Although the pathogenesis is not well understood, the increased portal blood flow impairs hepatic regeneration and induces hepatic dysfunction. The high portal flows cause a reciprocal decrease in hepatic arterial blood flow through accelerated adenosine washout and resultant hepatic artery constriction mediated via the hepatic arterial buffer response, which serves to regulate total hepatic blood flow within an acceptable range. Hepatic artery constriction results in bile duct ischemia and necrosis with bile leaks and parenchymal infarcts. In addition, endothelial cell injury results in thrombosis of small portal veins.

The clinical features of PHP syndrome are prolonged cholestasis, coagulopathy, and ascites within the first week after transplantation in the absence of other causes of ischemia. In severe cases, gastrointestinal (GI) bleeding, acidosis, hypoglycemia, encephalopathy, renal failure, and septic shock can occur. Doppler ultrasonography, angiography, and direct pressure measurements are used to document high portal flows and exclude other vascular complications.

The histologic features of SFSS can be divided into early and late phases of graft injury. Early histologic features are somewhat nonspecific and include centrilobular hepatocanalicular cholestasis, centrilobular steatosis, and mild ductular reaction with neutrophils. There is often evidence of portal vein and sinusoidal injury, including focal endothelial cell denudation along with portal and periportal hemorrhage (Fig. 20.10). Endothelial cell hypertrophy with subendothelial edema are late features, and patients may develop thrombosis of small portal vein branches with luminal obliteration or recanalization, nodular regenerative hyperplasia and biliary strictures. The high portal blood flow causes a reciprocal reduction in hepatic arterial flow, leading to ischemic cholangiopathy with bile leaks, bile abscesses, and parenchymal infarcts.

Portal hyperperfusion or SFSS is associated with increased morbidity and mortality and remains an important limiting factor for use of reduced size grafts. Treatment and prevention strategies are largely aimed at reducing portal flows and portal pressure while maintaining adequate portal flows to support liver regeneration. This may be achieved through techniques that reduce portal blood flow or divert a portion of the portal blood supply from the liver to the systemic circulation, including portal vein banding; splenectomy; splenic artery ligation or embolization; and splenorenal, portocaval or mesocaval shunts. Splanchnic vasoconstrictors such as octreotide or propranolol have also been used modify portal flows.

HEPATIC VENOUS OUTFLOW OBSTRUCTION OR CONGESTIVE HEPATOPATHY

Hepatic venous outflow obstruction (HVOO) is an uncommon yet serious posttransplant complication that results from impaired hepatic vein outflow from the transplanted liver caused by hepatic vein thrombosis or anatomical flattening or kinking of the hepatic vein due to graft positioning. Clinical signs of HVOO include ascites, pleural effusion, cholestasis, and liver enzyme abnormalities. Doppler ultrasonography shows absent or abnormal hepatic vein flow, and computed tomography shows nonopacified hepatic veins, luminal narrowing, or a geographic low attenuation area. Hepatic venography or manometry is used to confirm the diagnosis.

As in native livers, the histologic features vary with the severity and rapidity of the insult. The lobular parenchyma typically shows centrilobular sinusoidal dilation, hepatocyte atrophy, and sinusoidal congestion as well as focal, predominantly perivenular hepatocyte dropout (Fig. 20.11). Mild bile ductular reaction may

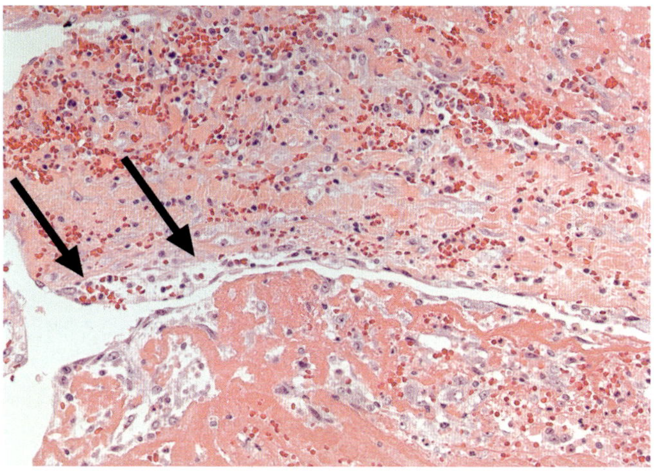

FIGURE 20.10

Denudation of the endothelial lining (arrows) in a portal vein in a case of small-fo-size disease.

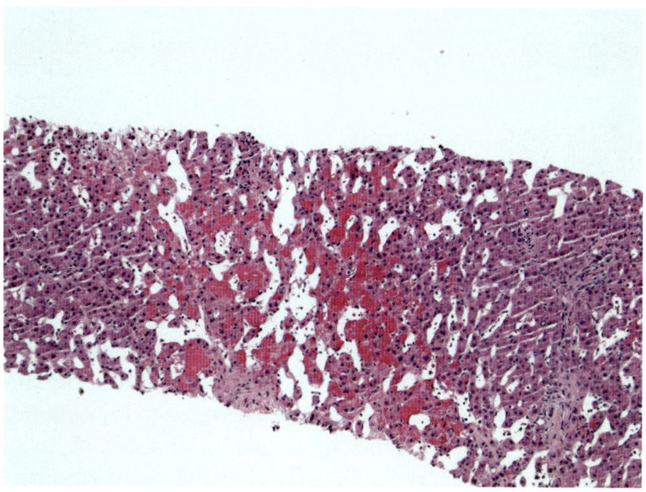

FIGURE 20.11

Venous outflow impairment revealing centrizonal sinusoidal dilation and congestion with focal hepatocellular dropout.

also be present. HVOO leads to graft dysfunction, graft loss, and increased patient mortality. Treatment strategies include medical management with diuretics, placement of vascular stents, surgical cavoplasty, and if these strategies fail, retransplantation.

BILIARY COMPLICATIONS

Biliary complications occur in up to 30 % of LT recipients and can present within the first week or several weeks to months after transplant. The most common types are anastomotic strictures, biliary leaks (which may be technical or ischemic), and intrahepatic strictures. Patients with biliary complications after LT may present with jaundice, fever, or abdominal pain. Laboratory testing reveals a cholestatic pattern of liver enzymes with bilirubin and ALP elevations.

Histologic features of biliary obstruction include neutrophil-rich portal inflammatory cell infiltrates with bile duct proliferation. Periductal edema is seen in some cases. The bile ducts may show mild features of injury, including biliary epithelial cells eosinophilia, nuclear overlapping, and pleomorphism (Fig. 20.12A). Hepatocellular or canalicular cholestasis may be evident, although this finding may be absent if the obstruction is incomplete. Although neutrophilic infiltration of bile ducts may be seen in obstruction, intraluminal collections of neutrophils are seen in acute ascending cholangitis (Fig. 20.12B).

In acute ischemic bile duct injury, there may be portal findings similar to those seen in obstruction, along with bile duct necrosis and marked biliary epithelial eosinophilia with formation of intraluminal eosinophilic bile duct casts. Large bile duct necrosis, bile leaks, and abscess formation may be seen in resection or explant specimens.

Biliary complications are a source of significant morbidity and mortality and are particularly problematic in living donor LT recipients. Anastomotic strictures are often corrected by dilation and stent placement. Intrahepatic strictures are difficult to treat and can lead to graft failure requiring retransplantation.

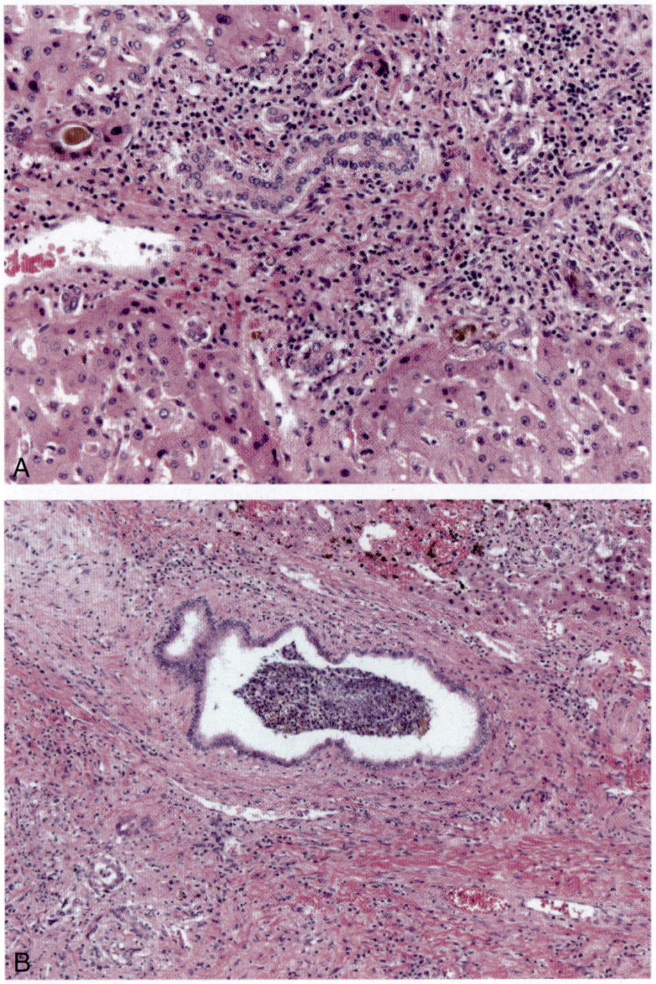

FIGURE 20.12

Biliary complications. **A**, Bile duct obstruction is characterized by bile ductular proliferation with accompanying neutrophils and stromal edema. **B**, Ascending cholangitis may complicate a subset of cases and should be considered when neutrophils are noted within the lumen of the bile ducts.

RECURRENT DISEASE

Recurrence of the liver disease that led to primary organ failure occurs at varying frequencies depending on the etiology (Table 20.7). The following section covers the most common forms of recurrent disease in liver allografts and describes features that help in differentiating these findings from acute rejection or CR.

TABLE 20.7

Post–Liver Transplantation Disease Recurrence Rates

	Peak	Frequency (%)
Hepatitis C	4–6 wk	>90[a]
Hepatitis B	Rare	<10
Autoimmune hepatitis	4–6 wk	20–30
PBC	>6 mo	20–50
PSC	>6 mo	20–30
NAFLD	>3–4 wk	20–40
Alcohol	>6 mo	10–30

[a]Hepatitis C recurrence rates may be decreasing because of increased use of antiviral regimens.

NAFLD, Nonalcoholic fatty liver disease; *PBC*, primary biliary cholangitis; *PSC*, primary sclerosing cholangitis.

TABLE 20.8

Histologic Features of Acute T Cell–Mediated Rejection Versus Recurrent Hepatitis C Infection in Liver Allograft

	Acute Cellular Rejection	Recurrent Hepatitis C
Portal inflammation	Mixed inflammation composed of large "activated lymphocytes," eosinophils, and scattered plasma cells	Chronic inflammatory infiltrate composed of small mature lymphocytes and sometimes lymphoid aggregates; the infiltrate typical spares the bile duct and veins
Bile duct injury	Often present; more prominent in early ACR	Uncommon; if present is focal and mild.
Endotheliitis	Often present; more prominent in early ACR	Uncommon
Lobular necroinflammatory activity	Uncommon; may be seen in severe ACR, mainly involving centrizonal perivenular regions	Common; often spotty distribution
Interface activity	Uncommon; if seen may be focal and in late ACR	Common; typically focal
Central perivenulitis	Often seen in moderate to severe ACR or isolated central perivenulitis or plasma cell–rich rejection	Uncommon

ACR, Acute T cell–mediated rejection.

Recurrent Hepatitis C

Recurrent viral hepatitis C is essentially universal among hepatitis C–infected recipients, although recent availability of highly effective direct-acting antiviral therapy has drastically reduced the burden of recurrent hepatitis C. Although hepatitis C tends to show more prominent hepatocyte injury versus the bile duct injury and endotheliitis of ACR, bile duct injury and endotheliitis can be seen in hepatitis C. Additional histologic findings are described in Table 20.8. Demetris et al. (2004) reported that errors were most often caused by overdiagnosis of rejection and suggested that at least 50% of bile ducts or central veins should be involved to establish a diagnosis of ACR in patients with hepatitis C. In general, the recommendation is to be conservative in these cases, and many patients fall in the category of "indeterminate for acute cellular rejection" when they demonstrate borderline ACR features.

Fibrosing Cholestatic Hepatitis

Fibrosing cholestatic hepatitis (FCH) is a virulent form of chronic viral hepatitis B or hepatitis C that occurs in immunocompromised hosts, including after liver or other organ transplantation. FCH is not necessarily considered a separate entity but a severe form of hepatitis C recurrence. Patients may present with jaundice, abdominal pain, and progression to acute hepatic failure over a period of weeks. Laboratory abnormalities demonstrate a predominant cholestatic profile of liver enzymes, with marked elevation of bilirubin, ALP, and GGT. Hepatitis C virus RNA by polymerase chain reaction (viral load) is significantly elevated, ranging in the millions IU/mL.

The biopsy findings include periportal sinusoidal fibrosis with diffuse hepatocyte swelling, lobular disarray, bile ductular reaction, and cholestasis (Fig. 20.13). Moreira et al. (2013) published a cohort of patients with hepatitis C recurrence and stratified patients' prognosis based on assessing the presence of ductular reaction, hepatocyte swelling, cholestasis, and fibrosis (Table 20.9). The main differential diagnosis is biliary obstruction. Features such as portal edema, bile duct dilation, bile infarcts, acute cholangitis, periductal fibrosis, and periportal copper deposition favor biliary obstruction over FCH.

The prognosis for patients with FCH C was poor before direct-acting antiviral therapy became available. Preliminary studies that have used newer direct antiviral agents suggest that most patients seem to respond favorably with full recovery and sustained virologic response.

Recurrent Primary Sclerosing Cholangitis

Primary sclerosing cholangitis recurs in 20% to 30% of cases with the classic features of bile duct injury, periductal fibrosis, and eventual bile duct loss and scarring. Recurrent PSC can cause diagnostic confusion with CR and other biliary complications. When present, obliterative arteriopathy is diagnostic of CR, and CR often lacks

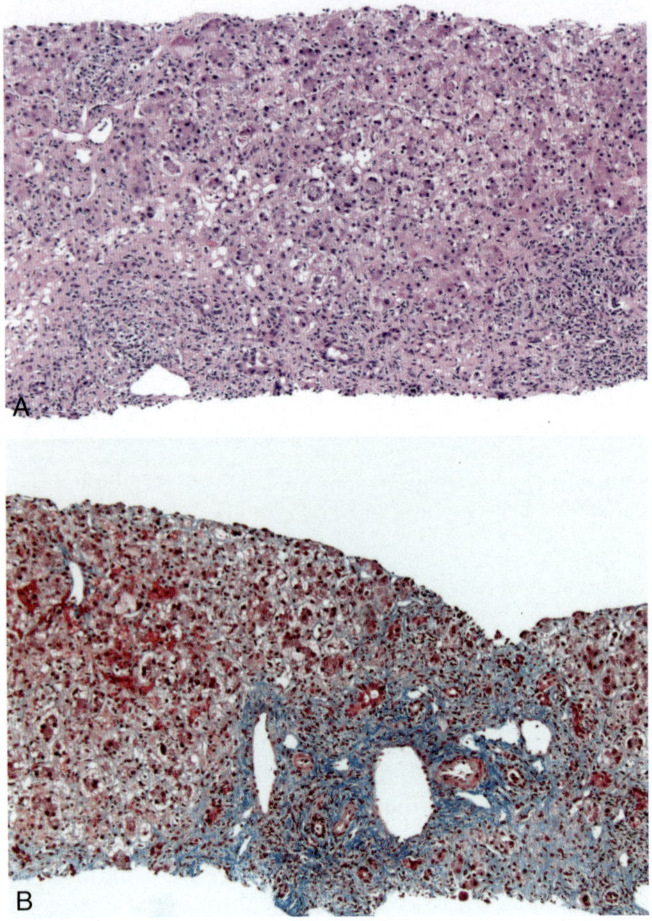

FIGURE 20.13

Fibrosing cholestatic hepatitis C. **A**, Histologic findings that suggest this diagnosis include bile ductular proliferation, canalicular cholestasis, and diffuse swelling of hepatocytes. **B**, The trichrome stain highlights periportal pericellular perisinusoidal fibrosis.

a ductular response. Arterial changes ("pruning") on imaging favor CR over PSC, and perivenular fibrosis is a feature of CR not seen in PSC. Unlike PSC, CR usually occurs in patients who have had severe, refractory, or multiple episodes of ACR; this clinical history can serve to be helpful in distinguishing the two scenarios.

Recurrent Primary Biliary Cholangitis

Recurrent PBC is seen in 20% to 50% of LT patients at 5 years after transplantation and exhibits the same histologic features of PBC as seen in the native liver. Most patients have positive antimitochondrial antibodies. In contrast to ACR, in which there is a rapid and persistent elevation of serum ALP, PBC is usually associated with a slow rise in ALP. In contract to the more mixed portal inflammatory cell infiltrates in ACR, biopsies from patients with recurrent PBC show patchy mononuclear inflammatory cell infiltrates. Collections of portal histiocytes or poorly formed granulomas may be found in association with injured ducts. Over time, patients may develop progressive fibrosis and features of chronic cholestasis. Although some histologic evidence of recurrent PBC is common, it is often an incidental finding, and recurrent PBC rarely results in cirrhosis or graft failure.

TABLE 20.9

Hepatitis Aggressiveness Score and Histologic Features Associated With Fibrosing Cholestatic Hepatitis

Histologic Findings
1. Prominent ductular reaction, at least focally expanding portal tracts, mimicking biliary obstruction
2. Prominent hepatocellular ballooning or swelling (enlarged hepatocytes with cytoplasmic rarefaction) and lobular disarray
3. Cholestasis (including at leas focal canalicular cholestasis)
4. Periportal sinusoidal fibrosis
FINAL SCORING INTERPRETATION
HAS 1: 0 of 4 features: nonaggressive hepatitis CHAS 2: 1–2 of 4 features: aggressive hepatitis CHAS 3: 3–4 of 4 features: fibrosing cholestatic hepatitis C

Adapted from Moreira RK, Salomao M, Verna EC, et al. The Hepatitis Aggressiveness Score (HAS): a novel classification system for post-liver transplantation recurrent hepatitis C. *Am J Surg Pathol*. 2013; 37(1):104–113.
HAS, Hepatitis Aggressiveness Score.

Recurrent Autoimmune Hepatitis

Autoimmune hepatitis recurs in 20% to 30% of patients and presents with clinical and histologic features identical to those seen in the native liver. The microscopic features include plasma cell–rich portal inflammatory cell infiltrates with well-established interface activity, lobular inflammation, hepatocyte "rosetting," and in a subset of cases, centrilobular perivenular necroinflammatory activity. The portal infiltrates are usually more mononuclear and often contain more plasma cells than those seen in ACR, although plasma cells are not a required feature. Interface hepatitis is often a prominent feature of recurrent AIH. Recurrent AIH is distinguished from the plasma cell hepatitis pattern of late ACR based on the history of AIH in the native liver. Patients with recurrent AIH, early ACR, and late ACR are all treated with heightened immunosuppression.

Recurrent Fatty Liver Disease

The reported recurrence rate of nonalcoholic fatty liver disease in allografts ranges between 10% and 40%. Recurrence may be related to the persistence of original risk factors for fatty liver disease (e.g., hyperinsulinemia, hyperlipidemia, obesity) and influence of immunosuppressive drugs, among others. Advanced fibrosis (bridging or cirrhosis) have been variably reported; the largest series (227 patients) reported a 5% risk of advanced fibrosis in 5 years. Most patients follow an indolent course without major complications or graft loss. Recurrent alcoholic liver disease is reported to occur in 10% to 30% of patients, and approximately 5% of patients die of recurrent alcohol-induced cirrhosis. Patients who relapse are at an increased risk of complications including ACR.

Posttransplant Lymphoproliferative Disorder

Posttransplant lymphoproliferative disorder (PTLD) represents a heterogeneous group of lymphoproliferative disorders associated with immunosuppression related to solid organ or hematopoietic cell transplant and often affecting extranodal organs such as the GI tract, lung, and liver. PTLD occurring after liver transplantation may present within the first month or decades after transplantation and affects 2% to 4% of adults and up to 20% of pediatric recipients. The vast majority are B-cell disorders, and most (80%) are EBV-driven processes. The pathogenesis of EBV-driven PTLD is attributed to the loss of T cell–mediated cytotoxicity against EBV-infected B cells because of immunosuppression. They comprise a spectrum ranging from EBV-driven polyclonal proliferations to EBV-positive or EBV-negative polymorphic and a monomorphic population of B or T or natural killer (NK) cells. Although less common overall, EBV-negative PTLD tends to occur in the later after transplant. The pathogenesis of EBV-negative PTLD is not well understood.

The clinical presentation is variable from asymptomatic patients to those that present with lymph node enlargement, fever, malaise, and hepatosplenomegaly. It typically occurs in the first year after transplantation. The histologic spectrum (Table 20.10) of lymphoid proliferation in PTLD ranges from nondestructive and polymorphic EBV-driven processes comparable to B-cell or (less commonly) T-cell lymphomas occurring outside of the setting of immunosuppression (see details in Chapter 19). Monomorphic PTLDs are categorized as B- and T- or NK cell PTLD and are classified according to the lymphoma they resemble. Classic Hodgkin lymphoma PTLD corresponds to a separate category within this spectrum.

TABLE 20.10

World Health Organization Categories of Posttransplant Lymphoproliferative Disorder

NONDESTRUCTIVE PTLD
- Plasmacytic hyperplasia
- Infectious mononucleosis
- Florid follicular hyperplasia

POLYMORPHIC PTLD

Monomorphic PTLD (B- and T- or NK cell types)
- Monomorphic B-cell PTLD
- DLBCL
- Burkitt lymphoma
- Plasma cell myeloma
- Plasmacytoma
- Others
- Monomorphic T- or NK cell PTLD
- Peripheral T-cell lymphoma, not otherwise specified
- Hepatosplenic T-cell lymphoma
- Other

Classic Hodgkin lymphoma PTLD

DLBCL, Diffuse large B-cell lymphoma; *PTLD*, posttransplant lymphoproliferative disorder.

It is important to distinguish these lymphoid infiltrates from "rejection-type" infiltrates of ACR. In PTLD, the lymphoid infiltrates are of B-cell origin (95% are B-cell lesions), but the lymphoid cells in ACR are T cells. This distinction is critical because treatment for PTLD consists of decreasing the immunosuppression and possibly adding an anti–B cell agent for more aggressive lesions, while treatment for ACR is increasing patient's immunosuppression level. Chromogenic in situ hybridization for EBV-encoded RNA is the preferred test in most laboratories for identifying EBV-infected cells. However, it is important to remember that identification of occasional EBV-positive cells in a liver allograft biopsy in the absence of a characteristic lymphoid or plasmacytic infiltrate should not be considered as diagnostic of PTLD.

Posttransplant lymphoproliferative disorder treatment includes reduction of immunosuppression, monoclonal anti-CD20 antibody (rituximab), and chemotherapy. Surgical resection is performed in some cases. The prognosis is highly variable and multifactorial, but some authors have reported that more than half of patients experience a complete response after treatment and a median overall survival period ranging from 37 to 50 months. Older studies reported mortality rates in the range of 25% to 60%, which has improved over the years with newer therapeutics options.

Opportunistic Infections

The more common infections affecting the LT recipient include wound infections, fungal infections, and viral infections. Fungal infections, usually from *Candida* spp. (Fig. 20.14), occur in up to 20% of LT recipients, most often affecting the mouth, esophagus, and urine.

Cytomegalovirus infection is the most common viral infection in this setting. It is most frequently seen in recipients who are CMV negative but receive an organ from a CMV-positive donor. CMV infection may affect the transplanted organ or in other sites. Typical viral inclusions can be seen in enlarged nuclei and cytoplasm of hepatocytes, biliary epithelial cells, endothelial cells, or stromal cells. The nuclear inclusions consist of an intranuclear mass separated from the nuclear membrane by a clear halo, creating an "owl's eye" effect. Cytoplasmic inclusions are granular and basophilic. Immunohistochemical staining can be helpful to identify or confirm the presence of viral inclusions.

Adenovirus and herpes simplex virus (HSV) infections are rare and tend to occur in LT recipients who are severely immunocompromised. Adenovirus hepatitis manifests as random foci of hepatocyte necrosis. Infected hepatocytes and biliary epithelial cells show characteristic basophilic, smudged intranuclear inclusions. HSV infection results in large areas of geographic necrosis that are randomly distributed throughout the parenchyma. The hepatocytes adjacent to these foci of necrosis show viral cytopathic effect characterized by chromatin margination, nuclear multinucleation, and molding. Immunohistochemical stains are available to assist identification of CMV, HSV, or adenovirus inclusions.

Epstein-Barr virus hepatitis is associated with portal and lobular inflammation with a characteristic sinusoidal "beading" pattern of the lymphocytic infiltrate. This feature can mimic the lobular hepatitis seen in some cases of late ACR. Chromogenic in situ hybridization for EBV-encoded RNA is used to diagnose EBV hepatitis.

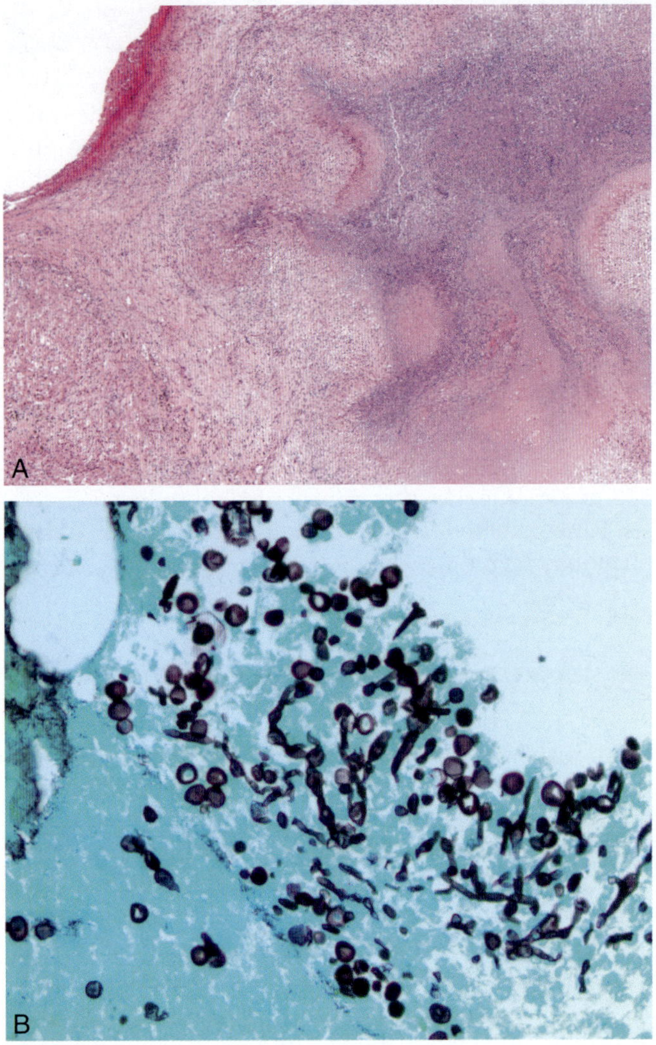

FIGURE 20.14

Opportunistic infections. **A**, Well-demarcated intrahepatic abscess with dirty central necrosis and organizing inflammation at the periphery. **B**, Gomori methenamine silver stain supports the diagnosis of *Candida* spp. as the underlying pathogen in this case.

SMALL BOWEL TRANSPLANTATION

Intestinal transplantation has evolved as one of the leading therapeutic options for patients with intestinal failure (IF) who are unresponsive to parenteral nutrition therapy. The main indications for intestinal transplantation that are approved by the Centers for Medicare & Medicaid Services include depletion of central venous access sites, multiple episodes of catheter-related sepsis, electrolyte disturbance, dehydration, and progressive cholestatic liver failure. Additional indications for intestinal and multivisceral transplant include diffuse portomesenteric thrombosis, malignancies limited to the abdominal compartment, and congenital motility disorders of the intestine. Per the Organ Procurement Transplant Network, a total of 22,914 intestinal transplants were performed between 1990 and 2017. This number is much lower compared with other solid organ transplants and has been steadily stabilizing over the recent years.

In children, intestinal transplant is commonly performed for conditions that result in short bowel syndrome (SBS), including necrotizing enterocolitis, intestinal atresia, volvulus, and motility disorders. In adults, the causes of SBS include Crohn's disease, mesenteric thrombosis, trauma, and desmoid tumors.

Most patients undergo isolated small bowel transplants in which the entire donor jejunum and ileum are anastomosed to the recipient proximal jejunum. An ileostomy is then created from the distal ileum of the allograft, with or without anastomosis of the distal small bowel with native colon. Combined liver–intestine graft is considered in patients with IF and concomitant IF-associated liver disease. Intestinal grafts can also be a component of multivisceral transplants that include stomach or colon in the liver–intestine allograft.

Allograft Dysfunction

The mechanisms of small bowel allograft dysfunction are related to multiple causes, including infection, rejection, chronic kidney disease, and PTLD. Histologic evaluation plays an essential role in evaluating the allograft status, especially with regard to infection, allograft rejection, and PTLD. In addition to clinical history and symptoms, the following information is critical while evaluating small bowel transplant biopsies: (1) location of the biopsy and its relation to stoma site, (2) native organ versus graft, and (3) endoscopic appearance of the mucosa and specific location of biopsies with respect to endoscopic findings (i.e., close to ulcer or relatively normal-appearing bowel).

Infection

Postoperative infection remains the most common complication and cause of allograft loss. These are mostly bacterial infections, although a subset of patients may also develop viral enteritis. Clinically, infectious enteritis often presents with increased stoma output and unexplained fever, thus mimicking allograft rejection. The common viruses that can affect small bowel allografts include EBV, CMV, rotavirus, adenovirus, and calicivirus. Histologic changes range from mucosal congestion, lamina propria edema, and focal neutrophilic epithelial injury to mucosal erosions and crypt abscesses. Crypt apoptotic activity is generally minimal and restricted to fragments with features of regenerating epithelium. As with other allografts, CMV and adenoviral infections are accompanied by viral cytopathic changes. The presence of scattered intranuclear glassy eosinophilic inclusions points to the diagnosis of adenoviral enteropathy (Fig. 20.15). IHC for CMV and adenovirus can be very helpful in this setting.

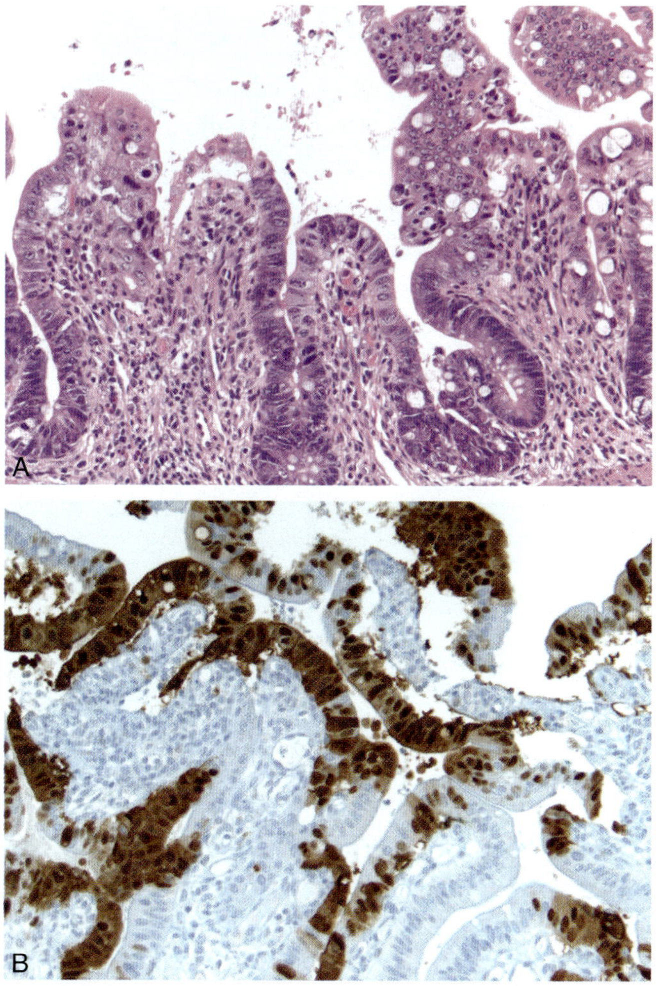

FIGURE 20.15

Adenovirus enteritis. **A**, The biopsy shows small bowel mucosa with villous architectural distortion and regenerative epithelial changes along with intranuclear basophilic inclusions. **B**, Immunohistochemical stain for adenovirus highlights the viral inclusion.

Rejection

In addition to biopsies performed in symptomatic patients, protocol biopsies are generally performed –two or three times a week for the first month and one to two times per week for the next 2 months. These intervals may vary depending on the transplant program. Because changes of rejection can be focal, a minimum of three biopsy fragments with ample number of crypts (at least 10) is considered as an adequate sample.

ACUTE CELLULAR REJECTION

Clinical Features

Acute cellular rejection is the leading cause of allograft loss in the first 2 months. Because the ileum has the highest concentration of lymphoid tissue in the gut, changes of rejection are most commonly observed in this region. Most patients present with fever, nausea, vomiting, abdominal pain, diarrhea, and distension.

Pathologic Findings

Acute Cell-Mediated Rejection

Endoscopically, the mucosal changes range from edema and hyperemia in the early phase of rejection to loss of vascular pattern and foci of erosion and ulcers in severe cases of rejection. The key parameter for diagnosing rejection is number of apoptotic bodies per 10 consecutive crypt cross-sections (apoptotic body count). Apoptotic bodies are characterized as fragmented nuclear debris within a cytoplasmic vacuole ("classical" exploding crypt cells).

Intraepithelial clusters of basophilic material account for the other form of crypt apoptosis. Although some investigators have studied the use of special stains such as cleaved caspase-3, the results have not been satisfactory. Therefore, routine hematoxylin and eosin–stained slides continue to be the gold standard for assessing features of rejection. One practical way of generating apoptotic body count is to scan the slide at low magnification and then select an area of highest concentration of apoptotic bodies. These foci usually tend to be in areas of epithelial injury or increased lamina propria inflammation. A high-power evaluation is then performed to generate the final count per 10 consecutive crypts.

Grading Acute T Cell–Mediated Rejection

The severity of rejection is graded based on the extent of mucosal injury, the amount of lamina propria inflammatory infiltrate, and the apoptotic body count (Table 20.11).

Negative for Rejection

The normal villous architecture is retained, and there is no increase in lamina propria inflammation. The apoptotic body count is less than 2 per 10 consecutive crypts.

Indeterminate for Rejection

The villous architecture may either be completely normal or there may be focal mild blunting of villi. The lamina propria is slightly expanded by a mixed population of cells composed of activated lymphocytes, small lymphocytes, neutrophils, and eosinophils. There is usually some accompanying epithelial injury with reactive changes. The apoptotic count is less than 6 per 10 consecutive crypts. A diagnosis of indeterminate for rejection is used when the features of rejection are quantitatively insufficient for a diagnosis of mild rejection or if other factors such as infection or nonrejection causes of mucosal injury are present in the biopsy.

Mild Acute Cellular Rejection

The villous architecture is usually distorted in fragments that show increased lamina propria inflammation. Apoptotic count is 6 or more per 10 consecutive crypts (Fig. 20.16). There may be accompanying reactive epithelial changes.

Moderate Acute Cellular Rejection

The villi are often congested and edematous and show moderate to marked architectural distortion. The lamina

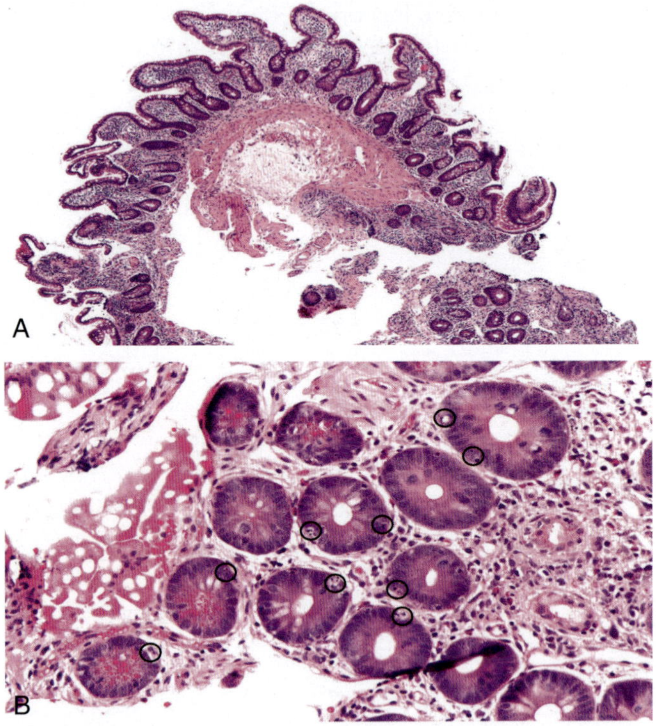

FIGURE 20.16

Small bowel allograft: mild acute cellular rejection. **A**, Low-magnification image shows slight villous distortion with expansion of the lamina propria by inflammatory infiltrate. **B**, Higher magnification image shows increased crypt apoptotic activity *(black circles)* at a rate of 9 per 10 consecutive crypts.

TABLE 20.11

Histologic Grading of Acute Cellular Rejection in Small Bowel Allografts

Grade of ACR	Apoptotic Body Count (per 10 consecutive crypts)	Degree of Lamina Propria Mixed Inflammation	Surface Epithelium
No ACR	<6/10; often <2–3/10	Normal; no activated lymphocytes	Intact
Indeterminate	<6/10; often 4 or 5/10	Focal increase	Intact
Mild	≥6/10	Mild to focal moderate increase	Intact
Moderate	Same as above with confluent apoptosis with or without crypt dropout	Moderate to severe increase	Erosions may be present
Severe	Same as above with extensive crypt dropout	Moderate to severe	Extensive erosions and/or ulcers

ACR, Acute T cell–mediated rejection.

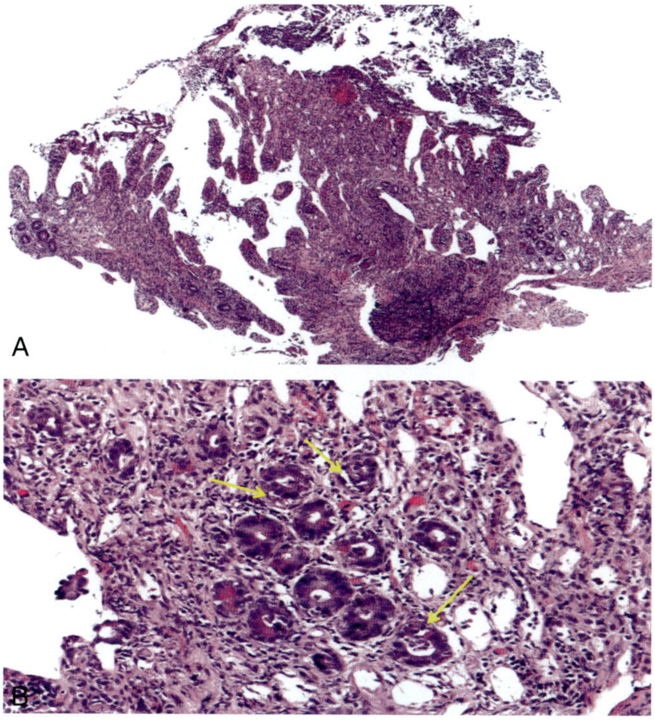

FIGURE 20.17

Small bowel allograft: severe acute cellular rejection. **A**, Low-magnification image shows ulcerated small bowel mucosa with granulation tissue and exudate. **B**, Higher magnification shows foci of crypt dropout and confluent apoptosis *(yellow arrows)*.

propria shows prominent mononuclear cell infiltrate with activated lymphocytes. The crypts show frequent apoptotic bodies, occasional confluent apoptosis, and focal dropout.

Severe Acute Cellular Rejection

There are moderate to marked increase in lamina propria inflammation and marked architectural distortion with crypt damage and erosion (Fig. 20.17). Extensive sloughing of the mucosa is accompanied by granulation tissue, in which case, the residual crypts should be carefully examined for changes of rejection.

ANTIBODY-MEDIATED REJECTION

Compared with other solid organ transplants, there are limited data on AMR in small bowel allografts, especially with regards to incidence and clinical significance of AMR. Preformed immunoglobulin (Ig) G antibodies in the first 2 weeks of transplant along with persistent mucosal congestion and hemorrhage should prompt work-up for AMR. Patients often have a strong crossmatch for T- or B-cell lymphocytotoxic antibodies. Other histologic findings include neutrophilic margination and fibrin thrombi (Fig. 20.18A) without neutrophilic or necrotizing arteritis. C4d immunohistochemical stain has not been validated for use in small bowel allografts. Nonetheless, the finding of diffuse C4d capillary staining (Fig. 20.18B) within lamina propria is abnormal and should raise concern for AMR in the appropriate clinical setting.

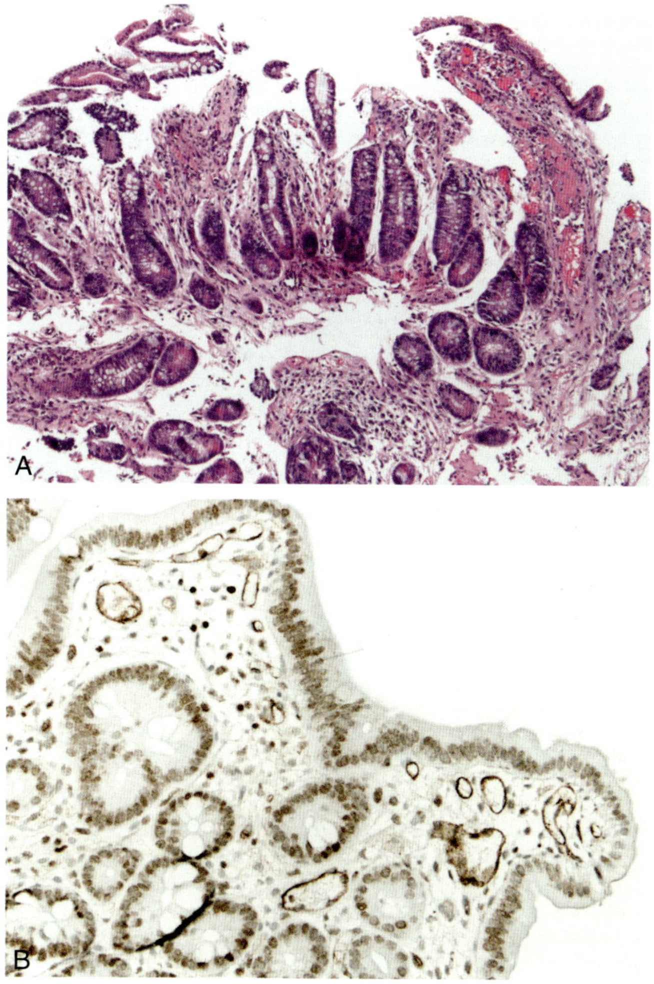

FIGURE 20.18

Small bowel allograft: antibody-mediated rejection. **A**, Small bowel mucosa shows mild architectural distortion and lamina propria congestion along with fibrin thrombus *(upper right aspect of image)*. **B**, C4d immunohistochemical stain shows diffuse staining of capillaries within the lamina propria.

CHRONIC REJECTION

Chronic rejection results in late allograft dysfunction and loss. Clinically, patients may present with nonspecific long-standing symptoms of diarrhea with nonhealing ulcers. These patients are often nonresponsive to antirejection medications. Almost always, there is history of repeated episodes of acute rejection. Endoscopically, the mucosal surface show flattened appearance, and focal ulcers may be present. Histologically, early changes are generally patchy in distribution and include mild fibrosis of the lamina propria and focal loss of crypts (Fig. 20.19A). Late changes of CR are characterized by lamina propria fibrosis, submucosal fibrosis, pyloric gland metaplasia, architectural distortion, and minimal apoptosis. The

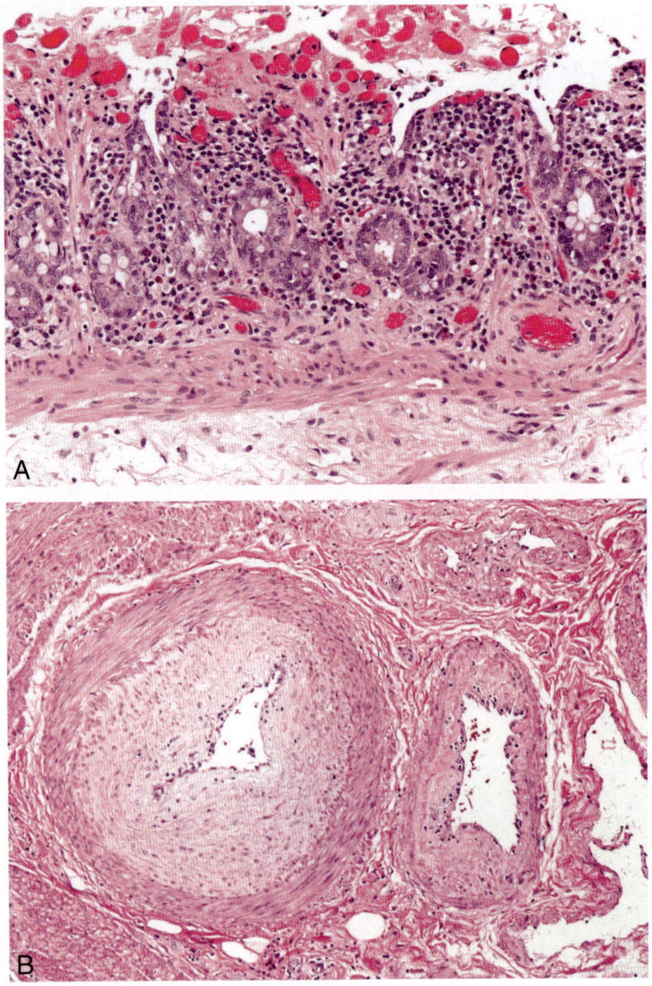

FIGURE 20.19

Small bowel allograft: Chronic rejection. **A**, Small bowel resection specimen with mucosal erosion, reactive epithelial changes, and lamina propria fibrosis. **B**, The sampled mesenteric vessels show obliterative arteriopathy characterized by myointimal hyperplasia of the arterial wall.

hallmark lesion of CR is allograft vasculopathy characterized by prominent intimal hyperplasia (Fig. 20.19B) of the mesenteric or submucosal arteries resulting in obliterative arteriopathy and hypoperfusion of the graft. Often, the biopsy samples may be noncontributory because the submucosal arteries are seldom sampled in these specimens.

Differential Diagnosis

In the early posttransplant period, it is important to distinguish infectious enteritis from acute cellular rejection because the management is different for both conditions. Both bacterial and viral enteritis can show increased crypt apoptotic activity. However, clinical findings such as involvement of intravenous lines, abdominal cavity, wounds, urinary tract, and respiratory tract suggest bacterial infection. Biopsies obtained from stomal ulcers can show mucosal erosions, ulcers, and granulation tissue, which are features that mimic severe rejection. However, the residual crypts in these biopsies typically do not harbor significant apoptotic activity. CR can mimic ischemic enteritis with features of lamina propria fibrosis and atrophic crypts. Clinical history of repeated episodes of rejection as well as mild increase in apoptotic activity favor CR over ischemia. Ultimately, clinical context is helpful in distinguishing these entities.

Prognosis and Therapy

Immunosuppressive therapy is the mainstay therapy for rejection and consists of tacrolimus and steroids with or without additional induction therapy with either cyclophosphamide or thymoglobulin. In some instances, azathioprine, mycophenolate mofetil, or sirolimus is added to the regimen. Patients with acute rejection episodes are treated with steroids and/or antilymphocyte antibodies (OKT3 or thymoglobulin). Per Organ Procurement and Transplantation Network/ Scientific Registry of Transplant Recipients annual data report 2017, 1- and 5-year survival rates for adult intestine–liver recipients were noted to be 66.7 % and 42.6 %, respectively. It was highest for pediatric intestine recipients (1- and 5-year survival rates, 86.2 % and 75.4 %, respectively).

Small Bowel Allograft Rejection–Fact Sheet

Definition

- Immunologic injury resulting in progressive graft dysfunction

Incidence

- Unknown

Morbidity and Mortality

- High morbidity in patients with sepsis

Gender, Race, and Age Distribution

- Occurs in all age groups
- No race predilection

Clinical Features

- Acute rejection
- Nausea, vomiting, abdominal pain, distension, diarrhea
- Increased stoma output
- Chronic rejection
- Long-standing diarrhea and nonhealing ulcers

Prognosis and Therapy

- Prognosis depends on recognizing features of allograft rejection and prompt treatment
- 1- and 5-year survival rates for adult intestine–liver recipients are 66.7% and 42.6%, respectively

Small Bowel Allograft Rejection—Pathologic Features

Gross Findings

- Acute rejection
  - Edema, hemorrhage in early or mild rejection; erosions and ulcers in severe rejection
  - Can be patchy and focal
- Chronic rejection
  - Flattened mucosa with or without ulcers

Microscopic Findings

- See Table 20.11

Differential Diagnosis

- Infectious enteritis
- Ischemic enteritis
- Peristomal biopsy changes

PANCREAS TRANSPLANTATION

From its inception in 1966 to 2014, more than 48,000 pancreas transplants were reported to the International Pancreas and Islet Transplant Registry. Of these, more than 29,000 were performed in the United States. Pancreas transplant is indicated primarily in patients with type 1 diabetes. Other indications include diabetes resulting from pancreatectomy performed for acute or chronic pancreatitis, pancreatic neoplasms, trauma, various pediatric genetic abnormalities, and patients with cystic fibrosis. Despite significant advances in surgical techniques, posttransplant immunosuppression, diagnosis of rejection on surveillance biopsies, better infection control regimens, and greatly improved long-term results, the rate of transplants performed in the United States has steadily decreased (≤20%) compared with non-US countries. This is likely related to improved medical management of diabetes, a decline in organ donor quality (more obese and older donors), and lack of consistent referral of transplant candidates for pancreas transplants from endocrinologists.

Types of Pancreas Transplants and Indications

Pancreas transplants can be broadly categorized as: (1) whole-organ transplants and (2) islet transplants. Whole-organ transplants are more commonly performed and are further classified as simultaneous pancreas and kidney transplant (SPK; 70%), pancreas after kidney transplant (PAK; 20%), and pancreas transplant alone (PTA; 10%).

Whole-Organ Transplants

The choice of type of pancreatic transplant often depends on the patient's renal function. Significant diabetic nephropathy or uremic type 1 diabetes often necessitate replacing both the kidney and pancreas to achieve better glycemic control and prevent further complications of diabetes such as neuropathy, diabetic gastroparesis, and retinopathy. In this type of transplant, both organs usually originate from cadavers. PAK transplants are performed in patients who have previously undergone a successful kidney transplant, and PTA transplants are indicated in patients with "brittle diabetes." In whole-organ transplant, exocrine secretions are managed either by intestinal or urinary bladder drainage. This is achieved by pancreaticoduodenal transplantation with anastomosis of donor duodenum to recipient small intestine or bladder. Although the pancreas graft survival rates of SPK transplants at 1 year are very similar for both methods of duct drainage (bladder drainage, 83%; enteric drainage, 82%), because of the unique metabolic and urologic complications in cases of bladder drainage, the latter are currently preferred.

Islet Cell Transplantation

Islet transplantation is a novel way of achieving optimal glycemic control without the inherent risks associated with whole-pancreas transplantation such as surgical risks and long-term immunosuppression. The procedure involves enzymatic separation of islets from exocrine pancreatic tissue using enzymes and implantation of isolated islets into the recipient liver via portal vein infusions. Other potential infusion sites include the subcutis, spleen, omentum, and renal capsule.

EVALUATING POSTTRANSPLANT NEEDLE CORE BIOPSIES

Allograft biopsies are obtained to evaluate status of the graft, especially in patients who show signs of acinar or islet cell injury, such as decreased urinary insulin and C-peptide levels, increased serum amylase, and lipase rejection. Irreversible rejection is still one of the leading causes of allograft loss. However, because of the poor specificity and sensitivity of these serologic markers, needle core biopsies have become the "gold standard" for evaluating pancreas grafts.

A biopsy should have at least three lobular areas and associated interlobular septa. The presence or absence of arterial branches should be documented because evaluation for arteritis is a crucial step of diagnosing rejection. In contrast, the presence of islets may be less critical in determining rejection because inflammation primarily affects exocrine pancreas before endocrine pancreas. The recommended steps for processing pancreas allograft biopsies are presented in Table 20.12.

TABLE 20.12

Recommended Steps for Processing Pancreas Allograft Biopsies

- Three slides for hematoxylin and eosin staining
- One slide for trichrome staining
- One slide for C4d immunohistochemical staining
- Five or more intervening unstained sections for additional stains as needed (i.e., hormone or viral markers)

Pancreas Allograft Rejection—Fact Sheet

Definition

- Immunologic injury resulting in progressive graft dysfunction

Incidence

- 15% to 21% at 1 year and 27% to 30% at 5 years

Morbidity and Mortality

- 4% at 1 year and 9% at 5 years

Gender, Race, and Age Distribution

- Occurs in all age groups
- No race predilection

Clinical Features

- Acute rejection
- Abdominal pain, fever
- Chronic rejection
- Abdominal pain

Prognosis and Therapy

- Prognosis depends on recognizing features of allograft rejection and prompt treatment
- Graft survival: 86% at 1 year and 54% at 10 years for simultaneous pancreas and kidney transplant recipients

Pancreas Allograft Rejection—Pathologic Features

Gross Findings

- Acute rejection
  - Edema, hemorrhage in early or acute rejection with or without necrosis
  - Can be patchy and focal
- Chronic rejection
  - Parenchymal fibrosis

Microscopic Findings

- See Table 20.13

Differential Diagnosis

- Infections
- Hemorrhagic necrosis caused by technical failure

Allograft Dysfunction

The mechanisms of allograft dysfunction have been broadly categorized as those related to technical failure and immunologic factors.

Technical Failure

Possible technical graft failures that can lead to removal of the graft include bleeding, thrombosis, infections, pancreatitis, and anastomotic leak. The rate of failure because of technical reasons is highest during the first year posttransplantation. In the early posttransplant period (usually within 1 month), one of the main causes of technical failure is massive vascular thrombosis. This irreversible event is often encountered by pathologists on whole explanted pancreas specimens with attached donor duodenal cuff. The thrombosis can be "idiopathic," characterized by recent thrombotic occlusion of large arteries, veins, or both. Histologic examination of the allograft shows ischemic necrosis without any parenchymal or vascular abnormality. In the setting of vascular thrombosis, it is prudent to exclude AMR, especially during the first month after transplantation.

Immunologic Factors

Immunologic injury, specifically acute rejection as a cause of graft loss is most frequent at 7 to 12 months after transplant and decreases after the first year. In contrast, CR as a cause of failure accounts for 20% to 30% of all graft failures after 1 year. Similar to other organs, histologic criteria for assessing allograft rejections were established at the 9th Banff conference on Allograft Pathology in 2007 and revised in 2015. These specific criteria are presented in Table 20.13.

Normal Allograft Biopsy

Normal allograft pancreas biopsies are usually encountered in the setting of protocol biopsies of well-functioning grafts. Normal allografts lack inflammatory infiltrates or exhibit very sparse inflammation composed of small, mature-appearing lymphocytes and rare plasma cells. This sparse inflammation is confined to the septae and typically spares the vessels, nerves, ducts, and acini. There are other clinical circumstances in which a biopsy may appear "normal." These include the late phase of recurrent autoimmune disease (i.e., after resolution of isletitis and disappearance of beta cells), drug toxicity, and acute AMR.

As in other solid organ transplants, two main mechanisms of graft rejection are recognized: cell-mediated rejection and AMR. It is crucial to differentiate the two forms of rejection because of significant therapeutic implications. Cell-mediated rejection therapy includes

TABLE 20.13

Diagnostic Categories of Pancreas Allograft Rejection: Banff Working Grading Schema

Diagnostic Category	Histologic Criteria
1. Normal	• No inflammation or Inactive septal, mononuclear inflammation not involving ducts, arteries, veins, or acini • Minimal fibrosis proportional to the size of enclosed structures (ducts and vessels) • No parenchymal atrophy or injury • No graft sclerosis
2. Indeterminate	• Active septal inflammation but overall features do not fulfill the criteria for mild acute rejection
3. Cell-mediated rejection	
ACUTE CELL-MEDIATED REJECTION	
Grade I: mild acute cell-mediated rejection	• Active septal inflammation composed of activated blastic lymphocytes and/or eosinophils • Venulitis • Ductitis*and/or* • Focal acinar inflammation (no more than two inflammatory foci per lobule with absent or minimal acinar cell injury)
Grade II: moderate acute cell-mediated rejection	• Multifocal (but not confluent or diffuse) acinar inflammation (≥3 foci per lobule) with spotty (individual) acinar cell injury and dropout *and/or* • Minimal intimal arteritis (with minimal [<25%] luminal compromise)
Grade III: severe acute cell-mediated rejection	• Diffuse, widespread acinar inflammation with focal or diffuse multicellular or confluent acinar cell necrosis *and/or* • Moderate or severe intimal arteritis (>25% luminal compromise) *and/or* • Transmural inflammation or necrotizing arteritis
4. AMR	Three diagnostic components: • C4d positivity in interacinar capillaries (≥1% of acinar lobular surface) • Serologic evidence of donor-specific antibodies (HLA or other antigens) • Histologic evidence of acute tissue injury One of three diagnostic components present: requires exclusion of AMR Two of three diagnostic components present: consider acute AMR Three of three diagnostic components present: definite acute AMR Histologic evidence of acute tissue injury: • **Grade I (mild acute AMR):** well-preserved architecture, mild interacinar monocytic–macrophagic or mixed (monocytic–macrophagic/neutrophilic) infiltrates with rare acinar cell damage (swelling, necrosis) • **Grade II (moderate acute AMR):** overall preservation of the architecture with interacinar monocytic–macrophagic or mixed (monocytic–macrophagic/neutrophilic) infiltrates, capillary dilation, interacinar capillaritis, intimal arteritis, congestion, multicellular acinar cell dropout, and extravasation of RBCs • **Grade III (severe acute AMR):** architectural disarray, scattered inflammatory infiltrates in a background of interstitial hemorrhage, multifocal and confluent parenchymal necrosis, arterial and venous wall necrosis, transmural or necrotizing arteritis, and thrombosis (in the absence of any other apparent cause)
5. Chronic active AMR	Features of category 3 and/or 4 with active chronic arteriopathy and/or category 6
6. Chronic arteriopathy	Fibrointimal arterial thickening with narrowing of the lumen • Inactive: fibrointimal arterial thickening with narrowing of the lumen • Active: infiltration of the subintimal fibrous proliferation by mononuclear cells (T cells and macrophages)Distinguish on the most affected artery: • Grade 0: negative; no narrowing of the luminal area • Grade 1: mild; ≤25% narrowing of luminal area • Grade 2: moderate; 26%–50% narrowing of luminal area • • Grade 3: severe; ≥50% narrowing of luminal area
7. Chronic graft fibrosis	• **Grade I (mild graft fibrosis):** expansion of fibrous septa; fibrosis occupies <30% of the core surface, but acinar lobules have eroded, irregular contours; the central lobular areas are normal • **Grade II (moderate graft fibrosis):** fibrosis occupies 30%–60% of the core surface. The exocrine atrophy affects the majority of the lobules in their periphery (irregular contours) and in their central areas (thin fibrous strands criss-cross between individual acini) • **Grade III (severe graft fibrosis):** the fibrotic areas predominate and occupy >60% of the core surface with only isolated areas of residual acinar tissue and/or islets present

Continued

TABLE 20.13
Diagnostic Categories of Pancreas Allograft Rejection: Banff Working Grading Schema

Diagnostic Category	Histologic Criteria
8. Islet pathology	• Recurrence of autoimmune diabetes mellitus (insulitis and/or selective β-cell loss) • Islet amyloid (amylin) deposition • Islet cell calcineurin inhibitor toxicity
9. Other histologic diagnosis	Pathologic changes not considered to be due to acute and/or chronic rejection (e.g., CMV pancreatitis, PTLD, bacterial or fungal infection, ischemic pancreatitis, recurrent autoimmune disease)

ACR, Acute T cell–mediated rejection; *AMR*, antibody-mediated rejection; *CMV*, cytomegalovirus; *HLA*, human leukocyte antigen; *PTLD*, posttransplant lymphoproliferative disorder; *RBC*, red blood cell.

corticosteroids and anti–T cell antibodies such as anti-thymocyte globulin and anti-CD3 monoclonal antibody. In contrast, treatment for patients with AMR targets circulating donor-specific antibodies with IVIg and plasmapheresis.

CELL-MEDIATED REJECTION

Acute Rejection

Rejection in pancreas allograft can be difficult to diagnose clinically. Patients present with clinical findings of fever and abdominal tenderness. Multiple serum markers are used to monitor graft function, including glucose, amylase, lipase, and C-peptide levels. Of these, lipase is the most specific. A pancreatic biopsy is performed in patients with elevated lipase levels and those who do not show evidence of vascular compromise or peripancreatic fluid collection on imaging.

Three grades of ACR (mild, moderate, and severe) are defined based on specific histologic lesions that predict progressively worse outcome.

Mild Acute T Cell–Mediated Rejection (Grade I)

This grade of rejection is defined by predominantly mononuclear septal inflammation composed of “activated blastic” lymphocytes admixed with variable numbers of eosinophils. These inflammatory cells extend into the ducts (ductitis) (Fig. 20.20) and subendothelial spaces of venules (venulitis) (Fig. 20.21). This is accompanied by mild (focal) acinar cell injury. The response to treatment approaches nearly 90%.

Moderate Acute T Cell–Mediated Rejection (Grade II)

This grade is characterized by multiple foci (three or more foci per lobule) of acinar inflammation with associated single-cell necrosis or dropout (Figs. 20.22 and 20.23). Occasionally, along with

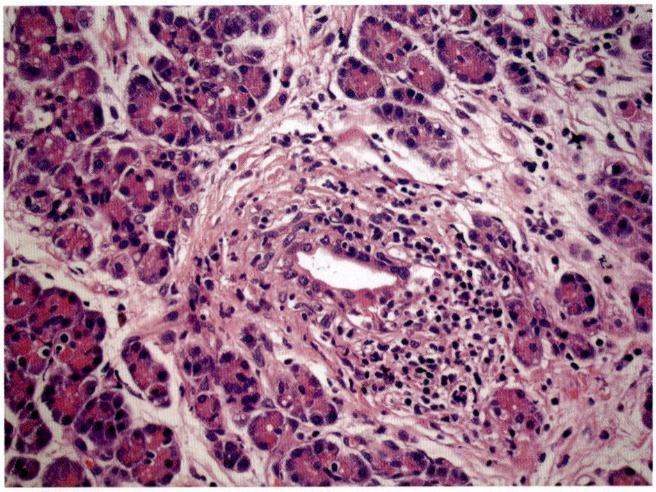

FIGURE 20.20
Hematoxylin and eosin–stained section of pancreas allograft biopsy (5 months posttransplant) with mild cellular rejection showing a polymorphous periductal inflammatory infiltrate composed of activated lymphocytes, small mature-appearing lymphocytes, and rare eosinophils. Lymphocyte-mediated duct epithelial damage (ductitis) is also noted.

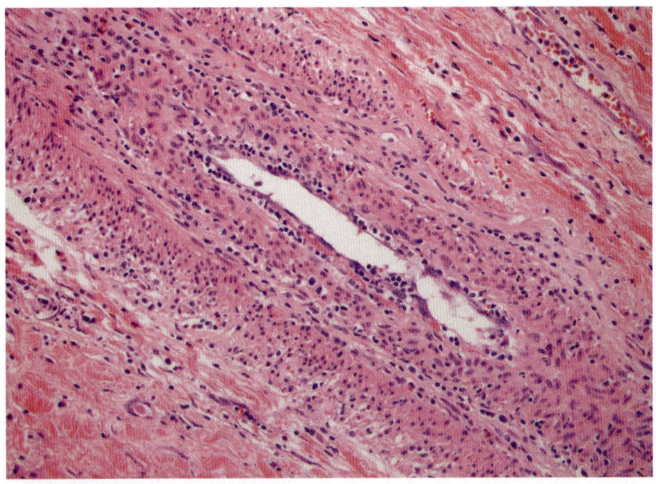

FIGURE 20.21
Hematoxylin and eosin–stained section of pancreas allograft biopsy (31 months posttransplant) with moderate acute cellular rejection characterized by a venous endothelial injury by activated lymphocytes.

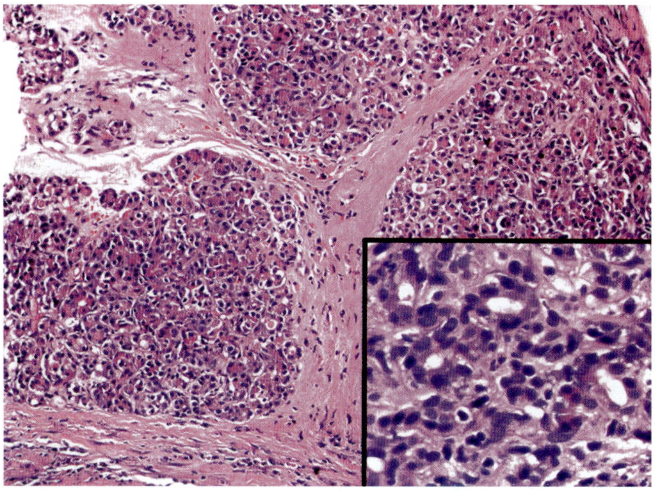

FIGURE 20.22
Hematoxylin and eosin–stained section of pancreas allograft biopsy (6 months posttransplant) with moderate cellular rejection showing marked interstitial fibrosis and lymphocyte-mediated acinar injury *(inset)*.

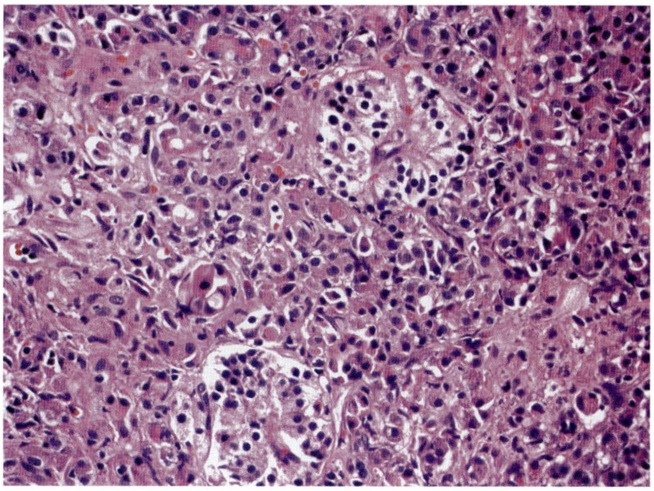

FIGURE 20.23
Hematoxylin and eosin–stained section of pancreas allograft biopsy (6 months posttransplant) with moderate cellular rejection showing diffuse lymphocyte-mediated acinar injury and destruction with focal dropout necrosis.

activated lymphocytes, eosinophils can be the predominant component of the inflammatory infiltrate. Alternatively, this pattern of injury may be diagnosed when minimal intimal arteritis (<25% luminal involvement) is identified (lymphocytes beneath the intima of a muscular artery but no endothelial activation or injury). In patients with grade II ACR, the response to antirejection therapy ranges from 71% to 85%.

Severe Acute T Cell–Mediated Rejection (Grade III)

This form of acute rejection is recognized histologically by three distinct lesions identified either in isolation or concurrently. Each of these lesions portends a poor prognosis. They include

1. Severe acinar inflammation and damage characterized by confluent, diffuse or extensive acinar inflammation associated with confluent necrosis. The inflammatory cells include activated lymphocytes and variable numbers of eosinophils and neutrophils. Interstitial edema and hemorrhage are indicators of severe tissue damage.
2. Moderate to severe intimal arteritis characterized by subintimal mononuclear cells as well as evidence of endothelial injury in the form of endothelial cell hypertrophy, fibrin leakage, neutrophil margination, macrophage activation, and activation of myointimal fibroblasts. These changes should involve more than 25% of the vascular lumen.
3. Arteritis (vasculitis) characterized by complete or partial circumferential necrosis often secondary to transmural arterial inflammatory infiltrates.

This form of rejection injury often manifests as hyperglycemia with poor response to antirejection regimens.

Antibody-Mediated Rejection

Primary humoral or AMR occurs in a recipient with preformed antidonor antibodies. The main risk factor is an ABO-incompatible graft. A diagnosis of AMR is based on three components: (1) histologic evidence of tissue injury, (2) complement deposition (C4d) positivity in interacinar capillaries (≥1% of acinar lobular surface), and (3) donor-specific antibodies in the serum. C4d staining in more than 5% of interacinar capillaries is typically present in cases of acute AMR. C4d staining is characterized as focal (>5%–50%) or diffuse (>50%), according to the extent of interacinar capillary staining in the lobular surface areas.

Grading Antibody-Mediated Rejection

Acute AMR typically occurs in the first few weeks after transplantation. The histologic criteria were recently outlined as follows.

Grade 1 (Mild Acute Antibody-Mediated Rejection)

Histologically, the pancreatic architecture is usually well-preserved. The inflammatory infiltrate is usually mild and composed of monocytic–macrophagic or mixed monocytic–macrophagic/neutrophilic infiltrates located between the acini. The acinar tissue shows rare foci of injury in the form of swelling or necrosis.

Grade 2 (Moderate Acute Antibody-Mediated Rejection)

The parenchymal architecture is intact. However, in addition to the interacinar inflammatory cell infiltrate, there are capillary dilation, interacinar capillaritis, intimal arteritis, congestion, multicellular acinar cell dropout, and extravasation of red blood cells.

Grade 3 (Severe Acute Antibody-Mediated Rejection)

The parenchymal architecture is distorted. In addition to scattered inflammatory infiltrates, there are interstitial hemorrhage, multifocal and confluent parenchymal necrosis, arterial and venous wall necrosis, transmural or necrotizing arteritis, and thrombosis.

CHRONIC REJECTION AND GRAFT FIBROSIS

Chronic Antibody-Mediated Rejection

This form of rejection is also referred to as chronic active AMR. Histologically, it has combined features of acute cell mediated or AMR along with chronic arteriopathy (see next section).

Chronic Arteriopathy

Arterial findings of rejection are seldom seen in needle biopsy samples. Sections from pancreatectomies performed for failed grafts with CR show extensive interstitial fibrosis or acinar atrophy along with the aforementioned obliterative arteriopathy (Figs. 20.24 and 20.25). This finding is more common after the second year posttransplantation. Chronic arteriopathy is characterized by the presence of fibrointimal arterial thickening with narrowing of the lumen (inactive). When the subintimal fibrous proliferation is infiltrated by mononuclear cells (T cells and macrophages), the lesion is defined as active chronic arteriopathy. The pathology report should specify how many medium and large arteries were sampled. Depending on the most affected artery, the arteriopathy is graded as grade 0, negative (no narrowing of the luminal area); grade 1, mild (≤25 % narrowing of the luminal area); grade 2, moderate (26 %–50 % narrowing of the luminal area); and grade 3, severe (≥50 % narrowing of the luminal area).

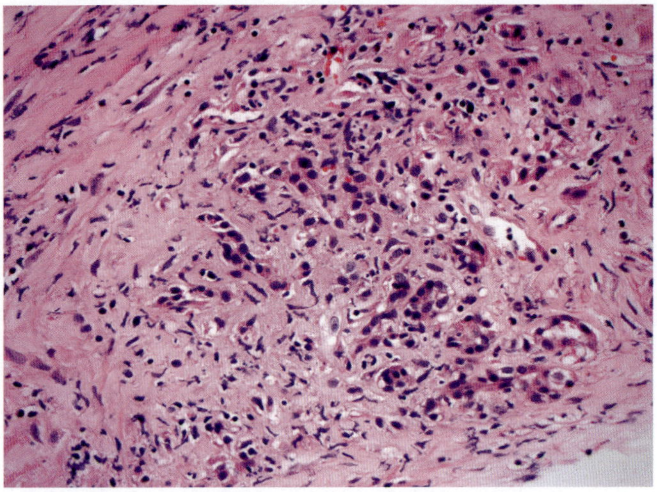

FIGURE 20.25

Hematoxylin and eosin–stained section pancreas allograft biopsy (13 months posttransplant) with extensive fibrosis and scattered parenchymal elements admixed with chronic inflammatory cells; changes are consistent with end-stage chronic rejection.

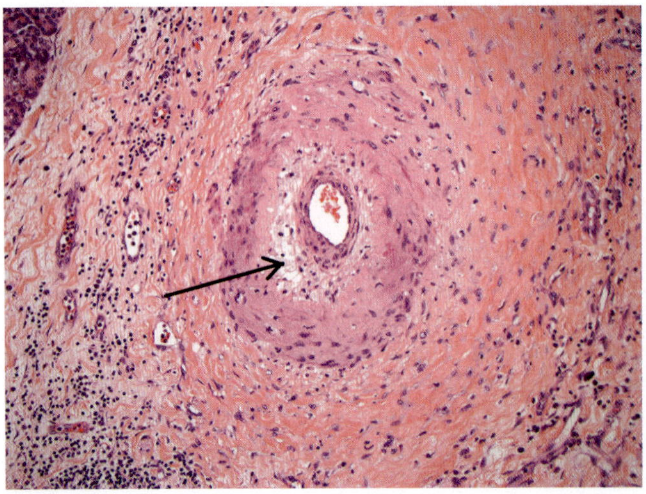

FIGURE 20.24

Hematoxylin and eosin–stained section of failed pancreatic transplant excision in a patient with simultaneous pancreas and kidney transplant showing chronic rejection with obliterative arteriopathy characterized by subintimal proliferation of fibroblasts, myofibroblasts, and smooth muscle cells with infiltration by mononuclear cells, including foamy histiocytes *(arrow)*.

CHRONIC GRAFT FIBROSIS

Chronic allograft rejection or graft sclerosis is semiquantitatively evaluated using a three-tier grading scheme as the extent of parenchymal loss and fibrosis corresponds with graft survival. The three stages of fibrosis correlate to less than 30 %, 30 % to 60 %, and greater than 60 % fibrosis in biopsy core samples. This is assessed in conjunction with the degree of lobular parenchymal atrophy ranging from preservation of acinar lobules with focal, irregular contours to stage II with atrophy affecting the center and periphery of lobules, eventually leading to stage III with marked reduction in the functional exocrine tissue (see Fig. 20.25). This grading scheme has significant prognostic value and should be applied to needle core biopsies (see Table 20.13).

Islet Pathology

As discussed earlier, biopsies with minimal inflammation should be distinguished from recurrence of autoimmune diabetes mellitus by performing stains for insulin and glucagon to assess β-cell loss. In addition, the islets are also prone to amyloid deposition and calcineurin inhibitor toxicity.

Differential Diagnosis of Acute Rejection

Acute T Cell–Mediated Rejection

The differential diagnosis for ACR includes peripancreatitis or superimposed infections such as CMV. However, these entities are seldom associated with venulitis, ductitis, or arterial inflammation. Extensive expansile inflammatory infiltrate requires differentiation from PTLD; the work-up of which described a previous section.

The histologic findings of early AMR can be quite subtle, with only mild inflammation in the biopsy samples. Biopsies with minimal or absent inflammation, especially in patients with hyperglycemia, should also be distinguished from other conditions such as recurrence of autoimmune diabetes. This distinction requires immunohistochemical assessment of the islets for the number and ratio of insulin-positive β cells and glucagon-positive α cells. Loss of β cells indicates recurrence of type 1 diabetes mellitus. Extensive hemorrhagic necrosis in severe AMR needs to be distinguished from thrombosis related to technical failure. Thrombosis related to technical failure typically occurs in the early transplant period as opposed to acute AMR, which occurs at a later time point. Furthermore, acute AMR is associated with arterial and venous endotheliitis of the small and large vessels. Thrombosis secondary to technical failure affects large arteries or veins (or both) without endothelial inflammation.

Prognosis and Therapy

In most cases, pulse steroid therapy and antilymphocyte therapy result in excellent treatment response in patients who are diagnosed with acute rejection. Multiple episodes of rejection may result in parenchymal fibrosis as well as disarray of the exocrine tissue. In early phases, islets are usually unaffected. However, eventually, ACR leads to diffuse graft fibrosis. Treatment of patients with AMR includes IVIg and plasmapheresis with or without rituximab. In patients who do not respond to this initial line of therapy, graft failure may occur in a short period of time (weeks or months) because of vascular thrombosis and necrosis. Pancreas transplant is associated with all-cause mortality rates of 4% at 1 year and 9% at 5 years. The graft survival rates are 86% at 1 year and 54% at 10 years for SPK recipients.

OTHER COMPLICATIONS

Pancreatitis and Peripancreatic Abscess Formation

Necrotizing infections as a result of bacterial or fungal infections can lead to parenchymal abscess formation, which may affect graft anastomoses. Biopsies from these allografts should be distinguished from rejection. In contrast to acute rejection, which shows preservation of overall parenchymal architecture, biopsies from patients with peripancreatic abscess show haphazard fibrotic bands usually obliterating septal structures.

Viral Infezzctions

Cytomegalovirus Pancreatitis

Cytomegalovirus pancreatitis manifests as multifocal, predominantly acinar inflammation composed of mononuclear cells associated with viral cytopathic changes within endothelial, stromal, or epithelial cells (Fig. 20.25). These changes can be easily confused with acute rejection, especially if not accompanied by diagnostic viral inclusions. Ancillary studies such as IHC, serology, and viral assays should be performed if there is strong clinical suspicion because early detection and diagnosis allow maintenance of good allograft function.

Epstein Barr Virus–Related Posttransplantation Lymphoproliferative Disorder

This disorder should be considered in the differential diagnosis of acute allograft rejection. The distinction is particularly important because the treatments for these conditions are exactly opposite (see Liver Transplantation section).

RECURRENCE OF PRIMARY DISEASE

Recurrence of type 1 diabetes mellitus is diagnosed when there is sudden or progressive loss of glycemic control associated with selective loss of beta cells in the graft and persistence of other types of islet cells, especially alpha cells. The destruction of beta cells is often associated with appearance of islet cell autoantibodies in serum (glutamic acid decarboxylase 65-kilodalton isoform [GAD-65] and islet antigen 2 [IA-2]). The reported overall incidences of posttransplant diabetes mellitus are nearly 17% for type 1 and 45% for type 2 diabetes. This is attributed to a combination of factors, which include increased pretransplant body mass index, higher pretransplant daily insulin dose, and the occurrence of acute rejection.

Another important source of posttransplant diabetes mellitus is islet cell damage induced by immunosuppressive agents such as tacrolimus. This is accompanied by morphologic changes such as cytoplasmic swelling and vacuolization of islet cells. Animal models as well as clinical studies have shown that this cell damage leads to hyperglycemia, which is dose related and reversible.

SUGGESTED READINGS

Liver Transplantation

Donor Biopsy Evaluation

1. Hubscher SG. Transplantation pathology. *Semin Liver Dis.* 2009;29:74–90.
2. Brown RS, Russo MW, Lai M, et al. A survey of liver transplantation from living adult donors in the United States. *N Engl J Med.* 2003;348:818–825.
3. Nocito A, Mohammad El-Badry A, Clavien P. When is steatosis too much for transplantation? *J Hepatology.* 2006;45:483–513.
4. Ploeg RJ, D'Alessandro AM, Knechtle SJ, et al. Risk factors for primary dysfunction after liver transplantation—a multivariate analysis. *Transplantation.* 1993;55:807–813.
5. Angele MK, Rentsch M, Hartl WH, et al. Effect of graft steatosis on liver function and organ survival after liver transplantation. *Am J Surg.* 2008;195:214–220.
6. Feng S, Goodrich NP, Bragg-Gresham JL, et al. Characteristics associated with liver graft failure: the concept of a donor risk index. *Transplant Proc.* 2009;41:975–979.
7. Müllhaupt B, Dimitroulis D, Gerlach JT, Clavien PA. Hot topics in liver transplantation: organ allocation--extended criteria donor--living donor liver transplantation. *J Hepatol..* 2008;48 (Suppl 1):S58–67.
8. Melin C, Miick R, Young NA, et al. Approach to intraoperative consultation for donor liver biopsies. *Arch Pathol Lab Med.* 2013;137(2):270–274.
9. Yersiz H, Lee C, Kaldas FM, et al. Assessment of hepatic steatosis by transplant surgeon and expert pathologist: a prospective, double-blind evaluation of 201 donor livers. *Liver Transplant.* 2013;19(4):437–449.
10. Neil DAH, Minervini M, Smith ML, et al. Banff consensus recommendations for steatosis assessment in donor livers. *Hepatology..* 2022;75(4):1014–1025.

Antibody-Mediated Rejection

11. Hubscher S. Antibody-mediated rejection in the liver allograft. *Curr Opin Transplant.* 2012;17:280–286.
12. Neuman UP, Neuhaus P. C4d immunostaining in acute humoral rejection after ABO blood group-incompatible liver transplantation. *Liver Transplant.* 2006;12:356–357.
13. O'Leary JG, Cai J, Freeman R, et al. Proposed diagnostic criteria for chronic antibody-mediated rejection in liver allografts. *Am J Transplant.* 2016;16(2):603–614.
14. Demetris AJ, Bellamy C, Hübscher SG, et al. 2016 Comprehensive update of the Banff Working Group on Liver Allograft Pathology: introduction of antibody-mediated rejection. *Am J Transplant.* 2016;16:2816–2835.
15. Lee BT, Fiel MI, Schiano TD. Antibody-mediated rejection of the liver allograft: an update and a clinico-pathological perspective. *J Hepatol.* 2021;75(5):1203–1216.

Acute and Chronic Cellular Rejection

16. Demetris AJ, Bellamy C, Hübscher SG, et al. 2016 comprehensive update of the Banff Working Group on Liver Allograft Pathology: introduction of antibody-mediated rejection. *Am J Transplant.* 2016;16:2816–2835.
17. Hubscher SG. Transplantation pathology. *Semin Liver Dis.* 2009;29:74–90.
18. International Panel Banff schema for grading liver allograft rejection: an international consensus document. *Hepatology.* 1997;25: 658–663.
19. Demetris AJ, Adams D, Bellamy C, et al. Update of the International Banff Schema for Liver Allograft Rejection: working recommendations for the histopathologic staging and reporting of chronic rejection. *An International Panel. Hepatology.* 2000;31(3): 792–799.
20. Demetris AJ, Adeyi O, Bellamy CO, et al. Liver biopsy interpretation for causes of late liver allograft dysfunction. *Hepatology.* 2006;44:489–501.
21. Demetris AJ, Eghtesad B, Marcos A, et al. Recurrent hepatitis C in liver allografts: prospective assessment of diagnostic accuracy, identification of pitfalls, and observations about pathogenesis. *Am J Surg Pathol.* 2004;28:658–669.
22. Krasinskas AM, Ruchelli ED, Rand EB, et al. Central venulitis in pediatric liver allografts. *Hepatology.* 2001;33:1141–1147.
23. Khettry U, Backer A, Ayata G, et al. Centrilobular histopathologic changes in liver transplant biopsies. *Hum Pathol.* 2002;33: 270–276.
24. Siddiqui I, Selzner N, Hafezi-Bakhtiari S, et al. Infiltrative (sinusoidal) and hepatitic patterns of injury in acute cellular rejection in liver allograft with clinical implications. *Mod Pathol.* 2015;28(9): 1275–1281.
25. Stevenson HL, Prats MM, Isse K, et al. Isolated vascular "v" lesions in liver allografts: how to approach this unusual finding. *Am J Transplant.* 2018;18(6):1534–1543.

"De Novo" Autoimmune Hepatitis or Posttransplant Plasma Cell Hepatitis

26. Aguilera I, Sousa JM, Gavilán F, et al. Glutathione S-transferase T1 mismatch constitutes a risk factor for de novo immune hepatitis after liver transplantation. *Liver Transplantation.* 2004;10(9): 1166–1172.
27. Fiel MI, Agarwal K, Stanca C, et al. Posttransplant plasma cell hepatitis (de novo autoimmune hepatitis) is a variant of rejection and may lead to a negative outcome in patients with hepatitis C virus. *Liver Transplant.* 2008;14:861–871.
28. Fiel MI, Schiano TD. Plasma cell hepatitis (de-novo autoimmune hepatitis) developing post liver transplantation. *Curr Opin Organ Transplant.* 2012;17(3):287–292.

Vascular Complications

29. Mourad MM, Liossis C, Gunson BK, et al. Etiology and management of hepatic artery thrombosis after adult liver transplantation. *Liver Transplant.* 2014;20(6):713–723.
30. daSilva RF, Raphe R, Felicio HC, et al. Prevalence, treatment and outcomes of the hepatic artery stenosis after liver transplantation . *Transplant Proc.* 2008;40:805–807.
31. Parrilla P, Sánchez-Bueno F, Figueras J, et al. Analysis of the complications of the piggy-back technique in 1,112 liver transplants. *Transplantation.* 1999;67(9):1214–1217.
32. Demetris AJ, Kelly DM, Eghtesad B, et al. Pathophysiologic observations and histopathologic recognition of the portal hyperperfusion or small-for-size syndrome. *Am J Surg Pathol.* 2006;30(8): 986–993.

Biliary Complications

33. Adeyi O, Fisher SE, Guindi M. Liver allograft pathology: approach to interpretation of needle biopsies with clinicopathological correlation. *J Clin Pathol.* 2010;63:47–74.

Recurrent Disease After Transplantation

34. Kotlyar DS, Campbell MS, Reddy KR. Recurrence of diseases following orthotopic liver transplantation. *Am J Gastroenterol.* 2006;101:1370–1378.
35. Hildebrand T, Pannicke N, Dechene A, et al. Biliary strictures and recurrence after liver transplantation for primary sclerosing cholangitis: a retrospective multicenter analysis. *Liver Transplant.* 2016;22(1):42–52.
36. Demetris AJ, Eghtesad B, Marcos A, et al. Recurrent hepatitis C in liver allografts: prospective assessment of diagnostic accuracy, identification of pitfalls, and observations about pathogenesis. *Am J Surg Pathol.* 2004;28:658–669.
37. Satapathy SK, Sclair S, Fiel MI, et al. Clinical characterization of patients developing histologically-proven fibrosing cholestatic hepatitis C post-liver transplantation. *Hepatol Res.* 2011;41(4): 328–339.

38. Moreira RK, Salomao M, Verna EC, et al. The Hepatitis Aggressiveness Score (HAS): a novel classification system for post-liver transplantation recurrent hepatitis C. *Am J Surg Pathol.* 2013;37(1):104–113.
39. Salomao M, Verna E, Lefkowitch JH, Moreira R. Histopathologic distinction between fibrosing cholestatic hepatitis C and biliary obstruction. *Am J Surg Pathol.* 2013;37:1837–1844.
40. Leroy V, Dumortier J, Coilly A, et al. Efficacy of sofosbuvir and daclatasvir in patients with fibrosing cholestatic hepatitis c after liver transplantation. *Clin Gastroenterol Hepatol.* 2015;13(11): 1993–2001.
41. Patil DT, Yerian LM. Evolution of non-alcoholic fatty liver disease recurrence after liver transplantation. *Liver Transplant.* 2012;18:1147–1153.
42. Yalamanchili K, Saadeh S, Klintmalm GB, et al. Non-alcoholic fatty liver disease after liver transplantation for cryptogenic cirrhosis or non-alcoholic steatohepatitis. *Liver Transplant.* 2010;16 :431–439.

Posttransplant Lymphoproliferative Disorders

43. Petrara MR, Giunco S, Serraino D, et al. Posttransplant lymphoproliferative disorders: from epidemiology to pathogenesis-driven treatment. *Cancer Lett.* 2015;369:37–44.
44. Swedlow S, Campo E, Pileri SA, et al. The 2016 revision of the World Health Organization classification of lymphoid neoplasms. *Blood.* 2016;127(20):2375–2390.
45. WHO Classification of Tumours of Haematopoeitic and Lymphoid Tissues Chapter 16. Immunodeficiency-associated lymphoproliferative disorders. *IARC.* 2017:453–462.

Opportunistic Infections

46. Bruminhent J, Razonable RR. Management of cytomegalovirus infection and disease in liver transplant recipients. *World J Hepatol.* 2014;6:370–383.

Small Bowel Transplantation

47. Matsumoto CS, Subramanian S, Fishbein TM. Adult intestinal transplantation. *Gastroenterol Clin North Am.* 2018;47(2):341–354 .
48. Ruiz P. Updates on acute and chronic rejection in small bowel and multivisceral allografts. *Curr Opin Organ Transplant.* 2014;19(3): 293–302.
49. Ruiz P, Takahashi H, Delacruz V, et al. International grading scheme for acute cellular rejection in small-bowel transplantation: single-center experience. *Transplant Proc.* 2010;42(1):47–53 .
50. Kesseli S, Sudan D. Small bowel transplantation. *Surg Clin North Am.* 2019;99:103–116.
51. Remotti H, Subramanian S, Martinez M. Small-bowel allograft biopsies in the management of small-intestinal and multivisceral transplant recipients: histopathologic review and clinical correlations. *Arch Pathol Lab Med.* 2012;136(7):761–771.
52. Parizhskaya M, Redondo C, Demetris A, et al. Chronic rejection of small bowel grafts: pediatric and adult study of risk factors and morphologic progression. *Pediatr Dev Pathol.* 2003;6(3):240–250.

Pancreas Transplantation

53. Loupy A, Haas M, Solez K, et al. The Banff 2015 Kidney Meeting Report: current challenges in rejection classification and prospects for adopting molecular pathology. *Am J Transplant.* 2017; 17(1):28–41.
54. Papadimitriou JC, Drachenberg CB. Distinctive morphological features of antibody-mediated and T-cell-mediated acute rejection in pancreas allograft biopsies. *Curr Opin Organ Transplant.* 2012;17(1):93–99.
55. Drachenberg CB, Torrealba JR, Nankivell BJ, et al. Guidelines for the diagnosis of antibody-mediated rejection in pancreas allografts-updated Banff grading schema. *Am J Transplant.* 2011;11(9):1792–1802.
56. Venturini M, Angeli E, Maffi P, et al. Technique, complications, and therapeutic efficacy of percutaneous transplantation of human pancreatic islet cells in type 1 diabetes: the role of US. *Radiology.* 2005;234:617–624.
57. Drachenberg CB, Odorico J, Demetris AJ, et al. Banff schema for grading pancreas allograft rejection: working proposal by a multi-disciplinary international consensus panel. *Am J Transplant.* 2008;8:1237–1249.
58. Drachenberg CB, Papadimitriou JC. The inflamed pancreas transplant: histological differential diagnosis. *Semin Diagn Pathol.* 2004;21:255–259.
59. Drachenberg CB, Papadimitriou JC, Farney A, et al. Pancreas transplantation: the histologic morphology of graft loss and clinical correlations. *Transplantation.* 2001;71:1784–1791.
60. Nakhleh RE, Sutherland DE. Pancreas rejection. Significance of histopathologic findings with implications for classification of rejection. *Am J Surg Pathol.* 1992;16:1098–1107.
61. Drachenberg CB, Klassen DK, Weir MR, et al. Islet cell damage associated with tacrolimus and cyclosporine: morphological features in pancreas allograft biopsies and clinical correlation. *Transplantation.* 1999;68:396–402.
62. Melcher ML, Olson JL, Baxter-Lowe LA, et al. Antibody-mediated rejection of a pancreas allograft. *Am J Transplant.* 2006;6: 423–428.
63. Dean PG, Kudva YC, Larson TS, et al. Posttransplant diabetes mellitus after pancreas transplantation. *Am J Transplant.* 2008;8 :175–182.
64. de Kort H, Munivenkatappa RB, Berger SP, et al. Pancreas allograft biopsies with positive c4d staining and anti-donor antibodies related to worse outcome for patients. *Am J Transplant.* 2010;10(7):1660–1667.

Index

Page numbers followed by "*f*" indicate figures, "*t*" indicate tables, and "*b*" indicate boxes.

A

Abdominal pain
- in actinomycosis, 272
- in celiac disease, 121
- in graft-versus-host disease, 140–141
- in intestinal lymphangiectasia, 147
- in mantle cell lymphoma, 626
- in mycophenolate mofetil colitis, 330
- in strongyloidiasis, 294
- in yersiniosis, 260

Abetalipoproteinemia, 137
Abscess, anal, 407–408
Acanthosis, glycogenic, differential diagnosis of, 16
Acetaminophen toxicity, 530–531, 532*f*–533*f*
Achalasia, esophageal, 22–24, 23*f*, 25*f*
Acid lipase deficiency, 549*t*, 550*t*
Acinar cell carcinomas (ACCs), 471, 478*f*
Acinar differentiation, tumors with (in pancreas), 476–484
- acinar cell carcinoma, 476–479
- acinar cell cystadenocarcinoma, 479
- acinar cell cystadenoma, 476
- mixed acinar–ductal and ductal–neuroendocrine carcinoma, 484
- mixed acinar–neuroendocrine carcinoma, 484
- mixed ductal–neuroendocrine carcinoma, 484
- pancreatoblastoma, 479–480
- serous cystadenocarcinoma, 482
- serous cystadenoma (SCA), 480–482
- solid-pseudopapillary neoplasm (SPN), 482–483

Acinar–ductal and ductal–neuroendocrine carcinoma, of pancreas, 484
Acinar–neuroendocrine carcinoma, of pancreas, 484
Actin, smooth muscle
- in gastrointestinal stromal tumors, 177
- in inflammatory myofibroblastic tumor, 203

Actinomyces infection, 219
Actinomycosis
- appendicitis in, 272
- colonic, 253*t*, 272–273
  - differential diagnosis of, 272–273

Acute antibody-mediated rejection, diagnosis of, 662*t*
Acute appendicitis, 213–215, 214*f*
- infectious causes of, 219–221

Acute cellular rejection (ACR), 663–668, 664*f*, 666*f*
Acute hepatitis pattern of injury, in liver, 489–490, 490*f*
- acute viral (hepatotropic) hepatitis, 491
- alcoholic liver disease, 509–513
- autoimmune hepatitis, 502–505
- chronic hepatitis pattern of injury, 496–498
- chronic viral hepatitis, 498–502

Acute hepatitis pattern of injury, in liver (*Continued*)
- fatty liver disease/steatohepatitis pattern of injury, 505
- nonalcoholic fatty liver disease, 505–509
- nonhepatotropic viral infections, 493

Acute intermittent porphyria (AIP), 553
Acute pancreatitis, 458–459, 458*f*
Acute versus chronic cholestasis, 512
Acute viral (hepatotropic) hepatitis, in liver, 491
"Adenocarcinoid" tumors, 237, 240
Adenocarcinoma, 155*f*
- of ampulla of Vater, 157–160, 157*f*
  - subtyping of, 159*t*
- of anus, differential diagnosis, 419–420
- colonic, 384*f*, 385*f*
- colorectal, 379–380, 384*f*. See also Colorectal cancer
- in Crohn's disease, 313–314
- differential diagnosis, 156
- of esophagus, 39–42
  - intramucosal, 38–39, 38*f*
- ex goblet cell carcinoid, 237, 239*f*
  - differential diagnosis of, 237
- of extrahepatic bile ducts, 444*f*, 445*f*, 451*f*
- gastric, 107–114
  - differential diagnosis of, 98–99
  - diffuse type of, 108
- infiltrating, 471*f*
- intestinal type of, 108, 108*f*
- invasive, of gallbladder, 441
- mucinous, 384*f*
- with Paget's disease of anus, 431
- signet ring cell, 385*f*
- small bowel, ampulla of Vater, 157–160, 157*f*, 159*t*
- of small intestine, 154–157
- tubular, 468*f*

Adenoid cystic carcinoma in esophagus, 47*f*
Adenoma, 225–226
- of appendix, 225*f*
- colorectal. *See* Adenomatous polyps
- differential diagnosis of, 226
- gastric, 101–104
  - differential diagnosis of, 101–104
  - foveolar-type, 102
  - intestinal-type, 102
- hepatic, 560–564, 561*f*, 562*f*, 562*t*
- pyloric gland, 104–106
- sessile serrated, 374–377
  - differential diagnosis of, 374–377

Adenomatosis, 564
Adenomatous polyps, 363–365, 364*f*, 365*f*, 384*f*
- carcinoma in situ, 366
- and colorectal cancer risk, 363–364
- differential diagnosis of, 367
- diffuse, 192
- familial, 192, 198, 337, 340*f*, 341*f*
  - differential diagnosis of, 341–343

Adenomatous polyps (*Continued*)
- flat, 364
- intramucosal adenocarcinoma, 366
- molecular features of, 366–367
- neuroendocrine proliferation in, 365–366
- tubular, 364
- villous, 364

Adenomyoma
- of gallbladder, differential diagnosis of, 438*f*
- gastric, differential diagnosis of, 98–99

Adenosquamous carcinoma, 471–472, 472*f*
Adenovirus enteritis, 677*f*
Adenovirus infection
- appendicitis in, 220–221, 221*f*
- of gastrointestinal tract, 247
- inclusions in, 220–221, 221*f*, 247

Advanced gallbladder carcinoma, 444–446
Aeromonas infection, 253*t*, 262, 263*f*
AIDS. *See* HIV infection
Alcoholic liver disease, 509–513
Alcoholic steatohepatitis (ASH), 505, 515*f*
"Almost normal" biopsy/nonspecific findings, in liver, 535–537, 535*t*, 536*f*
- hepatic granulomas, 537
- necrosis, 537–538

Alternative lengthening of telomeres (ALT) phenotype, 474
Amebiasis, 284*f*
Ampulla of Vater, adenocarcinomas of, 157–160, 157*f*
- subtyping of, 159*t*

Ampullary adenocarcinoma, 159*f*
- intestinal type, 159*f*, 159*t*
- pancreaticobiliary type, 159*f*, 159*t*

Ampullary adenoma, 157*f*, 160
Amyloidosis, 537
- esophageal achalasia in, 22
- gastric, 64–67, 82, 83*f*, 84*f*
  - differential diagnosis of, 75

Anal canal
- adenocarcinoma, 419
- anal tags in, 411–412
- anatomy and histologic landmarks of, 407
- Bowenoid papulosis, 427–428
- Bowen's disease, 426, 428*f*
- condyloma acuminatum of, 410–411, 424, 425*f*
- perianal high-grade squamous intraepithelial lesion, 426
- squamous cell carcinoma of, 415–416
- tumors and precursor lesions of, 412

Anal canal squamous intraepithelial lesion (ASIL), 412–413
Anal Crohn's disease, 409*f*
Anal fibroepithelial polyp. *See* Anal tag
Anal fistula tract, 408*f*
Anal gland adenocarcinoma, 419*f*
Anal squamous neoplasia, 412

Anal tag, 411–412
Ancylostoma duodenale, 292
Anemia, in gastric antral vascular ectasia, 84–85
Angina, intestinal, 145
Angiomyolipoma, of liver neoplasms, 598–600, 599*f*
Angiosarcomas, 602*f*
, malignant, 600–602
Anisakiasis, 295
  differential diagnosis of, 73
  gastritis in, 73, 295
Annular pancreas, 455
Anomalies of appendiceal anatomy, 211
Anorectum, syphilis of, 269
Antibody-mediated rejection (AMR), 661*f*
Antinuclear antibodies (ANAs), 502
Anti-smooth muscle antibodies (ASMAs), 502
α1-antitrypsin deficiency, 544
Antral vascular ectasia gastric, differential diagnosis of, 86*t*, 88
Anus
  Crohn's disease of, 408–409, 409*f*
  giant condyloma of Buschke-Lowenstein, 429–430
  hemorrhoids of, 410, 411*f*
  hidradenoma papilliferum of, 423, 424*f*
  melanoma of, 421, 422*f*
  non-neoplastic lesions in, 407–408
  Paget's disease of, 431, 432*f*
  squamous cell carcinoma of, 417*f*, 430*f*
  tags in, 410
  verrucous carcinoma of, 429–430
    differential diagnosis of, 426
APC gene/mutations, 198
Apoptotic cells, enterocytes in AIDS enterocolopathy, 249*f*
Appendiceal adenocarcinoma, 232
Appendiceal Crohn's disease, 217*f*
Appendiceal mucinous neoplasm, 224*f*
  high-grade, 228
  low-grade, 228
Appendicitis, 214*f*
  granulomatous, 218
  idiopathic granulomatous, 217*t*
  periappendicitis, 215–216, 215*f*
  ulcerative, 216
Appendix, 211
  chronic inflammatory disorders of, 217*t*
  in Crohn's disease, 214–218, 217*f*, 217*t*
  in cystic fibrosis, 211, 212*f*, 218–219, 219*f*
  deciduosis in, 221–223, 222*f*
  diverticula of, 211, 212*f*
  endometriosis of, 221–223, 222*f*
  epithelial neoplasms of, 223
  fibrous obliteration of lumen in, 211–213, 212*f*
  in gliomatosis peritonei, 221–222
  interval, 214–215, 214*f*
  invasive adenocarcinoma of, 232*f*
  mucinous neoplasms of, 229*f*, 234*f*, 240*f*
  neuroendocrine tumors of, 235
  retention cyst of, 230*f*
  serrated polyps of, 226, 227*f*
  in ulcerative colitis, 216
Arginase-1 immunohistochemistry, 590
Arteriosclerosis, differential diagnosis of, 84
Arthropathy, reactive, in *Campylobacter* infection, 259
Ascaris lumbricoides infection, 292, 293*f*
Aspergillosis, bowel infarction, 275*f*
Aspergillus infection, colonic, 275–276, 276*f*
  differential diagnosis of, 274*t*
ATP7B gene, 542
Atresia, esophageal, 17–19, 17*f*
  tracheoesophageal fistula with, 17–19, 18*f*
Atypical lipomatous tumor, of esophagus, 30–31
Atypical lymphocytes, 496
Autoimmune disorders
  gastritis, 64, 64*t*, 67*t*
    differential diagnosis of, 62, 67*t*
Autoimmune enteropathy, 133–135, 134*f*
  differential diagnosis of, 135
    microvillus inclusion disease (MVID), 135
Autoimmune hepatitis, in liver, 502–505, 502*t*
Autoimmune pancreatitis (AIP), 460–463, 461*b*, 461*f*, 462*b*

B

Bacterial enterocolitis, 252
Bacterial infections, of colon, 253*t*
Bacterial overgrowth syndrome, differential diagnosis of, 124
Balantidium coli organisms, 284
Bannayan-Riley-Ruvalcaba syndrome, 352
Barrett's esophagus, 32–34, 33*f*
  CK7/20 staining pattern in, 40
  differential diagnosis of, 1
  follow-up guidelines in, 38–39, 39*t*
  goblet cells in, 32, 33*f*
  high-grade dysplasia in, 35
    indefinite for dysplasia, 36, 36*f*
  intestinal metaplasia in, 37*f*
  low-grade dysplasia in, 37*f*
  negative for dysplasia, 35–36, 36*f*
  and reflux esophagitis, 1
Basidiobolus ranarum infection, 277
  differential diagnosis of, 278
Batts and Ludwig classification system, 497*f*, 498*f*
B-cell lymphoma(s)
  Burkitt lymphoma, 624*f*, 638–641
  diffuse large, 630–632, 631*b*, 631*b*–632*b*, 634*f*–635*f*
    differential diagnosis of, 640, 645
  extranodal marginal zone. *See* MALT lymphomas
Beckwith-Wiedemann syndrome, 575
Behçet's disease, differential diagnosis of, 131
Benign cystic lesions in pancreas, 456–458
  congenital cysts, 457
  duodenal diverticulum, 458
  simple mucinous cysts, 456–457
Benign lobular atrophy, 485*f*
Bevacizumab, 531
Bile duct adenomas (BDAdas), 579, 581*f*
Bile duct hamartomas (BDHs), 578, 579*f*
Bile duct injury, 532*f*–533*f*
Bile duct loss, 536–537
Bile duct margin, 486–487
Bile ducts, disorders of, 513
  Budd-Chiari syndrome, 523, 523*f*
  congestive (cardiac) hepatopathy, 524
  drug-induced liver injury, 530–531
  hepatoportal sclerosis, 528
  large duct obstruction, 513–516
  nodular regenerative hyperplasia, 527
  overlap syndromes, 522
  peliosis hepatis, 530, 530*f*
  portal vein thrombosis or obstruction, 526–527
  primary biliary cholangitis, 516–519
  primary sclerosing cholangitis (PSC), 519
  sinusoidal obstruction syndrome (SOS), 525
  vascular pattern of injury, 522–523
Bile ducts, extrahepatic
  botryoid embryonal rhabdomyosarcoma of, 453
  carcinoid tumors of, 452
  cystadenomas of, 452–453
Bile ducts in mesenchymal hamartoma, 598*f*
Biliary cholangitis, primary, 516–519
Biliary cirrhosis, 516*f*, 517*f*
Biliary cyst, 582*f*
Biliary cystadenomas. *See* Mucinous cystic neoplasms (MCNs)
Biliary intraepithelial neoplasia (BilIN) of gallbladder, 438–440
Biliary intraepithelial neoplasia–type changes, 444*f*
Biliary obstruction, 505
Biliary tumors bile duct hamartoma, 578–579
Bland cholestasis, 512–513, 513*f*
Bleeding
  in Dieulafoy's lesion, 88
  gastrointestinal
    in acute erosive/hemorrhagic gastritis, 53
    in chemical gastropathy, 56
    in gastric antral vascular ectasia, 84
    in schistosomiasis, 295
    in strongyloidiasis, 294
  in hemorrhoids, 410
  in mycophenolate mofetil colitis, 330
Boerhaave's syndrome, 26
Botryoid embryonal rhabdomyosarcoma, of extrahepatic bile ducts, 453
Bowenoid papulosis, 427–428
Bowen's disease, 432
Bronchogenic carcinoma, esophageal varices in, 25–26
Brunner's gland hyperplasia, 151–152, 152*f*, 463
  differential diagnosis of, 151–152
Budd-Chiari syndrome, 523, 523*f*
Burkitt lymphoma, 624*f*, 638–641, 641*b*
Buschke-Lowenstein giant condyloma, 429–430

C

C4d staining, 660–661, 661*t*, 679
Calcifying fibrous tumor, 186, 186*f*
  differential diagnosis of, 188
Calcinosis, gastric mucosal, 76
Caliber persistent artery, 88
Calymmatobacterium granulomatis infection, anal, 270–271
Campylobacter infections, 253*t*, 259, 259*f*
  and immunoproliferative small intestinal disease, 620–621
Campylobacter jejuni infection, 259*f*
Canalicular cholestasis, 513, 532*f*–533*f*
  and hepatocyte injury, 501*f*
Cancer development in Peutz-Jeghers syndrome, 346–347
Candida infection
  colonic, 273–275
    differential diagnosis of, 274*t*
  esophagitis in, 3, 14
Candida spp., 675–676
Capsulatum, histoplasma, 537*f*
Carbon tetrachloride, 532*f*–533*f*
Carcinoembryonic antigen (CEA), 569
Carcinoid tumors
  colorectal, 391–393, 392*f*
  differential diagnosis of, 195
  of extrahepatic bile ducts, 452
  gastric, 114–117

Carcinoma. *See also* Adenocarcinoma
adenosquamous, 472*f*
of anal canal, squamous cell, 415–416
of anus
differential diagnosis of, 431
squamous cell, 417*f*, 430*f*
verrucous, 426, 431
colorectal. *See* Colorectal cancer
of esophagus
intramucosal, 38–39, 38*f*
squamous cell, 42–45, 43*f*
of extrahepatic bile ducts
differential diagnosis of, 443*f*
fibrolamellar, 572–575
of gallbladder, 438–444
invasive, 446
gastric
intramucosal, 101
signet ring cell, differential diagnosis of, 99–100
in situ, 101
hepatocellular, 567–572, 568*f*. See also Hepatocellular carcinoma (HCC)
medullary, 472*f*
metastatic, 609*f*
undifferentiated, 472*f*
Cardiac-related venous congestion. *See* Congestive hepatopathy
Cast, esophageal mucosal, in caustic injury, 14–15, 15*f*
β-catenin, nuclear, in fibromatosis, 199, 199*f*
Caustic injuries of esophagus, 14–15, 15*f*
differential diagnosis of, 14–15
Cavernous hemangiomas (CHs), 557, 593*f*
CD10, 590
CD56, 589
CD system. *See* Immunohistochemistry
Celiac disease, 121–122
differential diagnosis of, 124, 645
extraintestinal disorders with, 121*t*
intestinal villi in, 121
lymphocytic gastritis in, 69
nonresponsive, 124–125
pathogenesis of, 122–124
refractory, 124–125
Cell-mediated rejection, 684–686
acute rejection, 684–685
mild acute T cell-mediated rejection, 684
moderate acute T cell-mediated rejection, 684–685
severe acute T cell-mediated rejection, 685
antibody-mediated rejection, 685–686
mild acute antibody-mediated rejection, 685
moderate acute antibody-mediated rejection, 685–686
severe acute antibody-mediated rejection, 686
Central perivenulitis, 664, 665*f*
Chagas disease, 25*f*
esophageal achalasia in, 22, 25*f*
Chancres, syphilitic, 269–270
Chemotherapy
esophagitis from, 9–11
mucositis from, 334–335, 334*f*
Chlamydia trachomatis infection, 270–271
Chloride levels in sweat in cystic fibrosis, 218
Cholangiocarcinoma (CC), 446–450, 451*f*, 583–584, 589*f*
of liver neoplasms, 586
peripheral/intrahepatic, 587*f*
Cholangitis lenta, 513
Cholate stasis, 512
Cholecystitis, 435, 436*b*
acute, 435–436, 438*f*
chronic, 435–437, 438*f*, 439, 444
differential diagnosis of, 441–443
eosinophilic, 435
epithelial changes in, 436, 438*f*
hyalinizing (of gallbladder), 436–437
xanthogranulomatous, 435–436, 437*f*, 439*f*
Choledochal cysts, 452
Choledocholithiasis, of gallbladder, 446
Choledocholiths, of gallbladder, 435–436
Choleliths, of gallbladder, 435–436
Cholestasis, 524
acute versus chronic, 512
bland, 513*f*
patterns and manifestations of, 512–513
Cholestatic pattern of injury, 512
Cholestatic steatohepatitis, 505
Cholesterolosis, of gallbladder, 435–436
Chronic antibody-mediated rejection, 686
Chronic arteriopathy, 686
Chronic ductopenic rejection, 668–669
Chronic graft fibrosis, 686–687
differential diagnosis of acute rejection, 687
acute T cell-mediated rejection, 687
islet pathology, 686–687
Chronic hepatitis pattern of injury, in liver, 496–498
Chronic inflammatory disorders, of appendix, 217*t*
Chronic pancreatitis, 459–460, 459*f*, 460*b*
Chronic passive venous congestion. *See* Congestive hepatopathy
Chronic rejection (CR), 670*f*
Chronic viral hepatitis, in liver, 498–502
Cinar cell cystadenoma, 477*f*
Cirrhosis, 553
Cloacogenic polyps of anus, inflammatory
differential diagnosis of, 372–373
Clonorchis sinensis, 448
Clostridial infection, of gut, 264
Clostridium difficile infection, 253*t*
differential diagnosis of, 255, 320–321
Coccidial infection, 287–288
Colitis
chemotherapy effect/mucositis, 334–335, 334*f*
collagenous, 315, 316*f*
collagenous gastritis with, 74
differential diagnosis of, 320–321
diversion, 323–324, 323*f*
diverticular disease-associated, 324–325, 324*f*, 325*f*
drug-induced, differential diagnosis of, 307–308
eosinophilic, 327–328, 327*f*
in Hirschsprung's disease, differential diagnosis of, 328
infections, differential diagnosis of, 307–308, 317
ischemic, 319–321, 320*f*
differential diagnosis of, 281, 307–308
lymphocytic, 318–319, 318*f*
differential diagnosis of, 317
mycophenolate mofetil, 330–331, 330*f*
nonsteroidal anti-inflammatory drug, 333–334
pseudomembranous, differential diagnosis of, 266, 294
radiation, 320–323, 322*f*
differential diagnosis of, 317
ulcerative, 301. *See also* Ulcerative colitis
Collagen in fibromatosis, 198
Collagenous disorders
colitis, 315, 316*f*
gastritis, 74, 75*f*
Collagenous sprue, 125, 126*f*
Colloid carcinoma, 471–472
Colon
AIDS enterocolopathy of, 249*f*
bacterial infections of, 253*t*
epithelial lymphocytosis of, 317
fibroblastic polyps of, benign, 189–191, 189*f*, 190*f*
fungus infections of, 273
herpesvirus infection of, 246*f*
smooth muscle tumors of, 176
submucosal leiomyoma, 177*f*
Colon cancer, metastatic, 609*f*
Colonic amebiasis, 284*f*
Colonic endometriosis, 390*f*
Colorectal cancer, 379–380, 384*f*
differential diagnosis of, 390
fungating, 381
hereditary nonpolyposis, 363
infiltrating adenomatous polyps, 379
medullary carcinoma, 385–386, 386*f*
mucinous, 383, 384*f*
necrotic material in, 384*f*
polypoid, 381
risk factors in, 363–364, 379
and serrated adenomas, 374–377
and serrated polyposis syndrome, 346
signet ring, 383, 385*f*
undifferentiated, 385–386
Colorectal carcinomas
HER2 immunohistochemistry in, 400, 401*f*
micropapillary carcinoma, 385, 385*f*
microsatellite instability testing of, 395–396
molecular oncology testing in, 400
molecular testing of, 395
morphologic features associated with microsatellite instability, 385–391
mucinous adenocarcinoma, 384*f*
signet ring cell adenocarcinoma, 385*f*
uncommon variants of, 383–385
Colorectal epithelial neoplasms, 363
adenocarcinoma, 379–380, 384*f*
adenomatous polyps, 363–365, 384*f*
colorectal carcinomas, 383–385
hyperplastic polyp (HP), 371–374, 371*f*, 372*f*
intramucosal adenocarcinoma and carcinoma in situ, 366
invasive adenocarcinoma versus misplaced epithelium, 369–370
Lynch syndrome, 380–383
malignant polyps, 367–369
microsatellite instability, morphologic features associated with, 385–391
molecular alterations, 378–379
neuroendocrine, 391–393, 392*f*
neuroendocrine neoplasms, 391–393
neuroendocrine proliferation in adenomatous polyps, 365–366
in polyposis syndromes, 337
serrated colorectal polyps, 371
serrated polyposis syndrome (SPS), 379
sessile serrated adenomas, 374–377
differential diagnosis of, 374–377
traditional serrated adenomas, 377–378, 378*f*
Colorectal polyps, 363
Combined hepatocellular–cholangiocarcinoma (HCC–CCs), 590–592, 591*f*
Common bile duct (CBD), 446
Common variable immunodeficiency, 132, 132*f*
differential diagnosis of, 132–133, 134*f*, 135
Condyloma, acuminata, differential diagnosis of, 270

Condyloma acuminatum, 410–411, 424, 425*f*
Congenital cysts, of pancreas, 457
Congenital tufting enteropathy, 136*f*
Congestive hepatopathy, 525*f*, 671–672
Congestive (cardiac) hepatopathy, in liver, 524
Constitutional MMR deficiency, 398
Conventional adenoma
  differential diagnosis, 156
  of small intestine, 154–157
Copper accumulation disorder, in liver, 542
  glycogen storage diseases, 546
  glycogenic hepatopathy, 552–553
  porphyrias, 553–555
  Wilson's disease, 542, 543*f*
Cord colitis syndrome, 332–333, 332*f*
Core antigen (HBcAg) immunohistochemistry, 501*f*
Cowden's syndrome, 352–357, 357*f*
  differential diagnosis of, 355
Cowdry's inclusions, in adenovirus infection, 220–221, 221*f*
C-reactive protein (CRP), 560
Crohn's disease, 9*f*, 137–138, 138*f*, 309
  anal, 408, 409*f*
    differential diagnosis of, 409–410
  appendix in, 214–218, 217*f*, 217*t*
  biopsy findings in, 310–311
  cytomegalovirus infection with, 243, 245*f*
  differential diagnosis of, 8–9, 139–140, 312–313
    in *Aeromonas* infection, 261
    in amebiasis, 284–285
    in cryptococcal infection, 281–283
    in cytomegalovirus infection, 245
    in diversion colitis, 322
    in ischemic colitis, 320–321
    in lymphogranuloma venereum, 270–271
    in NSAID colitis, 333
    in NSAID injury, 131
    in peptic duodenal disease, 128
    in shigellosis, 258
    in strongyloidiasis, 294
    in tuberculosis, 269
    in typhoid fever, 256–257
    in ulcerative colitis, 307–308
    in yersiniosis, 261, 261*f*
  endoscopy in, 309, 310*f*
  of esophagitis, 8–9
  gastric, 67–68, 68*f*
  gross appearance of, 310, 310*f*
  resection findings in, 311, 311*f*, 312*f*
Crohn's enterocolitis, 310*f*
  resection, 312*f*
Crohn's-like lymphoid response, 386*f*
Cronkhite-Canada syndrome (CCS), 357–360, 359*f*
  differential diagnosis of, 358
    in gastric hyperplastic polyps, 80, 95–96
    in Ménétrier's disease, 80
Cryptococcosis, colonic, 279*f*, 280–283
  differential diagnosis of, 274*t*
Cryptogenic cirrhosis, 505
Cryptosporidiosis, colonic, 288*f*
Cryptosporidium parvum, 435
Crypts, colonic
  in ischemic colitis, 320, 320*f*
  in mycophenolate mofetil colitis, 330
  in sessile serrated adenomas, 374–377
CTNNB1 gene, 480, 482
Cyclospora infection, 288–290
  differential diagnosis of, 290
Cystadenocarcinoma, 584
  of pancreas, 482
Cystadenoma
  hepatobiliary, 452–453
  of pancreas, 480–482
Cystic fibrosis, appendix in, 211, 212*f*, 218–219, 219*f*
Cystic mucinous duct lesion, 456–457
Cystic neoplasm, mucinous, 584
Cyst(s)
  congenital, of pancreas, 457
  epidermoid, of pancreas, 456
  esophageal, congenital, 18*f*
  lymphoepithelial (of pancreas), 456
Cytokeratins, 518. *See also* Immunohistochemistry
  in Barrett's esophagus, 40
  in gallbladder carcinoma, 446
  in gastric adenocarcinomas, 110–111
Cytomegalovirus, of gallbladder, 435
Cytomegalovirus hepatitis, 494
Cytomegalovirus infection, 676
  colon in, 244*f*, 245*f*
  Crohn's disease with, 243, 245*f*
  differential diagnosis of, 245
    in adenovirus infection, 248
    in chemotherapy effect/mucositis, 334
    in herpesvirus infection, 247
  esophagitis in, 3, 14
  gastritis in, 71*f*
    differential diagnosis of, 80
  in gastrointestinal tract, 243, 244*f*, 245*f*
Cytomegalovirus pancreatitis, 687
Cytoplasmic inclusions. *See* Inclusions, cellular

D

Davidson's disease, 135
De novo autoimmune hepatitis, 664
Deciduosis, appendiceal, 221–223
Deep sequencing. *See* Next-generation sequencing (NGS)
Desmin in gastrointestinal stromal tumors, 177
Desmoid fibromatosis, 198*f*, 199*f*
Desmoid tumors in familial adenomatous polyposis, 338
Developmental anomalies, of pancreas, 455
  annular pancreas, 455
  ectopic pancreas, 455
  pancreatic divisum, 455
Devon family syndrome, 360
Diabetes mellitus, hepatic glycogen. *See also* Glycogenic hepatopathy (GH)
Diarrhea
  in adenovirus infection, 247
  in *Aeromonas* infection, 263
  in AIDS enterocolopathy, 248
  in autoimmune enteropathy, 133
  in celiac disease, 121
  in *Clostridium difficile* infection, 263
  in *Escherichia coli* infection, 252
  in intestinal lymphangiectasia, 147
  in mantle cell lymphoma, 626
  in mycophenolate mofetil colitis, 330
  in necrotizing enterocolitis, 263
  in schistosomiasis, 296
  in shigellosis, 257
  in strongyloidiasis, 294
  traveler's, 252
  in typhoid fever, 255
  in ulcerative colitis, 301
  in yersiniosis, 260
Diastase resistance in granular cell tumors of anus, 431
Dietary factors in colorectal cancer, 363
Dieulafoy's lesion, gastric, 88
Diffuse large B-cell lymphoma, 630–632, 631*b*, 631*b*–632*b*, 634*f*–635*f*
  differential diagnosis of, 640, 645
Diversion colitis, 323–324, 323*f*
Diverticula
  appendiceal, 211, 212*f*
    in cystic fibrosis, 211, 218
  esophageal, 19–20, 21*f*
    differential diagnosis of, 18
  Zenker's, 20, 21*f*
Diverticular disease-associated colitis, 324–325, 324*f*, 325*f*
Donovan bodies in granuloma inguinale, 270–271
Doppler ultrasound study, 525
Downhill esophageal varices, 25–26
Down's syndrome, and celiac disease, 121
Doxycycline gastritis, 78
  differential diagnosis of, 78–79
Drug-induced disorders
  acute erosive/hemorrhagic gastritis in, 53, 54*f*
  chemical gastropathy in, 56
  colitis in, differential diagnosis of, 307–308, 312, 320–321
  iron pill gastritis in, 77
  NSAID injury in, 130–131
    differential diagnosis of, 131
    and peptic ulcer disease, 126, 129
  parietal cell hyperplasia from proton pump inhibitors, 92*f*
  pill esophagitis in, 11–12, 12*f*
Drug-induced liver injury (DILI), 489–490, 530–531, 532*f*–533*f*, 534*t*
Ductal adenocarcinoma, pancreatic, 471–474, 471*f*
Ductal cholestasis, 513
Ductal neoplasms, of pancreas, 464–466
  intraductal papillary mucinous neoplasm (IPMN), 466–469
  intraductal tubulopapillary neoplasm, 470–471
  mucinous cystic neoplasm, 469–470
  pancreatic ductal adenocarcinoma, 471–474
  pancreatic intraepithelial neoplasia, 464–466
  precursor lesions, 464
Ductal–neuroendocrine carcinoma, of pancreas, 484
Ductopenia, 536–537
Ductular cholestasis, 513
Ductular reaction or proliferation, 513
Duodenal adenoma, 154*f*
Duodenal diverticula, 458*f*
Duodenal diverticulum, of pancreas, 458
Duodenum
  gangliocytic paraganglioma in, 194, 195*f*
  "lipid hang-up" biopsy of, 128–129, 128*f*
  normal biopsy findings in, 127*f*
  peptic disease of, 126–129, 127*f*, 128*f*
    differential diagnosis of, 128
  well-differentiated neuroendocrine tumor of, 160*f*, 161*f*
Dysphagia, 440*b*
  in adenomatous polyps, 364–365
  in Barrett's esophagus, 35–38, 36*f*, 37*f*
  in caustic esophageal injury, 14–15
  colorectal epithelial, in sessile serrated adenomas, 374–377
  in Crohn's disease, 313–314
  differential diagnosis, 441–443
  in eosinophilic esophagitis, 4
  in esophageal diverticula, 19–20
  in esophageal motility disorders, 22–24
  of gallbladder, 437, 446–447
  gastric epithelial, 101–104
    differential diagnosis of, 103
  high-grade, 441*f*
  intestinal epithelial, 136
  low-grade, 440*f*
  in radiation esophagitis, 14
  in ulcerative colitis, 305–309, 306*f*

Dysplasia and early gallbladder carcinoma, 438–444, 442*b*
Dysplastic nodules (DNs), 564–567, 566*f*

E

Ectasia
  gastric antral vascular, 84, 85*f*, 86*t*
    differential diagnosis of, 84, 86*t*, 88
Ectopia, esophageal epithelial, 15*f*
Ectopic pancreas, 455
Ectopic pancreatic tissue in Meckel's diverticulum, 456*f*
Embryonal rhabdomyosarcoma, botryoid, of extrahepatic bile ducts, 453
Embryonal sarcoma of liver, 604–606, 606*f*
Encephalitozoon intestinalis infection, 288–289
Endocrine neoplasms. *See* Neuroendocrine tumors
Endometrioma of colon, 390
Endometriosis, 156
  appendiceal, 221–223, 222*f*
  colonic, 390*f*
Endoscopic retrograde cholangiopancreatography (ERCP), 446–447, 455
Endoscopy
  in Crohn's disease, 310, 310*f*
  in ulcerative colitis, 301, 302*f*
Endothelial lining, denudation of, 671*f*
Enema effect, differential diagnosis of, 317
Entamoeba histolytica infection, 283, 284*f*
Enteric (typhoid) fever, 255, 257*f*
Enteric ischemic disease, 142*f*, 145–147
Enteritis
  infectious, 147
  regional. *See* Crohn's disease
Enterobiasis, 290*f*, 291
Enterobius, appendicitis in, 220, 220*f*
Enterobius vermicularis, 220, 220*f*
Enterochromaffin-like cells, hyperplasia of in autoimmune gastritis, 62
Enterocolitis
  granulomatous. *See* Crohn's disease
  necrotizing, 264
    differential diagnosis of, 266, 328
Enterocolopathy in AIDS, 248, 249*f*
Enterocytes, apoptotic, in AIDS enterocolopathy, 249*f*
Enterocytozoon bieneusi infection, 288–289
Enteroendocrine cell dysgenesis, 136–137
Enteropathy
  autoimmune, 133–135, 134*f*
  gluten-induced. *See* Gluten-sensitive enteropathy
  in T-cell lymphoma, 125, 125*f*, 643–647, 644*f*–645*f*, 646*b*
  tufting, 136
Eosinophilic disorders
  cholecystitis, 435–436
  esophagitis, 4, 5*f*
    differential diagnosis of, 3, 6
  gastritis, 72, 74*f*
Eosinophilic esophagitis
  differential diagnosis of, 6
  endoscopy of, 5*f*
  of esophagus, 4–6
  intraepithelial eosinophils, 6*f*
Eosinophilic gastroenteritis (EGE), 143–144
  differential diagnosis of, 144
Eosinophilic inflammation, intact villi with, 119–120
Eosinophilic proctocolitis, 327–328, 327*f*
Epidermoid cyst, of pancreas, 456
Epidermoid cyst in an intrapancreatic accessory spleen (ECIPAS), 456
Epidermoid metaplasia, 16
Epithelial membrane antigen, luminal expression of, 589
Epithelial neoplasms of colorectum, 363
Epithelial tumors hepatocellular tumors focal nodular hyperplasia, 557
Epithelioid cells in gangliocytic paraganglioma, 195*f*
Epithelioid hemangioendothelioma (EHE), of liver neoplasms, 590, 602–604
Epithelioid inflammatory myofibroblastic sarcoma, 203*f*
Epithelium
  in cholecystitis, 436, 438*f*
  gastric, dysplasia of, 101–104
Epstein-Barr virus (EBV), of gallbladder, 444–445
Epstein-Barr virus hepatitis, 493, 495*f*, 496*f*, 676
Epstein-Barr virus infection and Burkitt lymphoma, 638*b*
Epstein-Barr virus–related posttransplantation lymphoproliferative disorder, 687
Erosive gastritis, acute, 53
Erythropoietic protoporphyria (EPP), 553
Escherichia coli infection, 252
  differential diagnosis of, 272–273
  enteroadherent, 252, 253*t*, 254*f*
  enterohemorrhagic, 252, 253*t*, 254*f*
    differential diagnosis of, 320–321
  enteroinvasive, 252
  enteropathogenic, 252, 253*t*
  enterotoxigenic, 252
Esophageal carcinoma, risk factors for, 34–35
Esophageal hyperkeratosis, 16
Esophageal neuroendocrine carcinoma, differential diagnosis of, 48
Esophageal papillomatosis, 30*f*
Esophagitis, 1–4, 2*f*
  differential diagnosis of, 3
  eosinophilic, 4, 5*f*, 6*f*
    differential diagnosis of, 3, 6
  graft-versus-host disease, 9
  infectious, 15*f*
    differential diagnosis of, 3, 6, 14–15
  inflammatory disorders, 1–2
    reflux esophagitis, 1
  pill, 11–12, 12*f*
    differential diagnosis of, 3, 11–12
  from radiation/chemotherapy, 9
  reflux, 1, 2*f*, 3*f*
    differential diagnosis of, 3, 6, 11–12, 14–15
Esophagitis dissecans superficialis, 12–14
Esophagus
  adenocarcinoma of, 39–42
  atresia of, 17–19, 17*f*
    tracheoesophageal fistula with, 17–19, 18*f*
  atypical lipomatous tumor, 30–31
  Barrett's, 32–34
  carcinoma of, intramucosal, 38–39, 38*f*
  caustic injuries of, 14–15, 15*f*
    differential diagnosis of, 14–15
  cysts of, congenital, 18*f*
  diverticula of, 19–22, 21*f*
  duplications of, 18*f*
  ectopias of, 15*f*
  eosinophilic esophagitis, 4–6
  gastroesophageal reflux disease (GERD), 1
  granular cell tumors of
    differential diagnosis of, 40–41
Esophagus (*Continued*)
  heterotopic sebaceous glands in, 15
  lichenoid esophagitis, 8
  lymphocytic esophagitis, 6–8
  motility disorders of, 22–24, 23*f*, 25*f*
  mucosal cast in caustic injury, 14–15, 15*f*
  neuroendocrine neoplasms of, 48
  non-neoplastic disorders of, 1
  papillomas of, squamous, 30–31, 30*f*
  perforations and tears in, 25–27
  polyps of, fibrovascular, 30–31
  polyps of, giant fibrovascular, 31*f*
  reflux esophagitis, 1, 2*f*, 3*f*
  salivary gland type tumors, 46
  secondary tumors of, 49–50
  squamous cell carcinoma of, 42–45, 43*f*
  squamous papillomas of, 29–30, 30*f*
  stenosis of, congenital, 19*f*
  stromal tumors in, 169
  structural abnormalities of, 17–19
    acquired, 19–22
    congenital, 17–19
  tumors of, 29
  undifferentiated carcinoma, 45
  varices in, 25–27, 26*f*
  webs and rings of, 19–22, 20*f*
Essile serrated polyp/adenoma (SSP/A), 375*f*, 376*f*
Ex goblet cell carcinoid, 237, 239*f*
Extended criteria, 657
Extrahepatic bile ducts, 446–448
  carcinoma of, 448–452, 449*b*, 450*b*
    invasive carcinoma, 450–451
    precursor neoplasia, 449–450
  inflammatory disorders of, 446–447, 447*b*, 448*b*
  intraductal papillary neoplasms of, 450*f*
  mesenchymal tumors of, 453
  mucinous cystic neoplasm of, 453*f*
Extrahepatic CC, 451–452

F

False-positive staining, 402
Familial adenomatous polyposis, 337, 340*f*, 341*f*
  differential diagnosis of, 341–343
Fatty liver disease, 505
  nonalcoholic, 505–509
Ferroportin disease (type B), 539*t*
Fibroblastic polyps of colon, benign, 189–191, 189*f*, 190*f*
Fibrolamellar carcinoma, of liver neoplasms, 572–575
Fibrolamellar hepatocellular carcinoma, 573*f*, 574*f*
Fibromatosis
  intraabdominal, 198–200, 198*f*
  mesenteric, 198*f*
    differential diagnosis of, 199
Fibrosarcoma, inflammatory, 202–205
Fibrosing cholestatic hepatitis (FCH), 498–501, 672–673
Fibrosing cholestatic hepatitis C, 502, 674*f*
Fibrosis, 533
  portal based, 501*f*
Fibrous obliteration, of appendix, 212*f*
Fissures, anal, 407–408
Fistulas
  anal, 407
  tracheoesophageal, esophageal atresia with, 17–19, 18*f*
Florid duct lesions, 515–517
Focal nodular hyperplasia (FNH), 557, 558*f*
Follicular lymphoma, 623–626, 624*f*
Food poisoning in *Salmonella* infection, 255

Foveola, gastric
in adenomas, 102
hyperplasia of, 95–96
differential diagnosis of, 95–96
metaplasia in peptic duodenitis, 127, 127*f*, 128*f*
Frozen section, 484–487, 486*f*, 487*f*
diagnosis of pancreatic ductal adenocarcinoma on, 485
of donor liver biopsy with steatosis, 658*f*
resection margins, evaluation of, 485–487
bile duct margin, 486–487
parenchymal margin, 485–486
tissue adjacent to superior mesenteric artery/hepatic artery, 487
Fundic gland polyps, 91–94, 92*f*
differential diagnosis of, 93, 95–96
Fungus infections
colonic, 273
differential diagnosis of, 274*t*

G

Gallbladder, 435–438
adenomyoma of, 438*f*
advanced gallbladder carcinoma, 444–446
carcinoma of, 435, 438–444
invasive, 449–450
cholecystitis of, 435
dysplasia and early gallbladder carcinoma, 438–444
early invasive lesions in, 442–443
gallbladder dysplasia and carcinoma, 437
invasive adenocarcinoma of, 445*f*
mesenchymal tumors of, 453
metaplasia of, 436
pyloric gland adenoma of, 442*f*
reactive changes in, 443*f*
undifferentiated gallbladder carcinoma, 445*f*
xanthogranulomatous cholecystitis of, 435–436, 437*f*, 439*f*
Gallbladder carcinoma, 446*b*
Gamma-glutamyl transferase (GGT), 511
Gangliocytic paraganglioma, 163, 163*f*, 194–196
Ganglioneuroma, 193*f*
differential diagnosis of
in neurofibroma, 192–194
in perineurioma, 192–194
Ganglioneuromatosis, diffuse, 192, 193*f*
Ganglionitis in esophageal achalasia, 23*f*
Ganglion-like cells in gangliocytic paraganglioma, 194, 194*f*, 195*f*
Gangrenous appendicitis, 214
Gardner's syndrome, 198, 338
Gastric adenocarcinoma
differential diagnosis of, 111
risk factors of, 107–108
Gastric amyloidosis, 82
differential diagnosis of, 84
Gastric amyloids, 64–67, 83*f*, 84*f*
differential diagnosis of, 75
Gastric antral vascular ectasia (GAVE), 57
Gastric carcinoma, gross appearance of, 108*f*
Gastric Crohn's disease, 68, 68*f*
Gastric foveolar-type metaplasia, 152*f*
Gastric heterotopia, 152–153, 152*f*
differential diagnosis of, 152
of small intestine, 152
Gastric heterotopia inlet patch, 15, 15*f*
Gastric peptic ulcer disease, 63
differential diagnosis of, 63
Gastric polyps, in stomach, 91
Gastric schwannoma, 187*f*, 188*f*
Gastric secondary tumors, 113
Gastric-type epithelium, 584
Gastric-type intraductal papillary mucinous neoplasm, 467*f*
Gastrin levels in Zollinger-Ellison syndrome, 80
Gastrinoma
in multiple endocrine neoplasia type I, 81
in Zollinger-Ellison syndrome, 81
Gastritis
acute erosive/hemorrhagic, 53, 54*f*
autoimmune, 64, 64*t*, 67*t*
chronic atrophic, and gastric carcinoids, 115
differential diagnosis of, 59, 62, 67*t*
collagenous, 74, 75*f*
colitis with, 74
differential diagnosis of, 75
cystica glandularis, differential diagnosis of, 95–96
cystica polyposa, 96–97
differential diagnosis of, 96–97
eosinophilic, 72, 74*f*
granulomatous, 67–68, 67*t*
differential diagnosis of, 67*t*
in gastric Crohn's disease, 67–68
in sarcoidosis, 68
Helicobacter heilmannii in, 61, 62*f*
Helicobacter pylori in, 57, 58*t*, 59*f*, 60*f*, 61*f*, 61*t*
infectious, 71
parasitic, 71, 79*f*
viral, 71*f*
ischemic, differential diagnosis of, 84
lymphocytic, 69, 70*f*
radiation, differential diagnosis of, 75
Gastroesophageal junction
inflammation of, 17
intestinal metaplasia of, 17
Gastrointestinal neoplasms
colorectal carcinoma, molecular testing of, 395
HER2 in colorectal carcinoma, 400
HER2 testing in upper gastrointestinal tract adenocarcinoma, 400–404
background and rationale, 400–401
immunohistochemistry, 402
in situ hybridization, 403
PD-1/PDL-1 in esophageal and gastric carcinomas, 403–404
specimen type, 402
mismatch repair function, assessment of, 395–400
future directions of molecular testing in colorectal carcinoma, 400
microsatellite instability-high carcinoma: sporadic versus lynch syndrome, 396–397
mismatch repair immunohistochemistry in, 397–399
polymerase chain reaction–based microsatellite instability testing, 395–396
RAS, extended RAS, and BRAF testing, 399–400
molecular testing of, 395
Gastrointestinal stromal tumors (GISTs), 156, 169–176, 171*f*
dedifferentiated, 173*f*
differential diagnosis of, 175
in glomus tumors, 195
in neurofibromas, 191–192
epithelioid, 173*f*
platelet-derived growth factor receptor-a (PDGFRA) in, 172*f*
risk defined in, 172–173
small intestinal, 172*f*
succinate dehydrogenase (SDH) in, 172*f*
Gastrointestinal tract
adenovirus infection of, 247
AIDS enterocolopathy of, 248
bacterial enterocolitis in, 252
bacterial infections
Sarcina ventriculi, 249–250, 250*f*
Tropheryma whipplei, 250–251
bacterial infections in, 249
clear cell sarcoma-like tumor of, 180–182
cytomegalovirus infection in, 243
herpesvirus infection of, 246–247
infectious disease of, 243
parasitic infections of, 283
viral infections of, 243
Gaucher disease, 549*t*, 550*t*
Genetic factors
in celiac disease, 122–123
in gastric adenomas, 101–104
in gastric cancers, 107–108
in multiple endocrine neoplasia type 2, 360
in neurofibromatosis type 1, 360
in squamous cell carcinoma of anus, 416–417
Giant fibrovascular polyp, 30–31, 31*f*
Gliomatosis peritonei, appendix in, 221–222
Glomus tumors, 196–198, 197*f*
gastric, differential diagnosis of, 116
Glutamine synthetase (GS) immunostain, 560
Gluten-sensitive enteropathy, 121
differential diagnosis of, 621–622
Glycogenated nuclei, 508
Glycogen storage diseases, in liver, 546, 547*t*
Glycogenic hepatopathy (GH), 552–553, 552*f*
GNAS mutations, 470
Goblet cell adenocarcinoma (GCA), 237, 238*f*, 239*f*
Goblet cell carcinoid (GCC), 237, 238*f*, 239*f*, 240*f*
differential diagnosis of, 237
Goblet cell–rich hyperplastic polyp, 373*f*
Goblet cells
in adenomatous polyps, 365
in autoimmune enteropathy, 134–135
in Barrett's esophagus, 32, 33*f*
carcinoid, 238*f*, 239*f*, 240*f*
differential diagnosis of, 237
in cystic fibrosis, 219, 219*f*
in Peutz-Jeghers syndrome, 347–348
Gonorrhea, 271
Graft-versus-host disease, 140–141, 142*f*
and adenovirus infection, 247
differential diagnosis of, 9, 245, 330, 334
Granular cell tumor, 179–180, 179*f*
anal, differential diagnosis of, 418
differential diagnosis of, 179–180
gastric, differential diagnosis of, 99–100
Granulocytic epithelial lesions, 460–461
in type 2 autoimmune pancreatitis, 462*f*
Granuloma, 532*f*–533*f*
in colonic tuberculosis, 269
in Crohn's disease of anus, 409–410, 409*f*
inguinale, differential diagnosis of, 270–271
in liver and common associations, 538*t*
Granulomatous appendicitis, 218
Granulomatous disorders
appendicitis, idiopathic, 217*t*
enterocolitis. *See* Crohn's disease
gastritis, 67–68, 67*t*, 68*f*, 69*f*, 70*f*
Groove pancreatitis, 153*f*
"Groove" pancreatitis, 462–463, 463*b*
Guillain-Barré syndrome in *Campylobacter* infection, 259
GVHD. *See* Graft-versus-host disease

H

Halo effect around yeast forms, 279*f*, 280
Halothane, 532*f*–533*f*
Hamartoma, 151–152
  differential diagnosis of, 151–152
  mesenchymal, 595, 597*f*
  pancreatic, 455–456, 457*f*
  "Schwann cell," 192
Hamartoma polyposis syndromes, 346–350
Helicobacter heilmannii gastritis, 61, 62*f*
Helicobacter pylori infection
  and diffuse large B-cell lymphoma, 630–632, 631*b*, 631*b*–632*b*
  and gastric cancer risk, 107
  gastritis in, 57, 58*t*, 59*f*, 60*f*, 61*f*, 61*t*
    differential diagnosis of, 54–55, 57, 59, 61–62, 71, 80
    and gastric xanthomas, 99–100
    lymphocytic, 69
  and gastroesophageal reflux disease, 15
  and immunoproliferative small intestinal disease, 620–621
  and MALT lymphomas, 614
    immunoproliferative small intestinal disease, 614
  and peptic duodenitis, 126, 128
Helminth infection, colonic, 290
Helminthic infections, 290
Hemangioendothelioma, epithelioid, 602–604
Hemangioma, infantile, 593–595, 596*f*
Hematopoietic stem cell transplantation (HSCT), 525
Hematoxylin
  and eosin-stained section of failed pancreatic transplant excision, 686*f*
  and eosin-stained section of pancreas, 684*f*
  and eosin-stained section of pancreas allograft biopsy, 686*f*
Hemochromatosis, 539*t*
Hemorrhagic gastritis, acute, 53
Hemorrhoids, 410, 411*f*
Hepatic adenoma (HA), of liver neoplasms, 557, 560–564, 561*f*, 562*f*
  classification of, 562*t*
Hepatic adenomatosis, 560–561
Hepatic angiomyolipomas, 598, 599*f*
Hepatic angiosarcoma (HAS), 600–601
Hepatic artery, tissue adjacent to, 487
Hepatic artery stenosis (HAS), 669–670
Hepatic artery thrombosis (HAT), 669–670, 671*f*
Hepatic granulomas, in liver, 537
Hepatic iron index (HII), 541
Hepatic lymphoma, primary, 606–607, 607*f*
Hepatic manifestations, glycogen storage diseases with, 547*t*
Hepatic mass lesions, 558*t*
Hepatic venous outflow obstruction (HVOO), 523, 671–672
Hepatis, peliosis, 530
Hepatitis
  acute viral (hepatotropic), 491
  autoimmune, 502–505
  viral, 491*t*
Hepatitis B core antigen (HBcAg), 501
Hepatitis B virus (HBV), 499
Hepatitis C virus (HCV) genotype 3 infection, 499
Hepatobiliary cystadenomas, 452–453, 584
Hepatoblastoma, of liver neoplasms, 575–578, 576*f*, 577*f*
Hepatocanalicular cholestasis, 513
Hepatocellular carcinoma (HCC), 557, 568*f*, 570*f*, 573*f*
  of liver neoplasms, 567–572
Hepatocellular–cholangiocarcinoma (HCC–CCs), of liver neoplasms, 590–592, 591*f*
Hepatocellular cholestasis, 513
Hepatocyte regeneration, 504*f*
Hepatoid carcinoma, 471–472
Hepatopathy, congestive, 524, 525*f*
Hepatoportal sclerosis (HPS), 527–528, 529*f*
Hepatosplenic T-cell lymphoma, 649–651, 650*f*, 651*b*
Herbal and dietary supplement (HDS), 531
Hereditary hemochromatosis (HH), in liver, 539
Hereditary mixed polyposis syndrome, 360, 360*f*
Hereditary non polyposis CRC syndrome. *See* Lynch syndrome
HER2 fluorescence in situ hybridization, 402*f*
HER2 in colorectal carcinoma, 400
Herpes simplex hepatitis, 495*f*
Herpes simplex virus (HSV) infection, 495, 676
Herpesvirus infection
  of colon, 246*f*
  differential diagnosis of
    in chemotherapy effect/mucositis, 334
    in esophagitis, 10
  esophagitis in, 3, 14
    differential diagnosis of, 10
  in gastrointestinal tract, 246–247
HER2 testing algorithm, 403*f*
HER2 testing in upper gastrointestinal tract adenocarcinoma, 400–404
  background and rationale, 400–401
  immunohistochemistry, 402
  in situ hybridization, 403
  PD-1/PDL-1 in esophageal and gastric carcinomas, 403–404
  specimen type, 402
Heterotopia
  gastric
    differential diagnosis of, 128
    in esophagus, 15*f*
  pancreatic, 97–99, 98*f*
    differential diagnosis of, 98–99
  sebaceous gland, in esophagus, 15*f*
Heterotopic sebaceous glands, in esophagus, 15, 15*f*
HFE mutation, 539
Hidradenoma papilliferum, 423, 424*f*
  differential diagnosis of, 423
High-grade appendiceal mucinous neoplasms, 228
  differential diagnosis of, 229–231
Hirschsprung's disease, colitis in, differential diagnosis of, 328
Histiocytic infiltrates in histoplasmosis, 279, 279*f*
Histiocytosis, Langerhans' cell, differential diagnosis of, 73
Histologic patterns of liver injury
  acute, 489–490
    acute viral (hepatotropic) hepatitis, 491
    alcoholic liver disease, 509–513
    autoimmune hepatitis, 502–505
    chronic hepatitis pattern of injury, 496–498
    chronic viral hepatitis, 498–502
    fatty liver disease/steatohepatitis pattern of injury, 505
    nonalcoholic fatty liver disease, 505–509
    nonhepatotropic viral infections, 493
  major, 489
Histoplasma capsulatum, 537*f*
Histoplasmosis, colonic, 278–280, 279*f*
  differential diagnosis of, 274*t*, 287
HIV infection
  adenovirus infection in, 247
  and AIDS enterocolopathy, 248, 249*f*
  anal condylomata in, 424
  in Burkitt lymphoma, 638
  coccidial infection in, 287–288
  cryptosporidiosis in, 288*f*
  salmonellosis in, 255
  and squamous cell carcinoma of anus, 417–418
HMB-45 stain in melanoma of anus, 421–422
HNF1α gene, 562–564
HNF1A-mutated adenomas (HAs), 563*f*
Homosexual men
  amebiasis in, 283
  anorectal syphilis in, 269
  gonorrhea in, 271
  herpetic proctitis in, 246
  infectious proctocolitis in, 270
  intestinal spirochetosis in, 271
Hookworms, 292
Human epidermal growth factor receptor 2 (HER2), 400
"Humoral" rejection. *See* Antibody-mediated rejection (AMR)
Hyalinizing cholecystitis (HC), of gallbladder, 435–437
Hyalinizing chronic cholecystitis, 439*f*
Hyperacute rejection, 660
Hyperbilirubinemia, 502
Hypereosinophilic syndrome, 73
Hyperplastic polyposis syndrome, 343
Hyperplastic polyp(s) (HP), 371–374
  colorectal, 371–374, 371*f*, 372*f*
    differential diagnosis of, 372–373
  gastric, 94–96, 95*f*
  goblet cell–rich, 373*f*
Hypersensitivity reactions, 531
Hypertension, portal
  duodenopathy in, 128
  esophageal varices in, 25–26
  gastropathy in, 86*t*, 87, 88*f*
Hypertrophied anal papilla. *See* Anal tag

I

Idiopathic duct-centric chronic pancreatitis, 460
Idiopathic inflammatory bowel disease, 299–300
Idiopathic posttransplant chronic hepatitis. *See* Posttransplant chronic hepatitis
IgG4 cholangitis, 520
IgG4-related esophageal disease, 9
IgG4 sclerosing cholangitis, 447
Ileal pouch enteritis, 314–315
  differential diagnosis of, 314–315
Ileitis
  backwash, 301–302
  terminal. *See* Crohn's disease
Ileocecal tuberculosis, 267
Ileum, 161
Immune checkpoint receptor inhibitor–associated colitis, 331–332
Immunohistochemistry
  in celiac disease, 121
  in deciduosis of gastrointestinal tract, 222–223
  in endometriosis of gastrointestinal tract, 222–223
  in fibroblastic polyps of colon, benign, 190
  in fibromatosis, 199, 199*f*
  in gastrointestinal stromal tumors, 171–172
  in lymphangioma, 205–206
  in MALT lymphomas, 616
  in neurofibroma, 191
  in PEComa, 207
  in perineurioma, 190
  in schwannomas, 178
  in smooth muscle tumors, 177

Immunoproliferative small intestinal disease, 614–616, 620–623, 622*b*
Incidental pigmentation, 148–149
  pseudomelanosis duodeni, 149*f*
Inclusions, cellular
  in adenovirus infection, 220–221, 221*f*, 247
    differential diagnosis of, 245
  Cowdry's, in adenovirus infection, 220–221, 221*f*
  in cytomegalovirus infection, 244, 244*f*
  herpetic, 246, 246*f*
  hyaline. *See* Mallory hyaline
  in microvillus inclusion disease, 135–136, 135*f*, 136*f*
  owl's eye, in cytomegalovirus infection, 244, 244*f*
Indeterminate for rejection, 665–666
Infantile hemangioendothelioma. *See* infantile hemangioma (IH)
Infantile hemangioma (IH), 593–595, 596*f*
Infectious disorders
  colitis in, differential diagnosis of
    in Crohn's disease, 312–313
    in diversion colitis, 322
    in eosinophilic proctocolitis, 328
    in lymphocytic colitis, 317
    in ulcerative colitis, 307–308
  enteritis in, 147
  esophagitis in, 14, 15*f*
    differential diagnosis of, 3, 6, 10–12
  in gastrointestinal tract, 243
  gastritis in, 71, 71*f*, 73*f*, 74*f*
Infectious enteritis, 147
Infiltrating adenocarcinoma, 471*f*
Inflammatory bowel disease, idiopathic, 299–300
Inflammatory disorders
  anal processes, 407–408
  bowel disease
    chronic, differential diagnosis of, 317
    Crohn's disease, 309
    pseudopolyps in, 351–352
    ulcerative colitis, 301
  cloacogenic polyps
    differential diagnosis of, 372–373
  colitides
    collagenous colitis, 315, 316*f*
    diversion colitis, 323–324, 323*f*
    diverticular disease-associated colitis, 324–325, 324*f*, 325*f*
    eosinophilic proctocolitis, 327*f*, 328
    ischemic colitis, 319–321, 320*f*
    lymphocytic colitis, 318–319, 318*f*
    mucosal prolapse/solitary rectal ulcer syndrome, 325–327, 326*f*
    radiation colitis, 320–321, 322*f*
  collagenous colitis, 316*f*
  pseudopolyps, differential diagnosis of, 351–352
Inflammatory fibroid polyp, 183*f*
  differential diagnosis of, 183–184
Inflammatory myofibroblastic tumor, 202–205
Injury, liver
  acute hepatitis pattern of, 489–490
    acute viral (hepatotropic) hepatitis, 491
    alcoholic liver disease, 509–513
    autoimmune hepatitis, 502–505
    chronic hepatitis pattern of injury, 496–498
    chronic viral hepatitis, 498–502
    fatty liver disease/steatohepatitis pattern of injury, 505
    nonalcoholic fatty liver disease, 505–509
    nonhepatotropic viral infections, 493
  major histologic patterns of, 489
Interface hepatitis, 499
  and lobular activity, 504*f*
Interlobular bile ducts in PSC, 521*f*
Interval appendix, 214–215, 214*f*
Intestinal disorders
  angina, 145
  metaplasia
    in Barrett's esophagus, 33*f*
Intestinal failure (IF), 676
Intestinal metaplasia, of gallbladder, 436
Intestinal-type neuroendocrine cells, 439*f*
Intestines
  large. *See* Colitis; Colon; Colorectal cancer
  small. *See* Small bowel disorders
Intracholecystic papillary neoplasm (ICPN) of gallbladder, 438–441
Intracholecystic papillary tubular neoplasm of gallbladder, 441*f*
Intraductal papillary mucinous neoplasm (IPMN), of pancreas, 466–469, 466*f*, 467*f*
Intraductal papillary neoplasm of the bile duct (IPNB), 449–450, 449*f*
Intraductal papillary neoplasms (IPNs), 584
Intraductal tubulopapillary neoplasm, of pancreas, 470–471, 470*f*
Intraepithelial neoplasia, pancreatic, 464–466
Intraluminal neutrophils, 514
Intrapancreatic spleen, of pancreas, 456
Invasive adenocarcinoma
  of gallbladder, 441
  versus misplaced epithelium, 369–370
Invasive carcinoma, of extrahepatic bile ducts, 450–451
Invasive mucinous adenocarcinoma, in polyp, 370*f*
Ipilimumab colitis, 331*f*
Iron-deficiency anemia in gastric antral vascular ectasia, 84–85
Iron overload, in liver, 540–541
Iron-related genes, common mutations in, 539*t*
Ischemia-reperfusion injury (IRI), 658
Ischemic colitis, 319–321, 320*f*
  differential diagnosis of, 320–321
    in radiation colitis, 320–321
    in ulcerative colitis, 307–308
Ischemic disease, enteric, 142*f*, 145–147
Islet cell transplantation, 681
Islets of Langerhans, 455–456
Isospora belli infection, 289
Ito cell hyperplasia, 537

J

Juvenile polyposis syndrome, 350–352, 353*f*–354*f*
  differential diagnosis of, 351–352

K

Kala-azar, 286
Kayser-Fleischer rings, 542
Keratinization, anal
  in condylomata, 424
  in squamous cell carcinoma, 415–416, 417*f*
  in verrucous carcinoma, 429–430
Keratoderma, nonepidermolytic palmoplantar, 35
Killian's triangle, 20
Klatskin tumor, 448
Klebsiella oxytoca infection, 267
Koilocytes in anal condylomata, 424
KRAS mutations, 400, 441, 450–451, 465, 476, 585
Kupffer cells, 492, 561

L

Lamina propria mucosae
  amyloid deposits in, 83*f*
  in autoimmune enteropathy, 134, 134*f*
  fibrosis in gastritis, 75
Langerhans' cell histiocytosis, differential diagnosis of, 73
Large duct obstruction, 513–516
Left-sided disease in ulcerative colitis, 301
Leiomyoblastomas, 172*f*
Leiomyoma, 176
Leiomyosarcoma, 176, 178*f*
Leishmaniasis, visceral, 286
  differential diagnosis of, 287
Leukemia
  chronic lymphocytic, anorectal herpetic inclusions in, 246*f*
  NK leukemia, differential diagnosis of, 649–650
Lichen planus, of esophagus, 8
Lichenoid esophagitis
  Crohn's disease, 8
  differential diagnosis of, 8
  graft-versus-host disease, 8
"Lipid hang-up" duodenal biopsy, 128–129, 128*f*
Lipogranulomas, 508
Liver
  acute hepatitis pattern of injury, 489–490, 490*f*
    acute viral (hepatotropic) hepatitis, 491
    alcoholic liver disease, 509–513
    autoimmune hepatitis, 502–505
    chronic hepatitis pattern of injury, 496–498
    chronic viral hepatitis, 498–502
    fatty liver disease/steatohepatitis pattern of injury, 505
    nonalcoholic fatty liver disease, 505–509
    nonhepatotropic viral infections, 493
  "almost normal" biopsy or nonspecific findings, 535–537, 535*t*, 536*f*
    hepatic granulomas, 537
    necrosis, 537–538
  bile ducts, disorders of, 513
    Budd-Chiari syndrome, 523, 523*f*
    congestive (cardiac) hepatopathy, 524
    drug-induced liver injury, 530–531
    hepatoportal sclerosis, 528
    large duct obstruction, 513–516
    nodular regenerative hyperplasia, 527
    overlap syndromes, 522
    peliosis hepatis, 530, 530*f*
    portal vein thrombosis or obstruction, 526–527
    primary biliary cholangitis, 516–519
    primary sclerosing cholangitis (PSC), 519
    sinusoidal obstruction syndrome (SOS), 525
    vascular pattern of injury, 522–523
  carcinoma of
    hepatocellular. *See* Hepatocellular carcinoma (HCC)
  copper accumulation disorder, 542
    glycogenic hepatopathy, 552–553
    glycogen storage diseases, 546
    porphyrias, 553–555
    Wilson's disease, 542, 543*f*
  embryonal sarcoma of, 606*f*
  major histologic patterns of injury, 489
  metabolic diseases, 538
    hereditary hemochromatosis (HH), 539
    iron overload, 540–541
    secondary iron overload, 541–542, 542*f*
  T-cell lymphoma, hepatosplenic, 649–651, 650*f*, 651*b*

Liver biopsy, 657
Liver disease, alcoholic, 509–513
Liver injury patterns, drug-induced, 534*t*
Liver necrosis, common entities associated with, 538*t*
Liver neoplasms
  angiomyolipoma, 598–600
  bile duct adenoma, 579
  biliary tumors bile duct hamartoma, 578–579
  cholangiocarcinoma (CC), 586
  combined hepatocellular–cholangiocarcinoma (HCC–CCs), 590–592, 591*f*
  dysplastic nodules (DNs), 564–567
  embryonal sarcoma of the liver, 604–606
  epithelial tumors hepatocellular tumors focal nodular hyperplasia, 557
  epithelioid hemangioendothelioma, 602–604
  fibrolamellar carcinoma, 572–575
  hepatic adenoma (HA), 560–564
  hepatoblastoma, 575–578
  hepatocellular carcinoma, 567–572
  infantile hemangioma (IH), 593–595
  macroregenerative nodules (MRNs), 564–567
  malignant angiosarcoma, 600–602
  mesenchymal hamartoma, 595
  mesenchymal tumors benign hemangioma, 592–593
  metastases, 607–611
  mucinous cystic neoplasm, 584
  polycystic liver disease, 583–584
  primary hepatic lymphoma, 606–607
  solitary biliary cyst, 580–583
Liver transplantation, 657
  acute cellular rejection, 663–668
    differential diagnosis of, 666–667
  antibody-mediated rejection, 660
    differential diagnosis of, 661–663
  biliary complications of, 672
  chronic ductopenic rejection, 668–669
    differential diagnosis of, 668–669
  complications of, 669–670
    hepatic artery stenosis (HAS), 669–670
    hepatic artery thrombosis (HAT), 669–670, 671*f*
  congestive hepatopathy, 671–672
  differential diagnosis of, 659
  hepatic venous outflow obstruction (HVOO), 671–672
  laboratory findings of, 658–660
  portal hyperperfusion (PHP), 670–671
  preservation/ischemia-reperfusion injury, 658
  pretransplant donor evaluation, 657–658
  recurrent disease, 672–676
    fibrosing cholestatic hepatitis (FCH), 673
    opportunistic infections, 675–676, 676*f*
    posttransplant lymphoproliferative disorder (PTLD), 675
    recurrent autoimmune hepatitis, 674
    recurrent fatty liver disease, 675
    recurrent primary biliary cholangitis, 674
    recurrent viral hepatitis C, 673
  small-for-size graft syndrome (SFSS), 670–671
Lobular disarray, 504*f*
Lobular neutrophils, 508
Low-grade appendiceal mucinous neoplasms, 228, 228*f*, 229*f*
  differential diagnosis of, 229–231
Low-grade B-cell lymphomas, 608*f*
Low-grade mucinous carcinoma, 233
Lye strictures of esophagus. *See* Esophagus, caustic injuries of
Lymphangiectasia, intestinal, 147, 148*f*
Lymphangioma, 205–206, 205*f*
  differential diagnosis of, 206
  of duodenum, 205*f*
Lymphocytic disorders
  colitis, 318–319, 318*f*
    differential diagnosis of, 318–319
  gastritis, 69, 70*f*
Lymphocytic esophagitis, 7*f*
  differential diagnosis of, 7
Lymphocytosis, colonic epithelial, 317
Lymphoepithelial cyst, of pancreas, 456
Lymphogranuloma venereum, colonic, 253*t*, 270–271
Lymphoma kinase, anaplastic, in inflammatory myofibroblastic tumor, 203, 203*f*
Lymphoma(s)
  of anus, differential diagnosis of, 419–420
  B-cell
    Burkitt lymphoma, 624*f*, 638–641
    diffuse large, 613, 630–632, 631*b*, 631*b*–632*b*, 634*f*–635*f*, 640
    extranodal marginal zone. *See* MALT lymphomas
  follicular, 623–626, 624*f*
  gastrointestinal, 613
  hepatic, 607*f*
  immunoproliferative small intestinal disease, 613, 620–623
  MALT lymphomas. *See* MALT lymphomas
  mantle cell, 624*f*, 626–629, 627*f*–628*f*
  NK lymphoma, differential diagnosis of, 649–650
  T-cell, 643–647, 646*b*
    enteropathy-associated, 125, 643–647, 644*f*–645*f*, 646*b*
    hepatosplenic, 649–651, 650*f*, 651*b*
Lymphomatosis polyposis, 360
Lymphoplasmacytic inflammation, intact villi with, 120
Lynch syndrome, 380–383, 395–397
Lysosomal storage diseases, 549*t*, 550*t*, 551*f*

M

Macrocephaly, multiple lipomas, and hemangiomata syndrome, 352
Macrophages
  tangible body, in Burkitt lymphoma, 623, 624*f*
Macroregenerative nodules (MRNs), 523–524, 564–567
Macrovesicular steatosis, 506*f*–507*f*, 532*f*–533*f*
Magnetic resonance cholangiopancreatography (MRCP), 446–447
Major histologic patterns of injury, in liver, 489
Malabsorptive disorders, 120
  celiac disease, 121–122
Malacoplakia, 220*f*
  in appendicitis, 219–220
  appendicitis in, 220*f*
Malignancies. *See* Neoplasms
Malignant angiosarcoma, of liver neoplasms, 600–602
Malignant colon polyp, lymphovascular invasion in, 369*f*
Malignant gastrointestinal neuroectodermal tumor, 180–182, 181*f*
  differential diagnosis of, 181–182
Malignant mesenchymoma. *See* Embryonal sarcoma of liver
Malignant polyps, 367–369
Mallory bodies. *See* Mallory-Denk bodies
Mallory-Denk bodies, 506–508, 515*f*
Mallory hyaline. *See* Mallory-Denk bodies
Mallory-Weiss syndrome, 26
MALT lymphomas, 613–620, 620*b*
  differential diagnosis of, 57–58
  immunoproliferative small intestinal disease, 613–623
Mantle cell lymphoma, 624*f*, 626–629, 627*f*–628*f*, 629*b*
Massive hepatic necrosis, 532*f*–533*f*
Massive parallel sequencing. *See* Next-generation sequencing (NGS)
Mast cell disease, differential diagnosis of, 73
Meckel's diverticulum, ectopic pancreatic tissue in, 456*f*
Medullary carcinoma, colorectal, 385–386, 386*f*, 471–472, 472*f*
Megamitochondria, 508
Melan-A stain in melanoma of anus, 421–422
Melanoma, of anus, 421, 422*f*
  differential diagnosis of, 418, 422
Melena in glomus tumors, 196
Ménétrier's disease, 79, 79*f*, 80*f*
  differential diagnosis of, 59, 80, 95–96, 358
Mesenchymal hamartoma, of liver neoplasms, 595, 597*f*, 598*f*
Mesenchymal sarcoma. *See* Embryonal sarcoma of liver
Mesenchymal tumors, 169
  fibroblastic polyps of colon, benign, 189–191, 189*f*, 190*f*
  fibromatosis, intra-abdominal, 198–200, 198*f*
  gangliocytic paraganglioma, 194–196, 194*f*, 195*f*
  ganglioneuroma, 192–194, 193*f*
    differential diagnosis of, 190–192
  glomus, 196–198, 197*f*
    gastric, differential diagnosis of, 116
  inflammatory fibrosarcoma/inflammatory myofibroblastic tumor, 202–205, 203*f*
  neurofibroma
    differential diagnosis of, 193
  perineurioma, 189–191, 189*f*, 190*f*
  schwannomas, 186–189, 187*f*, 188*f*
    differential diagnosis of, 191–192
  sclerosing mesenteritis, 200–202, 201*f*
  smooth muscle, 176–179, 177*f*
  stromal, 169–176. *See also* Gastrointestinal stromal tumors (GISTs)
Mesenchymal tumors benign hemangioma, of liver neoplasms, 592–593
Mesenchymal tumors of gallbladder and extrahepatic bile ducts, 453
Mesenteric artery/hepatic artery, tissue adjacent to, 487
Mesenteric disorders
  acute ischemia, 142*f*
  epithelioid tumors, 170, 172*f*
  fibromatosis, 198*f*
Mesenteritis, sclerosing, 200–202, 201*f*
Metabolic diseases, in liver, 538
  hereditary hemochromatosis (HH), 539
  iron overload, 540–541
  secondary iron overload, 541–542, 542*f*
Metachromatic leukodystrophy, 549*t*, 550*t*
Metaplasia
  of gallbladder, 436
    intestinal, 436
  gastric foveolar, in peptic duodenitis, 127, 127*f*, 128*f*
  intestinal
    in Barrett's esophagus, 33*f*
  pancreatic acinar, in gastric biopsies, 65
  Paneth cell, differential diagnosis of, 65

Metastases to colorectum, 390
Metastatic carcinoma, 609*f*
Metastatic colon cancer, 609*f*
Metastatic melanoma, 164*f*
Metastatic tumors, of liver neoplasms, 607–611
Metastatic well-differentiated neuroendocrine tumors, 610*f*
Methotrexate, Roenigk scoring system for, 534*t*
Michaelis-Gutmann bodies in malacoplakia, 99–100, 220*f*
Micropapillary carcinoma, 385, 385*f*
Microsatellite instability-high carcinoma (MSI-H), 380, 396–397
Microsatellite instability testing, of colorectal carcinoma, 395–396
Microsporidia infection, 288–289, 289*f*
Microvesicular steatosis, 506*f*–507*f*, 532*f*–533*f*
Microvillus inclusion disease (MVID), 135–136, 135*f*, 136*f*
Miscellaneous patterns of injury, in liver, 535
  "almost normal" biopsy/nonspecific findings, 535–537, 535*t*, 536*f*
  hepatic granulomas, 537
  necrosis, 537–538
Mismatch repair function, assessment of, 395–400, 396*t*
  immunohistochemistry interpretation, 396*t*
  microsatellite instability-high carcinoma, 396–397
  mismatch repair immunohistochemistry in, 397–399
  molecular testing in colorectal carcinoma, future directions of, 400
  polymerase chain reaction–based microsatellite instability testing, 395–396
  RAS, extended RAS, and BRAF testing, 399–400
Mismatch repair immunohistochemistry, 397–399
Mixed neuroendocrine–non-neuroendocrine neoplasm (MiNEN), 163–164
Mixed tumors, of pancreas, 483–484
  mixed acinar–ductal and ductal–neuroendocrine carcinoma, 484
  mixed acinar–neuroendocrine carcinoma, 484
  mixed ductal–neuroendocrine carcinoma, 484
MLH1 immunostain, 399*f*
MMR gene, 398
Model for End-Stage Liver Disease (MELD) score, 660
Molecular alterations, 378–379
Molecular oncology testing, in colorectal carcinoma, 400
Molecular pathways, for colorectal carcinogenesis, 380
Molecular testing in colorectal carcinoma, future directions of, 400
Motility disorders, esophageal, 22–24, 23*f*, 25*f*
MSH6 immunostain, 399*f*
MTOR (mammalian target of rapamycin) pathway, 474
Mucin
  extracellular
    in adenocarcinoma of anus, 419
  inspissated eosinophilic, in cystic fibrosis, 219, 219*f*
  stains in Paget's disease of anus, 432
Mucin-depleted hyperplastic polyp, 373*f*
Mucinous (colloid) adenocarcinomas, 383
Mucinous cystadenoma, 225
Mucinous cystic neoplasms (MCNs), 452–453, 585*f*, 586*f*
  of liver, 469*f*, 584
  of pancreas, 469–470
Mucinous cysts, simple
  of pancreas, 456–457
Mucinous neoplasms
  appendiceal, 229*f*, 234*f*, 240*f*
  carcinoma
    colorectal, 383, 384*f*
Mucinous non-neoplastic cyst, 456–457
Mucolipidoses, 549*t*, 550*t*
Mucopolysaccharidoses (MPS), 549*t*, 550*t*
Mucormycosis, colonic, 276, 277*f*
  differential diagnosis of, 274*t*
Mucosa-associated lymphoid tissue. *See* MALT lymphomas
Mucosal calcinosis, gastric, 76
Mucosal neuroma, differential diagnosis of, 191–192
Mucosal prolapse, 370*f*, 373*f*
  with solitary rectal ulcer, 325–327, 326*f*
Mucosal Schwann cell hamartoma, 191–192, 191*f*
  differential diagnosis of, 191–192
Muir-Torre, syndrome, 381
Multilocular lymphoepithelial cyst, 458*f*
Multiple endocrine neoplasia
  type I
    colorectal, 391
    gastrinomas, 81
  type II, 360
    multiple neuroma syndrome in, 360
  type IIB, diffuse ganglioneuromatosis in, 192, 193*f*
Multiple hamartoma syndrome. *See* Cowden's syndrome
Multiple neuroma syndrome, 360
Murphy sign, 435
Mycobacterial infection, of gut, 267–269
Mycobacterium avium-intracellulare complex infection, 268*f*
Mycobacterium avium-intracellulare infection
  of colon, 253*t*
    differential diagnosis of, 269
  differential diagnosis of, 99–100, 147
Mycobacterium tuberculosis infection. *See* Tuberculosis
Mycophenolate mofetil (MMF) colitis, 330–331, 330*f*
Myeloablative high-dose chemoradiation treatment, 525
Myofibroblastic tumor, inflammatory, 202–205, 203*f*
Myxoid stroma in IH, 595

N

Necrosis
  of colorectal cancer, 384*f*
  in liver, 537–538
Necrotizing disorders
  enterocolitis, 264
    differential diagnosis of, 266, 328
Necrotizing enterocolitis, 265*f*, 266*f*
Neisseria gonorrhoeae, 253*t*, 271
Nematode infections, 291
Neoplasia, of gallbladder, 437
Neoplasms
  "adenocarcinoid" tumors, 237, 240
  bronchogenic carcinoma, esophageal varices in, 25–26
  colorectal epithelial, 363. *See also* Colorectal epithelial neoplasms
  of esophagus, 29
    differential diagnosis of, 10
Neoplasms (*Continued*)
  mucinous. *See* Mucinous neoplasms
  in Peutz-Jeghers syndrome, 346–347
  small intestinal, 151
  of stomach, 91
Neoplastic cells, 603*f*, 604*f*
Neoplastic pancreatic ductal lesions, 464–474
  ductal neoplasms, 464–466
    intraductal papillary mucinous neoplasm (IPMN), 466–469
    intraductal tubulopapillary neoplasm, 470–471
    mucinous cystic neoplasm, 469–470
    pancreatic ductal adenocarcinoma, 471–474
    pancreatic intraepithelial neoplasia, 464–466
    precursor lesions, 464
Neuroendocrine carcinoma (NECs), 475–476
  of ampulla, 163–164
  of small intestine, 163–164
  of pancreas, 476
Neuroendocrine cells, 584
Neuroendocrine neoplasms, of esophagus, 48
Neuroendocrine tumor (NET), 161–162, 452*f*, 455–456. *See also* Carcinoid tumors
  appendiceal, 235
  colorectal, 391–393, 392*f*
    differential diagnosis of, 393
  differential diagnosis, 163
  gangliocytic paraganglioma, 163*f*
  gastric, 114–117
    differential diagnosis of, 98–99
  of pancreas, 474–476
    neuroendocrine carcinomas, 476
    well-differentiated, 474–476
  of small bowel, 162*f*
  of small intestine, 160–163
  tubular pattern of, 236*f*
  well-differentiated, 236*f*
Neurofibroma, 190
  differential diagnosis of, 190, 193
Neurofibromatosis type 1, 360. *See also* von Recklinghausen's disease
Neuroma, multiple, 360
Neutrophilic inflammation, intact villi with, 119
Neutrophils, 489
Next-generation sequencing (NGS), 400
Niemann-Pick disease, 549*t*, 550*t*
NK leukemia/lymphoma, differential diagnosis of, 649–650
Nocardia infection, differential diagnosis of, 272–273
Nodular regenerative hyperplasia (NRH), in liver, 523–524, 527, 528*f*
Nonalcoholic fatty liver disease (NAFLD), 499, 505–509, 506*f*
  pediatric, 508
Nonalcoholic steatohepatitis (NASH), 505
Noncirrhotic portal hypertension, 528
Nonhepatotropic viral infections, in liver, 493
Non-neoplastic diseases of pancreas, 455–458
  benign cystic lesions in pancreas, 456–458
    congenital cysts, 457
    duodenal diverticulum, 458
    simple mucinous cysts, 456–457
  developmental anomalies, 455
    annular pancreas, 455
    ectopic pancreas, 455
    pancreatic divisum, 455
  intrapancreatic spleen and epidermoid cyst, 456
  lymphoepithelial cyst, 456
  pancreatic hamartoma, 455–456

Non-neoplastic disorders, of colon, 299–335
Nonresponsive celiac disease, 124–125
Nonsteroidal anti-inflammatory drug-associated injury. *See* NSAID injury
NSAID injury, 130–131, 130*f*
colitis, 333–334
differential diagnosis of, 131
and peptic duodenal disease, 126, 129
Nuclear β-catenin in fibromatosis, 199, 199*f*
Nutcracker esophagus, 22

O

Obliterative phlebitis, 460–461
Odynophagia, in caustic esophageal injury, 14
in eosinophilic esophagitis, 4
in esophageal webs, 14
in radiation esophagitis, 14
Olmesartan-associated sprue-like enteropathy, 131–132, 132*f*
Omental stromal tumors, 169
Opisthorchis viverrini, 448
Opportunistic infections, 675–676, 676*f*
Overlap syndromes, in liver, 522
"Owl's eye" inclusions in cytomegalovirus infection, 244
Oxyntic gland adenoma, stomach
differential diagnosis of, 106

P

Paget cell, 431, 432*f*
signet ring type of, 431, 432*f*
Paget's disease of anus, 431, 432*f*
adenocarcinoma with, 431
differential diagnosis of, 432
Pain, abdominal. *See* Abdominal pain
Pancolitis, 301
Pancreas
acinar metaplasia in gastric biopsies, 65
frozen section, 484–487, 486*f*, 487*f*
bile duct margin, 486–487
pancreatic ductal adenocarcinoma diagnosis on, 485
parenchymal margin, 485–486
resection margins, evaluation of, 485–487
superior mesenteric artery/hepatic artery, tissue adjacent to, 487
heterotopia of, 97–99, 98*f*
differential diagnosis of, 65
neoplastic diseases, 464–474
intraductal papillary mucinous neoplasm (IPMN), 466–469
intraductal tubulopapillary neoplasm, 470–471
mucinous cystic neoplasm, 469–470
pancreatic ductal adenocarcinoma, 471–474
pancreatic intraepithelial neoplasia, 464–466
precursor lesions, 464
neuroendocrine tumors, 474–476
neuroendocrine carcinomas, 476
well-differentiated neuroendocrine tumors, 474–476
non-neoplastic diseases of, 455–458
congenital cysts, 457
developmental anomalies, 455
duodenal diverticulum, 458
intrapancreatic spleen and epidermoid cyst, 456
lymphoepithelial cyst, 456
pancreatic hamartoma, 455–456
simple mucinous cysts, 456–457
pancreatitis, 458–464
Pancreas (*Continued*)
acute pancreatitis, 458–459
autoimmune pancreatitis (AIP), 460–463, 462*b*
chronic pancreatitis, 459–460
pseudocysts, 463–464
tumors with acinar differentiation, 476–484
acinar cell carcinoma, 476–479
acinar cell cystadenocarcinoma, 479
acinar cell cystadenoma, 476
mixed acinar–ductal and ductal–neuroendocrine carcinoma, 484
mixed acinar–neuroendocrine carcinoma, 484
mixed ductal–neuroendocrine carcinoma, 484
pancreatoblastoma, 479–480
serous cystadenocarcinoma, 482
serous cystadenoma (SCA), 480–482
solid-pseudopapillary neoplasm (SPN), 482–483
Pancreas transplantation, 681
cell-mediated rejection, 684–686
mild acute antibody-mediated rejection, 685
mild acute T cell-mediated rejection, 684
moderate acute antibody-mediated rejection, 685–686
moderate acute T cell-mediated rejection, 684–685
severe acute antibody-mediated rejection, 686
severe acute T cell-mediated rejection, 685
chronic graft fibrosis, 686–687
differential diagnosis of acute rejection, 687
islet pathology, 686–687
chronic rejection and graft fibrosis, 686
chronic antibody-mediated rejection, 686
chronic arteriopathy, 686
posttransplant needle core biopsy, evaluation of, 681–684
allograft dysfunction, 682–684
immunologic factors, 682
normal allograft biopsy, 682–684
technical failure, 682
types of, 678
islet cell transplantation, 681
whole-organ transplants, 681
Pancreatic divisum, 455
Pancreatic ductal adenocarcinoma (PDAC), 455–456, 471*f*, 473*f*
Pancreatic hamartoma, 457*f*
Pancreatic heterotopia, 152*f*, 153
differential diagnosis, 153
groove pancreatitis, 153
of small intestine, 153
Pancreatic intraepithelial neoplasia (PanIiN) lesion, 465*f*
Pancreatic neuroendocrine carcinomas (PanNECs), 475–476
Pancreatic neuroendocrine tumors (PanNETs), 474, 475*f*
Pancreaticobiliary neoplasm, 160
Pancreatitis, 458–464, 687
acute, 458–459, 458*f*
autoimmune, 461*b*, 461*f*, 462*b*
autoimmune pancreatitis (AIP), 460–463, 462*b*
chronic, 459–460, 459*f*, 460*b*
paraduodenal/"groove," 462–463, 463*b*, 463*f*
pseudocysts, 463–464
Pancreatoblastoma, of pancreas, 479–480, 479*f*
Paneth cells, 439*f*
in adenomatous polyps, 365
in autoimmune enteropathy, 134–135
in gastric adenomas, 102
metaplasia of, differential diagnosis of, 65
in Peutz-Jeghers syndrome, 346–347
Papilloma, esophageal, squamous, 30–31, 30*f*
Papillomavirus infection and esophageal papillomatosis, 30*f*
Paraduodenal/"groove" pancreatitis, 462–463, 463*b*
Paraduodenal pancreatitis, 463, 463*f*
Paraganglioma, gangliocytic, 194–196
differential diagnosis of, 193, 195
Parasitic infection, 283
appendicitis in, 220
Enterobius vermicularis, 220, 220*f*
Parasitic infestations, eosinophilia in, 72, 74*f*
Parenchymal margin, 485–486
Parietal cell hyperplasia from proton pump inhibitors, 92*f*
Patchy glycogenosis, 508
Paucicellular inflammation, intact villi with, 120
PEComa, 206–209, 207*f*
differential diagnosis of, 208
Pediatric nonalcoholic fatty liver disease, 508
Pediatric steatohepatitis, 508*f*
Pedunculated ampullary adenoma, 160
Peliosis hepatis, in liver, 530, 530*f*
Penicillium marneffei infection, 280
Peptic duodenal diseases, 126–129, 127*f*, 128*f*
Peptic duodenitis, 152*f*
Peptic ulcer disease in Zollinger-Ellison syndrome, 80
Perforations, esophageal, 25–27
Perianal skin
squamous cell carcinoma of, 428–429, 429*f*
tumors and precursor lesions of, 423
Perianal squamous neoplasia, 412
Peribiliary glands, 487
Pericellular fibrosis, 515*f*
Perineurioma, 189–191, 189*f*, 190*f*
Periodic acid-Schiff reaction, in granular cell tumors of anus, 431
Periodic acid–Schiff (PAS) stain, 471
Periodic acid–Schiff with diastase (PAS-D) stain, 489
Peripancreatic abscess formation, 687
Peripheral/intrahepatic cholangiocarcinoma, 587*f*
Periportal hepatocytes, eosinophilic cytoplasmic inclusions in, 545*f*
Peutz-Jeghers syndrome, 346–348, 347*f*, 348*f*, 349*f*–350*f*
differential diagnosis of, 348–350
in Cronkhite-Canada syndrome, 358
in gastric hyperplastic polyps, 95–96
in juvenile polyposis syndrome, 351–352
Peyer's patches
in histoplasmosis, 279
in typhoid fever, 256
in *Yersinia* infection, 260
Phycomycosis, colonic, 276
Piecemeal necrosis, 499
Pigmented tumors in melanoma of anus, 421
PIK3CA mutations, 470
Pill esophagitis, 11–12, 12*f*
differential diagnosis of, 3, 11–12
Pinworms, 290*f*, 291
Plasma cell hepatitis, 664
Plasma cell–rich rejection, 664
diagnostic criteria for, 665*t*

Plexiform fibromyxoma, 185*f*
differential diagnosis of, 185
Plummer-Vinson syndrome, 20
and squamous cell carcinoma of esophagus, 34–35
Polycystic liver disease, 583–584, 583*f*
Polymerase chain reaction–based microsatellite instability testing, 395–396
Polypoid mucosal prolapse, 373*f*
Polyposis syndromes, 337
adenomatous, 337–343
classification of, 338*t*
Cowden's syndrome, 352–357, 357*f*
Cronkhite-Canada, 357–360
familial adenomatous, 340*f*, 341*f*
hereditary mixed, 360
hyperplastic, 343
juvenile, 350–352, 353*f*–354*f*
differential diagnosis of, 95–96
Peutz-Jeghers. *See* Peutz-Jeghers syndrome
serrated, 343–346
Polyp(s)
adenomatous, 363–365, 384*f*. See also Adenomatous polyps
of colon, benign fibroblastic, 189–191, 189*f*, 190*f*
esophageal, fibrovascular, 30–31
esophageal, giant fibrovascular, 31*f*
fundic gland, 91–94, 92*f*
differential diagnosis of, 91–94
gastric amyloidosis, differential diagnosis of, 57
gastric hyperplastic, 94–96, 95*f*
differential diagnosis of, 80, 94–96
hyperplastic, 371–374, 371*f*, 372*f*
differential diagnosis of, 372–373
inflammatory cloacogenic, differential diagnosis of, 372–373
neurofibroma, 190
Porcelain gallbladder, 435–437, 439*f*
Porphyria cutanea tarda (PCT), 553, 554*f*
Porphyrias, in liver, 553–555
Portal-based fibrosis, 501*f*
Portal hyperperfusion (PHP) injury, 670–671
Portal hypertension
duodenopathy in, 128
esophageal varices in, 25–26
gastropathy in, 86*t*, 87, 88*f*
Portal tracts, 527*f*
scattered mononuclear infiltrates within, 535–536
Portal vein thrombosis/obstruction, in liver, 526–527
Positive staining, 402
Posttransplant chronic hepatitis, 664
Posttransplant lymphoproliferative disorder (PTLD), 675
Posttransplant needle core biopsy, evaluation of, 681–684
allograft dysfunction, 682–684
immunologic factors, 682
normal allograft biopsy, 682–684
technical failure, 682
Precursor lesions, of pancreas, 464
Precursor neoplasia, of extrahepatic bile ducts, 449–450
Preservation/ischemia-reperfusion injury, 658
Primary biliary cholangitis (PBC), 516–519, 667
Primary biliary cirrhosis, 517*f*
Primary disease, recurrence of, 679
Primary hepatic lymphoma, of liver neoplasms, 606–607
Primary intestinal lymphangiectasia, 148*f*
Primary sclerosing cholangitis (PSC), 519*f*
of gallbladder, 446–447, 448*f*
in liver, 515–516, 519
Proctitis
herpetic, 246
syphilitic, 269
Proctocolitis, eosinophilic, 327–328, 327*f*
Prolapse, mucosal
with solitary rectal ulcer, 325–327, 326*f*
Proton pump inhibitors, parietal cell hyperplasia from, 92*f*
Protozoal infections, 283
Pruritus, anal, in enterobiasis, 291
Pseudocysts, 463–464, 464*f*
Pseudodiverticula, esophageal, differential diagnosis of, 21
Pseudodiverticulosis, diffuse esophageal intramural, differential diagnosis of, 21
Pseudomembranous colitis, 265
differential diagnosis of, 266, 294
Pseudomonas infection, differential diagnosis of, 272–273
Pseudomyxoma peritonei, 233–235, 234*f*
Pseudopolyps, inflammatory, differential diagnosis of, 351–352
Pseudotumor, 460–461
Pyloric antrum, vascular ectasia of, 84, 85*f*, 86*t*
differential diagnosis of, 86*t*
Pyloric gland, of gallbladder, 436
Pyloric gland adenoma, 104–106, 153–154, 154*f*
of small intestine, 153
Pyloric gland metaplasia, 439*f*

R

Radiation colitis, 321–323, 322*f*
differential diagnosis of, 322
Radiation-induced disorders
colitis, 320–321, 322*f*
differential diagnosis of, 317, 320–321
esophagitis, 9
gastritis, differential diagnosis of, 75
Rectum, solitary ulcer with mucosal prolapse, 325–327, 326*f*
differential diagnosis of, 326–327
Recurrent autoimmune hepatitis, 674
Recurrent fatty liver disease, 675
Recurrent hepatitis C, 669–670
Recurrent primary biliary cholangitis, 674
Recurrent primary sclerosing cholangitis, 673–674
Recurrent viral hepatitis C, 673
Reflux disease, gastrointestinal (GERD), 1, 2*f*, 3*f*
Reflux esophagitis, 1, 2*f*, 3*f*
Refractory celiac disease, 124–125
Rejection Activity Index, 665–666, 666*t*
Rendu-Osler-Weber disease, 593
Resection margins, evaluation of, 485–487
bile duct margin, 486–487
parenchymal margin, 485–486
superior mesenteric artery/hepatic artery, tissue adjacent to, 487
Reticulin stain, 528*f*
Rhabdomyosarcoma
botryoid embryonal, of extrahepatic bile ducts, 453
Rhodacoccus equi infection, 253*t*
Rhodanine/orcein stains, 518
Rhodococcus equi infection, 269
Rituximab, 531
RNF43 gene, 467
Roenigk grade, 533
Roenigk scoring system for methotrexate, 534*t*
Rokitansky-Aschoff sinuses, 436
in cholecystitis, 436, 438*f*, 442–443, 446
of gallbladder, 442–443, 446
Roundworms, 292, 293*f*
Rrokitansky-Aaschoff sinuses, 438*f*

S

Saccharomyces cerevisiae antibody, test for, 311–312
Salmonella infection, 253*t*, 255
differential diagnosis of, 256–257, 261
Sarcina infection, 249–250, 250*f*
differential diagnosis of, 250
Sarcoidosis
differential diagnosis of, 281–283
granulomatous gastritis in, 68, 69*f*
Sarcoma, embryonal, 604–606
Sausage-shaped pancreas, 460
Scattered mononuclear infiltrates within portal tracts, 535–536
Schatzki's ring, 20
Schistosomiasis, 295
granulomatous gastritis in, 67*t*, 69*f*
Schwann cell hamartoma, 192
Schwannomas, 186–189, 187*f*, 188*f*
differential diagnosis of, 191–192
esophageal achalasia in, 22, 24–25
lamina propria fibrosis in, 75
Sclerosing cholangitis, primary, 519
Sclerosing hyaline necrosis, 511
Sclerosing mesenteritis, 200–202, 201*f*
Sclerosis, hepatoportal, 528, 529*f*
Secondary iron overload, in liver, 541–542
Secondary tumors
differential diagnosis of, 50
of esophagus, 49–50
of small intestine, 164–167
Sentinel tag, anal, 407–408
Serous cystadenocarcinoma, of pancreas, 482
Serous cystadenoma (SCA), of pancreas, 480–482, 481*f*
Serrated adenocarcinomas, 383
Serrated adenomas
sessile, 374–377
differential diagnosis of, 372–373
traditional (colorectal), 377–378, 378*f*
Serrated colorectal polyps, 371
of appendix, 226, 227*f*
Serrated polyposis syndrome (SPS), 343–346, 344*f*, 379
differential diagnosis of, 346
dysplasia in, 345*f*
serrated polyps in, 345*f*
Serrated polyps
differential diagnosis, 156
of small intestine, 154–157
Sessile serrated adenomas, 374–377
differential diagnosis of, 372–373
Shigellosis, 253*t*, 257
differential diagnosis of, 258
Signet ring cell carcinoma, 471–472
colorectal, 383, 385*f*
gastric, differential diagnosis of, 99–100
Signet-ring type of Paget cell, 431, 432*f*
Simple mucinous cysts, of pancreas, 456–457, 458*f*
Sinusoidal lymphocytosis, 494
Sinusoidal obstruction syndrome (SOS), in liver, 525, 526*f*, 532*f*–533*f*

Sloughing esophagitis, 12–14, 13*f*
  differential diagnosis of, 13
Small bowel allografts
  acute cellular rejection in, 678*t*
  antibody-mediated rejection, 679*f*
  chronic rejection, 680*f*
  mild acute cellular rejection, 678*f*
  severe acute cellular rejection, 679*f*
Small bowel disorders, 119
  adenocarcinomas, of ampulla of Vater, 157–160, 157*f*, 159*t*
  autoimmune enteropathy, 134*f*
  bacterial overgrowth, 129–130, 129*f*
  celiac disease, 121–122
  clear cell sarcoma-like tumor, 180–182
  collagenous sprue, 125
  common variable immunodeficiency, 132
  Crohn's disease, 137–138
  enteric ischemic disease, 142*f*
  flattened villi pattern of, 119
  granular cell tumor, 179–180
  GVHD. *See* Graft-versus-host disease
  immunoproliferative small intestinal disease, 613, 620–623
  infectious enteritis, 147
  inflammatory fibroid polyp, 182–184
  intact villi pattern of, 119–120
  lymphangiectasia, 147–148, 148*f*
  malabsorptive disorders
    celiac disease, 120
  microvillus inclusion disease, 135–136, 135*f*, 136*f*
  neoplasms, 151
  nonresponsive celiac disease, 124–125
  nonsteroidal anti-inflammatory drug-associated injury, 130–131
  olmesartan-associated sprue-like enteropathy, 131–132
  pattern-based approach of, 120
  patterns of, 119–120, 120*t*
    flattened villi pattern, 119
    intact villi pattern, 119–120
  peptic duodenal diseases, 126–129, 127*f*, 128*f*
  plexiform fibromyxoma of, 184–186
  refractory celiac disease, 124–125
  sclerosing mesenteritis, 200–202, 201*f*
  smooth muscle tumors, 176–179
  stromal tumors, 169, 170*f*, 171*f*, 172*f*
  tropical sprue, 126
  Whipple disease, 147
Small bowel transplantation, 676–677
  acute cellular rejection, 677–679
  allograft dysfunction, 677
  antibody-mediated rejection, 679
  chronic rejection, 679–681
  differential diagnosis of, 680
Small-for-size graft syndrome (SFSS), 670–671
Small intestinal adenocarcinoma, 155–156
Small intestinal bacterial overgrowth, 129–130
Small intestinal inflammatory bowel disease, 137
Small intestine
  adenocarcinoma, 154–157
  adenoma and adenocarcinoma of ampulla of Vater, 157–160
  Brunner's gland hyperplasia, 151–152, 152*f*
  conventional adenoma, 154–157
  gangliocytic paraganglioma, 163, 163*f*
  gastric heterotopia, 152–153, 152*f*
  hamartoma, 151–152
  neuroendocrine carcinoma of small intestine, 163–164
Small intestine (*Continued*)
  neuroendocrine tumors of small intestine, 160–163
  pancreatic heterotopia, 152*f*, 153
  pyloric gland adenoma, 153–154, 154*f*
  secondary tumors of small intestine, 164–167
  serrated polyps, 154–157
Smoking
  and gastric adenocarcinoma, 107
  and peptic duodenal diseases, 129
Smooth muscle cells in glomus tumors, 196
Smooth muscle tumors, 176–179, 177*f*
Smudgy nuclear inclusions, 71*f*
Solid-pseudopapillary neoplasm (SPN), of pancreas, 482–483, 483*f*
Solitary biliary cyst, of liver neoplasms, 580–583
Solitary rectal ulcer syndrome, mucosal prolapse in, 325–327, 326*f*
  differential diagnosis of, 326–327
Somatostatin-producing NETs, 161
Spastic disorders, esophageal, 22–23
Sphincterotomy of the minor papilla, 455
Spindle cells
  in gangliocytic paraganglioma, 195, 195*f*
  in ganglioneuroma, 192, 193*f*
  in inflammatory myofibroblastic tumor, 203
  in obliteration of appendiceal lumen, 211–213
  in perineurioma, 189–190, 189*f*
  in smooth muscle tumors, 176–179, 177*f*
Spirochetosis, intestinal, 253*t*, 271, 272*f*
Spleen, hepatosplenic T-cell lymphoma, 649, 650*f*
Spleen, intrapancreatic (of pancreas), 456
Splendore-Hoeppli material in actinomycosis, 272
Sporadic versus lynch syndrome, 396–397
Sporadic versus Lynch syndrome, 396–397
S-100 protein
  in granular cell tumor of anus, 418
  in melanoma of anus, 421–422
Sprue
  celiac, 124
  collagenous, 125
  differential diagnosis of, 124
  nontropical, 124
  tropical, 126
Squamous cell carcinoma (SCC), 429*f*
  of anal canal, 415–416, 417*f*
    differential diagnosis of, 418–420, 430*f*
  colorectal, 383
  of esophagus, 42–45, 43*f*
  of perianal skin, 428–429, 429*f*
Squamous metaplasia, 584
Squamous papillomas, of esophagus, 29–30
  differential diagnosis of, 29–30
Steatohepatitis, 506*f*–507*f*
  pediatric, 508*f*
  pattern of injury, in liver, 505
Steatosis, 505–506
  congenital esophageal, 19*f*
  liver with, 510*f*
  macrovesicular, 506*f*–507*f*
  microvesicular, 506*f*–507*f*
Sterile acalculous cholecystitis, of gallbladder, 435
Stomach. *See also* Gastritis
  acute erosive/hemorrhagic gastritis, 53, 54*f*
  adenocarcinoma of, 107–114, 108*f*
  adenomas of, 101–104
Stomach (*Continued*)
  amyloidosis, 64–67, 83*f*, 84*f*
    differential diagnosis of, 75
  antral vascular ectasia of, 84, 85*f*, 86*f*, 86*t*
    differential diagnosis of, 88
  autoimmune gastritis, 64, 64*t*, 67*t*
  chemical gastropathy, 56
  collagenous gastritis, 74, 75*f*
  Dieulafoy's lesion of, 88
  doxycycline gastritis, 78
  dysplasia of, epithelial, 101–104
  eosinophilic gastritis, 72, 74*f*
  gastric amyloidosis, 82
  gastric carcinomas of, 100–101
  gastric Crohn's disease, 68
  gastric peptic ulcer disease, 63
  gastric polyps in, 91
  gastric secondary tumors of, 113
  gastritis cystica polyposa, 96–97
  glomus tumors of, 196–198, 197*f*
    differential diagnosis of, 116
  granulomatous gastritis, 67–68, 67*t*, 68*f*, 69*f*, 70*f*
  Helicobacter pylori gastritis, 57, 58*t*, 59*f*, 60*f*, 61*f*, 61*t*
  heterotopia
    differential diagnosis of, 128
    pancreatic, 97–99, 98*f*
  infectious gastritis, 71, 71*f*, 73*f*, 74*f*
  linitis plastica, 108, 108*f*
  lobular metastatic carcinoma of, 113*f*
  lymphocytic gastritis, 69, 70*f*
  Ménétrier's disease of, 79, 79*f*
  mucosal calcinosis of, 76
  neoplasms of, 91
  neuroendocrine tumors of, 100–101, 114–117
    differential diagnosis of, 116
  non-neoplastic disorders of, 53
  oxyntic gland adenoma of, 106–107
  polyps in
    fundic gland, 91–94, 92*f*
    hyperplastic, 94–96, 95*f*
  portal hypertensive gastropathy, 86*t*, 87, 88*f*
  pyloric gland adenoma, 104–106
  schwannomas in, 186–189, 187*f*, 188*f*
  stromal tumors in, 169, 170*f*, 171*f*, 172*f*
  syndromic gastric cancer of, 112
  xanthomas in, 99–100, 99*f*, 100*f*
  in Zollinger-Ellison syndrome, 80, 81*f*
Stress gastritis, acute, 53
Strictures
  in colonic tuberculosis, 267
  esophageal
    in caustic injuries, 14–15, 15*f*
    in eosinophilic esophagitis, 4
    in radiation injury, 9–10
Stromal tumors, gastrointestinal. *See* Gastrointestinal stromal tumors (GISTs)
Strongyloides stercoralis infection, 293–294
Strongyloidiasis, 294*f*
Submassive hepatic necrosis, 538*f*
Submassive/massive hepatic necrosis, 537–538
Sulfur granules in actinomycosis, 272
Surgical hepatitis, 489–490
Sweat chloride test for cystic fibrosis, 218
Synaptophysin
  in colorectal carcinoid tumors, 393
  in glomus tumors, 195
Syphilis, 269
Systemic mastocytosis, 328–330, 329*f*
  differential diagnosis of, 329
Systemic sclerosis, 24–25

T

Tags, anal, 410
Target lesion in aspergillosis, 275, 276*f*
T-cell lymphoma, 643–647, 646*b*
  enteropathy-associated, 125, 643–647, 644*f*–645*f*, 646*b*
  hepatosplenic, 649–651, 650*f*
Tears, esophageal, 25–27
Technetium-99 sulfur colloid scan, 558
Telangiectatic FNHs, 558–560, 562–564
Thyroid transcription factor 1 (TTF-1), 589–590
Torsion, appendiceal, 211
Toxic injuries, 532*f*–533*f*
Toxoplasma gondii infection, 288
Tracheoesophageal fistula, esophageal atresia with, 17–19, 18*f*
Traditional serrated adenomas (colorectal), 154*f*, 377–378, 378*f*
Trematodes, 295–296
Treponema pallidum infection, 269
Triangle of Killian, 20
Trichuris trichiura infection, 292
Trisomy 18, 575
Tropheryma whipplei, 250–251
Tuberculosis
  of appendix, 218
  of colon, 253*t*, 267
    differential diagnosis of, 269
Tubular adenocarcinoma, 468*f*
Tubulopapillary neoplasm, intraductal of pancreas, 470–471
Tubulovillous adenoma, 365*f*
Tufting enteropathy, 136
Tumor budding, 389*f*
Tumors. *See* Neoplasms
Tumors, metastatic, 607–611
Tumors with acinar differentiation, in pancreas, 476–484
  acinar cell carcinoma, 476–479
  acinar cell cystadenocarcinoma, 479
  acinar cell cystadenoma, 476
  mixed acinar–ductal and ductal–neuroendocrine carcinoma, 484
  mixed acinar–neuroendocrine carcinoma, 484
  mixed ductal–neuroendocrine carcinoma, 484
  pancreatoblastoma, 479–480
  serous cystadenocarcinoma, 482
  serous cystadenoma (SCA), 480–482
  solid-pseudopapillary neoplasm (SPN), 482–483
Turcot's syndrome, 338, 381
Tylosis, and squamous cell carcinoma of esophagus, 35
Type 2 autoimmune pancreatitis, granulocytic epithelial lesion in, 462*f*
Type 2 pediatric NAFLD, 508
Typhlitis. *See* Enterocolitis, necrotizing
Typhoid fever, 255, 257*f*
  differential diagnosis of, 256–257
Tyrosine kinase inhibitors, 531

U

Ulcerative colitis, 301
  appendix in, 216
  backwash ileitis in, 304*f*
Ulcerative colitis (*Continued*)
  biopsy findings in, 302–304, 303*f*
  chronic, 301*f*
  cytomegalovirus (CMV) infection in, 304*f*
  differential diagnosis of, 307–308
    in *Aeromonas* infection, 263
    in amebiasis, 284–285
    in Crohn's disease, 312–313
    in cryptococcosis, 281–283
    in diversion colitis, 322
    in diverticular disease, 325
    in radiation colitis, 320–321
    in shigellosis, 258
    in strongyloidiasis, 294
  dysplasia in, 305–309, 306*f*
  endoscopy in, 301, 302*f*, 303*f*
  gross findings in, 301–302, 302*f*
  invisible low-grade dysplasia in, 306*f*
  resection findings in, 303*f*, 304–305
  visible dysplasia in, 307*f*
Ulcer(s)
  in amebiasis, 283
  anal, 407
  of colon
    in candidiasis, 273
    in cytomegalovirus infection, 244*f*, 245*f*
    in mucormycosis, 276
    in tuberculosis, 267
  of gastrointestinal tract
    in cytomegalovirus infection, 243
  in herpetic colitis, 246
  in peptic duodenal disease, 126–129, 128*f*
  rectal, solitary, mucosal prolapse with, 325–327, 326*f*
Undifferentiated (anaplastic) carcinoma, 471–472
Undifferentiated carcinoma, 472*f*
  colorectal, 385–386, 386*f*
Undifferentiated carcinoma with osteoclast-like giant cells (UCOGC), 471–472
Undifferentiated gallbladder carcinoma, 445*f*
Undifferentiated sarcoma. *See* Embryonal sarcoma of liver
Unilocular cystic dilations of the bile duct, 452
Uphill esophageal varices, 25–26
Upper gastrointestinal tract adenocarcinoma, HER2 testing in, 400–404
  background and rationale, 400–401
  immunohistochemistry, 402
  in situ hybridization, 403
  PD-1/PDL-1 in esophageal and gastric carcinomas, 403–404
  specimen type, 402
Ursodeoxycholic acid, 519

V

Varices, esophageal, 25–27, 26*f*
Vascular ectasia, gastric antral, 84, 85*f*, 86*f*, 86*t*
  differential diagnosis of, 86*t*, 88
Vascular pattern of injury, in liver, 522–523
  common causes of, 522*t*
Veno-occlusive disease, 525, 532*f*–533*f*
Verrucous carcinoma of anus, 429, 430*f*
  differential diagnosis of, 426, 430*f*, 431
Vibrio cholerae infection, 262
  differential diagnosis of, 262
Viral hepatitis, 491*t*
  chronic, 498–502
Viral infections
  appendicitis in, 220–221, 221*f*
  nonhepatotropic, 493
  gastritis in, 71*f*
  of gastrointestinal tract, 243
Volcano lesions in *Clostridium difficile* infection, 265
Von Hippel-Lindau (VHL) syndrome, 460
Von Meyenburg complexes. *See* Bile duct hamartomas (BDHs)
Von Recklinghausen's disease, 360

W

Waldmann's disease, 148*b*
Warthin-Starry stain in spirochetosis, 271, 272*f*
Watermelon stomach, 84, 85*f*, 86*f*, 86*t*
  differential diagnosis of, 88
Webs, esophageal, 20*f*
Weibel-Palade bodies, 602
Well-differentiated neuroendocrine tumors
  of duodenum, 160*f*, 161*f*
  of pancreas, 474–476
Whipple disease, 147, 250–251
  differential diagnosis of, 147, 252
  in gastric xanthomas, 99–100
Whipworm, 292
Whole-organ transplants, 681
Wilson's disease, in liver, 502, 542, 543*f*
Worm infection, 291

X

Xanthogranulomatous cholecystitis
  of gallbladder, 435–436, 437*f*, 439*f*
Xanthogranulomatous disorders
  appendicitis, 214
  cholecystitis, 435–436, 437*f*, 439*f*
    differential diagnosis of, 441–443
Xanthomas, gastric, 99–100, 99*f*, 100*f*
  differential diagnosis of, 99–100
X-linked inheritance (IPEX) syndrome, 133–134

Y

Yeast forms, halo effect around, 279*f*, 280
Yersiniosis, 253*t*, 260, 261*f*, 263*f*
  differential diagnosis of, 261
    in Crohn's disease, 312–313
    in tuberculosis, 269
    in typhoid fever, 256–257

Z

Zenker's diverticulum, 19–20, 21*f*
Zollinger-Ellison syndrome, 80, 81*f*, 82*f*
  differential diagnosis of, 80–82
  gastric carcinoid tumors in, 114
  peptic ulcers in, 126
Zone 3 pericellular and perisinusoidal fibrosis, 511
Zygomycete infections, colonic, 277*f*
  differential diagnosis of, 274*t*